PHARMACOLOGIC BASIS
of NURSING PRACTICE

SIXTH EDITION

PHARMACOLOGIC of NURSING PRACTICE

JULIA B. FREEMAN CLARK, PhD
Health Scientist Administrator
National Institutes of Health
Bethesda, Maryland

SHERRY F. QUEENER, PhD
Professor of Pharmacology
Indiana University School of Medicine;
Associate Dean of the Graduate School
Indiana University
Indianapolis, Indiana

VIRGINIA BURKE KARB, RN, PhD
Associate Dean and Associate Professor
School of Nursing
University of North Carolina at Greensboro
Greensboro, North Carolina

 Mosby

A Harcourt Health Sciences Company

St. Louis   London   Philadelphia   Sydney   Toronto

Editor in Chief: Sally Schrefer
Acquisitions Editor: Jeanne Allison
Developmental Editor: Kristin Geen
Project Manager: Dana Peick
Designer: Pati Pye

SIXTH EDITION
Copyright © 2000 by Mosby, Inc.

NOTICE

Pharmacology is an ever-changing field. Standard safety precautions must be followed, but as new research and clinical experience broaden our knowledge, changes in treatment and drug therapy may become necessary or appropriate. Readers are advised to check the most current product information provided by the manufacturer of each drug to be administered to verify the recommended dose, the method and duration of administration, and contraindications. It is the responsibility of the appropriately licensed health care provider, relying on experience and knowledge of the patient, to determine dosages and the best treatment for each individual patient. Neither the Publisher nor the editor assume any liability for any injury and/or damage to persons or property arising from this publication.

The Publisher

Mosby, Inc.
A Harcourt Health Sciences Company
11830 Westline Industrial Drive
St. Louis, Missouri 63146

Printed in the United States of America

Library of Congress Cataloging-in-Publication Data

Freeman, Julia B.
    Pharmacologic basis of nursing practice / Julia B. Freeman, Sherry
F. Queener, Virginia Burke Karb. — 6th ed.
      p.   cm.
    Includes indexes.
    ISBN 0-323-00684-1
    1. Pharmacology. 2. Chemotherapy. 3. Nursing.   I. Queener,
Sherry F. II. Karb, Virginia Burke. III. Title.
    [DNLM: 1. Pharmacology Nurses' Instruction. 2. Drug Therapy
Nurses' Instruction.   QV 4 F855p 2000]
RC300.F72 2000
615' .1'024613—dc21
DNLM/DLC   99-35763

00 01 02 03 GW/VHP 9 8 7 6 5 4 3 2

CONTRIBUTORS

Lynn R. Willis, PhD
Chapter 7: Over-the-Counter Drugs and Self-Medication
& Alternative Therapies Boxes
Professor of Pharmacology
Indiana University School of Medicine
Indianapolis, Indiana

Julie S. Snyder, MSN, RN, C
Case Studies in Chapters 7, 9, 13, 14, 18, 20, 22, 24, 39,
52, 59, and 73
Faculty, School of Nursing
Louise Obici Memorial Hospital
Suffolk, Virginia

Pamela Wilde, RN, MS, CCRN
Case Studies in Chapters 26, 34, and 49
Associate Professor of Nursing
University of Alaska
Anchorage, Alaska

Betsy Atkinson Joyce, EdD, MSN, CPNP
Case Study in Chapters 44
Associate Professor, Family Health Nursing
Indiana University School of Nursing
Indianapolis, Indiana

REVIEWERS

David M. Baker, RPh, MBA, JD
Chair and Assistant Professor
Pharmacy Technology Department
Holyoke Community College
Holyoke, Massachusetts

Susan B. Battistoni, PhD, RN
Assistant Professor
Salisbury State University
Salisbury, Maryland

Julie Beshore Bliss, RN, EdD
Assistant Professor
William Paterson University
Montvale, New Jersey

Joan Parker Frizzell, PhD, RN
Assistant Professor
LaSalle University
Philadelphia, Pennsylvania

Thelma L. Halberstadt, EdD, RN
Professor of Nursing and
  Nursing I Coordinator
Northern Essex Community College
Lawrence, Massachusetts

Marlene Huff, PhD, MSN, BSN
Instructor, College of Nursing
University of Akron
Akron, Ohio

Elizabeth A. Jones, RN, MS
Associate of Science in Nursing Faculty
IVY Tech State College
Lafayette, Indiana

Donna M. Ketcham, MT (ASCP), MS
Instructor of Biology
Indiana-Purdue Universities at Fort Wayne
Fort Wayne, Indiana

Juliette Kruse, RN, MS
Clinical Instructor
San Francisco State University
San Francisco, California

Grace Labaj, MSN, PhD
Associate Dean and Professor
University of Mary Hardin-Baylor
Belton, Texas

Mary Ann Lavin, ScD, RN, CS, FAAN
Assistant Professor and Adult Nurse
  Practitioner
Saint Louis University
St. Louis, Missouri

Janet Mooney, MS, RN
Associate Professor of Nursing
Rock Valley College
Rockford, Illinois

Nancy O'Donnell, RN, MSN
Associate Professor, J. Sergeant
Reynolds Community College
Staff Nurse, Department of Pediatrics
Medical College of Virginia Hospitals
Richmond, Virginia

Margaret A. Tufts, MS, RNC
Assistant Professor
Quinnipiac College
Hamden, Connecticut

PREFACE

Pharmacology is a rapidly changing field. The dynamic nature of drug therapy and health care presents continual challenges. The role of the nurse becomes increasingly sophisticated as new drugs and new strategies are applied to patient care. *Pharmacologic Basis of Nursing Practice* effectively presents pharmacology in an understandable format. Emphasizing clear rationales for drug therapy, it relates the physiologic factors of disease processes to drug mechanisms.

NEW TO THIS EDITION

This sixth edition contains more than 110 new drugs that have been introduced during the 3 years since the last edition was published.

We have thoroughly revised specific content to include these new drugs in the tables and to integrate discussion of these agents in the text. The entire text has been reviewed and revised to keep up with current knowledge on drug mechanisms and therapeutic uses of agents.

The sixth edition features three new chapters: **Drugs to Treat Pancreatic and Gallbladder Diseases, Drugs to Treat Headaches,** and **Introduction to Cancer Chemotherapy.**

This edition also contains the following new features:

- **Case Studies** covering cultural, life span, community, and patient teaching considerations
- **Alternative Therapies** boxes
- **Home health and community content** highlighted throughout the text
- **References** section added to chapters when appropriate
- **Drug Classifications At-A-Glance** tear-out card for student reference and review
- **Key Drugs ▼** now listed in chapter openers
- Appendixes for **Metabolizing Enzymes, Drugs with Common Side Effects,** and **Answers to Case Studies**

Several features have been retained and enhanced from previous editions:

- **Application** and **Critical Thinking Questions** at the end of each chapter
- **Dietary Considerations, Geriatric and Pediatric Considerations, Drug Abuse Alerts,** and **Patient Problems** boxes
- **Research Highlights** include ten new boxes summarizing relevant research findings
- **Chapter Objectives, Overviews,** and **Key Terms** listed in chapter openers

GOALS

Our goal remains to provide an up-to-date, scientifically based pharmacology book that assists nursing students in studying drugs. Specifically, we seek to (1) present clearly the concepts of pharmacology that guide all drug use, (2) discuss the major drug classes with an emphasis on mechanisms of action, and (3) detail the nursing implications for drug administration throughout the nursing process. Our approach is to emphasize the rationale for drug therapy by relating the physiologic factors of disease processes to drug mechanisms. In addition to presenting a more thorough description of the scientific basis of drug action than do most nursing textbooks, this book carefully reviews pertinent physiologic fact so that students can readily see how drugs modify physiologic processes and apply this knowledge to nursing practice.

Because students often express frustration about trying to remember the large number of drugs they must learn, we have adopted a key drug approach that highlights the drugs that are most important in a particular drug class. We also strive to minimize students' difficulty by dealing with drug classes first and then emphasizing the similarities between drugs of a single drug class. Chapters are focused on the grouping of drugs according to their mechanism of action.

For the instructor, our goal is to provide a book that can be adapted to various curricula. This book is divided into 16 sections. Each section contains two or more chapters, and the chapters include distinct segments for different therapeutic situations. For example, antianginal drugs are covered in a section of the chapter on drugs that improve circulation, *Antianginals and Other Vasodilators.* This chapter is one of seven in the section titled, *Drugs Affecting the Cardiovascular and Renal Systems.* This organization allows the instructor to rearrange the order in which material is presented and gives students succinct sections to master.

ORGANIZATION

Section I, *How Drugs Work in the Body,* Section II, *Nursing Care Related to Drug Therapy,* and Section III, *How the Nervous System Controls Body Functions,* provide a solid foundation for applying pharmacologic principles and knowledge of medication administration to nursing management. Sections IV through XVI are devoted to drug category discussions, which are grouped by body system.

- Each chapter begins with **Objectives, Chapter Overview, Key Terms,** and **Key Drugs** and ends with **Application** and **Critical Thinking Questions** that apply chapter content to nursing practice.

Drug category chapters are presented in a streamlined, consistent format:

- First, the **Therapeutic Rationale** discussion provides a detailed review to set the stage for why certain drugs are used in the treatment of a specific disorder or disease and what these agents are supposed to do.

- Next, the **Therapeutic Agents** discussion presents individual drugs and explores them in detail. Key, or prototype, drugs are clearly identified. Key drugs are especially useful in programs in which pharmacology is integrated with another course in the curriculum. The **key drug approach** can be used to help students prioritize their study and compare the most important agents used within a drug class.

- Individual drugs are presented in a consistent drug monograph format that includes the following subheadings: **Mechanism of Action, Pharmacokinetics, Uses, Adverse Reactions and Contraindications, Toxicity,** and **Interactions.** The Therapeutic Agents section may be repeated within a chapter if more than one category of drugs is used to treat the disease or disorder under discussion.

- The **Nursing Process Overview** immediately follows the Therapeutic Agents discussion. This overview directly applies the nursing process to the content in the chapter with the five-step format of **Assessment, Nursing Diagnoses, Patient Outcomes, Planning/Implementation,** and **Evaluation.** The Nursing Process Overview provides a framework for applying pharmacologic knowledge to nursing practice. It is not meant to supplant the use of additional nursing textbooks or current nursing literature. The focus is on the pharmacologic factors rather than on the disease process itself within the five-step nursing process format.

- Next in the chapter, **Nursing Implications Summary** presents general guidelines for drug groups or specific therapies. It provides detailed, specific nursing interventions for each therapeutic agent, with emphasis on **Drug Administration** and **Nursing in the Community,** which encompasses important patient and family teaching points.

- At the end of each chapter is **Chapter Review,** which contains a series of **Application** and **Critical Thinking Questions.** Application questions help students test their comprehension of pharmacologic principles related to nursing. The more complex Critical Thinking Questions challenge students to conceptualize how pharmacologic principles are applied in nursing practice.

ANCILLARY PACKAGE

- **Instructor's Resource Manual.** This manual contains lecture strategies for each chapter and a test bank.
- **Student Learning Guide.** This resource contains worksheets for each chapter featuring review activities and case studies.
- **Mosby's Pharmacology Update.** This e-mail newsletter contains the latest on new drugs, drug news, feature articles, and more.
- **Mosby's Electronic Image Collection for Pharmacology.** This CD-ROM contains 150 full-color images for use in lectures.
- **Pharmacology Lecture Outlines in PowerPoint.** This innovative lecture tool, available on the Internet at

  www.mosby.com/pharm_ppt , features various

  drug classes and body systems.
- **Pharmacology Lecture Video.** Available to qualified adopters, this video discusses the Five Rights of Medication Administration.

ACKNOWLEDGMENTS

Special thanks to Lynne Pearcey, RN, PhD, Dean of the School of Nursing at the University of North Carolina, for her encouragement and support. Henry R. Besch, Jr., PhD, Chairman of the Department of Pharmacology and Toxicology at Indiana University School of Medicine, deserves special mention for the support he has given us during the development of all editions of this book. Mrs. Janie Siccardi, Administrative Assistant in the Department of Pharmacology and Toxicology, has greatly aided us in this effort. The continued contribution of Dr. Lynn R. Willis, Professor of Pharmacology at Indiana University School of Medicine, is also much appreciated.

Finally, we would like to thank two special colleagues who have lived with the book as long as we have. They are Dr. Stephen W. Queener, Senior Research Scientist, Eli Lilly and Company, and Dr. Kenneth S. Karb, Medical Oncologist, Greensboro, North Carolina.

Julia B. Freeman Clark
Sherry F. Queener
Virginia Burke Karb

CONTENTS

Drugs in the Body: Pharmacodynamics and Pharmacokinetics

OBJECTIVES

After studying this chapter, you should be able to do the following:

- *Explain the concept of drug receptors.*
- *Discuss mechanisms that produce unwanted drug reactions.*
- *Explain the factors that can influence enteral absorption of drugs.*
- *Discuss the advantages and disadvantages of common routes of administration.*
- *Explain how the elimination half-life of a drug influences the time required to attain a steady-state concentration when the drug is given on a regular schedule.*

CHAPTER OVERVIEW

Pharmacology is the study of how chemicals interact with living organisms to produce biologic effects. This book presents chemicals that produce therapeutically useful effects, chemicals referred to as *drugs*. This chapter focuses on classes of drugs to give information that forms the basis for understanding the actions of specific agents discussed in later chapters of this book.

MECHANISMS OF DRUG ACTION: PHARMACODYNAMICS

Drug Action is Determined by Where and How a Drug Interacts with the Body

Pharmacodynamics is the study of how drugs produce biologic effects by interacting with specific targets at the drug's site of action. The magnitude of the biologic effect produced by a drug is related to the effective concentration of the drug present at the site of action.

Sites of Drug Action

The site of action of a drug may be determined by many factors. A few drugs are administered in such a way that they enter the body fluid where they are intended to act. An example is an antacid, which enters the stomach, dissolves, and neutralizes excess stomach acid. Alteration of gastric pH is the only intended action of this drug. Other examples are drugs that accumulate in urine and alter urinary pH. By acidifying the urine with ammonium chloride or alkalinizing the urine with sodium bicarbonate, ion flow in the kidney is altered and drug excretion patterns are changed.

Certain classes of drugs are directed to their site of action because they are very lipid soluble and are thus able to interact with lipids and proteins in cell membranes. General anesthetic gases (discussed in Chapter 36) may act in this way. These agents alter properties of membranes by integrating into the lipid layers surrounding specific membrane proteins or by attaching to sites on membrane proteins that tend to attract lipidlike substances. Agents of this type are chemically diverse but share the property of being very lipid soluble.

The biologic activity of many drugs is directed to specific types of cells. This localization is possible because each type of cell possesses a unique array of proteins called **receptors**.

Drug Receptors

The idea of drug receptors is a key concept in pharmacology. The specific proteins called drug receptors are actually natural components of the body intended to respond to some chemical normally present in blood or tissues. For example, opioid receptors within the brain respond to morphine and related compounds from the opium poppy, but the natural function of these receptors is to bind to enkephalins and endorphins. These compounds produced in the brain are more potent than morphine in producing analgesia (see Chapter 32). Localization of opioid effects are ensured because only those cells possessing opioid receptors can respond to morphine.

The ability to bind to a specific receptor is determined by the chemical structure of the drug. This interaction is similar to a lock-and-key fit (Figure 1-1). A critical portion of the drug usually determines its ability to bind. Drugs that have similar critical regions but differ in other parts of the molecule might also be expected to have similar biologic activity (drugs A and B, see Figure 1-1). Drugs that differ in this critical region may not bind to the receptor at all (drug C, see Figure 1-1).

Specificity is the property of the receptor that lets it discriminate among generally similar compounds and bind only to those with the critical features. **Affinity** is the property that determines the strength of the binding of a compound to a receptor. When receptors are highly specific and have high affinity for the compounds that bind to them, very low concentrations of these compounds may show biologic activity. For example, hormones naturally present in the body act through specific receptors. Some of these hormones are found in the blood at concentrations of less than 1 picomole, or less than one part per trillion. Nevertheless, these tiny amounts are biologically effective because hormones are detected and bound by specific receptors.

Agonists and Antagonists

The ability to bind to the receptor and the capability of stimulating an action by the receptor are two different aspects of drug action. The ability to bind to the receptor is expressed as affinity. The capability of stimulating the receptor to some action is called **efficacy**.

Any compound, either natural or synthetic, that binds to a specific receptor and produces a biologic effect by stimulating that receptor is called an **agonist**. For example, norepinephrine produced in nerve terminals binds to specific proteins in the heart called beta$_1$-adrenergic receptors. Stimulation of these receptors causes the heart to beat faster. The synthetic drug isoproterenol acts on the same cardiac receptors and produces the same effects. Both norepinephrine and isoproterenol are therefore called agonists for the beta$_1$-adrenergic receptor (see Chapter 12). Agonists have both affinity for receptors and efficacy because they cause some action by the receptor (Figure 1-2).

Some drugs produce their action not by stimulating receptors but by preventing natural substances from stimulating receptors. These drugs are called **antagonists** (see Figure 1-2). For example, the drug propranolol blocks beta$_1$-adrenergic receptors and prevents agonists such as norepinephrine from stimulating the receptor normally. Propranolol therefore is classed as an antagonist of the action of norepinephrine. Antagonists have affinity for receptors but lack efficacy. When the receptor is occupied by an antagonist, the receptor cannot carry out its normal function.

Classifications of Receptors

Receptors may be classified according to their affinities for agonists or antagonists. For example, receptors in the adrenergic nervous system have been divided into two

Figure 1-1   Lock-and-key fit between drugs and receptors through which they act. Site on receptor that interacts with drug has definite shape. Those drugs conforming to that shape can bind and produce biologic response. In example, only shape along lower surface of drug molecule is important in determining whether drug will bind to receptor.

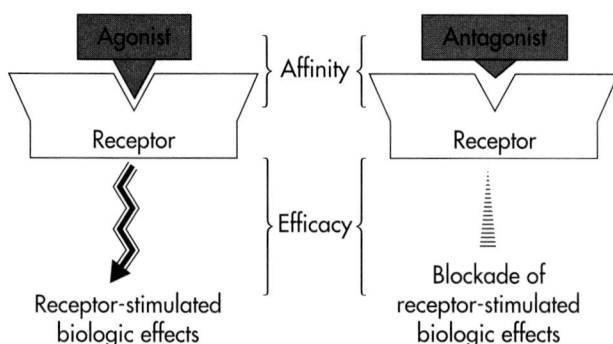

Figure 1-2   Biologic effects of agonists and antagonists. Agonists bind to the receptor and activate the processes linked to the receptor; thus agonists have both affinity and efficacy. Antagonists bind to the receptor but fail to activate it; therefore the biologic effect of an antagonist arises from blockade of normal receptor activity.

categories called alpha and beta, based on differing affinities for two natural agonists, epinephrine and norepinephrine (see Chapter 12).

Receptors may also be classified by location within the cell or on the cell membrane. Receptors on the cell membrane are typically on the outside of the cell, allowing the receptor to interact with substances in the extracellular fluid. One class of membrane-bound receptors regulates function of ion channels, either opening or closing channels as a result of binding to an agonist. This type of action produces a very rapid change in cell function. An example of this type of ion channel-linked receptor is the acetylcholine receptor in the cholinergic system (see Chapter 11).

Another type of membrane-bound receptor gains enzymatic activity when it binds an agonist. For example, the receptors for growth factors and for insulin (see Chapter 69) carry tyrosine kinase activity when the agonists are present. The actions of tyrosine kinase change various intracellular processes, including gene transcription, and thus change the function of cells over a period of hours.

Many receptors that are important for pharmacology are linked to a system of membrane proteins called *G proteins*. G proteins are capable of stimulating or inhibiting a wide array of activities, including adenylate cyclase (see Chapter 12) and calcium channels (see Chapter 13).

The ion channels, protein kinases, and G-protein systems linked to receptors are called *transducers* because they convert a signal from receptors outside the cell into an action inside the cell. An important feature of these transduction cascades is that they can amplify the signal received (Figure 1-3). For example, for each molecule of agonist bound to one beta-adrenergic receptor, 10,000 molecules of the internal messenger, cyclic adenosine monophosphate (cAMP),

may be produced. Therefore a few molecules of agonist circulating in blood can have profound effects on target cells.

Receptors that are inside the cell require that the agonist either diffuse into or be transported into the cell to produce its biologic effect. Thyroid hormones (see Chapter 67) and steroids (see Chapter 41) operate through receptors of this type. These receptors are activated in the cytoplasm by binding to agonists, but then move into the nucleus, where they influence gene transcription (Figure 1-4). This mechanism requires hours to days for full effects to be produced.

Drugs Do Not Create Functions but Modify Existing Functions within the Body

Drugs must always be considered in terms of the physiologic functions they alter in the body. In no case do drugs create a function in a tissue or organ. For example, the synthetic agent albuterol is a drug used to promote dilation of the bronchioles (see Chapter 12). Albuterol produces this effect by interacting with beta$_2$-adrenergic receptors. Thus, the drug does not create a new way for the bronchioles to dilate; albuterol simply acts through the existing mechanisms normally regulating bronchodilation.

To emphasize this principle, subsequent chapters on drug families start with a brief description of the normal physiology influenced by that group of drugs. This strategy

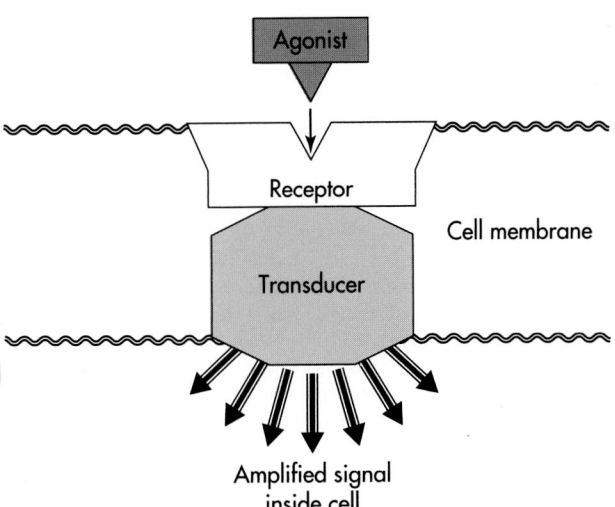

Figure 1-3   Amplification by transducers linked to receptors on the cell surface. One molecule of agonist bound to the receptor activates the transducer system, which generates an amplified signal involving many molecules inside the cell.

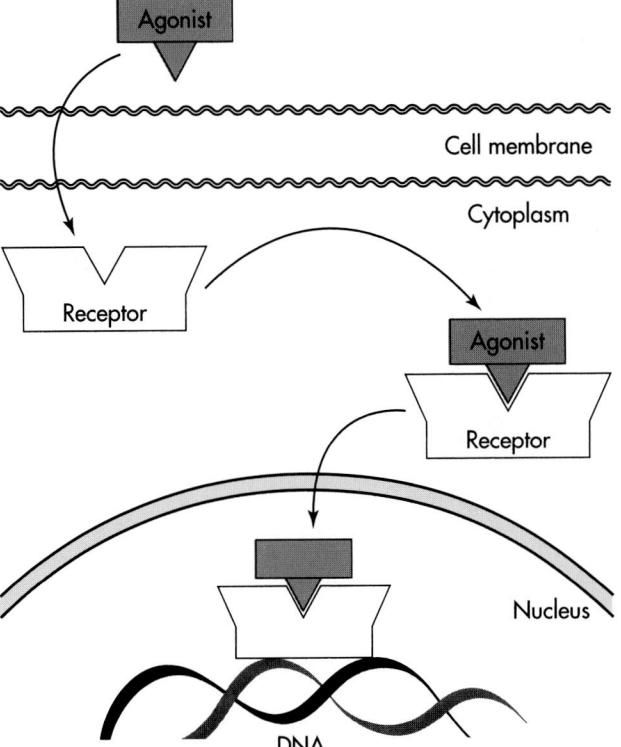

Figure 1-4   Mechanism of cytoplasmic receptors. Agonist enters the cell and binds to the cytoplasmic receptor. The activated receptor moves into the nucleus, where it influences gene transcription.

simplifies the learning process for pharmacology. For example, physiology teaches the function of beta-adrenergic receptors in regulating blood pressure, heart rate, and bronchodilation. Therefore, when a drug is noted to stimulate beta-adrenergic receptors, the clinical result of that stimulation is predictable from the known physiologic functions of those receptors.

No Drug Has a Single Action

The desired action of a drug is an expected, predictable response. Ideally, each drug would have the desired effect on one physiologic process and produce no other effect. However, all drugs have the potential for altering more than one function in the body. These unwanted actions are known as **side effects.** For example, the desired action of digitalis is to strengthen a failing heart, but at the same time it may cause erratic heartbeats, which is an undesirable side effect.

Predictable reactions arising from known pharmacologic actions of drugs account for 70% to 80% of all drug reactions. For example, barbiturates put a patient to sleep because they depress the central nervous system, but excessive depression of the central nervous system is lethal because the brain centers that control breathing are also depressed. Respiratory depression would therefore be an expected side effect when barbiturates are used at dosages that allow the drug to accumulate in the body. Other predictable side effects may occur at normal therapeutic dosages and are related to the secondary actions of the drug. For example, at normal therapeutic dosages barbiturates increase the drug-metabolizing activity of the liver. This ability is unrelated to the therapeutically desired activity of these drugs and actually leads to a number of interactions with other drugs.

Unpredictable reactions account for 20% to 30% of all drug reactions. Although experience shows that a certain

Table 1-1	**Forms of Medication**		
Form	Description	Form	Description
Capsules	Solid dosage forms for oral use in which medication is enclosed in gelatin shell that dissolves in stomach or intestine. Gelatin shell is colored to aid in product identification. Manufacturers use distinctive shapes for identifying their capsules.	Suspension	Finely divided drug particles that are suspended in suitable liquid medium before being injected or taken orally. Suspensions must not be injected intravenously.
Douche	Aqueous solution used as cleansing or antiseptic agent for part of body or body cavity. Douches are usually sold as powder or liquid concentration to be dissolved or diluted before use.	Sustained-action drugs	Form of medication altered so that dissolution is slow and continuous for extended period. Total dosage in sustained-action medication is greater than for regular formulations because drug is not all released at once.
Elixirs	Clear fluids for oral use that contain water and alcohol with glycerin and sorbitol or another sweetener sometimes added. Alcohol content of these preparations varies.	Syrups	Medication dissolved in concentrated solution of sugar such as sucrose. Flavors may be added to mask unpleasant taste.
Glycerites	Solutions of drugs in glycerin for external use. Solution must be at least 50% glycerin.	Tablets	Solid dosage forms shaped like disks or cylinders that contain, in addition to drug, one or more of following ingredients: binder (adhesive that allows tablet to stick together), disintegrators (substances promoting tablets dissolution in body fluids), lubricants (required for efficient manufacturing), and fillers (inert ingredients to make tablet size convenient).
Patches	Inner surface of the patch contacts skin and allows transdermal absorption of lipid-soluble drugs. The total amount of drug on the patch is very large, but typically only a small fraction is absorbed.		
Pills	Solid dosage forms for oral use in which drug and various vehicles are formed into small globules or ovoids. True pills are rare; most have been replaced by compressed tablets.	Enteric-coated drugs	Solid dosage forms for oral use. Medication in tablet form is coated with materials designed not to dissolve in stomach but to dissolve in intestine, where medication may be absorbed.
Solution	Liquid preparations, usually in water, containing one or more dissolved compounds. Solutions for oral use may contain flavoring and coloring agents. Injectable solutions must be sterile; solutions for intravenous injection must also be particle free.	Press-coated or layered drugs	Preformed tablet that has another layer of material pressed on or around it. This practice allows incompatible ingredients to be separated and causes them to be dissolved at slightly different rates.
		Tincture	Alcoholic or water-alcohol solutions of drugs.
Suppositories	Solid dosage forms to be inserted into body cavity where medication is released as solid melts or dissolves. Suppositories often contain cocoa butter (theobroma oil), which is solid at room temperature but liquid at body temperature, or glycerin, polyethylene glycol, or gelatin, which dissolves in secretions from mucous membranes.	Transdermal creams	Relatively lipid-soluble drugs that may be absorbed transdermally. Dosage is usually measured in inches of cream extruded from tube.
		Troches (also called *lozenges* or *pastilles*)	Solid dosage forms often shaped like disks or cylinders that contain drug, flavor, sugar, and mucilage. Troches dissolve or disintegrate in mouth, releasing medication such as antiseptic or anesthetic for action in mouth or throat. Troches dissolve more slowly than tablets.

percentage of the population may react to a drug in an un-usual manner, it is often impossible to predict which individual will show the reaction. Unpredictable drug reactions are of two types: idiosyncratic and allergic. Idiosyncratic reactions have no obvious cause and may relate to an undetected genetic difference from most of the population. Allergic reactions account for 6% to 10% of all drug reactions. An allergic reaction may be triggered by the drug in its original form or by a metabolite of the drug formed in the body.

Drug allergies range from mild skin reactions to potentially fatal reactions involving the cardiovascular and respiratory systems. *Anaphylaxis* is a severe, rare reaction marked by sudden contraction of the bronchioles and often by edema of the mouth and throat, which may completely cut off airflow to the lungs. In addition, blood pressure falls, and the patient may go into shock. These violent reactions may occur quickly, and aggressive therapy is required to save the patient's life.

Another serious drug allergy is called *serum sickness.* Symptoms include hives, pain in the joints, swollen lymph nodes, and fever. This reaction typically develops much more slowly than anaphylaxis, but it can nevertheless be life-threatening if not controlled.

Any patient can have an allergic reaction in response to any drug, but certain drugs are more prone to cause reactions. For example, penicillins are one of the more common causes of anaphylaxis, whereas iodides, sulfonamides, and phenytoin more commonly cause serum sickness. Patients receiving these agents should be closely monitored to detect early signs of allergic responses and thereby to protect them from injury.

Allergic reactions do not occur during the first exposure to a drug because time is required for the immune system to develop antibodies that cause these reactions (see Chapter 38). Documenting prior exposure to a drug is helpful but is not always easy. Patients do not always know the names of drugs they have received and are not always reliable sources of information on prior reactions to drugs. Moreover, persons may be unknowingly exposed to antibiotics or other drugs through food or milk if the drugs have been improperly used in animal medicine.

HOW DRUG DOSAGE RELATES TO DRUG ACTION: PHARMACOKINETICS

The Role of Route of Administration and Elimination

Drugs differ in their intrinsic ability to produce an effect, in their ability to penetrate to the site of action, and in their rate of removal from that site. **Pharmacokinetics** is the study of how drugs enter the body, reach their site of action, and are removed from the body. Both the pharmacokinetics and the pharmacodynamics of a drug determine how a drug is administered, how often it is given, and at what dosage.

CASE STUDY
Pharmacokinetics

James, who is taking 2.68 mg of clemastine every 12 hours for allergies, begins to complain of dry mouth, drowsiness, and unsteadiness after taking the drug for 4 days. His medication is then changed to one 2.68 mg tablet every 24 hours. After 1 week on the new regimen, James confides that the dry mouth and the other symptoms are less bothersome. He is concerned that 2 to 3 hours before it is time to take his next dose, he develops itchy eyes and congestion. In response, his dosing schedule is changed to one 1.34 mg tablet every 12 hours. On follow-up 3 weeks later, James reports good control of allergic symptoms and no recurrence of the original side effects.

1. How long will it take for a plateau concentration of clemastine to be achieved, if the half-life of clemastine is 12 hours?
2. Why was James switched from the standard dose of 2.68 mg every 12 hours to 2.68 mg every 24 hours?
3. What happens to the plateau concentration of this drug after the first dose change?
4. Why was James switched from 2.68 mg once daily to 1.34 mg twice daily?
5. What happens to the plateau concentration after the second dose change? What happens to the fluctuation in blood levels after the second dose change?

Factors Controlling Drug Absorption by Enteral Route

To be effective systemically, a drug must be present in body fluids or tissues in a free or available form. For most medications, less than the total amount of administered drug is ultimately available to produce effects on target tissues. The term **bioavailability** describes what proportion of the administered drug is available to produce systemic effects. If a drug has low bioavailability, most of the administered dose of the drug is lost or destroyed, never reaching the blood in a form that can be effective. Drugs that are freely and rapidly absorbed have a high bioavailability. The many factors that can influence bioavailability are discussed in the following sections.

Drug Dissolution. About 80% of drugs used in clinical practice are administered orally, primarily because of the ease and convenience of administration by this route. The drug may be given in liquid form or in a solid form such as a tablet or capsule (Table 1-1). To make this solid form, the drug is usually mixed with other compounds that serve various functions. Starches and other compounds may be added as inert fillers, especially when the actual amount of drug required per dose is too small to be conveniently handled. Adhesive substances called binders may also be added to allow a tablet to hold together after it is compressed in manufacture. Other compounds called disintegrators may be required to allow a tablet to absorb water and to break apart in the body. Lubricants are often added to prevent tablets from sticking to machinery during manufacture. These additions may make up most of the tablet. For example, in tablets containing 100,000 units of penicillin, the active ingredient, potassium penicillin, makes up only 11% of the tablet mass.

To be effective, the solid dose of a drug must break apart in the gastrointestinal tract and allow the drug to go into solution. Only dissolved drug is absorbed from the gastrointestinal tract into the blood. Because breakdown of the solid dosage form is required for absorption of drug, any variability in this process can affect how rapidly and completely the drug is absorbed. The formulation of a tablet or capsule affects dissolution rates. Tablets from different manufacturers that contain the same amount of active ingredient but different types and amounts of inert ingredients may not be identical in clinical action because each formulation may dissolve differently. Tablets may also change with age and conditions of storage. Older tablets tend to dry out and are harder to disintegrate, which leads to reduced bioavailability of the drug.

Gastrointestinal Tract. The presence of food influences the dissolution and absorption of drugs. For example, the antibiotic tetracycline should be given on an empty stomach because food blocks absorption of the drug. In contrast, the antifungal griseofulvin is best absorbed when taken with fatty foods.

Stomach acidity also influences absorption. For example, penicillins are not stable in acid, and part of the dose is destroyed rather than absorbed. There is considerable variation from person to person in gastric emptying times and therefore in the length of time a drug spends in stomach acid. In addition, the amount of acid in the stomach varies with the individual and the time of day. The very young and older adults have less stomach acid than middle-aged persons. Lower acidity may mean less drug is degraded and more is available to be absorbed.

Chemical Properties of the Drug. In addition to the physical state of the drug, its chemical nature determines how satisfactory oral administration will be. To pass through membranes lining the gastrointestinal tract, a drug must be relatively lipid soluble because the membranes themselves contain a high concentration of lipid. Ionic (charged) forms of drugs do not pass easily through these membranes. Many drugs can exist in an ionic state or in an uncharged lipid-soluble state, depending on the pH of the environment. This environment changes throughout the gastrointestinal tract (Figure 1-5). Stomach fluid is highly acidic. A drug such as aspirin, which is a weak acid, is converted from a charged to an uncharged form by the strong acid in the stomach. Because the uncharged form of the drug can readily diffuse

through the lipid membranes of the stomach cells, the drug is rapidly absorbed.

Enteric coatings on tablets or capsules protect some drugs that are sensitive to stomach acid (see Table 1-1). These coatings are inert at low (acidic) pH but soluble at higher (alkaline) pH. Therefore the drug passes through the stomach and is released in the intestine. Enteric coatings are also used for drugs that are highly irritating to the gastric mucosa.

Fluids in the small intestine are slightly alkaline. This higher pH favors absorption of weakly basic drugs because at this pH range weak bases are uncharged (see Figure 1-5). The small intestine also has an enormous surface area for drug absorption, which makes it a major site of absorption. However, some drugs, particularly proteins such as insulin or growth hormone, are destroyed in the small intestine by the action of digestive enzymes from the pancreas.

Drugs that are absorbed from the small intestine are transported by portal circulation directly to the liver before being circulated to the rest of the body (Figure 1-6). The liver may metabolize much of the drug before it can enter general circulation. The term **first-pass effect** refers to this process. Liver metabolism often inactivates drugs; when this happens, the first-pass effect lowers the amount of active drug released into systemic circulation. For example, morphine is very rapidly extracted from blood and metabolized by the liver; therefore, to achieve the same level of pain relief, it is necessary to administer six times more morphine orally than intramuscularly. In contrast, the related drug codeine is much less affected by the first-pass effect; therefore it takes only two times more codeine orally than intramuscularly to produce the same degree of pain relief. In these examples the larger oral doses compensate for the drug lost through inactivation by the liver.

The first-pass effect may be avoided by using other routes of administration, such as sublingual (drug dissolved under the tongue), buccal (drug dissolved between the cheek and gum), and rectal routes (see Figure 1-6). Drugs taken by these routes are absorbed directly across mucous membranes and rapidly enter the systemic circulation. The sublingual and buccal routes are useful when a palatable, highly lipid-soluble drug is involved. The rectal route is especially useful for unconscious patients. The best physical form for rectal use is a suppository that will melt at body temperature and release the drug for absorption (see Table 1-1).

Factors Controlling Drug Absorption by Parenteral Routes

Parenteral routes of drug administration require injection into the skin, muscle, or blood (see Chapter 5). Injection necessarily involves breaking the skin, and sterile technique must be used to prevent bacteria or viruses from gaining entry (Table 1-2). Special precautions often must be taken to avoid producing undue tissue damage from irritating drugs. These precautions may involve preventing the drug from contacting skin; some drugs require dilution before administration.

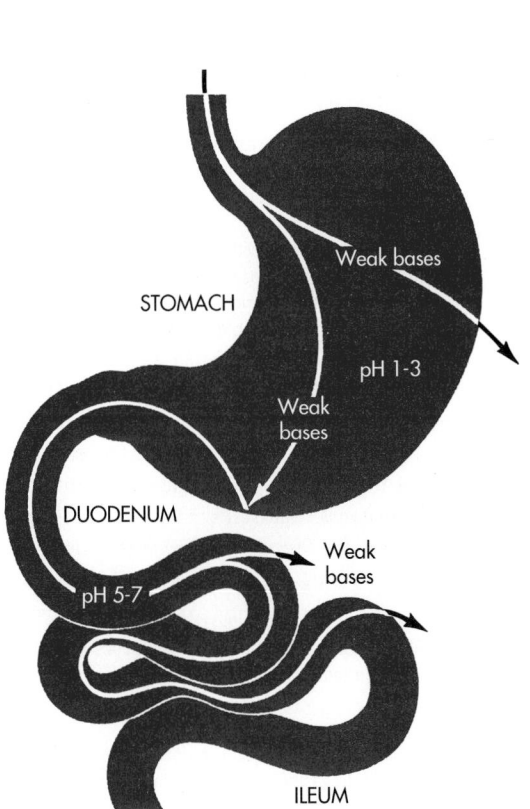

Figure 1-5   Effect of pH on ability of drugs to cross gastrointestinal membranes. The strongly acidic environment of stomach (pH 1 to 3) maintains weak acids in uncharged form, which is more easily absorbed. Weak bases remain charged in the stomach but are converted to uncharged forms as pH approaches neutrality (pH 7) or becomes slightly alkaline (pH 7 to 8).

Figure 1-6   Two circulatory pathways for materials absorbed from gastrointestinal tract. Materials absorbed from stomach, small intestine, or colon enter portal circulation, which perfuses liver before returning to heart. Materials absorbed from these sites are exposed first to action of liver microsomal enzymes and then are circulated to rest of body. In contrast, absorption through membranes lining mouth or rectum deliver material directly to systemic circulation.

Subcutaneous Injection. Subcutaneous injection (under the skin) is appropriate for small drug volumes and for drugs intended to be slowly absorbed (e.g., insulin). When very slow absorption is desired, drugs may be formulated as solid inserts that release the drug over prolonged periods. An example is the insert that releases hormones and provides birth control for months (see Chapter 70).

Intramuscular Injection. Intramuscular injection (into a muscle) is appropriate when large volumes of drug must be injected. Absorption from intramuscular sites is faster than from subcutaneous sites because muscles have a better blood supply than does skin. Absorption from subcutaneous or intramuscular sites can be hastened by applying heat or massage to the site to accelerate blood flow. Absorption can be slowed by decreasing blood flow to the injection site by applying ice packs or by the simultaneous injection of a drug such as epinephrine, which constricts blood vessels.

The forms of drugs intended for intramuscular or subcutaneous injection may be relatively insoluble. Some drugs are formulated specifically to dissolve slowly and therefore to be absorbed slowly from injection sites. These dosage forms are called *depot injections.*

Intravenous Injection. Intravenous injection (directly into a vein) requires special precautions. Drugs for intravenous use must always be in solution and can contain no particulate matter. Some drugs irritate the veins and cause thrombophlebitis if administered at too high a concentration. Other drugs must be injected slowly to avoid toxic concentrations of drug from reaching the heart or other vital organs. The intravenous route is valuable when drug concentrations must be maintained continuously, but potential harm to the patient is significant by this invasive route.

Special Injection Routes. A few drugs may be infected into very specific body sites. For example, local anesthetics may be injected into the spinal column to produce certain types of anesthesia. Other drugs may be injected directly into body cavities or joints.

Table 1-2   **Summary of Major Routes for Administration of Drugs**

Description	Advantages	Disadvantages
Aerosol		
Fine particles or droplets are breathed in.	Direct delivery to lung	Irritation of lung mucosa may occur. Special equipment is required. Patient must be conscious.
Buccal		
Drug is dissolved between cheek and gum and absorbed across mucous membrane.	Convenient Sterility not needed Direct delivery to general circulation	Not useful for drugs with unpleasant taste. Irritation to oral mucosa may occur. Patient must be conscious. Useful only for highly lipid-soluble drugs.
Inhalation		
Drug is inhaled as a gas.	Continuous dosing Patient may be unconscious.	Useful only for drugs that are gases at room temperature. Irritation of mucosa may occur.
Intramuscular		
Drug is injected into muscle mass.	Rapid absorption Soluble or insoluble drug forms Patient may be conscious or unconscious.	Sterile procedures are necessary. Minor pain is common. Irritation and local reactions may occur.
Intravenous		
Drug is injected directly into vein.	Direct control of drug concentration in blood Rapid attainment of effective blood levels	Sterile procedures are necessary. Risk of transient high drug concentrations is possible if injected too rapidly.
Oral		
Drug is swallowed and absorbed from stomach or small intestine.	Convenience Sterility not needed Economical	Unpleasant taste may cause noncompliance. Irritation to gastric mucosa may induce nausea. Patient must be conscious. Digestive juices may destroy drug. Absorbed drug enters portal circulation to liver, where it may be metabolized.
Subcutaneous		
Drug is injected under skin.	Patient may be conscious or unconscious.	Sterile procedures are necessary. Pain and irritation at site may occur.
Sublingual		
Drug is dissolved under tongue and absorbed across mucous membrane.	Convenient Sterility not needed Direct delivery to general circulation	Not useful for drugs with unpleasant taste. Irritation to oral mucosa may occur. Patient must be conscious. Useful only for highly lipid-soluble drugs.
Transdermal		
Drug is absorbed directly through skin.	Continuous dosing Sterility not needed Direct delivery to general circulation	Effective only for lipid-soluble drugs. Local irritation can occur. Discarded patches may pose danger of poisoning.

Such routes are used when conventional routes of injection do not allow high enough drug concentrations to be achieved at the desired site of drug action.

Factors Controlling Drug Persistence in Blood

After a drug has entered the blood, its ultimate fate is determined by the chemical properties of the drug and the way it is affected by blood and the tissues it contacts. Some drugs are metabolized by enzymes in blood. An example is succinylcholine. Drugs that persist in blood are usually bound to blood proteins rather than being simply dissolved directly in plasma.

The most important carrier protein is albumin, which is formed in the liver and released into the blood. Drugs bound to albumin or other carrier proteins remain in the blood because these proteins do not diffuse easily through capillary walls. Drug binding to albumin is a reversible process, and an equilibrium is established between drug that is bound to protein and drug that is free in solution. Only free drug is able to diffuse into tissues, interact with receptors, and

Table 1-3	Cytochrome P-450 Subgroups
Enzyme Subgroup	Drugs Metabolized
CYP1	acetaminophen
	caffeine
	theophylline
CYP2	codeine
	dextromethorphan
	naproxen
CYP3	acetaminophen
	cyclosporine
	estradiol
	theophylline

Table 1-4	Inducers and Inhibitors of Cytochromes P-450		
Induction		Inhibition	
Inducer	Enzyme	Inhibitor	Enzyme
Cigarette smoke	CYP1A	mexiletine	CYP1A2
Ethanol (chronic)	CYP2E1	quinidine	CYP2D6
Glucocorticoids	CYP3A4	ketoconazole	CYP3A

produce biologic effects. The same proportion of bound and free drug is maintained in the blood at all times. Thus, when free drug leaves the blood, some drug is released from protein binding to reestablish the proper ratio between bound drug and free drug.

The anticoagulant dicumarol is an example of a drug that binds to plasma protein. In blood 99% of this drug is bound to plasma albumin. Therefore only 1% of the blood content of dicumarol is free to diffuse to its site of action or to its sites of elimination. The net effect of binding to albumin is to create a reservoir of drug that is released to replenish free drug removed to other sites. In general, drugs that do not bind to plasma albumin remain in the body for shorter periods than do drugs that are tightly bound. A drug such as dicumarol, which is very strongly bound to albumin, remains in the body for up to 3 days. Drugs that are bound to plasma proteins are thus characterized by longer duration of action.

Factors Controlling Drug Distribution throughout the Body

High lipid solubility and low protein binding favor diffusion of a drug through membranes. All transport into tissues involves passing through lipid-containing membranes, a process that is difficult for water-soluble compounds but easy for lipid-soluble agents. High concentrations of free drug in blood also favors diffusion into tissues; high protein binding lowers free drug concentrations in blood and impedes diffusion into tissues.

Factors Controlling Drug Metabolism in the Body

Biotransformation is the ability of living organisms to modify the chemical structure of compounds. Many types of chemical transformations are carried out, but in general these reactions create water-soluble compounds that are more easily eliminated from the body by the kidneys. Biotransformation is sometimes divided into two phases. Phase I reactions include oxidation, hydrolysis, and reduction reactions. Phase II reactions, also called conjugations, combine a drug or metabolite with other chemicals such as acetate, glucuronic acid, glutathione, or sulfate.

The liver is by far the most important site for biotransformation of drugs, but it is not the only one. For example, the kidney is also capable of forming glucuronides and sulfates. Biotransformation may also be carried out by bacteria within the colon. This process may limit absorption of drug from the bowel after oral administration, or drug may diffuse from the blood into the bowel and be destroyed.

Biotransformation often inactivates drugs, but there are exceptions. For example, drugs such as codeine, diazepam, and amitriptyline are all converted by the liver into metabolites that are also active. A few drugs are not active until they are biotransformed by the liver. For example, the anticancer drug cyclophosphamide is inactive, but one of its metabolites produced in the liver is a highly reactive alkylating agent that is effective against cancer cells.

Phase I oxidation reactions are carried out by microsomal enzymes called cytochromes P-450. These enzymes have two important properties. First, the enzymes are relatively nonspecific, and therefore many drugs may be metabolized by the same enzyme system. Second, the liver can synthesize more enzyme if it is chronically exposed to certain drugs. This property means that the liver can increase its capacity to destroy a drug over a few days. This increase in microsomal enzyme content in the liver is called *enzyme induction.*

Three types of cytochromes P-450 carry out most of the oxidative reactions that inactivate drugs. These are designated as CYP1, CYP2, and CYP3. Within each family there are subgroups designated by capital letters and individual enzymes identified by number; for example, CYP3A is the subgroup that performs more than half of the known drug oxidation reactions and CYP3A4 is an individual member of this subgroup. Examples of common drugs metabolized by these enzymes are shown in Table 1-3.

The activities of cytochromes P-450 can be influenced by drugs or environmental chemicals. For example, cigarette smoke is a potent inducer of CYP1A (Table 1-4). Some drugs inhibit specific enzymes, creating a deficiency in the body's ability to eliminate other drugs that require that enzyme for elimination. For example, the antifungal ketoconazole raises the blood levels of many other drugs because ketoconazole inhibits CYP3A4, the most common of the drug metabolizing cytochromes P-450.

Factors Controlling Drug Elimination

The three main routes by which drugs may be eliminated from the body involve the liver, kidneys, and bowel.

Elimination in Feces. This route involves uptake of drug by the liver, release into bile, and elimination in feces. For some drugs, such as erythromycin and penicillins, the concentration of drug in bile may be much higher than its concentration in blood. Because between 600 and 1000 ml of bile is formed each day, this route of elimination may dispose of significant amounts of drug. However, drugs in bile enter the small intestine, where they may be reabsorbed into the blood, returned to the liver, and again secreted into bile. This secretion and reabsorption process is called *enterohepatic circulation.* Drugs that are extensively reabsorbed from the intestine after biliary secretion persist in the body much longer than drugs that remain in the lumen of the intestine and pass out with feces. If the reabsorbed drug is in an active form, the duration of action is prolonged.

Elimination in Urine after Metabolism by the Liver. The second route of elimination involves both liver and kidneys. Common biotransformations of drugs by the liver and other organs tend to form polar compounds, which can be more efficiently excreted by the kidneys. For example, a drug such as

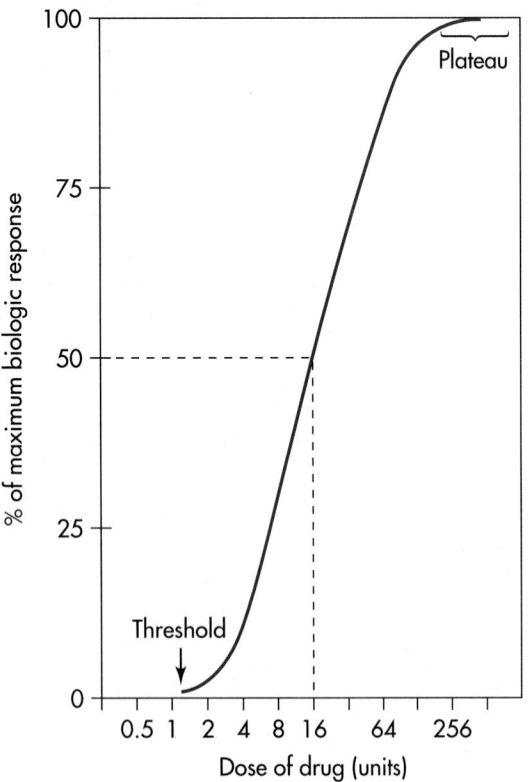

Figure 1-7 Log dose-response curve. Percent of maximum biologic response is plotted on linear scale on vertical axis. Dose of drug is plotted on logarithmic scale on horizontal axis. Threshold is dose of drug required to cause measurable response. Plateau is region of curve where increasing drug dose does not increase biologic response.

the antibiotic chloramphenicol normally enters glomerular fluid by passive diffusion but is reabsorbed from the tubules and reenters the blood. In the liver, however, chloramphenicol is transformed into chloramphenicol glucuronide. In this form the drug enters glomerular fluid, cannot be reabsorbed from the tubules, and hence is excreted in urine.

Various factors may influence the ability to metabolize drugs. For example, premature infants and neonates have immature livers that cannot perform certain biotransformations (see Chapter 2). Therefore these patients may accumulate drugs that must be metabolized in the liver before they can be excreted renally. Patients who have experienced hepatic damage, such as those who have chronic alcoholism, may also accumulate drugs normally excreted by this route.

Elimination in Urine without Metabolism by the Liver. Some drugs are not extensively metabolized anywhere in the body and are excreted unchanged in urine. This excretion may take place in one of two ways. Some drugs are excreted by passive diffusion into glomerular fluid. Other drugs are actively secreted by specific systems in the renal tubule. These active processes lead to more rapid drug elimination and allow much higher urinary concentrations of drug to be achieved. The antibiotic penicillin G is a good example of a drug that is actively secreted by renal tubules. Half of an intravenous dose of penicillin G can be eliminated in about 20 minutes by active tubular secretion. In contrast, an antibiotic such as tetracycline, which is eliminated primarily by passive diffusion in the kidneys, persists in the body for several hours.

Drugs that are normally excreted unchanged in urine accumulate in the body when there is a loss of renal function (see Chapter 2). Patients with renal disease often must have drug dosages lowered to compensate for the reduced ability of the kidneys to excrete the drug. Renal function declines with age even in healthy persons, and older adult patients may show a reduced ability to excrete drugs in their urine. Certain drugs, such as aminoglycoside antibiotics, are nephrotoxic and may directly damage the kidneys and thereby interfere with their own excretion.

Describing the Effects of Drugs in Patients

Dose-Response Curve

The relationship between the dose of drug and the response produced is described by an S-shaped (sigmoid) curve called the dose-response curve (Figure 1-7). This curve is created by plotting the observed response (on a linear scale) against the dose of the drug used to elicit that response (on a logarithmic scale).

The dose-response curve illustrates several important quantitative properties about drugs. First, there is a threshold for each drug-induced response. Doses of drug below that threshold will produce no observable effect. Second, the drug-induced response will reach a plateau rather than increase indefinitely. For example, the drug shown in Figure 1-7 produces its maximum response at a dose of about 256 units. Doubling the dose produces no detectable further effect. At lower drug concentrations, doubling the dose still does not double the effect. In this example the 50% maximum response is produced by a dose of 16 units, but twice that dose (32 units) produces only about 70%, not 100%, of the maximum response. In summary, the dose-response curve demonstrates that a finite dose is needed to cause a response and that doubling the dose does not double the response.

The dose-response curve in Figure 1-7 shows the magnitude of an effect of a drug on an individual (or average responses from several individuals). The same type of curve is produced when the drug response is instead defined as an all-or-none phenomenon (e.g., asleep versus awake) and the logarithm of the drug dose is plotted against the percentage of patients who show the drug effect at that given dose. The plateau for this curve is the drug dose at which all patients respond, and the threshold is the drug dose below which no patients respond. The recommended therapeutic dose of the drug is a dose at which most patients respond to the drug. Figure 1-8 shows this second type of dose-response curve.

Drugs produce multiple predictable biologic effects, and for each of these effects, a dose-response curve may be drawn. For example, the drug digitalis increases the force of contraction of a failing heart, but it also produces nausea, headaches, visual disturbances, and cardiac arrhythmias and ultimately triggers ventricular fibrillation. Each of these responses can be plotted as a dose-response curve (Figure 1-8). The dose-response curve for nausea lies close to the dose-response curve for therapeutic effect; therefore many patients receiving therapeutic doses of digitalis also experience nausea. With increasing doses of drug, more and more patients experience visual disturbances and arrhythmias. At drug concentrations well above normal therapeutic doses,

ventricular fibrillation occurs. These predictable drug reactions become an important part of patient care. For digitalis the visual disturbances are a warning that the concentration of drug in the patient is approaching toxic levels, which can cause cardiac arrhythmias and ventricular fibrillation.

Each drug may be described as relatively safe or relatively dangerous, based on dose-response curves such as those in Figure 1-8. For example, nausea is often associated with the use of digitalis because doses that produce nausea are only slightly greater than those that increase the force of contraction of the heart. Doses of digitalis that produce more serious reactions are only slightly higher than those that cause nausea. Digitalis therefore is a drug with a narrow margin of safety; doses must be rigorously controlled, and great care must be taken to keep blood levels of the drug within a very narrow range. In contrast, a drug with a wide margin of safety, such as penicillin G, may be given in doses greatly exceeding normal therapeutic doses without much danger of producing direct toxic effects.

Therapeutic Index. The relative safety of drugs is also sometimes expressed as a therapeutic index. The therapeutic index (TI) is the ratio of the dose of the drug lethal in 50% of a tested population (LD_{50}) to the dose of the drug therapeutically effective in 50% of the tested population (ED_{50}), or $TI = LD_{50}/ED_{50}$. These figures come from tests conducted in animals. A drug with a high therapeutic index has a wide safety margin; the lethal dose greatly exceeds the therapeutic dose. A drug with a low therapeutic index is more dangerous for patients because small increases over normal doses may be sufficient to induce toxic reactions.

Time Course of Drug Action

Drugs may enter the body by a number of routes, and all except the intravenous route take some time for the drug to enter the blood after administration. There is also a delay

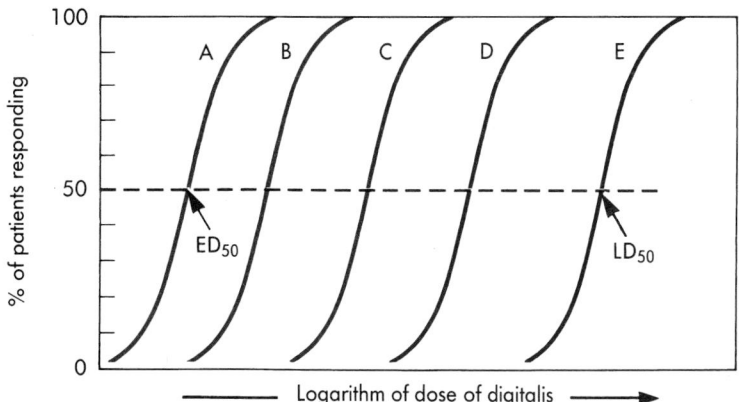

Figure 1-8   Log dose-response curves for effects of digitalis. Percent of patients responding to digitalis is plotted on vertical axis, and dose of digitalis is plotted on logarithmic scale on horizontal axis. These undesirable effects are all dose-related responses to digitalis. *Curve A,* strengthened force of contraction of heart produced by digitalis; *curve B,* nausea; *curve C,* visual disturbances; *curve D,* cardiac arrhythmias; *curve E,* ventricular fibrillation and death.

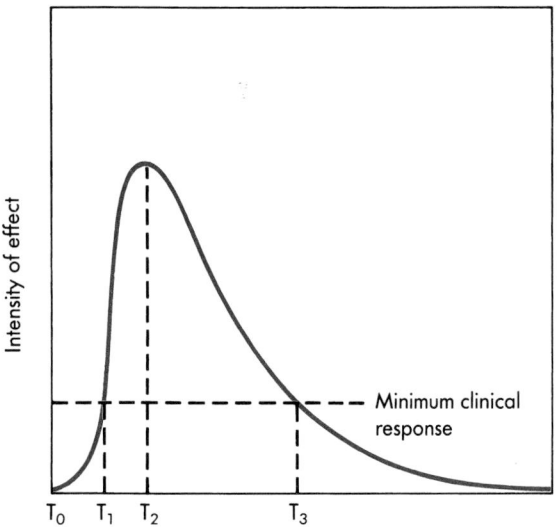

Figure 1-9   Time course of action of single dose of drug. Drug is administered at T_0. Time interval between T_0 and T_1 represents time of onset of action of drug. Peak action occurs at T_2. Time interval between T_0 and T_2 represents time for peak action. At T_3, drug response falls below minimum required for clinical effectiveness. Time interval between T_1 and T_3 represents duration of action of drug.

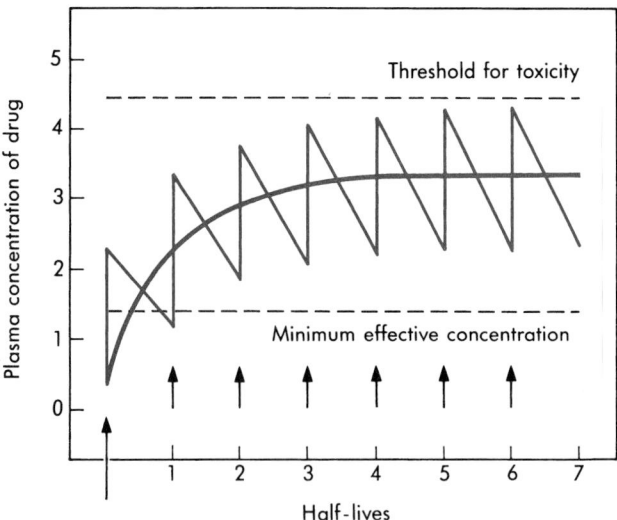

Figure 1-11   Plateau principle. In example, drug is administered once every elimination half-time for drug, as marked by arrows. Plasma concentration of drug rises and falls as drug doses are rapidly absorbed and slowly eliminated. Drug accumulates over time so that after four elimination half-times, average plasma concentration of drug has reached steady state. By adjusting the dose, average plasma concentration of drug may be adjusted.

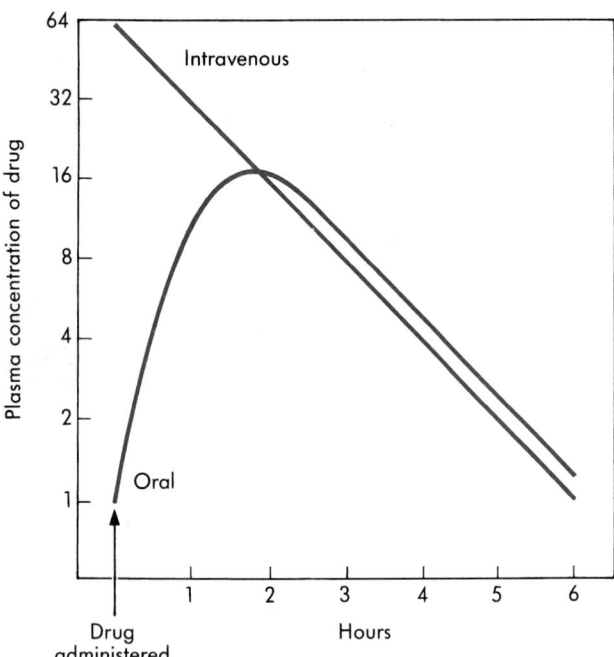

Figure 1-10   Absorption and elimination rates for drug administered by oral or intravenous route. Plasma concentration of drug is plotted on logarithmic scale on vertical axis.

between the time the drug enters the blood and the time it reaches its site of action. If the response to a single dose of a drug is measured over time, the pattern shown in Figure 1-9 is seen. The time for the **onset** of drug action is the time it takes after the drug is administered to reach a concentration that produces a response. As the drug continues to be absorbed, higher concentrations of drug reach the site of ac-

tion, and the response increases. As the drug is being absorbed, it is also subject to influences that tend to eliminate it from the body. Ultimately elimination dominates, and the concentration of drug in the body begins to fall. As a result the response will also begin to diminish. The time to peak effect is the time it takes for the drug to reach its highest effective concentration. The **duration** of action of a drug is the time during which the drug is present in a concentration large enough to produce a response. Onset and duration are determined by the rates of absorption and elimination.

Insulins are good examples of drugs for which an understanding of onset and duration of action is critical for successful drug therapy. Insulin lowers blood sugar levels, and the peak drug action must be planned to coincide with the absorptive period after meals when blood sugar levels rise rapidly. If insulin is injected at the proper dose but at the wrong time, a serious hypoglycemic (low blood sugar) reaction may endanger the patient.

Half-Life.   The concepts of onset and duration of drug action are also important for understanding the proper timing of administration of drugs given repeatedly for a course of therapy. The **half-life,** or elimination half-time, is how long it takes for elimination processes to reduce the blood concentration of drug by half. For example, the peak concentration of penicillin G in blood occurs a few moments after the drug is administered intravenously. Thereafter penicillin is rapidly excreted by the kidneys and disappears from blood. The length of time required for these processes to decrease the blood concentration of penicillin by 50% is the drug half-life, or elimination half-time, which for penicillin G is about 20 minutes. Therefore 20 minutes after an intravenous

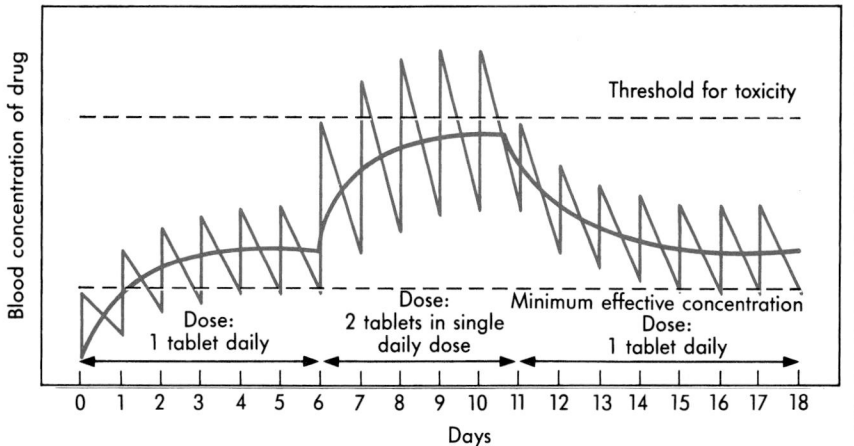

Figure 1-12   Plateau principle in practice. A patient receives a drug with a half-time of 24 hours. Increasing the dose of the drug from 1 to 2 tablets in single daily dose increases plateau concentration of drug. Return to previous dose reduces plateau concentration back to its former level.

dose of penicillin, only one half of the initial concentration of drug remains in the blood. After 40 minutes only one quarter of the initial concentration remains, and after 60 minutes only one eighth remains. During each succeeding 20-minute period, the remaining concentration decreases by half.

When drug absorption is not instantaneous, elimination competes with absorption, delaying the appearance of peak blood concentrations of drug. The drug shown in Figure 1-10 has a half-life of 1 hour. When the drug is given intravenously, the highest concentration is achieved on administration and decreases thereafter because of elimination processes. When the same dose is given orally, the drug is absorbed relatively slowly so that drug elimination is responsible for lowering the peak drug concentration that can be achieved. Once in the general circulation, however, the drug is eliminated in the same way, no matter what the initial route of administration.

Plateau Principle. When a drug is given repeatedly for therapy at fixed dosage intervals, its concentration in blood reaches a plateau and is maintained at that level until the dose or frequency of administration is changed. An example is shown in Figure 1-11, in which a rapidly absorbed drug is given at fixed intervals. The concentration of drug in blood fluctuates around a mean value, which approaches a plateau after four elimination half-times have passed; this leveling off happens regardless of the dose or frequency of administration, as long as these factors are constant. The actual dose of drug and frequency of dosage determine the plateau concentration of drug in the blood, but they do not determine how long it will take to reach that plateau.

An example of the plateau principle can be seen in a patient who is given a drug with a half-life of 24 hours. The patient takes 1 tablet at 8 AM every day. In 4 days the amount of drug being taken in each dose roughly equals the amount of drug eliminated each day; the plateau has been reached (Figure 1-12). The dose in this case is sufficient to produce clinically effective blood levels but is below the level that produces toxicity. On day 6 the patient decides to take 2 tablets instead of 1 tablet each morning. As a result the mean concentration of the drug in the blood rises, and after 4 days (four elimination half-times) a new plateau concentration is reached. At this new higher level some drug toxicity is seen. When the patient returns to the old dosage schedule of 1 tablet daily, the mean drug concentration returns to the original plateau concentration after 4 days (four elimination half-times) and is maintained until the dosage amount or intervals change.

This example illustrates the importance of maintaining regular dosage schedules and adhering to prescribed doses and dosage intervals. Timing and magnitude of the dose affect the peak concentration and the minimum (trough) concentration of the drug in blood. For many drugs these variations may not be critical, but for some the difference between a safe dose and a toxic dose is not great.

Monitoring levels of certain drugs in blood is a routine part of patient care in many settings. Direct assays for drugs allow physicians to adjust doses to ensure safe and effective blood levels of such drugs as gentamicin, amikacin, digitoxin, and phenytoin, which have a low therapeutic index. The nurse's responsibility in dealing with patients being monitored in this way may include drawing blood samples at specific times, such as at the peak or trough.

Nursing Process Overview

Drugs in the Body

Assessment

The material presented in this chapter forms the framework for subsequent specific information about drugs in each chapter. Study the mechanism of action of each drug class presented. Does this drug operate through specific receptors? Does it alter a body fluid or cell membranes? What are the anticipated effects? How does the typical patient manifest these effects?

Planning/Implementation

Consider the possible side effects of the action of the drug in tissues. For example, does the drug affect receptors in more than one organ or tissue? Note whether experience has indi-

cated that allergies or idiosyncratic reactions are common with the drug. How might the drug's half-life influence the patient's response? What is the drug's dosing schedule?

Evaluation

Consider the balance between the positive effects of the drug and the negative reactions to understand what place a drug has in clinical practice. For example, some highly effective drugs have limited clinical use because the side effects that they produce are unacceptable for most patients. Understanding the pharmacology of individual drugs thus becomes a rational process and is much more easily accomplished. Chapter 4 discusses the application of the nursing process to drug therapy.

 CHAPTER REVIEW

Application

1. How are drug actions localized to different sites in the body?
2. What is a drug receptor?
3. How do agonists and antagonists produce biologic effects?
4. How does affinity differ from efficacy?
5. What is the function of transducing systems linked to receptors on cell membranes?
6. What is the difference between a drug action and a side effect?
7. What are the two major types of unpredictable reactions to drugs that the nurse may encounter?
8. How are pharmacodynamics and pharmacokinetics helpful to the nurse in understanding the clinical use of drugs?
9. Describe how a drug in tablet form enters the blood after oral administration. What factors may influence absorption?

10. What is the first-pass effect? Does it apply to all routes of administration?
11. How does the binding of drugs to proteins in the blood influence the effect of the drug?
12. What is biotransformation?
13. What is enterohepatic circulation?
14. What information is expressed in a log dose-response curve?
15. What is the therapeutic index of a drug?
16. What is the onset time for a drug, and how does it differ from the duration of action of a drug? What is the half-life of a drug?
17. What is the plateau principle?

Critical Thinking

1. What are the advantages and disadvantages of subcutaneous, intramuscular, and intravenous routes of drug administration?
2. How may rates of biotransformation be influenced by enzyme induction? What implications can this have on drug interactions?

References

Edwards J: Guarding against adverse drug events, *Am J Nurs* 97(5):26-30, 1997.

Niederhauser VP: Prescribing for children: issues in pediatric pharmacology, *Nurse Pract* 22(3):16, 18, 23 passim, 1997.

Effects of Life Span, Genetics, and Medical Conditions on Drug Therapy

OBJECTIVES

After studying this chapter, you should be able to do the following:

- *Explain why fetuses and neonates may be more sensitive than adults to drugs.*
- *Discuss why certain drugs such as tetracyclines should be avoided in children.*
- *Explain why older adults may need reduced doses of drugs.*
- *Discuss why glucose-6-phosphate dehydrogenase deficiency increases the risk of hemolysis with certain drugs.*
- *Discuss what changes in drug dosage may be needed for patients with renal or hepatic impairment.*
- *Explain how drugs may interact in the body.*
- *Discuss the effects of alcohol or smoking on drug effects.*

CHAPTER OVERVIEW

Not all patients respond to a particular drug dosage in the same way because of biologic variation. This biologic variability is based on subtle physiologic differences among individuals. For example, absorption of oral drug doses can be greatly influenced by stomach acidity, gastrointestinal motility, pancreatic function, and intestinal bacteria. These processes vary greatly in most people. Likewise, individuals vary in the sensitivity of certain tissues to drugs. This variability may result from differences in the number or type of drug receptors, differences in permeability barriers, and many other factors. These factors are all difficult to assess and yet greatly influence the strength of drug effects. Although the exact causes of biologic variation may be unknown for an individual, general factors such as age, gender, genetic background, and overall health status can influence responses to drugs in predictable ways. These factors are the subject of this chapter.

EFFECTS OF AGE ON DRUG RESPONSE

Embryos and Fetuses

Developing embryos and fetuses are unintended targets of drugs and chemicals taken by their mothers. The effects of many drugs are benign or at least cannot be proved to be harmful, but a few drugs pose grave risks to the unborn. The degree of damage may be related to dose and length of exposure, but it is often also associated with the developmental stage of the fetus at the time of exposure. Table 2-1 summarizes the potential adverse effects of representative drugs.

Table 2-1 **Adverse Drug Effects During Pregnancy***	
Effect of Drug	**Drugs Known to Produce the Effect in Humans**
First-Trimester Effects on Embryonic Development	
Abortion	isotretinoin, quinine
Multiple anomalies involving craniofacial development	dicumarol, ethanol, isotretinoin, methotrexate, paramethadione, phenytoin, quinine, trimethadione
Neural tube defects	valproate
Goiter	iodide, methimazole, propylthiouracil
Abnormalities of reproductive organs	Androgens, diethylstilbestrol, estrogens, progestins
Inhibition of growth	methotrexate, tetracycline, tobacco smoke
Second- and Third-Trimester Effects on Fetal Development	
Abortion, mortality	heroin, isotretinoin, tobacco smoke
Mental retardation	dicumarol, ethanol
Altered cardiovascular function	Anticholinergic drugs, propranolol, terbutaline
Hearing loss and loss of balance	Aminoglycoside antibiotics
Hyperbilirubinemia	nitrofurantoin, sulfonamides
Hemolytic anemia	nitrofurantoin
Goiter	iodide, methimazole, propylthiouracil
Abnormalities of reproductive organs	Androgens, diethylstilbestrol, estrogens, progestins
Inhibition of growth	dicumarol, ethanol, heroin, methotrexate, tetracycline, tobacco smoke
Labor, Delivery, and Perinatal Period	
Increased mortality	Tobacco smoke, cocaine abuse
Altered cardiovascular function	Anticholinergic agents, caffeine, heroin, lidocaine, meperidine, propranolol, terbutaline
Gray-baby syndrome	chloramphenicol
Respiratory depression	diazepam, meperidine, morphine, phenobarbital, ethanol, tobacco smoke
Respiratory distress	reserpine
Bleeding	aspirin, dicumarol, indomethacin
Hypoglycemia	chlorpropamide, propranolol, tolbutamide
Hyperbilirubinemia	nitrofurantoin, sulfonamides
Hemolytic anemia	nitrofurantoin
Hyperirritability	cocaine

*This list does not include all drugs that affect fetal and neonatal function but is intended to give representative examples. The nurse should check sources of specific information about individual agents when drugs are administered to pregnant patients.

Drugs that are absorbed systemically have been labeled by the Food and Drug Administration (FDA) according to the level of risk to a fetus. These FDA pregnancy categories are summarized in Table 2-2, along with examples of drugs in each category. Discussions of individual drugs throughout the text also refer to the FDA pregnancy category.

Neonates

Premature infants and neonates may respond to medications quite differently from adults or older children. Many of these different responses are caused by immaturity of the liver and kidneys in infants. At birth the liver has low levels of many of the metabolizing enzymes that enable an adult liver to biotransform various types of compounds (Table 2-3). Before these metabolizing enzymes increase to adult levels during the first weeks or months of life, neonates are more vulnerable than adults to chemicals requiring detoxification in the liver.

The kidneys are also less efficient at birth than in adult life. Therefore excretion of many compounds takes longer in neonates than in adults. Failure to consider this reduced ex-

cretory capacity when calculating drug dosage can be important when certain drugs are administered to a neonate.

The antibiotic chloramphenicol illustrates the clinical effect of reduced detoxification and excretion in neonates. This potentially toxic drug is detoxified in the adult liver by the formation of chloramphenicol glucuronide, a metabolite that is efficiently excreted by adult kidneys. Unable to form the glucuronide or excrete the drug efficiently, neonates quickly accumulate chloramphenicol and experience potentially lethal toxicity. This deadly outcome is prevented by giving a reduced dose of drug that accounts for the reduced routes of elimination. The result is that less drug is required per kilogram of body weight to maintain effective levels of chloramphenicol in neonates than in adults.

Infants and Children

It is not safe to assume that any drug used in adults can also be used at adjusted doses in children. Many drugs have not been adequately tested in children, and therefore safe doses have not been established. This situation often occurs with new drugs. As more experience is gained, the drug may be

Table 2-2   FDA Pregnancy Categories

Category	Level of Risk with Drug Exposure	Examples
A	Controlled studies in women fail to demonstrate risk in the first trimester (and there is no evidence of risk in later trimesters), and possibility of fetal harm appears remote.	folic acid, thyroid hormones
B	Animal reproduction studies have not demonstrated fetal risk, but there are no controlled studies in pregnant women. Animal reproduction studies have shown adverse effect (other than decreased fertility) that was not confirmed in controlled studies on women in the first trimester. There is no evidence of risk in later trimesters.	amoxicillin, buspirone, cimetidine, fluoxetine, hydrochlorothiazide, metronidazole, piperacillin
C	Studies in animals have revealed adverse effects on fetus, and there are no controlled studies in women. In some cases, studies in women and animals are not available. Drugs in this category should be given only if potential benefit justifies risk to fetus.	alteplase, ciprofloxacin, codeine, isoproterenol, morphine, reserpine
D	There is positive evidence of human fetal risk, but the benefits for pregnant women may be acceptable despite the risk, as in life-threatening diseases for which safer drugs cannot be used or are ineffective. An appropriate statement must appear in the "warnings" section of the labeling of drugs in this category.	amikacin, captopril, midazolam, netilmicin, tobramycin
X	Studies in animals or humans have demonstrated fetal abnormalities; there is evidence of fetal risk based on human experience, or both. The risk of using the drug in pregnant women clearly outweighs any possible benefit. The drug is contraindicated in women who are or may become pregnant. An appropriate statement must appear in the "contraindications" section of the labeling of drugs in this category.	isotretinoin, lovastatin, methotrexate

made available for children and recommended dosages may be published, or the drug may be contraindicated in children. For example, tetracycline antibiotics are used safely by most adults, but these drugs should not be used in children. This class of antibiotics binds tightly to bones and may impede bone growth in very young children. Tetracycline antibiotics also bind to calcium salts in teeth and become permanently incorporated in teeth that are forming. Because children younger than 12 years old are constantly forming teeth, their teeth may become permanently discolored by tetracycline. These problems are avoided by limiting the use of tetracycline antibiotics to adults or children older than 12 years of age.

Children can be sensitive to drugs because development of some tissues is not complete until adulthood. For example, the fluoroquinolone antibiotics may damage cartilage, which can lead to deformities and changes in gait. The risk of this effect, which is most critical while cartilage is still developing, is sufficient reason to avoid using these drugs in children.

Children can also have special sensitivity to certain drugs. For example, aspirin is used safely by millions of adults but can cause a dangerous reaction in children who have a viral infection such as chicken pox. Although this reaction is uncommon, it is sufficient cause to avoid administering aspirin to children with fever.

Older Adults

Older adults are also especially at risk from many drugs. Several factors may be involved. Altered central nervous system function may mask signs of drug toxicity. Reduced renal function and changes in ratios of body water, body fat, and lean muscle mass can influence the distribution of a drug in the body and change rates of excretion. Older adult patients are more likely to be malnourished, which may alter serum

Table 2-3   Drug Metabolizing Enzymes That Change during Development

Activity in Enzyme	Fetus/Neonate	Age Adult Level Achieved
Phase I		
CYP1A2	Nearly absent	4 months; may be higher than adult in children from 1 to 2 years of age
CYP2C	Nearly absent	6 months; may be higher than adult in children from 3 to 4 years of age
CYP2D6	Nearly absent	3 to 5 years
CYP3A4	Low	6 to 12 months; may be higher than adult in children 1 to 4 years of age
CYP3A7	High	Begins to decline in the first week of life; very low in adults
Phase II		
Acetylase	Low	1 to 3 years of age
Glucuronosyltransferase	Low	6 to 18 months of age

albumin levels and influence drug binding. Older adults often have chronic diseases, and therefore they may be taking more than one drug, which increases their risk of drug interactions. For these reasons older adults need special attention to detect early signs of drug interactions or drug toxicity related to diminished excretory capacity, altered drug sensitivity, or altered drug distribution.

The aminoglycoside antibiotic gentamicin illustrates the type of drug likely to cause troublesome reactions in older adults. Aminoglycosides are excreted almost exclusively by the kidneys. Because renal function decreases with age, older adult patients excrete aminoglycosides at reduced rates. If the physician does not reduce doses to take this effect into account, aminoglycosides will accumulate. One of the early signs of toxicity may be partial loss of hearing or equilibrium, but loss of hearing or an unstable gait in an older adult patient may be mistaken for a sign of aging. Therefore the older patient may experience toxicity longer than a younger patient would because in the younger patient the same signs would be recognized immediately as **iatrogenic** (caused by a drug). Moreover, if an older person is taking an aminoglycoside and also taking a drug such as furosemide for hypertension, the risk of ototoxicity is increased because both aminoglycosides and furosemide cause this side effect.

Several other clinically important drugs illustrate how responses to drugs change in the elderly. For example, angiotensin-converting enzyme (ACE) inhibitors, a class of agents commonly used to treat hypertension, tend to accumulate in elderly patients, and the elderly tend to show a more marked decrease in blood pressure than younger adults with standard doses. Prazosin, another antihypertensive agent, has similar pharmacokinetics in young or older adults, but the older adults show a more dramatic fall in blood pressure for a given dose. These examples illustrate not only the need to adjust dosages properly for elderly patients but also the need to observe carefully for signs of excessive drug action in this age group.

EFFECTS OF GENETIC TRAITS ON DRUG THERAPY

Gender of the Patient

Men and women may respond differently to drugs. For example, metabolism of a drug such as propranolol occurs much more quickly in men than in women. As a result, when similar dosages are used, the levels of drug in the blood are about twice as high in women as in men. Similarly, the calcium channel blocker amlodipine lowers blood pressure more effectively in women than in men. Whether such differences exist for most drugs is unknown because specific trials to show differences based on gender have not been performed.

Men and women also respond differently to small amounts of ingested ethanol. In men a high level of the enzyme alcohol dehydrogenase exists in the stomach; this enzyme rapidly destroys significant amounts of the alcohol before it can be absorbed. In women the level of this enzyme is reduced and as a result more ethanol is absorbed, producing a higher blood level of the drug than the same dose produces in men.

Enzyme Changes Related to Ethnicity
Drug Metabolizing P-450 Enzymes

Different ethnic groups may respond differently to some drug classes. For example, blockers of the beta-adrenergic receptors are often used to control blood pressure, but African-American patients tend to respond less well to beta-blockers than do Caucasians; Chinese patients are much more sensitive to these drugs than either Caucasian or African-American patients. Asian populations also seem to respond to lower dosages of benzodiazepines and tricyclic antidepressants, two classes of drugs that are used extensively for mood disorders. The causes of these differences are beginning to be understood. For example, Asian populations tend to have a lower activity of the drug metabolizing enzyme CYP2D6, which acts on a variety of drugs, including the beta-blocker propranolol and the tricyclic amitriptyline (Table 2-4). Asian populations also have a higher proportion of individuals with the slow variant form of CYP2C19, an enzyme also acting on benzodiazepines and tricyclics. Both these changes lower drug metabolizing capacity, which tends to allow these drugs to accumulate unless dosages are reduced to accommodate the lowered metabolic capacity.

Acetylation

The rate of drug acetylation in the liver is another genetically determined trait that may affect the incidence of certain drug reactions (see Table 2-4). About half of Americans, both African-Americans and Caucasians, possess liver enzyme systems that acetylate drugs and other chemicals slowly, at rates less than half of those of the rest of the population. In contrast, slow acetylation occurs in about 20% of Chinese populations but is rare in Eskimos and Japanese populations.

Isoniazid, a drug used to treat tuberculosis, illustrates how the genetically determined ability to acetylate a drug can influence unwanted reactions. Isoniazid is inactivated primarily by acetylation and is eliminated in urine entirely as metabolites. In slow acetylators the half-life of the drug is about 3 hours, but in rapid acetylators it is only about 1 hour. Liver damage may be more common in rapid acetylators because the concentration of a hepatotoxic acetylated metabolite is

Table 2-4	Drug Metabolizing Enzymes with Known Genetic Variants		
Proportion of Variant in Populations of These Races:			
Metabolic Reaction	**African/Black**	**Asian**	**Caucasian**
Acetylation, slow variant	42%-65%	7%-22%	52%-62%
CYP2C19 oxidation, slow variant	Not established	12%-22%	3%-5%
CYP2D6			
Slow variant	1%-8%	1%	3%-10%
Intermediate activity		98%	
Normal activity	90%-98%		89%-96%
Super fast variant	ca. 1%-2%	ca. 1%	ca. 1%

high. Slow acetylation may be more closely associated with dose-related toxicity (neuropathy, depression of liver biotransformation enzymes) because the untransformed drug may accumulate in persons with this trait. Therefore dosages may need to be lowered for slow acetylators.

Glucose-6-Phosphate Dehydrogenase Deficiency

Some drug reactions are clearly linked to a particular genetic trait that is more prevalent in certain ethnic groups. For example, the enzyme glucose-6-phosphate dehydrogenase (G6PD) is abundant in tissues of most people. In red blood cells this enzyme plays a role in forming reduced nicotinamide-adenine dinucleotide phosphate (NADPH), which is needed to maintain active hemoglobin. As a result of a genetic alteration, some people lack adequate concentrations of G6PD in their red blood cells. Therefore NADPH is generated slowly. Under normal circumstances this alteration would not be critical, but if a person with this trait is exposed to chemicals that enhance the conversion of hemoglobin to methemoglobin (a relatively inactive form of hemoglobin), serious problems can arise. Lower levels of G6PD produce too little NADPH to fully reform active hemoglobin. When too much methemoglobin accumulates, red blood cells are destroyed.

G6PD deficiency is important for pharmacology because many drugs accelerate methemoglobin formation. Sulfonamides, antimalarial medications, and analgesic-antipyretic drugs (including aspirin) fall into this category. In a person lacking adequate G6PD activity, these drugs can cause life-threatening **hemolysis** (rupture of the red blood cells). The same drugs are relatively harmless in most people who possess adequate G6PD activity.

Certain populations have a high proportion of the gene that causes G6PD deficiency. For example, 13% of African-American men and 20% of African-American women may carry this gene. Sardinians also have an incidence of about 14%. More than half of Kurdish Jewish populations show G6PD deficiencies. This genetic difference from most of the American population places patients from these populations at greater risk for serious reactions with certain drugs. When these patients receive medications, they should be observed carefully for signs of toxicity.

Pseudocholinesterase Deficiency

Not all differences in drug handling are related to observable traits such as gender or ethnicity. Unsuspected genetic differences can produce unexpected reactions to drugs. For example, a small percentage of the population lacks pseudocholinesterase, an enzyme usually found in blood. People lacking this enzyme show no signs of this difference until they are exposed to drugs such as succinylcholine. Succinylcholine is a paralyzing agent used before surgery to relax muscles and allow easy tracheal intubation. In most people the drug is very short acting because it is destroyed by pseudocholinesterase. In people lacking this enzyme, succinylcholine stays in the blood, and the drug is very long

acting. These patients require artificial ventilation until the paralyzing effects of succinylcholine wear off, whereas most people recover within a minute and require no assistance.

EFFECTS OF MEDICAL CONDITIONS ON DRUG THERAPY

Renal Impairment

Renal function decreases with age, but it can also be diminished in younger people as a result of progressive hypertension, diabetes mellitus, or other causes. For many drugs excreted primarily through renal processes, dosages must be adjusted to compensate for reduced renal excretion. For example, cephalosporin antibiotics such as ceftazidime are excreted renally, and blood levels of the antibiotic are influenced by the degree of renal impairment. If reduced renal excretion is not taken into account, the drug may accumulate to toxic levels.

To adjust dosage to compensate for renal impairment, some measure of renal function must be made. A common measure of renal function is **creatinine clearance,** expressed in milliliters per minute (ml/min) or milliliters per second. Creatinine clearance is 100 to 120 ml/min when renal function is normal. Table 2-5 shows information from the package insert for the antibiotic ceftazidime. Note that if creatinine clearance is greater than 50 ml/min, no dosage adjustment is needed with this drug; the normal adult dose of 1 g every 8 hours can be given. If renal function is impaired, lower creatinine clearances are noted, and the dosage interval must be increased and/or the dose must be decreased. Note that if renal function is lost and the patient is undergoing hemodialysis, the dose is given only once in the interval between hemodialyses. Without renal excretion, blood levels of the drug persist for prolonged periods.

If direct measurement of creatinine clearance cannot be made, this value can be estimated from creatinine concentrations in the serum according to the following formula:

$$\text{Creatinine clearance (men)} = \frac{(140 - \text{Age}) \times (\text{Body weight in kg})}{72 \times \text{Serum creatinine}}$$

Table 2-5	Adjustment of Ceftazidime Dosage Based on Renal Function	
Creatinine Clearance (ml/min)	**Dosage**
>50	Usual adult dose (1 g q8h)
31-50	1 g q12h
16-30	1 g q24h
6-15	500 mg q24h
<5	500 mg q48h
Hemodialysis patients:	1 g after each hemodialysis period

The creatinine clearance for women is 85% of the value calculated by this equation. This formula is not as accurate as a direct determination of clearance, but measuring serum creatinine is much easier than measuring clearances and the accuracy of this calculation is adequate for most situations.

Alterations of Hepatic Function

Liver function may be diminished by drugs, infectious agents, and chronic alcohol consumption. These factors may make a patient much more sensitive than normal to toxicity from specific drugs. For example, the antituberculosis agent isoniazid causes clinical hepatitis in about 0.3% of healthy young adults who receive it for prophylaxis. In contrast, the incidence of acute hepatitis is 2.6% in patients who drink alcohol daily or who have significant liver disease.

Certain chemicals cause the liver to make more drug-metabolizing enzymes. This process, called **induction**, allows the liver to metabolize drugs more efficiently. For example, the anticonvulsant phenytoin can stimulate metabolism of the bronchodilator theophylline by inducing CYP3A4, one of the liver enzymes that metabolizes theophylline. As a result, the therapeutic effects of theophylline may be lost or diminished.

As a rule, drug dosage is not adjusted based strictly on measures of hepatic function. The common strategy is to monitor blood levels of the drug in question and adjust the dosage accordingly. In the example just given, for a patient receiving both phenytoin and theophylline, serum concentrations of both drugs should be monitored and the doses should be adjusted to maintain therapeutic concentrations.

Drug Interactions

Patients often have more than one condition for which they receive medical attention, and therefore they often take more than one medication at a time. This situation creates the possibility for drugs to interact. A **drug interaction** is any modification of the action of one drug by another drug. Interactions may either increase or decrease the action of the drugs involved. Drug **synergism** is a special interaction in which the effect of two drugs combined is greater than the effect expected if the individual effects of the two drugs independently were added together.

Drug interactions are commonly encountered in clinical practice and are sometimes planned as part of a therapeutic program. An excellent example is the treatment of chronic moderate hypertension, which often involves several drugs, each amplifying the action of the others to lower the blood pressure.

The negative aspect of drug interaction is that expected therapeutic results from a drug can be greatly affected by other drugs. This negative influence can be diminished if health care personnel are aware of major drug interactions, are thorough in determining which over-the-counter or prescription drugs a patient is taking, and give careful instructions to patients about drugs that interact with their prescribed medication.

Comprehensive lists of drug interactions have been published.

Pharmacokinetic Interactions

Drug interactions may arise when one drug alters the pharmacokinetics of another drug. For example, one drug may alter the dissolution, absorption, protein-binding activity, metabolism, or elimination of another drug. Pharmacokinetic interactions change the concentration of drug in the blood and at its site of action. For instance, if one drug decreases the absorption of a second drug, the concentration of the second drug is diminished and therefore the usual dose does not give the expected result. The same effect is produced if the metabolism or elimination of the second drug is increased by the first drug.

Some drugs also increase the concentration of other drugs, producing **potentiation**. Pharmacokinetic potentiation may arise because one drug increases the absorption or decreases the protein-binding activity, metabolism, or elimination of a second drug. The second drug is therefore present in higher concentrations than would be anticipated for the dose.

Pharmacodynamic Interactions

Drug interactions may also arise when one drug alters the pharmacodynamics of a second drug. If two drugs have the same action, drug potentiation results. An example is seen with vasodilators, which can lower blood pressure. A vasodilator such as hydralazine might be part of a therapeutic program for control of hypertension. Nitroglycerin is another vasodilator, but it is used to relieve angina. Patients who take hydralazine for hypertension and also take nitroglycerin for angina should anticipate a severe hypotensive response to nitroglycerin; they may need to lie down when taking the nitroglycerin to avoid fainting.

Drugs that are antagonists may produce pharmacodynamic interactions that diminish the response of both drugs at the usual therapeutic doses. An example is the beta-receptor antagonist propranolol, often used in patients with hypertension. If such a patient were to self-medicate for asthma, using an over-the-counter inhaler containing the adrenergic agonist epinephrine, a drug interaction could occur. Although in this example the therapeutic target for propranolol is the heart and that for epinephrine is the bronchioles, the two drugs would antagonize each other at all organs with beta-adrenergic receptors and neither drug would give the desired therapeutic effect.

ENVIRONMENTAL FACTORS AFFECTING DRUG THERAPY

Smoking

Environmental chemicals increasingly are being recognized as agents that cause significant drug interactions in some patients. For example, polycyclic hydrocarbons in cigarette smoke and chlorinated hydrocarbons in pesticides are active

Box 2-1 **Oral Administration of Selected Drugs**

Normally Taken on Empty Stomach with Full Glass of Water

acetaminophen	propantheline
aspirin	quinidine
cephalosporins	rifampin
erythromycin*	sulfonamides
isoniazid	tetracyclines*
penicillins	theophylline*

Normally Taken with Food to Improve Absorption

carbamazepine	lithium
cimetidine	nitrofurantoin*
griseofulvin†	propranolol
hydralazine	spironolactone
indomethacin*	

*Gastric irritation may require that the drug be taken with food, but absorption is delayed or diminished.
†This drug is taken with foods rich in fat for best absorption.

Table 2-6 **Drug Effects on Vitamin Metabolism**

Effect	Drugs
Interferes with absorption or action of folic acid, which can cause folate deficiency	Antibiotics, anticonvulsants, aspirin, clofibrate, ethanol, methotrexate, oral contraceptives
Depletes vitamin B_6	hydralazine, isoniazid, oral contraceptives
Interferes with absorption or action of vitamin B_{12}	Antibiotics, anticonvulsants, clofibrate, ethanol, oral hypoglycemics
Interferes with absorption or action of vitamin D	Antacids, anticonvulsants, mineral oil
Interferes with synthesis or absorption of vitamin K	Antibiotics, mineral oil

inducers of liver metabolic enzymes. People chronically exposed to these chemicals metabolize drugs such as the antiasthmatic medication theophylline more rapidly than normal. In these people the blood concentration of theophylline may be lower than desired unless dosage adjustments are made (see Chapter 28).

Alcohol (Ethanol)

Ethanol is a common cause of pharmacodynamic drug interactions. As a central nervous system depressant, ethanol acts synergistically with other drug classes that depress the central nervous system: antihistamines, sedative-hypnotics, antianxiety drugs, antidepressants, antipsychotics, general anesthetics, and narcotic analgesics. At low dosages the drowsiness characteristic of these drug classes is exaggerated by ethanol, but at higher dosages respiration can be dangerously depressed.

Food

Foods may interact with drugs and alter the effect of therapy, most obviously by altering the absorption of an orally administered drug. A few drugs are better absorbed or tolerated on a full stomach, but most drugs are absorbed more slowly or less completely when taken with food (Box 2-1). A few of these interactions may significantly diminish the clinical usefulness of the drug. For example, the antibiotic tetracycline forms insoluble precipitates with calcium and magnesium in food. This interaction lowers absorption of the drug so that insufficient amounts of the antibiotic enter the blood and therapy fails.

Some food-drug interactions directly antagonize the action of drugs in the body. For example, patients receiving a coumarin anticoagulant may lose the action of the drug if they ingest large amounts of leafy green vegetables and other foods high in vitamin K. Vitamin K directly antagonizes the action of the coumarins. Conversely, long-term administration of a drug may interfere with normal vitamin metabolism (Table 2-6). For example, long-term use of the antituberculosis drug isoniazid can deplete vitamin B_6 and cause neuritis. This complication can be prevented by administering vitamin B_6 supplement during isoniazid therapy.

Other food-drug interactions may arise when drugs interfere with normal mechanisms for removing noxious compounds from the body. For example, patients receiving monoamine oxidase inhibitors have a diminished ability to metabolize catecholamines and related compounds such as tyramine. When these patients eat foods with high concentrations of tyramine, such as aged cheese or red wine, they cannot eliminate the tyramine rapidly and it may accumulate, causing headache and hypertension.

Nursing Process Overview

Life Span, Genetics, Ethnic Background

Assessment

Assess the patient's age and weight. If the patient is an infant, was the child premature? Assess the patient's ethnic background. Take a family health history and check for allergies. Check laboratory work, especially renal function and liver function tests. Assess the patient's history of smoking or alcohol use.

Nursing Diagnoses

No diagnoses are based solely on the patient's age or background, but this information combined with an individualized assessment may provide the foundation for a nursing diagnosis.

Patient Outcomes

Information about the patient's age, gender, ethnic background, history of smoking or alcohol use, and existing medical problems will be reflected, if appropriate, in the dosage and

Continued

choice of drug prescribed. The patient will improve without serious adverse effects.

Planning/Implementation

Monitor the patient's vital signs and weight. Calculate dosages carefully, especially if the dosages are small for infants and children. Monitor intake and output if necessary to monitor renal function. Encourage the patient to limit smoking or stop if possible. Monitor parameters that would indicate improvement in the patient's condition, and consult with the physician when there are indications that the dosage of medication may be inappropriate for a specific patient situation. Develop and implement a teaching plan appropriate for the needs of the patient.

Evaluation

Ideally, there will be improvement in the patient's health status, with few side effects. Any side effects that do occur will be minor and diagnosed early. Adjustments in the dosage or drug will be made based on regular evaluation of the patient's condition.

Nursing Implications Summary

General Guidelines: Drug Therapy

➤ Include questions about alcohol consumption and tobacco use in the health history.

➤ Obtain a family history. What is the family's place of origin? Are the parents and grandparents still living? If not, what were the causes of death? Are siblings of the parents and siblings of the patient still living? Do they have any chronic health problems? Causes of death (if applicable)? Can the patient identify any chronic health problems in the family?

➤ Decide whether a diet history is indicated.

➤ Where is the patient employed? Is there work exposure to chemicals?

➤ Does the patient use over-the-counter remedies? Does the patient use home remedies or herbal remedies? Does the patient also use a healer, medicine man, or other traditional or native caregiver?

Neonates and Infants

➤ Monitor vital signs.

➤ Monitor fluid intake and output and body weight. Monitor laboratory work, including complete blood count (CBC), serum creatinine, blood urea nitrogen (BUN), and liver function tests.

➤ Double-check dosage calculations, especially if your math skills are not good or the dosage is unusually small.

➤ Use equipment that reduces the possibility of overdose or overload, such as minidrip tubing, volume-control devices in intravenous tubing, and rate-controlling devices.

➤ Have a colleague double-check intravenous drug dosages and volumes before administration.

Older Adults

➤ Monitor vital signs. Routinely check weight. Be alert to changes in mental status. Assess gait and balance.

➤ Monitor CBC, BUN, serum creatinine, liver function tests, serum drug levels, and other tests appropriate to the patient's medical history and medications.

➤ Ask the patient to bring all medications to the physician or nurse at each visit, or on a regular basis, so that they can be checked. Are all these medications still needed? Are there any nonprescription drugs that the patient is also taking?

 CHAPTER REVIEW

Application

1. What consideration should the nurse be aware of in administering drugs that require hepatic detoxification to a premature infant?

2. Why should the use of aspirin be avoided in a child with fever?

3. What major organ system involved in drug elimination is likely to have diminished function in normal older adults?

4. Why must biologic variability be considered in drug therapy?

5. What are some of the possible reasons for the observed differences in drug response seen among patients?

6. Why are persons of African or Mediterranean ancestry more likely than most other American populations to experience drug-induced hemolysis?

7. When is a dosage adjustment needed in patients with impaired renal function?

8. How may chronic alcohol consumption influence drug therapy?

9. What are drug interactions? What are the two major mechanisms by which they occur?

10. How can smoking, environmental chemical exposure, or dietary patterns influence the response of a patient to a drug?

Critical Thinking

1. Many years ago, mixed racial or ethnic marriages were more unusual, so most people were born of parents of the same general background. Today children of mixed backgrounds are more common, but this fact often cannot be determined by the child's appearance. What kinds of questions can the nurse ask while taking a patient history to help alert the health care team to possible genetic

traits that may be important to consider regarding medication use by the patient?

2. Consider the major industries in your local area. To what environmental hazards are people who work in these industries exposed? Are there known health problems associated with these agents? What are the signs and symptoms? How can you find out about these risks?

3. Some patients deny alcohol consumption even if they drink alcohol regularly; others report less alcohol intake than is true. Some patients may do the same when asked about smoking. When taking a health history, how can the nurse phrase questions to increase the likelihood of eliciting an accurate history of smoking or alcohol consumption?

4. Ethnic groups in the United States may retain traditional medicines; some may cause drug interactions. For example, the Chinese herbal Yin Zhi Huang alters enzymes involved in bilirubin metabolism. What ethnic groups are common in your area? What kind of traditional medications are used in these cultures? Is anything known about how they interact with western drugs?

References

Bertilsson L: Geographical/interracial differences in polymorphic drug oxidation, *Clin Pharmacokinet* 29:209, 1995.

Leeder JS, Kearns GL: Pharmacogenetics in pediatrics, *Pediatr Clin North Am* 44:55, 1997.

Rogers AS: The role of cytochrome P450 in developmental pharmacology, *J Adolescent Health* 15:635, 1994.

Legal Implications of Drug Therapy

OBJECTIVES

After studying this chapter, you should be able to do the following:

- *Discuss how drugs are tested for safety.*
- *Explain how a drug is determined to be effective for use in patients.*
- *Explain what controlled substances are.*
- *Discuss the role of nurses in drug testing.*

CHAPTER OVERVIEW

This chapter discusses the legal implications of drug therapy for nurses. Patients receiving medications have always faced certain risks, which include the possibility that the medication (1) will not produce the beneficial effect claimed by those who make and sell the drug, (2) may be directly harmful, or (3) may be improperly administered. Modern drug legislation is designed to reduce or eliminate these risks to patients.

ESTABLISHMENT OF SAFETY AND EFFICACY OF DRUGS

History of Drug Development

The earliest medical practice depended on various natural products that, by trial and error, were discovered to have certain effects on the body. For example, ancient Egyptians knew that parts of the poppy plant could be used to relieve pain, a remedy first recorded in the Ebers papyrus in 1500 BC. Equally ancient is the use of parts of the ephedra shrub by the Chinese, who called the preparation ma huang. In the New World, South American Indians used bark from the cinchona tree to relieve symptoms of malaria. Even in more recent times, natural products were used for medical practice. For example, in 1785 a British physician named Withering described the use of the leaf of the foxglove plant to relieve a certain type of edema that had previously resisted all therapy.

Until the mid-1800s, natural products were the only medicinal agents available. The most common medications were made from plants and called *botanicals*. Most botanicals have been replaced as chemists have identified the active ingredients in these crude products. The active ingredients are the chemicals in the crude preparation that are responsible for producing the biologic effect of the medicinal agent. For example, the poppy plant relieves pain because it contains opium. Ma huang produces its effects on the heart, lungs, and other organs because it contains ephedrine, an agent that stimulates the sympathetic nervous system. Similarly, the quinine in cinchona bark relieves the symptoms of malaria, and the digitalis in foxglove leaves relieves edema associated with heart failure.

Identification of the active ingredient in a crude medicinal agent has two benefits. First, the amount of active ingredient can be measured in the crude preparation, allowing effective dose standardization. For example, the digitalis content of foxglove leaves varies from plant to plant. A dosage based on the amount of leaf taken may actually contain a variable amount of digitalis and may therefore have variable biologic effects. Because the biologic activity of a drug is related to the dose of the active ingredient, dosages based on the digitalis content should have a more predictable biologic effect.

The second benefit of identifying the active ingredient of a medicinal agent is that the chemical structure and properties of the active drug are revealed. This knowledge can lead to better ways of isolating the active material from natural sources. After the structure of an active agent is known, chemists may also be able to synthesize it. Ephedrine is an example of a drug that is now chemically synthesized in a simple process that has replaced the more complicated procedure of isolating the drug from plant materials.

Standardization of Agents

Recognizing the relationship between drug dosage and biologic effect produced, most nations have adopted codes for standardizing the content of medicinal agents. Drugs sold in the United States must comply with the standards established in the *United States Pharmacopeia* (*USP* 23) and the *National Formulary* (*NF* 18). The *USP* contains chemical and physical information on all active ingredients used in medications. For example, the *USP* classifies aspirin as an antipyretic (fever-reducing), analgesic (pain-reducing) agent. A variety of tablet sizes is described, containing amounts of aspirin ranging from 65 to 650 mg. To meet *USP* standards, tablets must contain between 95% and 105% of the amount of aspirin indicated on the label. Thus an aspirin tablet labeled 500 mg must contain between 475 and 525 mg of aspirin. The aspirin used in these tablets must meet the chemical and physical standards listed for that compound in the *USP*. This information is most useful for pharmaceutical manufacture.

Recognizing the need for authoritative information on the clinical use of drugs, the *USP* also publishes *Drug Information for the Health Care Professional*. This work attempts to present the consensus on clinical indications and doses for each drug, as well as useful information on side effects, interactions, and comparisons with other agents. This work in three volumes, referred to collectively at the *USPDI*, is published yearly and updated regularly.

Standards for medicinal agents vary among countries. In Canada the current *Compendium of Pharmaceuticals and Specialties (CPS)* indexes available agents and contains monographs on specific drugs. The *British Pharmacopoeia* is the standard reference for the United Kingdom. It also includes information from the *European Pharmacopoeia* and is updated yearly with published addenda. An *International Pharmacopoeia* published by the World Health Organization (WHO) includes drug methods and standardizations.

The information in these references is indexed by generic, or nonproprietary, names. The **generic name** applies to the drug, no matter who manufactures or markets it. Trade, or proprietary, names belong to a specific company. For example, cefuroxime sodium is the generic name for a specific antibiotic; this single compound is sold under the **trade names** of Zinacef by Glaxo, Inc., and Kefurox by Eli Lilly & Co.

Legislation

Drug manufacturing and sale are regulated by state and federal agencies. For federal laws to apply, a drug must enter interstate commerce. A drug totally manufactured within a single state and sold only in that state would not be subject to the federal drug laws. Very few drugs fall into this category.

The first effective federal drug law in the United States was passed in 1906 (Table 3-1). This law was intended to protect citizens from adulterated medicines and medications that contain harmful ingredients not listed on the label. Each new law passed since that time has been intended to overcome specific problems that have arisen. For example, in the early 1900s, a certain patent medicine was advertised as a cure for cancer. The federal government sought to force the manufacturer to stop using the false advertisement. However, the drug label on the bottle accurately named the contents of the medicine. Under the 1906 law, accurate labeling of contents was all the government could require. When the Sherley Amendment was added in 1912, both advertising claims and contents of the drug label could be controlled.

The Food, Drug, and Cosmetics Act of 1938 added the requirement that a drug had to be safe before it could be marketed. Before 1938, a company was not responsible for the safety of the drugs it manufactured and sold. For example, in 1937 more than 100 people died from taking a product that was sold as an "elixir of sulfanilamide." The cause of death was not sulfanilamide but the propylene glycol used to dissolve the drug. The amazing fact is that no one had tested the toxicity of propylene glycol before using it in this

 DIETARY CONSIDERATIONS

Modern Botanicals

The use of many ancient botanicals such as ma huang and opium poppy was rationalized when efficacy of the active ingredients was proven in modern trials. In recent years a thriving industry has grown up around modern botanical preparations such as St. John's Wort, ginseng, and extract of *Gingko biloba*, for which much less convincing data exists despite potential pharmacologic effects on various body systems. Thus these agents are sold as dietary supplements, which are not subject to the same level of oversight given to medicinal agents. There is no industry-wide quality control to ensure that levels of active ingredients are standardized, and there is no requirement to prove efficacy. These preparations are discussed in Chapter 7, "Over-the-Counter Drugs and Self-Medication." Individual preparations are discussed in Alternative Therapies boxes appearing in appropriate chapters related to their active ingredients or proposed biologic effect.

Table 3-1	**Federal Drug Legislation in the United States**	
Date	**Title of Law**	**Major Provisions**
1906	Pure Food and Drug Act	Established *USP* and *NF* as official standards.
		Set standards for proper drug labeling.
1912	Sherley Amendment	Prohibited fraudulent claims for therapeutic effects of drugs.
1914	Harrison Narcotic Act	Regulated importation, manufacture, sale, or use of opium, cocaine, marijuana, and other drugs likely to produce dependence.
1938	Food, Drug, and Cosmetic Act	Required that a drug be proven safe before it was marketed.
1941-1945	Amendments to Pure Food and Drug Act	Required biologic products used as drugs (e.g., insulin) to be certified on a batch-by-batch basis by a government agency.
1952	Durham-Humphrey Amendment	Defined legend drugs (must be marked "Caution: Federal Law prohibits dispensing without prescription").
		Restricted right of pharmacist to distribute legend drugs.
1962	Kefauver-Harris Amendment	Required proof of efficacy for a drug to remain on market.
		Authorized FDA to establish official names for drugs.
1970	Comprehensive Drug Abuse Prevention and Control Act (or Controlled Substances Act)	Classified drugs by abuse potential and medical usefulness.
		Regulated manufacture, distribution, and sale of controlled substances.
1983	Orphan Drug Act	Protected companies for 7 years against competition on nonpatentable orphan drugs.
1984	Drug Price Competition and Patent Term Restoration Act	Drugs introduced after 1962 eligible for shortened drug application.
		Generic drugs are more easily introduced.
		Established guidelines for bioequivalence.
		Restored up to 5 years patent protection for time used in drug development.
1986, 1988	National Childhood Vaccine Injury Act	Private health care providers are required to keep records on adverse events following immunization.
1987	Prescription Drug Marketing Act	Bans diversion of prescription drugs from legitimate channels.
		Restricts reimportation of drugs from other countries.
1988	Food and Drug Administration Act	Establishes FDA within Department of Health and Human Services.
		Sets mechanism for appointing Commissioner of Food and Drugs.

medication. Under the law in 1937, however, the company responsible for this disaster could be charged only with mislabeling the drug because an elixir is by definition an alcohol solution.

One major provision of legislation currently controlling drug marketing and use in the United States is that a drug must be effective in treating the medical condition for which it is recommended (see Table 3-1). The requirement for proving effectiveness and safety has increased the amount of drug testing done by companies that develop new drugs. As a result fewer new drugs enter the market, and more time and money are required to place a drug on the market. On the other hand, drugs that do enter the market are much more reliable medications than they were in the past.

One class of drugs especially affected by the great cost of drug development is known as orphans. **Orphan drugs** are medicines that have not been profitable to develop and market, either because the market is too small (e.g., drugs used for treatment of rare diseases) or because patent protection has expired on the drug. Under provisions of the Orphan Drug Act (1983), companies can recover much of their development costs for orphan drugs. Companies that develop and market nonpatentable orphan drugs are also protected from competition by an Food and Drug Administration (FDA) policy that limits approval for an orphan drug to one company for the first 7 years. Orphan drugs are listed in an appendix of *Drug Information for the Health Care Professional.*

Another provision of current laws is that pharmaceuticals be produced by good manufacturing practices. Under this provision of the Food and Drug Act, the FDA inspects manufacturing facilities and oversees the production of medications. Good manufacturing practices are general procedures, not specific processes, and may vary widely from company to company.

Legislation adopted in 1984 set guidelines for bioequivalence of drugs and streamlined application processes so that approval of generic drugs was facilitated. When a drug is first introduced, it is sold only by the company that developed it or by others licensed to sell it. The developer's control of the drug is protected for 17 years by patents. After that time other companies can make and sell the drug if they have met FDA requirements for good manufacturing processes and have satisfied bioequivalence standards. For example, the antibiotic clindamycin was discovered by Upjohn and sold under the trade name Cleocin. Sales were protected by Upjohn's patent rights to the compound, but when the patent expired, several other companies applied for the right to manufacture and market the drug. These companies cannot use the trade name Cleocin, but they can sell the generic compound clindamycin. These generic preparations of clindamycin currently share the market with the original drug.

Under existing drug laws, several federal agencies are involved in regulating drug trade. In addition to official government agencies, a number of private organizations contribute advice or expertise to the government on matters

Table 3-2	Organizations Involved in Drug Regulation in the United States		
Name	Common Abbreviation	Function	
Department of Health and Human Services	HHS	Secretary of HHS is a cabinet-level officer whose duties include designating official names for drugs sold in the United States and overseeing the Public Health Service.	
Drug Enforcement Administration	DEA	Agency created within Department of Justice by the Controlled Substances Act of 1970 as the sole drug enforcement arm of the U.S. government.	
Federal Trade Commission	FTC	Regulates advertisement of medications aimed at the general public (not medical personnel).	
Food and Drug Administration	FDA	Guarantees safety, purity, effectiveness, and reliability of drugs sold in the United States; regulates advertising of medications to medical personnel.	
National Academy of Sciences–National Research Council	NAS–NRC	NAS is a private organization composed of scientists in the United States; NRC is the research arm of NAS.	
Public Health Service	PHS	Funds clinical research and is responsible for maintaining basic research programs under the National Institutes of Health.	
Pharmaceutical Manufacturers Association	PMA	This private organization representing the companies where most drugs are developed functions as an advisory group to the FDA and as a lobbying group to Congress.	
United States Adopted Names Council	USAN	This private group advises the secretary of HHS on appropriate official name for each new drug.	
United States Pharmacopeial Convention	USP	This group of experts sets standards for medications (published in the *USP*) and establishes consensus on drug uses (published in the *USP Drug Information* volumes).	

concerning medicines. These organizations are listed and described in Table 3-2.

DRUG TESTING

The development of new drugs and biologicals is a major industry in the United States. To meet the current standards set by drug legislation, a detailed format is followed to test drugs as they are developed for market. This format is described in this section. The final stage of drug development is testing in humans. Nurses play an important role in drug testing trials.

Assessment of Safety of Drugs

All medications intended for human use must undergo extensive toxicity testing in at least two species of animals. The toxicity tests must include acute and chronic studies. Acute toxicity tests assess the short-term effects of extreme doses of the drug. The intent of these tests is to identify organs or tissues that may be sensitive to the drug. The acute tests also allow researchers to determine how dangerous the drug might be in cases of overdose in humans.

Chronic toxicity tests assess the effects of prolonged dosage with the experimental agent. Several exposure levels are usually tested, with at least one group of animals receiving dosages far in excess of those expected to be used in humans. After prolonged exposure to the test drug, the animals undergo extensive pathologic and histologic examinations to detect any effects on organs or tissues. Significant toxicity observed in animals is usually sufficient cause for abandoning development of a drug.

Chronic toxicity tests are the stage at which a drug is usually tested for carcinogenic (cancer-inducing) effects. The carcinogenic effects of compounds may also be assessed by the Ames test, which measures mutagenicity (the ability to cause mutations) in bacteria. Because many chemicals that are mutagens are also carcinogens, this test can help predict which drugs may be carcinogenic. This bacterial test is less expensive and faster than chronic toxicity tests in animals, which may last months or years.

Drugs are also tested for their effects on pregnant animals and on fetuses. Drugs that cause fetal abnormalities are called teratogens. Some drugs are very dangerous to fetuses at certain stages in embryonic development but relatively harmless to adult animals or more mature fetuses. The stage of fetal development in which the fetus is most sensitive to drugs or toxins is the first third of fetal life. A tragic example of this sensitivity occurred with the drug thalidomide. Thalidomide is a sleep medication that was widely marketed in Europe during the 1960s. The drug was not dangerous to adults, but when used by women in the early stages of pregnancy, it inhibited proper development of fetal limb buds. The result was a number of babies born with tiny nonfunctional limbs—a tragedy that could have been prevented by more extensive drug testing. Thalidomide was, in fact, not marketed in the United States because insufficient information was available to satisfy FDA guidelines for new drugs.

Efficacy of Drugs

After an experimental drug has been tested for toxicity in animals, the manufacturer may file with the FDA a "notice of claimed investigational exemption for a new drug (IND)." The chemical structure of the new drug is included, partly to prove that the drug really is new. All the toxicity data in animals, data on drug absorption and metabolism, and data on the expected biologic activity of the drug must be included. The manufacturer or licenser must justify the tests that will be conducted in human subjects.

Phase I, the first testing of a drug in humans, is carried out on a small number of healthy volunteers. The purpose of this phase is to identify a safe dosage range for the drug in most persons and to establish how well the animal studies correlate with the results in humans. For example, drug absorption in humans may differ from that observed in certain animal species. Therefore it may be necessary to repeat certain studies in humans. Occasionally an unexpected side effect may appear at this stage of testing. For example, alterations of mood may not be easily recognized in experimental animals and yet may be severe enough in humans to prevent further development of an experimental drug.

Phase II, the second stage of testing in humans, involves clinical trials on patients. Clinical trials may take many forms, but they all are designed to answer the question, "Is this drug an effective treatment for a defined medical condition?" To answer this question, a relatively large number of patients must be studied, and the results must be analyzed in an objective manner, usually with statistical methods.

The **double-blind design** is one highly effective format for a clinical trial. In this type of study, patients are randomly assigned to treatment groups or are assigned so that groups have the same average age, the same proportion of men and women, or some other desired characteristic. One group receives the drug to be tested. Another group receives a placebo, which contains no pharmacologically active ingredient. The drug and the placebo should be in the same form so that they cannot be told apart by sight or taste. The placebo-treated group of patients serves as a control and allows researchers to assess how many patients would improve without therapy. The term *double-blind* refers to the fact that during the experiment neither the patients nor the medical personnel dispensing the medication know which patients are receiving the test drug and which are receiving the placebo. In some studies the control group receives the therapy that is currently accepted as the best available for the condition being tested, rather than a placebo. This type of control allows researchers to compare the efficacy of a new drug to that of existing therapy.

Patients who receive placebo in clinical trials and show clinical improvement may be of two types. The first type includes patients whose disease has gone into spontaneous remission during the course of the clinical trial. For example, spontaneous remission is commonly observed in some depressive diseases and in certain types of arthritis. The second type includes patients who improve while receiving placebo simply as a result of receiving medical attention rather than an effective drug. For example, as many as 30% of patients with mild pain report significant relief when they are given a placebo. With drugs affecting mood, response to placebo is observed in an even higher percentage of patients.

The **placebo effect** (clinical improvement in response to placebo) is a complication in clinical trials and makes the task of evaluating the role of a particular drug in therapy more difficult. The existence of such an effect, however, emphasizes the importance of sympathetic human contact in relieving a patient's suffering. A patient who responds to placebo should by no means be considered to have been suffering from an imaginary complaint. We now understand the normal mechanisms by which the body induces analgesia (see Chapter 32) and realize that these internal mechanisms may be regulated by the central nervous system and affected by emotional states. Therefore the attention and support given to patients may alter their emotional state and allow these natural mechanisms to improve the patient's clinical condition.

After a drug has been proved effective in controlled clinical trials, the manufacturer may request the FDA to release the drug for testing at several sites on large numbers of patients. This is phase III of the evaluation process. During the first round of clinical trials the total number of patients tested may be small. When the drug is released into limited circulation, it may be tested in a few thousand patients. This larger number of patients allows assessment of rare complications of drug therapy that could not be predicted from more limited trials. Before a tested drug is finally released for interstate marketing, its developer must file a new drug application (NDA) with the FDA. The NDA includes all data available on toxicity of the new drug, its use in patients, and results of clinical trials. If the FDA rules that the drug has been proved safe and effective and that claims made for the drug in the package insert and other professional advertising are supported by the results of clinical trials, the drug may be released for sale in interstate commerce.

The procedure for testing drugs as outlined in the preceding discussion was a careful, conservative approach that often took many years to complete. In 1985 the FDA streamlined procedures to bring new drugs into the marketplace more rapidly. The agency reduced the number of case reports required in the application but increased requirements for postmarketing surveillance. All serious adverse effects must be reported to the FDA within 15 days; all adverse effects must be reported every 3 months for the first 3 years and yearly thereafter. Forms for reporting these reactions are published regularly as part of the *FDA Drug Bulletin* and other publications. The FDA can also be accessed electronically (http://www.fda.gov/opacom/index/index2.html).

Further pressure for more rapid movement of drugs into clinical tests arose as the acquired immunodeficiency syndrome (AIDS) epidemic began. Without treatment, AIDS patients live a very short time. For these patients and for others with conditions for which no effective therapy exists, a new procedure was created to allow experimental agents to be used on a wider scale than was previously possible. This process releases drugs for use in patients who meet set criteria, even though the drug is not yet on the market. For example, while didanosine was in trials against human immunodeficiency virus (HIV), it was available for use in AIDS patients more than 12 years of age who had symptomatic HIV infection, were intolerant to the standard drug zidovudine, and were unable to enroll in a phase II trial because of geographic location.

Drug Efficacy Study Implementation

All drugs introduced after the Kefauver-Harris Amendment in 1962 went through the extensive testing just described and were proved effective and safe. Drugs already on the market in 1962 posed a special problem because they had been tested primarily for safety and not efficacy. The Drug Efficacy Study Implementation (DESI) was implemented to bring all drugs up to the same standard. Drugs were rated using the system shown in Table 3-3. Drugs rated as ineffective were removed from the market. Drugs listed as possibly effective or probably effective required reformulation or retesting to stay on the market.

Rights of the Patient in Drug Testing

Anyone involved in assessing the clinical usefulness of a new drug is bound by certain moral and legal constraints. No one may be coerced into receiving a drug that is under investigation. All drug studies must be done on volunteers who have read, understood, and signed informed consent forms. The law requires that all potential hazards associated with use of the drug be explained clearly to the patient. The patient or volunteer must not be promised unrealistic benefits from therapy. The patient must also be free to withdraw from the study at any time without fear that his or her level of medical care will be compromised.

Although compliance with these constraints may seem a simple matter, there are complications in practice. For example, some people believe that experimental drugs are always better than currently used drugs. These people may not have realistic expectations, despite having been told the properties of the drug being tested. Another problem concerns patients who are intimidated by medical personnel and afraid to refuse to participate in a drug study. These patients may confide their fears to an accessible and sympathetic nurse. It is the duty of the nurse to assist such patients in making their true feelings known.

Nurses assist patients in many ways throughout drug testing, including acting as an advocate for the patient. The nurse assesses whether the patient understands the possible benefits and limitations of the drugs being tested and the testing protocol. During testing the nurse assesses the patient for benefits, fears, drug side effects, and changes in the underlying health problem. Finally, the nurse supports the patient's decisions about participation in drug testing. This may be a difficult process because the nurse may disagree with the patient's decision but must support it.

Table 3-3	**DESI Rating System**
Rating	**Description**
Effective	Substantial evidence exists to show that drug is effective treatment for defined medical condition.
Probably effective	Some evidence exists, but more is needed to prove drug effective.
Possibly effective	Minimum evidence exists to suggest that drug may be effective.
Ineffective	Controlled trials failed to show that drug is more effective than placebo.
Ineffective as a fixed combination	Individual components of medication might be effective alone at appropriate doses, but no evidence suggests that all components of medication are necessary to effect.
Effective but	Qualification to use of drug is made, which must be added to labeling.

Nursing Process Overview

Nurses and Drug Testing

Laws governing the role of the nurse in drug testing vary. In the United States each state's nurse practice act regulates all aspects of nursing practice for that state. Examine the laws governing practice to determine the extent to which nurses are allowed to participate in drug testing in your state, province, or country.

Assessment

Assess all patients in a thorough, individualized manner.

Nursing Diagnoses

Nursing diagnoses are based on individualized patient assessment. In the early stages of drug testing, the major focus may be to identify and describe commonly encountered drug side effects.

Planning/Implementation

Patient management in a drug testing study may differ from that in a normal clinical situation. For example, the nurse should be certain that the institution where the study is taking place permits the nurse to administer investigational drugs. Some institutions require that the person conducting the experiment (study) actually administer the experimental

Continued

drugs. The nurse should also determine whether a nurse is legally allowed to obtain informed consent. Some institutions do not permit anyone but the principal investigator to obtain informed consent from the patient.

Evaluation

Evaluation of patients receiving experimental drugs may be a major component of the research in a drug testing program. In many cases, thorough evaluation, including detailed patient histories, laboratory tests, and radiographic evaluation, is carried out by the physician or researcher. Nevertheless, the nurse should continue to evaluate patients in a manner consistent with good nursing practice. The extent to which nursing evaluations become part of the permanent record of the experiment depends on the institution and the protocols established by the investigator.

CONTROLLED SUBSTANCES

Addiction

Certain substances can alter normal functions of the human body so profoundly that the body becomes dependent on that substance and experiences physical harm if it is withdrawn. This condition is physical addiction or dependence (see Chapter 8). Narcotic analgesics and some general depressants may cause this type of dependence. Substances such as cocaine and marijuana, although not producing clear evidence of physical addiction, cause psychologic addiction.

Regulation of Controlled Substances

Because substances that produce physical or psychologic addiction clearly have the capacity to harm their users, they have been regulated extensively. The original legislation in the United States was the Harrison Narcotic Act of 1914. This law restricted importation of many of these addictive substances. One of the major aims of the Pure Food and Drug Act of 1906 and the Harrison Act was to prevent the sale of patent medicines that contained no active ingredient except one of these addicting agents.

The Harrison Act did not eliminate the problem of illicit drug use and addiction. This legislation was replaced by a more comprehensive law in 1970, the Controlled Substances Act. In addition to supplying guidelines for defining drug dependency and establishing education and treatment programs, this law clearly classifies drugs based on abuse potential and clinical usefulness and specifies the restrictions that apply to each type of controlled drug. The drug schedules are described in Table 3-4.

Drugs in each schedule defined by the Controlled Substances Act are regulated by rules appropriate to them. For example, schedule I substances have no approved medical use and are banned. Schedule II drugs are controlled at every stage from initial manufacture through distribution and final use. By law, no prescription for a schedule II drug may be refilled. Physicians must be licensed to prescribe these drugs and must keep accurate records to ensure that the medications are used strictly for legitimate purposes. Likewise, pharmacies must be specially licensed and keep accurate records for schedule II drugs.

Drugs in schedules III, IV, and V are less dangerous than those in schedule II. For the most part this greater safety results from inherent properties of the chemicals in these schedules, but some chemicals appear in more than one schedule. For example, codeine used alone as an antitussive is a schedule II drug. However, medications that contain codeine compounded with aspirin, acetaminophen, or other agents are schedule III drugs, even when the total dose of codeine is the same as that used in schedule II preparations. One reason that these compounded forms of codeine are less likely to be abused is that adverse symptoms from overdoses of the other ingredients discourage abuse of these mixtures. Codeine also appears in several cough syrups that are on schedule V. The recommended single dose of codeine for

Table 3-4	**Classification of Controlled Substances**	
Classification	Description	Specific Substances
Schedule I	Drugs that have high potential for abuse and no accepted medical use. Containers marked C-I.	heroin, lysergic acid diethylamide (LSD), peyote, marijuana
Schedule II	Drugs with high potential for abuse but accepted medical use. Dependence may include physical and psychologic dependence. Containers marked C-II.	amobarbital, amphetamine, codeine, meperidine, methadone, hydromorphone, morphine, opium, phenazocine, methylphenidate, secobarbital
Schedule III	Medically accepted drugs that may cause dependence but are less prone to abuse than drugs in schedules I and II. Containers marked C-III.	codeine-containing medications, butabarbital, paregoric
Schedule IV	Medically accepted drugs that may cause mild physical or psychologic dependence. Containers marked C-IV.	chloral hydrate, chlordiazepoxide, diazepam, meprobamate, phenobarbital
Schedule V	Medically accepted drugs with very limited potential for causing mild physical or psychologic dependence. Containers marked C-V.	Drug mixtures containing small quantities of narcotics, such as over-the-counter cough syrups containing codeine

adults in these schedule V medications is 5 or 10 mg, whereas the doses found in schedule II or III forms are 15 to 60 mg. This lower dose in cough medications is responsible for the schedule V classification.

Important provisions of the Controlled Substances Act and related rules are reprinted in Volume III of the *USPDI*.

Nursing Process Overview

Controlled Substances

Because of the addictive potential of many controlled substances, legal restraints have been placed on the use of these drugs in medical practice. These regulations, as well as the special nature of the drugs, add a special burden and responsibility for the nurse.

Assessment

Controlled drugs may be used for pain relief, cough suppression, and other uses. Observe whether an individual displays signs and symptoms that make the use of the controlled substance appropriate. Anticipate side effects that occur regularly with some controlled substances.

Nursing Diagnoses

- Constipation related to frequent use of narcotic analgesics
- Altered comfort: nausea related to narcotic use

Planning/Implementation

When administering controlled substances, the nurse has legal and nursing responsibilities. The legal responsibilities include ensuring that controlled substances (schedules II through IV, United States) are kept under lock and key. These substances are available only to authorized personnel. Because all the material must be accounted for, records on the use of these substances must be kept. Unauthorized use of controlled substances must be reported to the proper authority.

The nurse must also be aware of institutional policies regarding the use of these drugs. For example, for schedule II drugs (United States), the physician may need to renew the order for narcotics every 48 hours, that is, a 'standing order' for a narcotic is prohibited. A nurse who administers the drug after the 48-hour period without obtaining a renewal order is in violation of institutional policy. There are comparable national and institutional restrictions related to Canadian narcotics and schedule G drugs. Specific uses for controlled substances are discussed in the appropriate chapters.

Evaluation

Evaluate the patient's response to the medication. The dosage of many controlled substances may be adjusted based on patient response and the severity of any side effects.

CANADIAN DRUG LEGISLATION

Food and Drugs Act

Drug regulation is carried out through the Health Protection branch of the Canadian government. Under this branch the Drugs Directorate oversees the bureaus that deal with specific areas of regulation, such as prescription drugs, nonprescription drugs, biologicals, drug research, and control of drug quality. Updates and other current information can be obtained via the Health Canada web site (http://www.hc-sc.gc.ca/hpb/drugs/drhtmeng/index.html).

Under the Food and Drugs Act of 1953, drugs are divided into categories (Table 3-5). When approved for sale, all Canadian drugs are assigned a six-digit number preceded by the letters GP (proprietary drug) or DIN (over-the-counter drug). In addition, each prescription drug must be well marked with a symbol to identify the schedule to which it belongs. Regulations covering the various schedules of drugs differ, making the clear identification system important. Drugs listed in schedule F are sold only by prescription, with refills limited to 6 months. Drugs in schedule G are called controlled drugs and have more stringent controls regulating the number and timing of refills for prescriptions. Certain controlled drugs are called designated drugs because their use is restricted to specific conditions described by law.

The Food and Drugs Act in Canada also protects citizens from contaminated, adulterated, and unsafe drugs. To ensure drug quality, the law requires inspection of manufacturing facilities, calls for analysis of drug samples by government laboratories, and maintains an active monitoring system to detect adverse reactions to drugs. Drug labeling is also closely controlled so that false, misleading, and deceptive labels are prohibited. Drugs may not be advertised to the general public as cures for alcoholism, cancer, heart disease, infectious diseases, and other specific conditions.

Narcotic Control Act

The Narcotic Control Act (1961) regulates the manufacture, distribution, and sale of narcotic drugs, establishing this group as separate from drugs regulated under the Food and Drugs Act. Regulations spell out specific provisions of this act and are often revised in response to changing needs.

All steps in the manufacture, distribution, and sale of narcotics are subject to stringent regulation. Possession of these drugs for any reason other than those related to medical use as described in the legislation is an offense subject to severe penalties. Dispensers of these drugs must be licensed by the government and must maintain extensive records documenting the sources of and recipients for all drugs and the amounts and dates for all transactions. As in the United States, nurses may possess narcotics or controlled and restricted drugs only when authorized by a physician's order to administer the drug to a patient or when authorized to act as official custodian of drugs for a specific unit of a health care facility.

Table 3-5   **Canadian Drug Classifications**

Classification	Description	Specific Substances
Nonprescription Drugs		
Proprietary medicines	Drugs that may be widely purchased for self-treatment of symptoms of minor self-limiting diseases; identified by six-digit code preceded by letters *GP*	Cough drops, medicated shampoos, minor pain relievers
Over-the-counter drugs	Drugs available in pharmacies, used on advice of health professional for control of minor self-limiting diseases; identified by six-digit code preceded by letters *DIN*	Laxatives, cough syrups, cold remedies, sinus preparations, certain vitamins
Prescription Drugs		
Schedule F	Drugs that may not be used except after professional consultation; identified by *Pr* on label	Hormones, antibiotics, tranquilizers
Schedule G	Drugs that affect central nervous system (e.g., stimulants, sedatives); identified by *C* on label	Amphetamines, barbiturates
Narcotics	Drugs used mostly for relief of pain but have significant psychotropic activity; identified by *N* on label	Cannabis (marijuana), cocaine, codeine, morphine, opium, phencyclidine
Restricted Drugs		
Schedule H	Drugs with no recognized medical use and significant danger of physiologic and psychologic side effects; available only to institutions for research	Lysergic acid diethylamide (LSD), *N,N*-diethyltryptamine (DET), *N,N*-dimethyltryptamine (DMT), 4-methyl-2, 5-dimethoxyamphetamine (STP, DOM)

Development of New Drugs in Canada

New drugs are evaluated in Canada by a sequence of tests similar to those used in the United States. Promising drugs undergo preclinical testing in three mammalian species, including one nonrodent species, to determine threshold doses that produce toxicity or death. The next stage is a clinical pharmacology trial similar to phase I trials in the United States. During clinical pharmacology trials the drug is given to healthy human volunteers to establish safety for doses that might be used clinically. If the drug is proved safe and if manufacturing processes produce a pure and uniform preparation for human use, the manufacturer may apply for permission to distribute the drug to qualified investigators who will test it in patients. This stage of testing is similar to phase II in the United States. Before the drug can be released for general use, extensive documentation concerning formulation, labeling, packaging, clinical data on humans, and test data on animals must be filed and evaluated. All new drugs are monitored after being placed on the market. The drug is released from controls required for a new drug only after extensive information has documented the safety of a new drug when used in normal medical practice.

Nursing Implications Summary

General Guidelines: Legal Implications of Drug Therapy

➤ Become familiar with the nurse practice acts that govern practice in your setting. These acts are written in legislative language, so ask questions as needed to clarify the meaning of all components.

➤ Stay informed of agency policies related to dispensing, administering, and accounting for drugs. Observe deadlines and expiration dates of orders. Maintain vigilance in working with controlled and scheduled drugs.

➤ Consult the current literature, the pharmacist, and the physician to learn about new drug preparations. Ask questions as needed to clarify changes in protocols for administration of drugs.

➤ Assess each patient individually, and ask "Is this the right drug in the right dose for this patient?" See Chapter 4 for additional information.

➤ Be familiar with policies regarding the role of the nurse with investigational drugs. Serve as the patient's advocate in working with patients involved in drug studies.

CHAPTER REVIEW

Application

1. What is the "active ingredient" of a medicinal preparation?
2. What is the purpose of the *United States Pharmacopeia* and the *National Formulary*?
3. What is the *USPDI* and what kind of information does it contain?
4. Outline the steps involved in getting a new drug approved in the United States or Canada.
5. What is a clinical trial? Describe a clinical trial following the double-blind design.
6. What is the placebo effect?
7. What is the purpose of the informed consent form?
8. What is a treatment IND?
9. What are controlled substances? What are some nursing implications related to administering a controlled substance?
10. What special precautions are required for handling controlled substances?
11. Define the schedules used for controlled substances in the United States.

Critical Thinking

1. Suggest two explanations for the placebo effect observed in drug trials. How might the nurse use knowledge of the placebo effect to attempt to improve the patient's response to a medication?
2. In your current clinical setting, find out if controlled substances are regularly administered. Where are they stored? Who has access to these drugs? How is their use recorded? What steps are taken if there is a discrepancy; that is, the amount in stock is not the same amount as the record indicates there should be in stock?
3. Call or write to your State or Provincial Board of Nursing. Find out what happens to a nurse who steals a controlled substance for personal use.

Reference

Tranter J: The patient's rights in clinical research, *Prof Nurse* 12(5):335-337, 1997.

Application of the Nursing Process to Drug Therapy

OBJECTIVES

After studying this chapter, you should be able to do the following:

- *Discuss the use of the nursing process with patients receiving medications.*
- *Explain the five rights of drug administration.*
- *Describe the factors that influence patient compliance with drug therapy.*
- *Discuss legal constraints on the administration of drugs.*
- *Describe the nurse's role when medication errors occur.*

CHAPTER OVERVIEW

The focus of this chapter is the use of the nursing process in administering drugs. This chapter includes a discussion of the classic steps in the nursing process. In addition, it elaborates on the issues that the nurse should consider in preparing and administering drugs. This chapter complements Chapter 3, "Legal Implications of Drug Therapy"; Chapter 5, "Drug Administration"; and Chapter 7, "Over-the-Counter Drugs and Self-Medication."

THE NURSING PROCESS AND PHARMACOLOGY

Assessment

Assessment involves gathering data about the patient. This database is important in the treatment of the patient. The assessment forms the baseline against which changes will be compared. It also allows the nurse to develop an individualized care plan for the patient.

The physical assessment should be complete yet tailored to the patient's needs and the severity of the presenting health problems. The history of the present health problems includes a drug history (Figure 4-1). Information from the drug history helps the nurse better understand the patient's previous drug use, attitudes about drugs, and knowledge about drugs. In addition, the nurse can learn about any over-

the-counter (OTC) drugs the patient may be using and about his or her current lifestyle, including smoking, drinking alcoholic beverages, and dietary habits.

Another component of the assessment comes from laboratory results, radiology reports, and results of other diagnostic testing. These data may confirm existing health problems or provide a baseline against which the nurse can later check for deviations or improvement, possibly related to the drugs administered.

Nursing Diagnoses

A **nursing diagnosis** is a statement of a health problem or potential problem that a nurse is licensed and competent to treat. The nurse derives nursing diagnoses by analyzing the data obtained in the patient assessment. No nursing diagnoses apply solely to drug administration. The diagnoses

Name _____

Age _____   Date _____

Major health problems: _____

_____

Other health problems requiring medications: _____

_____

1. Medications used for major health problems
   These questions are only a guide. The patient's comments may lead the examiner to pursue certain topics in more detail.
   What medicines are you currently taking?

Medicine	Dose	Frequency	Comments

   Are you having problems with any of these medicines? *Go through each medicine, asking the following questions:*
   a. Are you able to take this drug the way it is ordered? What time(s) each day do you take it?
   b. Are you having any side effects? *Use words that the patient can understand, such as "Are there reasons you cannot take this medicine?" or "Are there any problems with taking this medicine?"*
   c. Do you think this drug is helping? *For example, "Is your blood pressure pill helping your blood pressure?"*
   d. If appropriate, ask about cost: *"Some patients find that this medicine is very expensive. Has the cost of this drug been a problem?"*
   e. If appropriate, ask about side effects patients may be reluctant to discuss. *For example, "Some people find this drug causes difficulty maintaining erections. Have you had that problem while taking this drug?"*
   f. If appropriate, ask about ability to obtain refills: *"Do you have any problems getting refills for this drug?" "Do you have any problems picking up your refills at the drugstore?"*
   Note anything that might be important in teaching this patient about medications: drugs that should be refrigerated or left at room temperature, dangers of putting drugs in unlabeled containers, importance of storing drugs out of reach of small children, etc.

2. General drug use
   How do you take care of the following problems/conditions? What medicines do you use for them?
   "How often do you take the medicine?" "Does it work?" "When did you last take it?"
   a. Pain: headache, muscle pains, toothaches? *Expand as needed for each patient.*
   b. Gastrointestinal system: constipation, diarrhea, upset stomach, heartburn?
   c. Skin conditions: psoriasis, athlete's foot, dry skin? *Ask about special shampoos and creams.*
   d. Nervous, mental, or emotional disorders: nervousness, being unable to sleep, upset?
   e. Reproductive system: birth control pills, female hormones, menstrual pain, backache?
   f. Nutritional deficiencies: iron, vitamins, bran, yeast, diet supplements, weight loss products, etc.?
   g. Upper respiratory tract, eye, and nose: What do you do for a cold? Cough? Stuffy nose? Sinus problem? Do you take nosedrops? Use nasal spray? Eyedrops?
   h. Other: special teas, liniments, plasters, soda, herbal remedies, drugs made from roots? *Knowledge of local custom is helpful in this category.*

3. General health habits
   a. Do you smoke? How much? Do you chew tobacco? How much?
   b. How much whiskey (beer, wine) do you drink? (Response may not be accurate.)
   c. How often do you do drugs on a recreational basis? (Response may not be accurate. Remain nonjudgmental.)
   d. Do you follow any special diet (low salt, diabetic, low protein, etc.)? Are you a vegetarian? *In some cases a complete diet history might be warranted.*
   e. Where do you work? What kinds of work have you done in the past? Have you lived anywhere else in the country?
   f. Are you allergic to anything? Are there any medicines you cannot take? Why?
   g. Which immunizations have you received? When did you last have a tetanus shot?

Figure 4-1   Sample drug history.

reflect an analysis of the entire patient and the patient's needs, which may include aspects of drug administration.

The wording of the nursing diagnoses is specific, established by the North American Nursing Diagnoses Association (NANDA). NANDA has met regularly since 1973 to refine the list of NANDA-approved nursing diagnoses. The most recent listing is published when it is updated. With regard to medication administration, several points about nursing diagnoses should be made. The only nursing diagnosis that can be applied in all situations of drug administration is that of a knowledge deficit. Most patients who are to receive a new drug therapy have some knowledge deficit, but it may be minimal. Careful assessment may reveal that other diagnoses are more appropriate.

A nursing diagnosis that encompasses an entire health problem may be more appropriate than one that focuses on the drug therapy alone. For example, for the diabetic patient who must take insulin, a nursing diagnosis of "risk for altered health maintenance related to lack of knowledge of diabetes mellitus, management, and signs and symptoms of complications" would allow for a more detailed plan than a diagnosis that focuses on insulin alone.

Side effects that are commonly encountered or are very serious may form the basis for some nursing diagnoses. For example, narcotic analgesics cause constipation. When these narcotics are used for only two or three doses, the constipation may be minimal. When narcotics are used in large doses for extensive periods, as for some patients with cancer, it would be appropriate to include in the plan a nursing diagnosis that comes from knowledge of the drug and the side effect of constipation. Thus for a patient with cancer who is receiving frequent or large doses of narcotics, a nursing diagnosis of "at risk for constipation related to narcotic use for pain relief" may be appropriate. For a patient on a diuretic known to contribute to potassium loss, "at risk for elec-

trolyte abnormalities (hypokalemia) related to furosemide therapy" may be appropriate.

Nursing diagnoses may describe a problem for which additional data are needed. Consider the patient who must take moderate to large doses of corticosteroids. These drugs have the side effects of weight gain and development of a characteristic round face (moon face). A nursing diagnosis might be "possible self-concept disturbance related to physical changes secondary to prednisone therapy."

It would be easy to develop extensive lists of at risk for and possible diagnoses related to any known side effect of drug therapy. However, it is more prudent to use such diagnoses for serious or commonly encountered problems. Remember that each patient is unique, and therefore a problem for one patient will not necessarily be the same for another.

Sometimes patients are at risk for a potential complication that cannot be prevented or treated with nursing measures alone. In such a situation the patient may have, instead of or in addition to nursing diagnoses, one or more collaborative problems. Consider an acutely ill patient with diabetes. The patient may have the potential complication (PC) of hypoglycemia or hyperglycemia.

Patient Outcomes

Patient outcomes describe the goal(s) of therapy in terms of the patient. The outcomes should be objective or measurable so that it will be possible to determine whether the outcomes have been achieved. For example, an outcome for the patient receiving regular morphine might be as follows: "The patient will have a bowel movement at least every 48 hours." Each nursing diagnosis should have at least one patient outcome. Patient outcomes should be developed with the patient and family. Such collaboration helps the patient understand what the health care team is trying to achieve and provides an opportunity to teach the patient.

If the patient has one or more potential complications that are collaborative problems, the goals may be worded in terms of the nurse: "The nurse will manage and minimize episodes of hypoglycemia or hyperglycemia."

Planning/Implementation

Planning involves developing an outline of nursing interventions needed to treat the nursing diagnoses. The plan should spell out the nursing interventions that should be used by members of the team. These interventions may be carried out on a daily timetable, or deadlines for accomplishing components of the plan may be identified. Thus an intervention to check the stool for occult blood should be done each time a patient has a bowel movement. Another intervention might be to "increase ambulation by walking 10 feet more each time the patient is up; by Tuesday the patient should be able to walk to the end of the hall and back." This intervention includes a goal within the intervention.

The **implementation** phase is the carrying out of the plan. In this phase the nurse must incorporate the steps of the plan

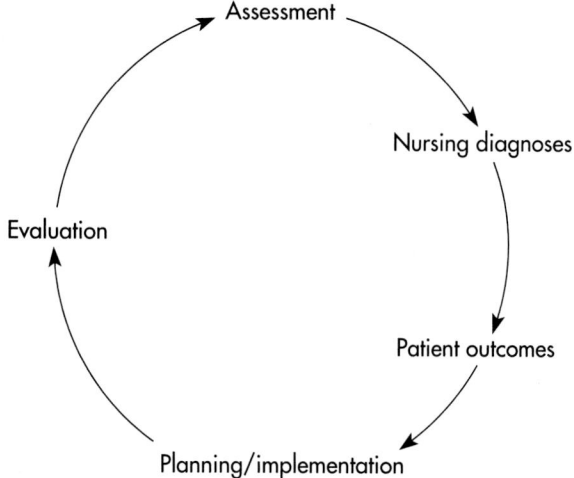

Figure 4-2 The nursing process as a continuous activity.

in the patient's daily routine. It is often during this phase that the nurse or the patient begins to identify changes that need to be made. For example, the nurse may see that the plan is unreasonable, the goal (patient outcome) is not realistic, or the patient is not ready for such detailed instruction.

Evaluation

Evaluation, although listed as the final step of the nursing process, takes the nurse back to the first step of assessment. During evaluation the nurse determines whether the plan is working. Is the patient displaying the desired patient outcomes? What should be modified in the plan? What additional data are needed? Are the drugs working as planned? Are side effects developing? What new problems have occurred?

The **nursing process** is often presented in a linear fashion:

Assessing $\rightarrow$ Diagnosing $\rightarrow$ Planning/implementing $\rightarrow$ Evaluating

However, it often occurs in a circular fashion (Figure 4-2). Working closely with the patient, the nurse may assess the patient and begin to develop nursing diagnoses. As more information is needed, the nurse obtains additional assessment data. In developing the plan and implementing it, the nurse constantly evaluates its feasibility and success. While evaluating the plan, the nurse continues to assess. The nursing process is a systematic, organized way of approaching the patient and developing a plan for health care.

THE FIVE RIGHTS OF DRUG ADMINISTRATION

Traditionally, the teaching of principles of drug administration has centered around the **five rights of drug administration** (Box 4-1): the right drug, via the right route, in the right dose, at the right time, and to the right patient. Although at first glance it might seem that these rights should be easy to achieve, the day-to-day practice of nursing requires thoughtful attention to these rights at all times.

The Right Drug

The right drug suggests that the patient receive not only the prescribed drug but also the right drug for the specific health problem being treated. The nurse must pay careful attention to drug orders and medication labels while preparing drugs and be familiar with the health care problems for each patient. To know if a prescribed drug is appropriate, the nurse must know and understand the patient's health problems

and be current in pharmacologic knowledge. The rest of this book provides basic material about drugs, but in practice the nurse must also regularly consult printed materials and other health care professionals for additional information. Some of these sources are discussed in Chapters 3 and 7.

The Right Route

To ensure that the patient receives prescribed medications via the right route, the nurse must know each medication that is administered. The student may have difficulty understanding how or why a nurse could administer a medication via the wrong route, but in a busy nurse's day, errors can occur easily. For example, an experienced nurse who usually works in the coronary care setting was asked to work for a day in the surgical intensive care unit. The nurse, accustomed to administering morphine intravenously for cardiac pain, administered all parenteral pain medications intravenously in the surgical intensive care setting, even those ordered via the intramuscular route. Fortunately, in this true incident, the nurse discovered the errors and reported them, and no harm came to the patients.

The Right Dose

Administering the right dose of medication is extremely important. Not only must the nurse double-check calculations for mathematic accuracy, the nurse also must ask, "Is this dose appropriate for the size and age of the patient?" This responsibility emphasizes the need for current knowledge about drugs and usual dosage ranges. Although the administration of an incorrect dose is serious for any patient, it can be especially serious in the pediatric patient, for whom prescribed doses are often small. A review of dosage calculations can be found in Chapter 6.

The Right Time

Ensuring that the patient receives drugs at the right time may be difficult. Often the health care team must weigh the information available about the pharmacokinetics and pharmacodynamics of drugs (see Chapter 1) against the patient's lifestyle and potential for compliance. In the critical care setting, where one nurse may care for one or two patients, drugs are administered at evenly spaced intervals throughout a 24-hour period. The nurse, although usually very busy, can concentrate on administering medications to a few patients. However, on a busy general care unit the nurse may have 20 or more patients who must receive drugs, and these patients may be coming and going to the radiology department, physical or occupational therapy, or surgery. In addition, most patients would prefer not to be wakened at night to receive medications. In the home it is even easier for the patient to forget to take a dose or to be less careful about the interval between doses. Another factor in the home setting is general lifestyle. For example, patients who work a night shift and sleep during the day may need help determining the right time to take drugs.

Box 4-1	**The Five Rights of Drug Administration**

The right drug
The right route
The right dose
The right time
The right patient

Other factors that influence the right dosage time include whether the patient is receiving multiple drugs, whether a drug can be taken on an empty or full stomach, and whether a prescribed drug can be taken with other medications. To ensure that a patient receives drugs at the right time, the nurse must know about the patient, the health care problems, and the drugs.

The Right Patient

Finally, the right patient must receive the drug. The nurse must check the patient's identity each time a drug is administered. Not only should the patient be Ms. Smith, but it must be the right Ms. Smith. The right patient also means that the right drugs were prescribed for the right patient, and thus the nurse is back to the first of the five rights of drug administration.

PATIENT EDUCATION AND MEDICATIONS

One of the major goals of nursing care in drug administration is preparing the patient and family for a return to independent functioning in the home or community. The patient, when able, will take over the role of self-administration of medications. No one can guarantee that the patient will take a medication exactly as directed and derive the expected benefits of drug therapy. However, careful patient assessment, planning, and teaching by the nurse can help the patient better understand prescribed medications and how to use them safely.

Attitudes about Medications

All patients come to the health care system with preexisting ideas and attitudes about who should take medications, whether medications are generally helpful, what the meaning of sickness and health is, and what to expect of the health care team. Additional factors include personal beliefs, attitudes and opinions of family and friends, religious and cultural beliefs, and the influence of the media about certain kinds of medications. The public may not even use the same vocabulary as the health care team. For example, a nurse or physician may use the words drug, medicine, or medication interchangeably; but these words may have different connotations to the patient.

To be successful in preparing the patient for self-management, the nurse needs to assess the patient's attitudes about medicines. This is done by asking questions or developing an assessment tool, by remaining attuned to the patient's response to medications in the health care setting, and by attempting to validate these impressions with the patient. The nurse in the hospital or institution is generally in control of the medication situation, and the patient can avoid becoming very involved in the self-medication plans. The nurse in the home is given many more clues about patient attitudes about medication administration. Any plan for teaching patients about drugs will be more successful if it is compatible with the patient's existing beliefs and attitudes. It is possible to change attitudes and beliefs, but doing so requires careful planning and is difficult.

Box 4-2 Safe Medication Use: Points to Review with All Patients

- Take drugs prescribed for you; do not borrow drugs from others or share your drugs with others.
- Take only the dose prescribed. If you feel the dose is too large or too small, check with the physician before adjusting the dose or frequency of doses.
- When a new drug is prescribed, find out what to do if a dose is missed. Do not double-up for missed doses. Take a missed dose as soon as it is remembered, unless it is within 2 hours of the next regularly scheduled dose. Resume the regular dose schedule.
- When a new drug is prescribed, find out how to take it in relation to meals or other drugs you may be taking. Some drugs should be taken with meals or food, whereas others should be taken on an empty stomach.
- Each time a new drug is prescribed, find out why you are taking it and what the common side effects are. Never hesitate to call the doctor if an unexpected sign or symptom develops; it may be related to the medications you are taking.
- Store your medications properly. Usually, this means in a dry place (not in the bathroom, where steam and moisture may cause medicines to deteriorate and lose strength). Do not mix different pills in the same container, such as a pill box for your pocket or purse. This may cause the medicines to lose their strength, and without labels, you may take the wrong drug by accident.
- Write down the names of the drugs you are taking, and take this list with you when you visit the doctor, nurse, dentist, podiatrist, ophthal-

mologist, osteopathic physician, chiropractor, or clinic. Keep all your health care providers informed of all the drugs you are taking, even those you purchase over the counter.
- Keep drugs out of the reach of children. Use childproof caps if there are children in your home. Never refer to medications as candy.
- Read the label each time you take a dose of medicine to make sure you are taking the drug you think you are taking. Sometimes two different drugs look alike or their containers look alike.
- Wear a medical identification tag, bracelet, or necklace listing your chronic health problems and medication allergies.
- Keep track of your prescription drugs. Try not to run out of them on the weekend or during holidays, when it may be difficult to get a prescription refilled. If your drug supply is getting low, call the physician's office. Be prepared to give the nurse the name of the drug and dose and the name of the pharmacy and its telephone number where you wish to have the prescription filled.
- Keep the telephone number of the local poison control center near your telephone. Keep ipecac in your home but out of the reach of children. This drug can be used to make a person vomit if a drug was taken that should not have been. Never use ipecac unless the poison control center or your doctor says you should.
- If you become pregnant, notify the physician immediately: many medications should not be used during pregnancy, and the doctor may want to change your prescriptions.

General Principles to Teach about All Medications

Regardless of the specific drugs prescribed for a patient, there are some general principles about drugs to teach all patients (Box 4-2). Instruct patients to keep all drugs out of reach of children and to keep the drugs in the original labeled containers. Decorative pill boxes are attractive, but many patients fill them with several different types of drugs. This practice provides great potential for error, and if pills are left for weeks or months in these boxes, it may hasten decomposition of some drugs. At the same time, using labeled pill boxes may be a useful way to help some patients remember to take their drugs each day (Box 4-3). Remind patients to use childproof caps unless they cannot remove them without assistance. Even so, children must be protected from access to drugs. Explain that, ideally, all drugs should be stored in a locked container, out of reach of children.

Emphasize that medications should be taken only as ordered. Patients should not double up on medication to catch up when a dose has been missed. Remind patients not to share medications with family or friends. Warn patients that altering the dose amount does not improve the effect; two pills are not better than one. Explain that if any medication is left after a health problem has been treated, it should be discarded. Emphasize that drugs purchased over the counter should be treated with the same degree of respect as other medications; they are not to be considered less seriously because they have not been prescribed by a physician or dispensed by a pharmacist.

Instruct patients to keep all health care providers informed of all drugs they are taking. Patients taking multiple drugs should keep a list of drugs and dosages, preferably with them at all times, and check it regularly to see if it is current. Encourage patients with chronic conditions or severe allergies to wear a medical identification bracelet or necklace listing the allergy, medical condition, or type of medication used.

Teach all individuals, especially parents of young children, to keep the number of the local poison control center near the telephone in the event of ingestion of a toxic amount of drugs or exposure to or ingestion of other toxic substances. Teach children that drugs are not for playing with and that they are not candy. This rule applies to all drugs, including vitamins, birth control pills, laxatives, and other prescription and nonprescription substances (see Box 4-2 and the Pediatric and Geriatric Considerations boxes).

 PEDIATRIC CONSIDERATIONS

Assessment of Medication Use in Homes with Young Children

- Where are medications kept in the house? The kitchen? The bathroom? On the kitchen table?
- Are there prescription or over-the-counter medications that are out of date? Can you work with the family to discard them?
- Ask the caregiver to demonstrate preparing medications. Can the caregiver manipulate the equipment? Are oral suspensions shaken before the dose is poured? Are medications that should be refrigerated stored in the refrigerator?
- Is the caregiver able to monitor and record the patient's weight, pulse, blood glucose, or other parameters appropriate to the health condition?
- Is there anything about the general environment that might place the patient at risk?
- Are there medications within easy reach of a young child?
- Does the family have ipecac in the house? Do they know what it is for and how to use it? Is the number of the nearest poison control center posted near the telephone?

Box 4-3 Helping Patients Remember to Take Their Pills

As a rule, keeping several different unlabeled medications in a single container can cause problems: confusion about which drug is which, with the potential for error in self-medication, and over the long term, some medications may cause others to decompose more rapidly. At the same time, strategic use of different kinds of pill containers may be useful in assisting patients to remember to take their pills. Many kinds of pill containers, often inexpensive, that can be used in a variety of ways are available at the drugstore:

- *The pill box with an alarm:* Have patients keep doses of "hard to remember" drugs in them, such as medicines that must be taken an hour before meals, and set the alarm accordingly, or use them for patients who must remind themselves during a busy work day to take medications.
- *The pill container with a compartment for each day of the week:* These are often available in different colors. Use one box (that contains seven compartments) for the patient who loses track of whether pills have been taken. Have the patient fill the box at the beginning of the week; each day is labeled, and by the end of the week, the pills should be gone. Or, for the patient with many drugs, use three or four of these

boxes, in different colors: the morning medicine goes in the yellow box, the midday doses in the blue box, the late afternoon doses in the green box, and so on.

- *The large box with 28 compartments: morning, noon, evening, and nighttime doses for 7 days:* The patient or family member can fill the box once a week for the patient.
- *Is there a substitute in the home that could be used, especially if the patient has limited funds?* An egg carton? A clean fishing tackle tray? Old small spice jars that have been carefully washed and relabeled, one per day? What else?
- *Points to consider in choosing these pill box reminders:* Are the days of the week clear and legible (elderly patients may have difficulty seeing some kinds of writing)? Are the compartments large enough to hold all the medication for that time period? Does the patient have sufficient dexterity to open the box? Who will fill the box? Where will it be kept (i.e., available to patient, but out of reach of children)? Will the patient remember oral liquids, eye drops, transdermal patches, and so on, that will not fit in the box? Even with a reminder system, some patients have trouble remembering; will this system work for your patient?

GERIATRIC CONSIDERATIONS

Assessment of Medication Use in Older Adult Patients

- How does the patient keep track of when medications are due and whether they have been taken each day?
- Ask the patient to tell you how he or she manages medications each day.
- Where are medications kept in the house? The kitchen? The bathroom? On the nightstand?
- Are there over-the-counter (OTC) medications or herbal remedies in the home that the patient uses regularly but forgot to mention?
- Are there prescription or OTC medications that are out of date? Can you work with the patient to discard them?
- Ask the patient to demonstrate preparing medications. Can the patient manipulate the equipment? Can the patient see the syringe or medicine dropper well enough to prepare the correct dose? Can the patient see well enough to test blood glucose?
- Is the patient able to monitor and record his or her weight, pulse, or other parameters appropriate to the health condition?
- Consider the medications the patient is supposed to take. Is there anything about the general environment that might place the patient at risk? For example, are there small bottles of ear medicine, glue, or other items kept close to the place where eye drops are kept? If the patient taking a diuretic gets up at night to urinate, is the way to the bathroom uncluttered? Is there a night-light or hall light that can be left on so the patient can see?
- If the patient must administer injectable medications, are there satisfactory arrangements for discarding contaminated needles, syringes, or intravenous equipment?
- If possible, look in the refrigerator and the kitchen cabinets. Is the patient's diet adequate?

Information about a Specific Drug

To teach a patient about a specific drug, the instructional approach should be tailored to the needs and abilities of the patient. Careful patient assessment and analysis form the foundation of the teaching plan. Figure 4-1 illustrates a sample drug history that may provide data for use in developing a teaching plan. It can also be incorporated into the general health history recorded for all patients. The drug history questions should be modified as needed.

Teach the patient what the name and dosage of the prescribed drug are, why the drug is being used, and what the anticipated benefits of the drug are. Discuss the potential side effects in sufficient detail so that the patient will be able to list the most commonly encountered side effects. Whether the more serious (sometimes fatal, but also more rare) side effects should be discussed in detail depends on the patient and the situation. Instruct all patients and caregivers about whom to call (e.g., physician or nurse practitioner) if anything unexpected occurs.

If the patient must make any management decisions, review them carefully with the patient. Examples include changes in dose strength or frequency, depending on the patient's response to the medication, or home treatment of commonly encountered side effects. Have the patient practice any measurements that would be made at home (e.g., taking and recording pulse and checking blood glucose).

Inform the patient of any special considerations related to the dose, such as whether to take the drug on an empty or full stomach, whether to avoid milk, or whether to avoid taking two particular drugs simultaneously. If a new drug administration technique is involved, ascertain that the patient can demonstrate how to do this safely and accurately. Include appropriate general principles related to drug use.

Finally, provide the patient with information about how and when follow-up will occur and how to call for help or additional information. It is often advisable and helpful to have one or more family members present if the instruction is lengthy and complicated. In addition, provide written instructions when possible. It also may be helpful to refer the patient to a community-based nursing agency for follow-up in the home.

Patient Compliance

Even when the nurse has developed and implemented what seems to be a complete and individualized teaching plan, patient compliance may be poor. Some of the many possible reasons for this include the following:

- The patient or family misunderstands the directions.
- Poor vision or hearing leads to errors in understanding or reading medication labels.
- The patient cannot get the prescription refilled because it must be renewed by the physician, the patient cannot get to the pharmacy, or the patient cannot afford the cost.
- The patient becomes confused by the number of medications being taken and takes the drugs in incorrect amounts and at wrong times.
- The patient cannot manage the new route of administration in the home without help (e.g., self-injection).
- The patient is unable to accept a particular diagnosis (e.g., the teenager with diabetes who does not check blood glucose in the morning before insulin administration or who injects insulin too late in the day).
- Intolerable side effects occur, and the patient is too embarrassed to mention them to anyone (e.g., sexual impotence).
- Side effects occur that cause the patient to feel worse than the health problem alone did. This is a common problem with some drugs, such as antihypertensives.

The nurse who is in the patient's home may find clues to noncompliance. For example, too many pills may remain in the bottle at the end of the month, or the patient may be unable to describe how to take the prescribed medications. In the office or hospital setting, it may be more difficult for the nurse to find these clues. Only the lack of congruence between objective data and subjective response (e.g., the patient describes taking the antihypertensive, but the blood pressure remains high) may give the nurse a clue. The nurse must use careful nonjudgmental questioning to find out whether there is a problem and to help the patient find a way to better manage the health problem (i.e., by taking the drug).

The nurse must be creative in finding ways to help patients (Box 4-4). Some commonly tried methods include making a special calendar with items that the patient must check off when the dose is taken or putting the pills into color-coded cups or containers that correspond to a specific mealtime. The doses of a medication may be prepared for 7 days and left with the patient who has difficulty preparing the dosage form. Pill containers with an alarm are also available; these can be set to go off each time a patient is scheduled to take a dose of drug. In other situations compliance can be improved by adjusting the dosage, changing the time the drug is to be taken, or even changing the drug. Consult the physician about such adjustments. Finally, remember that patients have the right to choose whether or not and how they will take their medications. Some simply choose not to comply.

REGULATIONS AND DRUG ADMINISTRATION

Personnel: Who Does What?

Many people may be involved in the prescription, preparation, and administration of a drug to a patient. Generally, physicians prescribe drugs. Their authorization to prescribe is granted through licensing and medical practice acts. Other individuals can also prescribe drugs, including dentists and oral surgeons, osteopathic physicians, podiatrists, nurse practitioners, midwives, and physician's assistants. However, the degree of independence of practice that these and other health care practitioners may exercise varies with the laws of the state, province, or nation. This issue introduces the first of many points that the nurse must consider before administering a drug: Who has prescribed the drug, and does that person have the legal right to do so in that setting?

In the institutional setting, safeguards are often created to prevent unauthorized prescription of drugs. For example, to be granted privileges to practice in a hospital, a physician must present appropriate credentials, proof of licensure, and other documents required by that hospital.

After a nurse has worked on a nursing unit for several weeks, he or she will know the physicians, which also helps reduce the chance of errors related to who may prescribe. Even in the hospital the nurse ascertains the role of each person on the health care team. For example, in some teaching hospitals it is customary for medical students to be acting interns with clinical rotations (they may have other titles also). Although these individuals are not yet licensed, they may be caring for patients under the supervision of licensed preceptors (physicians). The nurse must be clear about the legal

---

> ### Box 4-4 Inability to Read
>
> If a patient cannot read, the standard written instructions will not be helpful. Some patients who cannot read are frank about this limitation and will let the nurse know immediately. Others have managed to keep this information secret from friends and family and may be reluctant to tell the nurse. Actions that *may* indicate that the patient cannot read include the following:
> - Not filling out the menu when in the hospital
> - Not reading the newspaper, if available
> - Professing fatigue and asking family members present to read instructions or the menu
> - When asked if instructional materials have been read, indicating fatigue or forgotten glasses or stating something such as "I'll read them after my husband [wife] gets here"
> - Not recording weight or pulse or blood glucose results at home
>
> If the nurse suspects that the patient cannot read, or has limited reading skills, the nurse should include pictures or icons of some kind on instructional materials. A medication chart that combines pictures that represent times of the day, with a drawing of the medication, will be more helpful to the patient. The pharmacist may be able to help by providing one dose of each medication that can be pasted onto the instruction sheet. Another family member may be willing and able to fill daily pill boxes for the patient.

---

ramifications of administering drugs prescribed by a nonlicensed individual.

When looking for guidance about who may prescribe and whose prescriptions must be administered, the nurse can consult the nurse practice act (or comparable professional practice act) for that state, province, or nation. The written policies of the employing agency or institution also provide guidance. Finally, nurses must consider their own moral and ethical codes of conduct in deciding whether to administer a specific drug to a patient. The nurse always has the personal right to refuse to administer a medication. For example, a nurse may refuse to give an ordered medication if the nurse's professional judgment indicates that the dose is excessively high. The nurse must notify the physician and the nurse in charge about the decision not to administer the medication.

It is important to remember that the legal constraints the nurse must consider may have little meaning to the patient. This situation is faced more often in the home, where the patient may wish to have the nurse administer a medication or home remedy prescribed or recommended by someone not recognized by the nurse practice act.

Pharmacists, who usually dispense medication, are licensed to do so and are governed by legal statutes. Pharmacies often employ aides or technicians to help fill prescriptions, but these individuals function under the supervision of the registered pharmacist. The pharmacist is an excellent source of information about drugs for the nurse or the patient but is often underused in this role.

Registered nurses can administer medications within the legal framework of the nurse practice act. Licensed practical nurses and licensed vocational nurses also have practice acts that regulate the role they play in drug administration. In some areas, pharmacists, medication technicians, medical students, emergency medical technicians, or others may administer drugs as employees of an institution or agency. Various students may be permitted to administer drugs in an agency, institution, or other setting if they are supervised. This category includes students participating in nursing, medical, physician assistant, emergency medical technician, and other educational programs. As the health care system changes, the responsibilities of individuals in various settings may also change. Therefore nurses must stay current with the various roles of members of the health care team. In the home the patient and family administer drugs.

Institutional Policies and Practices

The nurse practices within not only the legal framework of the nurse practice act but also the policies and procedures of the employing agency. The nurse is responsible for reading carefully any written information that defines restrictions or expectations of practice within the employing agency structure. The nurse should not blindly adhere to policy that is in direct conflict with legal guidelines or reasonable ethical and moral standards, but neither should the nurse practice outside the role defined by the agency.

In some agencies, verbal orders for drugs may be taken only by registered nurses. Students, licensed practical nurses, and others may not take these orders (Box 4-5). Some institutions prohibit the nurse from obtaining the patient's informed consent for investigational drugs; they may require this consent to be obtained only by the physician. In other settings the physician alone may administer investigational drugs. Medication orders written by medical students may be administered only after they are cosigned by a licensed physician. Such policies often develop as an interpretation of the law or to prevent anticipated problems.

Box 4-5 Verbal Medication Orders

Steps you should follow when taking a verbal medication order include the following:
1. If possible, have the patient's chart and medication records at hand.
2. Write down the order as it is dictated by the physician. (This may be done on scrap paper.)
3. Have the physician spell any unclear words.
4. Clarify any unclear part of the order.
5. Read the order back to the physician, including the patient's name and room number; the drug, dose, frequency, route of administration, and any other information given in the order; and the physician's name.
6. Glance at the other medications that the patient is receiving. If a question arises about the new medication ordered and the other medications the patient is currently receiving, ask the physician at that time.
7. Transcribe the order to the patient's record, noting the physician's name, your name, the date, and the time of day. Also note whether the order was given in person or by telephone.

Certain procedures in an agency are often developed in response to previous problems or errors. Examples include the requirements that all heparin and insulin doses be checked by two nurses before they are administered, that any parenteral drugs administered to pediatric patients be checked by two nurses before being administered, and that narcotics be counted at the end of each shift by two nurses, one from the ending shift and one from the beginning shift.

It may not be necessary for the nurse to know exactly *why* a policy or procedure has been developed. It is important for the nurse to practice within policy and procedure guidelines and, if the guidelines need to be changed, to work through the appropriate channels to change them. The beginning nurse may view these dos and don'ts as time-consuming, and some probably are not as important as others. However, all were designed to ensure safe patient care. Careless nursing practice can result in harm to the patient and malpractice suits. Failure to adhere to stated policies and procedures may weigh against the nurse in determination of legal liability.

Medication Errors

All medications are ordered, prepared, and administered with the best intentions. However, errors do occur with surprising frequency. What is an error? Defining an error is not always easy. It is clear that an error has occurred if a patient receives the wrong drug, if a patient is overmedicated, or if a prescribed drug is omitted. Other situations may be less clear-cut but also involve an error. Consider the following examples. A patient receives tetracycline with a glass of milk (tetracycline should not be administered with milk). A patient in the radiology department receives his 10 AM drugs at noon. Through an error in calculation, another patient receives the correct drug at the correct time but in half the ordered dose.

Some institutions differentiate between an error and an incident. Others define any deviation from policy and procedure as an error. This variability emphasizes the need for the nurse to know and adhere to the standards of practice defined by the nurse practice act, the policies and procedures of the employing agency and institution, and common sense.

The times at which drugs are administered in a hospital or institution are established by that setting; they are usually part of the policies and procedures. In addition, there is usually an explicit definition of what is meant by administering a drug on time. For example, a drug to be administered at 10 AM is considered to be on time if it is administered any time between 9:30 AM and 10:30 AM. The way a particular patient unit or entire institution handles deviations from the "a half hour before to half hour after" rule influences whether the time at which a particular drug is administered is called an error. Because the times for qid, bid, and qd are set by custom or policy, they also can be readjusted.

Another factor that affects the time is the drug itself and how frequently it is ordered. Consider the following situations. A vitamin ordered for qd, customarily given at 10 AM, is forgotten and given at 2 PM. Most agencies would not consider this an error and would not notify the physician. Insulin ordered for qd is administered at 10 AM instead of before breakfast (when it should be given). This is an error. Another drug is ordered to be given qid. On a particular unit, that schedule is customarily 10 AM, 2 PM, 6 PM, and 10 PM. A nurse misreads the medications record and administers it at 8 AM. Depending on the medication, the nurse's action may not be considered an error because the dosage times could be readjusted to 8 AM, 12 noon, 4 PM, and 8 PM.

Causes of Errors

There are many causes of the errors associated with administering medications. The following situations are examples:

- A drug is ordered for the wrong patient (i.e., written on the wrong patient's chart).
- The wrong dosage is ordered.
- The correct drug or dosage is ordered, but because of poor penmanship, the wrong drug or dosage is dispensed.
- An error in calculating the dosage is made, so the patient receives the wrong dosage.
- A drug is given via the wrong route.
- The patient's identity is not checked, and the wrong patient receives the drug.
- The first person who administers a drug fails to record it immediately afterward. A second person, checking the patient's chart, thinks that the drug has not been administered and so administers a dose. The patient has received a double dose.

What to Do if an Error Occurs

A professional accepts responsibility for his or her actions. If you think an error in drug administration has occurred, take the following steps. First, check the patient. Obtain any subjective or objective data appropriate to the patient's condition. If the patient received the wrong drug or the wrong dosage, assess the individual for the effects of the drug. For example, if too large a dose of antihypertensive was administered, take the patient's blood pressure, and then put the patient to bed. Notify the nurse in charge and the physician. Fill out any error forms required by the institution. Continue to monitor the patient. Modify your personal nursing practice, if needed, to help avoid the error in the future.

Two points need to be emphasized. The student or beginning practitioner may lack experience in handling an error or in deciding what is an error. If unsure, the practitioner should always report any problem associated with drug administration to the nurse in charge and to the physician. There are students and nurses in practice who want to avoid filling out incident forms or medication error forms because they believe that admitting that an error has occurred will be detrimental to their employment or student status with the institution or agency. However, records of errors help insti-

tutions develop new policies, procedures, and systems that will reduce the overall incidence of errors. No hospital or agency wants to continue to employ nurses who make repeated errors, especially of a careless nature, but most institutions recognize that anyone can make an occasional error.

Students sometimes fear that they will be sued for malpractice if an error occurs. There is no way to guarantee that a nurse will not be sued. However, if an error occurs but steps are taken to assess the patient and reverse the effects of the error as soon as the error is discovered, it will be difficult to argue that the nurse had a pattern of irresponsible behavior. Nurses must remain vigilant in all nursing care activities to provide the best quality, careful nursing care.

How to Avoid Medication Errors

The basis of avoiding errors is using and acting on common sense. Read and adhere to institutional policies and procedures; do not try shortcuts. Read each order carefully, asking yourself whether this drug makes sense for this particular patient at this dosage. Look up any drug or dosage that seems questionable in a standard drug reference. Never assume that the physician was right, the pharmacist was right, or the previous nurse who administered the drug was right if there is any question in your mind. Be especially careful in taking verbal or telephone orders because it is easy to misunderstand what is said (see Box 4-5).

Double-check all dosage calculations. If you still feel uneasy about a drug amount, have a colleague or the pharmacy double-check it. If a dose seems unusually large or small, double-check it. For example, if the order was for 10 mg (1 tablet) of a drug, but through an error in recording, it is noted as 100 mg, the dose would require 10 tablets, an unusually large amount for a patient. The other extreme also can happen. For example, the dose of ferrous sulfate (an iron preparation) for an adult may be listed as 30 mg. To administer that dose would require 1/10 of a 300 mg tablet, an impossible task.

If possible, avoid distractions while preparing medications. Check each label three times: when taking the drug out of the drawer or cabinet; when checking the medications record, computer, or Kardex for the dose and time; and again at the bedside just before administering the drug. Leave medications in their labeled containers until you are at the bedside. Always check the patient's identity carefully. If the patient asks any questions that indicate a possible error, assume that the patient is right, and double-check. Examples include statements such as the following: "That doesn't look like my usual morning pill," "I already took that—the other nurse gave it to me earlier today," or "The doctor said I would have a different pill today."

Ask the patient about a history of allergies before administering any new drug. Finally, check each patient within a short period after administering medications. Administering medications is just one of many nursing responsibilities, but it can be one of the most dangerous if done carelessly.

Nursing Process Overview

The Nursing Process with Drug Therapy

Assessment

Assessment includes gathering all the subjective and objective pertinent data about a patient, physically assessing the patient, and evaluating laboratory, radiographic, and other data. Throughout assessment the nurse analyzes the data and formulates nursing diagnoses.

Nursing Diagnoses

Nursing diagnoses are derived from the assessment data. With the possible exception of "knowledge deficit," no single nursing diagnosis fits all situations related to drug therapy.

Patient Outcomes

Patient outcomes describe in measurable terms the goals of therapy in relation to the patient.

Planning/Implementation

The nurse develops the plan in response to the assessment of patient needs and the knowledge of the treatment plan. The plan should include goals and specific steps to reach the goals. The patient or family is included in the plan development. Implementation involves carrying out the plan. Planning and implementation should include individualizing the approach to fit the unique needs of the patient.

Evaluation

Evaluation involves determining the success of the plan and its implementation. The step includes determining whether the goals for the patient have been reached. It involves deciding whether the goals were appropriate for the patient. Finally, evaluation focuses on revising the overall plan.

CHAPTER REVIEW

Application

1. What are the steps of the nursing process?
2. Discuss how medication administration fits into the nursing process.
3. What are the five rights of drug administration?
4. List the basic teaching points about safe medication use that should be taught to all patients.
5. In the settings where you practice, who may prescribe drugs? Who prepares them? Who administers them?
6. What is the difference between the nurse practice act (or other legal statutes) and institutional policies and procedures?
7. What are some examples of medication errors?

Critical Thinking

1. What kinds of information about drugs should be included in the patient teaching plan?
2. What are some factors that influence patient compliance?
3. When the nurse discovers that a medication error has occurred, what should be done? Find the incident/error report form for your agency. What kinds of information must the nurse provide when an error has occurred?
4. Ask some of the nurses you work with if they have ever made a medication error. Why do they think the error occurred? What was the patient outcome?

References

Hansen M, Fisher, JC: Patient-centered teaching from theory to practice, *Am J Nurs* 98(1):56, 58, 60, 1998.

Katz J: Back to basics: providing effective patient teaching, *Am J Nurs* 97(5):33-36, 1997.

Keegan L: Alternative & complementary therapies, *Nursing* 28(4):50-53, 1998.

Kelly M: Medications and the visually impaired elderly, *Geriatr Nurs* 17(2):60-62, 1996.

OBJECTIVES

After studying this chapter, you should be able to do the following:

- *Describe three drug administration systems.*
- *Give examples of information about drug administration that must be recorded on the patient's record.*
- *Give examples of how administration of drugs to children or older adults may require more individualized planning.*
- *Describe how to administer drugs via a variety of routes.*

CHAPTER OVERVIEW

This chapter emphasizes drug administration. Drug therapy is only a part of total patient care, but for drug therapy to be successful, it must be carried out properly. The patient has the right to receive the right drug, in the right dose, at the right time, via the right route.

The administration of drugs to patients is an opportunity for the nurse to continue to assess the patient's condition, to teach the patient in preparation for self-management of the health condition, to participate in discharge planning with the patient, and to evaluate the effectiveness of the care plan being implemented by the health care team. The reader should also study Chapter 4 carefully for information about the application of the nursing process to drug therapy.

DRUG ADMINISTRATION SYSTEMS

At least three drug administration systems are in use today. In the **unit-dose system** each dose of medication is individually wrapped, labeled, and supplied to the patient's unit in sufficient quantity to last 24 hours. On the patient unit, each patient has a designated drawer, box, or container, and the exact number of ordered doses of medications for a 24-hour period is placed in that container by the pharmacy daily. The nurse prepares each patient's medications, as ordered, from the supply in the patient's medication drawer. There are several advantages to this system, including that the medication remains in a labeled container until the nurse is at the bedside, thus reducing the chance of mixing up drugs; patients can be billed by exactly the number of medication doses that are taken, and unauthorized use of medications is decreased.

In the **stock drug system** each patient unit is supplied with large-quantity stock containers of the drugs commonly used in that setting or institution. The nurse administering a drug takes the order sheet, Kardex, or medication card to the medication room and prepares the dose of the drug from the stock supply, usually putting the dose into a small medicine cup. The advantages of this system are that the pharmacy need not restock the floor stock daily, calculation and preparation of doses require fewer pharmacy personnel because these duties are performed by the nurses, and stat and new orders can be filled immediately because the stock drugs are on the unit. A disadvantage of this system is that medication errors are more common.

A third drug administration system gaining more widespread use is the **computer-controlled dispensing system.** In this system, medications are supplied to the unit in a locked cabinet or cart. To obtain a dose for the patient, the nurse enters the patient's name or hospital identification number, and the nurse's personal identification number or security code. The system delivers the dose of medication, records it, and bills the patient's account. This system is especially helpful for the management and control of narcotics on the unit.

Most institutions combine their systems. The nurse must learn as much as possible about the drug administration systems in use to be efficient in preparing and administering medications.

RECORDING DRUG-RELATED INFORMATION

Recording drug administration is an important responsibility of the nurse. Forms for recording drug administration vary among agencies or institutions, but some general points usually do apply. The nurse should record that a dose was given as soon after administering the dose as possible. If a dose of medication is omitted, the reason must be noted, usually in the nurses' notes, on the form designated by the agency, or in the computer. Most institutions also require that doses given significantly early or late be accompanied by a notation explaining why. These records are legal documents, and information recorded on them should be accurate, and if handwritten, legible.

Information related to the route of administration or to the drug itself may need to be recorded. Examples include the blood glucose level, measured before a sliding-scale insulin dose is administered; the site of an injection; and the location of a topical nitroglycerin preparation.

Another important kind of information relates to individualized patient care, including the assessment, management, and evaluation of a specific patient. Assessment data might include the subjective and objective information that led the nurse to conclude that a prn drug was needed. Information related to the management of a patient, such as the patient's tolerating physical therapy best when a prn analgesic is administered 1 hour before therapy, becomes part of the care plan. Another kind of drug management information relates to the actual techniques of administration. An example of this kind of information is that the patient will take the drug more easily if it is crushed and mixed with applesauce.

Information related to the patient's response to the medication and the effectiveness of the drug (evaluation) should also be recorded. The exact location in the record and the amount of detail the nurse should include vary with the agency. Most of the forms in the patient's record are legal documents; therefore information recorded must be accurate, complete, and signed by the nurse.

ADMINISTERING DRUGS TO CHILDREN

Some drugs have been widely used in neonates and infants, and therefore dosage regimens are well documented; however, many drugs have not been studied in this population. Children are not simply small adults. Because of the small size and immature organs of neonates and infants, doses may be small and must be carefully calculated. Not only must the dose be correct, but also, because fluid overload can easily occur, the volume of medications being administered must be monitored closely. Finally, the child may be unable or unwilling to take prescribed medications.

A developmental approach should be used in administering drugs to children. A tentative plan is prepared for drug administration based on knowledge of growth and development for different age groups. The plan is initially tentative because the child's chronologic age may not match the developmental age. As the nurse develops rapport with the child, effective individualized approaches can be noted in the care plan.

To understand the developmental approach, think about a 2-year-old child who is to receive an injection and an oral medication. First, consider the available information about the child's general level of functioning, motor ability, interactions with other children, vocabulary, and ability to conceptualize. Then consider theories of child development such as those of Erickson, Freud, and Piaget for guidance.

The 2-year-old child, in Erickson's framework, is in the stage of autonomy versus shame and doubt. Behaviors characteristic of this stage include negativism, difficulty making choices, separation anxiety, and ritual. The child shows pride in performing well, is able to feed self, and has a limited understanding of time. Involve family members, if available. The child's mother or caregiver may be helpful in suggesting approaches that have worked well in the past. A few nursing approaches for children include giving simple directions; describing honestly what will occur but not until shortly before administering the medications; and asking the child to administer the oral drug. Do not ask, "Do you want to take your medicine?" because the answer is often "No!" If possible, give the child a choice of beverage to accompany taking the oral drug, but limit the choice (e.g., milk or apple juice). Follow the same pattern each time drugs are administered. Use firmness and consistency. Be prepared with adequate but nonthreatening assistance to restrain the child for the injection. Give positive feedback when the child cooperates and assists, provide comfort as needed, and encourage family members to do the same. Children of this age often want to assist or cooperate but need guidance in how to do so.

Remember that children vary, and although a developmental approach provides guidance, it does not replace individualized assessment and planning. Children also differ from adults in their ability to understand and accept the intrusive nature of many of the routes of drug administration. The young child may be terrified of receiving eardrops because the child cannot see what the nurse is doing to the ears. Injections are painful, and young children may have unrealistic fears (e.g., that their insides will come out of the hole created by the needle). Simply applying a bandage over the injection site may eliminate this fear. These examples may be difficult for the adult caregiver to understand because adults have learned how to reason. Adults may also dislike injections, even fear them, but they understand that the injection is fast and for their overall benefit.

Children's level of comprehension is very concrete until the early teens. Thus children may have difficulty understanding why an injection in the thigh could help their earache. Children also have trouble understanding time relationships and thinking about long-term consequences. Thus long-term drug therapy for treating diabetes, tuberculosis, or seizures may be difficult for the young child to understand.

A few additional guidelines related to techniques of administration include the following. Do not dilute medications in a large volume of liquid or food; if the child does not finish eating all of it, the nurse does not know how much medication has been consumed. Do not disguise medications in a favorite or essential food; the child may be unwilling to eat that food again. Do not try to trick the child into taking medications; be honest but caring in approaching children. Never administer an intramuscular injection to a sleeping child.

Use drawings, simple stories, coloring books, and toys dealing with medications and hospitalization. Explain the steps of administering the drug to preschool and young school-age children in a manner appropriate for their age. Allow children to play out their feelings. In a setting where children are often treated, have available a toy box containing items such as small dolls, medicine cups, and plastic syringes without needles to allow children to pretend, before or after medications are administered.

Do not underestimate the child's ability to understand or adjust to medication administration. At early ages many children can begin to accept responsibility for medication administration, especially for chronic health problems. For example, children 6 to 8 years old can be taught to self-administer insulin correctly.

There are other potential problems with medication administration and children. Some of these relate to the home environment. Problems that might place a child at risk include the following:

- Using medications originally prescribed for an adult in the household, without verification from a physician that the drug or dose is appropriate for the child
- Leaving medications within easy reach of young children, with the potential that a child will overdose
- Inaccurately measuring dosages, which might occur, for example, if spoons of different capacities are used to measure doses
- Using a medication prescribed for one child to treat others in the family when a definitive diagnosis on the other children has not been made
- Parents or caregivers lacking knowledge that some medications should not be used in children in certain situations, for example, administering aspirin to treat fever in a child with chicken pox
- Referring to medications as "candy," which may cause children to not understand the serious nature of medications

The nurse who can visit the family in the home may be able to identify some of these problems, if they exist, and work with the family to correct them.

ADMINISTERING DRUGS TO OLDER ADULTS

Older adult patients can also present special care considerations for the nurse. As discussed in Chapters 1 and 2, the physiologic changes that accompany aging influence the patient's response to medications. Medication use among the older adults is generally higher than among younger groups. As many as two thirds of Americans older than age 65 take at least one prescription drug; of these, at least one-third take three or more drugs. Physiologic changes that may occur in older adults have been outlined earlier in this book. However, there is great variability in the older adults. Some individuals at age 65 show marked physiologic changes, whereas others in their eighties or nineties show few physiologic changes. Some older adults take many medications, whereas others take few or none.

Individualized assessment and planning are important when working with older adults. One role for the nurse is to make certain that all medications ordered for a patient are still necessary. Sometimes as side effects to one drug develop, an additional drug is prescribed to treat them. Side effects to the second drug develop, and these are treated with a third drug. It may be difficult for the physician, the nurse, and the patient to understand what the drug regimen is designed to do.

Another problem occasionally encountered with older adults is the use of several health care providers who may not be communicating with one another about the patient. A patient may have an ophthalmologist, a cardiologist, a podiatrist, and a urologist, each prescribing treatments and drugs. The patient may unknowingly be at risk for overmedication and drug interactions.

Even if multiple medications are appropriately indicated and prescribed, patients can have difficulty managing a complicated medication regimen that may include drugs to be taken before and after meals, some once a day, others more often during the day, with the dose of other drugs changing based on the day of the week or the day of the month. If a complicated drug regimen is combined with the effects of chronic disease, possible poor nutrition, or other problems,

it is not surprising that some older adult patients are at great risk from their medications.

Some older adults remain vigorous, physically active, and mentally alert. However, many have one or more physical problems that make medication use difficult or potentially hazardous. For example, cataracts and glaucoma are both more prevalent in older adults, as are alterations in vision from strokes and other neurologic problems. Other patients have vision problems resulting from a general decline in visual acuity that has evolved over the years. Vision problems in older adults may make reading drug labels and package inserts and preparing the correct dose of a medication difficult. Alterations in vision may make it difficult for patients to read test results correctly or to monitor their weight (because they cannot read the scale). Hearing may decline in some patients. Alterations in hearing may place older adults at risk for misunderstanding verbal instructions about how to take medications correctly.

Physical dexterity may be altered in some patients. Arthritic changes, paralysis secondary to stroke, or other problems may make it difficult for older adults to manipulate items such as pill bottles, syringes, blood glucose testing equipment, and small pills or tablets.

Many older adults live on fixed low incomes, and medications are expensive. Older adult patients who would like to take their medications as ordered may have difficulty be-

---

RESEARCH HIGHLIGHTS

Too Many Medications, Too Little Money: How Do Patients Cope?

—Chubon CSJ, Schulz RM, Lingle EW, Coster-Schulz MA: Public Health Nurs *11(6)4:412-415, 1994.*

PURPOSE
In South Carolina, Medicaid pays for three prescriptions a month for Medicaid recipients. Many Medicaid recipients need more than three prescribed medications per month. The purpose of this study was to explore what patients who have multiple prescribed drugs do when the cost of only three of their prescriptions is provided.

METHOD
This was a qualitative pilot study with a convenience sample. Pharmacists in two small towns helped identify Medicaid recipients taking more than three prescribed medications. Prospective participants were contacted in writing. Those willing to participate were paid $20. Subjects were interviewed in the participant's home by an experienced public health nurse. Subjects showed their medications to the nurse and discussed how they managed. Interview results were analyzed for common themes and unique experiences.

RESULTS
This study included 19 subjects: 17 women and 2 men. One subject was a child, but the others were adults. Of the subjects, 14 were over age 60. The mean age of the adults was 68.7 years. The mean number of drugs prescribed during the preceding year was 7.6. Medical diagnoses reported included dia-

betes, hypertension, heart disease, chronic lung disease, cancer, and asthma.

Subjects reported taking the following actions when they were faced with a prescription medication not paid for by Medicaid: (1) paid out of pocket (100%), (2) obtained medication in other ways (58%), (3) got money from someone else (42%), (4) did not get the medicine at all (42%), (5) changed the way medicine was taken (37%), and (6) took another person's medicine (11%). Those who obtained the medication in other ways reported receiving samples from the physician or obtaining medications from the pharmacist on credit until they could pay. Those who got money from someone else usually identified their children as a source of this additional money, although one person had taken out a loan to buy prescriptions. Prescriptions not filled included ones for digoxin, glyburide, furosemide, albuterol sulfate, metaproterenol sulfate, and sulindac.

IMPLICATIONS
Nurses working with patients on Medicaid or patients with limited resources for obtaining prescription medications should assess patients carefully to see if the drugs are being used as prescribed. Patient teaching may need to include guidelines about which medications can be omitted if necessary. Nurses should also use opportunities to advocate for their patients and to contact legislators and policy makers about the needs of patients.

cause they cannot afford the medication or cannot physically get to the drugstore to pick up their prescription. Some patients may not be able to afford the drug in the dosing frequency prescribed; therefore they try to save money by taking doses only half as often as ordered (see the Geriatric Considerations box).

Some older adults may also be poorly nourished. This situation may be due to lack of money, difficulty getting to the store, or difficulty eating certain foods (because of lacking teeth or having poorly fitting dentures). Still other reasons may be lack of knowledge about a well-rounded nutritious diet or lack of energy or interest in cooking regular meals (e.g., if the person lives alone). If the patient is poorly nourished, the serum albumin level may be low, causing a potential problem in the effects of protein-bound drugs. Poor nutritional status may place the patient at risk for side effects from some drugs.

Another problem that older adults face is having family or health care team members assume that a decline in their condition represents a natural part of aging, without adequate patient assessment. Weakness, loss of balance, confusion, memory loss, slurred speech, fatigue, and loss of appetite are but a few symptoms that could be due to drug side effects and should not be attributed to aging.

Older adult patients must be approached as adults. Older adults who have taken many drugs over the years may have established elaborate rituals associated with taking drugs. The ritual may involve factors such as the time of day, the order in which the drugs are taken, or the fluid used to swallow the drugs. Ask patients about their usual practices before rushing in at 10 AM to administer a handful of drugs. When possible, allow patients to continue their usual routine.

Older adults may also be more sensitive to nausea as a side effect. This sensitivity combined with the potential interaction of a large quantity of drugs may compound the nausea. It may be necessary to readjust the dosage schedule to spread out the prescribed medications over the course of the day. Also, if the patient must drink 6 to 8 ounces of fluid or more to take all the medications, they should not be administered just before a meal. After drinking a full glass of liquid, the patient may not feel like eating.

DRUG ADMINISTRATION SCHEDULES

In the hospital or nursing home the nurse determines the times to administer the medications. In the home the patient must do it. Scheduling may be difficult, and it may require incorporating many of the following adjustments (among others):

- Multiple daily doses of the same drug should be evenly spaced throughout the 24 hours to help maintain serum drug levels (see Chapter 1).
- Drugs with known interactions should not be administered at the same time (e.g., cholestyramine with digoxin).
- Drugs that interact with specific foods should not be given concurrently with those foods (e.g., tetracycline and milk).
- For best effect, some drugs work best if given before or after a meal (e.g., sucralfate).
- Some drug doses must be scheduled early in the day for appropriate effect (e.g., insulin).
- The patient's sleep should not be interrupted any more than necessary. At home the patient may not get up to take any medications during the night.
- In the hospital some drugs are arbitrarily scheduled at a time during the day to allow for the return of laboratory results (e.g., warfarin).

When a patient is taking many medications, scheduling can be a challenge for the nurse and an even greater challenge for the patient.

Patients with multiple chronic health problems may need to take several drugs simultaneously. The combination of drugs or the total amount of fluid needed by the patient to swallow the drugs may be nauseating. If the patient refuses to take all the medications, tires before all the drugs are taken, or becomes too nauseated to take all the drugs, the nurse must ensure that the more necessary drugs are taken first and the less necessary ones are left until last. Consider a patient receiving a cardiotonic, an antihypertensive, a diuretic, a potassium replacement, a vitamin, and an iron supplement at 10 AM. All of these drugs are necessary for management of the patient's condition. However, the nurse may decide that the cardiotonic, antihypertensive, diuretic, and potassium replacement are of greater priority. This is not to suggest that the nurse can simply decide not to administer

---

 GERIATRIC CONSIDERATIONS

Reducing Drug Costs

Prescription drugs can be costly. Possible ways to reduce costs for patients include the following:

- Ask the physician if the drug can be prescribed in the generic form.
- Shop around (via telephone) for the best buy. Pharmacies vary in their prices.
- If the prescription is for a new drug, ask the physician for a few samples, or ask the pharmacist to fill part of the prescription (e.g., to give you 10 tablets of the 100 ordered tablets) until you see whether this drug causes serious side effects.
- If a drug must be taken for an extended period, is there any organization through which drugs can be purchased at a reduced cost? For example, through the American Association of Retired Persons (AARP), members can buy large quantities of AARP medicines at reduced rates. However, these drugs must be ordered through the mail, so this service is most helpful with drugs that will be needed on a long-term, continuing basis.

certain medications but that the nurse is often required to exercise judgment and make decisions on short notice. A better long-term solution to this multiple drug problem might be to schedule the vitamin and the iron supplement at a time when the patient is taking fewer drugs and will then have less difficulty in taking all that are ordered. See Chapter 4 for additional discussion of medication scheduling.

TECHNIQUES FOR ADMINISTERING DRUGS

Box 5-1 lists the steps to be followed in administering all drugs. For more detailed descriptions or additional illustrations, see nursing fundamentals textbooks.

Stay informed about agency policies regarding infection control and guidelines from the Centers for Disease Control and Prevention. Wear gloves when administering medications if there is a chance of exposure to body fluids. Follow agency guidelines for disposing of contaminated needles and always be vigilant in working with needles. Keep up to date on immunizations (e.g., hepatitis B immunization) and follow agency guidelines if a needle stick occurs.

Oral Route

Drugs are most commonly administered via the oral route. This route is safe, convenient, and acceptable for most patients and medications.

B o x 5-1   General Steps in Drug Administration

1. At the start of the workday, review each patient's record, noting the medical and nursing diagnoses, current problems, relevant laboratory findings, and plan of health care.
2. Compare the physician's original order against the working tools (may be medication Kardex, medication cards, computer printout, or computer screen—whatever is used in that setting to guide the nurse in preparing drugs).
   a. Check for accuracy of transcription: Drug name? Drug dose? Route of administration? Frequency of administration?
   b. Check for appropriateness of the order. Does this drug make sense for this patient? Is this dose in the usual range for a patient of this age and weight?
   c. Other: Have any automatic expiration dates passed? Are there new laboratory values to be considered, such as serum electrolyte levels, serum drug levels, culture reports, or renal or liver function studies?
3. Look up any new drugs or check any drug information that is unclear.
4. Check the medication supply.
   a. Is stock bottle supply adequate for the shift? If not, reorder from the pharmacy.
   b. Check each patient's drawer or box of drugs. Are the drugs present?
   c. Are any missing drugs in the refrigerator, on the back of the medication cart, at the bedside? Where else?
   d. Are there sufficient supplies to prepare and administer the drugs (straws, water cups, medication cups, spoons, mortar and pestle, syringes)?
5. Review the specific drugs. Are there any special assessments to be made or data to check before any drug is administered? Examples might include measurement of apical pulse, blood pressure, temperature, weight, urine, or blood test.
   a. Organize equipment that might be needed.
   b. Make a list if necessary.
6. Check care plans (if not already done) to note personal preferences, previous problems, and nursing care approaches. Make a list of items to remember, such as applesauce, juices, coffee, crackers, yogurt, jelly sandwich, ice cream, or other foods to disguise flavors.
7. Just before preparing the drugs, wash hands.
8. Check the working tool and obtain the medication. Read the label carefully, checking the drug, the dose, and the route of administration.*
9. Pour or prepare the dose. If from a stock bottle, read the label again before replacing the bottle. If from a unit dose, check the label; do not remove the drug from the package.

10. Prepare all medications for that patient. If preparing medications in the medication room, prepare the medications for all the patients who are to receive them.
11. Go to the bedside, and identify the patient (if possible, use all three methods):
    a. Call the patient by name. (Be especially careful if there is more than one patient on the unit with the same last name.)
    b. Ask the patient to state his or her full name.
    c. Check the patient identification band. (This may be the only possible way to identify the infant, small child, or confused adult.)
12. Assess the patient.
    a. Note any changes since you last saw the patient.
    b. Obtain any objective data needed before administering the drugs, such as apical pulse, blood pressure, or breath sounds.
    c. Obtain any appropriate subjective information.
    d. If you did not previously know the patient or if new drugs are being administered, check on history of allergy.
13. If the data obtained in step 12 were not acceptable, withhold the corresponding drugs. For example, if the patient is hypotensive, withhold the antihypertensive until you discuss the patient's situation with the physician. Other drugs may be given if the patient's condition is satisfactory.
14. Draw the curtain or otherwise ensure privacy, if needed.
15. Administer the medications, helping the patient as needed. If the medicines are in unit-dose packages, open the packages. Make certain the patient takes the medication. Do not leave any medications at the bedside unless authorized by a physician's order or written institutional policy.
16. Assist the patient to return to a comfortable position.
17. Wash hands.
18. If using a medication cart and the medication record is kept with the cart, immediately record that the drugs were given. If using a different system, administer all medications, then return to the medication record and record that the drugs were given.
19. Depending on the drug, the patient and the usual policies and procedures, notify appropriate individuals (e.g., nurse in charge, physician) about doses that were withheld.
20. Record other appropriate information such as data obtained during assessment, drugs withheld and why, and changes in the patient's condition.
21. Make appropriate additions to the care plan.
22. Check on the patient at appropriate intervals to evaluate the response to drug therapy.

---

*The next few steps vary slightly, depending on whether the drugs are prepared in the medication room, such as with a stock drug system, or in the patient's room, such as with a medication cart and unit-dose system.

After carefully checking and preparing the medications ordered, identify the patient, help the patient sit upright (if possible), and then hand the medications and a glass of water or other preferred liquid to the patient. The patient then puts the pills, tablets, or capsules in the mouth and swallows them with the offered fluid. The patient should drink enough fluid to ensure that the medication reaches the stomach. Drugs that lodge in the esophagus can cause irritation and burning and may result in poor absorption. Approximately 4 ounces of fluid is usually sufficient, but encourage the patient to drink more unless contraindicated. Patients who are not sitting upright may need additional fluid to ensure that the medication has reached the stomach.

Ensure that the medication was swallowed and is not being hidden in the patient's mouth. Although this situation is rare, it can occur with confused individuals or those with certain psychiatric problems. After the patient swallows the drug, record that the medication has been taken.

Many patients have difficulty swallowing whole tablets or capsules. Break scored tablets along the lines indicated. It may be possible to separate the halves of capsules and pour out the powdered drug into another liquid or soft food such as applesauce. Crush tablets and mix with water or food. Especially with children, use as little applesauce or other food as possible. Otherwise, the child may feel full or refuse the rest of the applesauce, and the nurse has no way of knowing how much of the prescribed dose was actually consumed. See Box 5-2 for a list of drug forms that should not be crushed or chewed. If in doubt, consult the pharmacist before crushing tablets or breaking open capsules.

Children sometimes take medications wrapped in a jelly sandwich. Another way to encourage the child is to give the medication in a cup and follow it with a "chaser" of water, milk, or carbonated beverage in another medication cup. Children like the small cups and are not overwhelmed with a large volume of fluid. When choosing a food or fluid to give a child to help disguise or take medications, do not select items with high sugar content if the medication must be taken regularly because the item may contribute to dental caries. For children with diabetes, use sugar-free foods.

Although in some institutions the pharmacy will send crushed dosage forms to the nursing unit, it is usually the nurse's responsibility to crush the medication. There are several ways to do this. Some agencies supply pill crushers in the nursing unit. A mortar and pestle may be used. Be sure that these implements are clean and dry before use, and wash away any remaining drug residue and dry them after preparing the dose. It may be possible to place the tablet inside a plastic or paper medication cup and then place a second cup over the pill. Any handy blunt instrument can then be used to crush the tablet between the layers of the cups. Alternatively, place the pill between two metal spoons and crush it. Also, some unit-dose packages are sturdy enough to allow the pill or tablet to be crushed in the package. Regardless of how the drug is crushed, be careful to check that all the powdered drug is brushed into the cup that you give the patient.

As an alternative to crushing medications, obtain a liquid form of the drug. Many drugs are available in liquid forms as **suspensions** or solutions. Make substitutions carefully; be sure to consult the physician and pharmacist. For example, a sustained-release form of a drug might be available in tablet form, but the only liquid preparation available may not be a sustained-release form; therefore dosage frequency may require adjustment.

It is generally easy to measure the prescribed dose in a capsule or tablet form, but liquid preparations require more care. If the drug is in suspension form, shake the container thoroughly before pouring the dose. Inadequate shaking of suspensions can result in the patient receiving a small dose from the top of the bottle and a large dose near the bottom of the bottle, as the unsuspended particles of drug collect. In the institutional setting, medication cups are usually provided for measuring the prescribed dose unless the drug is supplied in the unit dose from the pharmacy. Place the medication cup on a flat surface or hold it upright at eye level to check that the correct dose has been poured. The base of the meniscus should be at the level of the desired dose (Figure 5-1). For small amounts of liquids or odd quantities, measure the dose with a syringe. It is not acceptable to estimate 2 ml or 12.5 ml of a drug.

In the home, patients usually use household tablespoons and teaspoons for measuring dosages. Encourage patients to use the same spoon each time because household spoons are not standardized and switching spoons may result in varying

---

Box 5-2   Drug Forms That Should Not Be Crushed or Chewed

- Enteric-coated tablets
- Sustained-release forms. These often have the following suffixes attached to the drug name:
  - Dur (duration)
  - SR (sustained release)
  - CR (controlled or continuous release)
  - SA (sustained action)
  - Contin (continuous)
  - LA (long acting)
- Trade names that imply sustained release such as spansules, extentabs, and extencaps
- Trade names with the bid (twice a day) abbreviation in the name, such as Theobid, Lithobid, and Cardabid
- Liquid-containing capsules, although occasionally it may be acceptable to puncture the capsule and squeeze out the contents; consult the pharmacist or manufacturer
- Sublingual or buccal tablets

The name alone may not provide enough information. Consult the pharmacist if in doubt. Some forms that look like sustained forms are not, and vice versa. Some capsules containing small, slow-release pellets may be opened, and the pellets may be sprinkled on applesauce or gently mixed into liquid or food, but they should not be crushed or dissolved.

Scored tablets may be broken along the scored line but should not be chewed or crushed.

dosages. Tell patients to read the pharmacy label to see whether liquid forms must be stored in the refrigerator.

The use of a liquid form of a drug does not guarantee patient cooperation in taking the drug. Many liquid forms, especially tinctures and elixirs, are unpleasant tasting. Patients may be more willing to take a crushed tablet in food than to take the drug in the liquid form. Some patients may take liquid forms better through a straw placed near the back of the mouth. If the preparation can stain teeth, use a straw so the medication is delivered to the back of the throat, bypassing contact with the teeth. Cut the straw in half to make it easier for children to manage.

The use or particular property of a drug may influence the sequence of oral drug administration. For example, Xylocaine Viscous, an oral preparation of lidocaine hydrochloride, is prescribed to produce relief of oral discomfort; it accomplishes this by producing local anesthesia. Administer this drug last if several drugs are being administered simultaneously because this drug may interfere with swallowing. Administer drugs via the sublingual or buccal route last, after drugs that are swallowed.

Record on the patient medication Kardex or care plan anything unique about the administration of medications to each patient.

Figure 5-1 Reading meniscus. Meniscus is caused by surface tension of solution against container walls. Surface tension causes formation of concave or hollowed curvature on solution surface. Read level at lowest point of concave curve.

Sublingual, Buccal, Troche, Lozenge, and Lingual Spray Forms

Sublingual drugs are in tablet form but are placed under the tongue to dissolve. The most commonly prescribed sublingual drugs are the nitrates and nitrites for anginal heart pain. Instruct the patient to let the tablet dissolve under the tongue. Tell the patient not to drink any fluid, eat, or smoke while the drug is dissolving. This route of administration may be new to the patient, so make certain that the patient understands how to use drugs taken sublingually. Teach family members to administer drugs via this route when the patient is unable to do so, if appropriate for the patient's situation.

Teach patients to hold **buccal tablets** between the cheek and the gum and allow them to dissolve. Alternate cheeks with each dose of medication to minimize the chance for irritation of the mucosa. Report any oral irritation to the physician. Dissolve **troches** and **lozenges** in the mouth. These drug forms are usually designed to allow for slow release of the drug over several minutes. Avoid drinking, eating, or smoking until troches, lozenges, sublingual tablets, or buccal tablets have dissolved.

Another oral form is the **lingual spray.** Teach patients to spray one or two jets from a small canister into the mouth, under the tongue (as prescribed). The canister delivers a specific dose with each jet.

Feeding Tubes

Most medications that can be administered orally also can be administered via feeding tubes. Liquid preparations are preferred, but some medications can be finely crushed and mixed with sufficient water to ensure complete passage of the drug to the stomach (see Box 5-2). Before administering any drug via a tube, verify that the tube is in the correct place. Refer to appropriate texts of nursing fundamentals for details about the care of patients with feeding tubes. If the drugs do not form a solid precipitate, mix them together and administer. Otherwise, administer the drugs one at a time,

Figure 5-2 Drug mixing vial. **A,** Remove protective cap from vial. **B,** Push rubber plunger on top of vial. This action forces small rubber plug between upper and lower compartment into lower compartment, which allows powder and diluent to mix. Rotate vial between hands to speed mixing. Clean top of plunger with alcohol. **C,** Insert needle of syringe into plunger and withdraw dose. For best results needle must go straight into plunger.

followed by a small amount of water (about 30 ml) to flush the drug through the tube, to help maintain the patency of the tube, and to ensure that subsequent drugs do not precipitate with residue remaining in the tube from an earlier drug. Do not mix the drugs with the tube feeding itself. After the final drug is administered, clear the tube with water. Include the amount of fluid used to flush the tubing in the totals for the patient's fluid intake.

Parenteral Medications: Injections

The word *parenteral* means outside the intestines, but in common use it is usually limited to injections. There are many kinds of injections, which are named by indicating the site at which the medication is deposited. Intradermal, intramuscular (IM), intravenous (IV), and subcutaneous injections are all commonly used in everyday practice. Other injection sites, often used only by the physician, include intracardiac (usually reserved for resuscitation efforts), intrathecal (into the subarachnoid space via lumbar or ventricular puncture), and intraarticular (into a joint). The term *hypodermic* is being replaced by subcutaneous.

There are advantages and disadvantages associated with parenteral administration. This route is used in patients who have difficulty swallowing, who are not alert, or who lack an adequate gag reflex. It can be used for a patient unwilling or unable to take other, usually oral, medications. (If multiple doses are required, IV administration is usually preferred in children because it is less intrusive.)

Insulin, heparin, and some other medications may be administered only parenterally. On the other hand, drugs administered via this route are generally considered irretrievable. With IM injections a slight chance of infection exists because the integrity of the skin is broken. Inadvertent administration into the vascular space is also possible, although rare. Damage to muscles and nerves can also occur. IM injections are also uncomfortable.

Carefully calculate and prepare the prescribed dose. Many injectable medications are dry powders and must be reconstituted before administration. Although the pharmacy can do this, sometimes the nurse must do it. Carefully read the manufacturer's information regarding reconstitution of dry medication. There may be restrictions on what fluids may be used for reconstitution, or the diluent may be supplied by the manufacturer.

Not only must the correct diluent be used, but also the correct amount of diluent must be added to the dry powder. Beginners often find it difficult to understand the instructions related to reconstitution. For example, one form of penicillin states that certain amounts of diluent may be added to the 1,000,000-unit vial to provide the dilutions listed, stating, "Add 9.6 ml, 4.6 ml, or 3.6 ml to provide 100,000 units, 200,000 units, or 250,000 U/ml, respectively." Another vial used for some drugs combines the diluent and powder in a single glass vessel containing two compartments (Figure 5-2). Mix the diluent and powder in the closed vial before withdrawing the dose. Consult the pharmacist or

---

RESEARCH HIGHLIGHTS

Defining Unnecessary Disinfection Procedures for Single-Dose and Multiple-Dose Vials
—Buckley CT, Dudley SM, Donowitz LG: Am J Crit Care 3(6):448, 1994.

PURPOSE

Agency procedures describing techniques for drug preparation vary. This study was designed (1) to evaluate the need for cleansing the top of a single-dose medication vial and (2) to compare the effectiveness of cleaning the top of multiple-use vials with alcohol versus povidone-iodine and alcohol.

SAMPLE AND METHODOLOGY

The rubber stoppers of five single-dose vials from each of 20 packages (N = 100) were cultured after the top of the vial was removed. The rubber stoppers of 87 previously used multiple-dose vials of antibiotics from the refrigerator of the neonatal intensive care unit were cultured. All of these vials had been routinely cleaned using this technique: cleansing with a povidone-iodine pad, allowing the vial to sit for 3 minutes, and then wiping with 70% isopropyl alcohol to remove the povidone-iodine. After a change in institution practice to cleaning multiple-use vials with alcohol-only, 100 multiple-use vials that had been cleansed in this manner were cultured.

FINDINGS

Of the 100 single-dose vials cultured, 99% of the surfaces were sterile. One culture was positive for three colonies of *Staphy-*

lococcus epidermidis. Of the multiple-dose vials cleaned with povidone-iodine followed by alcohol, 83 (95%) were sterile. Of the multiple-use vials cleaned with alcohol only, 100% of the surface cultures were sterile.

IMPLICATIONS

This study supports the view that the rubber stopper of single-use drug vials is sterile when the cap is removed and thus needs no further disinfection. With multiple-use vials, what seems like a more thorough procedure (cleaning with two agents instead of one) may not be more effective. The time involved in cleaning multiple-use vials and the cost of two agents were not necessary in this institution. Cleaning multiple-dose vials with alcohol only was more effective than using two agents. Two limitations identified by the authors of this study were that all the multiple-use vials contained antibiotics and all were stored in the refrigerator.

CRITICAL THINKING: Are there procedures you have been taught that could be reevaluated? Are there measures in your agency that could be streamlined without compromising patient care? How could these be tested?

a nursing supervisor with questions about reconstituting powder for injection (see the Research Highlights box on unnecessary disinfection procedures).

Write the date, time of reconstitution, and concentration on the vial of reconstituted medication. Many institutions also require that the nurse initial the vial and put the patient's name on it. Reconstituted medications are often stored in the refrigerator. Many vials are provided in single-dose concentrations; however, in pediatric settings, where the prescribed dose may be quite small, the nurse may use only a portion of the contents of a medication vial. Remember to read the label before using stored medications and observe expiration dates. Once reconstituted, many medications may be safely used for a short period, but follow agency policy.

Not all medications for injection are supplied in vials. Many come in small glass ampules, from which a single dose is withdrawn, and the ampule is discarded (Figure 5-3). A small metal saw may be supplied with the ampules. If supplied, use the saw and make two to three passes across the neck of the ampule. Do not saw through the glass, but make a scored line as a guide for breaking the ampule. To protect your fingers from getting cut, wrap the ampule in a piece of gauze or paper towel before opening it. Sharply snap the top off the ampule. Use a filter needle on the syringe, if one is available, to prevent small slivers of glass from entering the syringe. After withdrawing the dose, replace the filter needle with the needle for the injection.

Other medications are provided in prefilled syringes. The advantage of these syringes is fast and easy preparation. However, they are also more expensive. Most agencies stock prefilled syringes for narcotics and for selected other situations when drugs must be immediately available, such as the emergency drug box or resuscitation cart. Techniques for loading and activating prefilled products vary with manufacturer. Consult the manufacturer or agency about devices used in any individual setting. See Figure 5-4 for an illustration of one kind of prefilled syringe.

The choice of syringe and needle to be used depends on the information obtained from assessment of the patient, the route of administration to be used, the characteristics of the fluid to be injected (e.g., aqueous or oil based), and the volume of medication to be delivered. Sample syringe sizes include 1-ml tuberculin and insulin syringes and 2.5-, 5-, and 10-ml syringes. Larger syringes are available but are rarely used for medication administration via the parenteral route. Use tuberculin syringes, marked in 0.01-ml gradations, for small volumes. Insulin syringes are available in 0.5- or 1-ml volumes, although some institutions stock an insulin syringe with a maximum volume of 25 or 35 U. Do not substitute tuberculin and insulin syringes for each other.

Needles vary in length and gauge, from ³/₈ inch to 3 inches or more in length and from 14 gauge (large lumen) to 28 gauge (small lumen). Most institutions limit the variety of needles and syringes in stock. Use smaller lumen (larger gauge) needles for intradermal injections. Administer subcutaneous injections with a ¹/₂- or ⁵/₈-inch, 23- or 25-gauge needle. Administer IM injections with a 19- or 21-gauge, 1¹/₂- to 2-inch needle; a 16- or 18-gauge needle may also be used (Box 5-3).

Figure 5-3   **A,** Examples of scored and ringed glass ampules. **B,** Hold ampule upright and gently flick top to shake medication into bottom of ampule. **C,** Hold vial with alcohol wipe or gauze and snap off top. **D,** Withdraw medication from bottom half of ampule.

After preparing the ordered dose and choosing the appropriate needle and syringe, go to the patient's bedside to administer the injection. Check the patient's name band to verify identity, draw the curtain or otherwise ensure privacy, explain what is going to happen, and assist the patient to assume the necessary position. If the patient is unable or unwilling to assist in positioning, bring someone to assist you. Put on gloves, assess the injection site, locate the anatomic landmarks, and smoothly administer the injection. Help the patient return to a comfortable position. Dispose of the syringe and needle according to the procedures of the agency; usually there is a container for contaminated "sharps" at the bedside or in the bathroom. Do not recap needles. Record

that the medication has been given, noting the location so that injection sites can be rotated. Check the patient again to make certain no untoward effects have occurred and to evaluate whether the drug is working as anticipated.

Record any aspects of the injection that are unique to the patient on the medication Kardex or patient care plan. You can find more detailed information about drawing up medications, handling equipment, and administering injections in a text of nursing fundamentals. Practice in giving injections is important for students to become accurate, efficient, and confident.

In recent years there have been efforts to improve equipment to minimize the possibility of needlestick injury. One development has been the addition of a protective shield over the syringe. After the medication is administered and the needle withdrawn from the skin, slide the protective sheath over the needle. Box 5-4 discusses needleless injections using a pressure-jet device. Another needleless syringe is illustrated in Figure 5-5.

Intradermal Injection

An **intradermal injection** is made just below the epidermis, or outer layer of skin (Figure 5-6). Such an injection is used for allergy testing and for administration of local anesthetics. Use a small-bore needle and a small-volume syringe,

---

Box 5-3   Preparation of Oil-Based Medicines for Intramuscular Administration

Oil-based medicines are released more slowly because it takes the oil longer to be absorbed from the muscle than aqueous solutions. Administer oil-based medicines via the intramuscular route only, never intravenously.

- Heat the unopened vial or ampule in warm water for several minutes to decrease oil viscosity.
- Roll the vial vigorously between the hands to resuspend the medication, which is usually an inconspicuous film on the side of the ampule. Resuspension is adequate when no particles of medication remain on the bottom or sides of the vial. Failure to shake or roll the vial sufficiently results in inaccurate dosage and erratic absorption.
- Draw up the correct dose into a syringe fitted with a large-bore (19- to 21-gauge), 1½-inch needle (for an adult), and administer the dose immediately, before the oil cools.
- Inject the medicine, exerting slow, even pressure on the plunger. Attempting to inject too rapidly can cause pressure to increase within the syringe, and the needle and syringe may separate, causing loss of medication.
- Use large muscle masses, such as the buttock, thigh, or ventrogluteal site. In infants and small children, use the vastus lateralis muscle.
- The oil base can produce palpable lumps because it is absorbed slowly. Record injection sites, rotate them, and avoid the deltoid muscle.

Box 5-4   Will We Ever Get Rid of Injections?

Traditional injections are uncomfortable to the patient and, because a needle is involved, pose the possible risk to the nurse of needlestick injury. Research to develop needleless injections continues. One device currently available is the pressure-jet device, which forces medication through the skin into the subcutaneous tissue. Research indicates that it delivers insulin accurately and safely, and the insulin is absorbed more rapidly because of the way it is dispersed into the tissue. Acceptance of insulin therapy is greater when needles are not involved. Children especially are happier with a needleless system. The pressure-jet device costs more than traditional syringe and needle systems.

Cartridge

Administration device

Figure 5-4   Prefilled medication cartridge and holder.

Figure 5-5   Example of a needleless system that may be used to inject medication into intravenous infusions.

Figure 5-6   Comparison of angle of insertion and location of deposition of medication for intramuscular, subcutaneous, and intradermal injections. Note: for subcutaneous injection, a 45-degree angle is often used in thin or emaciated patients. Always assess the patient and follow your institution's policy.

such as a 1-ml tuberculin syringe. The volume injected is usually small, less than 0.5 ml. Commonly used sites for allergy testing are the medial surface of the forearm and the back.

Put on gloves, then clean the skin surface with alcohol. Allow the surface to dry or wipe off the alcohol with a sterile sponge. Hold the skin taut with one hand. With the other hand, hold the syringe at a 10- to 15-degree angle, with the needle bevel up, and gently but smoothly puncture the skin until the bevel is completely under the skin surface. Inject the prescribed amount or an amount that creates a raised **wheal** resembling a mosquito bite. If a wheal is not produced or if the site bleeds, the injection is probably too deep and should be repeated. If several injections are given in the same site (e.g., on the same forearm), label them with a pen, especially if the reaction is to be checked at 48 hours.

Subcutaneous Injection

Use a **subcutaneous injection** to place medication below the skin into the subcutaneous layer (see Figure 5-6). Limit the volume of a subcutaneous injection to less than 1 ml, and use a ½- or ⅝-inch, 23- or 25-gauge needle. Insert the needle at a 45-degree angle, although it may be inserted at a 90-degree angle if the patient has heavy subcutaneous tissue

or the nurse has pinched the subcutaneous tissue between thumb and fingers, holding the subcutaneous tissue up from the underlying muscle tissue. The usual injection technique is used. Put on gloves, choose the site, cleanse it with alcohol, let the alcohol dry or wipe it off with a sterile sponge, hold the skin taut, insert the needle, and aspirate for blood. If no blood is present, gently but smoothly inject the medication. Alternatively, put on gloves, cleanse the skin as described, then gently pinch the subcutaneous tissue between the thumb and the other fingers. Insert the needle, aiming it for the pocket created between the subcutaneous tissue being pinched and the tissue below.

The two medications most commonly administered via this route are heparin and insulin, and controversy continues about specific aspects of their administration. For additional discussion about the administration of these two drugs, consult Chapters 20 and 69. The usual sites for subcutaneous injection are illustrated in Figure 5-7.

Intramuscular Injection

Intramuscular injection is familiar to most students and patients. Immunizations and some antibiotics are administered via this route. Because the muscle layer is below the subcutaneous layer of skin, a longer needle is used, usually

Figure 5-7 Commonly used subcutaneous injection sites.

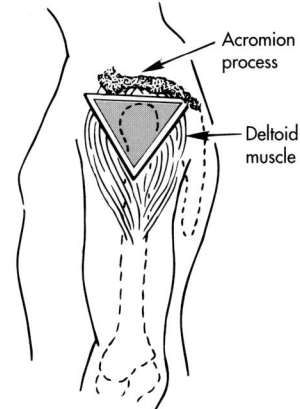

Figure 5-8 Deltoid muscle injection site roughly forms inverted triangle, with acromion process as base. Muscle may be visible in muscular patients.

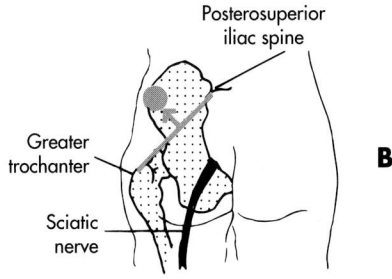

Figure 5-9 Two accepted methods for defining dorsogluteal injection site. **A,** Patient's buttocks can be divided on one side into imaginary quadrants. Center of upper outer quadrant should be used as injection site. **B,** Nurse locates site by palpation of posterosuperior iliac spine and greater trochanter, then draws imaginary line between them. Injection site up and out from that line should be used.

1½ inches, often of large lumen size, such as 19 or 21 gauge. Insert the needle at a 90-degree angle (see Figure 5-6). Consider the viscosity of the medication to be injected, the muscle to be used, and the patient's size and age in choosing the needle. A common error of beginning students is to choose too short a needle for administration of a medication to an overweight adult via a large muscle mass such as the vastus lateralis or dorsogluteal area.

The intramuscular technique is the same as other injection techniques previously outlined. Carefully prepare the ordered medication. Take the syringe to the bedside, and check the name band to verify the patient's identity. Draw the curtain or otherwise ensure privacy. Assist the patient to assume the necessary position. Identify appropriate anatomic landmarks to help define the injection site. Put on gloves, cleanse the skin, and let it dry. Hold the skin taut or gently pinch the skin. Swiftly insert the needle at a 90-degree angle, aspirate for blood, and if no blood is present, gently but smoothly inject the medication. If blood oozes after the needle is withdrawn, apply gentle pressure and a bandage if needed. Help the patient assume a comfortable position. Dispose of needle and syringe as directed by agency policy and then record that the medication has been given. Finally, check the patient again.

The **deltoid muscle,** located on the upper arm, is the site used for intramuscular injection of certain immunizations. It forms a triangular shape, with the base of the triangle along the acromion process and its peak ending about one third of the way down the upper arm (Figure 5-8). In muscular patients the deltoid muscle may be clearly visible. In other patients it may be necessary to palpate it. This muscle is small in children, many smaller-than-average patients, and older adults, so it can accommodate only small volumes of injected fluid (e.g., 1 ml). Depending on the patient's clothing, bruises or needle marks may be visible, which may be unacceptable to the patient. The radial nerve is nearby. The advantage of the deltoid muscle is that it is easily accessible.

The **dorsogluteal site** is made up of several gluteal muscles, although the gluteus medius is the muscle most often used for injections. As indicated in Figure 5-9, there are two ways to define this site. One way is to divide the buttocks on one side into imaginary quadrants and administer the injection in the upper outer quadrant. The second method is to locate the posterosuperior iliac spine and the greater trochanter of the femur and then draw an imaginary line between them. Give the injection up and to the side of this line. It is important to have a clear view of the area to help define the landmarks. Have the patient lie down, with the toes pointed inward, which helps foster muscle relaxation and thus decreases discomfort. Do not use this site for children younger than 3 years because the muscles are not yet well developed and because of the proximity of the sciatic nerve. In most ambulatory adults the dorsogluteal muscles are well developed and can accommodate an injection volume up to 5 ml if necessary, although any volume greater than 3 ml may be uncomfortable to the patient.

The **Z-track technique** can be used with any intramuscular injection, although it was first described for administration of an iron preparation that stains the skin if it leaks out. The dorsogluteal site is most commonly used for injections requiring the Z-track technique. After preparing the drug, measure the ordered amount of drug into the syringe, draw 0.1 to 0.3 ml of air into the syringe, and then change the needle. Follow the usual technique for identifying the patient, wearing gloves, cleansing the site, and so on. When administering drugs via the Z-track method, pull the skin taut to one side, causing the layers of skin to slide sideways. While the skin is pulled laterally, insert the needle, then inject the medication and the small amount of air smoothly and slowly. Pause for 10 seconds before removing the needle. Withdraw the needle, then allow the skin to relax (Figure 5-10). This

process disrupts the track created by the needle, preventing seepage and possible skin discoloration caused by the medication. Do not massage or rub the site.

Both the **vastus lateralis muscle** and the **rectus femoris muscle** are found in the thigh. As shown in Figure 5-11, the two muscles lie side by side. Place one hand on the patient's upper thigh and one hand on the lower thigh. The area between your hands should represent the middle third of the thigh and the middle third of the underlying muscle. The vastus lateralis is lateral to midline, whereas the rectus femoris is in the midline. The vastus lateralis is the preferred injection site for children because it is well developed and has few major nerves that could be injured. This site is also satisfactory for adults. The rectus femoris is most often the site chosen by adults who self-administer intramuscular injections because it is easily accessible. The acceptable volume for injection in these sites varies with the patient's age and the size of the muscle, but up to 5 ml may be administered in one injection to the well-developed adult.

To define the **ventrogluteal muscle,** create a V between the index finger and the remaining three fingers. Place the palm on the greater trochanter of the femur, with one side of

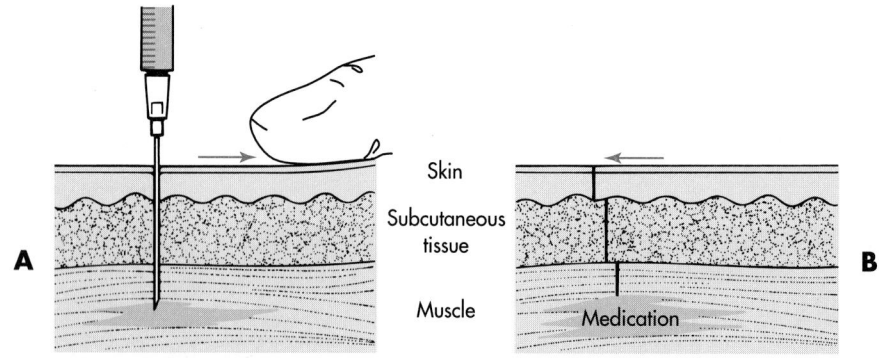

Figure 5-10   **A,** In Z-track intramuscular injection, skin is pulled laterally, then injection is administered. **B,** After needle is withdrawn, skin is released. This technique helps prevent medication from leaking.

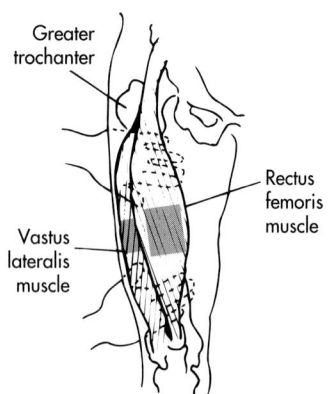

Figure 5-11   To define vastus lateralis and rectus femoris muscle sites, place one hand below patient's greater trochanter and one hand above patient's knee. Space between two hands defines middle third of underlying muscle. Rectus femoris muscle is on anterior thigh; vastus lateralis muscle is on lateral thigh.

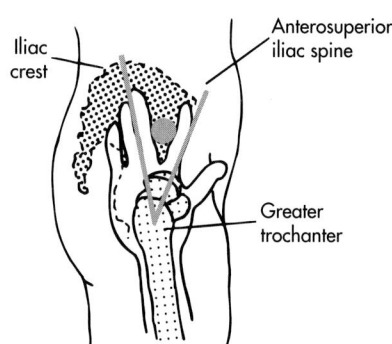

Figure 5-12   To locate ventrogluteal muscle injection site, place palm of hand on greater trochanter of femur. Make a V with fingers, with one side running from greater trochanter to anterosuperior iliac spine and other side running from greater trochanter to iliac crest.

the V extending from the greater trochanter to the iliac crest and the other side running from the greater trochanter to the anterosuperior iliac spine (Figure 5-12). This muscle may accommodate up to 5 ml of drug in adults.

Intravenous Injection

The administration of drugs directly into the vascular system via the IV route is widely used today for a variety of reasons. If an IV infusion line is already in place, IV infusion is easy. Drugs begin to take effect immediately. IV injection avoids side effects caused by intramuscular injection. On the other hand, errors can be serious, even fatal, because medications administered via this route take effect quickly and are irretrievable. The possibility of infection resulting from direct access to the vascular system is also present.

In some settings the IV team or designated nurses perform venipunctures and establish the IV infusion. If no designated team exists, many agencies or state nurse practice acts require special instruction, classes, and supervised practice in venipuncture techniques before nurses are permitted to perform this technique in their usual setting. Become familiar with the specific practices and policies of your agency or institution.

First, inspect the forearms and choose the venipuncture site. Figure 5-13 illustrates the location of veins commonly used in the forearm. Figure 5-14 illustrates the location of veins on the dorsal aspect of the hand. Other veins, such as those in the feet, are used only if absolutely necessary; some agencies may require a specific physician order if they are used. Thrombophlebitis is more common with venipuncture of the lower extremities. Scalp veins are used in infants. If the patient may need repeated venipunctures, choose a distal site rather than a proximal one. The rationale is that with each subsequent venipuncture the site should be moved more proximally (i.e., closer to the major vessels of the chest).

After choosing a site and preparing the necessary equipment (needle, intracatheter, heparin well, tubing, blood collection devices, medication, and tape), apply a tourniquet several inches above the expected insertion site. Put on gloves, and palpate the vein to further define its location. Then cleanse the skin with alcohol, povidone-iodine solution, or other cleansing agent. Allow the area to dry or wipe it with a sterile sponge. With one hand, stabilize the extremity and the vein; with the other hand, hold the venipuncture needle bevel up. Approach the insertion site at a slight angle, about 10 degrees. Puncture the skin and then the vein. Experienced nurses can feel the vein wall being punctured. If blood appears in the tubing or syringe, release the tourniquet. Slowly inject the medication into the vein, draw the blood, or secure the infusion device to the forearm, depending on the reason for the venipuncture.

To remove any needle or tubing from a vein, put on gloves, carefully remove any securing tapes and dressing, place a sterile sponge over the insertion site, and apply gentle pressure. With the other hand, swiftly withdraw the needle or catheter, pulling straight back from the angle of insertion; then apply firm pressure for 2 to 5 minutes to prevent bleeding or bruising. Apply a bandage over the insertion site. Dispose of any needles and syringes according to agency procedures. Record any medication that has been administered, and check the patient again. Further elaboration of these techniques can be found in texts of nursing fundamentals and agency procedure manuals. In addition, the Centers for Disease Control and Prevention in Atlanta have established guidelines for preventing infections in venipuncture and IV infusions.

Figure 5-13 Veins of medial aspect of forearm commonly used for venipuncture.

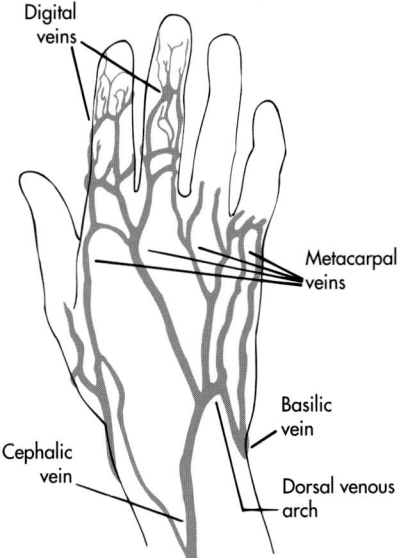

Figure 5-14 Major veins of dorsum of hand.

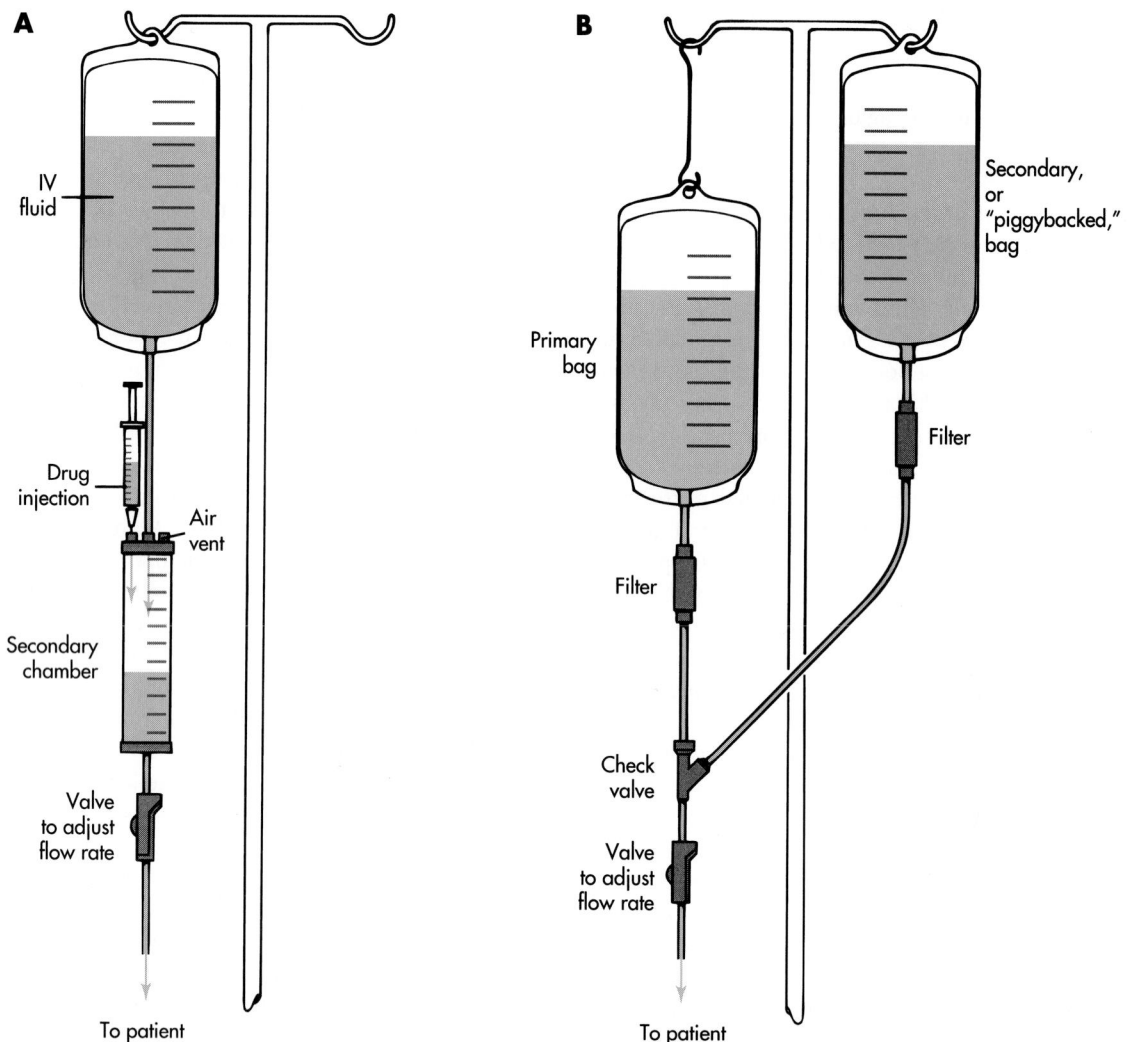

A

IV fluid

Drug injection

Air vent

Secondary chamber

Valve to adjust flow rate

To patient

B

Primary bag

Secondary, or "piggybacked," bag

Filter

Filter

Check valve

Valve to adjust flow rate

To patient

Figure 5-15   Example setups for intermittent drug infusion. **A,** Drug is injected into secondary chamber, where it may be further diluted with IV fluid. Upper fluid reservoir may be temporarily closed while drug infuses. **B,** Secondary, or "piggybacked," bag containing drug diluted in 50 to 100 ml of fluid is hung at level higher than primary bag. Contents of higher bag will infuse first, then contents of lower bag resume infusing. Check valve prevents medication from flowing into primary bag. Note that both lines have a filter.

Heparin Lock. Nurses may administer IV medications via a **heparin well** or **heparin lock.** This device consists of a needle attached to a short length of tubing capped by a piece of resealable rubber. The needle is placed in the vein; the device is then secured to the forearm. Its advantage is that medication can be administered via the IV route, but the patient does not need to be attached to continuous IV infusions or have repeated venipunctures for each dose of medication. Heparin wells are helpful in children who require IV medications but not additional fluids. When not receiving a dose of medication, patients are not restricted by long IV tubing.

Heparin may be administered via heparin well, as described in Chapter 20. One method for administering other medications by intermittent infusion via heparin well is to insert and secure the heparin well and then prime it with 1 ml of a 10-U/ml heparin solution. Solutions of 10 U/ml are available in prepackaged syringes or multiple-dose vials, or the pharmacy or the nurse can mix the heparin with normal saline solution to achieve the desired concentration. Each time a drug is administered, put on gloves, cleanse the rubber insertion site with alcohol or another cleansing agent, flush the well with 1 to 2 ml of normal saline solution (this step may be omitted if the drug to be administered is compatible with heparin), administer the prescribed medication via push or infusion, flush the well with 1 to 2 ml of normal saline solution, then fill the well with 1 ml of the solution containing 10 U/ml heparin. The purpose of leaving the heparinized solution in the well is to prevent blood from clotting in the needle. Many agencies have found that normal saline solution left in a heparin well is as good as a dilute heparin solution in maintaining patency of the heparin well. Follow the institution's policies and procedures.

Intravenous Tubing. Another way to administer IV medications is via tubing already in place for the patient who is receiving constant IV fluids. At least two variations should be noted. The nurse must frequently administer a small amount, usually less than 5 ml, of drug. This is often called **IV push** drug or bolus injection. Prepare the drug, and verify the patient's identity. Then locate an injection site on the IV tubing. Put on gloves, then cleanse the site with alcohol or another solution. Inject 2 ml of normal saline solution (this step may be omitted if the IV push drug is compatible with the fluids infusing). Administer the ordered drug, and then administer another 2 ml of normal saline. Readjust the ongoing infusion to provide the ordered rate. Most commercially available IV tubings have check valves, or one-way valves, as part of the tubing (Figure 5-15). If a check valve is not present, however, clamp the tubing above the injection site before administering the drug and proceed as outlined previously. If there is no check valve or if the tubing is not clamped, the injected medication will go in the direction of lower pressure, which may be up toward the bag or bottle of fluid instead of down toward the patient. Avoid this situation. When the medication goes toward the large bag or bottle of fluid, the patient does not receive the complete dose until the bag is empty; drugs administered after that dose may not be compatible with the drug remaining in the fluid line.

The second method of giving IV drugs is to administer an intermittent infusion of medication. The drug is prepared and diluted in a larger volume of fluid, at least 50 to 100 ml in adults, which is usually administered for 20 to 60 minutes. This volume can then be administered in several ways. One method is to add the drug to an in-line device such as a burette or volume-limiting device and then fill the device with 50 to 100 ml of the infusing IV fluid. The ongoing fluids are temporarily stopped, the diluted drug is allowed to infuse, and then the ongoing fluids are continued. Commercially available infusion tubing that has two ports for hanging IV bags or bottles may also be used. These tubing systems have an identified port for attaching the primary fluids and a secondary port for attaching the intermittently administered volume containing the drugs (see Figure 5-15).

The third method of administering IV drugs is to prepare the drug in a small volume of fluid and then attach IV tubing and a needle. Prime the tubing by running sufficient fluid through the tube to eliminate any air. Insert the needle into an identified insertion site on the tubing of the ongoing infusion after the site has been cleansed. The initial or primary infusion is clamped, the bolus containing the drug is allowed to infuse, then the continuous fluids are restarted. You may then discard the secondary infusion tubing and needle. To be effective and efficient, become familiar with the equipment and procedures used in your agency.

Many agencies are switching to **needleless equipment** to minimize the chance of needlestick injury. Although a needle must be used to puncture the skin, once an IV access is established, medications may be administered and continu-

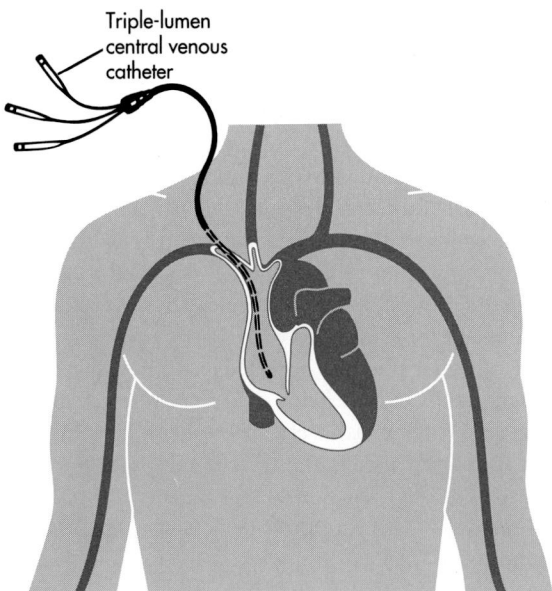

Figure 5-16 Triple-lumen central venous catheter in place.

ous infusions started and stopped without the need to use needles. The end of the heparin well, the access ports along IV tubing, and the ports on multilumen catheters are fitted with ports that allow a syringe without a needle to be attached for the purpose of administering medications. These ports may have a sterile cap on them. Follow agency policy regarding cleaning the caps. Many agencies have a mix of equipment. The advantage of needleless ports in preventing the possibility of injury is obvious (see Figure 5-5).

Central Venous Catheters and Multilumen Catheters. **Central venous catheters** are inserted for venous access in many patients. In this case, *central* refers to a large, more central vein, close to the heart, as opposed to a smaller, more peripheral vein. Several kinds of venous access devices exist. To provide correct nursing care, it is important to find out what kind of device is being used in each patient and for what purposes it is being used. One type of device is a **nontunneled catheter,** intended usually for 10 to 14 days of use. It may be a single or multilumen catheter, inserted into the subclavian or internal jugular vein, with the tip advanced into the superior vena cava, or further, depending on the intended use of the device (Figure 5-16). The catheter may be used for hemodynamic monitoring as well as medication administration. Another type of device is a **tunneled catheter** such as the **Broviac, Hickman,** or **Groshong** catheter. The tip of the catheter is inserted into the internal or external jugular or cephalic vein, and the tip rests in the superior vena cava. The other end is tunneled through the subcutaneous tissue for 5 to 8 cm and exits through a small skin incision in the chest. With care these catheters can remain in place for months to years.

Another type of device is an **implanted infusion port** (implanted **vascular access port,** or VAP) such as the Infusa-A-Port or Port-A-Cath, both top entry designs, and the S.E.A. Port, a side-entry design. With these devices a reservoir, or port, is implanted subcutaneously against a bony structure such as along the ribs of the chest wall. The port is attached to a catheter, typically a Hickman or Groshong catheter, which is tunneled subcutaneously to the selected vein. The implanted infusion port is designed to withstand 1000 to 2000 punctures by a needle. These devices can remain in place for months to years.

Recently, **peripherally inserted central catheters (PIC catheters, or PICCs)** are being used more often. As the name implies, the catheter is inserted peripherally, usually in the basilic or cephalic vein in the antecubital space. The catheter is threaded through the vein so that the tip rests in the superior vena cava. With care these devices can remain in place for months or longer.

Each of these catheters and ports, except the PIC catheter, must be inserted by the physician. Some states and some agencies will permit specially trained nurses to insert PIC catheters. All these devices can be used to withdraw blood samples, as well as to administer blood products, hyperalimentary products, and medications. Because the distal end of the catheter is in an area of high blood flow and volume, it permits infusion of large volumes of fluids. Also, central venous catheters allow administration of more irritating fluids and drugs than can be administered via peripheral IV lines. There is always the risk of infection or of introducing air with such catheters, especially when those with multiple ports are used.

Usually, care for the catheter and the insertion site is more rigorous for a centrally placed catheter than for a standard peripherally placed catheter. (A PIC catheter is a central line, even though it is inserted peripherally.) For example, cleansing of an injection port on a peripheral catheter may be done with an alcohol swab, whereas the port on a central line may require cleansing with a povidone-iodine solution. Also, there may be special dressing change procedures for the dressing covering the catheter insertion site. Follow agency procedures. Monitor the patient for signs of infection such as fever, redness at the insertion site, and increased white blood cell count.

For multilumen catheters, care of the ports not in use is important to keep the lumens patent. Follow agency procedure. Different types of catheters may require different protocols. One protocol is to change the cap on each port weekly or when it appears worn. Wear sterile gloves during cap changes, and discard contaminated caps carefully. Irrigate the ports not in use with 2.5 ml of heparinized solution (10 U/ml of heparin) every 12 to 24 hours. Irrigate a port after each intermittent infusion is given via that port. If blood is drawn via a port, irrigate the port after the sample is obtained. Cleanse the insertion site every 48 hours.

With an implanted infusion port, the skin must be punctured with a needle each time the patient must receive medication; however, there is no daily cleansing procedure as there is with the partially implanted catheters. To use an implanted device, put on sterile gloves and cleanse the site with a povidone-iodine solution (or as agency protocol directs). With one hand, palpate and locate the injection site. After the device is defined and stabilized with one hand, use the other hand to puncture the skin and septum with a noncoring needle (Figure 5-17). The noncoring needle is designed to prevent excessive damage to the rubber septum and has a deflected point and a side opening to prevent damage to the septum. The needle may be bent 90 degrees to facilitate attaching infusions. Push the needle in far enough to feel it touch the back of the device. Aspirate blood to help determine patency, and then inject saline to flush the system. The device may be used to obtain blood samples, administer constant or intermittent infusions, or inject medica-

Figure 5-17   Implanted infusion device. **A,** Side view illustrating needle inserted through skin and top of infusion device. Distal end of device is in vein. **B,** Use one hand to secure device before inserting needle.

tions. After use, flush the device with a heparinized solution. Review the manufacturer's directions and request guidance in using these devices until comfortable with their use and operation.

Drug Pumps. Several types of drug pumps for slowly injecting a medication are now available for patients' home use. Cancer chemotherapy, narcotic infusion for severe pain, and insulin therapy are common uses of drug pumps. One such device is the autosyringe pump, which consists of a syringe with a battery attachment for slow injection. This device injects the medication subcutaneously or attaches to an implanted infusion port such as the Port-A-Cath or a partially implanted catheter such as a Hickman catheter. Follow the manufacturer's instructions when preparing and using a drug pump and have the patient give a return demonstration before discharge. Handbooks for home IV therapy that illustrate various equipment and procedures for using drug pumps, tubing, filters, and ports in the home setting are now available.

Information about calculation of infusion rates is included in Chapter 6. Additional general guidelines for care of the patient receiving an IV infusion are given in Chapter 17.

Rectal Medications

Administering medications via the rectal route is an alternative for patients who are nauseated or unable to swallow. Drugs are usually in the form of a suppository or enema.

The procedure for administering medication by enema is the same as that for any enema. Because the goal is to have the patient retain the medication for as long as possible, a small-volume enema is administered. After preparing the medication and any other necessary equipment, go to the bedside and verify the patient's identity. Explain briefly what will be done. Then draw the curtain or otherwise ensure privacy. Position the patient on his or her left side. Place adequate protective covering on the bed. Put on gloves, and lubricate the applicator or tubing tip with water-soluble jelly or lubricant (Figure 5-18). Separate the patient's buttocks with one hand, and ask the patient to take a deep breath. Use the other hand to insert the tubing or tip the desired distance. Administer the medication slowly to avoid stimula-

tion and immediate expulsion. Withdraw the applicator, and gently hold the buttocks together until the patient's immediate urge to defecate has subsided. Wash the patient's buttocks, and assist the patient in returning to a comfortable position. Instruct the patient to try to hold the medication at least 30 minutes (or as indicated by the nature of the medication).

Suppositories are medications that have been mixed with cocoa butter, glycerin, or other substances that allow them to remain solid at room temperature but permit them to melt and release the medication when they contact the warm rectal mucosa. Suppositories are stored in the refrigerator to keep them firm. If a suppository is too soft to insert easily, run it under cold water (if foil wrapped) or place it in the refrigerator to help harden it before administering. The general procedure for administration is similar to that for the enema. Wear a finger cot or glove for inserting the suppository. Moisten the suppository with a water-soluble lubricant. Insert the suppository about a finger's distance into the rectum in adults, past the anal sphincter (Figure 5-19). If the suppository is not inserted far enough, it will be uncomfortable to the patient and will be quickly expelled. It may be necessary to place a small gauze pad over the anus to absorb oozing medication after the suppository has been inserted. If the suppository was intended to cause defecation, the patient may defecate as soon as the urge occurs. Unless the medication was prescribed to stimulate defecation, instruct the patient to retain the suppository as long as possible and to report when it is expelled.

Vaginal Medications

Vaginal medications can take the form of douches or irrigations, creams, or suppositories. The patient may be able to choose the form she prefers.

Many women are familiar with over-the-counter douche preparations and may feel comfortable with their use. For best effect, administer douches with the patient lying down. Moisten the tip of the tubing or applicator with water or a water-soluble lubricant. Insert the applicator or end of the tubing about 2 inches initially. Then advance it another 1 to 2 inches as the fluid is allowed to run in by gravity. A text on

Figure 5-18   Administering single-dose enema. Position patient on his or her left side, and place protective covering on bed. **A,** After donning gloves, remove cover from tip. Apply water-soluble lubricant if tip is not already lubricated. **B,** Gently insert applicator tip and squeeze bottle to propel medication into patient's rectum.

Figure 5-19   Inserting suppository. After positioning patient and removing suppository from package, don non-sterile gloves. **A,** Lubricate suppository with water-soluble lubricant. **B,** Insert suppository past anal sphincter.

Figure 5-20   **A,** Nitroglycerin ointment and papers for measuring doses. **B,** Gently squeeze out a line of ointment along paper guide for prescribed length. **C,** Apply ointment to patient's skin. Clear plastic wrap may be applied over site to increase absorption and keep ointment from staining clothing.

fundamentals of nursing offers more complete information about douching.

Insert vaginal suppositories by pushing them in with a gloved finger or with an applicator supplied by the manufacturer. The suppository may be lubricated with water or a water-soluble lubricant before being administered. It is important to place the suppository high in the vaginal vault, or

the patient will expel it rapidly. The patient may be able to self-administer the suppository and may prefer to do so.

If the patient is taking a dose once daily, insert the vaginal suppository just before the patient goes to sleep so that it will remain in the vaginal vault all night and not drain out or be expelled. If the dose is given more than once daily, instruct the patient to remain lying down for a short period af-

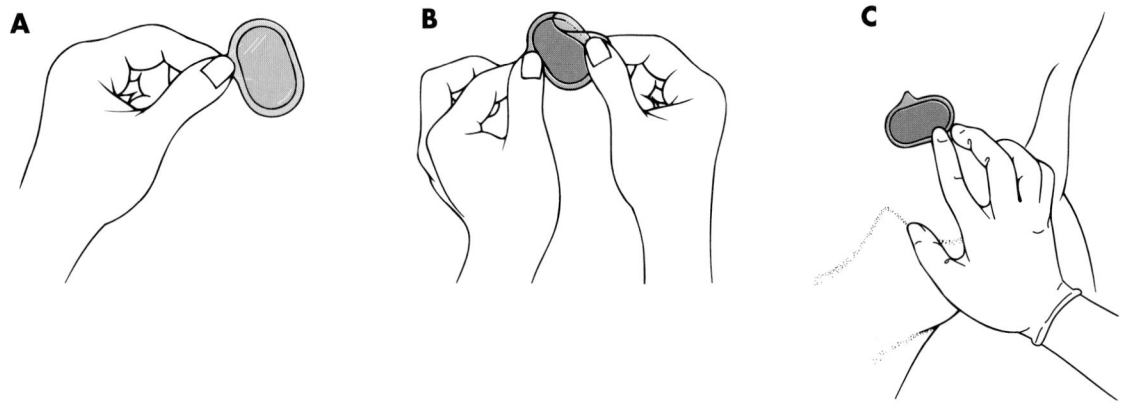

Figure 5-21 Transdermal patch. **A,** Hold patch by small wing. **B,** Remove protective backing. **C,** Place patch on chosen skin site and press into place. Sites should be changed or alternated with each successive dose.

ter administration so that the medication will not be quickly lost. Instruct the patient to continue the medication even during the menstrual period and to avoid the use of tampons while taking vaginal medications. It is usually necessary for the patient to wear a sanitary napkin during the course of therapy.

Insert vaginal creams with the applicator supplied by the manufacturer. The same guidelines outlined under vaginal suppositories apply. Creams are generally messier than suppositories, and patients may not accept them as well. If the applicator is reused for several doses, wash and dry it after each dose.

Skin Application

Many medications are applied to the skin, but it is such an easy and common route of administration that the nurse or patient may inadvertently become too casual about it. Some topical preparations, such as emollients for dry skin, may be applied liberally, as needed. However, most skin medications must be measured and applied as ordered to prevent the patient from receiving too large a dose. Avoid direct contact with the medication to prevent sensitization and to avoid the effects of the medication. Wear gloves and apply the medication with applicators, gauze, or cotton balls; or make certain that the medication is applied directly from the measuring guide, as is done with topical nitroglycerin preparations (see Chapter 15). Depending on the medication, rotate application sites and avoid applying the medicine to abrasions, cuts, or other areas where the skin is not intact. Some topical preparations require dressings. If in doubt, ask the physician about the goals of therapy and consult the pharmacist to determine the most effective method of administering the drug.

Nitroglycerin ointment is one type of skin application (Figure 5-20). The dose is ordered in inches, and the ointment is supplied with small papers printed with a 2-inch measuring guide. Squeeze out an even line of ointment of the prescribed length. Place the paper ointment-side down on the patient. Avoid rubbing in the ointment, although it is usually permissible to press the paper guide sufficiently to

spread out the dose. Clear plastic wrap may be ordered to be placed over the paper and ointment to facilitate absorption and prevent staining of clothing.

Another form for topical application is the single-dose, adhesive-backed delivery system, or transdermal patch (Figure 5-21). Examples include several types of nitroglycerin preparations, estrogen, and a scopolamine preparation. Refer to the manufacturer's literature for guidelines about the specific product. Review instruction sheets with the patient; these provide illustrations and additional information. Information includes the preferred location for application, frequency of changing, and the effect of swimming or bathing on the delivery system.

Eye Medications

Eye medications are usually in the form of drops or ointments. Eyedrops are supplied in small volumes because each dose is contained in 1 or 2 drops. Avoid contaminating the dropper. Each patient should have a separate bottle of eyedrops. Before administering eyedrops, be certain which eye is to be medicated (if not both). A common source of errors is confusion about the abbreviations for left eye (OS), right eye (OD), and both eyes (OU). Have the patient lie down or sit with the head tilted back. With your hand holding the dropper, place your hand on the patient's cheek or forehead to stabilize your hand and help prevent injury to the eye. Use the thumb (or fingers) of your other hand to gently pull down the lower lid; it may be necessary to use a small gauze sponge or cotton ball to help do this and avoid contaminating the eye. Drop the dose into the lower conjunctival sac, never onto the eyeball.

Use the following modification of technique when administering eyedrops to patients who blink easily. Place the patient in the supine position, with the head turned to one side, about 45 degrees from midline. The eye to receive the eyedrops should be uppermost. With the eye closed, drop the prescribed dose on the inner canthus of the eye. Have the patient slowly turn from the side to midline, then toward the other side, while blinking. The eyedrops will move via gravity and surface tension into the conjunctival sac.

Eye ointments are applied much the same way as eyedrops. Squeeze a thin line of ointment onto the lower conjunctival sac, close the eye, and gently rub the eyelid to help distribute the dose (Figure 5-22).

Another drug form available for eye medications is the sustained-release insert. Place the insert into the upper or lower conjunctival sac. The medication is released slowly, over several days. Because the unit may fall out at night, instruct patients to make sure that the insert is in place every morning. The unit is designed to be replaced weekly. Consult the manufacturer's literature and patient instruction sheet for specific guidelines about new drug forms.

Caution patients to read labels carefully, especially on refilled prescriptions. Only medications labeled for ophthalmic use should be put into the eye. Eyedrops should be kept in a safe place, away from other similarly shaped containers. Occasionally patients have inadvertently put glue or other toxic substances in their eyes because they did not read the label or depended on feel to select the bottle or tube of medication. Many eye medications cause blurred vision, so warn patients not to drive or engage in other dangerous activities immediately after using eye medications.

Nosedrops and Sprays

To instill nosedrops, have the patient lie down with the head over the edge of the bed (Figure 5-23). Support the patient's head with one hand while instilling the drops with the other. When the patient's head is in the midline, the nosedrops primarily reach the ethmoid and sphenoid sinuses; turning the patient's head toward the side will facilitate having the drops reach the maxillary and frontal sinuses. Have the patient remain in this position briefly, and then, if possible, bend over into a head-down position to help distribute the drug. Tell the patient to avoid blowing the nose for several minutes so that the medication will not be expelled.

Administering nose spray requires that the patient inhale via one nostril while occluding the other and squeezing a spray applicator. It is usually easier for the patient to self-administer nose spray than for the nurse to do it. Remove the applicator from the nostril before releasing the pressure on the other nostril to avoid pulling sensitive nasal mucosa to the applicator opening. Have the patient keep the head upright or tilted slightly back. Many nose sprays are available over the counter, especially nasal decongestants (see Chapter 7). Caution the patient to use these sprays only as needed, for as short a period as possible, and only as directed.

Ear Medications

Most ear medications are in the form of drops. Have the patient lie down with the affected ear up. Keep the medication at body temperature. In adults or children older than 3 years, pull the top of the ear up and back to straighten the ear canal, then gently instill the prescribed number of drops. If the patient is a child younger than 3 years, pull the ear down and straight back (Figure 5-24). Have the patient remain with the affected ear up for 10 minutes to allow the medicine to disperse. Place a medication-soaked cotton ball plug gently and loosely in the ear to prevent oozing; a dry cotton ball will absorb the medication. If it is necessary to treat the other ear, repeat the procedure with the other ear after the 10-minute waiting period.

Endotracheal Tubes

Occasionally it is necessary to administer drugs via an endotracheal tube. Use this route only if necessary and only if specified by the physician. Drugs typically administered via this route include epinephrine, atropine, lidocaine, and surfactants. Dilute the prescribed dose in 5 to 10 ml of sterile water or saline solution. Attach a long needle or soft

Figure 5-22 Administering ophthalmic ointment. To instill ointment, gently pull lower lid down as patient looks upward. Squeeze ophthalmic ointment into lower sac. Avoid touching tube to eyelid. Wear gloves to avoid contact with body fluids.

Figure 5-23 Administering nosedrops. Have patient gently blow nose. Open medication and draw liquid up to calibration on dropper. Instill medication. Have patient remain in position for 2 to 3 minutes. Repeat on other side if necessary. Wear gloves to avoid contact with body fluids.

catheter to the syringe. Auscultate the lungs to verify placement of the endotracheal tube. The patient should remain in the supine position. Instruct the patient to hyperventilate for three to five breaths. Remove the ventilator or resuscitation bag, and inject the medication through the endotracheal tube as deeply as the catheter or needle permits. Do not puncture the tube with the needle. Reattach the resuscitation bag or ventilator, and tell the patient again to hyperventilate for three to five breaths. Assess the patient's response to the medication.

Intraosseous Infusion

Intraosseous infusion may be used in emergency situations in children when an IV infusion cannot be started. In this technique a special needle is inserted into a large bone. Proper placement of the needle must be verified through aspiration of bone marrow. Drugs, fluids, or blood can then be infused. Although establishing an intraosseous infusion is easier than starting an IV infusion for small children and infants, several potential hazards, including infection, are associated with this technique. If this technique is used in your agency, request instruction in its use and carefully review the protocol and procedure.

Implanted Dosage Forms

Some drugs may be delivered by subcutaneous implantation, a procedure usually performed by the physician. The female contraceptive levonorgestrel (Norplant) is administered this way. See Figure 70-1 for an illustration of this form. The advantage is that the drug is slowly released over months to years, so the patient does not need to remember to take daily or more frequent doses. Disadvantages include the need for a minor surgical procedure to administer new doses, the possibility of small scar formation, and the possibility that the patient may forget to return for subsequent doses. In addition, it is difficult to discontinue the medication (remove the implant) once inserted.

Inhalation

A few drugs are administered via inhalation. For best results this method requires a cooperative patient who can inhale deeply and can manage the psychomotor tasks of using the equipment and preparing the medication. Often, however, the patient is a child or anxious or hypoxic because of the condition being treated, such as asthma.

In the hospital or institutional setting, inhalation therapy is fairly common, in the form of oxygen therapy via nasal cannula, nasal catheter, or some form of face mask. Other drugs may also be administered via intermittent positive-pressure breathing (IPPB) machines or nebulizer. Trained respiratory therapists may be available to provide assistance.

Several inhalation drug delivery systems, such as metered-dose inhalers and turboinhalers, are available. Each system has advantages and disadvantages. Carefully review the literature supplied by the manufacturer, including the patient instruction sheet. Do not attempt to do a teaching session with the patient who is short of breath or anxious. Make certain that patients show a satisfactory return demonstration before concluding that they can use the prescribed drug correctly. Remind patients to keep handheld nebulizers and other equipment clean to prevent contamination and infection. Instruct patients to use the product only as ordered to prevent side effects, drug overdose, and drug dependency. See Chapter 28 for an illustration of a metered-dose inhaler. Figure 5-25 illustrates how the patient can estimate the amount of drug remaining in a canister. This method is helpful for patients using metered-dose inhalers or nitroglycerin lingual spray forms.

Other Drug Delivery Systems

New drug delivery systems are constantly being developed. The nurse faced with an unfamiliar delivery system should consult the manufacturer's literature and the patient instruction sheet that often accompanies the dosage form.

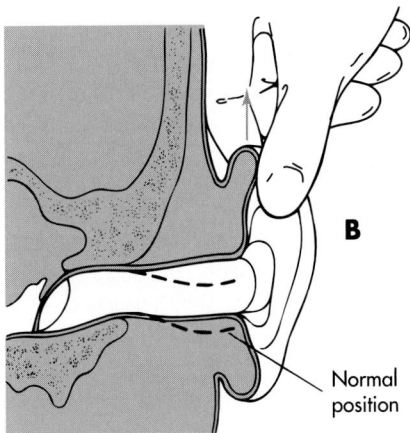

Figure 5-24   Straightening ear canal for administration of ear medication. Patient is lying on side with ear up. **A,** For child younger than 3 years, pull ear down and straight back. **B,** For all others, pull top of ear up and back. Wear gloves to avoid contact with drainage.

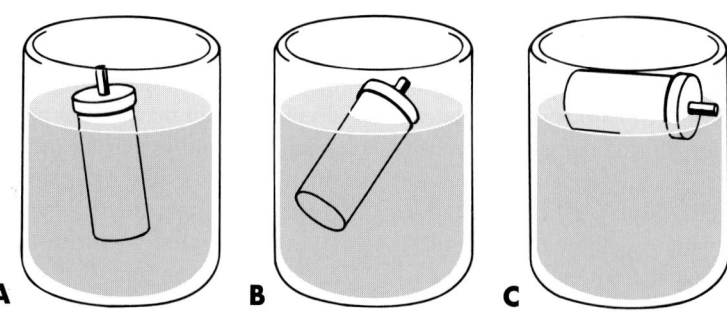

Figure 5-25 Checking canister for medication. This check could be done for metered-dose inhaler (see Chapter 28) or canister with nitroglycerin spray. **A,** Canister is full. **B,** Canister is partially full. **C,** Canister is nearly empty. This method of estimating how much medication remains is satisfactory for most drugs. Read manufacturer's instructions, however, because number of sprays used per canister must be counted for some drugs.

Nursing Process Overview

Drug Administration

Assessment

When assessing a patient, ask why this patient might need a prescribed drug. Identifying the reason for each prescription helps the nurse detect inadvertent errors in which the wrong drug may be administered.

Obtain objective and subjective data from the patient to aid in determining the need and effectiveness of drug use. Determine any patient preferences about drug use and incorporate these if possible. Determine the developmental level of children to aid in planning nursing care approaches.

Nursing Diagnoses

Not all patients require the formulation of nursing diagnoses as a consequence of drug therapy. Most patients are not knowledgeable about a specific drug at the start of drug therapy. Other diagnoses may develop as the patient develops side effects, is unable to manage self-administration, or has collaborative problems as potential complications.

Patient Outcomes

The patient will improve as a result of the efforts of the health care team, and medications may be one part of therapy. The patient will experience no serious side effects of drug therapy, or the side effects will be diagnosed quickly and handled effectively.

Planning/Implementation

Implementing the therapeutic plan involves proper administration of the prescribed medications. The nurse should seek information about specific drugs from a variety of sources, including the physician, the pharmacist, and current printed materials. For a student nurse the prospect of learning about all the medications to be administered is likely to be overwhelming. After a nurse is in practice, however, repeated administration of medications facilitates development of a basic understanding of commonly used drug categories.

Not only must the nurse know about the prescribed medications, but the nurse must also exercise caution that the prescribed medication is what the patient actually receives. Thus medications should remain in labeled packages or containers until they are administered.

The patient has a right to receive the medication in the correct dose. Regardless of how drugs are supplied to the patient care unit, check labels carefully and double-check all dosage calculations. Some nurses have difficulty with the mathematic calculations necessary for determining correct doses; have a colleague verify dosage calculations rather than possibly subjecting the patient to an incorrect dose of medications. Consult the pharmacy for additional help. Successful drug therapy may depend on the proper timing of drug doses, as discussed in Chapter 1. To ensure that the patient receives each drug via the right route of administration, check that the route of administration ordered for each drug is appropriate for that drug. Learn how to administer medications via each route.

Develop a sense of suspicion whenever a medication order seems to be out of the ordinary. Double-check a dose of medication that seems unusually large or small. When at the bedside, if the patient seems hesitant to take the medication, stating that it is new or not what is usually taken, double-check the physician's orders before administering the medication. Record that a patient has received a medication as soon as possible after administration to avoid inadvertent duplicate administration by other members of the health care team.

Evaluation

The major question during evaluation is whether the medication is working as expected. The nurse must know what was expected of the medication, have initial baseline data about the patient, and know what parameters to assess to determine whether the drug is working as desired. Determine whether there were any problems associated with the route, time, or dose of medication, and make appropriate notation on the Kardex, care plan, or computerized patient record.

CHAPTER REVIEW

Application

1. Describe the differences between a unit-dose system, a stock drug system, and a computer-controlled dispensing system.
2. In your practice settings, where is information about medications recorded?
3. What are some problems you may encounter in administering drugs to older adult patients? to children?
4. For each of the routes of medication administration listed below, answer the following questions:
   a. What are advantages and disadvantages of this route?
   b. Are there considerations unique to older adult patients or children with this route of administration?
   c. How is a drug administered via this route?
      - Oral route: pills, capsules, tablets
      - Oral route: suspensions, tinctures, elixirs, syrups, and solutions
      - Oral route: sublingual tablet, buccal tablet, troche, lingual spray, lozenge forms
      - Oral drugs through feeding tubes

- Intradermal injections
- Subcutaneous injections
- Intramuscular injections
- Intravenous injections
- Z-track intramuscular injections
- Rectal enemas and suppositories
- Vaginal douches, creams, suppositories
- Skin applications: creams, ointments that must be measured, transdermal patches
- Eyedrops and eye ointments
- Nosedrops and sprays
- Eardrops
- Drugs via inhalation

Critical Thinking

1. Which is used in your practice setting: unit-dose system, a stock drug system, or a computer-controlled system? If your agency is not using a computer-controlled system but there is an agency in your community that is, can you arrange to visit the agency to see this system in use?
2. How can you use theories of Erikson, Freud, or Piaget as a guide in administering medications to children?

References

Angeles T: How to prevent phlebitis, *Nursing* 27(1):26, 1997.

Angeles T: Removing a nontunneled central catheter, *Nursing* 28(5):52-53, 1998.

Beyea SC, Nicoll LH: Back to basics: administering IM injections the right way, *Am J Nurs* 96(1): Contin Care Extra Ed: 34-35, 1996.

Brooks K: Reducing epidural catheter infections, *Nursing* 27(4):15, 1997.

Covington TP, Trattler MR: Bull's eye! Finding the right target for I.M. injections, *Nursing* 27(1):62-63, 1997.

Easing the discomfort of venipuncture, *Nursing* 28(3):30, 1998.

Gever MP: Transdermal patches. What's in a brand name? *Nursing* 28(5):58-59, 1998.

Hall JC: Low-profile gastrostomy devices, *Nursing* 27(6):62-64, 1997.

Hussey VM, Poulin MV, Fain JA: Effectiveness of lidocaine hydrochloride on venipuncture sites, *AORN J* 66(3):472, 1997.

Intravenous therapy handbook, *Nursing* 26(10):48-51, 1996.

Johns T: Intravenous filters, panacea or placebo? *J Clin Nurs* 5(1):3-6, 1996.

Knight J: Inserting an insulin catheter, *Nursing* 28(2):58-60, 1998.

Konick-McMahan J: Full speed ahead with caution: pushing intravenous medications, *Nursing* 26(6):26-32, 1996.

Krupp KB, Heximer B: Going with the flow. How to prevent feeding tubes from clogging, *Nursing* 28(4):54-55, 1998.

Macklin D: How to manage PICCs, *Am J Nurs* 97(9):26-32, 1997.

Masoorli S: Managing complications of central venous access devices, *Nursing* 27(8):59-63, 1997.

Masoorli S: Removing a PICC? *Nursing* 28(3):56-57, 1998.

Mayo DJ, et al: The effects of heparin flush on patency of the Groshong catheter: a pilot study, *Oncol Nurs Forum* 23(9):1401-1405, 1996.

McConnell EA: Administering an I.V. push injection through an existing peripheral line, *Nursing* 26(8):24, 1996.

McConnell EA: Administering intradermal injections, *Nursing* 26(2):18, 1996.

McConnell EA: Admixing drugs in a syringe, *Nursing* 28(5):20, 1998.

McConnell EA: Giving medications through an enteral feeding tube, *Nursing* 28(3):66, 1998.

McConnell EA: Inserting a nasogastric tube, *Nursing* 27(1):72, 1997.

McConnell EA: Using transdermal medication patches, *Nursing* 27(7):18, 1997.

Metheny N, Wehrle MA, Wiersema L, Clark J: Testing feeding tube placement: auscultation vs. pH method, *Am J Nurs* 98(5):37-43, 1998.

Ouwendyk M, Helfery M: Central venous catheter management: how to prevent complications, *ANNA J* 23(6):572-579, 1996.

Posanza CP: Special delivery: using a syringe pump to administer I.V. drugs, *Nursing* 27(9):43-45, 1997.

Ritter J: Using invasive medical devices safely, *Nursing* 28(5): 32hn12, 32hn15-32hn16, 1998.

Sansivero GE: Maintaining a PICC line: what you should know, *Nursing* 27(4):14, 1997.

Schmieding NJ, Waldman RC, Desaulles C: Nasogastric tubes: insertion, placement, and removal in adult patients, *Gastroenterol Nurs* 20(1):15-19, 1997.

Wise MA: Understanding needle-free access devices, *Nursing* 27(7):32, 1997.

Calculating Drug Dosages

OBJECTIVES

After studying this chapter, you should be able to do the following:

- *Define common abbreviations used in drug orders, such as gtt, prn, and PO.*
- *Perform calculations based on the strength of solutions of drugs.*
- *Calculate drug dosages based on the patient's body weight.*
- *Calculate infusion rates for drugs administered intravenously.*
- *Calculate pediatric drug dosages.*

CHAPTER OVERVIEW

Chapters 1 and 5 discussed routes by which a drug may be given to a patient and the importance of careful control of drug levels in the body. Administering the proper drug dose by the appropriate route is the first step in ensuring that the desired drug concentration appears in the blood. This chapter focuses on how to calculate drug dosages.

Students with good arithmetic skills can readily solve problems of the level included in this chapter, but many students initially experience difficulty because they have forgotten the basic rules of arithmetic and algebra. If you have trouble with the practice problems in this chapter, you should consult one of the many review texts on drug dosage calculations.

CALCULATING DRUG DOSAGES: ROLE OF THE NURSE

Nurses share moral and legal responsibility with physicians and pharmacists in administering drugs. In many hospitals, pharmacists calculate and prepare drugs for administration to patients, according to the physician's order. This practice does not remove responsibility from the nurse who gives the drug to the patient. The nurse must verify that the right drug at the proper dose has been prepared (see Chapter 5). Therefore the nurse must be familiar with the forms of drugs and able to recognize common medications.

Nurses should also question a physician's order for a drug when that order seems inappropriate. For example, the nurse should question a drug dose that is outside the normal clin-ical dosage range. Nurses have access to several sources of information about specific drugs, including pharmacists, package inserts supplied by the manufacturer, and references (see Chapter 3).

READING DRUG ORDERS

Physicians and pharmacists sometimes use a system of abbreviations in writing orders or prescriptions. These abbreviations are derived from Latin and Greek words and phrases. Although Latin and Greek are no longer used in medical writing, use of the phrases persists through custom. Therefore nurses must be familiar with common abbreviations (Table 6-1). Many of the abbreviations explain how to administer a drug. For example, a physician's order might

Table 6-1	Pharmaceutical Abbreviations
Abbreviation/Phrase	Translation
ad lib (ad libitum)	Freely; as much or as often as wanted
aa (or $\overline{aa}$) (ana)	Of each
ac (ante cibum)	Before meals
bid (bis in die)	Twice daily
$\overline{c}$ (cum)	With
gtt (guttae)	Drops
hs (hora somni)	At bedtime
non rep (or non repetat) (non repetatur)	Do not repeat
od (oculus dexter)	Right eye
os (oculus sinister)	Left eye
ou (oculus uterque)	Both eyes
pc (post cibum)	After meals
PO (per os)	By mouth
PR (per rectum)	By rectal route
prn (pro re nata)	According to circumstances
qs (quantum suffict [satis])	As much as is necessary
qd (quaque die)	Every day
qh (quaque hora)	Every hr
q4h	Every 4 hr
qid (quarter in die)	4 times daily
ss (or $\overline{ss}$) (semis)	One half
stat (statim)	Immediately
tid (ter in die)	3 times daily

Table 6-2	Common Systems of Units	
System	Unit of Mass	Unit of Volume
Metric	Gram (g)	Liter (L)
Apothecary	Grain (gr)	Minim (m)
Household	Pound (lb)	Pint (pt)

Table 6-3	Equivalents within Metric System	
Units of Mass		Units of Volume
1 kg = 1000 g		1 L = 1000 ml
1 g = 1000 mg		1 ml = 1000 μL
1 mg = 1000 μg		1 ml = 1 cc

read "penicillin G 100,000 U q3h, PO." This order would be translated as "100,000 units (U) of penicillin G are to be given every 3 hours (q3h) by mouth (PO)."

Pharmaceutical abbreviations can be confusing, and the nurse must be certain that the physician's intent is clearly understood. Among the most troublesome are the abbreviations ad lib and prn. A drug given prn is given at the prescribed interval if the patient requires the drug. For example, after surgery a patient might have the following order on the chart: "Morphine 10 mg q4h, prn." Every 4 hours the nurse should assess the patient; if the patient is comfortable, the nurse may postpone the dose. According to the drug order, morphine may be given less often than every 4 hours but not more often. In contrast, a medication prescribed ad lib is given whenever the patient needs it. Such abbreviations are used as medical shorthand to save time in communicating between medical personnel. If the use of an abbreviation creates any uncertainty, the physician or the pharmacist should be consulted for clarification.

UNITS OF DRUG DOSAGE

In clinical practice, nurses encounter situations in which they must translate a physician's order for a certain drug dosage into the proper number of tablets or the proper volume of drug for an individual patient. This section is intended to illustrate how to handle these problems with skill and confidence.

Before addressing the technique for solving dosage problems, students must be familiar with various systems of units. The metric system (Table 6-2) is an international system that is most commonly used for drug dosage calculations. The primary units nurses must be familiar with are units of mass and volume because most problems to be solved are expressed in units of drug mass and drug volume.

The primary unit of mass within the metric system is the **gram** (g). With the use of prefixes, this unit can be adjusted to express thousands of grams (1 kilogram [kg] = 1000 g) or thousandths of grams (1 milligram [mg] = 0.001 g). The prefixes *deci-* and *centi-,* meaning $^1/_{10}$ and $^1/_{100}$, respectively, are used less often. The primary unit of volume within the metric system is the **liter** (L). With prefixes, the liter is commonly divided into thousandths (1 L = 1000 milliliters [ml]) and less commonly into millionths (1 L = 1,000,000 microliters [$-\mu$L]) or hundredths (1 L = 10 deciliters [dl]). The milliliter (ml) is the metric volume unit that is equivalent to the older unit, the cubic centimeter (cc). These relationships are summarized in Table 6-3.

The metric system possesses many advantages in terms of ease of calculation and convenience of units. Nevertheless, other units of mass are sometimes encountered. For instance, body weight may be given in pounds rather than kilograms. Another instance is the grain (gr), the unit of mass in the apothecary system. This older system was retained for a few drugs, such as aspirin and morphine, that have been used medically for decades, but dosages of these drugs are now most commonly calculated in milligrams. Equivalents between the metric system and other less commonly used systems are listed in Table 6-4.

Abbreviations for the various units are not entirely standardized in the medical literature. For example, gram may be abbreviated Gm, gm, or g. One set of abbreviations has been adopted for use throughout this book. Table 6-5 summarizes the abbreviations in use for various units.

The nurse in practice deals with solutions of drugs daily. A solution is a given mass of solid substance dissolved in a known volume of fluid (weight/volume, or w/v) or a given volume of a liquid substance dissolved in a known volume of another fluid (volume/volume, or v/v). The concentration of a w/v solution is always expressed as units of mass per units of volume. Common concentration units are g/ml, g/L, and

mg/ml. Concentrations are also commonly expressed as percentages, based on the definition of a 1% solution as 1 g of solid/100 ml of solution. Proportions are also used as expressions of concentrations. For example, 1:1000 designates a solution containing 1 g/1000 ml of solution. Blood levels of certain metabolites are often expressed as mg% (mg/100 ml) of solution. The term mg/100 ml is equivalent to mg/deciliter (dl); that is, a 1 mg% solution is the same as a 1 mg/dl solution. The relationship between the various expressions of concentration is illustrated in Table 6-6.

Table 6-4 Conversion between Measurement Systems

Apothecary		Metric
15 grains (gr)	=	1 g*
1 dram (dr)	=	4 g
15 minims (m)	=	1 ml
1 fluid dram (f dr)	=	4 ml

Household		Metric
1 teaspoon (t)	=	5 ml
1 tablespoon (T)	=	15 ml
1 fluid ounce (f oz)	=	32 ml (or 30 ml)†
1 pint (pt)	=	480 ml (or 500 ml)†
1 quart (qt)	=	960 ml (or 1000 ml)†
1 gallon (gal)		3.85 L (or 4 L)†
1 pound avoirdupois (lb)		0.46 kg‡

*Two factors have been used for converting grains to milligrams. Older conversion factor is 65 mg = 1 gr. This factor is basis for aspirin and acetaminophen formulations (i.e., a 5-gr aspirin tablet contains 325 mg of aspirin). More recently agreed-on conversion factor is 60 mg = 1 gr. This new conversion factor is easier to use for drugs (e.g., morphine) that are commonly administered in small doses (fractions of grains). For example, 1/4 gr of morphine equals 15 mg when new conversion factor is used. It is important to remember that these factors are simply estimates agreed on for ease of calculation. All problems presented in this book use conversion 15 gr = 1000 mg.
†Values in parentheses have been used because they are more easily measured in most clinical glassware.
‡This conversion is equivalent to 1 kg = 2.2 lb.

Table 6-5 Abbreviations Summary

Unit	Abbreviation Used in This Text	Other Acceptable Abbreviations
Gram	g	Gm, gm
Milligram	mg	mgm
Microgram	μg	mcg
Liter	L	l
Milliliter	ml	cc*

*Used for gases only.

CALCULATIONS

Calculating the Strength of Drug Solutions

To calculate the concentration of a drug solution, use the following equation:

$$\text{Concentration} = \frac{\text{Mass of drug}}{\text{Volume of solution}}$$

If you know any two of these quantities, you can solve directly for the third, provided all the quantities are expressed in the same system of units. Therefore as a first step in the solution of any problem, it may be necessary to convert units from one system to another, as seen in Example 1.

Example 1
Prepare 1 L of a 5% solution.
You know:
  1. Volume of solution (1 L)
  2. Concentration (5%)
To solve:
  1. Convert all quantities to the same system of units:

$$5\% = 5 \text{ g}/100 \text{ ml}; 1 \text{ L} = 1000 \text{ ml}$$

  2. Substitute the known quantities into the equation:

$$5 \text{ g}/100 \text{ ml} = \text{Mass of drug}/1000 \text{ ml}$$

  3. Solve for mass of drug:

$$\text{Mass} = \frac{1000 \times 5 \text{ g}}{100 \text{ ml}} = 50 \text{ g}$$

In other words, if 50 g of the drug is dissolved in enough diluent to make a final volume of 1 L, the result is a 5% solution.

Table 6-6 Equivalents of Concentration Expressions

%	Ratio	g/L	g/dl	mg/ml	mg/dl	μg/ml
10	1:10	100	10	100	10,000	100,000
1	1:100	10	1	10	1,000	10,000
0.1	1:1,000	1	0.1	1	100	1,000
0.01	1:10,000	0.1	0.01	0.1	10	100
0.001	1:100,000	0.01	0.001	1	10	
0.0001	1:1,000,000	0.001	0.0001	0.001	0.1	1

Example 2

What is the strength of a 2-L solution containing 10 g of drug?
You know:

1. Mass of drug (10 g)
2. Volume of solution (2 L)

To solve, substitute the known quantities into the equation:

$$\text{Concentration} = \frac{10\ \text{g}}{2\ \text{L}} = \frac{5}{\text{L}}$$

The strength of this solution could be expressed equally well as 0.5% (0.5 g/100 ml) or as a 1:200 solution (see Table 6-6).

Example 3

How much of a 2% solution can be prepared with 6 g of drug?
You know:

1. Concentration (2%)
2. Mass of drug (6 g)

To solve:

1. Convert all quantities to the same system of units:

$$2\% = 2\ \text{g}/100\ \text{ml}$$

2. Substitute the known quantities into the equation:

$$2\ \text{g}/100\ \text{ml} = 6\ \text{g}/\text{Volume of solution}$$

3. Solve for volume of solution:

$$\text{Volume} = \frac{6\ \text{g} \times 100\ \text{ml}}{2\ \text{g}} = 300\ \text{ml}$$

Self-Test for Proficiency in Drug Calculations

After thorough study of the previous section, you should be able to work the following problems. Check your answers and see the calculations worked out at the end of this chapter.

Set 1: Conversions of Units and Expressions of Concentration

1. A solution is labeled 1:50. Express this concentration in the following units:
   a. g/L
   b. mg/ml
   c. %
   d. mg%
   e. μg/ml
2. The body weight of a patient is given as 150 lb. What is the body weight expressed in kilograms?

Calculating the Strength of Diluted Solutions

The preceding examples have all dealt with weight/volume problems. In examining volume/volume problems, the basic equation can be modified slightly and the problems can be solved in much the same way as before. The equation becomes as follows:

(Concentration of solution) $\times$ (Volume of solution) =
(Concentration of stock) $\times$ (Volume of stock)

Stock or **stock solution** is a concentrated form of a drug that must ordinarily be diluted before use. With the use of this equation, calculations are performed as shown in the following examples.

Example 4

Prepare 500 ml of 1% solution from a 1:25 stock.
You know:

1. Volume of solution (500 ml)
2. Concentration of solution (1%)
3. Concentration of stock (1:25)

To solve:

1. Convert all quantities to the same system of units:

$$1\% = 1\ \text{g}/100\ \text{ml}$$
$$1{:}25 = 4\ \text{g}/100\ \text{ml}$$

2. Substitute the known quantities in the equation:

$$\frac{500\ \text{ml} \times \text{g}}{100\ \text{ml}} = \frac{4\ \text{g}}{100\ \text{ml}} \times \text{Volume of stock}$$

3. Solve for the unknown:

$$\frac{500\ \text{ml} \times 1\ \text{g}}{100\ \text{ml}} \times \frac{100\ \text{ml}}{4\ \text{g}} = 125\ \text{ml}$$

Example 5

How much of a 0.5% solution can be prepared from 10 ml of a 20% solution?
You know:

1. Concentration of solution (0.5%)
2. Volume of stock (10 ml)
3. Concentration of stock (20%)

To solve:

1. Convert all quantities to the same system of units:

$$0.5\% = 0.5\ \text{g}/100\ \text{ml}$$
$$20\% = 20\ \text{g}/100\ \text{ml}$$

2. Substitute the known quantities in the equation:

$$\frac{0.5\ \text{g}}{100\ \text{ml}} \times \text{Volume of solution} = \frac{20\ \text{g}}{100\ \text{ml}} \times 10\ \text{ml}$$

3. Solve for the unknown:

$$\text{Volume of solution} = \frac{20\ \text{g}}{100\ \text{ml}} \times \frac{10\ \text{ml} \times 100\ \text{ml}}{0.5\ \text{g}} = 400\ \text{ml}$$

Self-Test for Proficiency in Drug Calculations

After thorough study of the previous section, you should be able to work the following problems. Check your answers and see the calculations worked out at the end of this chapter.

Set 2: Dilution of Stock Solutions

1. A stock solution of a drug contains 10,000 U/ml.
   a. Calculate the amount of stock that must be included in 500 ml of infusion fluid if a 150-lb

patient is to receive 20,000 U of drug in this volume.

b. Calculate the concentration of the diluted drug.

2. Prepare 1 quart of a 2% solution from a 1:10 stock.

3. How would you prepare 1 gallon of a 5% solution from a 50% solution?

Calculating Drug Dosages

All the examples thus far have dealt with the preparation of a drug for administration. The next step is the use of those materials to fulfill the physician's drug order for a patient. The equation is as follows:

Body weight × Dosage = Volume of drug × Drug concentration

A drug dosage is expressed as units or mass of drug per body weight of patient. For example, 0.1 g of drug/kg body weight is a drug dosage expression, but 0.1 g of drug is not. For example, occasionally a physician may order a dose of 500 mg of an antibiotic with the understanding that 500 mg is the appropriate dose for the standard 70-kg patient (Box 6-1). More accurate dosages, of course, must be calculated for persons who deviate greatly from the normal weight range or when highly toxic drugs are involved. Common types of problems in drug dosage are presented in the following examples.

Example 6

A 100-kg patient is to receive a dose of 4 U/kg body weight. How many milliliters of the 100 U/ml stock solution are required?

You know:

1. Drug dosage (4 U/kg body weight)
2. Patient body weight (100 kg)

---

3. Concentration of the drug to be administered (100 U/ml)

To solve:

1. Substitute the known quantities in the equation:

$$100 \text{ kg} \times \frac{4 \text{ U}}{\text{kg}} = \text{Volume of drug} \times 100 \text{ U/ml}$$

2. Solve for volume of drug:

$$\text{Volume of drug} = 100 \text{ kg} \times \frac{4 \text{ U}}{\text{kg}} \times \frac{1 \text{ ml}}{100 \text{ U}} = 4 \text{ ml}$$

Example 7

The attending physician has left orders for infusion with 25,000 U of a drug in 0.5 L of normal saline solution. The drug is supplied as 50,000 U/ml stock solution. What volume of the drug stock would you use to make up the 0.5 L drug solution for administration? What is the dosage if the patient weighs 100 kg?

To solve:

1. Set up the following proportion to calculate the volume of stock to be added to make the infusion mixture:

$$\frac{25,000 \text{ U}}{\text{ml of stock}} = \frac{50,000 \text{ U}}{1 \text{ ml}}$$

$$\text{ml of stock} = 0.5 \text{ ml}$$

2. Dosage is defined as the amount of drug per unit of body weight.

Therefore the dosage is:

$$\frac{25,000 \text{ U}}{100 \text{ kg}} = \frac{250 \text{ U}}{\text{kg}}$$

Box 6-1 The Standard Patient, or Who Is the 70-kg Man, and Why Is He in All My Dosage Problems?

If we deal with an intravenous drug, we can measure the dosage very accurately and deliver an exact dose calculated in milligram of drug per kilogram of body weight. If we deal with a tablet, how can we achieve the same accuracy of dosage? The answer is that we cannot, in any practical way. The solution to this problem was to adopt a 70-kg, or approximately 150-lb, man as the standard patient and include the appropriate amount of drug for that patient into the standard oral dosage form. For example, penicillin V tablets contain either 250 or 500 mg of drug; therefore a 70-kg man would receive a dosage of 3.6 or 7.2 mg/kg (250/70 or 500/70). These dosages are within the target range for this drug. What if the patient is a small woman who weighs 110 lb? This patient weighs only 50 kg (110 lb/2.2 lb per kg) and would receive dosages of 5 to 10 mg/kg (250/50 or 500/50). For a safe drug like penicillin, these dosages may still be in a safe range, but for other medications, small female patients may be more prone to some side effects because they receive larger doses relative to their body weight than do larger patients. Some adjustment of dosage may be possible with scored tablets that can be broken in half or with oral solutions, but even with solutions, there is a limit to how accurately a patient can measure fractions of a teaspoon to adjust the dose of the medication.

Self-Test for Proficiency in Drug Calculations

After thorough study of the previous section, you should be able to work the following problems. You can check your answers and see the calculations worked out at the end of this chapter.

Set 3: Drug Dosages

1. A 70-kg patient is to receive 1.2 g of a drug administered in a 3-ml volume. What is the concentration of the drug solution administered to the patient, and what is the drug dosage?

2. A 60-kg patient is to receive 600 mg of a drug administered in a 2-ml volume. What is the drug dosage?

3. A certain drug is dispensed in tablets marked 250 mg. The drug package insert says that the dose of the drug is not to exceed 10 mg/kg. If a 60-kg adult patient receives 2 tablets, will the dosage exceed what the manufacturer considers safe?

4. A certain patient is to receive a drug at a dose of 5 mg/kg. The drug is supplied in a vial marked 500 mg/ml. What volume of drug from the vial should be administered to a 70-kg patient?

5. A certain drug is known to cause thrombophlebitis when given intravenously at high concentrations. Therefore the package insert says the drug must be infused at a concentration of less than 10 mg/ml. A 50-kg patient is to receive 500 mg of the drug by intravenous (IV) infusion. What is the drug dosage, and what volume will need to be infused?

Calculating Infusion Rates

Many drugs must be administered intravenously by slow infusion rather than as a rapid bolus injection. Large volumes of fluids of various types are also given by IV infusion. Disposable infusion sets are available from several manufacturers. These sets are commonly calibrated to deliver 10, 12, 15, 20, 50, or 60 drops/ml (abbreviated gtt/ml) of fluid. The nurse in practice can find the calibration, or drop factor, for any particular infusion set by examining the package in which it is supplied. Usually a hospital has only two sizes available to minimize confusion: one regular, or macrodrip, set of 10, 12, or 15 gtt/ml; and one pediatric, or microdrip, set of 50 or 60 gtt/ml.

Calculations of infusion rates can be carried out with the following equation:

$$\text{gtt/min} = \frac{\text{gtt/ml calibration}}{60 \text{ min/hr}} \times \frac{\text{Total ml to be administered}}{\text{Total hours of infusion}}$$

The use of this formula is illustrated in the following examples.

Example 8

A physician's order reads "3500 ml 5% dextrose in water IV in 24 hours." What is the correct infusion rate if the infusion set delivers 60 gtt/ml?
You know:
1. gtt/ml calibration (60 gtt/ml)
2. Total amount to be administered (3500 ml)
3. Total length of infusion (24 hr)
To solve, substitute the known quantities in the equation:

$$\text{gtt/min} = \frac{60 \text{ gtt/ml}}{60 \text{ min/hr}} \times \frac{3500 \text{ ml}}{24 \text{ hr}} = 145 \text{ to } 146 \text{ gtt/min}$$

Example 9

To give 50 ml of antibiotic solution IV in 30 minutes, what should the infusion rate be in drops per minute? The infusion set is calibrated for 60 gtt/ml.
You know:
1. Total amount to be administered (50 ml)
2. Total length of infusion (0.5 hr)
3. gtt/ml calibration (60 gtt/ml)
To solve, substitute the known quantities in the formula:

$$\text{gtt/min} = \frac{60 \text{ gtt/ml}}{60 \text{ min/hr}} \times \frac{50 \text{ ml}}{0.5 \text{ hr}} = 100 \text{ gtt/min}$$

Example 10

If an infusion set calibrated for 15 gtt/ml is running at a rate of 45 gtt/min, how much time will be required to infuse 1 L of fluid?
You know:
1. gtt/ml calibration (15 gtt/ml)
2. Total volume to be administered (1000 ml = 1 L)
3. Flow rate (45 gtt/min)
To solve, substitute the known quantities in the equation:

$$45 \text{ gtt/min} = \frac{15 \text{ gtt/ml}}{60 \text{ min/hr}} \times \frac{1000 \text{ ml}}{\text{Hours of infusion}}$$

The formula can be rearranged to solve for the number of hours:

$$\text{Hours of infusion} = \frac{15 \text{ gtt/ml}}{60 \text{ min/hr}} \times \frac{1000 \text{ ml}}{45 \text{ gtt/min}} = 5.55 \text{ hr}$$

Self-Test for Proficiency in Drug Calculations

After thorough study of the previous section, you should be able to solve the following problems. You can check your answers and see the calculations worked out at the end of this chapter.

Set 4: Calculating IV Infusion Rates

1. The physician's order reads "1000 ml of D5W IV in 8 hours." What is the correct infusion rate if the administration set delivers 10 gtt/ml?
2. To give 50 ml of antibiotic solution intravenously in 30 minutes, what should the infusion rate be in drops per minute if the infusion set is calibrated to deliver 10 gtt/ml?
3. Half a liter of normal saline solution is to be infused over 5 hours. The infusion set delivers 20 gtt/ml. What should the rate of infusion be?
4. The physician's order reads "1000 ml D5W in 24 hours." If the infusion set calibration is 60 gtt/ml, how many drops per minute should be administered?
5. An infusion of 500 ml of IV fluid is to be carried out over 3 hours. What infusion rate must be used with an infusion set delivering 10 gtt/ml?

Calculating Pediatric Dosages

Calculation of pediatric dosages requires special knowledge of each drug and how it interacts with the unique metabolism of the infant (see Chapter 2). Some drugs may be given to children and infants in doses that are in the same proportion to body weight as the doses used in adults. Other drugs must be given in greatly reduced doses because the infant is more sensitive or is incapable of metabolizing the drug as rapidly as an adult. Physicians take these considerations into account when determining recommended pediatric doses. For many drugs the pediatric doses listed in various drug reference publications include a statement indicating that the dosage may be calculated for children according to their

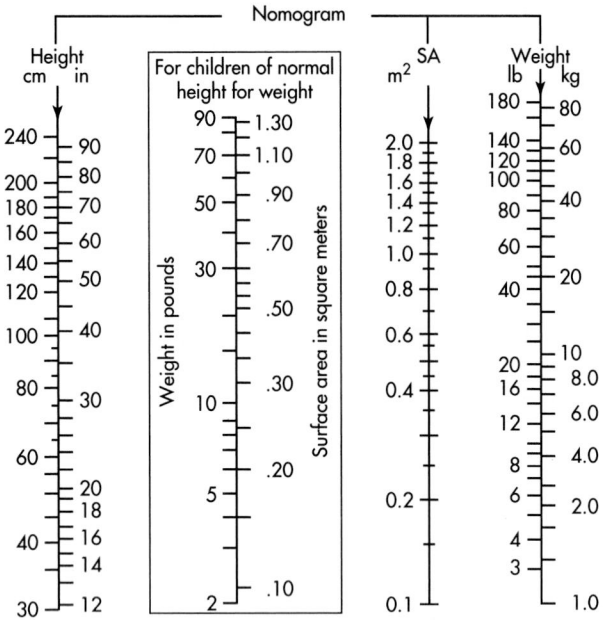

Nomogram

Figure 6-1   Nomogram for calculating body surface area. Place a straight edge from the patient's height in the left column to his weight in the right column. The point of intersection on the body surface area column indicates the body surface area (SA) in m². *(From Behrman RE, Kliegman R, Jensen HB, editors: Nelson's textbook of pediatrics, ed 16, Philadelphia, 2000, WB Saunders.)*

body weight, for example, but should not exceed a stated upper limit.

Several methods for calculating pediatric dosages exist. Three methods are presented here. The first method, called **Young's rule,** is based on the age of the child and applies to children between 1 and 12 years of age. The equation is as follows:

$$\text{Child's dose} = \frac{\text{Age of child in years}}{\text{Age of child in years} + 12} \times \text{Adult dose}$$

The use of Young's rule is illustrated in the following example.

Example 11

What is the appropriate dose of aspirin for a 3-year-old child? A normal adult dose is 650 mg.
You know:
Adult dose (650 mg)
To solve, substitute the known quantities in the equation:

$$\text{Child's dose} = \frac{3 \text{ years}}{3 + 12} \times 650 \text{ mg} = \frac{1}{5} \times 650 \text{ mg} = 130 \text{ mg}$$

A second method for calculating pediatric dosages is based on a comparison of the child's weight to the average weight of an adult. This formula, which applies to all ages of children, is called **Clark's rule.** The equation is as follows:

$$\text{Child's dose} = \frac{\text{Weight of child in pounds}}{150 \text{ pounds}} \times \text{Adult dose}$$

The use of Clark's rule is illustrated in the following example.

Example 12

What is the appropriate dose of aspirin for a 30-lb child if the normal adult dose is 650 mg?
You know:
  1. Weight of the child (30 lb)
  2. Adult dose (650 mg)
To solve, substitute the known quantities in the equation:

$$\text{Child's dose} = \frac{30 \text{ lb}}{150 \text{ lb}} \times 650 \text{ mg} = 130 \text{ mg}$$

Note that Clark's rule and Young's rule give the same answer when the child is not much lighter or heavier than the normal weight for age. The 30-lb 3-year-old child used in examples 11 and 12 is near the normal weight for that age. Clark's rule is considered the more accurate of the two rules because it will adjust dosage for a child who does deviate from normal weight.

The most accurate method of calculating pediatric dosage is based on the **body surface area** of the child's body relative to that of an adult. Surface area is obviously more difficult to measure than age or weight. Measurements under laboratory conditions yield 1.7 square meters (m²) as the average body surface area for an adult. Measurements taken under similar conditions with children have allowed the construction of charts, and nomograms that relate the child's body weight to surface area. An example of such a nomogram is shown in Figure 6-1. The equation used for the drug dose calculation is:

$$\text{Child's dose} = \frac{\text{Surface area of child in m}^2}{1.7 \text{ m}^2} \times \text{Adult dose}$$

The use of the formula is illustrated in the following example.

Example 13

What dose of meperidine (Demerol) does a child weighing 10 kg require?

The adult dose of meperidine is 50 mg. To calculate the dosage on the basis of body surface area, determine from Figure 6-1 the surface area that corresponds to a body weight of 10 kg and height of 25 inches. That value is 0.46 m². With that information you can solve the problem.
You know:
  1. Surface area of child (0.46 m²)
  2. Adult dose (50 mg)
To solve, substitute these values in the equation:

$$\text{Child's dose} = \frac{0.46 \text{ m}^2}{1.7 \text{ m}^2} \times 50 \text{ mg} = 13.5 \text{ mg}$$

Self-Test for Proficiency in Drug Calculations

After thorough study of the previous section, you should be able to work the following problems. Check your answers and see the calculations worked at the end of this chapter.

Set 5: Calculating Pediatric Doses

1. A physician orders the antibiotic cephalexin for a 25-lb child. The normal adult dose for this drug is 250 mg qid. Use Clark's rule to calculate the dose for this child. Does the prescribed dose fall within the recommended dose of 6 to 12 mg/kg listed in the package insert?

2. You are to give a 5-year-old child phenobarbital. The adult dose is 60 mg. Use Young's rule to calculate the approximate dose for the child.

3. A 10-year-old child who weighs 70 lb and is 5 feet in height requires codeine sulfate. The normal adult dose is 30 mg. Use body surface area to calculate the appropriate dose for this child.

4. You must give aspirin to a 4-year-old child. Adults take 325 or 650 mg of aspirin, depending on the severity of the pain to be relieved. Use Young's rule to calculate the appropriate dose for the child, based on the maximum adult dose.

5. A 12-kg infant 85 cm in height is to receive atropine. The normal adult dose is 0.3 mg (300 μg). What is the appropriate dose for this infant, based on body surface area?

6. You are to give penicillin G to a 40-lb child. The adult dose is 300,000 U. Use Clark's rule to calculate the child's dose.

Nursing Process Overview

Calculating Drug Doses

Assessment

The patient and ordered medications should be assessed individually. Is the drug appropriate? What is the usual dose, and is the dose ordered within the normal range? Is there anything about the patient that would indicate that an ordered dose is too large or too small?

Planning/Implementation

Calculate dosages systematically. Have a colleague check calculations if the dose seems unusual or if the mathematic calculations are difficult. Do a "common sense" check also: 2 tablets might make sense, but 20 tablets? If an intramuscular (IM) dose is calculated at 7 ml, is there an error? Most IM doses do not exceed 2 ml. A dose can be too small; for example, should a calculated IV dose of 0.02 ml be 0.2 ml or 2 ml?

Evaluation

Is the patient achieving the desired result? Are there side effects? Are they severe? What data indicate a prescribed dose is too large or too small? What should be recorded?

ANSWERS TO SELF-TEST FOR PROFICIENCY IN DRUG CALCULATIONS

At the end of each section in the text, there are questions designed to assist the student in developing proficiency. The correct answer for each self-test question is given below, followed by the calculation.

SOLUTIONS TO SET 1

1. The solution is labeled *1:50*. Ratio is defined as g:ml, with both usually expressed as whole numbers. Therefore 1 g/50 ml is the expression of concentration. You may now readily carry out the other conversions required. The answers are given first, followed by the calculation.

   a. *20 g/L:* 1 g/50 ml = ? g/1000 ml. (Remember that 1 L = 1000 ml.) ? g = (1000 ml × 1 g)/50 ml = 20 g/L.

   b. *20 mg/ml:* 1 g = 1000 mg. Therefore: 1000 mg/50 ml = ? mg/1000 ml; ? mg = (1000 ml × 1 mg)/50 ml = 20 mg/ml.

   c. *2%:* Percentage is defined as g/100 ml. Solving by proportion: 1 g/50 ml = ? g/100 ml. Therefore: ? g = (1 g × 100 ml)/50 ml = 2 g. Thus the solution of 2 g/100 ml is 2%.

   d. *2000 mg%:* mg% is defined as mg/100 ml. Solving by proportion: 1 g/50 ml = ? mg/100 ml. Therefore: ? mg = (1000 mg × 100 ml)/50 ml = 2000 mg. Thus the solution of 2000 mg/100 ml is 2000 mg%.

   e. *20,000 μg/ml:* 1 mg = 1000 μg. Therefore: 20 mg/ml = 20,000 μg/ml.

2. From Table 6-4, you find that 1 lb = 0.46 kg. Therefore solving by proportion: 0.46 kg/1 lb = ? kg/150 lb. Thus: ? kg = (0.46 kg × 150 lb)/1 lb = 69 kg.

SOLUTIONS TO SET 2

1. a. *2 ml:* Calculate the *amount of stock* that contains 20,000 U. Solving by proportion:

$$\frac{10,000 \text{ U}}{1 \text{ ml}} = \frac{20,000 \text{ U}}{? \text{ ml}}$$

$$? \text{ ml} = \frac{(1 \text{ ml}) (20,000 \text{ U})}{10,000 \text{ U}} = 2 \text{ ml}$$

   b. *40 U/ml:* Diluted drug is 20,000 U in 500 ml, so

$$\frac{20,000 \text{ U}}{500 \text{ ml}} = 40 \text{ U/ml}$$

2. *Dilute 200 ml of 1:10 stock to 1 qt (1000 ml):* 1:10 stock is 1 g/10 ml; 1 qt = 1000 ml; 2% solution is 2 g/100 ml. To make 1 qt of 2% solution would require:

$$\frac{2 \text{ g}}{100 \text{ ml}} = \frac{? \text{ g}}{1000 \text{ ml}}$$

? g = (2 g × 1000 ml)/100 ml = 20 g. To get 20 g from the 1:10 stock:

$$\frac{1 \text{ g}}{10 \text{ ml}} = \frac{20 \text{ g}}{? \text{ ml}}$$

? ml = (20 g × 10 ml)/1 g = 200 ml

3. *Add 400 ml of the 50% stock solution to 3600 ml of water:* 1 gal = 4000 ml, a 5% solution = 5 g/100 ml, and a 50% solution = 50 g/100 ml. Therefore the volume of stock solution to be added equals:

$$\frac{(5 \text{ g}/100 \text{ ml}) \times 4000 \text{ ml}}{(50 \text{ g}/100 \text{ ml})} = 400 \text{ ml}$$

Note that this volume is to be mixed with 3600 ml of water for the final volume of the solution to be 1 gallon.

SOLUTIONS TO SET 3

1. *The concentration is 0.4 g/ml, and the dosage is 17 mg/kg:*

$$\text{Concentration} = 1.2 \text{ g}/3 \text{ ml} = 0.4 \text{ g/ml}$$

$$\text{Dosage} = 1.2 \text{ g}/70 \text{ kg} = 0.017 \text{ g/kg} = 17 \text{ mg/kg}$$

2. *Dosage is 10 mg/kg:*

$$\text{Dosage} = 600 \text{ mg}/60 \text{ kg} = 10 \text{ mg/kg}$$

3. *Dosage = 8.33 mg/kg. Therefore the dose as prescribed should be within the accepted safety limits:*

$$\frac{2 \text{ tablets}}{\text{Dose}} \times \frac{250 \text{ mg}}{\text{Tablet}} = \frac{500 \text{ mg}}{\text{Dose}}$$

Therefore: 500 mg/60 kg = 8.33 mg/kg.

4. *0.7 ml:* (5 mg/kg) × 70 kg = 350 mg drug in each dose. Therefore:

$$\frac{350 \text{ mg}}{500 \text{ mg/ml}} = 0.7 \text{ ml volume from the vial}$$

5. *Dosage = 10 mg/kg and the minimum infusion volume is 50 ml:*

$$\text{Dosage} = \frac{500 \text{ mg}}{50 \text{ kg}} = 10 \text{ mg/kg}$$

$$\text{Minimum infusion volume} = \frac{500 \text{ mg}}{10 \text{ mg/ml}} = 50 \text{ ml}$$

SOLUTIONS TO SET 4

1. *20 to 21 gtt/min:*

$$\text{gtt/min} = \frac{10 \text{ gtt/ml}}{60 \text{ min/hr}} \times \frac{1000 \text{ ml}}{8 \text{ hr}} = 20 \text{ to } 21 \text{ gtt/min}$$

2. *16 to 17 gtt/min:*

$$\text{gtt/min} = \frac{10 \text{ gtt/ml}}{60 \text{ min/hr}} \times \frac{50 \text{ ml}}{0.5 \text{ hr}} = 16 \text{ to } 17 \text{ gtt/min}$$

3. *33 to 34 gtt/min:*

$$\text{gtt/min} = \frac{20 \text{ gtt/ml}}{60 \text{ min/hr}} \times \frac{500 \text{ ml}}{5 \text{ hr}} = 33 \text{ to } 34 \text{ gtt/min}$$

4. *41 to 42 gtt/min:*

$$\text{gtt/min} = \frac{60 \text{ gtt/ml}}{60 \text{ min/hr}} \times \frac{1000 \text{ ml}}{24 \text{ hr}} = 41 \text{ to } 42 \text{ gtt/min}$$

5. *27 to 28 gtt/min:*

$$\text{gtt/min} = \frac{10 \text{ gtt/ml}}{60 \text{ min/hr}} \times \frac{500 \text{ ml}}{3 \text{ hr}} = 27 \text{ to } 28 \text{ gtt/min}$$

SOLUTIONS TO SET 5

1. *Dosage prescribed = 3.8 mg/kg, which is less than the suggested lower limit of 6 mg/kg:*

$$\text{Child's dose} = (25 \text{ lb} \times 250 \text{ mg})/150 \text{ lb} = 42 \text{ mg}$$

$$25 \text{ lb} \times 0.46 \text{ kg/lb} = 11 \text{ kg}$$

$$\text{Dosage} = 42 \text{ mg}/11 \text{ kg} = 3.8 \text{ mg/kg}$$

2. *17.6 mg:*

$$\text{Child's dose} = \frac{5 \text{ years}}{5 + 12 \text{ years}} \times 60 \text{ mg} = 17.6 \text{ mg}$$

3. *19.8 mg:* According to the nomogram, the body surface area of this child = 1.12 m².

$$\text{Child's dose} = (1.12 \text{ m}^2/1.7 \text{ m}^2) \times 30 \text{ mg} = 19.8 \text{ mg}$$

4. *2.5 gr:*

$$\text{Child's dose} = \frac{4 \text{ years}}{4 + 12} \times 650 \text{ mg} = 162 \text{ mg}$$

5. *0.01 mg:* According to the nomogram, the body surface area of this infant = 0.54 m².

$$\text{Child's dose} = \frac{0.54 \text{ m}^2}{1.7 \text{ m}^2} \times 0.3 \text{ mg} = 0.01 \text{ mg}$$

6. *80,000 U:*

$$\text{Child's dose} = \frac{40 \text{ lb}}{150 \text{ lb}} \times 300,000 \text{ U} = 80,000 \text{ U}$$

Over-the-Counter Drugs and Self-Medication

Lynn Roger Willis

OBJECTIVES

After studying this chapter, you should be able to do the following:

- *Explain the difference between over-the-counter medications and prescription drugs.*
- *Explain the differences in federal rules that govern the promotion and sale of herbal remedies and conventional over-the-counter medications.*
- *Describe the advantages and disadvantages of fixed combinations of active ingredients.*
- *Explain the proper use of effective classes of over-the-counter agents.*
- *Discuss the dangers associated with continuous use of over-the-counter agents such as laxatives and sleeping medications.*

CHAPTER OVERVIEW

As health professionals, nurses focus on medications ordered for the patient by the physician. It is important to remember that patients also self-medicate, using a wide array of over-the-counter drugs. In certain circumstances over-the-counter medications may significantly influence the effects of prescribed agents. This chapter summarizes the properties of most classes of over-the-counter agents. Later chapters discuss how prescription drugs influence the same body systems.

REGULATION OF OVER-THE-COUNTER DRUGS

Over-the-counter (OTC) medications are medicinal agents deemed safe enough for self-use and sale without a prescription. Products intended for the self-medication have been sold in the United States since colonial times. Until the early twentieth century, however, no restrictions governed the contents, potency, purity, safety, efficacy, sale, or advertising of these nostrums, patent medicines, tonics, or remedies. Consequently, some were of marginal safety at best and most provided no obvious therapeutic benefit. Most of these early nostrums were harmless and ineffective, but many contained alcohol, narcotics, or other dangerous drugs in unspecified quantities. Thus they often posed serious risks to an unsuspecting public.

Some control of the patent medicine industry was achieved with passage of the first Pure Food and Drug Act of 1906 (see Chapter 3). This act required that package labels accurately list the ingredients of medicinal products. Any substance present but not listed on the label was deemed an adulterant. A later amendment to the act, the Sherley Amendment (1912), forbade false and fraudulent labeling claims. In 1938 a new Food and Drug Act was enacted. It required proof of safety for all medicinal products intended for sale. In 1952 the Durham-Humphrey Amendment to the 1938 Act specified (1) drugs safe enough for sale without a prescription (over the counter) and (2) drugs deemed sufficiently dangerous or unsuitable for self-medication to require sale by prescription only.

Present control of OTC drugs stems from the Kefauver-Harris Amendment of 1962, which required proof of efficacy and safety and lack of **teratogenicity** (the ability to cause birth defects). This amendment affected all drugs introduced after 1962 and all drugs that had entered the market since 1938. To meet the conditions of this amendment, the Food and Drug Administration (FDA) convened several panels of experts to review the classes of OTC drugs and assign each to one of the following categories:

Category I: Recognized as safe and effective for the claimed therapeutic indication

Category II: Not recognized as safe and effective

Category III: Additional data needed to decide safety or effectiveness

Drugs assigned to category I can be sold to the general public. Those in category II cannot. Drugs in category III, if generally recognized as safe, may be sold even though the evaluation of their safety and effectiveness has not been completed.

Since this review process began, many unsafe or ineffective OTC drugs and products have disappeared from the market. Others have undergone labeling changes or have had their formulations redesigned. However, because manufacturers are not required to indicate on the product label whether the drugs in their products are in category I or III, OTC products cannot be assumed to be effective simply because their sale is permitted. Some consumer interest groups have objected to the sale of drugs in category III, apparently in the belief that a drug should be considered unsafe and ineffective unless proven otherwise. Such groups have also challenged the assignment of other drugs to category I. Until the FDA review panels have completed their work, the therapeutic benefit of some OTC drugs will remain questionable.

COMMON PROPERTIES OF OVER-THE-COUNTER DRUGS

Small Doses

Today's manufacturers of OTC remedies are particularly concerned with the safety of their products. The toxicity of a drug varies in direct proportion to the dose administered; that is, the larger the dose, the greater the risk of toxicity. Thus most OTC products contain small, sometimes less-than-therapeutic, amounts of active ingredient. As such, they may serve as little more than **placebos** (inactive substances usually presented in the guise of an active medicine), especially for such subjective complaints as minor pain, itching, and sleeplessness. For such indications, proof that a drug is effective may be difficult to establish, even when adequate dosage is provided.

Combination of Ingredients

Many OTC products contain several drugs. The drugs may be totally different, or they may be of the same or similar pharmacologic classification. When drugs are combined, adverse interactions may occur. Although the risk of interactions is low for the drugs in a given product, it is not so low when other drugs are taken simultaneously.

OTC products with several ingredients are called **fixed-combination products**; that is, the doses of the drugs in the product are fixed within the tablet or other dosage form and cannot be altered. For example, if a tablet contains 4 mg of antihistamine and 60 mg of decongestant, a patient who needed to increase the antihistamine dosage would also have to take more of the decongestant. Complete control of drug dosage is possible with readily available single-drug products, and such products can often be purchased less expensively than the heavily advertised combination products. By understanding the pharmacology of the drugs in OTC products and the specific needs of the patient, the nurse can advise a rational method of product selection.

HERBAL REMEDIES AS OVER-THE-COUNTER DRUGS

Herbs and herbal remedies are now used by large numbers of people as adjuncts to or substitutes for conventional medicines. Such remedies are widely available in pharmacies, health food stores, and grocery stores and by mail order. Some herbal remedies may be useful and devoid of serious side effects, but others may provide no therapeutic benefit at all. Some clearly have the potential to cause serious harm.

Herbal Remedies and the FDA

Legally speaking, at least in the United States, medicinal herbs are used as foods, not drugs. This is because to sell an herbal remedy as a drug, a manufacturer must provide the FDA with evidence that the remedy is safe and effective for the intended use. Most marketers of herbal remedies have not provided such evidence, mostly because of the huge expense involved in doing so (through lengthy clinical trials) and because herbal remedies, having been used for centuries, cannot be patented. Consequently, most herbal remedies are marketed under the auspices of the FDA as nutritional or dietary supplements, not as drugs. In that setting, the law forbids the appearance of any therapeutic claims on the product labeling. If such claims appear, the manufacturer is liable to prosecution for marketing unapproved drugs.

The problems inherent in marketing as food what in reality are drugs are obvious. If the law does not provide for objective evaluation of the therapeutic claims for such products, the door opens wide for promoters and manufacturers to make exaggerated and even false claims aimed at increasing sales while ignoring potential side effects and toxicity. Until recently, most such promotion occurred through channels that were not easily policed by the FDA (e.g., word-of-mouth, mail-order catalogs). In 1993, however, responding to rampant promotional abuses for herbal and other unproven remedies, the FDA appeared ready to remove herbal remedies from the market altogether. This produced a public outcry on behalf of herbal remedies, fueled in large part by the health food industry, and led Congress to pass the Dietary Supplement Health and Education Act of 1994. This law permits the sale of herbal remedies as dietary supplements so long as therapeutic claims do not appear on the label. The label may contain a statement describing the product's role in some aspect of human health, and information presenting a balanced view of the available scientific information can be provided with the product. Importantly, the law requires that the FDA must prove that an herbal remedy is unsafe before the agency can remove it from the market.

Herbal Remedies and the Nurse

The Dietary Supplement Health and Education Act of 1994 effectively places a huge number of herbal remedies on a therapeutic par with conventional OTC remedies; but unlike the case for the conventional remedies, the Act does not require manufacturers of herbal remedies to provide evidence of product safety and effectiveness. Accordingly, if nurses are to provide helpful information about herbal remedies to their patients, they must understand the legal differences between herbal remedies and conventional OTC drugs and be prepared to look beyond the information provided by manufacturers for the most credible information. Sadly, this information is not always easy to find.

Currently, the most authoritative information available on the safety and effectiveness of herbal remedies is in the German medical literature. This information, which exists as monographs for individual herbal drugs, is being translated into English and will be published as a compendium. Each monograph describes available information on safety and effectiveness derived from laboratory and clinical investigations. This compendium will be available through the American Botanical Council. In the interim, helpful and authoritative information on herbal remedies can be obtained through reference librarians and such organizations as the American Pharmaceutical Association, the American Botanical Council, and the Herb Research Foundation.

Because herbal remedies for sale in the United States are not FDA-approved drugs, their labeling cannot be relied on to provide proper instructions for use and appropriate cautionary warnings; they have no FDA-enforced standards of quality. This means that products may contain subtherapeutic amounts of herbal constituents and that potential users can rely only on the good reputation of the manufacturer for reliability. The nurse should especially remind prospective users of herbal remedies that regardless of their classification as "dietary supplements," these remedies are in fact drugs of largely unproven safety, especially for pregnant or nursing mothers and for young children and infants, none of whom should be taking these remedies without medical supervision.

Herbal Remedies Go Beyond the Scope of OTC Drugs

OTC drugs are deemed safe enough to use for self-medication of conditions that do not ordinarily require the attention of a physician. Some herbal remedies (e.g., laxatives for constipation) have a long history of reliability and safety in this regard. More recently, other herbal remedies have come to public attention for use in treating potentially more serious, not-so-easily-diagnosed conditions such as depression (St. John's Wort), benign prostatic hypertrophy (saw palmetto), cirrhosis of the liver (milk thistle), and vascular insufficiency (ginkgo biloba). Although evidence of effectiveness supports to varying degrees such uses for these remedies, one can question the wisdom of self-medicating to treat or prevent such conditions.

MAJOR CLASSES OF OVER-THE-COUNTER DRUGS

The classes of OTC drugs chosen for discussion in this chapter include analgesic drugs, cold and cough remedies, and sleep aids; their component drugs are discussed in other chapters. Also discussed are ophthalmic products, acne treatments, sunscreens, topical antiinfectives, and hemorrhoidal products. Newly added to this chapter, and elsewhere in this book, is mention of specific herbal remedies that, based on existing, credible data, may provide a potentially effective and safe addition to the list of drugs currently used for various conditions.

Analgesics

Aspirin, acetaminophen, ibuprofen, naproxen, and ketoprofen are the most effective OTC analgesic drugs available. Nearly all OTC analgesic products intended for internal consumption contain one of these drugs. Aspirin, ibuprofen, naproxen, and ketoprofen belong to a larger class of drugs called **nonsteroidal antiinflammatory drugs** (NSAIDs). These drugs inhibit the synthesis of prostaglandins by inhibiting cyclooxygenase. This action may be related to the mechanism by which they produce analgesia. Acetaminophen is chemically unrelated to these four drugs. Its mechanism of action differs from that of NSAIDs, and it can be used by people who cannot tolerate NSAIDs. The complex pharmacology of these drugs is discussed in detail in Chapter 31.

▼ aspirin

Aspirin in doses of 650 mg relieves minor pain and reduces fever in most adults. Larger doses (as in "extra-strength" products) provide little additional relief for most people. Aspirin also relieves the pain and inflammation of arthritic disorders; however, this effect requires doses substantially greater than approved OTC doses, which should not be taken without supervision.

Aspirin produces numerous side effects. Although it normally presents no problem for individuals who take the drug

CASE STUDY
Over-the-Counter Medications

Jane is a 25-year-old secretary who is home after an emergency appendectomy. She is able to take care of her basic needs, and her mother, who lives nearby, helps her with meals. The physician prescribed two medications for the postoperative period: Keflex 500 mg every 6 hours and Vicodin 1 to 2 tablets every 4 hours prn for pain.

When you call Jane for a 4-day postoperative check, you ask her about the medications she is taking. She says she has developed the flu and has been taking the following for the last 3 days:

- Sinutabs without Drowsiness, 2 tablets twice a day (acetaminophen 500 mg and pseudoepinephrine 30 mg per tablet)
- Excedrin, 1 tablet, twice a day for headache (aspirin 250 mg, acetaminophen 250 mg, and caffeine 65 mg per tablet)
- Excedrin P.M., 1 tablet at bedtime for sleep (acetaminophen 500 mg and diphenhydramine 38 mg per tablet)
- Vicodin, 1 tablet, every 4 hours while awake for pain (acetaminophen 500 mg and hydrocodone bitartrate 5 mg per tablet). She takes 4 tablets per day.

Jane complains that she has been feeling a bit nauseated and has no appetite; she attributes these feeling to the flu. She says she thinks she needs to take Tylenol tablets for her fever, which is 102° F.

1. While reviewing her medications, what is your answer about the Tylenol or her fever?
2. What is the maximum recommended dosage for acetaminophen in 24 hours? How many milligrams did she take yesterday, if she has taken what she has told you? Is there a concern?
3. Explain the effect of acetaminophen on the liver at this dosage.
4. What suggestions would you make about her medication regimen?

only occasionally, it may be troublesome for those who take it regularly or are particularly sensitive to it. For example, aspirin inhibits platelet aggregation. As little as one 650-mg dose of aspirin may double the bleeding time for several days. Aspirin also irritates the stomach lining, sometimes causing pain, discomfort, and on occasion, localized bleeding, which can cause the loss of 5 to 10 ml of blood in the stool each day. The bleeding is ordinarily of no consequence with occasional use of the drug, but those who take aspirin for prolonged periods may develop iron deficiency anemia resulting from long-term blood losses. Individuals with a history of peptic ulcer or intestinal bleeding or those who are taking anticoagulant drugs should not take aspirin.

Various dosage forms for aspirin are available, reflecting efforts by manufacturers to overcome some of the problems it causes. Aspirin is available in buffered, effervescent, and enteric-coated tablets to minimize gastric irritation. Timed-release tablets are available for persons who must take aspirin regularly. Because aspirin is unstable in aqueous solution, liquid forms are not available.

▼ acetaminophen

Acetaminophen is as effective as aspirin at relieving minor aches and pains and reducing fever. Maximum analgesic and antipyretic effectiveness are achieved in most adults with 650 mg of either drug. Larger doses (as in "extra-strength" products) provide little, if any, additional relief for most people, but they appear to be more effective than usual doses in some people. Unlike aspirin, acetaminophen does not relieve the pain and inflammation of arthritic disorders.

Acetaminophen (Datril, Tylenol, and other brands) is remarkably free of side effects when used according to directions. It does not affect blood clotting, nor does it irritate the stomach lining. Rarely, acetaminophen causes an allergic reaction, often a skin rash, but hepatotoxicity is the most serious adverse effect of acetaminophen. Patients who take large overdoses of the drug, such as in a suicide attempt, can die of hepatotoxicity, but the potential for serious hepatotoxicity also exists for patients who merely exceed the recommended maximum dosage of 4 g in 24 hours. Patients who do not eat regularly (e.g., those who fast) and who consume alcohol more than occasionally are especially at risk of hepatotoxicity from acetaminophen and should be so advised.

▼ ibuprofen, naproxen, and ketoprofen

Ibuprofen (Advil, Nuprin) has been available OTC since 1984, **naproxen** (Aleve) was granted OTC status in 1994, and **ketoprofen** (Actron) was added to the OTC list in 1995. These NSAIDs (see Chapter 31) were approved for OTC sale largely because they have a somewhat wider margin of safety than either aspirin or acetaminophen, especially in cases of overdose.

All three of these drugs are recommended for people who cannot tolerate aspirin, but this recommendation requires rather narrow interpretation. People who are allergic to aspirin are also likely to be allergic to these drugs. Similarly, these drugs can irritate the gastric mucosa and may cause gastrointestinal bleeding. The drugs are often promoted as less likely than aspirin to cause gastric irritation, but some people may find them as troublesome as aspirin in this regard. For such people, acetaminophen remains the preferred alternative. No therapeutic advantage is gained by taking any of these drugs, including aspirin and acetaminophen, together; indeed, doing so increases the risk of adverse effects.

Although ibuprofen, naproxen, and ketoprofen are usually superior to aspirin or acetaminophen for relieving certain types of pain, such as that associated with menstrual cramps, dental work, and severe muscle strains, they are no more effective than aspirin or acetaminophen against most other types of mild pain and generally are more expensive.

Cold Remedies

Most of the available OTC cold remedies (e.g., Contac, Novahistine) contain a sympathomimetic drug to relieve nasal and sinus congestion, an antihistamine to dry excessive nasal secretions, or an analgesic drug to relieve minor aches and pains. Some products also contain caffeine, vitamins, a laxative, or other substances. A few products contain only a single drug, usually a sympathomimetic or an antihistamine, but most cold remedies are combination products.

Sympathomimetic drugs relieve nasal stuffiness and congestion by constricting the blood vessels in swollen nasal membranes, decreasing local blood flow and swelling. When the swelling is relieved, the breathing passages open. The sympathomimetic drugs commonly included in OTC cold remedies as decongestants are phenylephrine, phenylpropanolamine, and pseudoephedrine. These drugs are available in many products, and their pharmacologic characteristics are discussed in Chapter 30. Phenylephrine is the least reliable of the three because stomach acid reduces its activity, and its absorption into the blood is often erratic.

Sympathomimetic drugs can cause stimulation of the central nervous system (CNS) and generalized vasoconstriction. As a result the side effects of irritability, nervousness, insomnia, headache, and hypertension can occur. Individuals with high blood pressure, thyroid disease, or heart disease are cautioned against taking these drugs unless directed to do so by their physician. The vasoconstrictive effects of sympathomimetics are intensified by monoamine oxidase inhibitors (e.g., Marplan, Nardil), which may be prescribed to treat depression (see Chapter 59) and may cause alarming and dangerous elevations of blood pressure and threat of stroke.

The rationale for including an antihistamine in a product intended to treat symptoms of the common cold is not based on antagonism of histamine receptors. Unless the cold is causing the increased release of histamine, such as occurs in allergic rhinitis, antagonism of histamine receptors will be of no use (see Chapter 29). Instead, antihistamines are included in OTC cold remedies largely because of their anticholinergic action, which reduces secretion of mucus by the nasal and bronchial mucosa and produces a drying effect. This effect, however, is not strong, especially at approved OTC doses.

The therapeutic index of antihistamines is high, and little risk of serious toxicity exists for adults. The most prominent side effects of antihistamines are drowsiness and sedation. These effects occur with all OTC antihistamines and doses. They pose a potentially serious threat to operators of motor vehicles or persons in hazardous occupations, and they are intensified by the concurrent use of alcohol or other CNS depressants. Cold remedies that are promoted as "nondrowsiness formulas" generally do not contain an antihistamine.

Cough Remedies

If a cough accompanies a cold, it may be productive or nonproductive. A productive cough removes phlegm from the lower respiratory tract and generally should not be suppressed. A nonproductive cough is dry and, because of local irritation caused by the rapid movement of air, may be self-perpetuating. Nonproductive coughs can be safely suppressed and relieved with an OTC cough suppressant (antitussive) drug. Expectorants are also included in many OTC cough remedies. The detailed pharmacologic properties of expectorants and antitussives are discussed in Chapter 30.

Expectorants

The use of expectorants in clinical medicine is controversial. The controversy stems partly from a lack of objective evidence that expectorant drugs are effective and partly from confusion concerning the expected effect of an expectorant drug. By one definition, an expectorant should promote the expulsion of mucus, phlegm, and fluid from the lungs and bronchial passages; that is, it should enhance the productiveness of a cough. By another, it should relieve a dry, irritating cough by causing the secretion of soothing and protective mucus in the airway. There is little evidence to suggest that expectorant drugs are any better than placebo for promoting the expulsion of phlegm or relieving a cough.

Guaifenesin is the only expectorant approved for use in OTC cough remedies. It stimulates the reflex production of bronchial secretions by irritating the gastric mucosa. At higher dosages it causes nausea and vomiting.

Cough Suppressants

Three antitussive drugs have been approved for OTC status by the FDA: codeine, dextromethorphan, and diphenhydramine. Each relieves coughs by suppressing the cough reflex center in the brain.

Codeine once was the most widely used antitussive agent, but because it is an opioid narcotic, it can cause psychologic and physical dependence; thus its popularity has waned. In truth, the risk of dependence with codeine is much less than that for morphine, and it is virtually nonexistent when the drug is used in recommended doses for short periods. Nevertheless, none of the other drugs in this class has a potential for dependence, and they have proved to be more popular among consumers.

The side effects most often associated with the use of codeine are nausea, constipation, and drowsiness. The drowsiness is caused by depression of the CNS and is intensified by other CNS-depressants (e.g., barbiturates, alcohol, antihistamines). Codeine should not be taken with any other CNS-depressant. Poisoning with codeine causes respiratory depression.

Abuse of OTC cough preparations that contain codeine has been a problem in the United States, and varying restrictions on their sale have been enacted by state legislatures. These restrictions range from a limit on the quantity that can be purchased by an individual to complete prohibition of sale without a prescription.

Dextromethorphan is a nonnarcotic cough suppressant with about the same antitussive potency and efficacy as codeine. Dextromethorphan suppresses the cough reflex center in the brain, but it does not cause dependence or respiratory depression. Side effects are uncommon and generally mild, consisting largely of drowsiness and gastrointestinal upset. Overall, dextromethorphan is the best choice for cough suppression, and the great majority of OTC antitussive products contain it.

Diphenhydramine, an antihistamine, is also an effective cough suppressant. It is nonnarcotic and therefore does not cause dependence. In adults the drug suppresses coughs at a dosage of 25 mg every 4 hours. Drowsiness commonly occurs at this dosage, however, and severely limits the usefulness of this drug for many people. Paradoxically, diphenhydramine may cause stimulation, not sedation, in small children. This effect and its high propensity to cause drowsiness in adults makes it the least useful of the approved antitussive drugs.

Decongestant Nosedrops and Nasal Sprays

Several sympathomimetic drugs are available without a prescription as nosedrops and nasal sprays for the symptomatic and temporary relief of nasal congestion. These drugs include phenylephrine, ephedrine, and naphazoline, which are short-acting decongestants that are used as frequently as every 3 or 4 hours, and xylometazoline and oxymetazoline, which are long-acting decongestants that are used only two or three times a day.

Topical decongestants have advantages over oral decongestants, but there are also some serious disadvantages. Because the drops and sprays apply the drugs directly to the congested nasal membranes, the onset of action and relief of congestion occur rapidly. In addition, only small amounts of the drugs need be administered because they are applied locally. Therefore the incidence and severity of systemic side effects (e.g., elevated blood pressure) are reduced. On the other hand, the intense localized vasoconstriction in the nasal mucosa can cause "rebound congestion," in which the congestion that returns when the effect of the drug has dissipated may be worse than the congestion that existed in the first place. A vicious cycle can then develop in which the drug that originally relieved congestion now becomes the cause of it. If unrecognized, this cycle of futile treatment can lead to chronic nasal stuffiness that will no longer respond to the decongestant drugs. Rebound congestion probably cannot be totally avoided when topical decongestants are used, but it can be minimized if the drugs are used only sparingly and strictly according to directions.

Nasal sprays are most convenient for adults and older children, and nosedrops are often preferable for use in young children. Topical decongestants should not be given to children younger than 2 years except as directed by a physician.

Sleeping Aids

Insomnia disrupts the restful nights of nearly everyone from time to time. Some people have difficulty falling asleep; others may awaken in the middle of the night and be unable to go back to sleep. The cause of sleep difficulties may be physiologic or psychologic. In most cases the difficulties are temporary.

A wide variety of common remedies for sleeplessness may be tried. They include warm baths, a dull book, a glass of warm milk, or a cup of decaffeinated or herbal tea. In severe cases of insomnia the assistance of a physician may be sought, and a powerful sedative-hypnotic drug may be prescribed (see Chapter 57). Many people fear the addictive properties of these drugs, but they find little or no relief from home remedies. Between these extremes lies the OTC sleeping aid.

The FDA severely restricts the number of drugs that can be sold as OTC sleeping aids. OTC sleeping aids may contain an antihistamine alone or an antihistamine with aspirin or acetaminophen. Diphenhydramine is the only antihistamine recognized by the FDA as safe and effective for use as an OTC sleeping aid. Doxylamine, another antihistamine, may legally be sold in OTC sleeping remedies, but its safety and clinical effectiveness are still under investigation.

Antihistamines have utility as OTC sleeping aids because of their tendency to cause drowsiness. This tendency, plus a wide margin of safety, lends credence to marketing claims for the effectiveness of antihistamines in the treatment of occasional insomnia. An analgesic drug is included in some preparations on the assumption that mild nighttime pain may contribute to sleeplessness. Clinical comparisons of antihistamines with placebo in sleep laboratories tend to reinforce the claims of effectiveness, but some authorities remain doubtful.

The most common side effects produced by antihistamines are drowsiness or dizziness, although young children, older adults, and patients with CNS dysfunction may exhibit signs of stimulation at therapeutic doses. The sedating effects of these drugs are additive with ethanol and other CNS depressants, and the potential for poisoning exists when an acute overdose of the antihistamine is taken with another depressant drug. Other side effects of antihistamines include blurred vision, tinnitus, and dry mouth.

It is important for nurses to assess the cause of sleeplessness and the need for a sleeping aid. If mild pain is keeping someone awake, relief of the pain with aspirin or acetaminophen will often be sufficient to allow sleep to occur. If anxiety is the cause, antihistamine-induced drowsiness may be helpful, but it may also be no more effective than a glass of warm milk or a warm bath, although more expensive. Wise nursing counsel may be the most effective remedy for patients with mild insomnia.

Ophthalmic Products

OTC ophthalmic products are intended only for symptomatic, short-term relief of mild self-limiting conditions

RESEARCH HIGHLIGHTS

Insomnia, Alcohol, and Over-the-Counter Drug Use in Old-Old Urban Women

—*Johnson JE:* J Comm Health Nurs *14(3):181-188, 1997.*

PURPOSE

Older adults often complain of a need for more sleep. In addition, elderly people purchase and use large numbers of OTC medications, some of which may be to aid in sleeping. Historically, alcohol has been used as a sedative. A previous study by this researcher summarized the use of alcohol and OTC drugs by rural elderly women. This exploratory study was designed to examine the use of alcohol and OTC medications used as sleep aids by urban women over the age of 85.

METHODS

A structured interview was used to administer a two-part questionnaire for this study. Part 1 of the instrument assessed demographic data and information about general health. Part 2 of the instrument addressed sleep patterns, alcohol and OTC medication use to improve sleep, awareness of hazards associated with these substances, and the reasons for seeking health care for sleep problems. Subjects were 155 volunteer women ranging in age from 85 to 99, with a mean age of 90.3, who lived in an urban center in the western United States.

RESULTS

All participants reported at least one chronic illness, with arthritis, vision loss, and hearing impairment the most commonly reported conditions. The average number of medications taken each day was 1.8 (range 1 to 4), with 57% (n = 89) using prescription medication daily. Analgesics, antiinflammatories, and sedatives or tranquilizers were the most commonly used prescription medications used daily. All respondents reported difficulty sleeping. The majority of women (n = 130, 84%) used alcohol regularly, with 91 (70%) indicating they had a drink before bedtime. Of the women who used alcohol before bedtime, 77 (85%) also used OTC medication, and 33 combined alcohol and OTC medications each night. When asked about hazards associated with the use of alcohol, OTC medications, or both for sleep, 129 (83%) were unable to describe any.

IMPLICATIONS

This study supports the finding that the elderly complain of difficulty sleeping. This suggests that nurses working with elderly women should anticipate this as a problem, assess for it, and teach patients about appropriate strategies for inducing sleep. The lack of knowledge of possible hazards associated with mixing alcohol and OTC medications suggests that health care providers may not be screening elderly women for drug and alcohol use or may not be teaching enough about OTC medications. Finally, interviews with these volunteers indicated several teaching needs, such as risks associated with alcohol use and antiinflammatory drugs, and alcohol and sedatives or tranquilizers.

CRITICAL THINKING: Alcohol will induce sleep, but the quality of sleep may be worse. What are some of the objective and subjective patient problems associated with the sleep that follows alcohol consumption? What are other strategies a nurse could suggest to a patient who identifies trouble sleeping? What questions would you use in assessing possible difficulties in sleeping?

---

such as eye fatigue, tearing, redness, or the itching and stinging associated with allergic or chemical conjunctivitis. The products are sold as eyewashes, artificial tears, and decongestants. Conditions involving marked eye pain or blurred vision require attention by a physician.

All OTC ophthalmic products must be clear, odorless, colorless, and sterile solutions with a pH and tonicity similar to that of natural tears. They must also contain preservatives to help maintain sterility. Sterility cannot be maintained indefinitely, however, and bacterial contamination may be transferred to the eye if cloudy, discolored, or outdated solutions are used.

OTC ophthalmic products contain a variety of nonmedicinal ingredients. Tonicity adjusters (e.g., dextran, glycerin) prevent excessive tearing that can dilute and wash away active ingredients. Antioxidants and stabilizers (sodium bisulfite, metabisulfite) prevent the chemical alteration of the ingredients. Buffers (e.g., boric acid) maintain the pH of the solution within a range of 6 to 8. Solutions of higher or lower pH may irritate the eyes. Wetting agents (polysorbate 80) reduce surface tension. Preservatives (e.g., benzalkonium chloride) prevent bacterial growth. Viscosity-increasing agents (gelatin, polyethylene glycol) spread the solution over the eye.

Decongestant ophthalmic products contain a sympathomimetic drug (hydrochloride forms of ephedrine, naphazoline, phenylephrine, or tetrahydrozoline). Local application of one of these drugs to the eye promptly relieves the symptoms of allergic conjunctivitis. By constricting dilated blood vessels in the white of the eye, they also relieve the bloodshot look and restore the normal white color to the eyes. Sympathomimetic drugs also stimulate the adrenergic receptors affecting pupillary size and may cause dilation of pupils (mydriasis). Therefore these products should not be used by persons with narrow-angle glaucoma.

Problems may occur with decongestant ophthalmic products. Rebound congestion can occur by the same mechanism as described previously for topical nasal decongestants. It can be minimized or avoided by using the medicine only occasionally and strictly according to directions. In addition, these products will be ineffective if the cause of the symptoms is within the eyeball. The medicine may mask a bacterial infection.

Acne Medications

Acne vulgaris often afflicts adolescents. For them, prevention and treatment of even mild attacks of the disease, with its unsightly pimples and scars, are given high priority. The pimples and skin eruptions of acne are called comedones. They contain sebum, which is produced by the sebaceous glands of the hair follicles, and epithelial cells shed by the infundibulum of the follicle. Acne is associated with excessive production of sebum, which impairs the normal washout of infundibular cells as they are shed. The cells become compacted and plug the follicle, which then becomes distended with accumulated sebum and cells. The condition is relieved by removal of the plug by lancing the comedone or by the natural growth of the hair, which brings the plug to the surface. This form of acne, called noninflammatory, is not usually associated with scarring. Scarring is more likely to occur with the inflammatory form of the disease, which is characterized by pustule formation and local inflammation. In the inflammatory form, comedones do not open at the skin surface to relieve the pressure within the hair follicle. An inflamed follicle may rupture beneath the skin surface and spread sebum, cells, and bacteria to surrounding tissues. Noninflammatory acne can be treated with OTC products, but inflammatory acne should be referred to a physician.

External factors may contribute to the development of acne. These factors include personal hygiene, diet, and self-image. Personal hygiene combats excessive skin oiliness, but compulsive and vigorous cleansing of the skin has not proved to be more effective in preventing acne than normal washing. Because bacterial infection is not ordinarily associated with acne, the use of antibacterial soaps and antiseptic solutions is neither necessary nor recommended.

The role of diet in acne is controversial. Chocolate has long been condemned as a causative factor, but there is no evidence of a cause-and-effect relationship between chocolate and acne. Similarly, evidence does not support the need for dietary restrictions of sweets, nuts, and greasy foods. Until a clearer understanding of acne and its cause emerges, individual trial and error with diet, hygiene, and other factors should neither be excluded nor discouraged.

Desquamating Agents

Noninflammatory acne is treated symptomatically. Treatment consists of removing excess sebum from the skin by washing and promoting the production and turnover of new skin to prevent closure of the pilosebaceous orifices of the hair follicle. The skin should be washed with warm water, mild soap, and a soft washcloth, no more than three times daily. The washing and rubbing produce some drying and peeling of the skin. Closure of the pilosebaceous orifices can be prevented by the topical application of mildly irritating agents, which promote desquamation (peeling) and stimulate growth of new skin cells.

OTC desquamating agents include sulfur (2% to 10%), resorcinol (1% to 4%), and salicylic acid (0.5% to 2%). Resorcinol and salicylic acid often appear in alcoholic solutions that dry quickly and do not leave a visible film. Some products contain all three agents. Dosage forms of these drugs include creams, lotions, gels, and liquids. Ointment bases tend to be greasy and messy. Some soaps include desquamating agents, but this formulation is irrational because rinsing and drying remove the agents from the skin.

Benzoyl peroxide is a stronger irritant and desquamating agent than is sulfur, resorcinol, or salicylic acid. Used in concentrations of 5% to 10%, it generally produces mild stinging and warming of the skin. For most acne problems, benzoyl peroxide is probably no more effective than the milder agents and should be used only after the milder irritants and faithful adherence to a regular skin-washing schedule have been unsuccessful. Benzoyl peroxide is highly irritating and should not contact the eyelids, neck, or lips. Its use should be discontinued if severe and prolonged stinging or irritation occurs.

More serious forms of acne require treatment with medications available only by prescription. Antibiotics may be used topically or orally in small doses. Isotretinoin may be effective in severe cases when the patient is unresponsive to other therapy.

Sunscreen Products

The sun emits principally two types of ultraviolet radiation, UVA and UVB. UVA radiation causes tanning of the skin. UVB radiation causes sunburn. Sunburn occurs when UVB radiation damages small blood vessels in the skin, causing them to become leaky and congested. Many people incorrectly consider sunburn a harmless, although painful, price to pay for a seasonal tan.

UVA radiation tans the skin by stimulating production of the dark pigment, melanin. The darkness of the tan depends on how much melanin is produced. People who do not tan easily do not produce enough melanin. Melanin absorbs UVA and UVB radiation and protects the skin from harmful effects of ultraviolet radiation. Naturally dark skin contains more melanin than pale skin and is correspondingly better protected.

The harmful effects of ultraviolet radiation can be serious, permanent, and potentially life-threatening. These effects, including premature aging and wrinkling of the skin and skin cancer, occur after years of repeated exposure and may occur without significant episodes of sunburn. Sunscreens diminish the harmful consequences of ultraviolet radiation by absorbing or reflecting it. Used correctly, they prevent sunburn and premature aging of the skin and reduce the risk of skin cancer. Chemical sunscreens selectively absorb and screen out most of the harmful burning radiation but permit tanning radiation to reach the skin. Physical sunscreens scatter and reflect all ultraviolet radiation. They prevent sunburn well, but they also prevent tanning.

Twenty-one chemical sunscreens have been approved by the FDA. Those most commonly available include aminobenzoic acid, cinoxate, homosalate, menthyl anthranilate, oxybenzone, and padimate O. Sunscreen products may contain one or several of these agents. Physical sunscreens include titanium oxide and zinc oxide in ointments and creams. They are intended for complete coverage of small areas of sunburn-prone skin such as the nose and lips.

Not all suntan products contain sunscreens. Some contain cosmetically appealing but otherwise inactive ingredients such as cocoa butter, mineral oil, and lanolin. None of these ingredients prevents sunburn or promotes tanning.

Some drugs, cosmetics, and soaps sensitize a person's skin to ultraviolet radiation and cause it to burn more easily than usual. Examples of such photosensitizing drugs include tetracycline antibiotics (see Chapter 47) and diuretics (see Chapter 14). Photosensitivity reactions are triggered by UVA radiation. Most sunscreens absorb little, if any, of this radiation and will not prevent it. Those that do block UVA radiation include menthyl anthranilate and oxybenzone.

The effectiveness of sunscreens is rated by the **sun protection factor (SPF)**, which is listed on the product label. The SPF relates the amount of time it takes a person to get a mild sunburn without sunscreen protection to the time required after a sunscreen has been applied to the exposed skin. For example, skin that ordinarily burns after 30 minutes of exposure to the sun will, if treated with a sunscreen with an SPF of 4, be able to stay in the sun for 2 hours (4 times as long) before it burns to the same degree. A sunscreen with an SPF of 8 protects 8 times as long (4 hours). Products with SPFs greater than 8 screen out tanning and burning radiation. Therefore persons who desire a tan should not use a sunscreen with an SPF higher than 8. Products with higher SPF values (some go as high as 50) screen out nearly all tanning and burning radiation. These products offer approximately equal protection from the radiation and differ only in the length of time that they allow a person to stay exposed to the sun. In some cases the higher SPF is of marginal value. For example, a sunscreen with an SPF of 15 would let someone who normally burns in 60 minutes stay in the sun for 15 hours. This would extend the time of protection into the night.

The choice of SPF depends on how easily a person burns or tans. The FDA recommends products with an SPF of 8 or more for people who always burn and never tan, 6 to 7 for those who always burn and seldom tan, 4 to 5 for those who burn moderately and tan gradually, 2 to 3 for those who burn minimally and always tan well, and 2 for those who rarely burn and tan profusely.

Sunscreens should be applied at least 30 minutes before each exposure to the sun to allow the chemicals time to penetrate the skin. Some products, such as aminobenzoic acid, should be applied 1 to 2 hours before exposure. No sunscreen or suntan product will promote a deeper tan than a person's skin can naturally produce. If skin does not readily produce melanin, it will never tan as well as skin that readily produces the pigment.

Topical Antiinfective Drugs

Serious infections of the skin require systemic antiinfective agents that are available by prescription. In certain situations, minor infections of the skin may respond to topical application of agents directly at the site of infection. Drugs used in this way tend to be too toxic for systemic use, but in the small doses used topically they are safe enough to be available without a prescription.

Antifungal Products

Several common tineal (fungal) infections of the skin generally respond to self-medication with OTC products, although responsiveness depends on the strain of fungus, the site of infection, and the severity and duration of the infection. Microorganisms most often responsible for superficial tineal infections in humans are *Trichophyton*, *Microsporum*, *Epidermophyton*, and *Candida* species. OTC products are effective only for acute superficial infections. Chronic and extensive infections respond slowly, if at all, and often require the attention of a physician. Fungal infections of the toenails or fingernails and those that have penetrated the hair shafts generally respond poorly to OTC antifungal products. The nurse should exercise care in selecting or recommending OTC antifungal medications. If the condition involves an apparent tineal infection of the foot (athlete's foot), groin, or scalp, reasonably rapid results can be expected from OTC products. Patients with suspected fungal infections of other body regions should be referred to a physician.

OTC antifungal preparations include keratolytic agents, fungistatic agents, and fungicides. Keratolytic preparations include selenium sulfide and Whitfield's ointment (containing benzoic acid [6%] and salicylic acid [3%]). These agents irritate the skin and cause peeling of the superficial layers to expose deeper sites of infection to other antifungal compounds. Selenium sulfide stops cellular growth when it is applied in concentrations of 1% to 2%. It is a common and effective ingredient in antidandruff preparations.

Fungistatic agents include fatty acids and salicylanilide. Sodium propionate and undecylenic acid are fungistatic fatty acids. Sodium propionate is effective in 1% solution and 5% ointment. Undecylenate is effective as the acid (5%) and as the zinc salt (20%). It is commonly used as an ointment, powder, or spray for the relief of athlete's foot.

The fungicidal drug tolnaftate is effective against most superficial fungal infections except *Candida* species. Tolnaftate is sold as powder, liquid, cream, spray, or gel (all 1%). Relief of itching occurs within several days, but complete suppression of the infection generally requires 2 to 3 weeks of treatment. If the skin is rough and scaly, prior treatment with a keratolytic agent to remove the scales improves the effectiveness of tolnaftate.

Antibacterial Products

The antibacterial drugs available without a prescription include bacitracin, neomycin, polymyxin B, tetracycline, chlortetracycline, and oxytetracycline. The FDA OTC Panel on Antimicrobial Drugs recognizes skin-wound antibiotics and skin-wound protectants. The former includes products for the treatment of overt skin infections; the latter refers to products with antibiotics added to prevent the subsequent infection of a wound and the growth of organisms in the product. All OTC antibiotics sold as skin-wound antibiotics were classified in category III. All but neomycin were classified in category I for use as skin-wound protectants.

When used as directed, the OTC topical antibiotics are generally safe. However, their low concentration in the available products makes their effectiveness against skin-wound infections questionable. Bacitracin, neomycin sulfate, and polymyxin B sulfate are nephrotoxic if absorbed systemically. With ordinary topical use, such toxicity is rare. In view of the questionable topical efficacy of the drugs and their potential toxicity, their use is not recommended.

Hemorrhoidal Products

Environment, heredity, and posture have contributed to the incidence of a number of painful anorectal disorders, the most prevalent of which is hemorrhoids. Hemorrhoids are varicosities produced by increased pressure in the hemorrhoidal veins. Upright posture, hypertension, coughing, pregnancy and labor, physical exertion, straining during defecation, and rectal carcinoma can contribute to hemorrhoids. These varicosities, which can occur within or outside the anorectal line, are associated with itching, burning, inflammation, and swelling. Mild pain and discomfort are common; however, bleeding, prolapse of an internal hemorrhoid, and severe chronic pain require the attention of a physician.

OTC products for treating anorectal disorders are intended for the symptomatic relief of pain, itching, and burning. They contain a variety of pharmacologic agents, including local anesthetics, vasoconstrictors, antiseptics, astringents, emollients or lubricants, keratolytics, anticholinergics, and a variety of miscellaneous agents such as counterirritants and wound-healing agents.

The FDA OTC Panel on Hemorrhoidal Drug Products has ruled on the efficacy of these agents. Antiseptics, wound healers, and anticholinergics all have been classified as category II (ineffective) hemorrhoidal products. Local anesthetics have been judged effective for relief of the itching and burning of hemorrhoids. Of the many local anesthetics available, only two are safe and effective: benzocaine (5% to 20%) and pramoxine hydrochloride (1%). Ephedrine sulfate, epinephrine hydrochloride, and phenylephrine hydrochloride are vasoconstrictor drugs that have been judged effective for the symptomatic relief of hemorrhoidal itching and swelling, although conclusive evidence of effectiveness

on swollen hemorrhoidal tissue itself is lacking. Presumably, the vasoconstrictor drugs directly constrict the vascular smooth muscle in the anorectal area.

A variety of emollients or lubricants (protectants) have been recommended for use in hemorrhoidal preparations. These include calamine, cocoa butter, cod liver oil, glycerin, mineral oil, petrolatum, shark liver oil, and zinc oxide. All can be administered to the rectum externally and internally except glycerin, which is intended for external use only. Petrolatum may be the most effective of these agents. To be effective, the total protectant concentration of an OTC hemorrhoidal product should be 50%.

Mildly keratolytic agents such as aluminum chlorhydroxy allantoinate relieve the itching and burning of hemorrhoids. Their usefulness is confined to the external anal tissues. Stronger agents, such as resorcinol and sulfur, are not recommended.

Astringents coagulate skin cell protein, thereby protecting underlying skin cells from dehydration and irritation. Calamine, zinc oxide, and hamamelis water (witch hazel) have been judged effective for the relief of hemorrhoidal itching, irritation, and pain. Calamine and zinc oxide may be applied externally or internally to anorectal tissue, whereas hamamelis water is for external use only. Antiseptics are no more effective than washing with soap and water for the prevention of anorectal infections. Antiseptics may adversely alter the normal bacterial flora in that region.

Anticholinergic drugs (e.g., atropine; see Chapter 11) are of dubious value in OTC hemorrhoidal preparations. These drugs are not absorbed through the skin and, if applied to the external anal tissues, do not relieve itching or pain. They can be absorbed across the rectal mucosa, however, and in sufficient dosage can interfere with autonomic nerve function throughout the body. There is no evidence that a local or systemic anticholinergic effect is of any value in treating hemorrhoids.

A counterirritant drug distracts from the discomfort of itching, irritation, and pain by stimulating local nerve endings to provide a sensation of warmth, tingling, or coolness. Counterirritation forms the therapeutic basis for the relief of minor muscle aches and pain by OTC remedies that provide deep-heating and penetrating warmth. These remedies do not directly affect muscles. Instead, their effects are localized to the skin, where they stimulate local sensory nerve endings. However, because no sensory nerves occur in the rectal mucosa, there is no rational basis for including a counterirritant in an internal hemorrhoidal preparation. A counterirritant may provide temporary relief of pain and itching if applied externally to the anorectal region. Menthol is the only recommended counterirritant for external hemorrhoidal preparations.

Wound-healing agents include an extract of brewer's yeast, skin respiratory factor (SRF), cod liver oil, and vitamins A and D. No convincing evidence of their effectiveness as wound healers exists; until such evidence emerges, their value in treating hemorrhoids is questionable.

OTC products for the treatment of hemorrhoids and other mild anorectal disorders are provided in a variety of dosage forms, including ointments, creams, suppositories, pads, and foams. Ointments (oil base), creams (water soluble), and gels are equally effective in delivering active ingredients to the affected areas. Devices such as the pile pipe, a tube having lateral exit ports, are useful for applying the medication directly into the rectum. Suppositories are not particularly useful for the treatment of hemorrhoids. They may slip beyond the affected site, releasing their active ingredients in contact with healthy mucosa. In addition, with suppositories the degree of coverage of the affected area may be erratic and cannot be controlled. Finally, relief of painful symptoms is delayed with suppositories because suppositories must melt to release their active ingredients. Foams provide no advantages over ointments or creams and foams are much more messy to use.

Personal hygiene and normal bowel habits are important in the successful treatment of hemorrhoids. Many physicians recommend taking sitz baths or soaking with astringent solutions as an adjunct to the use of OTC products for the relief of mild itching and burning sensations. In addition, the diet should be adjusted to avoid either excessively loose or compact stools.

Nursing Process Overview

Over-the-Counter Drugs

OTC, or nonprescription, drugs and herbal remedies do not form a major part of the clinical responsibilities of the practicing nurse. Nevertheless, the nurse is often sought as a source of information on these agents. The following presentation is one suggestion for a method of patient counseling about nonprescription medications.

Assessment

Because the patient is involved in self-care, assist the individual to clearly state what condition or symptoms are to be treated. For example, if the individual is seeking a medication to treat the symptoms of a cold, lead the person to consider exactly what symptoms require treatment. For some persons a cough might be the most outstanding symptom, whereas for others it might be nasal congestion or headache.

Nursing Diagnoses

Knowledge deficit related to not knowing how to self-medicate for minor health problems.

Patient Outcomes

The patient will have symptomatic relief of the problem being treated, with no side effects.

Planning/Implementation

After leading the patient to define exactly what symptoms are to be treated, teach the patient what types of medications are available to treat these symptoms. Suggest that fixed combinations of ingredients are more difficult to use because dosages are impossible to regulate for each component of the combination. More control may be gained by using single agents at appropriate doses as necessary for defined symptoms. Suggest other sources of information about nonprescription drugs, such as the pharmacist.

Evaluation

Effectiveness of the treatment is evaluated by the patient involved in self-care. If the patient seeks advice because therapy is unsuccessful, have the patient consider whether the proper medication was administered for the symptom to be controlled and if the correct dose was used.

Nursing Implications Summary

General Guidelines: OTC Drugs

➤ If asked about OTC remedies, first assess the patient. What symptoms or problems require treatment? What has the patient used successfully in the past?

➤ Remember that many patients do not consider drugs purchased without a prescription as true drugs; that is, if questioned about medications they are taking, they may not think to include OTC preparations.

➤ As a part of assessment, ask specifically about medicine purchased at the drugstore or health food store. It may be helpful to include some leading questions such as "Do you take any cold medicines, cough syrups, vitamins, or other medicines that you can buy without a prescription?" or "Do you use any herbal remedies?" It may also help to know of local health problems or habits. For example, in an area where there are frequent high pollen counts, causing frequent allergy problems, ask questions about allergies and what the patient uses to relieve allergy symptoms.

➤ In asking how a patient uses OTC drugs, try to frame questions in a nonjudgmental way to learn about actual use patterns. Most patients want to use medications correctly and will welcome instruction about drug use but not if they feel defensive about their current practices.

Nursing in the Community

➤ Point out to patients that many OTC preparations contain multiple drugs. Encourage patients to consider purchasing products that contain only the drug needed. This may be difficult because the ingredients for a product may

Continued

Nursing Implications Summary—cont'd

be listed in generic names, which are not usually familiar to patients.

➤ Ideally, the nurse would accompany the patient to the drugstore and review product labeling during the instruction. In the absence of this possibility, suggest that the patient talk over the medication needs with the pharmacist. In addition, the pharmacist can help the patient choose the least expensive but most effective product available at that store.

➤ If visiting the patient's home, ask to see the boxes or containers for OTC medications and herbal remedies. Read the packaging and use it as a basis for teaching the patient.

➤ Talking about OTC drug use may provide the ideal opportunity to review general safe practices regarding drug use (see Box 4-2 on safe medication use [p. 38]).

➤ Suggest that the patient periodically look over all the medications in the house and discard those that look discolored or crumbled or that have passed the expiration date. Emphasize to patients the need to discard medications in a way that children or animals cannot find them and take them. Small amounts of liquids can be poured down the sink or toilet, and a few remaining tablets or capsules can be flushed also. If there is a large quantity of medication, consider checking with a local pharmacy or poison control center for guidance about proper disposal.

➤ Encourage patients who are not obtaining relief from appropriate OTC medications to seek medical care for the problem.

CHAPTER REVIEW

Application

1. The present laws that regulate the OTC drug industry have evolved from which law?
2. What classes of drugs did the Durham-Humphrey Amendment to the 1938 law create?
3. What does the Kefauver-Harris amendment to the 1938 law require?
4. How do the Federal Food and Drug Laws distinguish between herbal and conventional OTC remedies?
5. What are the categories used by FDA review panels on OTC drugs to classify drugs?
6. List the advantages and disadvantages of fixed-ratio combination drug products.
7. Which analgesics are available without a prescription?
8. What are the ingredients of OTC cold remedies?
9. What are the major side effects of antihistaminic drugs?
10. What are the OTC expectorant drugs?
11. What are the available OTC cough suppressants?
12. What drugs are available in OTC sleeping aids?
13. What are the classes of ingredients in OTC ophthalmic products?
14. What precautions should be exercised in the use of OTC ophthalmic products? How might you teach patients about these precautions?
15. What are the commonly available OTC drugs for treatment of acne?
16. What is the difference between chemical and physical sunscreens?
17. What is sun protection factor (SPF)?
18. OTC antifungal products include which drugs?
19. What is the difference between keratolytic, fungistatic, and fungicidal drugs?
20. Which antibiotics are currently available in OTC preparations?
21. What are the ingredients of OTC hemorrhoidal products and what are their actions?

Critical Thinking

1. A friend twists her ankle playing tennis and asks you what medication she should take for pain. What factors should you consider in advising her?
2. What factors should you consider in choosing a cold remedy?
3. You have a cold and bad cough. What factors should you consider in buying a cold remedy and cough suppressant?
4. Give some examples of situations in which an analgesic should be used at bedtime.
5. How do you advise a male client who says he thinks he has an enlarged prostate gland and asks if he should use an herbal remedy that was recommended for this condition on television?
6. Your roommate is distressed by her acne. She is willing to let you advise her. Develop a plan to treat her acne.
7. In addition to applying sunscreen, what other measures can be used to limit skin exposure to the sun?
8. Develop a plan of care that includes nonmedication measures to treat hemorrhoids in a pregnant woman.

Chapter 8

Issues of Drug Abuse

OBJECTIVES

After studying this chapter, you should be able to do the following:

- *Define drug use, misuse, abuse, and dependence.*
- *Identify the characteristics of an individual that may increase the risk of drug abuse.*
- *Identify the characteristics of drugs that may increase the potential for drug abuse.*
- *Recognize why certain drugs are attractive to specific individuals.*
- *Describe current drug abuse treatment modalities.*
- *Describe medications that are used in withdrawal and treatment.*
- *Apply the nursing process to care of patients who abuse drugs.*

CHAPTER OVERVIEW

This chapter defines drug use, misuse, abuse, and dependence. Drug abuse is described in terms of risk factors for the individual and the abuse potential of specific drugs. The most commonly used drugs are discussed, including prescription drugs and alcohol. Current concepts of treatment and medications used in treatment and withdrawal are described.

OVERVIEW OF DRUG ABUSE

This chapter focuses on substances that are commonly used and abused, including legal drugs, such as prescription medications, alcohol, and tobacco, and illegal or illicit drugs, such as marijuana and cocaine. All drugs have the potential for abuse.

Nurses encounter patients with a variety of conditions. Often the physical or mental condition is related, directly or indirectly, to drug abuse. It is important that nurses routinely assess drug use/abuse in an initial workup and continue to consider its possibility throughout their care of the client. When drug abuse is part of the health care problem and is not addressed, care is incomplete, increasing the likelihood of recurrence. Underlying drug abuse may be a factor in as many as 40% of hospital admissions.

Current Definitions: Drug Abuse and Drug Dependence

Differentiating between drug misuse, abuse, and dependence is not simple. It is based on patterns of use, such as amount and frequency. Defining these terms is complicated by legal definitions. By legal definition, any use of an illicit or illegal drug is considered abuse. In health care the effects of drugs on the body and on the behavior of the individual are the concern.

Drug use occurs on a continuum from experimentation, infrequent use, regular use, abuse with resulting health and social problems, and dependence characterized by loss of control. Both drug abuse and drug dependence are diagnostic terms defined by the American Psychiatric Association's *Diagnostic and Statistical Manual (DSM)*. The current version, *DSM-IV*, identifies the abused drug of choice as part of the diagnosis.

Drug abuse occurs when the individual's drug use becomes problematic, causing social and personal difficulties that stem from the drug use.

Diagnostic criteria for drug abuse are evaluated during a 12-month period. The patient's impairment must involve one or more of the following: (1) failure to fulfill major role obligations at work, school, or home; (2) use in physically hazardous situations; (3) recurrent substance-related legal problems; or (4) use despite persistent or recurrent social or interpersonal problems as a result of use.

Drug dependence is diagnosed when physiologic effects appear and/or when loss of control over the drug and its use becomes increasingly apparent.

Diagnostic criteria for drug dependence include the presence of at least three of the following factors within a 12-month period: (1) tolerance; (2) withdrawal; (3) substance taken in larger amount or longer period than intended; (4) persistent, unsuccessful efforts to cut down; (5) an increased amount of time spent procuring, using, or recovering from the effects of the substance; (6) other previously important activities are avoided or reduced because of substance use; and/or (7) continued use despite knowledge of a problem.

Use and abuse are complicated by legal issues. Some drugs are legal, whereas others are illegal. Both legal and illegal drugs can be used to meet the criteria for abuse or dependence. Some drugs such as tobacco and alcohol are legal for persons who meet certain criteria, such as age. Legality is not a diagnosis, but legal difficulties are one criterion for a diagnosis. In addition, legal problems can be an external condition that encourages the individual to recognize the problem and seek treatment. For example, legal difficulties such as repeatedly driving under the influence of drugs, particularly alcohol, can result in a drunk-driving charge, and the individual may be given a choice between incarceration or treatment. A charge of possession of an illegal drug also can result in individuals recognizing how out of control their use is.

Risk Factors for Drug Abuse

The common neuroanatomic link underlying addiction lies in a small cluster of brain neurons called the nucleus accumbens. These neurons release the neurotransmitter dopamine. Drugs causing addiction share the property of causing the release of dopamine by the nucleus accumbens. The entire neural network is called the mesolimbic reward system. Addiction results from a combination of dopamine rush in the mesolimbic reward system and other complex neural actions governing behavior.

Not everyone who experiments with a drug develops personal and social complications or loses control of drug use. Why this happens to some individuals and not to others is a question that is not fully understood and the topic of much research. When this question is better answered, both prevention and treatment of drug abuse will benefit.

Although no one knows exactly who will develop a drug abuse problem, some characteristics of those who are at higher risk for abuse have been identified. Individual risk factors for drug abuse can be categorized as genetic, environmental, or a combination of the two.

Genetic Risk Factors

Research has identified that one risk factor for drug abuse is a family history of abuse, particularly by a mother, father, or sibling. The genetic component of alcohol abuse in particular has been well documented with twin and adoption studies. For instance, either twin with alcoholism in the biologic family background is more likely to become alcohol dependent when adopted into a nondrinking environment than either twin with no alcoholism in the biologic family background adopted into a drinking environment. Genetic risk is greater than environmental risk.

Environmental Risk Factors

The family environment is a major risk factor for drug abuse. A child who grows up with a drug-abusing parent receives both role modeling and interpersonal experiences that may promote eventual drug abuse either during adolescence or adulthood. Family relationships are distorted to accommodate the drug-abusing parent.

Coping skills are another modifier of risk. These skills reflect how an individual adapts his or her behavior in response to demands. Ineffective coping or coping strategies overwhelmed by stress are a major risk factor for drug abuse. Drugs are often used as a temporary measure to decrease the psychologic discomfort caused by high stress or poor coping strategies. This situation is promoted in our society by advertising that features alcohol and nicotine as a means of coping with stress. Individuals who model this behavior put themselves at risk for abuse by managing stress indirectly through drugs rather than directly through constructive action to decrease stress and cope.

Personal crises are a risk factor. Coping skills are tested during situational or maturational crises. Situational crises are those that result from specific stressors such as job loss, divorce, and death. Maturational crises are a result of reaching new development stages such as adolescence or young adulthood. These situational crises increase the risk for drug use and abuse when used to decrease the pressure, stress, or emotional pain. Sometimes the health care system facilitates abuse. For example, stress may produce physiologic symptoms for which a health care provider prescribes a minor tranquilizer. This type of drug is subject to abuse when used over an extended time in place of learning new and more effective coping strategies.

Ready access to drugs is another risk factor. Drug abuse by health care professionals is a source of professional and societal concern. Licensed health care professions have become increasingly active in identifying and addressing substance abuse among their members in recent years. For nurses, in particular, some of the risk factors for substance abuse include a family history of substance abuse, a history of health problems, and a history of depression. The availability of drugs and a professional culture in which a drug is offered for every problem encourage nurses to self-medicate, thereby increasing their risk of abuse. Nurses recovering from drug dependence often say that their use began with prescription pain medications for an injury and progressed to abuse and dependence. Many professional organizations now sponsor peer assistance organizations that help identify substance abuse and resources for treatment, and monitor the professional on return to employment.

GENERAL CHARACTERISTICS OF ABUSED DRUGS

Drugs that produce a pleasurable effect, such as an elevated mood, euphoria, or a calming effect, are most likely to be abused. Drugs that do not produce a mood-altering effect are rarely intentionally abused. One exception is anabolic steroids, which are abused because of their muscle-building effects.

The National Institute of Drug Abuse sponsors the National Household Survey of Drug Use, which contacts randomly selected households in the United States to provide comprehensive information on current drug use in the United States. The data in Table 8-1 describe drug use during the month before the 1997 survey. The table graphically indicates that the most widely used drugs in 1997 were alcohol and nicotine and the most widely used illegal drug was marijuana. Of the subjects, 6% claimed illicit use of a drug in the previous month, and a little over 1% stated that they had used psychotherapeutic drugs in a nonmedical manner in the previous month. The survey did not include caffeine.

Route of Administration

In general, the more rapidly a route delivers the substance to the brain, the greater the effect and the higher the addictive potential of the drug. For example, cocaine powder is usually taken intranasally (snorted), and crack cocaine is smoked. Although the nasal mucosa is highly vascular and snorting allows rapid blood-brain transfer, inhalation is a faster route. This shorter time appears to be a factor in the highly addictive nature of nicotine in cigarettes.

The route of administration may be of particular concern in its own right. One example is intravenous (IV) drug use with its danger of spreading infection, particularly human immunodeficiency virus (HIV)/acquired immunodeficiency syndrome (AIDS), when IV materials are shared. IV use also exposes the individual to cellulitis and scarred or sclerosed veins. Ingestion of alcohol often causes damage to the gastrointestinal tract. The intranasal use of cocaine can cause deterioration of the nasal septum. These pathologic signs provide external clues to drug use.

Table 8-1	Drug Use in the United States in the Month Preceding the National Household Survey of Drug Use, 1997
Drug Use	**All Ages over 12 years (%)**
Any illicit use	6.4
Any illicit drugs other than marijuana	2.6
Nonmedical use of any psychotherapeutic	1.2
Alcohol	51.8
Binge Drinking	14.9
Nicotine—cigarettes	29.6
Nicotine—smokeless tobacco	3.2
Marijuana/hashish	5.1
Total cocaine	0.7
Crack cocaine	0.3
Analgesics	0.7
Inhalants	0.4
Stimulants	0.3
Tranquilizers	0.4
Hallucinogens	0.8
Sedatives	0.1
Phencyclidine (PCP)	0.1
Heroin	0.2

Data from Substance Abuse and Mental Health Services Administration, Office of Applied Studies; Table 5B at URL: http//www.samhsa.gov/oas.

Tolerance

Tolerance concerns the effect of the drug on the body over time. Tolerance has occurred when it takes increasing amounts of the drug to achieve the same physiologic or psychologic effect. Although tolerance is particularly characteristic of opiates, prolonged use of alcohol, barbiturates, and benzodiazepines also leads to tolerance.

Cross-tolerance describes a physiologic characteristic in which developing a tolerance to one drug also increases the tolerance to a related category of drugs. Tolerance to alcohol, a central nervous system (CNS) depressant, results in cross-tolerance to other CNS depressants such as benzodiazepines and many anesthetic agents. The tolerant individual may require a higher dosage of anesthesia to achieve the desired level of surgical anesthesia. This is one reason why it is important to have a thorough drug history before any care is given.

Withdrawal

Drugs that produce tolerance, a physiologic change caused by the presence of the drug, also produce symptoms when the drug is withdrawn, particularly when it is withdrawn abruptly. **Withdrawal** symptoms are characteristic of the drug class and are often the opposite of the drug's action. Alcohol, a CNS depressant, produces withdrawal symptoms characterized by hyperactivity. Conversely, when cocaine, a CNS stimulant, is withdrawn, one of the effects is depression and a loss of feeling and pleasure. These withdrawal effects are neurologic rebound effects; because the neurons have adjusted their neurotransmitters to the presence of the drug, when the drug is withdrawn, the body overproduces neurotransmitters or lacks the balancing effect of the drug. The withdrawal symptoms characteristic of alcohol, benzodiazepines, and barbiturates are the most dangerous and require careful monitoring. Individuals vary greatly in their potential for and range of withdrawal symptoms.

Dependence

Physical dependence follows tolerance when the lack of the drug produces withdrawal symptoms. Physiologic dependence was once considered the essential factor in drug dependence; however, recent *DSM* criteria recognize both physical and psychologic characteristics in a diagnosis of drug dependence.

Psychologic dependence describes the psychologic need to continue drug use. Psychologic tolerance is the individual's psychologic attachment to the drug, including the behaviors surrounding acquiring and using the drug and the feeling state accompanying use. This complex set of feelings and behaviors is reinforced through use and experience with the drug, and these behaviors make giving up drug use more difficult. Psychologic dependence is often related to the use of the drug to reduce stress, which eventually becomes the only means of stress reduction. As an understanding of neurophysiology and neurotransmitters increases, the boundary between physical and psychologic dependence blurs.

CHARACTERISTICS OF SPECIFIC DRUGS

The major characteristics of commonly abused drugs are summarized in Table 8-2.

▼ caffeine

Caffeine may be the most widely abused drug in the United States, although the effects of this abuse are much less obvi-

ous and are usually less harmful than those produced by other abused drugs. Caffeine abuse often takes place unwittingly. Consider the following example:

> John has a cup of coffee while dressing in the morning and a second cup at breakfast. At work he consumes another cup of coffee at the 10:30 AM coffee break. At lunch John drinks two glasses of iced tea. During his afternoon coffee break, he has a chocolate bar and a cola. Before he leaves work, John takes two Excedrin for a headache. At dinner he drinks two cups of tea. Before bed John takes two more Excedrin. Why is John unable to sleep? John cannot sleep because he ingested about 1 g of caffeine during this typical day.

Most people are aware of the caffeine content of coffee, which ranges from 80 to 150 mg per cup. Less well known is the fact that tea, colas, chocolate, and some nonprescription medications (e.g., Excedrin) also contain caffeine. In the example given, John took more than $\frac{1}{2}$ g of caffeine in these forms.

Ingestion of more than 500 mg of caffeine daily produces a variety of CNS effects and cardiovascular reactions. Irritability or nervousness is a common complaint, along with sleep disturbances. Patients may report heart palpitations or say that their heart is "racing." These descriptions may suggest premature ventricular contractions and tachycardia, common symptoms of chronic caffeine toxicity. Diarrhea and gastrointestinal irritation often accompany chronic overdosage with caffeine. Patients complaining of symptoms such as these should be questioned about their caffeine intake. The person taking the history should ask specifically about individual beverages, foods, and medications that contain caffeine to make an accurate estimate of intake. The caffeine content of commonly ingested substances is presented in Table 8-3.

Whether true psychologic dependence on caffeine can occur is questionable, but many people have great difficulty in eliminating caffeine from their diet. Nevertheless, patients with peptic ulcer disease should avoid caffeine. Pregnant

Table 8-2	**Major Characteristics of Commonly Abused Drugs**					
Drug	Primary Route(s)	Dependency		Desired Effect	Withdrawal Effect	Treatment
		Physiologic	Psychologic			
caffeine	Ingestion	Yes	Yes	Mild stimulation	Headaches	None
alcohol	Ingestion	Yes	Yes	Euphoria	Tremors	Benzodiazepines
nicotine	Inhalation, buccal	Yes	Yes	Relaxation	Irritability	None
marijuana, hashish	Inhalation, ingestion	No	Yes	Relaxation	None	None
Opioids	Injection, ingestion	Yes	Yes	Euphoria	Yes	Methadone
Inhalants	Inhalation	No?	No?	Euphoria	None	None
cocaine	Inhalation, smoking	No?	Yes	Euphoria	Depression	None
Amphetamines	Ingestion, injection	No	Yes	Euphoria	Depression	Tapering dose
Hallucinogens	Ingestion, smoking	No	No	Distorted perception	None	None
phencyclidine (PCP)	Smoking, ingestion	No	No	Euphoria	None	None
Benzodiazepines	Ingestion, injection	Yes	Yes	Relaxation	Tremors, seizure	Tapering dose
Barbiturates	Ingestion, injection	Yes	Yes	Euphoria, relaxation	Yes	Phenobarbital

women may wish to avoid caffeine because it freely passes to the fetus. Any person who ingests more than 200 mg of caffeine daily should be encouraged to reduce his or her caffeine intake to avoid the subtle onset of chronic toxicity.

▼ alcohol

Alcohol is a CNS depressant. It is widely available, relatively inexpensive, and comes in a variety of forms, such as beer, wine, wine coolers, and distilled spirits. In the United States alcohol is commonly served in social settings, where it is thought to promote conviviality. Heavy drinking over time can produce psychologic dependence, particularly in those genetically predisposed. Physical damage most commonly appears in the liver and brain. The alcohol withdrawal syndrome can be serious, characterized by tremors, changes in level of consciousness, with progression to seizures and delirium tremens, which are life-threatening conditions. These withdrawal symptoms are treated with a decreasing dose of benzodiazepines, most often chlordiazepoxide (Librium) or diazepam (Valium). The patient must be carefully observed, and supportive therapy must be given as necessary for respiratory, cardiovascular, and seizure complications. Alcohol use and abuse are discussed in detail in Chapter 57.

▼ nicotine

Nicotine is both a stimulant and a depressant. It may be the drug with the highest addiction potential; that is, there is a high risk that someone who begins to use a nicotine product will progress to becoming physically dependent on this drug. The initial effect of nicotine is physical stimulation, but this stage is then replaced by a relaxation effect. Nicotine is commonly used by smoking, although smokeless tobacco products, such as chewing tobacco, are also widely used.

Because nicotine produces tolerance, the user must keep increasing the amount of drug used to derive the same effect. Nicotine produces physiologic and psychologic dependence. Once dependent, an individual finds it extremely difficult to abstain. Withdrawal symptoms include craving, restlessness, decreased concentration, and hyperirritability.

Nicotine has only recently come to be seen as a drug, which represents a change in thinking about tobacco and both its abuse potential and social acceptability. Nicotine use contributes to a variety of serious health problems, including lung cancer, hypertension, and cardiovascular disease. It is estimated that 80% of American smokers have attempted to quit smoking at some time. More than 90% of those who do quit, do so "cold turkey." There are also organized programs to assist smokers in quitting, and both nicotine chewing gum and transdermal patches are available to use in combination with other interventions. The antidepressant drug bupropion (Wellbutrin) has recently been shown to help people quit smoking. Organized programs have about a 20% to 30% success rate for 1 year abstinence. However, many smokers "quit" several times before finally achieving long-term cessation.

▼ marijuana

Marijuana and its stronger version hashish are not easily classified. Both are derived from the marijuana plant, but hashish is more concentrated. The active ingredient is tetrahydrocannabinol, also known as THC. Marijuana is usually consumed by inhalation or ingestion. The primary effect is relaxation and a sense of well-being accompanied by a distortion in one's sense of time. Tolerance for some of the physiologic effects can develop over time, and physical dependence has been demonstrated in animals at high dosages. Physical dependence in humans has not been clearly demonstrated. Marijuana may produce a psychologic dependence that is manifested by daily use. Long-term use can produce an amotivational syndrome characterized by apathy and loss of motivation. Marijuana is stored in the fat cells of the body and released gradually; therefore in heavy smokers such syndromes may be related to the presence and continuous slow release of the drug in the body. Withdrawal symptoms are mild and rarely require medical intervention.

▼ cocaine

Cocaine is a stimulant drug. It is available in a white powder that is used intranasally (snorted) or in a less expensive solid form, crack cocaine, that can be smoked or injected intravenously. Either form produces an intense, short-lived euphoric high. Physical dependence on cocaine is unclear. However, with high dosages of crack cocaine, withdrawal is characterized by an initial dysphoric reaction followed by

Table 8-3	Caffeine Content of Commonly Ingested Substances
Substance	**Caffeine Content**
Foods and Beverages	
Coffee	
Brewed	80-150 mg/5 oz cup
Instant	85-100 mg/5 oz cup
Decaffeinated	2-4 mg/5 oz cup
Tea, brewed	30-75 mg/5 oz cup
Cocoa	5-40 mg/5 oz cup
Cola soft drinks*	35-60 mg/12 oz bottle or can
Nonprescription Medications	
Analgesics (Anacin and Vanquish)	32 mg/tablet
Excedrin	65 mg/tablet
Cold Medications	
Dristan AF	16.2 mg/tablet
Korigesic	30 mg/tablet
Stimulants	
Nodoz	100 mg/tablet
Vivarin	200 mg/tablet

*Many soft drinks other than colas contain caffeine as an additive. The label reveals the presence of caffeine but not the amount.

depression, craving, prolonged sleep, and anhedonia (the inability to experience pleasure). Cocaine overdose produces a medical emergency consisting of hypertension, tachycardia, seizures, dyspnea, and ventricular arrhythmias.

▼ Amphetamines

Amphetamines are stimulants often taken initially to increase alertness or to stay awake. Continued use can progress from pills to IV use, which is more potent and dangerous. Methamphetamine is readily synthesized illegally. Recent use of methamphetamine has turned to smoking of methamphetamine base crystals ("ice"). Amphetamine users often switch to a depressant drug to "come down" from the stimulant effects of the amphetamines and to get needed rest. These dramatic, drug-controlled physiologic changes often cause the individual to become exhausted and physically debilitated. Such polydrug use can also lead to dependency on both types of drugs. Prolonged amphetamine use produces a physiologic withdrawal characterized by depression. Amphetamines are described in Chapter 60.

▼ Inhalants

Inhalants are substances such as airplane glue, gasoline, and cleaning products with vapors that produce a "high." Inhalation produces rapid neurologic effects, and many of the inhalants are neurotoxic. In addition, inhalation allows little dose control. The substance is often kept in a plastic bag that is then placed over the face and the vapors inhaled, which creates a real potential for asphyxiation. Inhalant use is most common in children and adolescents. However, health care professionals such as dentists and anesthesia personnel may abuse nitrous oxide.

▼ Hallucinogens

Hallucinogens alter perceptions and thought processes. Most hallucinogens are smoked or ingested. LSD (D-lysergic acid diethylamide) is a hallucinogen that was popular in the 1960s and is becoming available again. Other hallucinogens include mescaline (peyote) and psilocybin, which are derived from mushrooms, and synthetic drugs such as MDA (3,4 methylenedioxy amphetamine) and MDMA (3,4 methylenedioxy methamphetamine), which are amphetamine derivatives with hallucinogenic properties. Although physical and psychologic dependence are not characteristic of hallucinogens, behavior is unpredictable and may put the individual in danger.

PCP (phencyclidine) is an anesthetic agent that is used and abused for its hallucinogenic properties. It is smoked sometimes in conjunction with marijuana cigarettes. Individuals who use PCP may experience altered sensation and decreased sensitivity to pain and may exhibit violent behavior.

▼ Opioids

Opioids include drugs derived from the opium poppy and their synthetic derivatives. Many opioids are excellent analgesics (see Chapter 32). Heroin is an opioid available in a fine white powder that can be dissolved and administered intravenously or subcutaneously (skin popping). The drug produces a euphoric response. Unlike other opioids, heroin is illegal in the United States. Its addiction potential is very high with regular use because the individual rapidly develops increasing tolerance to the drug and must use more to achieve the same effect. Both physical and psychologic dependence develop as the individual becomes dependent not only on the drug but on the whole lifestyle that goes with use of the drug. There is a predictable set of withdrawal symptoms that occurs with heroin and other opioids. The individual experiences rhinitis, nausea, and diarrhea, then muscle cramps, twitching, and tremors. This syndrome lasts 3 to 5 days but may last longer. Although the withdrawal syndrome is very uncomfortable, it is not physiologically dangerous.

Prescription drugs are legally available only by prescription from a licensed health care provider. Patients often believe that any drug prescribed by a health care practitioner is unquestioningly safe. These patients are not aware of the addictive potential of some drugs. If they have a problem with use, they may not discuss it with their health care provider. Patients may not take the medication appropriately, using too much, taking it too often, or taking it at inappropriate times. Providers may not collect enough information about the other drugs the patient is using or past experiences with drugs. Special problems include adding new medications to treat the side effects of other drugs, lacking knowledge of usual side effects, and multiple caregivers prescribing drugs in isolation.

Drugs that produce physical or psychologic addiction are extensively regulated in the United States and Canada, as described in Chapter 3. Three categories of controlled prescription drugs were included in the Household Survey: opioids (see preceding discussion), benzodiazepines, and barbiturates.

Benzodiazepines

Benzodiazepines are categorized as minor tranquilizers or antianxiety agents and were initially developed to treat short-term anxiety. They were at one time widely prescribed, particularly for women. The drugs were overused for their relaxation effects. It was found that when benzodiazepines are used over time physical and psychologic dependence result. Withdrawal symptoms, including tremors, anxiety, and potential for seizures, can occur after heavy, prolonged use. To avoid withdrawal after prolonged use, the dosage must be tapered gradually. Benzodiazepines are discussed in Chapter 57.

Flunitrazepam (Rohypnol) is a fast-onset diazepam that produces prolonged sedation, a feeling of well-being, and short-term memory loss. It is not sold in the United States or Canada but is smuggled illegally from Mexico and other countries. Because small amounts are effective and the drug is odorless, colorless, and tasteless, small amounts may be added to drinks and taken unknowingly. This drug is implicated in "date rapes" in which the victim does not remember the event because of the amnesia-producing effect of the drug.

Barbiturates and Sedatives

Barbiturates and other sedatives comprise another category of prescription drugs subject to abuse. These drugs are prescribed for sleeplessness but also produce relaxation and euphoria. They can be taken by ingestion or injection, rapidly produce tolerance, and result in both physical and psychologic dependence. Withdrawal is characterized by hypotension, fever, and delirium and can result in seizures. As with benzodiazepines, tapering the drug, especially by substituting a long-acting barbiturate such as phenobarbital, is recommended. Barbiturates and sedatives are covered in Chapter 57.

Polydrug Abuse

Many drugs are used in combination, either concurrently (together) or sequentially (first one, then the next). Alcohol is more likely to be used alone than any other drug, and it is also commonly used in combination with other drugs because of its easy availability. Polydrug use also may occur because an individual is unable to locate the drug of choice and uses an available substitute or because the individual likes the combination. Alcohol and other depressants are often used concurrently. Sometimes an individual may use a second drug to counteract the effects of the first; for example, a depressant drug is used to "come down" from a stimulant. This behavior is a pattern of alternating use.

When either of these patterns has occurred over a long time, withdrawal is more complicated because the individual needs to withdraw from two drugs that often produce opposite effects.

TREATMENT FOR DRUG ABUSE

Treatment Programs

Treatment for substance abuse is currently undergoing great change as the health care system itself changes. The predominant model for treatment developed experientially is based on the program at Hazelden, Minnesota (near Minneapolis). This program, a 28-day inpatient model, became known as the "Minnesota Model." The Minnesota Model is based on Alcoholics Anonymous (AA) and often uses recovering individuals as counselors. Twelve-step groups, of which AA is the prototype, are self-help groups in which members, who are all recovering from alcohol or drug dependence, join together to offer each other support and direction. Twelve-step groups are not considered treatment but are often adjuncts to treatment and in some cases are the only modality used by an individual.

Withdrawal Treatment

A thorough history of drug use and tests of body fluids for drugs at admission are essential measures to make sure that all abused drugs are identified so that a safe plan of withdrawal can be instituted.

Medications used to treat withdrawal symptoms are administered to reestablish physiologic homeostasis. The need for withdrawal treatment depends on the specific drug abused, how much and how long it was abused, and the physical and psychologic characteristics of the individual. Withdrawal effects vary greatly from individual to individual depending on these factors. This variation seems to reflect differences in neurologic response among individuals. A history of prior withdrawal experiences is extremely helpful because it can identify former problem areas that are likely to recur. This is particularly true with alcohol.

The most dangerous substances for withdrawal are the CNS depressants: alcohol, benzodiazepines, and barbiturates, all of which produce physiologic tolerance. Severe alcohol withdrawal syndrome is called delirium tremens (DTs). DTs begin as tremors and agitation, progress to hallucinations and delirium, and sometimes result in death. History is an important predictor of withdrawal symptoms; this information should be routinely collected on admission. Careful monitoring of vital signs and mental status is crucial because early withdrawal symptoms are reflected in the vital signs as increased blood pressure and pulse and in an altered mental status. Early intervention with medications can prevent initiation of DTs; the alcohol withdrawal syndrome is very difficult to stop once started. Benzodiazepines used for alcohol withdrawal vary, but diazepam (Valium) and chlordiazepoxide (Librium) are often used on a schedule of decreasing dosage over 3 to 5 days. However, increasingly benzodiazepines are used on an as-needed basis for patients who experience symptoms or have a history of severe withdrawal.

Barbiturate withdrawal is managed through a decreasing dosage of a long-acting barbiturate, usually phenobarbital, over several days, depending on the dosage the patient was using before treatment. The potential for seizures is high during barbiturate withdrawal because the drugs themselves decrease seizure potential.

Benzodiazepine withdrawal is usually managed by decreasing the dosage of diazepam over several days or weeks.

Opioid withdrawal can be treated in several ways. Methadone is a long-acting opiate that can be administered once daily to prevent withdrawal symptoms. The use of methadone as a replacement drug for opiates has long been the treatment of choice; however, recent data suggest that this approach may increase the likelihood of relapse to opioid use. Other alternatives are the use of clonidine to relieve symptoms or the use of buprenorphine over 5 to 8 days.

Treatment of withdrawal from stimulant dependence depends on the symptoms. Withdrawal from cocaine may result in a state of depression and loss of feeling and pleasure that requires treatment with antidepressants. Amphetamine withdrawal may result in either depression or an amphetamine-induced psychosis. These effects are treated with an antidepressant or antipsychotic medication, respectively, until the specific symptoms are under control.

Because many drugs interact, both in effect and tolerance, withdrawal from a combination of drugs, particularly combinations of CNS depressants, deserve particular caution in treatment. It may be necessary to manage withdrawal from each drug sequentially, particularly with alcohol and barbiturates or alcohol and benzodiazepines. Sequential withdrawal means to withdraw one drug while continuing the use of the other until the individual's condition is stabilized from the first withdrawal. Then withdrawal from the other drug is initiated.

Medication to Promote Abstinence

Medications used in treatment are oriented toward helping the individual achieve and maintain abstinence from drugs.

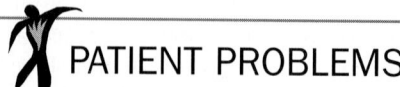

PATIENT PROBLEMS

Alcoholism

Patients often deny alcohol abuse. The CAGE is a series of four questions that can be easily inserted into any assessment tool. To help remember the questions, the first letter of a key word in each question is highlighted and spells "CAGE." One "yes" response suggests a possible alcohol problem. More than one "yes" response makes it highly likely that a problem exists. However, a problem may exist even if all answers are "no" but there have been drinking-related problems with a job, relationships, health, or the law. This tool can be readily reworded for drug abuse.

- Have you ever felt you ought to **c**ut down on your drinking?
- Have people **a**nnoyed you by criticizing your drinking?
- Have you ever felt bad or **g**uilty about your drinking?
- Have you ever had a drink first thing in the morning to steady your nerves or get rid of a hangover? (**e**ye-opener)

From Mayfield D, McLeod G, Hall P: The CAGE questionnaire: validation of a new alcoholism instrument, *Am J Psychiatry* 131:1121-1123, 1974.

None of the medications is meant as treatment alone but rather as an adjunct to an ongoing program of recovery. There is a growing recognition that relapses should not be accepted as failure but should be seen as a temporary setback in an ongoing program.

Antabuse is used to promote abstinence in alcohol-dependent patients. When taken daily, Antabuse produces extreme nausea if the individual uses alcohol. Antabuse is used primarily to discourage impulse drinking and to help patients gain confidence in their ability to abstain.

Naltrexone is sometimes used with opiate users. It blocks the binding sites for opiates so that, if used, the opiate does not produce a euphoria or "high," which is the psychologic reinforcement for opiate use. Naltrexone is a long-acting medication that can be given in a daily dose. A new use of naltrexone is in the treatment of alcohol abuse. It appears that naltrexone may decrease craving for alcohol.

Methadone is used as part of a maintenance program. Patients who have been stabilized on a maintenance dose of methadone receive methadone daily, under clinic supervision, for an indefinite period. Methadone becomes a long-term substitute for the opioid, and the patient must attend the clinic daily for methadone and for periodic urine screening for other drugs. The use of methadone maintenance is controversial. Those who favor methadone maintenance for long-term use with opioid abusers believe that it allows the patient to lead a productive life, particularly one free of crime, until the individual is ready to achieve abstinence. Those who oppose methadone maintenance do so because the drug use continues, although under controlled conditions. Achieving full abstinence from opiates in methadone maintenance programs has been rare after long-term treatment.

Levo-alphaacetylmethadol (LAAM), like methadone, is a long-acting opioid that needs to be taken only every other day. It was approved for use in the maintenance treatment of opioid dependence in 1993 but is not widely used.

Nursing Process Overview

Drug Abuse

Assessment

Include questions about drug use or abuse in the initial patient assessment. This approach is important to (1) avoid withdrawal symptoms, (2) identify underlying reasons for physiologic findings, (3) assist with appropriate medication or anesthetic choice for a patient, and (4) determine appropriate referral and treatment for the patient.

A tool commonly used for screening that can be easily inserted into any assessment tool is the CAGE (see the Patient Problems box on Alcoholism). It consists of four questions that can identify alcohol or other drug abuse. This is one of many assessment tools available in the literature. Keep in mind the possibility of substance abuse whenever physical or other findings suggest drug involvement. Remember that some patients will not respond honestly to assessment questions about the use of drugs or alcohol. Use open-ended questions and maintain a nonjudgmental approach. Obtain a thorough drug history with all patients. Identify all current medications, both prescribed and over-the-counter. Include the specific drugs, dosage, how often taken, and for how long. When the information is unclear or inconsistent, return to the questions later. Some patients may need to write down the names of their drugs or bring in their medication bottles. A "red flag" for possible prescription drug abuse is multiple prescriptions or multiple prescribers. This may be more common in older adults, who tend to have multiple and chronic health problems. They may not be aware that their prescribed drugs have associated risks.

During treatment, continue to assess the patient's behavior and mental status. Some patients may use drugs to treat a mental health problem such as depression that may reappear or intensify when drug use is terminated.

Nursing Diagnoses

A variety of nursing diagnoses may be indicated for patients who are intentionally or unintentionally abusing drugs. Common nursing diagnoses for patients who experience withdrawal from drugs are (1) sensory-perceptual alteration, (2) alteration in comfort, and (3) potential for injury.

Patient Outcomes

Outcomes for patients who abuse drugs are related to (1) safe withdrawal from drugs, (2) stabilization of physical conditions aggravated by drug abuse, and (3) appropriate referral for treatment for the drug abuse if appropriate.

Planning/Implementation

Nursing responses to patients who abuse drugs include developing an understanding of how drug abuse is part of the patient's lifestyle. This understanding from the patient's point of view helps the nurse determine what treatment and other resources would be most acceptable to the patient.

Patients who abuse drugs often need basic information about their drug of abuse, its characteristics, and problems associated with the drug. This information may be new to the patient. Explain withdrawal symptoms and any treatment of the withdrawal. The nurse should be familiar with withdrawal symptoms related to the specific drug and closely monitor the patient through vital signs and mental status for changes consistent with withdrawal. There are several assessment scales for withdrawal from alcohol that quantify withdrawal symptoms, one of which is the CIWA, Clinical Institute Withdrawal Assessment Scale.

Teach the patient about current drug abuse treatment programs and their rationale to help the patient decide on the type and format of treatment that will be most helpful. Include a discussion of the disease concept of drug abuse and the role of 12-step groups in treatment and follow-up.

Educate family members and significant others so that they can provide support and encourage the patient to seek further appropriate treatment.

There are various books on prescription medications that are written for the lay public and can be suggested to help adults for whom prescription drug abuse has been partly inadvertent. Discuss aspects of medication administration such as timing, missed doses, and side effects and validate that the patient understands the information. Also teach patients about the issues involved in multiple drug use and in combining drugs with alcohol.

Evaluation

The patient should be able to state an understanding of how drug abuse was involved in this health care episode and plan for further treatment if indicated. The patient's family should also be able to explain this information. The patient should understand any withdrawal symptoms experienced and their relationship to the drug abuse. The patient should understand the use of any prescription medications.

CHAPTER REVIEW

Application

1. What are the criteria for diagnosing drug abuse? for drug dependence?
2. What are some of the environmental risk factors for drug abuse?
3. Abused drugs tend to produce what kinds of mood changes?
4. What commonly abused drug has the highest addiction potential?
5. Which prescription drugs are most commonly abused?

Critical Thinking

1. Describe the interrelationship between tolerance, withdrawal, and dependence.
2. Describe withdrawal treatment for CNS depressants.
3. Contact a local hospital or your State or Provincial Board of Nursing. Inquire about the number of nurses involved in drug abuse during the last year. What kinds of consequences were there for their actions? What kinds of assistance are there for nurses who have abused drugs?

References

Coombs RH: Addicted health professionals, *J Subst Misuse Nurs Health Soc Care* 1(4):187-194, 1996.

Kinney J: *Clinical manual of substance abuse*, ed 2, St Louis, 1996, Mosby.

Kowalski SD: Self-esteem and self-efficacy as predictors of success in smoking cessation, *J Holistic Nurs* 15(2):128-142, 1997.

Simmons DH: Caffeine and its effect on persons with mental disorders, *Arch Psychiatr Nurs* 10(2):116-122, 1996.

Smith DE, Seymour RB: Cannabis and cannabis withdrawal, *J Subst Misuse Nurs Health Soc Care* 2(1):49-53, 1997.

Wewers ME, Ahijevych KL: Smoking cessation interventions in chronic illness, *Ann Rev Nurs Res* 14:75-93, 1996.

Chapter 9

Care of the Poisoned Patient

OBJECTIVES

After studying this chapter, you should be able to do the following:

- *Discuss the importance of the field of clinical toxicology.*
- *Differentiate between toxicodynamics and toxicokinetics.*
- *Explain the rationale for nonspecific antidotes to poisons: decontamination, emesis and lavage, activated charcoal, and cathartics.*
- *Describe the basis for specific antidote categories: competitive antidotes, chelates, antibodies, and agents that produce metabolic alterations.*
- *Differentiate between diuresis and dialysis.*
- *Summarize nursing care implications for drugs discussed in this chapter.*

CHAPTER OVERVIEW

Toxicology is the study of poisons. A poison is a chemical substance that injures or kills when introduced into the body. There are literally thousands of potential poisons. Drugs, household and industrial chemicals, plants, pesticides, carbon monoxide, and heavy metals are the major agents of poisoning seen in clinical practice.

Poison control centers, located in communities throughout the United States, are usually identified in local telephone books. These centers provide the lay public and health professionals with information about the appropriate first aid and clinical management of suspected poisoning. Poisondex is a computerized database of more than 650,000 substances and includes information about most medicines and consumer products. Large poison control centers may also offer specialized poison treatment and consultation. Educational services such as professional training and poison prevention education for the public may also be offered.

Each year approximately 1.5 million cases are handled by poison control centers. More than 90% of all poisonings occur at home. Children younger than 3 years of age are the most common victims. These statistics highlight the tendency of young children to ingest pills, cleaning agents, and plants. Pills that are particularly attractive and troublesome to children include chocolate-flavored laxatives and vitamins (particularly those with iron given to pregnant women).

Children are also at risk for gradual poisoning by lead in the environment (see Pediatric Considerations box).

The U.S. mortality rate from poisoning of all types has recently been reported at approximately 12,000 deaths per year. Of these, about half are suicides and half are accidental. Less than 50 deaths per year are considered homicides.

Clinical toxicology is the study of care of the poisoned patient. Poisoning can be acute, subacute, or chronic, depending on the dose, length of exposure, and extent of tissue injury. In this chapter the primary emphasis is on the acutely poisoned patient. Acute poisoning is usually the immediate and direct result of a single excessive dose. Acute poisoning in children is most commonly caused by the ingestion of plants, drugs, or household products. In adults acute poisoning is often the result of a drug overdose. About 70% of adult drug overdose cases involve a central nervous system (CNS) depressant, commonly alcohol (23%) or a benzodiazepine (24%). Alcohol and benzodiazepines greatly potentiate the toxic effects of each other or other CNS depressants.

PEDIATRIC CONSIDERATIONS

Lead Poisoning

THE PROBLEM

Lead is considered the leading environmental problem for American children. Low levels of lead in the bodies of children can decrease IQ, cause reading and learning disabilities, reduce attention span, and cause behavioral problems. About 900,000 children under the age of 6 years are estimated to have more lead in their blood than is considered safe (10 μg/dl). Lead poisoning is defined by blood levels greater than 25 μg/dl. Common sources of exposure include lead in old house paint, in dust and soil from paint chips, in industrial emissions, and from some water pipes.

SOLUTIONS

- Test children between 6 months and 2 years old for lead. One child in nine under 6 years old has enough lead in the blood to place him or her at risk.
- If levels of lead are high, test the home environment and water for lead.
- Of all private housings built before 1980, 75% contain some lead paint. Renovations are especially likely to throw off dust high in lead. Radiators, stair trim, door and window trim, and baseboards are most likely sources inside the house. Old exterior paint is even more likely to be high in lead.
- Lead solder is another common source of environmental lead.

CASE STUDY

Lead Poisoning: Detection and Treatment in Children

As part of your nursing school community project, you are to visit area day-care centers and present information to the caregivers and the parents on the prevention of lead poisoning.

1. Find an Internet source of information for this topic.
2. What are potential sources of lead exposure for children?
3. Describe the adverse effects of lead poisoning (acute and long-term).

One of the children in the center has been diagnosed with acute lead poisoning. She is to receive edetate calcium disodium. The child weighs 12 kg.

4. Calculate the dosage for this medication and this child. What is the preferred route?
5. What must be monitored during chelation therapy with this medication?

THERAPEUTIC RATIONALE: TOXICODYNAMICS AND TOXICOKINETICS

The general principles of toxicology are those of pharmacology extended to excessive doses. (The principles relating drug dosage to drug action are discussed in Chapter 1.) The same factors that control pharmacokinetics and pharmacodynamics also apply to toxicology.

Toxicodynamics describes the harmful effects that a poison produces on the body. The graded dose-response curves described in Chapter 1 relate to both toxic effects and therapeutic effects. Therefore the symptoms of poisoning reflect the dosage of the poison. Treating the poisoned patient is often complicated because the dose of the poison is seldom known with any accuracy and the identity of the poison itself may not be known. Therefore a thorough assessment of the patient is especially important in cases of poisoning. If the nature of the poison is known, the severity of the symptoms shown by the patient will be important in monitoring the course of treatment. If the nature of the poison is unknown, the symptoms become vital in suggesting the nature of the poison. The application of toxicodynamics to the poisoned patient is demonstrated in Table 9-1, which lists symptoms and gives the common poisons that can cause them.

Toxicokinetics deals with the action of a poison in the patient as a function of time. It encompasses the absorption, distribution, localization, biotransformation, and elimination of the poison. However, the kinetics of a drug overdose is not necessarily the same as that of the therapeutic dose because a large dose of drug may saturate and overwhelm one or more of the mechanisms controlling absorption, distribution, biotransformation, and elimination of therapeutic concentrations of the drug. Moreover, normal physiologic processes, such as heart rate, blood pressure, and respiration, may be compromised and thereby alter the disposition of the drug overdose. In this chapter toxicokinetics is presented as embodying the major steps in the care of the acutely poisoned patient. These steps include nonspecific antidotes to remove poison not yet absorbed, specific antidotes to counteract a few select poisons, and occasionally, diuresis or dialysis.

THERAPEUTIC AGENTS: CARE OF THE ACUTELY POISONED PATIENT

Nonspecific Antidotes

For a summary of information on nonspecific antidotes, refer to Table 9-2.

Decontamination

Decontamination is the removal or neutralization of a toxin. If the toxin is present on the clothing, skin, or eyes (e.g., insecticide spray), the clothing should be removed and the skin scrubbed well with soap and water. The eyes should be washed with a copious amount of warm water. If the patient has inhaled a noxious gas, he or she should be given fresh air

Table 9-1   Physical Symptoms Produced by Common Poisons

Symptoms	Poisoning Agent	Symptoms	Poisoning Agent
Mental and Motor Symptoms		Hypotension—cont'd	aspirin
Drowsiness, coma	acetaminophen		muscarine
	Alcohols		Nitrates, nitrites
	Antihistamines		Opioids
	carbon monoxide		Sedative-hypnotics
	insulin		Tranquilizers
	Opioids (e.g., codeine)	Oliguria, anuria	carbon tetrachloride
	Salicylates		ethylene glycol
	scopolamine		Heavy metals
	Sedative-hypnotic drugs		methanol
	Tranquilizers		Mushrooms
	Tricyclic antidepressants		Petroleum distillates
Excitation, twitching, convulsions	aminophylline	**Oral and Gastrointestinal Symptoms**	
	atropine	Acetone odor	acetone
	CNS stimulants		alcohol
	carbon monoxide		Salicylates
	cyanide	Almond odor	cyanide
	Local anesthetics	Garlic odor	Arsenic
	Organophosphate insecticides		Dimethyl sulfoxide
	Phenothiazines		Phosphorus
Agitation, delirium	Alcohols		Organophosphate insecticides
	aminophylline	Dry mouth	amphetamine
	atropine		Antihistamines
	Lysergic acid diethylamide (LSD)		atropine
	lead		Opioids
	marijuana		Phenothiazines
	phencyclidine (PCP)	Excessive salivation	arsenic
	physostigmine		Corrosives
Paralysis	Foods containing *Clostridium botulinum* (botulism)		mercury
	Heavy metals		Mushrooms
Ataxia (motor incoordination)	Alcohols		Organophosphate insecticides
	Anticonvulsants	Heavy vomiting	aminophylline
	carbon monoxide		Corrosives
	Hallucinogens		Food poisoning
	Heavy metals		Heavy metals
	Hydrocarbons		Salicylates
	Sedative-hypnotics	**Pupillary Symptoms**	
	Tranquilizers	Dilated pupils	Alcohols
Cardiovascular and Renal Symptoms			Anticholinergics
Increased pulse rate	Alcohols		Antihistamines
	amphetamine		CNS depressants
	aspirin		CNS stimulants
	atropine	Constricted pupils	Mushrooms
	cocaine		Organophosphate insecticides
	Parasympatholytics		Opioids
	Sympathomimetics	Nystagmus	Sedative-hypnotics
Decreased pulse rate	digitalis	**Dermatologic Symptoms**	
	Opioids	Jaundiced skin	arsenic
	Parasympathomimetics		carbon tetrachloride
Hypertension	amphetamine		Mushrooms
	Sympathomimetics		naphthalene
Hypotension	Alcohols		
	aminophylline		

CNS, Central nervous system.

Table 9-1 **Physical Symptoms Produced by Common Poisons—cont'd**

Symptoms	Poisoning Agent	Symptoms	Poisoning Agent
Flushed skin	alcohol Antihistamines Anticholinergics	Depressed respiration	alcohol Opioids Sedative-hypnotics Tranquilizers
Cherry-red skin	Carbon monoxide Cyanide Nitrites	Wheezing	Mushrooms Opioids Organophosphate insecticides Petroleum distillates
Pulmonary Symptoms			
Rapid breathing	amphetamine Carbon monoxide methanol Petroleum distillates Salicylates		

Table 9-2 **Nonspecific Antidotes**

Antidote	Trade Name	Administration/Dosage	Comments
Emetics			
ipecac	Ipecac syrup*	ORAL (in 8 oz water): *Children 6 mo-1 yr*—5-10 ml; *children 1-12 yr*—15 ml; *adults*—30 ml. Vomiting within 30 min in 90% of patients. May repeat dose after 20-30 min if no vomiting has occurred.	Give only to conscious patient who has gag reflex and is not likely to aspirate vomitus. Do not give when vomitus will itself be injurious (e.g., acids, bases, hydrocarbons). Encourage patient to drink water. Water distends stomach and makes it more susceptible to action of ipecac syrup. Walking also helps induce vomiting. Average return of stomach contents is 20%-60%. Keep vomitus for analysis.
Gastric Lavage			
Water 0.45% saline 0.9% saline		BY GASTRIC TUBE: *Young children*—10 ml/kg; *adults*—300 ml.	If patient is in deteriorating condition, unconscious, prone to seizures, or lacking a gag reflex, nasotracheal intubation is necessary before lavage to protect airway. Use large-bore (28 to 40-Fr Ewald or Burke orogastric lavacutor) tubing to allow aspiration of tablets. Keep first wash for analysis. Continue washings until return is clear (2-20 L). Administering more than recommended volume distends stomach and may induce vomiting.
activated charcoal	Acta-Char Charcoaid Charcodate† Insta-Char* Liqui-Char	ORAL OR BY GASTRIC TUBE: *Children*—15-30 g in 4-8 oz water; *adults*—25-50 g in 8-16 oz water.	Administer as slurry within first hours of poisoning, after induced vomiting (charcoal will inactivate ipecac) or gastric lavage. Do not use with acetylcysteine in management of acetaminophen poisoning. Do not use magnesium citrate as cathartic.
activated charcoal and sorbitol	Actidose with Sorbitol Charcoaid Charcodate† Insta-Char with Sorbitol Liqui-Char with Sorbitol	ORAL: *Adults, adolescents*—50 g of activated charcoal as a single dose; *children 1-12 yr*—25-50 g of activated charcoal as a single dose.	Sorbitol prevents constipation from activated charcoal. Do not use for multiple-dose therapy because of excessive catharsis due to sorbitol. However, activated charcoal with sorbitol may be alternated with activated charcoal only.
Cathartics			
magnesium sulfate 10% solution	Epsom salts	ORAL: *Children*—1-2 ml/kg; *adults*—150-250 ml.	Do not use magnesium salts if patient has renal failure.

*Available in Canada and the United States.
†Available in Canada only.

Continued

Table 9-2 **Nonspecific Antidotes—cont'd**

Antidote	Trade Name	Administration/Dosage	Comments
magnesium citrate, 10% solution		ORAL: *Children*—1-2 ml/kg; *adults*—150-250 ml.	Do not use citrate if activated charcoal has been given.
polyethylene glycol 3350 and electrolytes	CO-Lav Colyte* GoLYTELY* Peglyte†	ORAL: *Adults, adolescents*—240 ml every 10 min, up to 4 L, or until fecal discharge is clear; *children*—25-40 ml/kg/hr until fecal discharge is clear. NASOGASTRIC TUBE: *Adults, adolescents*—20-30 ml/min (1.2-1.8 L/hr); *children*—same as oral dose.	Onset of action: 30-60 min. Negligible absorption or renal excretion. Cleans the bowel by fluid overload with an osmotically balanced solution. Also used preoperatively or before gastrointestinal examination.

*Available in Canada and the United States.
†Available in Canada only.

DRUG ABUSE ALERTS

Ipecac Syrup

BACKGROUND
Normally ipecac syrup is administered to induce vomiting in a case of acute poisoning. Ipecac syrup is readily obtained at a drugstore. Chronic administration of ipecac is abuse. Such abuse occurs in some child abuse cases and in some cases of eating disorders. In eating disorders, ipecac syrup may be taken to purge ingested food.

PHARMACOLOGY
Emetine HCl (ipecac alkaloid) is a safe drug for inducing vomiting in emergency home use. Administered chronically, however, it can produce many chronic symptoms. These may not be readily associated with abuse. Most of these symptoms relate to distorted electrolyte imbalances that arise from continual vomiting and loss of gastric fluids. The active alkaloid of ipecac also has a direct depressive action on heart and skeletal muscle.

HEALTH HAZARDS
Symptoms of continued ipecac administration include chronic diarrhea and vomiting, muscle weakness, colitis, cardiomyopathy, fever, edema, and electrolyte disturbances. Therapy for ipecac abuse is supportive while ipecac is discontinued.

or oxygen to breathe. When a poison or drug overdose has been swallowed, much of the substance usually remains unabsorbed for some time. In treating poisoned patients it is common to flush the poison from the gastrointestinal tract. Such techniques as induced vomiting (emesis), gastric lavage, administration of activated charcoal, and catharsis are appropriate to help eliminate a drug overdose that has been swallowed. The dosages for these nonspecific antidotes are listed in Table 9-2.

Emesis and Lavage

The stomach is emptied by either emesis or gastric lavage. There are three major points that determine whether vomiting or gastric lavage should be used. First, induction of vomiting is not appropriate when the patient might aspirate the vomitus. Therefore this method is contraindicated when the patient is lacking normal reflex control of gagging and vomiting, is unconscious, or is having seizures. Second, vomiting is not indicated when the regurgitated material can be damaging to the esophagus or lungs. Such material includes acids, bases, and nonaromatic or nonhalogenated hydrocarbons (oils and solvents). Third, induction of vomiting can take 20 to 30 minutes and therefore should not be used when time is critical.

The emetic of choice is **ipecac syrup,** which induces vomiting within 30 minutes in 90% of treated patients. With this agent, 20% to 60% of the stomach contents can be emptied. Emetics such as salt water (sodium chloride), mustard water, and copper sulfate are considered dangerous and ineffective. When vomiting is induced, the vomitus should be saved for analysis. See the Drug Abuse Alerts box for information on ipecac syrup abuse.

Gastric lavage is the preferred method of emptying the stomach in adults. The airway is first protected by an endotracheal tube. Use of a large-bore tube such as an Ewald or Burke tube allows tablets to be retrieved. Gastric lavage is less successful in children because a small-bore tube must be used. Tablets from some drug formulations partially deteriorate and then coalesce in the stomach to form a mass of undissolved drug that is too large to be washed out and yet is poorly soluble. Lavage is continued until the return is clear. It is important to note that the first wash is saved for analysis.

▼ activated charcoal

After emesis or lavage a slurry of **activated charcoal** may be administered through the lavage tube or a nasogastric tube, or it may be given orally. Because activated charcoal will absorb and inactivate ipecac, it should not be given until after vomiting has occurred. Activated charcoal absorbs a number of drugs and chemicals and thereby prevents their absorption into the body. The charcoal itself, with absorbed chemicals, is eliminated in the feces. Administration of activated charcoal is most effective if given within the first few hours of poisoning. Although activated charcoal may be used to remove acetaminophen, the activated charcoal should be removed if acetylcysteine is administered. The antidote for acetaminophen is acetylcysteine, which is absorbed by activated charcoal.

Cathartics

Cathartics are the final common treatment of acute poisoning. The primarily use of cathartics is to prevent constipation after administration of activated charcoal. The preferred cathartic for this use is sorbitol. Cathartic salts may be used, but magnesium sulfate is contraindicated if there is impairment of renal function. Magnesium citrate should not be used after charcoal administration because the citrate can displace poisons from charcoal. Oil-based cathartics such as mineral oil and castor oil are not used in treating poisoned patients because these oils can speed systemic absorption of some poisons. Cathartics are especially indicated when enteric-coated tablets have been ingested, when poisoning occurred 1 hour or more previously, or when hydrocarbons have been ingested.

Whole bowel irrigation with a solution of electrolytes and polyethylene glycol formulated for bowel cleansing and administered orally or through a gastric tube may be used to promote evacuation of poison objects such as iron tablets, enteric-coated medications, drug-filled packets for illicit transport, and foreign bodies.

Specific Antidotes

A **specific antidote** is one that directly reverses the toxic action of the poison. In only 5% of poisoning cases is there a specific antidote (Table 9-3). Two specific antidotes, naloxone and flumazenil, are especially important in emergency department situations. They can be both diagnostic tools and potential treatments. Administration of naloxone (Narcan) to a patient who is comatose from an overdose of an opioid (heroin, morphine, pentazocine, propoxyphene) reverses the sedation within 2 minutes. Administration of flumazenil (Mazicon) to a patient who is comatose from an overdose of a benzodiazepine (e.g., chlordiazepoxide or diazepam) reverses the sedation within 1 minute.

Competitive Antidotes

At the receptor a specific antidote may compete for the toxin. **Naloxone** displaces narcotics (opioids) at the opioid receptor. Unlike other opioids, naloxone does not depress the respiratory center; therefore the occupation of the opioid receptor by naloxone protects against respiratory depression. Flumazenil is an antagonist of benzodiazepines, reversing the cognitive, psychomotor, hypnogenic, and electroencephalographic effects of benzodiazepines. Oxygen in high concentration competes with carbon monoxide in binding to hemoglobin to restore oxygenation. **Atropine** blocks the muscarinic receptor from the acetylcholine accumulated in anticholinesterase poisoning.

Chelates

Another category of action of specific antidotes is chelates, compounds that form a nontoxic complex with the toxin. Poisoning by heavy metals in particular is treated with chelates, which form a nontoxic complex with the metal; this complex is quickly eliminated, usually in the urine. Accumulation of the heavy metal is thereby reversed. Dimercaprol complexes arsenic, copper, lead, and mercury. Penicillamine, a drug used to treat rheumatoid arthritis and lupus (see Chapter 42) also complexes copper, lead, and mercury. Deferoxamine is a specific chelate for iron (see Chapter 22). Ethylenediaminetetraacetic acid (EDTA) is the chelate used for lead or cadmium intoxication.

Antibodies

In a few instances treatment with specific antibodies to the poison is possible. Antibodies to digoxin are available to counteract toxic levels of this important cardiac drug. These antibodies reverse the cardiac toxicity by complexing the digoxin and lowering the large pool of digoxin that is bound to plasma albumin. The digoxin then is not free to act. Antivenoms are antibodies for certain snake and spider venoms.

Metabolic Alterations

Specific antidotes may alter the metabolism of a toxin. Ethanol inhibits the biotransformation of methanol and ethylene glycol to toxic metabolites, particularly formic acid. Thiosulfate enhances the transformation of cyanide to the relatively nontoxic thiocyanate. Acetylcysteine restores the sulfhydryl groups of the liver after depletion by acetaminophen metabolism. Sulfhydryl groups protect the liver from toxic metabolites of acetaminophen. Physostigmine inhibits acetylcholinesterase, the enzyme that normally degrades acetylcholine. This action allows acetylcholine concentrations to rise at the synapses and compete with anticholinergic drugs blocking these receptors. This reversal by acetylcholine restores function in anticholinergic poisoning by drugs that either are anticholinergic, such as atropine or scopolamine, or have anticholinergic actions, such as antihistamines, tricyclic antidepressants, and antipsychotic drugs. Used as an antidote, pralidoxime reactivates acetylcholinesterase after it has been inactivated by an anticholinesterase poison. The poison is freed in an inactive form to be eliminated.

Diuresis and Dialysis
Diuresis

Diuresis can be used to hasten elimination of poisons excreted primarily by the kidneys. It is used when the level of poison in the blood is at a potentially fatal concentration, when the patient is in a coma, and when the patient other-

Text continued on p. 108

Table 9-3   Specific Antidotes

Antidote	Poison	Administration/Dosage	Comments
Cholinergic Poisoning			
atropine	Anticholinesterase Organophosphates Physostigmine	INTRAVENOUS: *Children*—0.02 mg/kg; *Adults*—1-2 mg. This is initial dose. Repeat every 20 min until copious secretions are controlled.	Blocks muscarinic receptors to prevent peripheral actions of excessive concentrations of neurotransmitter, acetylcholine. See Chapter 11 for more information about actions of acetylcholine and how atropine blocks actions of acetylcholine. Muscarinic symptoms for which atropine is given include nausea, vomiting, diarrhea, sweat, increased bronchial and salivary secretions, and slow heart rate (bradycardia).
pralidoxime chloride (PAM)	Anticholinesterase Organophosphates	*Organophosphate poisoning:* BY INFUSION in 100 ml saline over 15-30 min: *Children*—20-40 mg/kg; *adults*—1-2 g. A second dose can be given in 1 hr. *Carbamate (neostigmine, pyridostigmine) poisoning:* INTRAVENOUS: *Adults*—1-2 g initially, followed by 250 mg every 5 min as necessary to reverse cholinergic crisis.	Reactivates enzyme acetylcholinesterase after inactivation by irreversible anticholinesterases or organophosphates. This allows acetylcholine to be degraded and relieves paralysis (overstimulation) caused by accumulated acetylcholine. Pralidoxime acts mainly outside CNS. In organophosphate poisoning, pralidoxime is given to restore neuromuscular function, especially to relieve paralysis of respiratory muscles. Atropine is given concurrently (see above) to relieve depression of respiratory center and to reverse muscarinic stimulation. In overdose by carbamate anticholinesterases (neostigmine, pyridostigmine and ambenonium, drugs for myasthenia gravis), pralidoxime antagonizes effects of these drugs on neuromuscular junction.
physostigmine salicylate (Antilirium)	Antimuscarinic anticholinergic	INTRAVENOUS OR INTRAMUSCULAR: *Adults*—0.5-2 mg. INTRAVENOUS: *Children*—0.5 mg by slow (1 min) infusion. Repeat if needed at 5- to 10-min intervals until desired effect, or 2 mg total dose, is reached.	Reversible anticholinesterase that increases concentration of acetylcholine at its receptor sites. Reverses both CNS and peripheral anticholinergic effects. Useful for reversing toxic anticholinergic effects caused by overdose of atropine and other belladonna alkaloids, tricyclic antidepressants, phenothiazines, and antihistamines. Central anticholinergic effects include anxiety, delirium, disorientation, hallucinations, hyperactivity, seizures, and in extreme cases, coma, medullary paralysis, and death. Peripheral anticholinergic toxic effects include fast heart rate (tachycardia), fever, mydriasis (dilated pupils), vasodilation, urinary retention, decreased secretions, and decreased gastrointestinal motility.
Sedative-Hypnotic/Opioid Poisoning			
ethanol	methanol ethylene glycol	INTRAVENOUS: *Adults*—0.6 g/kg + 7-10 g over 1 hr; then 10 g/hr maintenance; *children*—0.6 g/kg + 4-5 g over 1 hr; 5 g/hr maintenance.	All three alcohols are metabolized by aldehyde dehydrogenase. Ethanol is preferred substrate and thereby blocks metabolism of methanol and ethylene glycol to toxins formaldehyde and formic acid (both alcohols) and oxylate (ethylene glycol). Ethanol is given in additional loading dose to achieve blood level of 100 mg/dl.
flumazenil (Mazicon)	Benzodiazepines	INTRAVENOUS: *Adults*—initially 0.2 mg administered over 30 sec; if desired level of consciousness is not obtained, a further dose of 0.3 mg may be administered over another 30 sec. Additional doses of 0.5 mg may be administered over 30 sec at 1-min intervals to a cumulative dose of 3 mg. If patient relapses, repeat doses at 20-min intervals as needed, but no more than 1 mg at a time and no more than 3 mg per hour.	Reversible antagonist of benzodiazepine receptor. Reverses cognitive, psychomotor, hypnogenic, and electroencephalographic effects of benzodiazepines. Because flumazenil increases level of consciousness in cases of benzodiazepine overdose even in presence of alcohol intoxication, flumazenil helps in diagnosis. Symptoms of poisoning with barbiturates, alcohol, and phenothiazines are not affected. However, flumazenil may worsen toxicity of tricyclic antidepressants. Flumazenil is also used to improve recovery from surgical sedation with benzodiazepines.
fomepizole (Antizol)	ethylene glycol	INTRAVENOUS: *Adult*—15 mg/kg body weight initially, followed by 10 mg/kg body weight every 12 hr for 4 doses, then 15 mg/kg body weight every 12 hr until ethylene glycol concentration decreases to less than 20 mg/dl.	New drug. Reversible inhibitor of alcohol dehydrogenase to decrease formation of toxic metabolites. The metabolite oxalate is toxic to the kidneys. Each dose of fomepizole should be administered over 30 min.

CNS, Central nervous system.

Table 9-3   Specific Antidotes—cont'd

Antidote	Poison	Administration/Dosage	Comments
naloxone (Narcan)	Narcotics (opioids), including pentazocine, propoxyphene, diphenoxylate	INTRAVENOUS (May also give intramuscularly or subcutaneously): *Adults*—0.4-2 mg. Additional doses are repeated at 2- to 3-min intervals until patient responds or until 10 mg is given. *Children*—0.01 mg/kg with 0.1 mg/kg as subsequent dose.	Reversible antagonist of opioid receptor. Useful for reversing narcotic depression, including respiratory depression. Naloxone is preferred because it is pure opioid antagonist and causes no respiratory depression of its own. Naloxone is effective within 2 min and has duration of action of 1-4 hr. Because most opioids have a longer duration of action, effects of naloxone may wear off and patient may relapse, requiring additional naloxone.

Specific Metabolic Poisons

Antidote	Poison	Administration/Dosage	Comments
acetylcysteine (Mucomyst)	acetaminophen	ORAL: 140 mg/kg as 5% solution mixed with soda, water, or grapefruit juice. Follow with 17 maintenance doses of 70 mg/kg every 4 hr.	Acetylcysteine restores sulfhydryl groups depleted by acetaminophen metabolism. This prevents toxicity to liver produced by metabolites of acetaminophen. Acetylcysteine should not be given with activated charcoal because charcoal absorbs it.
amyl nitrite sodium nitrite sodium thiosulfate (Cyanide Antidote Package)	cyanide	*Amyl nitrite:* Crush ampule on gauze and have patient inhale vapor. *Sodium nitrite:* Inject 10 ml of 3% solution after IV line is established. *Sodium thiosulfate:* Inject 50 ml of 25% solution after administration of sodium nitrite.	Cyanide has almond odor. Toxicity of cyanide is caused by its blockage of enzymes using oxygen in mitochondria (cytochrome oxidase), thereby depressing cellular respiration. Inhibition of cytochrome oxidase depends on binding of cyanide to ferric iron in cytochrome oxidase. Nitrite converts ferrous iron in hemoglobin to ferric iron, producing methemoglobin. This large pool of ferric iron in blood competes with cytochrome oxidase for cyanide, thereby restoring cellular respiration. Thiosulfate accelerates conversion of cyanide to relatively nontoxic thiocyanate, which is readily excreted in urine.

Metal Poisoning

Antidote	Poison	Administration/Dosage	Comments
deferoxamine mesylate (Desferal)	iron	INTRAMUSCULAR, CONTINUOUS SUBCUTANEOUS, OR SLOW INTRAVENOUS: *Adults*—1 g initially, 0.5 g at 4 and 8 hr. Additional doses if needed, up to 6 g daily. For IV, do not give at rate greater than 15 mg/kg/hr. Administer IM if possible. *Children*—50 mg/kg IM or IV every 6 hr up to 15 mg/kg/hr by continuous IV. Maximum dosage: 6 g/24 hr or 2 g/dose.	Chelates iron and thereby prevents iron from entering cells and inhibiting chemical reactions. Chelate of iron and deferoxamine is rapidly excreted in urine, removing iron from body.
dimercaprol (BAL)	arsenic gold mercury lead	INTRAMUSCULAR: Because dimercaprol is oil, give deep intramuscularly only. *Mild arsenic or gold poisoning:* 2.5 mg/kg 4 times daily, 2 days; 2 times, day 3; once daily, 10 days. *Severe arsenic or gold poisoning:* 3 mg/kg 4 hr for 2 days, 4 times day 3; twice daily 10 days. *Mercury poisoning:* 5 mg/kg initially; 2.5 mg/kg 1.2 times daily for 10 days. *Acute lead poisoning:* 4 mg/kg alone initially, then at 4-hr intervals with calcium disodium edetate (administered at separate site). Maintain for 2-7 days.	Dimercaprol is a sulfhydryl compound that chelates arsenic, gold, and mercury and promotes their excretion in urine. Dimercaprol also reactivates affected sulfhydryl enzymes. Peak plasma concentrations occur 30-60 min after administration. Excretion is complete in 4 hr. Dimercaprol is not very effective for poisoning caused by antimony and bismuth. It is contraindicated in iron, cadmium, and selenium poisoning because chelates are more toxic, especially to kidney, than metal alone. Alkalinization of urine protects kidney from breakdown of dimercaprol-metal complex in acid urine. Common side effects of dimercaprol are rise in blood pressure with tachycardia (fast heart rate) and burning sensation of lips, mouth, and throat.
edetate calcium disodium (calcium disodium versenate)	lead	INTRAVENOUS: 50-75 mg/kg/day in 3-6 doses, each dose administered over at least 1 hr. Can continue for up to 5 days. Wait 2 days before resuming therapy for additional 5 days. INTRAMUSCULAR: Preferred route for children. Give 35 mg/kg twice daily. After 3-5 days, discontinue for 4 days or more.	Calcium-bound to EDTA is displaced by lead and resulting chelate is excreted in urine (50% in 1 hr: 95% in 24 hr). EDTA can produce toxic effects, including renal damage and irregularities in cardiac rhythm. Doses must be carefully monitored.
penicillamine (Cuprimine, Depen)	copper lead zinc mercury	ORAL: *Adults*—1-1.5 g daily in 4 divided doses on empty stomach for 1-2 mo; *children*—30-40 mg/kg daily or 600-750 mg/m² daily for 1-6 mo.	Penicillamine chelates copper, lead, zinc, or mercury, promoting their excretion in urine. Side effects include allergic reactions (principally rashes) and loss of sweet and salt tastes. Severe side effects include bone marrow depression and renal toxicity.

wise has stable cardiovascular, respiratory, and renal function. Fluid diuresis, achieved with a potent loop diuretic such as furosemide, increases the glomerular filtration rate and thereby decreases the renal tubular reabsorption of the poison. Osmotic diuresis with mannitol or urea prevents reabsorption of the poison in the kidney by creating an osmotic load that effectively flushes the kidney tubule.

Alkalinization of the urine with sodium bicarbonate enhances the excretion of weak acids such as aspirin and phenobarbital by maintaining them in their ionized form, which is not reabsorbed readily. Similarly, acidification of the urine with ammonium chloride or ascorbic acid aids the excretion of weak bases such as amphetamine or phencyclidine by maintaining them in their ionized form, which is not reabsorbed. Diuretics are discussed fully in Chapter 14.

Dialysis

Dialysis is indicated in cases of extreme poisoning or renal failure when the poison is dialyzable. For instance, the anticoagulant warfarin and the cardiac glycoside digitoxin are tightly bound to protein in the blood and therefore are not successfully removed by dialysis.

Hemodialysis is a highly technical and complex procedure in which the blood is shunted from the body and through tubing immersed in a physiologic buffer. Any chemical present in the blood but not in the buffer diffuses into the buffer because of the concentration gradient. The blood so dialyzed, or "washed," is continuously returned to the body. Salicylate, methanol, and ethylene glycol are especially effectively removed by hemodialysis.

Hemoperfusion is a technique in which the blood is pumped from a venous catheter through a column of absorbent material and returned to the patient. Anticoagulation with heparin is necessary to prevent the patient's blood from clotting in the cartridge. Hemoperfusion is effective for high-molecular-weight poisons with poor water solubility because the cartridge has a large surface area for absorption. Drugs cleared more rapidly through hemoperfusion include salicylates, phenytoin, ethchlorvynol, phenobarbital, theophylline, and carbamazepine.

Peritoneal dialysis is the simplest dialysis technique, but unfortunately, it is the most inefficient in removing most drugs. In peritoneal dialysis, physiologic buffer is introduced into the abdomen and left there for several hours before being drained and replaced. Because the gastrointestinal tract has a rich blood supply, the blood is dialyzed as it flows through the normal gastrointestinal network.

Nursing Process Overview

Treatment of Poisoning

Assessment

Patients who have been exposed to poisons or who have ingested poisons may enter the health care system in any condition, from the child who is alert, oriented, and feeling fine after ingesting a handful of children's vitamins, to the patient who requires resuscitation or is comatose and unable to provide any information about the toxic substances. Obtain a complete baseline assessment, including vital signs, mental status, blood pressure, weight, serum electrolyte levels, liver and renal function studies, blood gases, and electrocardiogram. The health history should include information about the poison(s) ingested (how much, when, what efforts have been tried as treatment) and preexisting health problems.

Nursing Diagnoses

- Anxiety related to treatment and/or possible outcome of treatment
- Altered comfort: nausea and vomiting from use of ipecac
- Ineffective airway clearance related to drug overdose with potential for aspiration

Patient Outcomes

The patient will recover from the poisoning episode with no ill effects. The nonspecific or specific antidote will successfully treat the poisoning, vomiting will end, and the patient will not aspirate and will be alert enough to clear airway. Suicidal patients will begin psychiatric care.

Planning/Implementation

Establish and maintain a patent airway with adequate ventilation. Other measures might include supportive care of the unconscious patient, administration of nonspecific or specific antidotes, and hospitalization for further observation or treatment. Monitor vital signs, blood pressure, and electrocardiogram as needed. Initiate and maintain intravenous therapy, monitor intake and output, monitor laboratory work (blood gases, liver and renal function studies, serum levels of suspected toxins and/or antidotes), insert a nasogastric or orogastric tube for gastric lavage, or induce vomiting as ordered. Monitor mental status. Keep the patient and the family informed of actions being taken and their effect.

Evaluation

Effective treatment for overdose or exposure to toxins occurs when the poisonous substance is eliminated and the patient returns to normal without experiencing side effects associated with the poison or treatment. Most antidotes will not be administered on an outpatient basis. Before discharge, instruct the patient and the family about continuing care or observations required. If appropriate, give instructions about removing toxic substances from the home or workplace. Refer the patient to social services or a community-based nursing care agency if appropriate. Provide positive reinforcement about psychiatric care if recommended for the patient.

Nursing Implications Summary

General Guidelines: Care of the Poisoned Patient

➤ Thoroughly assess any patient suspected of having ingested a toxic substance or a toxic amount of a generally nontoxic substance. If the patient's condition obviously requires emergency treatment, the initial assessment may be abbreviated until the patient is stabilized, then further assessment should be performed. Assess blood pressure and vital signs; neurologic examination; level of respiratory effort; presence of cyanosis; breath sounds; electrocardiogram; complete visual inspection, including nose and mouth; blood gases; serum electrolytes; renal and liver function tests; and weight. Obtain a detailed history from the patient and family about the suspected toxic agents, including the amount, when the substance was ingested, efforts made to induce vomiting or dilute the substance, the patient's age, and any coexisting medical problems. Save any samples of the toxic substance, vomitus, or stool; label carefully and send to the laboratory for analysis.

➤ Work quickly and efficiently to administer prescribed antagonists or other treatments, but remain calm. Reassure the patient and family that everything possible is being done. Families of children may be especially upset. Nurses who work in settings where overdoses or toxic ingestions are commonly seen (e.g., emergency departments, some occupational health settings) should know the following: location of emergency equipment for intubation, assisted ventilation, and resuscitation; telephone number of the nearest poison control center; location of reference guides to emergency treatment of overdoses; location of antidotes, antagonists, and equipment (e.g., lavage tubes) used in that setting; and general procedures to be followed in treating overdoses.

➤ Prevention of overdose is preferable to treatment for overdose; however, preventive health teaching is usually not appropriate during treatment of acute overdose. Nurses who work with patients or families in situations that involve drugs or toxic chemicals should review general safety measures on a regular schedule. Teaching points to review with patients and families to help prevent accidental ingestion of medicines or toxic household chemicals include keeping medications out of the reach of children, the incompetent, or the confused; keeping medications in a locked cabinet; keeping household products out of reach of children; keeping drugs and chemicals in clearly and correctly labeled containers; using safety latches on cabinets and drawers; never referring to medicines as candy; treating all medicines with respect; using childproof caps when children are in the environment; using drugs only as prescribed; and never doubling or increasing the dose of any drug unless specifically directed to do so by the physician. Teach patients never to borrow medications prescribed for another person.

➤ Ipecac is available in small quantities without a prescription and should be kept in the home (out of the reach of children) for emergency treatment of overdose. However, teach families to call the poison control center before administering ipecac to ascertain that inducing vomiting is appropriate for the ingested substance. Teach patients to keep the number of the poison control center handy near the telephone.

➤ Instruct patients or families calling for emergency help to bring a sample of the drug or toxic substance and any vomitus to the emergency department when they bring the patient.

ipecac
Drug Administration/Nursing in the Community

➤ Ipecac may be purchased without prescription and may be kept in the home. Do not administer ipecac until directed to do so by the physician or poison control center. Any ipecac remaining after a dose has been administered should be discarded. Check expiration dates.

➤ Have the patient drink a full glass of water (8 oz) after taking the ordered dose ($\frac{1}{2}$ to 1 full glass for a child). A frightened child may do better if the water is administered before the ipecac. Avoid milk products. Generally, if vomiting does not occur after the first dose, the dose is repeated in about 20 minutes. If vomiting does not occur after the second dose, take the patient to the emergency department. Do not give this drug to infants younger than 6 months of age. Children 6 months to 1 year of age should be treated in the emergency department.

➤ If the physician has also prescribed activated charcoal, give ipecac syrup first and administer the activated charcoal after vomiting has ceased. Do not induce vomiting in anyone who is drowsy because this may lead to aspiration. Save vomitus and send it to the laboratory for analysis.

activated charcoal
Drug Administration

➤ Activated charcoal is most effective when administered within 30 minutes of ingestion of the poison. The mixture is unattractive. Put it into an empty soft-drink can to administer it to children. Mix charcoal with water or a small amount of fruit juice. Do not mix with ice cream, milk, sherbet, or chocolate syrup because these foods will decrease the ability of the charcoal to absorb the toxin. Activated charcoal adsorbs ipecac; do not administer these simultaneously. If multiple doses of activated charcoal are ordered, preparations that contain sorbitol should not be used for each dose because the total amount of sorbitol may cause diarrhea; alternate sorbitol-containing preparations with activated charcoal that does not contain sorbitol. Caution patients that activated charcoal may cause feces to turn black.

Cathartics
Drug Administration

➤ See Chapter 24 for additional information about saline cathartics. Do not use sodium salts if the patient has a history of heart disease. Do not use magnesium salts if the patient has a history of renal failure. Do not use magnesium sulfate if activated charcoal has been administered.

Continued

Nursing Implications Summary—cont'd

atropine
➤ See Chapter 11 for additional information about atropine.

pralidoxime chloride
Drug Administration
➤ Review the information presented in Table 9-3. Keep a suction machine and intubation equipment readily available when using this drug. See Chapter 42 for a discussion of myasthenia gravis. Keep edrophonium, atropine, syringes, and a tourniquet handy when working with patients with myasthenia gravis. Monitor patients carefully. Side effects of pralidoxime may mimic effects of ingested substances: dizziness, blurred vision, diplopia, drowsiness, nausea, tachycardia, hyperventilation, and muscle weakness.

physostigmine salicylate
Drug Administration
➤ Review the information presented in Table 9-3. Monitor vital signs and blood pressure. Treat overdose of physostigmine with atropine, which should be kept at the bedside. Because the drug has a short duration of action (30 to 60 minutes), it may be necessary to repeat doses. Monitor the patient carefully. Physostigmine may be administered intravenously undiluted. Administer at a rate of 1 mg or less over 1 to 3 minutes (adults) or 0.5 mg per minute (children). Too rapid intravenous (IV) administration may cause convulsions, difficulty breathing, and bradycardia.

ethanol
Drug Administration
➤ Ethanol can be administered intravenously or via orogastric or nasogastric tube. Orally, a 20% solution is preferred to reduce the risk of gastritis, but if needed, any blended whiskey can be used. If the patient's condition warrants it, oral administration is preferred because the IV route is limited to 5% and 10% solutions. Monitor blood ethanol levels during therapy. Monitor vital signs, blood pressure, and electrocardiogram. When using ethanol for treatment of overdose, keep a suction machine and equipment for intubation and resuscitation at the bedside.

flumazenil
Drug Administration
➤ Flumazenil may be administered via direct IV push at a rate of 200 μg over 30 seconds. It may also be diluted in D5W, normal saline, or 0.45% sodium chloride and 2.5% dextrose. See the manufacturer's literature for information about admixing with other drugs. Monitor level of consciousness and vital signs, especially respirations. Have a suction machine at the bedside. Anticipate the possibility of needing an artificial airway and ventilatory and circulatory support. Have drugs readily available to treat seizures. Monitor electrocardiogram and oxygenation via pulse oximetry. If resedation occurs, it may be necessary to repeat doses. Flumazenil is also discussed in Chapter 57.

Nursing in the Community
➤ Flumazenil is used in an acute-care setting. If flumazenil has been used as part of outpatient surgery or procedures, warn the patient not to resume regular activities for at least 18 to 24 hours after discharge because psychomotor and memory deficits may persist that long. Give postdischarge instructions in writing to the patient and a responsible caretaker.

naloxone
Drug Administration
➤ Monitor respirations. Naloxone should promptly increase the respiratory rate and volume. If it does not, then respiratory depression is probably not the result of narcotic overdose, or multiple agents were consumed or injected. Keep intubation and resuscitation equipment and drugs readily available if the patient manifests respiratory depression.
➤ Monitor vital signs and blood pressure. Naloxone has a relatively short half-life, and the dose may need to be repeated. Remember that in narcotic addicts this drug may precipitate withdrawal symptoms. Monitor neonates carefully. Naloxone may be used to treat neonatal respiratory depression, which may be present if narcotic analgesics were administered in large doses during labor and delivery or if the mother is a narcotic addict. If the mother is an addict, naloxone will precipitate withdrawal symptoms in the infant. Naloxone is also discussed in Chapter 32.

acetylcysteine
Drug Administration
➤ Review Table 9-3 and see Chapter 30. Monitor vital signs and blood pressure. Side effects from acetylcysteine are rare; they include nausea, vomiting, and increase in blood pressure. Acetylcysteine has a bad odor; doses must be diluted before administration. The manufacturer's insert provides information about volumes of diluent to use per dose. Try chilling doses and have the patient take doses through a straw placed in a cup or container that is tightly capped. Doses vomited within 1 hour of administration must be repeated; check with the physician.

Cyanide Antidote Package
Drug Administration
➤ This combination of drugs (amyl nitrite, sodium nitrite, sodium thiosulfate) is recommended for cyanide poisoning and also for treatment of overdose with sodium nitroprusside (see Table 9-3 and Chapter 13). Side effects are rare. Monitor vital signs and blood pressure.

deferoxamine mesylate
Drug Administration
➤ Monitor blood pressure, vital signs, fluid intake and output, and serum iron levels. Rapid intravenous administration may cause hypotension, tachycardia, erythema, and urticaria. Anaphylactic reactions are rare, but keep epinephrine

Nursing Implications Summary—cont'd

and intubation and resuscitation equipment handy. In cases of acute iron poisoning, treat with deferoxamine in addition to lavage and/or induction of emesis, maintain a patent airway, control shock (IV fluids, vasopressors), and correct acidosis (administer sodium bicarbonate or other drugs).

➤ Intramuscular injection is the preferred parenteral route. Reconstitute powder with 2 ml of sterile water for injection for each 500-mg vial; use 8 ml for each 2-g vial. Dissolve all powder before injecting the dose. After subcutaneous injection some patients experience a local histamine-like reaction.

➤ Reserve IV injection for patients who exhibit signs of shock. Reconstitute powder as just described, then further dilute with normal saline solution, dextrose injection, or lactated Ringer's injection. Administer at a rate not exceeding 15 mg/kg/hr.

Nursing in the Community

➤ Advise patients receiving long-term therapy to have regular ophthalmic examinations.

➤ Usually discontinue chelation therapy during pregnancy. Advise women considering pregnancy to consult the physician.

➤ Warn patients that deferoxamine may turn urine red.

dimercaprol
Drug Administration

➤ Review Table 9-3. Monitor vital signs, blood pressure, and fluid intake and output. Monitor the blood urea nitrogen (BUN), serum creatinine, and serum electrolytes. Do not administer medicinal iron to patients receiving dimercaprol.

➤ To avoid skin contact with the drug when preparing doses, wear gloves. Keep the urine alkaline to facilitate chelation, and monitor the urine pH. For detailed instructions in preparing oil-based suspensions, see Chapter 5.

Nursing in the Community

➤ Inform patients that the drug may produce a garliclike odor to the breath. Inform parents that some children have a fever during therapy.

edetate calcium disodium
Drug Administration

➤ Read the physician's orders carefully. Do not confuse edetate calcium disodium (used to treat lead poisoning) with edetate disodium (used to treat hypercalcemia). Assess urine output before administering. Because the chelate is excreted in the urine, patients with oliguria or renal disease may be unable to tolerate this drug. Monitor vital signs, blood pressure, BUN, urinalysis, serum electrolytes, serum creatinine, fluid intake and output, and electrocardiogram. Edetate calcium disodium interferes with the duration of action of zinc insulin preparations. Patients with diabetes who are receiving zinc insulin may need a change in dosage or drug while they are receiving edetate calcium disodium.

➤ IV injection is the preferred route of administration in children and in individuals with lead encephalopathy, although patients in the latter group must be monitored carefully for increased intracranial pressure.

➤ For intramuscular use, lidocaine or procaine may be added to the reconstituted solution to help prevent pain at the injection site (check with the physician or pharmacy). Assess the mouth and gums for development of sores. These sores should subside after drug therapy. Zinc replacement may be necessary between courses of therapy with edetate calcium disodium.

penicillamine
➤ Review Table 9-3. Penicillamine is also used to treat rheumatoid arthritis, as discussed in Chapter 42.

CHAPTER REVIEW

Application

1. What do the terms *toxicology* and *clinical toxicology* mean?
2. What is toxicodynamics, and why is it important clinically?
3. What is toxicokinetics, and why is it important clinically? How does toxicokinetics differ from pharmacokinetics?
4. How does the health professional use nonspecific antidotes in treatment of acute poisoning?
5. What is the role of cathartics in treating acute poisoning? Which drugs are recommended? Why?
6. What specific antidotes would the health professional consider for each of the following categories: competitive antidotes, chelates, antibodies, metabolic alterations?
7. When is diuresis indicated in treating acute poisoning? What is meant by fluid and osmotic diuresis and alkalinization and acidification of the urine? When may these processes be helpful?
8. When is dialysis indicated in treating cases of acute poisoning?

Critical Thinking

1. Determine whether your community has a poison control center. What services are offered by this center? Where is the number in the telephone directory?
2. Why is patient assessment so important in treating poisoning?
3. Contrast the uses of emesis and gastric lavage in emptying the stomach. What is the drug of choice for inducing vomiting? Why?
4. It is recommended that households with children have on hand a small quantity of ipecac. What are important teaching points about this drug?
5. When is the administration of activated charcoal indicated? When is it not indicated?
6. Differentiate between hemodialysis, hemoperfusion, and peritoneal dialysis.
7. What are important teaching points for promoting safety and decreasing the possibility of poisoning in the household?

Reference

Valladares P: Comparing clinical management of overdoses, *Emerg Nurse* 4(1):6-8, 1996.

Chapter 10

Introduction to Autonomic Pharmacology

OBJECTIVES

After studying this chapter, you should be able to do the following:

- *Differentiate between the motor nervous system and the autonomic nervous system.*
- *Distinguish between acetylcholine, norepinephrine, and epinephrine.*
- *Describe the divisions of the autonomic nervous system: sympathetic and parasympathetic.*
- *List the effects on tissues of sympathetic (adrenergic) stimulation and parasympathetic (cholinergic or muscarinic) stimulation.*
- *Describe the "fight or flight" response.*

CHAPTER OVERVIEW

A separate introductory section on autonomic pharmacology has been a feature of this textbook from its beginning. This format introduces the student to key concepts in autonomic pharmacology and asks the student to concentrate first on mechanisms and effects before proceeding to drugs and therapeutics. Many different classes of drugs, used for a variety of therapeutic purposes, affect the nervous system at some level. Some of these drugs are designed to alter the function of some portion of the nervous system, whereas others alter functions of the nervous system as a side effect. A review of the anatomy and biochemical function of the nervous system is necessary to understand the mechanisms of these drugs and the array of side effects they produce. This chapter presents that review. Chapter 11 reviews the mechanisms of cholinergic drugs and inhibitors, and Chapter 12 reviews the mechanisms of adrenergic drugs and inhibitors. The purpose of Chapters 11 and 12 is to introduce the student to the spectrum of mechanisms and therapeutic uses for drugs that affect these two neurotransmitters. The student is cautioned not to be concerned initially with actual drugs listed because these drugs, their therapeutic uses, and the implications for nursing are all discussed in detail in the following chapters. However, the student will find the detailed classification of drugs by mechanism useful as a review later in the course of study.

OVERVIEW OF THE PERIPHERAL NERVOUS SYSTEM

Role of the Peripheral Nervous System

The nervous system is divided into the central nervous system and the peripheral nervous system. The **central nervous system** includes the brain and spinal cord. The functions of these structures are twofold: first, to monitor, convey, and process signals from sensory receptors throughout the body by way of ascending neuronal pathways and, second, to sequence information and convey signals to initiate or to modify body actions.

The neurons that relay information from the central nervous system to the rest of the body are called **efferent neurons.** The ascending sensory neurons and the efferent neurons form the **peripheral nervous system.** The peripheral nervous system plays a dual role by collecting information from throughout the body for processing by the central ner-

Figure 10-1   Synthesis, release, and termination of neurotransmitters. **A,** Acetylcholine. *(1)* Choline is taken up by neuron and *(2)* used to synthesize acetylcholine, which *(3)* is stored in vesicles. On stimulation of neuron *(4),* some vesicles merge with membrane to discharge acetylcholine into synapse, where acetylcholine diffuses to *(5)* its receptor to activate cell, or to *(6)* acetylcholinesterase, enzyme that degrades acetylcholine. Plasma cholinesterases *(7)* can also degrade acetylcholine. **B,** Norepinephrine. *(1)* Tyrosine is taken into neuron and in three reactions is converted to norepinephrine, which is *(2)* stored in vesicles. On stimulation of neuron *(3),* some vesicles merge with membrane to discharge norepinephrine into synapse, where it diffuses to *(4)* its receptor to activate cell. Most of norepinephrine is *(5)* taken up by neuron through receptor mediated process and reused. Some norepinephrine is degraded by *(6)* mitochondrial enzyme monoamine oxidase (MAO) or *(7)* enzyme catechol *O*-methyltransferase (COMT) found in most body tissues.

vous system and by relaying information from the central nervous system to coordinate bodily responses. The peripheral nervous system is subdivided into the motor nervous system and the autonomic nervous system.

Neurotransmitters and Receptors

All neurons use neurotransmitters to contact neurons and other cells. A **neurotransmitter** is a chemical that is synthesized in the nerve cell and stored inside vesicles (sacs) in the terminal. When the neuron is stimulated, some of the vesicles merge with the nerve terminal membrane and quantities of neurotransmitter are released. There is a space between the neuron and the cell with which the neuron is communicating. This space is the synaptic cleft or synapse. The neurotransmitter molecules diffuse across the synapse and occupy specific receptors on the next cell. The function of the receptor is to recognize a specific neurotransmitter and to initiate a cellular response to that neurotransmitter. The binding of the neurotransmitter to its receptor is reversible. When the neurotransmitter diffuses away from the receptor, the stimulation of the cell is terminated.

Two neurotransmitters, acetylcholine and norepinephrine, are the neurotransmitters of the peripheral nervous system. A given class of neurons, however, will use only one of these neurotransmitters. The synthesis and degradation of each neurotransmitter are discussed first. A description of where each neurotransmitter is found in the peripheral nervous system and the responses produced follows.

▼ acetylcholine

Acetylcholine is synthesized in the nerve terminal by the enzyme choline acetylase from choline and an acetate molecule activated by coenzyme A (Figure 10-1). This acetylcholine is packaged in vesicles. On stimulation of the nerve, some of the vesicles release acetylcholine into the synapse, where the acetylcholine diffuses to the opposing membrane and binds at the specific receptors for acetylcholine. In addition, the opposing membrane contains the enzyme acetylcholinesterase, which degrades acetylcholine to acetate and choline. The acetylcholinesterase is very active, and the half-life of the acetylcholine released is only a few milliseconds. Any acetylcholine that diffuses from the synapse into the blood is degraded by nonspecific cholinesterases in the blood or tissues. Thus, when released, acetylcholine produces a response in the next cell by way of the acetylcholine receptor and/or is rapidly degraded by the membrane-bound enzyme acetylcholinesterase or by nonspecific cholinesterases in the blood plasma.

▼ norepinephrine and the neurohormone epinephrine

Norepinephrine is synthesized in the nerve terminal from the amino acid tyrosine (see Figure 10-1). Norepinephrine is a neurotransmitter because it is released from a neuron to act on an adjacent cell. The chromaffin cells of the adrenal medulla also synthesize norepinephrine but convert 80% to

85% of the norepinephrine to epinephrine. These adrenal stores of epinephrine and norepinephrine are released into the blood on stimulation of the adrenal medulla in response to stress. **Epinephrine** is called a neurohormone because it is released into the blood to produce effects at distant sites.

Most norepinephrine is not degraded after release. Instead, it is taken back up into the neuron from which it was released and stored again in granules. This process is called **reuptake.** Two enzymes can degrade norepinephrine and epinephrine. Monoamine oxidase (MAO) is located in the mitochondria of most cells, including nerve terminals that release norepinephrine. Catechol *O*-methyltransferase (COMT) is found in the cytoplasm of most cells. Both MAO and COMT are found in large concentrations in the liver and kidney. Any norepinephrine that diffuses into the blood or any epinephrine in the blood is quickly degraded by the liver and/or kidney. No drugs are used that interfere with COMT, but in later chapters we shall see that drugs that inhibit MAO are used for treating depression, hypertension, and parkinsonism. Epinephrine and norepinephrine are metabolized to the common product vanillylmandelic acid (VMA). Because VMA is excreted in the urine, the measurement of VMA in collected urine is used as an index of sympathetic activity.

The main features of the peripheral nervous system and its neurotransmitters acetylcholine and norepinephrine are reviewed as a preparation for discussing drugs that act by modifying neurotransmitter action within the peripheral nervous system. The motor nervous system is discussed first and then the more complex autonomic nervous system.

MOTOR NERVOUS SYSTEM

The motor (somatic) nervous system is under both conscious and unconscious control to initiate muscle contraction (Figure 10-2). A motor neuron has a cell body in the spinal cord and contacts a striated muscle at a specialized region, the neuromuscular junction. Motor neurons are found in several cranial nerves and in all spinal nerves. Stimulation of a motor neuron releases acetylcholine at the neuromuscular junction, and the muscle cell reacts to acetylcholine by contracting. Stimulation of a motor neuron may arise as a result of a willed impulse originating in the brain and transmitted to the appropriate neuron in the spinal cord or, unconsciously, as a reflex. A reflex is initiated by sensory input (i.e., heat, touch, pressure, pain) that is transmitted to the spinal cord and then out to the motor neurons without processing by the brain.

AUTONOMIC NERVOUS SYSTEM

Divisions of the System

The role of the **autonomic nervous system** is to monitor and control internal body functions such as cardiac output, blood volume, blood composition, blood pressure, and digestive processes, primarily by modifying the tone of tissue smooth muscle and the quantity of tissue secretions (see Figure 10-2). The autonomic nervous system has two distinct efferent divisions: the **parasympathetic (cholinergic) nervous system** and the **sympathetic (adrenergic) nervous system.** Both divisions commonly act on a given organ but produce opposite responses. This activity is highlighted in Table 10-1, in which the prominent effects of the two divisions on key tissues are summarized. For example, the parasympathetic division slows the heart rate, whereas the sympathetic division increases the heart rate. This dual antagonistic innervation is a hallmark of the autonomic nervous system; it allows full control of organ function according to bodily requirements. This antagonism is a result of two distinct kinds of receptors, adrenergic receptors and cholinergic receptors, coexisting on the same organ. In general, activation of the cholinergic receptor produces the opposite cellular response from activation of the adrenergic receptor.

Autonomic Tone

The concept of autonomic tone is also important. Although a minimal but constant release of each neurotransmitter affects each tissue, one branch of the autonomic nervous system is dominant and sets the tone of that tissue to coordinate with other tissues. The sympathetic nervous system provides the dominant tone for the cardiovascular system; therefore the magnitude of cardiac and blood pressure responses reflects predominantly the degree of sympathetic tone, which is itself determined and coordinated within the central nervous system. Parasympathetic control of the cardiovascular system is primarily that of a reflex decelerator system to protect against rapid rises in cardiovascular function. On the other hand, parasympathetic tone is coordinated within certain brain centers to dominate visual, digestive, and eliminatory functions and to determine the intensity of these responses. The role of the sympathetic nervous system is primarily that of an override mechanism to depress these functions in times of stress.

Preganglionic and Postganglionic Neurons

Each efferent division of the autonomic nervous system is a two-neuron system. The first neuron (preganglionic neuron) has its cell body in the brainstem or spinal cord and

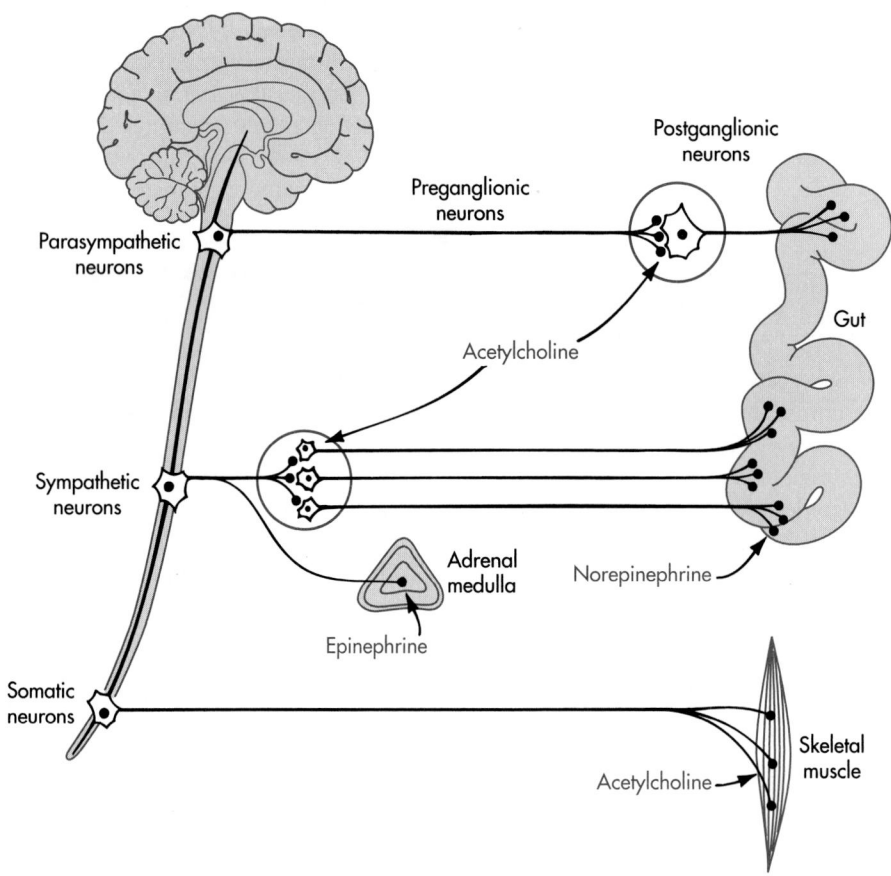

Figure 10-2 Neurotransmitters of autonomic nervous system. Acetylcholine and norepinephrine are released from neurons as indicated to act on adjacent cells. Epinephrine is released from adrenal medulla into blood to act throughout body. The parasympathetic neurons originate mainly in the brainstem with axons in cranial nerves III, VII, IX, X, and XI although a few neurons originate in the lower spinal cord with axons in sacral nerves II, III, and IV. The sympathetic neurons originate in the thoracic and lumbar parts of the spinal cord. Somatic (motor) neurons arise from all parts of the spinal cord.

terminates outside the spinal cord in a special nervous tissue, a ganglion (see Figure 10-2). The first neuron sends a projection out of the spinal cord (preganglionic fiber) that contacts a second neuron (postganglionic neuron) within the ganglion. The neurotransmitter for the synapse in the ganglion is acetylcholine. The second neuron has its cell body in a ganglion and by means of a postganglionic fiber innervates an internal organ, usually modifying the action of involuntary muscle such as smooth muscle or cardiac muscle.

Role of acetylcholine, norepinephrine, and epinephrine

The most important pharmacologic difference between the parasympathetic and the sympathetic nervous systems is that the final postganglionic transmitter is different for the two divisions. The preganglionic neurotransmitter at the synapses within the ganglia for both divisions is acetylcholine. However, the parasympathetic nervous system also uses acetylcholine as a postganglionic neurotransmitter. Therefore the parasympathetic nervous system is often called the cholinergic nervous system.

The sympathetic nervous system uses norepinephrine as the postganglionic transmitter. The sympathetic nervous system has another component, the neurohormone epinephrine. Epinephrine is released from the adrenal medulla as a reaction to stress. The adrenal medulla acts like a postganglionic neuron because it is innervated by a preganglionic fiber and on stimulation releases epinephrine. Epi-

nephrine is carried by the blood throughout the body, where epinephrine not only activates tissue receptors for norepinephrine but also activates additional receptors more specific for epinephrine itself. The sympathetic nervous system is also called the adrenergic nervous system. The term *adrenergic* comes from the British word for epinephrine, adrenaline. (Norepinephrine is also called noradrenaline.) The identity of the neurotransmitter at the various sites of the peripheral nervous system is diagrammed in Figure 10-2.

Characteristics of the Autonomic Nervous System

Functional Characteristics

Certain characteristics readily distinguish the parasympathetic and the sympathetic nervous systems functionally. These characteristic functions are listed in Table 10-1. The parasympathetic nervous system has dominant control over "regulatory" processes of the body, whereas the sympathetic nervous system provides immediate adaptation for "fight or flight." Indeed, the easiest way to remember the actions of the sympathetic nervous system (and by contrast the parasympathetic nervous system) is to review the "fight or flight" adaptations: the eyes dilate so that vision is improved even in dim light, the bronchioles dilate to let air flow to and from the lungs more readily, the heart beats faster and with greater strength to supply blood to muscle, the visceral blood vessels are constricted but muscle blood vessels are dilated

Table 10-1	**Autonomic Nervous System Actions**	
Tissues	**Parasympathetic (Cholinergic or Muscarinic) Response**	**Sympathetic (Adrenergic) Response**
Eye	Constriction (miosis)	Dilation (mydriasis)
	Accommodation (focus on near objects)	
Glands	Increased salivation (copious, watery)	Increased sweating*
	Increased tears and secretions of respiratory and gastrointestinal tract	Increased salivation (thick, contains proteins)
Heart	Decreased rate (negative chronotropy)	Increase rate (positive chronotropy)
	Decreased strength of contraction (negative inotropy)	Increased strength of contraction (increased contractility or positive inotropy)
	Decreased conduction velocity through the atrioventricular node (negative dromotropy)	Increased conduction velocity through atrioventricular node (positive dromotropy)
Bronchioles	Smooth muscle constriction (restricts airways)	Smooth muscle relaxations (opens airways)
Blood vessels	Constriction of vessels in heart (not a prominent effect in humans)	Dilation of vessels in salivary gland and erectile tissues
	Dilation of vessels in heart and skeletal muscle	Constriction of vessels in skin, viscera, salivary glands, erectile tissues, kidney
Gastrointestinal tract		
Smooth muscle	Contraction	Relaxation
Sphincters	Relaxation	Contraction
Urinary bladder		
Fundus	Contraction	Relaxation
Trigone and sphincter	Relaxation	Contraction
Uterus		Contraction
Liver		Glycogenolysis

*Acetylcholine is the neurotransmitter for this sympathetic response. This is the exception to the rule that norepinephrine is the postganglionic neurotransmitter.

so that the increased blood flow can meet the demands of cardiac and skeletal muscle for oxygen and nutrients, digestive and excretory processes are slowed, and the liver breaks down stored glycogen to provide glucose for fuel. All these responses represent actions of the sympathetic nervous system.

Anatomic Characteristics

The parasympathetic and the sympathetic nervous systems also differ in their anatomy. The postganglionic neurons of the two systems derive from distinct areas of the spinal cord. The efferent neurons for part of the parasympathetic nervous system arise in the lower area of the brain. These parasympathetic cell bodies include the respiratory and circulatory centers of the medulla, which control cardiovascular and gastrointestinal processes. The remainder of the preganglionic neurons of the parasympathetic nervous system arise from the sacral portion of the spinal cord and allow parasympathetic control of digestive, excretory, and reproductive processes. In contrast, the preganglionic neurons of the sympathetic nervous system all arise in the thoracic and lumbar regions of the spinal cord. Also, the number of postganglionic to preganglionic neurons is highly characteristic of each division. In the parasympathetic nervous system each preganglionic neuron contacts one or two postganglionic neurons so that there is discrete neuronal control over organ function. In contrast, the sympathetic nervous system may have 20 or more postganglionic neurons in contact with each preganglionic neuron so that the action on stimulation of preganglionic neurons is diffuse, in keeping with the "alarm" nature of the sympathetic nervous system.

Role of Other Autonomic Neurotransmitters

An expanded view of the autonomic nervous system is evolving. First, the concept that a neuron makes only one kind of neurotransmitter has proven incorrect. Current evidence indicates that in addition to either norepinephrine or acetylcholine, other chemical messengers such as peptides, eicosanoids, or purines may be co-released. These messengers act to modulate the response to the neurotransmitter. For instance, VIP (vasoactive intestinal peptide) appears to be co-released with acetylcholine from parasympathetic fibers that innervate blood vessels and exocrine glands. In this case, VIP acts to synergize the action of acetylcholine to stimulate vasodilation or secretion. A second evolving concept is that nonadrenergic, noncholinergic neurons control smooth muscle activity in many tissues. Purinergic nerves using adenosine triphosphate (ATP) as the neurotransmitter have shown in the gastrointestinal tract, the genitourinary tract, and some blood vessels. Endothelial cells of the inner layer of blood vessels act as modulators of autonomic and hormonal messengers. In particular, endothelial cells release nitric oxide. Nitric oxide has emerged as the important agent causing vasodilation of vascular smooth muscle. This has opened up new research for understanding atherosclerosis and inflammation.

CENTRAL NERVOUS SYSTEM: COMMENTS

The brain and spinal cord are more complex in their neuronal organization than is the peripheral nervous system. This complexity is necessary because information must be processed rather than just transmitted. This processing is accomplished in two ways. First, a given neuron may send out many axonal projections and thereby form synaptic junctions with many different neurons. This arrangement serves to send a flow of information to several areas for further processing. Second, a given neuron can receive information from more than one neuron. Thus dendrites from a given neuron may have synaptic junctions with axons from many neurons. This arrangement serves to collect information from different sources.

Neurotransmitters

The central nervous system uses a number of neurotransmitters. In addition to acetylcholine and norepinephrine, the central neurotransmitters that will be encountered in discussing central nervous system pharmacology in later chapters include dopamine, serotonin, epinephrine, histamine, gamma-aminobutyric acid (GABA), glycine, and enkephalins. Some neurotransmitters, in particular GABA and glycine, are inhibitory rather than excitatory. The neuronal response to these neurotransmitters is to develop a more negative resting potential with a decreased likelihood of firing rather than to depolarize more readily and fire.

Correlation of Function with Neurotransmitters

In the past few years nerve tracts have been described in the brain and characterized by their neurotransmitter content. These nerve tracts have cell bodies in different areas of the brain to collect information, but the neurons then converge and form synaptic junctions with many neurons in other regions of the brain. Through surgery or chemical destruction of specific nerve tracts, it has been possible to associate control of mental and motor behavior with some of the nerve tracts and their neurotransmitters. Examples include a role for norepinephrine in the control of sympathetic tone (see Chapter 13), acetylcholine and dopamine in the central coordination of muscle movement (see Chapters 62 and 63), a role for dopamine in psychosis (see Chapter 58), a role for dopamine and serotonin in depression (see Chapter 59), and the role of enkephalins in analgesia (see Chapter 32). A current goal in neuropharmacology is to identify how drugs modify behavior through their modification of neurotransmitter synthesis, storage, release, action, and inactivation.

CHAPTER REVIEW

Application

1. What are neurotransmitters?
2. What is the synthesis, storage, release, and termination of action of acetylcholine and norepinephrine?
3. What are the two divisions of the autonomic nervous system? How are they involved in dual antagonistic innervation and in determining autonomic tone?
4. Describe the neurons of the autonomic nervous system and those of the motor nervous system with respect to anatomy and identity of the neurotransmitter used.

Critical Thinking

1. Describe the "flight or fight" adaptations of the sympathetic nervous system. What objective data would you expect to find?
2. What would be the objective change in heart rate that you might see if you administer a drug that blocks the adrenergic stimulation?
3. What would be the effect on secretions (glands) of administering a drug that blocks the cholinergic stimulation?

Chapter

11

Mechanisms of Cholinergic Control

OBJECTIVES

After studying this chapter, you should be able to do the following:

- *Differentiate between muscarinic and nicotinic receptors.*
- *Describe the difference between direct- and indirect-acting cholinomimetic drugs.*
- *Explain the difference between reversible and irreversible acetylcholinesterase inhibitors.*
- *List three therapeutic uses of cholinomimetic drugs.*
- *Describe three kinds of cholinergic antagonists.*
- *Describe six therapeutic uses of muscarinic receptor antagonists (atropine).*

CHAPTER OVERVIEW

This chapter is intended to be read twice during a course in pharmacology. The beginner should read the chapter for the mechanisms and therapeutic applications but should not be overly concerned with the drugs given as examples. Later, in a course in pharmacology, the student can return to this chapter to review the mechanism of action of these drugs.

In this chapter the basis of selective action of cholinergic drugs is explained. The emphasis is on how the therapeutic activities of these drugs arise from their selective action on classes of receptors for acetylcholine. Cholinergic drugs achieve their effects through stimulation and inhibition of receptors. The organ systems most prominently affected include the eye, gastrointestinal system, and muscle.

POPULATIONS OF CHOLINERGIC RECEPTORS AS DEFINED BY DRUG ACTION

In Chapter 10, three distinct populations of receptors for acetylcholine in the peripheral nervous system were presented: receptors on striated muscle at the neuromuscular junction, receptors on postganglionic neurons within the ganglia, and receptors on other innervated tissues.

Muscarinic Receptors

The distinction between acetylcholine receptors is not just anatomic. Chemical differentiation is made with **muscarine,** a chemical found in certain mushrooms, which mimics the effects of acetylcholine by slowing the heart rate or stimulating smooth muscle when applied to those tissues. Muscarine produces no effect when applied to skeletal muscles or to ganglia. Muscarine mimics acetylcholine only at the postganglionic receptors. The parasympathetic postganglionic receptors are therefore called **muscarinic receptors.**

As a cholinergic agonist, muscarine is a laboratory tool. It is encountered clinically only as a toxin responsible for acute mushroom poisoning. (Another kind of mushroom poisoning exists in which symptoms take several hours to appear.) The symptoms of acute mushroom poisoning appear within an hour or so of ingestion and consist of generalized parasympathetic overstimulation that includes glandular stimulation (sweating, tearing, salivation), an overactive gastrointestinal system (nausea, cramps, diarrhea), cardiovascular symptoms (flushed skin, slow heart rate), constricted pupils, and excessive urination.

The molecular basis of muscaric receptors has been clarified. Five types of muscarinic receptors have been identified through molecular cloning. These five types (M1 to M5) can be grouped into two subclasses based on which G-protein set (see Chapter 1) is linked to the receptor. M1, M3 and M5 belong to one subclass in which the G-protein set mediates Ca^+-dependent smooth muscle contraction and secretion. M2 and M4 belong to another subclass in which the G-protein set mediates inhibition of adenylate cyclase, activation of certain potassium membrane channels, and suppression of the voltage gated calcium channels. M1 receptors are found primarily in ganglia and some secretory glands. M2 receptors are found primarily in the heart and smooth muscle. M3 and M4 are found in smooth muscle and secretory glands. All five types are found in the central nervous system (CNS).

Nicotinic Receptors

Nicotine, found in tobacco, is another cholinergic agonist. Nicotine is the laboratory agent that mimics the effects of acetylcholine at the skeletal muscle and ganglionic receptors. Therefore the **nicotinic receptors** are the ganglionic and neuromuscular receptors for acetylcholine. Nicotine is not an effective agonist for acetylcholine at the muscarinic receptors.

The molecular biology of the nicotinic receptors is quite distinct from that of the muscarinic receptors. Five subunits make up a nicotinic receptor. The nicotinic receptor found in muscle has four different subunits, with only the alpha subunit appearing twice. Far more variable are the nicotinic receptors found in ganglia and in the CNS. These receptors are also pentamers. Although they are composed of only alpha and beta subunits, there are eight subtypes of alpha subunits and three subtypes of beta subunits. A variety of different nonmuscular nicotinic receptors is therefore found. However, all nicotinic receptors act by the same basic mechanism. When activated, the receptor is a pore in the membrane through which sodium and potassium ions can diffuse rapidly down their concentration gradients. The receptor is activated when acetylcholine binds to an alpha subunit and changes the conformation to allow opening of the pore.

DIRECT- AND INDIRECT-ACTING CHOLINOMIMETIC DRUGS

Drugs that mimic the action of acetylcholine act by one of two mechanisms: directly, by mimicking acetylcholine (these drugs are chemically related to acetylcholine), or indirectly, by inhibiting acetylcholinesterase (these drugs allow acetylcholine to remain intact longer because its degradation is inhibited).

Acetylcholine itself is not commonly used as a therapeutic agent because it produces too many responses and because it is too rapidly degraded in the blood. Rarely, acetylcholine is used topically in eye surgery. Carbachol (Carbacel) and pilocarpine (Pilocar) are examples of direct-acting cholinomimetic drugs used principally in ophthalmology. Bethanechol (Urecholine) is the only direct-acting cholinomimetic drug used systemically.

Reversible and Irreversible Acetylcholinesterase Inhibitors

The acetylcholinesterase inhibitors can be subdivided into the reversible inhibitors and the irreversible inhibitors. The reversible inhibitors, as the name implies, bind to the enzyme reversibly, and therefore the drug effect wears off as the drug is eliminated from the body, usually in a few hours. Examples of reversible inhibitors of acetylcholinesterase include physostigmine (Eserine), pyridostigmine (Mestinon), and neostigmine (Prostigmin).

The **irreversible inhibitors** form a permanent covalent bond with acetylcholinesterase, and the enzyme must be completely replaced before the drug effect wears off, a process requiring days to weeks. The most common examples of irreversible acetylcholinesterase inhibitors are the organophosphate compounds, which include potent drugs for constricting the pupil (miotics): demecarium (Humorsol), echothiophate (Phospholine), and isoflurophate (Floropryl); the insecticides parathion and malathion; and several agents developed for chemical warfare. It is interesting to note that the antidote for poisoning by an irreversible acetylcholinesterase inhibitor is pralidoxime (PAM), which is itself an acetylcholinesterase inhibitor. PAM, however, is able to compete with the enzyme for the phosphate group of the inhibitor, thereby eliminating itself and the inhibitor from the enzyme, reversing the "irreversible" inhibition.

Therapeutic Uses of Cholinomimetic Drugs

Cholinomimetic drugs are used clinically for three effects in the peripheral nervous system:

1. To restore muscle tone in patients with myasthenia gravis or in surgical patients treated with tubocurarine. This is a nicotinic effect at the neuromuscular junction. The drugs used to increase muscle strength are all acetylcholinesterase inhibitors. Cholinomimetic drugs acting at the neuromuscular junction are discussed in Chapters 37 and 42.

2. To constrict the pupil (miosis), a muscarinic effect that is used in ophthalmology. Cholinomimetic drugs administered to act in the eye are described in Chapters 73 and 74.

3. To stimulate an atonic bladder or intestine. This is a muscarinic effect. Cholinomimetic drugs affecting the gastrointestinal system are discussed in Chapter 23.

Table 11-1 reviews the receptor specificity for a few of the cholinomimetic drugs discussed in detail in other chapters. No clinical use is made of drugs stimulating nicotinic

Table 11-1 Receptor Specificity of Selected Cholinomimetic Drugs at Therapeutic Doses

Generic and Trade Names	Muscarinic Receptor	Nicotinic* (Neuromuscular Receptor)	Therapeutic Uses
Direct-Acting			
bethanechol (Urecholine)	+	0	Stimulates atonic bladder or intestine
pilocarpine (Pilocar and others)	+ (topical)		Causes miotic reaction (constriction of pupil)
Indirect-Acting: Reversible Inhibitors of Acetylcholinesterase			
edrophonium (Tensilon)	(+)	+	Diagnoses myasthenia gravis; differentiates myasthenic crisis from cholinergic crisis
physostigmine (Eserine)	+ (topical)		Causes miotic reaction (constriction of pupil)
pyridostigmine (Mestinon)	(+)	+	Restores muscle strength in myasthenia gravis
Indirect-Acting: Irreversible Inhibitors of Acetylcholinesterase			
demecarium (Humorsol)	+ (topical)	(+) Near eye	Causes miotic reaction (constriction of pupil)
pralidoxime (Protopam)	+	+	Reactivates acetylcholinesterase

*+, Stimulation; (+), stimulation; at high concentrations, of muscles near eye; 0, no stimulation.
†No drugs are used therapeutically that primarily stimulate nicotinic-ganglionic receptors. Stimulation of nicotinic-ganglionic receptors is a toxic effect of cholinomimetic drugs.

receptors of the ganglia. Ganglia are involved in so many responses that their stimulation by drugs is clinically useless.

CHOLINERGIC ANTAGONISTS

Anticholinergic Drugs

As illustrated in Figure 11-1, each group of receptors for acetylcholine is characterized by a drug that blocks the action of acetylcholine at that type of receptor by occupying the receptor and preventing cholinergic action. Because each class of acetylcholine antagonist acts on a discrete receptor population, clinical use of each class of antagonist differs greatly. Table 11-2 reviews receptor specificity of a few cholinergic receptor antagonists discussed in detail in other chapters.

Neuromuscular Receptor Antagonists

Tubocurarine primarily blocks the receptors for acetylcholine at the neuromuscular junction and thereby causes muscular relaxation or paralysis. Antagonists of the neuromuscular cholinergic receptor are used chiefly as an adjunct to anesthetics and are discussed in Chapter 37.

Ganglionic Receptor Antagonists

The receptors for acetylcholine in the ganglia are blocked by hexamethonium, thus blocking transmission for both parasympathetic and sympathetic impulses. Antagonists like hexamethonium lack much specificity in the response produced. Limited use of drugs antagonizing the action of acetylcholine in the ganglia is made in treating severe cases of hypertension. One such drug, trimethaphan, is discussed in Chapter 13, along with the other antihypertensive drugs.

Muscarininc Receptor Antagonists

Atropine and scopolamine are the prototypes of drugs that block acetylcholine at the muscarinic receptors. These are the parasympathetic postganglionic receptors for acetylcholine on the heart, smooth muscle, and exocrine glands.

Atropine is an alkaloid originally derived from the leaves of the deadly nightshade, or Atropa belladonna, which belongs to the potato family. Several other plants also contain atropine and a related drug, scopolamine. These two drugs are often referred to as belladonna alkaloids. Many references to the use of these plants as medicinal agents are found in ancient medical literature. To this day, atropine remains the most useful and widely versatile of the antimuscarinic drugs.

Therapeutic Uses

1. Muscarinic receptor antagonists block secretions. Salivation is readily blocked by atropine. Indeed, one classic side effect of atropine is a dry mouth (xerostomia). Secretions in the respiratory tract are also inhibited by atropine. This inhibition of bronchial and salivary secretions is the desired effect when atropine is administered as a preanesthetic agent before surgery. The drying effect of atropine reduces secretions that may be involuntarily aspirated when the patient is drowsy or unconscious. Atropine and related drugs are moderately effective in depressing gastric acid secretion in patients with peptic ulcers. The role of cholinergic antagonists in treating gastrointestinal disorders is discussed in Chapter 23. Large doses of atropine and scopolamine dilate the blood vessels in the skin, especially around the face and particularly in children, thus producing a pronounced blushing. The mechanism for this vasodilation is not clear, but because sweating is inhibited by atropine, this flush may represent

Table 11-2   Receptor Specificity of Selected Cholinergic Receptor Antagonists (Anticholinergics) at Therapeutic Doses*

Generic and Trade Names	Muscarinic Receptor	Nicotinic (Ganglionic) Receptor	Nicotinic (Neuromuscular) Receptor	Therapeutic Uses
atropine	−	0	0	Produces mydriasis (dilated pupil) and cycloplegia (paralysis of accommodation): eye topical; reduces gastric acid secretion and gastrointestinal motility and tone of bladder and ureter: systemic use
homatropine methyl-bromide (Homapin)	−	0	0	Reduces gastrointestinal hypermotility and gastric acidity
ipratropium (Atrovent)	−	0	0	Relaxes bronchial smooth muscle
propantheline (Pro-Banthine)	−	0	0	Controls gastrointestinal hypermotility, gastric acidity, and hypermotility of genitourinary and biliary tracts
scopolamine	−	0	0	Same as atropine
succinylcholine (Anectine)	0	0	−	Relaxes skeletal muscle (depolarizing)
trimethaphan (Arfonad)	0	−	0	Lowers blood pressure in selected cases of hypertensive crisis
tropicamide (Mydriacyl)	− (topical)			Produces mydriasis (dilated pupil) and cycloplegia (paralysis of accommodation)
tubocurarine (Tubarine)	0	(−)	−	Relaxes skeletal muscle (nondepolarizing)

* −, Inhibition; (−), inhibition at high concentrations; 0, no inhibition.

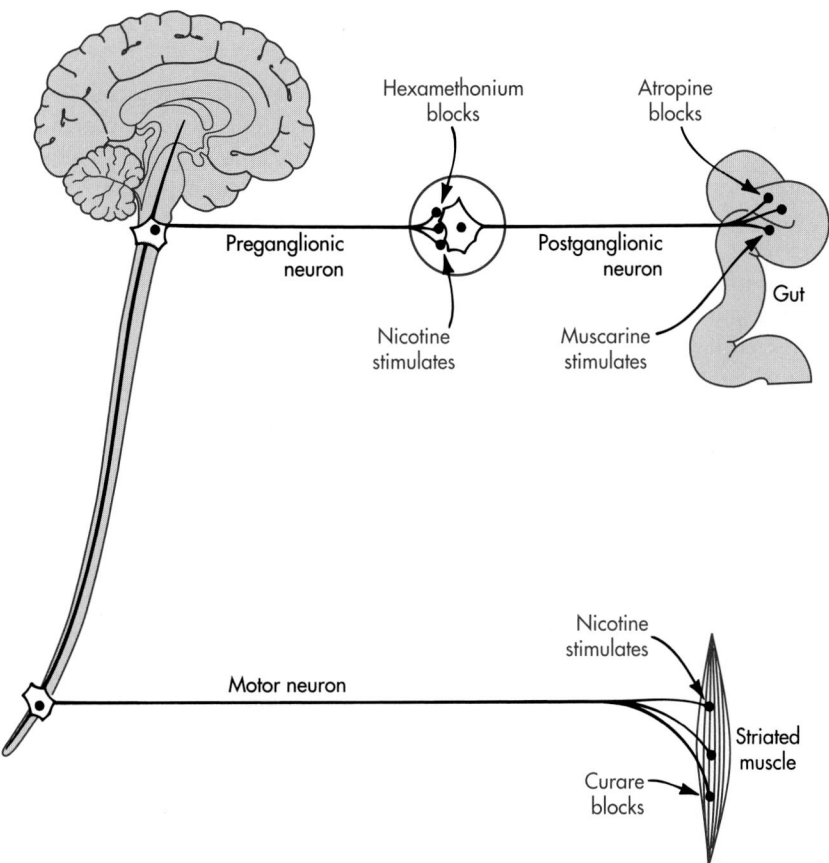

Figure 11-1   Acetylcholine is peripheral neurotransmitter at three receptor populations. Each receptor population is characterized by an agonist and an antagonist. Muscarine is agonist and atropine is antagonist of parasympathetic postganglionic (muscarinic) receptors. Nicotine is agonist and hexamethonium is antagonist of parasympathetic preganglionic (nicotinic) receptors. Nicotine is agonist and tubocurarine is antagonist of neuromuscular junction (nicotinic) receptors.

a mechanism to dissipate heat and a fever may be noted.

2. These agents depress an overactive gastrointestinal tract. A prominent antimuscarinic effect of atropine is to inhibit the tone and motility of smooth muscle. The gastrointestinal smooth muscle is very sensitive to atropine. Drugs affecting gastrointestinal motility are discussed in Chapter 23.

3. Muscarinic receptor antagonists dilate the eye (mydriasis) and paralyze accommodation (cycloplegia). Atropine is applied by drops to the eye to block the actions of acetylcholine. The result of this antagonism is dilation of the pupil, caused by relaxation of the circular muscles of the iris, and blurred vision, associated with paralysis of accommodation. This mydriasis and cycloplegia allow measurements of lens refraction, examination of the retina, and aid in the healing of some infections. Drugs affecting the eye are discussed further in Chapters 73 and 74. Atropine taken orally will also reach the eye. Photophobia (sensitivity to light) as a result of the dilation and blurring of vision (caused by the cycloplegia) are common side effects of oral administration of atropine.

4. These agents increase the heart rate. Atropine is administered to increase the heart rate by antagonizing the acetylcholine released by the vagus nerve at the atrioventricular node of the heart (see Chapter 19).

5. These agents relax bronchial smooth muscle. Ipratropium alleviates bronchospasm, which is common in many pulmonary diseases.

6. These agents treat toxicity of cholinergic agents. The most common cause of cholinergic toxicity is overexposure to insecticides such as malathion and parathion, which are organic phosphate acetylcholinesterase inhibitors. Atropine will reverse the muscarinic effects (i.e., salivation, tearing, diarrhea, bradycardia) but will not reverse the neuromuscular paralysis. PAM, which regenerates acetylcholinesterase at all sites, is therefore the drug of choice.

Side Effects

Side effects may occur in addition to therapeutic effects. The side effects of atropine are extensions of the actions just described. The expected cardiovascular effect is an increase in the heart rate (tachycardia), although a slowing of the heart rate (bradycardia) may be noted with small doses administered intravenously. Dilated pupils and blurred vision are accompanied by an intolerance of the eye to light (photophobia) and, sometimes, eye pain. In addition to dry mouth and constipation, patients may experience nausea and vomiting. Urinary hesitancy or retention is common. The skin is dry and flushed, and some patients may develop a fever from the inability to dissipate heat through sweating.

Side effects produced by anticholinergics in the CNS vary. Atropine, particularly in an overdose, produces generalized excitement, which in the toxic state may result in hallucinations. In contrast, although scopolamine can produce hallucinations, scopolamine also produces sleepiness, sedation, and amnesia.

Other Uses

Drugs that are muscarinic receptor antagonists have other uses unrelated to peripheral muscarinic receptors. Many anticholinergic drugs also have effects in the CNS. Scopolamine, unlike atropine, is effective in preventing motion sickness. Some drugs have antitremor activity and are used to relieve certain tremors called extrapyramidal motor effects caused by Parkinson's disease, other diseases, and some drugs. Anticholinergic drugs used in the treatment of parkinsonism are discussed in Chapter 62.

 CHAPTER REVIEW

Application

1. What are muscarine and nicotine, and how do they relate to receptors for acetylcholine?
2. What are the three prototype acetylcholine antagonists, and with which receptor population is each associated?
3. What are the five actions of atropine that the nurse would see as useful therapeutically?

Critical Thinking

1. Contrast the mechanisms of direct- and indirect-acting cholinomimetic drugs. How might this knowledge about a drug influence the frequency of patient assessment?
2. Compare and contrast the three therapeutic uses of cholinomimetic drugs with regard to the receptor stimulated.
3. What atropine-like (anticholinergic) side effects might the nurse anticipate that a patient would experience? How would you assess each effect you have listed?
4. Develop an argument for and against classifying nicotine, as found in cigarettes, as a drug.

Mechanisms of Adrenergic Control

OBJECTIVES

After studying this chapter, you should be able to do the following:

- *Define catecholamine.*
- *Discuss alpha₁-, alpha₂-, beta₁-, and beta₂-adrenergic receptors and the effect of stimulation of these receptors.*
- *Relate the activity of the beta-adrenergic receptors to the "fight or flight" concept mentioned in Chapter 10.*
- *Describe the role of cyclic adenosine monophosphate (cAMP) in stimulation of the beta-receptors.*
- *Define directly mimicking and indirect-acting adrenergic drugs.*
- *Explain the four mechanisms by which drugs interfere with adrenergic activity.*

CHAPTER OVERVIEW

Like Chapter 11, this chapter is intended to be read as an introduction at the beginning of a course in pharmacology and again later as a review. When reading this chapter as an introduction, pay attention to the mechanisms and their associated effects. The drugs given as examples and their classification by mechanism of action will be of interest when the chapter is reviewed later.

This chapter explains the basis of selective action of adrenergic drugs. Emphasis is given to showing how the therapeutic activities of these drugs arise from their selective action on classes of receptors for norepinephrine and epinephrine. These drugs achieve their effects through stimulation or inhibition of receptors. The organ systems most prominently affected include the eye, bronchial smooth muscle, blood vessel smooth muscle, and the heart.

CATECHOLAMINES AND THEIR RECEPTORS

Naturally Occurring Catecholamines

Dopamine, norepinephrine, and **epinephrine** are naturally occurring **catecholamines** that function as neurotransmitters and neurohormones. Dopamine is derived from the amino acid tyrosine and is the chemical precursor of norepinephrine:

Tyrosine → Dopamine → Norepinephrine → Epinephrine

All three catecholamines are important neurotransmitters in the central nervous system (CNS). As described in Chapter 10, in the autonomic nervous system norepinephrine

125

is the sympathetic postganglionic neurotransmitter, and epinephrine is the neurohormone released from the adrenal medulla in reaction to stress. Dopamine plays a minor role as a neurotransmitter in the autonomic nervous system but a major role as a neurotransmitter in the central nervous system.

The therapeutic use of an **adrenergic drug** depends on whether it acts on alpha$_1$-, alpha$_2$-, beta$_1$-, or beta$_2$-receptor. Catecholamines themselves are relatively or completely ineffective when taken orally because they are rapidly destroyed in the gastrointestinal tract or by the liver, whereas many noncatecholamines can be taken orally. A variety of drugs that are relatively specific for activating a given receptor type and thereby directly mimic some portion of norepinephrine or epinephrine action have been synthesized. A few adrenergic drugs act indirectly by causing the release of norepinephrine. Selected adrenergic drugs are listed in Table 12-1.

Classes of Adrenergic Receptors and Responses

Isoproterenol was the first synthetic catecholamine to be studied. The existence of two classes of adrenergic receptors was proposed in the late 1940s to explain the different physiologic effects elicited by norepinephrine, epinephrine, and isoproterenol. **Alpha-receptors** are those receptors for which norepinephrine and epinephrine are equally potent, but isoproterenol is less potent. **Beta-receptors** are those receptors for which isoproterenol is more potent than or as potent as epinephrine or norepinephrine. Molecular cloning has shown that all adrenergic receptors are closely related proteins. There are two major classes of alpha-receptors: alpha$_1$-

and alpha$_2$-receptors. Each class has three subtypes. There are three subtypes of beta-receptors: beta$_1$-, beta$_2$-, and beta$_3$-receptors. The three major classes of adrenergic receptors, alpha$_1$, alpha$_2$, and beta, differ in their mode of signal transduction.

Signal Transduction and Second Messengers

The identification of hormones and neurotransmitters as molecules released to act at other, sometimes distal sites, raises the question of how the agents effect change once they are bound to their specific receptors. This is the problem of **signal transduction.** The first system to be well characterized was that of the beta-receptor.

In the 1950s Earl Sutherland began the work of elucidating how epinephrine causes glycogenolysis (breakdown of glycogen to glucose) in the dog liver. He and his colleagues subsequently showed that epinephrine acts by binding to what we now recognize as the beta$_2$-receptor on the liver cell membrane. When the beta$_2$-receptor is occupied, there is a structural change that activates the membrane-bound enzyme adenylate cyclase.

As illustrated in Figure 12-1, this structural change is complex. When occupied, the beta-receptor activates a transducer protein called G$_s$ (s = stimulatory protein). G$_s$ then activates adenylate cyclase. The active portion of adenylate cyclase is inside the cell. The enzyme catalyzes the conversion of adenosine triphosphate (ATP) to pyrophosphate (PP) and cyclic adenosine 3′,5′-monophosphate (cAMP). cAMP is the key to the intracellular action of epinephrine. Epinephrine is the hormone released to signal the cell to act. **cAMP** is the "second messenger" that translates the presence

				Central	
Generic and Trade Names	Alpha-Receptor	Beta$_1$-Receptor	Beta$_2$-Receptor	Nervous System	Main Therapeutic Uses
Catecholamines					
dobutamine (Dobutrex)	0	+	0	0	Increases cardiac contractility with little increase in heart rate or conductivity
dopamine (Intropin)	(+)I	(+)I	0	0	Dilates renal arteries at low doses by activating dopamine receptors and preventing kidney shutdown in shock
epinephrine	+	+	+	(+)	Treats anaphylactic shock
isoproterenol (Isuprel)	0	+	+	(+)	Improves bronchodilation for asthma
norepinephrine, levarterenol (Levophed)	+	+	0	(+)	Counteracts hypotension of spinal anesthesia
Noncatecholamines					
albuterol (Ventolin, Proventil)	0	0	+	0	Improves bronchodilation
amphetamine	+I	+I	0	+	Stimulates respiration; counteracts narcolepsy
ephedrine	+I,D	+I,D	+	+	Improves bronchodilation; reduces nasal congestion
metaraminol (Aramine)	+I,D	+I,D	0	0	Counteracts hypotension of spinal anesthesia
midorine (ProAmatine)	+	0	0	0	Treats orthostatic hypotension
naphazoline (Privine)	+	0	0	0	Nasal decongestant (local spray)
phenylpropanolamine	+I,D	+I,D	+	(+)	Nasal decongestant (systemic)
ritodrine (Yutopar)	0	0	+	0	Stops premature labor

+I, Indirectly acting (releases norepinephrine); *+ (or D),* directly action on receptors; *(+),* effect is modest except at high concentration; *0,* no effect.

of epinephrine at the cell surface to the internal machinery of the cell. Many cAMP molecules are formed as a result of each receptor occupation, amplifying the epinephrine signal. cAMP produces cellular effects by stimulating other enzymes. The enzymes present in the cell that can be stimulated by cAMP determine the cellular response. In the liver the response is the breakdown of glycogen. In the heart the response is an increase in heart rate, force of contraction, and conduction speed. In smooth muscle the response is relaxation. All three subtypes of beta-receptors act through adenylate cyclase.

Recently it has been shown that the alpha$_2$-receptor is also linked to the adenylate cyclase. When occupied, the alpha$_2$-receptor activates a transducer protein called G$_i$ (i = inhibitory protein). G$_i$ then inhibits adenylate cyclase activity. Therefore the beta-receptors (beta$_1$ and beta$_2$) and the alpha$_2$-receptor have opposite effects.

Activation of the alpha$_1$-receptor uses a different second messenger. This activation also initiates interaction with a G-protein called G$_q$, but the result is activation of mechanisms that elevate intracellular calcium. The increased cytosolic concentration of calcium changes the activity of certain enzymes. The changes in enzymatic activities account for the actions produced by the activation of the alpha$_1$-receptor.

Two more features of the cAMP system need to be highlighted. First, epinephrine is not the only hormone that stimulates the formation of cAMP. Most polypeptide hormones are known to work through cAMP. Important exceptions are insulin, growth hormone, and prolactin. Each hormone has its specific receptor on its target tissues. This is why each hormone can have tissue-specific actions while using the same second-messenger system. Second, cAMP is rapidly degraded by the enzyme phosphodiesterase to 5'-adenosine monophosphate (AMP). A few drugs have been identified that inhibit phosphodiesterase and thereby produce elevated cAMP concentrations. The main drug of this type is theophylline and its dimer, aminophylline. Such drugs are used to produce vasodilation in cerebral ischemia and, more important, to treat asthma by promoting bronchial dilation (see Chapter 28).

Alpha$_1$-Adrenergic Receptors

Alpha$_1$-receptors account for the primary responses elicited by norepinephrine released from sympathetic postganglionic neurons. Epinephrine is as potent as norepinephrine in stimulating alpha$_1$-receptors.

The general role of the alpha$_1$-receptor is to stimulate contraction of smooth muscle. The most prominent systemic effect is an increase in blood pressure resulting from the constriction of blood vessels, mainly arterioles. The blood vessels controlled by alpha$_1$-receptors are those that service the internal organs, mucosal surfaces, and skin. Blood

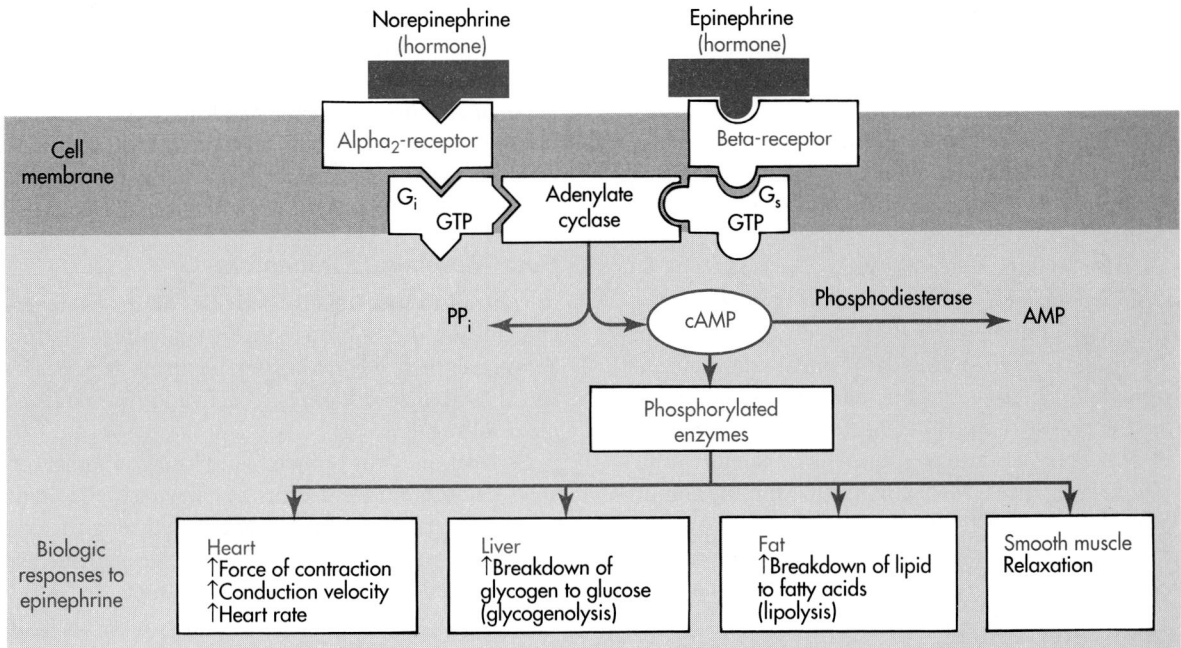

Figure 12-1 Second-messenger concept. Binding of hormone at cell surface initiates a series of reactions that modify activity through phosphorylation of key enzymes and thereby modify cellular responses. Cyclic adenosine monphosphate *(cAMP)* is second messenger because it carries message that hormone is at cell surface and translates this message into action by stimulating a phosphorylating enzyme (cAMP-dependent protein kinase). Cellular responses to epinephrine characteristic for a given organ are given as examples of biologic responses mediated through cAMP. Note that while the beta-adrenergic receptor acts through a stimulatory G protein *(G$_s$)* to promote production of cAMP, alpha$_2$-adrenergic receptor acts through an inhibitory G protein *(G$_i$)* to suppress production of cAMP. ATP is substrate for adenylate cyclase, with cAMP and pyrophosphate *(PP$_i$)* being products. G proteins are regulated by binding and hydrolysis of guanosine triphosphate *(GTP)*.

pressure is in part a reflection of the degree of constriction of these blood vessels because blood pressure is determined by cardiac output and peripheral resistance to blood flow in blood vessels.

Specific physiologic effects resulting from stimulation of alpha$_1$-receptors include the following:

1. Contraction of the radial muscles of the iris. The radial muscles are arranged like the spokes of a wheel so that contraction causes dilation of the pupil (mydriasis). Adrenergic drugs used therapeutically for this effect are discussed in Chapters 73 and 74.
2. Constriction of arterioles and veins, which causes an increase in blood pressure. Adrenergic drugs that are used to raise the blood pressure are discussed in Chapter 16.
3. Contraction of smooth muscle sphincters in the stomach, intestine, and bladder.
4. Contraction of the uterus (in women) and stimulation of ejaculation (in men).
5. Decreased secretions from the pancreas.
6. Breakdown of glycogen in the liver (glycogenolysis) and synthesis of glucose (gluconeogenesis).

Drugs mimicking the adrenergic effects listed in items 3 through 6 are not used therapeutically.

Therapeutic use is made of local vasoconstriction by epinephrine and some other alpha$_1$-adrenergic receptor agonists. Nasal decongestion may be achieved by local application of a vasoconstrictive drug (see Chapter 30). Drug absorption from parenteral sites is slowed when a drug is injected along with a vasoconstricting agent. Local anesthetics in particular will have a longer duration of action when injected with epinephrine to slow systemic absorption.

Alpha$_2$-Adrenergic Receptors

The existence of a second class of alpha-receptors, the **alpha$_2$-receptors,** was experimentally proved in the 1970s. Alpha$_2$-adrenergic receptors play an important role in regulating vascular tone peripherally and centrally. Specific effects attributed to alpha$_2$-receptors include the following:

1. Inhibition of norepinephrine release. Alpha$_2$-receptors are found presynaptically on sympathetic neuronal terminals. These presynaptic alpha$_2$-receptors inhibit further release of norepinephrine when they are stimulated. Presynaptic alpha$_2$-receptors therefore function as a negative feedback system to limit the amount of norepinephrine released from the neuron.
2. Platelet aggregation. Alpha$_2$-receptors are found on platelets where their activation causes platelets to aggregate.
3. Systemic vasoconstriction. Alpha$_2$-receptors are also found on the smooth muscle of the blood vessels that determine blood pressure: the resistance vessels. Like alpha$_1$-receptors, alpha$_2$-receptors mediate vasoconstriction to increase resistance and thereby increase blood pressure. However, alpha$_2$-receptors are not located next to alpha$_1$-receptors where the sympathetic postganglionic nerve terminates on the blood vessel, but at other sites along the blood vessel. The alpha$_2$-receptors on the blood vessel are believed to mediate vasoconstriction to blood-borne dopamine and catecholamine.
4. Blood flow to the skin. Alpha$_2$-receptors also control blood flow in the skin. Activation of alpha$_2$-receptors results in vasoconstriction. The fact that cold potentiates activation of alpha$_2$-receptors may explain the etiology of Raynaud's disease. This condition is characterized by intense cutaneous vasoconstriction, leading to pain and, in the extreme, loss of digits. The therapeutic potential of drugs acting at alpha$_2$-receptors remains to be developed.
5. CNS control of sympathetic tone. The antihypertensive drugs clonidine, guanfacine, and methyldopa have been found to stimulate the alpha$_2$-receptor. The antihypertensive activity of these drugs comes from activation of alpha$_2$-receptors in the CNS. This activation suppresses sympathetic activity.

Beta$_1$-Adrenergic Receptors

The **beta$_1$-receptors** are stimulated by norepinephrine and by epinephrine, but isoproterenol is a more potent stimulant than either of these drugs. Physiologic responses to activation of beta$_1$-receptors is important in controlling cardiac function.

There are three cardiac effects. Activation of the beta$_1$-receptor in the conducting tissue of the heart speeds the repolarization of the cells. An increase in heart rate (positive chronotropic effect) and an increase in impulse conduction speed (positive dromotropic effect) are the two consequences. Stimulation of the beta$_1$-receptors in the ventricular muscle increases the force of contraction (positive inotropic response). Drugs acting on beta$_1$-receptors that are used for stimulating the heart under certain restricted conditions are presented in Chapter 16.

Beta$_2$-Adrenergic Receptors

In contrast to their relative activities on the beta$_1$-receptors, epinephrine and isoproterenol are equipotent in stimulating **beta$_2$-receptors,** whereas norepinephrine is a weak stimulant. Physiologic responses to activation of beta$_2$-receptors include the following:

1. Dilation of the bronchioles. The relaxation of bronchial smooth muscle decreases airway resistance and makes it easier to breathe. Drugs acting through activation of beta$_2$-receptors are used to treat patients with restricted airways, primarily caused by asthma or chronic obstructive lung disease. These drugs are discussed in Chapter 28.
2. Relaxation of uterine smooth muscle. Drugs acting through activation of beta$_2$-receptors, such as ritodrine and terbutaline, are used to stop premature labor by relaxing the pregnant uterus (see Chapter 71).
3. Dilation of the blood vessels in the skeletal muscle, brain, and heart. Activation of these beta$_2$-receptors causes vasodilation and shunts blood to the skeletal muscle, brain, and heart.

4. Breakdown of glycogen in the liver (glycogenolysis) and synthesis of glucose (gluconeogenesis). Note that these also are alpha$_1$-adrenergic effects. No therapeutic use is made of these actions.

Beta$_3$-Adrenergic Receptors

Stimulation of the beta-receptor of fat tissue induces lipolysis, the breakdown of stored fat. This activity used to be attributed to the beta$_1$-receptor, but molecular cloning has revealed a separate beta-receptor. The fatty acids that are released can then be used as energy sources by the heart and liver. No therapeutic use is made of drugs mimicking this adrenergic effect.

Systemic Effects of Activation of Beta-Adrenergic Receptor

The value of the responses to beta-receptors can be appreciated by recalling the "fight or flight" nature of the sympathetic nervous system discussed in Chapter 10. The heart rate and cardiac output increase because epinephrine reinforces the action of norepinephrine on the beta$_1$-receptors. Blood is shunted to muscle, brain, and heart, where stimulation of beta$_2$-receptors results in vasodilation, and from the skin and abdominal organs, where stimulation of alpha$_1$-receptors causes vasoconstriction. Epinephrine also stimu-

lates the liver to break down glycogen to glucose, and it stimulates the fat cells to break down lipid to fatty acids to provide readily available energy sources for the body.

DRUGS INHIBITING ADRENERGIC ACTIVITY

Table 12-2 lists selected drugs that interfere with peripheral adrenergic activity and the therapeutic use of these drugs. Several different drug mechanisms interfere with adrenergic activity. These mechanisms include the following:

1. Blockade of alpha-adrenergic receptors
2. Blockade of beta-adrenergic receptors
3. Depletion of peripheral neuronal stores of norepinephrine
4. Inhibition of peripheral sympathetic activity through an action in the CNS

Each of these mechanisms are discussed further in regard to the spectrum of physiologic effects produced.

Blockade of Alpha-Adrenergic Receptors

Drugs that block of alpha$_1$-receptors are used primarily in the treatment of hypertension. Prazosin, doxazosin, and terazosin act selectively to antagonize norepinephrine at the alpha$_1$-receptors. A person with normal blood pressure taking one of these drugs would experience little change in

Table 12-2   Selected Drugs Inhibiting Adrenergic Receptor Activity

Generic and Trade Names	Alpha-Receptor	Beta$_1$-Receptor	Beta$_2$-Receptor	Central Nervous System (CNS)	Main Therapeutic Uses
Alpha-Adrenergic Receptor Antagonists					
phenoxybenzamine (Dibenzyline)	−	0	0	0	Treats vasospastic disorders of digits (Raynaud's syndrome); treats hypertension related to pheochromocytoma
prazosin (Minipress)	−	0	0	0	Treats chronic hypertension; benign prostatic hyperplasia
Beta-Adrenergic Receptor Antagonists					
atenolol (Tenormin)	0	−	0	0	Treats chronic hypertension; prophylactic for angina
betaxolol (Betoptic)	0	−	0	0	Treats glaucoma (topical)
esmolol (Brevibloc)	0	−	0	0	Controls supraventricular tachycardia
labetalol (Trandate, Vescal)	−	−	0	0	Treats chronic hypertension; prophylactic for angina
metoprolol (Lopressor)	0	−	0	−	Cardioselective; treats chronic hypertension; prophylactic for angina
propranolol (Inderal)	0	−	−	−	Treats chronic hypertension; prophylactic for angina, migraine and cardiac arrhythmias
timolol (Blocadren, Timoptic)	0	−	−	0	Treats chronic hypertension; glaucoma (topical)
Drugs Depleting Neuronal Stores of norepinephrine					
guanadrel (Hylorel)	I	I	I	0	Treats severe chronic hypertension
reserpine (Serpasil)	I	I	I	−	Treats chronic hypertension
Drugs Inhibiting Sympathetic Activity Through CNS Action					
methyldopa (Aldomet)	−CNS	0	0	−	Treats chronic hypertension
clonidine (Catapres)	−CNS	0	0	−	Treats chronic hypertension; treats withdrawal symptoms
guanabenz (Wytensin)	−CNS	0	0	−	Treats chronic hypertension

−, Inhibition; *0*, no effect; *I*, indirect inhibition resulting from depletion of norepinephrine stores; −*CNS*, decrease in peripheral sympathetic tone through action in central nervous system.

blood pressure as long as the person is lying down. However, any sudden shift to the upright position causes orthostatic (postural) hypotension because the blockade of the alpha$_1$-receptors prevents the vasoconstriction necessary to redistribute blood flow. Therefore in orthostatic hypotension the blood pools in the legs and drains from the head, causing fainting. Other effects characteristic of blockade of the alpha$_1$-receptors include a pinpoint pupil (miosis), nasal stuffiness, or inhibition of ejaculation (in men).

The uses and pharmacokinetics of the alpha$_1$-receptor antagonists in the treatment of hypertension are discussed in Chapter 13. Blockade of alpha$_1$-receptors in the base of the bladder and prostate reduces the resistance to urine flow. This has led to the use of alpha$_1$-blockers to improve urinary flow with benign prostatic hyperplasia.

No drugs that specifically block alpha$_2$-receptors in the periphery are widely used. Tolazoline is the only specific alpha$_2$-blocker available, but is used mainly in arteriography and to treat persistent pulmonary hypertension of the newborn. Phentolamine, used in the short-term control of severe hypertension associated with the tumor pheochromocytoma, blocks alpha$_1$- and alpha$_2$-receptors equally.

Blockade of Beta-Adrenergic Receptors

The physiologic effects of beta-receptor antagonists can be anticipated by considering the functions of the beta-receptors. In the healthy person, blockade of the beta$_1$-receptors in the heart causes little change at rest but limits the increase in cardiac functions normally elicited by exercise and hypertension. Conditions improved by beta$_1$-receptor blockade include angina, hypertension, and some cardiac arrhythmias. Recently, propranolol, metoprolol, and timolol have been found to be effective treatment for patients with angina to prevent recurrent heart attacks.

Beta-blockers are effective in treating hypertension as single agents. They also act in an additive fashion when combined with diuretics to lower blood pressure. Also, when a beta-blocker is given with a vasodilator drug, the beta-blocker inhibits the reflex activation of the heart caused by the drop in blood pressure. Therefore a beta-blocker combined with a diuretic and vasodilator is especially effective in treating hypertension. The use of beta-blockers in the therapy of hypertension is discussed in Chapter 13.

Propranolol (Inderal) was the first beta-receptor antagonist approved for clinical use in the United States. It blocks both beta$_1$- and beta$_2$-receptors and is used to treat hypertension, angina, and cardiac arrhythmias. In addition, propranolol is an effective prophylactic in the treatment of migraine headaches, although the mechanisms involved are unclear. A number of non-selective beta-blockers are now widely used in clinical practice, primarily for the treatment of hypertension, angina, cardiac arrhythmias, and glaucoma.

Blockade of beta$_2$-receptors limits bronchiole dilation and therefore can severely compromise pulmonary function in patients with asthma. This effect has led to the development of beta$_1$ selective antagonists (**cardioselective antagonists**) such as atenolol (Tenormin) and metoprolol (Lopressor).

Timolol (Timoptic), betaxolol (Betoptic), levobunolol (Betagan), and metipranolol (OptiPranolol) are examples beta-receptor antagonists that are effective in treating glaucoma by reducing the production of aqueous humor in the eye. They are discussed with other ophthalmic drugs in Chapter 73.

Depletion of Peripheral Neuronal Stores of norepinephrine

Guanethidine (Ismelin) and reserpine (Serpasil) are antihypertensive drugs that deplete norepinephrine from peripheral neurons.

Guanethidine is taken up into the postganglionic sympathetic nerve terminals, where it then prevents the release of norepinephrine. After several days the neuronal content of norepinephrine is depleted. Guanadrel is a more recent drug that has the same mechanism of action.

Reserpine also causes a depletion of norepinephrine stores not only in the periphery but also in the brain. The central action of reserpine is believed to contribute in a major way to the depression of sympathetic tone with this agent.

Reserpine and guanethidine are useful in treating chronic hypertension (see Chapter 13) and Raynaud's disease (see Chapter 15).

Inhibition of Peripheral Sympathetic Activity Through Central Nervous System Action

The CNS also plays a major role in the control of sympathetic activity through vasopressor centers in the brainstem. Stimulation of alpha$_2$-receptors in the vasomotor center results in a decreased sympathetic outflow. Several antihypertensive drugs act through this central mechanism. These antihypertensive drugs include clonidine (Catapres), methyldopa (Aldomet), guanabenz (Wytensin), and guanfacine (Tenex). The role of these drugs in the treatment of hypertension is described in Chapter 13.

 # CHAPTER REVIEW

Application

1. Which are the three naturally occurring catecholamines, and where are they found?
2. What does the "second messenger" (cAMP) do?
3. What are the four major drug mechanisms that inhibit adrenergic activity? What therapeutic use is made of each of these actions?

Critical Thinking

1. What physiologic actions does the nurse associate with stimulation of the alpha$_1$-adrenergic receptor? of the alpha$_2$-adrenergic receptor? of the beta1-adrenergic receptor? of the beta$_2$-adrenergic receptor? What changes in objective data would you expect to see with each of these?

Antihypertensive Drugs

OBJECTIVES

After studying this chapter, you should be able to do the following:

- *Discuss the factors that control blood pressure.*
- *List lifestyle modifications that may be used to help reduce blood pressure.*
- *Discuss the drug classes that may be used for initial drug therapy for hypertension.*
- *Describe modifications in antihypertensive therapy that may be needed for special populations: African-Americans, older adults, pregnant women, and patients with coexisting cardiovascular disease.*
- *Develop a plan of nursing care for patients who receive one or more of the following drug groups: beta-blockers, alpha$_1$-blockers, sympatholytics, centrally acting antihypertensives, angiotensin-converting enzyme inhibitors, calcium channel blockers, and other vasodilators.*
- *Develop a plan of nursing care for a patient with a hypertensive emergency being treated with diazoxide, sodium nitroprusside, or trimethaphan.*
- *Develop a teaching plan for a patient who has orthostatic hypotension or who needs to reduce sodium intake.*

CHAPTER OVERVIEW

Hypertension is generally defined as a resting systolic blood pressure greater than 140 mm Hg or a diastolic blood pressure greater than 90 mm Hg, or both, in an adult. In the United States it is estimated that this condition may apply to 50 million persons. High blood pressure reflects an increased tone of the arteries and arterioles. Renal, endocrine, or neurogenic diseases are found to be the cause of hypertension in 10% of patients with hypertension. The hypertension in these patients is treated by focusing on its cause. No primary cause of the hypertension can be found in the remaining 90% of patients with hypertension; this condition of unknown origin is called **essential hypertension.**

INTRODUCTION

The patient with hypertension may have no symptoms of this disease but will have an increased risk of stroke, blindness, and heart and renal disease after 10 years or more of sustained high blood pressure that produces vascular and organ damage. The prevalence of hypertension is higher in older adults than in younger adults, higher in men than in women during the young adult and early middle-age range, but higher in women than men from middle age onward. Hypertension is more common in African-Americans, in those from the southeastern United States, and in poor and less educated individuals.

Effective drug therapy for hypertension has been available for two decades. Throughout this period, for patients controlling their hypertension with therapy, mortality from coronary heart disease has decreased by 50% and that from stroke by 57%. Also during this time, evidence from epidemiologic studies has accumulated to show that a systolic blood pressure greater than 120 mm Hg and/or a diastolic blood pressure greater than 80 mm Hg is associated with increased risks or morbidity, disability, and mortality. This chapter presents the drugs used to control hypertension and the rationale for their use.

THERAPEUTIC RATIONALE: HYPERTENSION

Physiology of Hypertension

The major factors that regulate blood pressure are diagrammed in Figure 13-1. These factors center around those that influence the circulating volume through adjustments of body salt and water (renal mechanisms) and those that influence the activity of the heart and blood vessels (cardiovascular mechanisms). Vasoactive peptides play a role in mediating renal and cardiovascular mechanisms.

Renal Mechanisms

The kidney plays an important role in maintaining blood pressure through control of the salt and water content of the body (see Chapter 14). A decrease in blood pressure stimulates the release of renin from the kidney. Renin release is partly controlled by beta-adrenergic receptors. Renin is a proteolytic enzyme that acts on a protein in the blood to produce the peptide angiotensin I. Angiotensin I is rapidly converted to angiotensin II, a small peptide that is a potent vasoconstrictor and therefore increases blood pressure. Angiotensin II also acts on the adrenal cortex to stimulate the secretion of aldosterone.

Aldosterone is the mineralocorticoid hormone that acts on the kidney to decrease the excretion of sodium and to increase potassium excretion. The resulting sodium retention expands the plasma and extracellular fluid volumes, which contribute to the elevation of blood pressure.

Cardiovascular Mechanisms

Within the blood vessels, the blood pressure depends on the cardiac output and the resistance to blood flow in the blood vessels. Baroreceptors in the aorta and carotid sinus monitor the blood pressure and send the information to the brain. The brain integrates this information and adjusts the heart rate and resistance of the blood vessels, largely

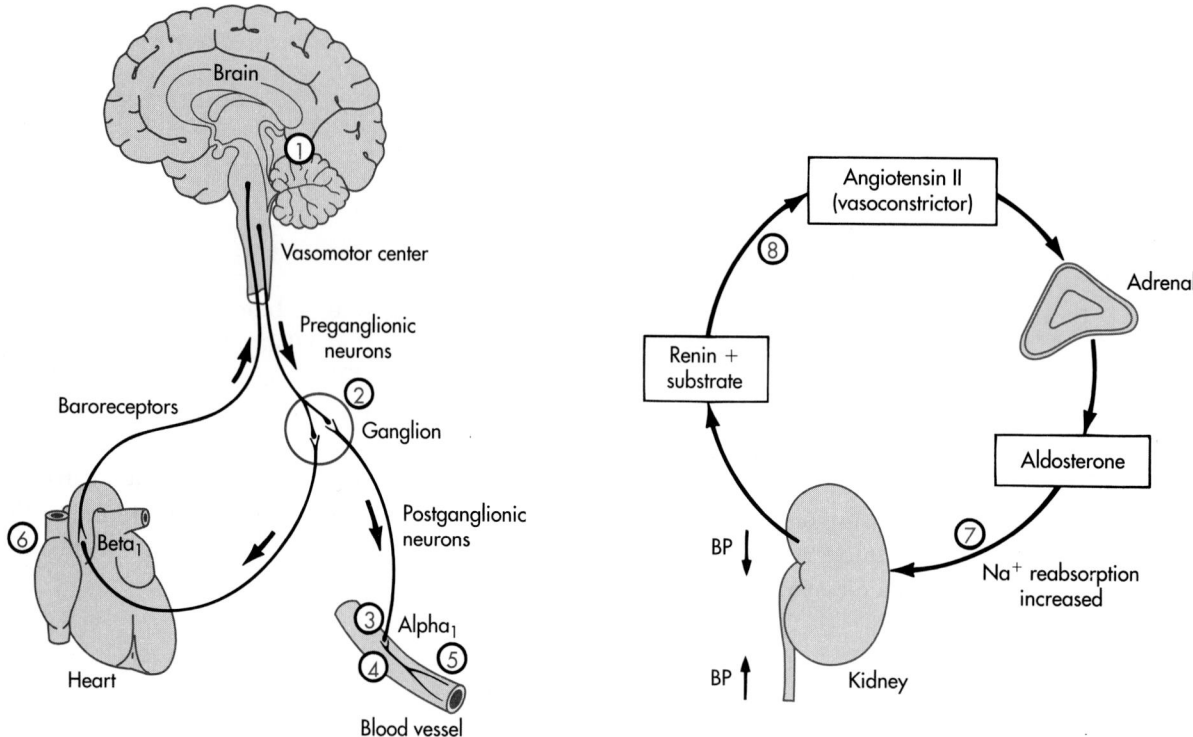

Figure 13-1   Numbers in diagram refer to mechanisms by which various antihypertensive drugs appear to act. *1,* Drugs acting centrally to depress sympathetic tone: clonidine, methyldopa, guanabenz, reserpine. *2,* Drug blocking ganglionic receptor for acetylcholine: trimethaphan. *3,* Drugs interfering with norepinephrine synthesis, storage, or release: guanethidine, guanadrel, reserpine. *4,* Drugs (a) blocking alpha-adrenergic receptor: prazosin, phenoxybenzamine, phentolamine, labetalol or (b) blocking angiotensin II receptor: losartan. *5,* Drugs directly dilating smooth muscle: hydralazine, minoxidil, sodium nitroprusside, diazoxide, calcium channel blockers. *6,* Drugs decreasing cardiac output: beta-blockers, calcium channel blockers. *7,* Drugs blocking sodium reabsorption: diuretics. *8,* Drugs inhibiting angiotensin II formation: ACE inhibitors.

through the sympathetic nervous system, to fine-tune the blood pressure. The vasomotor center in the medulla is a major center in the brain that controls blood pressure. As the neurotransmitter of the sympathetic nervous system, norepinephrine raises blood pressure by stimulating the $beta_1$-receptors of the heart to increase cardiac output and by stimulating the $alpha_1$-receptors of the blood vessels, causing constriction and increasing resistance to blood flow. By contrast, in the central nervous system (CNS), norepinephrine is the neurotransmitter for nerve tracts that ultimately decrease blood pressure.

Vasoactive Peptides

Cell-to-cell communication often involves the release of specific peptides from one tissue to communicate at different diverse sites and coordinate a response. Angiotensin II was the first vasoactive peptide to be well characterized. Its role as a potent vasoconstrictor mediating the renal control of blood pressure is described in the previous section. However, other vasoactive peptides have been characterized in recent years as well. Some peptides act as vasoconstrictors: vasopressin, endothelins, and neuropeptide Y. Other peptides act as vasodilators: bradykinin and related kinins, natriuretic peptides, vasoactive intestinal peptide, substance P, neurotensin, and calcitonin gene-related peptide. At this time, only drugs controlling angiotensin II are used as antihypertensives. These drugs are the angiotensin-converting enzyme (ACE) inhibitors and the angiotensin II receptor blockers, described later in this chapter.

Therapeutic Options for Hypertension

Lifestyle Modifications

Habits and lifestyle affect blood pressure. The first line of both prevention and treatment of hypertension is making lifestyle modifications. Counseling the hypertensive individual to control weight and sodium intake (see Dietary Considerations box), to give up smoking and excessive alcohol consumption, and to exercise regularly is important in blood pressure management. Altering these habits and lifestyle risk factors can reduce blood pressure. For the mildly hypertensive individual, these changes may be the only treatment needed. Even if drug therapy is required, modification of these lifestyle factors will be additive and reduce the level of drug intervention required.

Lifestyle modifications for prevention and management of hypertension have been developed from a study of how dietary changes in patients with hypertension affect blood pressure. The effective modifications for decreasing blood pressure include the following:

- Lose weight if overweight
- Limit alcohol intake: 1 oz ethanol for men; 0.5 oz for women and lighter weight people
- Increase aerobic physical activity: 30-45 min most days
- Reduce sodium intake to 6 g sodium chloride
- Maintain adequate potassium, calcium, and magnesium

- Stop smoking
- Reduce intake of dietary saturated fat and cholesterol

Antihypertensive Therapy

There has been an explosion of new drugs for the treatment of hypertension. Table 13-1 outlines those drugs that have a role in the treatment of hypertension. Agents that depress sympathetic tone encompass several adrenergic mechanisms because adrenergic drugs can lower blood pressure by decreasing the activity of the sympathetic nervous system peripherally or centrally. (Drug mechanisms that modify the activity of the sympathetic nervous system are reviewed in Chapter 12.) A variety of agents also alter vascular tone. Figure 13-1 shows the sites of action of antihypertensive drugs.

Choices for Therapy

The Joint National Committee on Detection, Evaluation, and Treatment of High Blood Pressure updated and published its

---

 DIETARY CONSIDERATIONS

Sodium and Hypertension

Excessive intake of sodium is associated with fluid retention and hypertension in some individuals. The first step in decreasing sodium intake is to stop adding salt to food while cooking or to cooked food during meals. The next step is to eliminate processed foods that contain a large amount of added sodium, including the following:

- Relishes and pickles
- Salted popcorn, nuts
- Sauerkraut
- Bouillon cubes
- Salted crackers
- Potato chips, pretzels
- Canned, frozen, or dehydrated soup
- Bread, rolls, bran, bran flakes
- Processed cheese, cheese spreads
- Canned meat such as tuna and Vienna sausages
- Salt-cured meat such as bacon, ham, corned beef, salt pork, luncheon meats, frankfurters, and sausage
- Seasonings such as garlic or onion salts, or prepared mustard; meat extracts and tenderizers such as monosodium glutamate, soy sauce, and Worcestershire sauce; catsup; steak sauce; and cooking with salt pork or bacon grease

Instruct patients to read food ingredient lists and to limit or avoid foods containing salt, baking soda, monosodium glutamate, baking powder, and sodium compounds such as sodium benzoate, sodium citrate, sodium propionate, sodium alginate, sodium sulfite, sodium hydroxide, disodium phosphate, and sodium saccharin. Finally, instruct patients to limit or avoid foods naturally high in sodium such as milk, eggs, meat (including fish and poultry), cheese, beets and greens, carrots, celery, chard, spinach, kale, and white turnip roots.

Table 13-1 Categories of Antihypertensive Drugs

Type	Drugs	Antihypertensive Action
Drugs for Initial Therapy		
Diuretics		
Thiazide-type	hydrochlorothiazide See also Table 14-3	Reduces body salt and water; decreases arterial blood pressure; may reduce plasma volume. Often a diuretic alone is effective as the only antihypertensive agent. Diuretics counteract fluid retention caused by other antihypertensive drugs and/or enhance the action of most antihypertensive drugs.
Loop	furosemide torsemide	More potent than the thiazide-type. May need higher dosages for patients with renal impairment or congestive heart failure.
Potassium sparing	amiloride spironolactone triamterene	Used mainly in combination with other diuretics to reverse or avoid hypokalemia; may cause hyperkalemia when combined with potassium supplements or ACE inhibitors.
Adrenergic Inhibitors		
Beta-blocker	atenolol betaxolol bisoprolol metoprolol nadolol oxprenolol propranolol sotalol timolol	Decreases cardiac output; decreases plasma renin activity. Preferred for patients with angina or after a heart attack. Atenolol, betaxolol, bisoprolol, and metoprolol are cardioselective and at low dosages should not aggravate asthma.
Beta-blocker with intrinsic sympathetic activity	acebutolol carteolol penbutolol pindolol	Mechanism is the same as other beta-blockers. Intrinsic sympathetic activity is an advantage for patients with bradycardia and those with diabetes mellitus because they have fewer metabolic side effects.
Alpha-beta-blocker	carvedilol labetalol	Acts like beta-blocker with alpha$_1$ blockade for vasodilation. May cause postural effects.
Alpha$_1$-blocker	doxazosin prazosin terazosin	Blocks postsynaptic alpha$_1$-receptors on arterioles to cause vasodilation. Orthostatic hypotension common. Used less commonly by themselves; more commonly combined with a diuretic.
Angiotensin-Converting Enzyme (ACE) Inhibitors	benazepril captopril enalapril fosinopril lisinopril moexipril quinapril ramipril trandolapril	Blocks formation of angiotensin II, a potent vasoconstrictor, and prevents degradation of the vasodilators bradykinin and certain prostaglandins. Especially useful in treating congestive heart failure, hypertension with left ventricular hypertrophy and renovascular hypertension of diabetes and scleroderma.
Angiotensin II Antagonists	irbesartan losartan valsartan	Blocks receptor for angiotensin II, preventing vasoconstriction.
Calcium Channel Blockers	amlodipine diltiazem felodipine isradipine nicardipine nifedipine nisoldipine verapamil	Blocks inward movement of calcium ion across cell membranes, resulting in smooth muscle relaxation (vasodilation). Diltiazem and verapamil also block slow calcium channels in the heart.
Supplemental Antihypertensive Agents		
Centrally Acting Alpha$_2$-Agonist	clonidine guanabenz guanfacine methyldopa	Stimulates alpha$_2$-receptors in the brain that inhibit peripheral sympathetic pathways.

Table 13-1 Categories of Antihypertensive Drugs—cont'd		
Type	Drugs	Antihypertensive Action
Drugs Interfering with Storage and/or Release of norepinephrine	guanadrel guanethidine reserpine and related drugs	Guanadrel and guanethidine inhibit catecholamine release from peripheral neurons; reserpine deplete tissue stores of catecholamines.
Direct Vasodilators	hydralazine minoxidil	Acts directly on vascular smooth muscle; not recommended in the presence of other cardiovascular disease.

recommendations in 1997 (JNC VI). The Committee updated the classification of hypertension to normal, high normal, and three stages:

CLASSIFICATION OF BLOOD PRESSURE FOR ADULTS (>18 YR)

CATEGORY	SYSTOLIC	DIASTOLIC
Normal	<130	<85
High normal	130-139	85-89
Stage 1	140-159	90-99
Stage 2	160-179	100-109
Stage 3	≥180	≥110

The JNC VI report strongly encourages lifestyle modification as the important step in addressing hypertension. For many people, lifestyle modification can prevent high blood pressure. For those with high-normal blood pressure or stage 1 hypertension, lifestyle modification should be the primary therapy.

Treatment of hypertension has become more aggressive. Drug therapy is recommended for patients whose blood pressure is in the high-normal range (130/85 to 139/89 mm Hg) if they also have diabetes, cardiovascular disease, target organ damage, or more than one major risk factor. Accumulated evidence shows that even high-normal hypertension is associated with an increased incidence of cardiovascular disease and stroke, especially when risk factors are present.

The Committee recommends that initial therapy of hypertensive patients be customized based on a risk stratification for cardiovascular disease. Having one or more of the six major risk factors identified for hypertension is one component of the risk stratification. The six risk factors are smoking, high blood cholesterol or triglycerides, diabetes, age older than 60 years, being a man or a postmenopausal woman, and having a history of cardiovascular disease. The risk stratification also factors in whether the patient has clinical cardiovascular disease (left ventricular hypertrophy, angina or prior myocardial infarction, prior coronary revascularization, or heart failure) and whether there is target organ damage (stroke or transient ischemic attack, nephropathy, peripheral arterial disease, or retinopathy).

Risk Group A. Risk group A are those with no risk factors and no clinical cardiovascular disease or organ damage. These patients should be treated initially with counseling and follow-up for lifestyle changes. Risk group A patients need drug therapy if they fall into stage 2 or 3 hypertension or if they are stage 1 and have not responded to lifestyle modifications after 1 year.

Risk Group B. Risk group B are those who have one or more major risk factor but do not have diabetes, clinical cardiovascular disease, or organ damage. Most hypertensive patients are in risk group B. These patients are advised to adopt lifestyle changes, but only patients with stage 2 or 3 hypertension are also started on drug therapy. Patients with stage 1 hypertension, 140/90 to 159/99 mm Hg, are started on drug therapy if their blood pressure does not fall into normal ranges with lifestyle modifications.

Risk Group C. Risk group C are those with diabetes, clinical cardiovascular disease, or target organ damage. These patients are begun immediately on drug therapy. However, they are also counseled on lifestyle changes because they may lower the dose of drugs needed and thereby reduce side effects of drug therapy.

Initial Drug Therapy

Drug therapy is generally advised for patients who have stage 1 or stage 2 hypertension, especially those with risk factors and with a blood pressure remaining at or above 140/90 mm Hg for 12 months despite attempts to change lifestyle factors. In general, drug therapy for hypertension is standard. Yet therapy is changing as more is being learned about hypertension and as new drugs become available. Current drug therapy is based on a treatment algorithm in which drug classes are substituted or added until blood pressure is brought under control.

Initial drug therapy begins with the administration of a single drug from one of several drug classes. Diuretics and beta-blockers are the preferred classes because these have been proven effective in many clinical trials. Other drug classes may be used, especially when beta-blockers and diuretics are ineffective. These drug classes include ACE inhibitors, calcium antagonists, alpha$_1$-receptor blockers, and the alpha-beta-blocker.

Diuretics. The most common choice is an oral diuretic, usually a thiazide or thiazide-like diuretic. Hydrochlorothiazide and chlorthalidone have been found effective in clinical trials. Diuretics are especially effective as single agents for African-American patients with hypertension. Diuretics inhibit renal tubular reabsorption, causing diuresis that leads to reduction of body salt and water (extracellular fluid). The loss of extracellular fluid is associated with reduction of arterial blood pressure, but the mechanism of this hypotensive action remains obscure. This hypotensive effect is not seen in normotensive patients. The volume depletion also produces a reduction in plasma volume, although it is not clear that this reduction persists after the first month of therapy. In addition, many antihypertensive drugs cause fluid retention, an action that limits their antihypertensive effect. Diuretics are therefore commonly given with other antihypertensive drugs. Diuretics are discussed in Chapter 14.

Beta-Blocker. Instead of a diuretic, a beta-blocker may be given as the first drug. Hypertensive individuals with high plasma renin levels are especially responsive to beta-blockers and generally unresponsive to diuretics because beta-blockers inhibit the release of renin from the kidney. Unfortunately, renin levels cannot be reliably or readily determined at present. In general, however, Caucasian hypertensive patients in the younger age groups have high renin levels, whereas African-American hypertensive patients in the older age groups have low renin levels. A beta-blocker is also indicated for patients who have coronary artery disease. Beta-blockers have been shown to have a protective effect against sudden death in individuals who have had a heart attack, whereas diuretics may, through a lowering of potassium levels, increase the vulnerability of the compromised heart to sudden failure.

Calcium Channel Blockers. Calcium channel blockers are another choice as initial therapy. These agents act by preventing the entry of calcium into the smooth muscle layer of blood vessels. This action diminishes the contraction of the blood vessels and results in vasodilation. Calcium channel blockers decrease hypertension without causing reflex sympathetic stimulation or fluid retention. These drugs are especially effective as single agents for older adult patients, those with angina, and those with low plasma renin activity. Calcium channel blockers are tolerated by all age groups.

ACE Inhibitors. ACE inhibitors are effective in treating most forms of hypertension and for treating congestive heart failure. The ACE inhibitors are another choice for initial therapy suitable for all age groups, but they are more effective in Caucasian than in African-American patients. ACE inhibitors block the formation of the potent vasoconstrictor, angiotensin II. The antihypertensive response is not associated with an increase in heart rate or cardiac output. ACE inhibitors are especially indicated for the hypertensive patient with heart failure.

Alpha₁-Blockers. Alpha₁-blocking agents are occasionally used as the initial antihypertensive agent. This drug class has a beneficial effect on hyperlipidemia. A limitation is the orthostatic hypotension characteristic of these agents. The alpha-beta-blocker is also occasionally used as the initial drug.

After 3 to 6 months, the response of the patient is evaluated. If the response is inadequate, the drug dosage may be increased, another drug may be substituted, or a second drug from a different class may be added. The most common two-drug regimen involves the addition of an adrenergic inhibitor to diuretic therapy. The adrenergic inhibitor is commonly a beta-blocker. The choice of therapy will depend on how the patient tolerates the various side effects of the drug classes. A patient with stage 3 hypertension often requires a combination of two or three drugs to achieve control of blood pressure. The centrally acting alpha₁-agonists, the peripheral-acting adrenergic antagonists, and the direct-acting vasodilators are other choices for combination therapy.

Drug therapy can rarely be discontinued after the blood pressure is brought into a normal range; however, the drug dosage can often be reduced with time. This reduction is important because antihypertensive drugs can produce uncomfortable side effects, whereas the hypertension itself may not produce uncomfortable symptoms, a situation that can make patient compliance with drug therapy difficult. Obesity and high salt intake are factors that aggravate hypertension. If a patient reduces weight and salt intake, drug requirements often may also be reduced.

Antihypertensive Therapy for Special Patient Populations

African-American Patients

Hypertension is more prevalent in African-Americans; it develops at an earlier age and is more severe than in Caucasians. In general, African-American hypertensive patients respond best to diuretics or calcium channel blockers as monotherapy. ACE inhibitors and beta-blockers are generally less effective as single agents for African-American patients than for Caucasian patients. However, in combination with diuretics, ACE inhibitors and beta-blockers are equally effective in Caucasian and African-American hypertensive patients. Other antihypertensive drug classes, the calcium antagonists, alpha₁-blockers, and the alpha-beta-blocker, are equally effective in both racial groups. African-Americans have a higher prevalence of salt sensitivity, obesity, and smoking. These are risk factors that can be modified with lifestyle changes.

Asian Patients

Patients of south Asian background are generally more responsive to various antihypertensive medications than are Caucasians.

Older Adult Patients

Approximately two thirds of the U.S. population aged 65 years or older has hypertension. Studies have shown that treating older adult patients with an elevated systolic pressure but normal diastolic pressure with diuretics decreases the incidence of both strokes and heart attacks. The development of heart failure was reduced by 50%. Older patients who had already had a heart attack benefited the most, with an 80% reduction in heart failure.

Older patients are more sensitive to diuretics, beta-blockers, and the orthostatic hypotensive effects of other antihypertensive drugs. The starting dose for older patients should be about half that listed for younger adults. All classes of antihypertensive agents are effective in older adult patients, but only diuretics and beta-blockers have been used in clinical trials and have been shown to reduce cardiovascular disease and death.

Pregnant Patients

Hypertension during pregnancy imposes risk for both the mother and the fetus. Four diagnostic categories are recognized: chronic hypertension, preeclampsia-eclampsia, chronic hypertension with superimposed preeclampsia, and transient hypertension. Preeclampsia is a pregnancy-specific condition that develops primarily in first pregnancies after 20 weeks' gestation. It is characterized by increased blood pressure and is accompanied by proteinuria, edema, and occasionally abnormalities of coagulation and liver function. Eclampsia is the convulsive phase. Diet and bed rest are the first line of treatment for preeclampsia, but if high blood pressure persists, methyldopa, hydralazine, and beta-blockers have each proved effective in controlling blood pressure and improving fetal survival. If hypertension is unrelated to pregnancy, treatment should continue, although aggressive antihypertensive therapy is discouraged. However, ACE inhibitors are contraindicated during pregnancy because serious neonatal problems, including renal failure and death, have been reported when women have taken these drugs during pregnancy. Methyldopa, the most extensively evaluated antihypertensive agent used during pregnancy, has few adverse effects. Beta-blockers also appear safe when used during the latter part of the pregnancy. They may be associated with growth retardation of the fetus if used early in the pregnancy.

Patients with Diabetes

Hypertension is a major risk factor for kidney and cardiovascular problems in patients with diabetes. Diabetic patients should be started on drug therapy even if their blood pressure is only in the high-normal range. Because beta-blockers tend to mask hypoglycemic symptoms, ACE inhibitors, alpha-blockers, calcium channel blockers, and diuretics in small doses are preferred. Diabetic patients with any evidence of kidney failure should be treated with ACE inhibitors. These drugs have been shown to have a protective effect in kidney failure. A recent study comparing enalapril (an ACE inhibitor) and nisoldipine (a calcium channel blocker) in diabetic adults showed that the two drugs were equally effective in controlling hypertension. However, patients taking nisoldipine were seven times more likely to have a heart attack. This study has raised concerns about the safety of calcium channel blockers for diabetic patients.

Patients with Asthma or Chronic Airway Disease

In general, beta-blockers and alpha-beta-blockers should not be used in patients with asthma because these drugs also block bronchiole dilation.

Patients with Coexisting Cardiovascular Disease

Cerebrovascular Disease. Hypertension should be treated in a patient with cerebrovascular disease, but treatment may be suspended immediately after a stroke. Orthostatic hypotension should be avoided as a side effect of antihypertensive therapy.

Coronary Artery Disease. Beta-blockers or calcium antagonists, especially those that reduce the heart rate, are useful for patients with angina. However, short-acting calcium antagonists, especially the short-acting formulation of nifedipine, have negative effects on the heart and should not be used. Beta-blockers without intrinsic sympathomimetic activity are drugs of choice for patients who have had a myocardial infarction because these agents have been shown to reduce the risk of a subsequent attack and death.

Cardiac Failure. ACE inhibitors, alone or in combination with digoxin or diuretics, are effective in reducing mortality caused by progressive congestive heart failure. The new alpha-beta-blocker carvedilol has been shown effective when added to therapy with ACE inhibitors, digoxin, and diuretics. If ACE inhibitors are not effective or not tolerated, the vasodilator combination of hydralazine and isosorbide dinitrate may be effective. In general, calcium antagonists are contraindicated; however, amlodipine and felodipine are safe when combined with ACE inhibitors, diuretics, and digoxin for patients with angina, hypertension, and heart failure.

Left Ventricular Hypertrophy. Hypertrophy results from cardiac adaptation to the increased afterload imposed by elevated blood pressure. Antihypertensive therapy, especially the combination of a diuretic and ACE inhibitor, is effective in reducing increased left ventricular mass. Direct-acting vasodilators may worsen the condition and should not be used. Weight loss and salt restriction are beneficial.

Peripheral Vascular Disease. Hypertension is a major risk factor for atherosclerosis and aneurysms. However, there have been no studies to show whether controlling blood pressure alters the course of these diseases.

THERAPEUTIC AGENTS: DRUGS ALTERING PERIPHERAL SYMPATHETIC ACTIVITY

Antihypertensive drugs that alter peripheral sympathetic activity include antagonists (blockers) of both the alpha-

Text continued on p. 142

Table 13-2 Drugs for Treatment of Chronic Hypertension

Generic Name	Trade Name	Administration/Dosage	Comments
Beta-Blockers (Beta-Adrenergic Receptor Antagonists)			
acebutolol hydrochloride	Monitan† Sectral*	ORAL: *Adults*—400 mg once a day or in two divided doses. Maintenance dose range: 400-800 daily to control hypertension. Reduce dose by 50%-75% for patients with renal failure. Do not exceed 800 mg/day in elderly. FDA pregnancy category B.	Cardioselective drug. Moderate intrinsic sympathetic activity. Indications: hypertension. Nonlabeled indications: angina, supraventricular arrhythmia, and ventricular tachycardia, hypertrophy cardiomyopathy, myocardial infarction, mitral valve prolapse, thyrotoxicosis, anxiety.
atenolol	Apo-Atenolol† Novo-Atenol† Tenormin*	ORAL: *Adults*—25-50 mg/day initially, increased gradually to 50-100 mg after 2 wk if necessary; dosage reduced for patients with impaired renal function: 50 mg/day when creatinine clearance is 15-35 ml/min; 50 mg every 2 days when creatinine clearance <15 ml/min. FDA pregnancy category D.	Cardioselective drug. Indications: hypertension, angina, myocardial infarction. Nonlabeled indications: supraventricular arrhythmia and ventricular tachycardia, hypertrophy cardiomyopathy, mitral valve prolapse, thyrotoxicosis.
betaxolol	Kerlone	ORAL: *Adults*—10 mg/day initially, doubling after 1-2 wk if needed. Elderly may require less or more than usual adult dose. Reduce dosage in half for patients with renal function impairment undergoing hemodialysis. FDA pregnancy category C.	Cardioselective drug. Indications: hypertension, glaucoma.
bisoprolol	Zebeta	ORAL: *Adults*—5 mg/day initially, doubling after 1-2 wk if needed. Elderly may require less or more than usual adult dose. Reduce dosage in half for patients with bronchospastic disease. FDA pregnancy category C.	Cardioselective drug. Indication: hypertension.
carteolol	Cartrol	ORAL: *Adults*—2.5 mg/day initially, adjusting to 10 mg if needed. Elderly may require less or more than usual adult dose. Dosage intervals are increased for patients with impaired renal function: 48 hr if creatinine clearance is 20-60 ml/min; 72 hr if creatinine clearance is <20 ml/min. FDA pregnancy category C.	Nonselective drug. Moderate intrinsic sympathetic activity. Indication: angina.
carvedilol	Coreg	ORAL: *Adults—Hypertension:* 6.25 mg twice a day, with food. May gradually increase up to 25 mg twice a day if needed and tolerated. FDA pregnancy category C.	Nonselective drug with alpha$_1$-blocking activity, no intrinsic sympathomimetic activity. Indications: control of hypertension, adjunct for congestive heart failure.
labetalol hydrochloride	Trandate* Normodyne	ORAL: *Adults*—100 mg twice a day; adjust in 100-mg increments every 2 or 3 days as needed. Maintenance: 200-400 mg twice daily. INTRAVENOUS: *Adults*—20 mg injected slowly over 2 min with additional 40- or 80-mg injections at 10-min intervals until desired blood pressure or 300 mg total; alternatively, infuse at 2 mg/min for desired effect of 50 to 300 mg. FDA pregnancy category C.	Nonselective beta-blocker; selective alpha$_1$-beta-blocker. Indication: control of hypertension.
metoprolol tartrate	Apo-Metoprolol† Betaloc† Lopressor Novometoprol† Toprol-XL	ORAL: *Adults*—50 mg every 12 hr initially, increased if necessary to no more than 120 mg every 8 hr; extended release, 100-400 mg once a day. Elderly may require less or more than usual adult dose. FDA pregnancy category C.	Cardioselective drug. Indications: hypertension, angina, myocardial infarction. Nonlabeled indications: supraventricular arrhythmia and ventricular tachycardia, hypertrophy cardiomyopathy; mitral valve prolapse, thyrotoxicosis, vascular headache, anxiety.
nadolol	Corgard* Syn-Nadolol†	ORAL: *Adults*—40 mg/day initially, increased if necessary by 40-80 mg each week to maintenance daily dose of 80-320 mg. Elderly may require less or more than usual adult dose. Dosage intervals are increased for patients with impaired renal function: 24-36 hr if creatinine clearance is 31-50 ml/min; 24-48 hr if creatinine clearance is 10-30 ml/min; 40-60 hr if creatinine clearance is <10 ml/min. FDA pregnancy category C.	Nonselective drug. Indications: hypertension, angina. Nonlabeled indications: supraventricular arrhythmia and ventricular tachycardia, hypertrophy cardiomyopathy, myocardial infarction, mitral valve prolapse, thyrotoxicosis, vascular headache.
oxprenolol hydrochloride†	Trasicor†	ORAL: *Adults*—20 mg 3 times/day initially; may increase by 60 mg/day every 1-2 wk if necessary. Total usual	Nonselective drug. Moderate instrinsic sympathetic activity. Indication: hypertension.

MI, Myocardial infarction.
*Available in Canada and United States.
†Available in Canada only.

Table 13-2 Drugs for Treatment of Chronic Hypertension—cont'd

Generic Name	Trade Name	Administration/Dosage	Comments
oxprenolol hydrochloride† —cont'd		daily dose: 120-320 mg. Extended release, for maintenance, 120-320 mg/day in the morning.	Nonlabeled indications: angina, hypertrophic cardiomyopathy, myocardial infarction, tremors, mitral valve prolapse.
penbutolol	Levatol	ORAL: *Adults*—20 mg once a day. FDA pregnancy category C.	Nonselective drug. Moderate sympathetic activity. Indication: hypertension. Nonlabeled indication: angina.
pindolol	Novo-Pindol† Syn-Pindolol† Visken*	ORAL: *Adults*—5 mg 2 times/day; may increase by 10 mg/day every 2-3 wk if necessary; usual daily dose: 45-60 mg. FDA pregnancy category B.	Nonselective drug. Most intrinsic sympathetic activity of all beta-blockers. Indication: hypertension. Nonlabeled indications: angina, hypertrophic cardiomyopathy, mitral valve prolapse.
propranolol	Apo-Propranolol† Detensol† Inderal* Novopranolol†	ORAL: *Adults*—40 mg 2 times/day, increase gradually if needed to 120-240 mg/day. FDA pregnancy category C. *Children*—0.5-1 mg/kg/day in 2-4 divided doses. *For pheochromocytoma:* ORAL: *Adults*—20 mg 3 times/day to 40 mg 3 or 4 times/day for 3 days before surgery, given with alpha-adrenergic blocking medication. FDA pregnancy category C.	Nonselective drug. Indications: hypertension, arrhythmias, hypertrophic cardiomyopathy, myocardial infarction, pheochromocytoma, vascular headache, tremors. Nonlabeled indications: anxiety, thyrotoxicosis, mitral valve prolapse, neuroleptic-induced akathisia.
sotalol hydrochloride	Betapace Sotacor†	ORAL: *Adults*—80 mg 2 times/day, increasing 80 mg 2 times/day at weekly intervals as needed. Maintenance: 160 mg 2 times/day. FDA pregnancy category B.	Nonselective drug. Indications: hypertension, angina, arrhythmias. Nonlabeled indications: hypertrophic cardiomyopathy, myocardial infarction, thyrotoxicosis, anxiety, mitral valve prolapse.
timolol maleate	Apo-Timol† Blocadren*	ORAL: *Adults*—10 mg 2 times/day initially, may increase weekly as needed; maintenance: 20-40 mg/day. FDA pregnancy category C.	Nonselective drug. Indications: hypertension, myocardial infarction, vascular headache. Nonlabeled indications: angina, hypertrophic cardiomyopathy, pheochromocytoma, tremors, anxiety, thyrotoxicosis, mitral valve prolapse.

Alpha₁-Blockers (Alpha₁-Adrenergic Receptor Antagonists)

Generic Name	Trade Name	Administration/Dosage	Comments
doxazosin mesylate	Cardura*	ORAL: 1 mg/day at bedtime; maintenance: may increase every 2 wk, doubling dose, to 16 mg/day if needed. FDA pregnancy category C.	Indication: hypertension. Nonlabeled indications: benign prostatic hypertrophy. Favorable side effect is the lowering of cholesterol and triglyceride levels.
prazosin hydrochloride	Minipress*	ORAL: *Adults*—Initial dose 0.5 mg 2 or 3 times/day for 3 days; maintenance: adjust gradually to 6-15 mg/day divided in 2 or 3 doses. FDA pregnancy category C.	Indication: hypertension. Nonlabeled indications: Raynaud's phenomenon (vasospasticity in digits), benign prostatic hyperplasia, toxicity of ergot alkaloids. Favorable side effect is the lowering of cholesterol and triglyceride levels.
terazosin hydrochloride	Hytrin*	ORAL: *Adults*—Initial dose 1 mg at bedtime; maintenance: adjust gradually to 1-5 mg/day. FDA pregnancy category C.	Indications: hypertension, benign prostatic hyperplasia. Favorable side effect is the lowering of cholesterol and triglyceride levels.

Alpha₁-, Alpha₂-Blockers (Nonspecific Alpha-Adrenergic Receptor Antagonists)

Generic Name	Trade Name	Administration/Dosage	Comments
phentolamine mesylate	Regitine Rogitine†	*Prevention of dermal necrosis:* Add 10 mg to each liter of norepinephrine intravenous solution; in event of extravasation of intravenous norepinephrine, infiltrate 5-10 mg in 10 ml normal saline. *Before surgery for pheochromocytoma:* ORAL: *Adults*—50 mg every 4-6 hr. *Children*—25 mg every 4-6 hr. INTRAMUSCULAR, INTRAVENOUS: *Adults*—5 mg. FDA pregnancy category C. *Children*—1 mg.	Indications: prevent or control hypertension from pheochromocytoma before and during surgery, reverse ischemia and prevent necrosis of the skin after IV administration or extravasation of norepinephrine.
phenoxybenzamine hydrochloride	Dibenzyline	ORAL: *Adults*—10 mg/day. May be increased by 10 mg/day to maximum dose of 60 mg/day. FDA pregnancy category C. *Children*—0.2 mg/kg body weight up to 10 mg, once a day.	Irreversible inhibitor. Indications: control of hypertension and sweating from pheochromocytoma prior to surgery. Nonlabeled indication: Treatment of urinary symptoms associated with benign prostatic hypertrophy.

Continued

Table 13-2   Drugs for Treatment of Chronic Hypertension—cont'd

Generic Name	Trade Name	Administration/Dosage	Comments
Sympatholytic Drugs			
deserpidine	Harmonyl	ORAL: *Adults*—250-500 mg in a single or divided dose daily. FDA pregnancy category C.	Rauwolfia alkaloid. Indication: control of hypertension. Nonlabeled indication: Raynaud's phenomenon.
guanadrel	Hylorel	ORAL: *Adults*—5 mg twice daily initially; may increase to 20-75 mg/day divided into 2-4 doses. FDA pregnancy category B.	Depletes norepinephrine in sympathetic neurone. Indication: control of severe hypertension.
guanethidine monosulfate	Apo-Guanethidine† Ismelin*	ORAL: *Adults*—10-12.5 mg/day initially; may increase to 25-50 mg/day. FDA pregnancy category C. *Children*—200 μg/kg body weight or 6 mg/square meter body surface daily.	Depletes norepinephrine in sympathetic neurone. Indications: control of severe hypertension, renal hypertension.
Rauwolfia serpentina	Raudixin Rauval Rauverid	ORAL: *Adults*—50-200 mg in a single or divided dose daily. FDA pregnancy category C.	Rauwolfia alkaloid. Indication: control of hypertension. Nonlabeled indication: Raynaud's phenomenon.
reserpine	Novoreserpine† Reserfia† Serpasil† Serpalan	ORAL: *Adults*—100-250 mg/day. FDA pregnancy category C. *Children*—5-20 μg/kg body weight 150-600 μg/square meter body surface daily.	Rauwolfia alkaloid. Indication: control of hypertension. Nonlabeled indication: Raynaud's phenomenon.
Angiotensin-Converting Enzyme (ACE) Inhibitors			
benazepril hydrochloride	Lotensin	ORAL: *Adults*—10 mg/day; may increase to 20-40 mg/day in a single or divided dose. FDA pregnancy category C (first trimester) and D (second and third trimesters).	Inhibits production of angiotensin II, a potent vasoconstrictor. Indication: control of hypertension. Nonlabeled indications: congestive heart failure, hypertension of scleroderma.
captopril	Capoten*	ORAL: *Adults—Antihypertensive:* 12.5 mg 2 or 3 times/day; may double dose after 1 or 2 wk. *Left ventricular dysfunction (post-MI):* Initial dose of 6.25 mg; then 12.5 mg 3 times/day; may increase gradually to 25 mg 3 times/day. *Diabetic nephropathy:* 25 mg 2 times/day. *Congestive heart failure:* 12.5 mg 2 or 3 times/day; may increase gradually to 50 mg/day. FDA pregnancy category C (first trimester) and D (second and third trimesters). *Children*—300 μg/kg body weight 3 times/day. *Newborns*—10 μg/kg body weight 2 or 3 times/day.	Inhibits production of angiotensin II, a potent vasoconstrictor. Indications: control of hypertension, congestive heart failure, left ventricular dysfunction post-MI, diabetic nephropathy. Nonlabeled indication: hypertension of scleroderma.
enalapril maleate	Vasotec*	ORAL: *Adults—Hypertension:* 5 mg/day initially; may increase after 1-2 wk; maintenance: 10-40 mg/day divided into 1 or 2 doses. *Congestive heart failure, left ventricular dysfunction:* 2.5 mg 1 or 2 times/day; may increase to 5-20 mg/day as 1 or 2 doses. FDA pregnancy category C (first semester) and D (second and third trimesters). INTRAVENOUS (Enalaprilat): *Adults*—1.25 mg administered over 5 min; may repeat in 6 hr. FDA pregnancy category C (first trimester) and D (second and third trimesters).	Inhibits production of angiotensin II, a potent vasoconstrictor. Indications: control of hypertension, congestive heart failure, left ventricular dysfunction. Nonlabeled indication: control of hypertension of scleroderma.
fosinopril sodium	Monopril	ORAL: *Adults*—10 mg once a day; may increase to 20-40 mg. FDA pregnancy category C (first trimester) and D (second and third trimesters).	Inhibits production of angiotensin II, a potent vasoconstrictor. Indication: control of hypertension. Nonlabeled indication: control of hypertension of scleroderma.
lisinopril	Prinivil* Zestril*	ORAL: *Adults—Hypertension:* 10 mg once a day; may increase to 20-40 mg. *Congestive heart failure:* 2.5-5 mg/day; may increase to 10-20 mg/day. FDA pregnancy category C (first trimester) and D (second and third trimesters).	Inhibits production of angiotensin II, a potent vasoconstrictor. Indications: control of hypertension, congestive heart failure. Nonlabeled indication: hypertension of scleroderma.
moexipril	Univasc	ORAL: *Adults*—7.5 mg once a day, 1 hr before a meal; may increase up to 30 mg/day. FDA pregnancy category C (first trimester) and D (second and third trimesters).	Inhibits production of angiotensin II, a potent vasoconstrictor. Indication: control of hypertension.
quinapril hydrochloride	Accupril	ORAL: *Adults*—10 mg once a day; may increase to 20-80 mg. FDA pregnancy category C (first trimester) and D (second and third trimesters).	Inhibits production of angiotensin II, a potent vasoconstrictor. Indication: control of hypertension. Nonlabeled indications: congestive heart failure, hypertension of scleroderma.

MI, Myocardial infarction.
*Available in Canada and United States.
†Available in Canada only.

Table 13-2   Drugs for Treatment of Chronic Hypertension—cont'd

Generic Name	Trade Name	Administration/Dosage	Comments
ramipril	Altace	ORAL: *Adults*—2.5 mg once a day; may increase to 20 mg. FDA pregnancy category C (first trimester) and D (second and third trimesters).	Inhibits production of angiotensin II, a potent vasoconstrictor. Indication: control of hypertension. Nonlabeled indications: congestive heart failure, hypertension of scleroderma.
trandolapril	Mavik	ORAL: *Adults*—1 mg once a day in non–African-American patients and 2 mg once a day in African-American patients; may increase up to 4 mg/day. FDA pregnancy category C (first trimester) and D (second and third trimesters).	Inhibits production of angiotensin II, a potent vasoconstrictor. Indication: control of hypertension.

Angiotensin II Receptor Blockers

Generic Name	Trade Name	Administration/Dosage	Comments
irbesartan	Avapro	ORAL: *Adults*—150 mg once a day; may increase to 300 mg. FDA pregnancy category C (first trimester) and D (second and third trimesters).	Blocks receptor for angiotensin II. Indication: control of hypertension.
losartan potassium	Cozaar	ORAL: *Adults*—50 mg once a day; may increase to 100 mg. FDA pregnancy category C (first trimester) and D (second and third trimesters).	Blocks receptor for angiotensin II. Indication: control of hypertension.
valsartan	Diovan	ORAL: *Adults*—80 mg once a day; may increase to 320 mg. FDA pregnancy category C (first trimester) and D (second and third trimesters).	Blocks receptor for angiotensin II. Indication: control of hypertension.

Calcium Channel Blockers

Generic Name	Trade Name	Administration/Dosage	Comments
amlodipine besylate	Norvasc	ORAL: *Adults*—5 or 10 mg once a day. FDA pregnancy category C.	Vasodilation from blocking of calcium ion flow in smooth muscle membranes. Indications: control of hypertension, angina.
diltiazem hydrochloride	Cardizem*	ORAL: *Adults*—30 mg 3 or 4 times/day initially; may increase gradually. Maximum: 360 mg/day. FDA pregnancy category C.	Vasodilation from blocking of calcium ion flow in smooth muscle membranes. Indications: hypertension, angina, supraventricular tachycardia.
felodipine	Plendil* Renedil†	ORAL: *Adults*—5 mg once a day; up to 10 mg. FDA pregnancy category C.	Vasodilation from blocking of calcium ion flow in smooth muscle membranes. Indications: control of hypertension, angina.
isradipine	DynaCirc	ORAL: *Adults*—2.5 mg 2 times/day; may increase gradually to 20 mg/day. FDA pregnancy category C.	Vasodilation from blocking of calcium ion flow in smooth muscle membranes. Indication: control of hypertension.
nicardipine hydrochloride	Cardene*	ORAL: *Adults*—20 mg 3 times/day. FDA pregnancy category C.	Vasodilation from blocking of calcium ion flow in smooth muscle membranes. Indications: control of hypertension, angina.
nifedipine	Adalat* Apo-Nifed† Novo-Nifed† Nu-Nifed† Procardia	ORAL: *Adults*—10 mg 3 times/day. Maximum: 120-180 mg/day. FDA pregnancy category C.	Vasodilation from blocking of calcium ion flow in smooth muscle membranes. Indications: control of hypertension, angina.
nisoldipine	Sular†	ORAL: *Adults*—20-40 mg once a day. FDA pregnancy category C.	Vasodilation from blocking of calcium ion flow in smooth muscle membranes. Indication: control of hypertension.
verapamil hydrochloride	Calan Isoptin* Novo-Veramil† Nu-Verap† Verelan	ORAL: *Adults*—80-120 mg 3 times/day. Maximum daily dose: 480 mg. *Extended release:* 240 mg once a day; may increase weekly to 240-480 mg/day. FDA pregnancy category C. *Elderly*—40 mg 3 times/day initially. *Children*—4-8 mg/kg body weight daily in divided doses.	Vasodilation from blocking of calcium ion flow in smooth muscle membranes. Indications: hypertension, angina, supraventricular tachycardia. Nonlabeled indications: hypertrophic cardiomyopathy, vascular headache.

Other Vasodilators

Generic Name	Trade Name	Administration/Dosage	Comments
hydralazine hydrochloride	Apresoline* Novo-Hylazin†	ORAL: *Adults*—10 mg 4 times/day for 2-4 days, then 25 mg 4 times/day; may increase to 50 mg 4 times/day after 1 wk. *Children*—750 μg/kg body weight or 25 mg/square meter body surface daily in divided in 2-4 doses.	Direct-acting vasodilator. Indications: severe hypertension; hypertensive crisis. Nonlabeled indication: congestive heart failure.

Continued

Table 13-2 **Drugs for Treatment of Chronic Hypertension—cont'd**

Generic Name	Trade Name	Administration/Dosage	Comments
hydralazine—cont'd		INTRAVENOUS, INTRAMUSCULAR: *Adults*—10-40 mg, repeated as needed. FDA pregnancy category C. *Children*—1.7-3.5 mg/kg body weight or 50-100 mg/ square meter body surface daily, divided into 4-6 doses.	
minoxidil	Loniten*	ORAL: *Adults*—5 mg/day as one or divided dose. Maintenance: 10-40 mg/day. *Children*—200 μg/kg body weight daily as 1 or 2 doses, up to 50 mg/day. FDA pregnancy category C.	Direct-acting vasodilator. Indication: severe hypertension.

Centrally Acting Antihypertensive Drugs

Generic Name	Trade Name	Administration/Dosage	Comments
clonidine hydrochloride	Catapres* Dixarit†	ORAL: *Adults*—100 μg twice a day initially; may increase to 600 μg/day in divided doses. TRANSDERMAL: *Adults*—Begin with system delivering 100 μg/day for 1 wk; may increase dosage delivered weekly to 300 μg/day. FDA pregnancy category C.	Decreases central sympathetic outflow. Indication: control of hypertension. Nonlabeled indications: diagnosis of pheochromocytoma, prophylaxis for vascular headaches, treatment of vasomotor symptoms of dysmenorrhea or menopause, aid in opioid withdrawal and nicotine withdrawal, treatment of Giles de la Tourette's syndrome.
guanabenz acetate	Wytensin	ORAL: *Adults*—4 mg 2 times/day initially; may increase every 1-2 wk by 4-8 mg/day. Maximum: 32 mg/day. FDA pregnancy category C.	Alpha$_2$-agonist; acts centrally to decrease sympathetic outflow. Indication: control of hypertension.
guanfacine hydrochloride	Tenex	ORAL: *Adults*—1 mg daily at bedtime initially; may increase in 3-4 wk to 2 mg/day. Maximum: 3 mg daily. FDA pregnancy category B.	Decreases central sympathetic outflow. Indication: control of hypertension.
methyldopa	Aldomet* Apo-Methyldopa† Dopamet† Novomedopa†	ORAL: *Adults*—250 mg 2-3 times/day initially; may adjust after 2-day intervals. Usual maintenance dose: 500 mg/day; maximum dose: 3 g/day. *Children*—10 mg/kg body weight or 300 mg/square meter body surface daily divided into 2-4 doses. Maximum daily dose: 65 mg/kg body weight or 3 g, whichever is less. FDA pregnancy category B. INTRAVENOUS INFUSION: *Adults*—250-500 mg in 100 ml 5% dextrose over 30-60 min; may repeat in 6 hr. FDA pregnancy category B. *Children*—5-10 mg/kg body weight in 5% dextrose over 30-60 min; may repeat in 6 hr.	Decreases central sympathetic outflow. Indications: control of hypertension; hypertensive crises (IV).

*Available in Canada and the United States.
†Available in Canada only.

and beta-adrenergic receptors and drugs that interfere with the storage and/or release of norepinephrine, the adrenergic neurotransmitter. Each of these drug classes is discussed separately, and they are summarized in Table 13-2.

Beta-Blockers

General Characteristics

Mechanism of Action

Beta-blockers are more precisely the beta-adrenergic receptor antagonists. Beta$_1$-adrenergic receptors are found principally in heart and fat tissue, stimulating heart function and lipolysis, respectively. Beta$_2$-adrenergic receptors mediate bronchodilation and peripheral vasodilation. The antihypertensive action of beta-blockers is not entirely clear, but it appears to result from the decreased cardiac output and inhibition of renin production by the kidney. The decreased cardiac output is a result of the inhibition of the beta$_1$-adrenergic receptors to decrease heart rate, contractility, and automaticity.

One goal in the development of new beta-blockers has been to develop cardioselective agents, drugs specific for the beta$_1$-receptor. The adverse side effects associated with blockade of beta$_2$-receptors include bronchospasm, prolongation of insulin-induced hypoglycemia, and aggravation of peripheral vascular insufficiency. However, the superiority of the cardioselective beta-blockers for avoiding these complications is marginal.

Another goal in the development of new beta-blockers has been to find drugs with some intrinsic sympathetic activity (partial agonists), as seen in acebutolol, carteolol, oxprenolol, and pindolol. These drugs should produce less cardiac depression and should be safer for patients with compromised cardiac function. The issue of improved safety remains to be proved.

Pharmacokinetics

The available beta-blockers do not differ in their antihypertensive effect. However, they do differ in their physiologic distribution and metabolism. Dosages of each of the drugs must be individualized for the patient. Some of the drugs must be given two or more times a day, whereas others require only once-a-day administration. Beta-blockers are metabolized by the liver and excreted in the urine.

Uses

Beta-blockers have been proven effective as antihypertensive agents when used alone or with a diuretic. They are most effective when given as a sole drug to hypertensive patients with high plasma renin levels. These patients are principally young white patients. Older African-American hypertensive patients tend to have low plasma renin concentrations and respond better to a diuretic alone or to a diuretic given with another type of sympathetic depressant.

A beta-blocker is needed when a direct-acting vasodilator, such as hydralazine or minoxidil, must be added to the therapy. These vasodilators alone cause a reflex increase in cardiac output because of their marked hypotensive effect. This reflex cardiac stimulation is blocked by the beta-blocker.

Beta-blockers are also used in the treatment of angina (see Chapter 15) and certain arrhythmias (see Chapter 19) and after myocardial infarction. The use of these drugs after myocardial infarction is intended to prevent sudden death resulting from electrical abnormalities in the recovering heart. Specifically, atenolol, metoprolol, oxprenolol, propranolol, and timolol have been approved for use in reducing the incidence of sudden death after a heart attack.

Adverse Reactions and Contraindications

Clinical trials have shown beta-blockers to be well tolerated and effective in the treatment of hypertension. Adverse effects are reported in 10% of patients and are usually mild. The most common side effects are sleep disturbances, fatigue, cool extremities, reduced exercise tolerance, tingling in the fingers or toes, gastrointestinal (GI) upset, bronchospasm, depressed mood, and sexual dysfunction (impotence in men).

Patients with abnormal cardiovascular function are the most likely to encounter more serious side effects, such as pulmonary edema, hypotension, cardiac failure, and an atrioventricular nodal block.

Beta-blockers should not be discontinued abruptly because such an action may exacerbate angina, myocardial infarction, or ventricular arrhythmias. Instead, the dosage should be reduced gradually over 1 to 2 weeks with careful monitoring of the patient for these possible complications.

Beta-blockers are used with caution in patients whose health status could be worsened by this class of drugs; specific conditions include poor cardiac function, asthma, peripheral vascular disease, and diabetes. Blockade of beta-receptors can compromise cardiac function, induce bronchospasm, and inhibit peripheral vasodilation. Hypoglycemia normally elicits the discharge of epinephrine. The effects of this released epinephrine will not be noticed easily in a patient who is taking a beta-receptor blocking drug. This is an important point for those patients with diabetes mellitus who are taking insulin or an oral hypoglycemic drug.

Toxicity

Symptoms of overdose include severe dizziness or fainting, hypotension, irregular or slow heartbeat, difficulty in breathing, bluish-colored fingernails or palms of the hands, and seizures. These symptoms require treatment that includes gastric lavage and administration of activated charcoal followed by supportive therapy for specific symptoms.

Interactions

The therapeutic effects of beta-blockers are inhibited by cocaine, by sympathomimetic agents such as the bronchodilators, by xanthines such as theophylline, and by the centrally acting antihypertensive drugs clonidine and guanabenz. The hypotensive actions of beta-blockers are potentiated by most other antihypertensive agents. The calcium channel blockers diltiazem and verapamil are more likely than other drugs of their class to cause significant bradycardia when given with beta-blockers.

Allergen immunotherapy or the use of allergenic extracts for skin testing is not recommended for patients taking beta-blockers. The beta-blockers increase the potential for serious systemic reactions or anaphylaxis. They also impair glycemic control in diabetic patients taking insulin or oral hypoglycemic agents.

Specific Beta-Blockers

acebutolol

Acebutolol (Sectral) is an intermediate-acting cardioselective beta-blocker with moderate intrinsic sympathomimetic activity. It is indicated for treating hypertension and arrhythmias. It is taken orally and moderately well absorbed. Acebutolol is metabolized by the liver, but the drug is mostly excreted unchanged, both in the urine and in the feces through enterohepatic circulation. The dosage is reduced for patients with renal function impairment.

▼ atenolol

Atenolol (Tenormin) is a long-acting cardioselective beta-blocker. It is indicated for treating angina and hypertension and to prevent sudden death after a myocardial infarction. It is also used as a prophylactic for the treatment of migraine. Poorly absorbed from the GI tract, the drug is poorly metabolized by the liver and excreted in the urine. The time between doses must be increased in patients with impaired renal function.

betaxolol

Betaxolol (Kerlone) is a long-acting cardioselective beta-blocker structurally related to metoprolol. It is indicated for treating hypertension. It is well absorbed after oral administration and metabolized by the liver. Doses should be decreased in patients with renal impairment and for older adults. Betaxolol is also available for ophthalmic administration to treat glaucoma.

bisprolol

Bisoprolol (Zebeta) is a long-acting cardioselective beta-blocker. It is indicated for the treatment of hypertension. It is well absorbed after oral administration and metabolized by the liver.

carteolol

Carteolol (Cartrol) is a long-acting nonselective beta-blocker with moderate intrinsic sympathomimetic activity. It is indicated for the treatment of hypertension. The drug undergoes minimal hepatic metabolism and is largely excreted unchanged in the urine. The dosage interval must be increased for patients with impaired renal function. Carteolol is available in an ophthalmic preparation for the treatment of glaucoma.

carvedilol

Carvedilol (Coreg) is an alpha-beta-blocker with vasodilator properties. This drug is being primarily tests for the treatment of congestive heart failure.

labetalol

Labetalol (Normodyne, Trandate) has both alpha- and beta-receptor antagonist activities. The decrease in heart rate is not as pronounced with labetalol as with other beta-blockers. The alpha-antagonist effect is more prominent with labetalol than the beta-antagonist effects, and a decrease in peripheral resistance is probably the major therapeutic effect. Labetalol is especially useful for treating hypertensive patients who also have angina. Orthostatic hypotension may be experienced early in therapy.

An intravenous (IV) preparation of labetalol is available for hypertensive emergencies, especially hypertensive encephalopathy, hypertension associated with extensive burns, and hypertension in patients with coronary artery disease or recent heart attack.

metoprolol

Metoprolol (Lopressor, Betaloc) is a short-acting cardioselective beta-blocker. It is indicated for the treatment of angina and hypertension and to prevent sudden death after a myocardial infarction. It is also used as a prophylactic for the treatment of migraine. It is well absorbed from the GI tract and readily metabolized by the liver. Dosages do not need to be modified with hepatic or renal function impairment. Extended-release and injectable forms are available.

nadolol

Nadolol (Corgard) is a long-acting nonselective beta-blocker. It is indicated for the treatment of angina and hypertension and is also used as a prophylactic for the treatment of migraine. It is not well absorbed from the GI tract, and up to one fourth of the dose may be excreted in the feces. Absorbed drug is excreted unchanged in the urine. The time between doses must be increased in patients with impaired renal function.

oxprenolol

Oxprenolol (Trasicor) is a short-acting nonselective beta-blocker with intrinsic sympathomimetic activity. It is indicated for the treatment of hypertension. It is well absorbed and metabolized by the liver. Oxprenolol is available in Canada but not in the United States. An extended-release form is available.

penbutolol

Penbutolol (Levatol) is a long-acting nonselective beta-blocker with intrinsic sympathomimetic activity. It is indicated for the treatment of hypertension. It is well absorbed and metabolized by the liver; the metabolites are excreted in the urine.

pindolol

Pindolol (Visken) is a short-acting nonselective beta-blocker with significant intrinsic sympathomimetic activity. It is indicated for the treatment of hypertension and is also used to treat angina. It is well absorbed when taken orally. Pindolol is metabolized by the liver, but about half the dose is excreted unchanged in the urine.

propranolol

Propranolol (Inderal), a nonselective beta-blocker, is the oldest of the clinically used beta-blocking drugs. It is well absorbed orally and readily metabolized by the liver. Propranolol is short acting but is available in extended-release forms. It is also available as an oral solution and in an injectable form. Propranolol has several approved indications in addition to those as an antianginal, antiarrhythmic, and antihypertensive agent. These indications include prophylactic treatment

---

CASE STUDY

Hypertension: Compliance Issues and Lifestyle Modifications

Mr. Todd is a 48-year-old African-American who was diagnosed with hypertension 6 months ago. He is a salesman for a busy company and travels often to meet with potential customers. During his follow-up visit, Mr. Todd confesses that he still eats out often with his clients because it is "part of my job." He admits that he has not tried to reduce his salt intake, and he drinks one or two cocktails during these dinner meetings. His weight is unchanged from 3 months ago; he is 42 pounds over his ideal body weight. He states that he sometimes "forgets" to take his medication because he does not "feel better" while taking it but actually feels more tired and has had some "other" problems too. He is currently taking 80 mg of nadolol (Corgard) daily along with daily 5 mg dose of hydrochlorothiazide. His blood pressure is 150/98 mm Hg at this time.

1. Is there a reason for this combination of medications for Mr. Todd?
2. What "other" problems might Mr. Todd be experiencing?
3. Explain additional lifestyle modifications that may help Mr. Todd.
4. Mr. Todd asks if he will be able to discontinue the medications if he loses weight and maintains a normal blood pressure. What is your answer to him?

against sudden death after a myocardial infarction, adjunct to the treatment of the adrenal tumor pheochromocytoma, treatment of tremors, and prophylaxis for migraine.

sotalol

Sotalol (Sotacor) is a very long-acting nonselective beta-blocker. It is moderately well absorbed and poorly metabolized by the liver. Most of the drug is excreted unchanged in the urine. Patients with renal failure should be given the drug less frequently. In the United States sotalol is approved for the treatment of cardiac arrhythmias but not approved for the treatment of hypertension. However, sotalol is approved as an antianginal and antihypertensive agent in Canada.

timolol

Timolol (Blocadren, Apo-Timol) is a short-acting nonselective beta-blocker. It is well absorbed from the GI tract and metabolized by the liver. Timolol is approved for use in treating hypertension, as prophylactic treatment for vascular headache, and against sudden death after a myocardial infarction. An ophthalmic formulation is available for the treatment of glaucoma.

Alpha₁-Blockers

General Characteristics

Mechanism of Action

Alpha₁-adrenergic receptors are found on vascular smooth muscle, where they mediate vasoconstriction in response to sympathetic nerve stimulation. Blockade of these receptors therefore results in vasodilation. Both arterioles and veins dilate, reducing the total peripheral resistance.

Pharmacokinetics

Alpha₁-blockers are taken orally one or more times a day, depending on the drug. The major pharmacologic difference between the alpha₁-blockers is their duration of action. They are metabolized by the liver, and metabolites are excreted in the urine.

Uses

Alpha₁-blockers are largely used as second or third drugs in the treatment of hypertension. A favorable side effect is a reduction in cholesterol and triglyceride levels. Moreover, reflex tachycardia is not common, in contrast with other classes of direct vasodilators. A diuretic is usually necessary because the alpha₁-adrenergic blockers tend to cause fluid retention.

Alpha₁-blockers are also useful in treating benign prostatic hyperplasia. These drugs reduce the tone of the prostatic smooth muscle, thereby decreasing pressure on the urethra and allowing urine to pass more freely.

Adverse Reactions and Contraindications

The most common side effects are dizziness, light-headedness, palpitations, and fainting caused by orthostatic hypotension. Therefore the dosage is often started low and raised gradu-ally to allow patients to develop some tolerance to the orthostatic hypotension. Other complaints may include weakness, fatigue, drowsiness, blurred vision, nasal congestion, nausea, edema, and weight gain.

Because blood pressure is lowered to a degree that can interfere with the perfusion of blood in the heart, attacks of angina may be precipitated by alpha₁-adrenergic blockers.

Interactions

Antiinflammatory drugs tend to cause fluid retention, which may be worsened with alpha₁-adrenergic blockers. Alcohol has a vasodilator effect that increases the risk for dizziness and fainting.

Specific Alpha₁-Blockers

doxazosin

Doxazosin (Cardura) is indicated for the treatment of hypertension and benign prostatic hypertension. It can be taken just once a day. This drug is well absorbed orally. The main hypotensive effect is apparent after 2 hours. The drug is highly protein bound and degraded in the liver.

prazosin

Prazosin (Minipress) has a shorter duration of action than the other alpha₁-blockers. It is commonly given with a diuretic when used for the treatment of hypertension. Because marked orthostatic hypotension may occur when the drug is first administered, the dosage is started low or given at bedtime.

▼ terazosin

Terazosin (Hytrin) is effective alone or with a diuretic in treating hypertension. The drug is long acting. It is also approved for treating benign prostatic hyperplasia.

Alpha₁-, Alpha₂-Blockers

phenoxybenzamine

Mechanism of Action

Phenoxybenzamine (Dibenzyline) is an irreversible and nonselective blocker of alpha-adrenergic receptors.

Pharmacokinetics

Phenoxybenzamine is given orally. The onset of action takes several hours. Because the drug combines irreversibly with alpha-adrenergic receptors, the effect is cumulative over a week with daily dosing. The duration of action is prolonged 3 to 4 days after a single dose. Phenoxybenzamine is metabolized by the liver with renal and biliary excretion of metabolites.

Uses

Phenoxybenzamine is used to control the high blood pressure caused by the elevated plasma levels of epinephrine in patients with the adrenal tumor pheochromocytoma when they are not yet ready for surgical removal of the tumor. Phenoxybenzamine is also used to dilate blood vessels in the skin, as in the treatment of Raynaud's phenomenon, in which there is a prominent neurogenic vasoconstriction of the blood vessels of the skin, particularly in the hands and feet (see Chapter 15).

Adverse Reactions and Contraindications

The prominent side effect of phenoxybenzamine is orthostatic hypotension (see Patient Problems box). Reflex tachycardia, nasal congestion, and GI upset are other common side effects of phenoxybenzamine resulting from its alpha-adrenergic antagonist activity.

Interactions

A major source of drug interactions with phenoxybenzamine is overstimulation of beta-adrenergic receptors by drugs such as epinephrine, which have both alpha- and beta-adrenergic receptor agonist activity. The blockade of alpha-receptors allows beta-receptor activation to go unopposed. Tachycardia is

---

PATIENT PROBLEMS

Orthostatic Hypotension

THE PROBLEM
The blood pressure drops markedly as the individual moves from lying to sitting or sitting to standing position.

SIGNS AND SYMPTOMS
Dizziness, light-headedness, weakness, and syncope (fainting)

ASSOCIATED OR CONTRIBUTING FACTORS
Long periods of standing; hot weather; hot showers or baths; ingestion of alcohol; exercise, especially when followed by immobility; and dehydration

PATIENT AND FAMILY EDUCATION
- Tighten calf muscles regularly while standing, or take a break to walk around frequently.
- If possible, sit instead of standing at work.
- Reduce the temperature of baths and showers.
- Wear support stockings. In severe cases tailor-made waist-high stockings may be needed.
- Avoid the use of alcohol.
- Move slowly from lying to sitting position. Hold on to something to provide support while moving from lying to sitting or standing position.
- Maintain adequate fluid intake to avoid dehydration, especially in the summer or if perspiring profusely.
- If the problem is severe, consult the physician. A change in drug or dose may be needed.

ADDITIONAL NURSING CARE MEASURES
- Monitor the blood pressure with patient lying, sitting, and standing. To document hypotension, check both arms.
- Supervise ambulation. Instruct patients with marked hypotension to call for assistance when moving from a reclining to a standing position.
- See Chapter 16 for information about drug treatment of orthostatic hypotension.

---

exaggerated. The vasodilator activity of drugs (as of the opioids) is exaggerated in the presence of phenoxybenzamine.

phentolamine

Mechanism of Action

Phentolamine (Regitine, Rogitine) is a short-acting and reversible alpha-adrenergic receptor antagonist. The major effects of phentolamine are vasodilation resulting from blockade of alpha$_1$-adrenergic receptors and cardiac stimulation believed to be associated with blockade of the presynaptic alpha$_2$-adrenergic receptors. (The presynaptic alpha$_2$-adrenergic receptors are associated with uptake of norepinephrine; see Chapter 12.)

Pharmacokinetics

Phentolamine is not well absorbed orally; IV administration is used.

Uses

Phentolamine has specific clinical uses as a vasodilator. One use is to lower blood pressure in patients with a tumor of the adrenal medulla that secretes large amounts of epinephrine (the tumor is called a pheochromocytoma). Another use is to lower blood pressure in patients who are being treated with a monoamine oxidase inhibitor and are suffering from the "cheese reaction," a hypertensive crisis that can be reversed with phentolamine. (See Chapter 59 for a discussion of the "cheese reaction.") A third use is to treat patients who are being withdrawn from the antihypertensive drug clonidine and may suffer a temporary hypertensive crisis.

A major use of phentolamine is to infiltrate a site where levarterenol (norepinephrine) or metaraminol has leaked into the tissue surrounding the infusion site. Commonly, 10 mg phentolamine mesylate is added to each liter of IV fluid containing norepinephrine. Phentolamine reverses the profound vasoconstriction that can otherwise cause tissue death.

Phentolamine, usually with papaverine, may be used in the treatment of impotence. The drugs are administered intracavernosally within 2 hours of intercourse.

Adverse Reactions and Contraindications

Side effects of the systemic use of phentolamine include hypotension, a rapid heart rate (tachycardia) as a reflex response of the body to the hypotension, nasal congestion associated with the vasodilation, and general GI upset. Caution should be used in administering phentolamine to patients with angina, coronary insufficiency, or a history of heart attacks.

Interactions

Phentolamine antagonizes the vasopressor action of sympathomimetic drugs such as dopamine, epinephrine, and phenylephrine.

Sympatholytic Drugs

Sympatholytic drugs are those drugs that interfere with the storage and/or release of norepinephrine. The drugs in longest use are the rauwolfia alkaloids. Because these drugs cause a variety of side effects, they are no longer in wide use but may prove effective in cases refractory to the newer drugs.

guanethidine

Mechanism of Action

Guanethidine (Ismelin) is a postganglionic adrenergic blocking agent. It enters peripheral sympathetic neurons; it is taken into the cell by the same mechanism as for the re-uptake of norepinephrine. Inside the neuron guanethidine blocks norepinephrine release. Guanethidine does not cross the blood-brain barrier and therefore produces no central effects. Because norepinephrine is not available for release from peripheral sympathetic neurons, both peripheral vascular resistance and cardiac output are decreased.

Pharmacokinetics

The effects of guanethidine may take 1 to 2 weeks to reach the maximum therapeutic response to a given dosage regimen. Moreover, the effects of guanethidine persist for 7 to 10 days after therapy is discontinued.

Uses

Guanethidine is a very potent antihypertensive drug that is restricted for use in controlling severe hypertension. It is also indicated in the treatment of renal hypertension, including that secondary to pyelonephritis, renal amyloidosis, and renal artery stenosis.

Adverse Reactions and Contraindications

A number of uncomfortable side effects arise from the depletion of peripheral norepinephrine stores. Orthostatic (postural) hypotension is a special problem with guanethidine therapy. The tone of blood vessels is diminished by guanethidine, and if the patient moves suddenly from a reclining to a standing position, the appropriate vascular changes cannot take place quickly enough for proper blood redistribution to occur. The blood stays in the periphery and drains from the head on standing, resulting in fainting. Patients taking guanethidine must be instructed to change body positions slowly. Other side effects resulting from the depletion of norepinephrine include a slow heart rate (bradycardia) and diarrhea. This diarrhea, which occurs after meals, can be severe and of an explosive nature. In men failure of erection or ejaculation may arise as a result of the loss of vascular tone. Guanethidine also causes sodium retention; therefore a diuretic is administered concurrently.

Contraindications for guanethidine therapy include the presence of angina, cerebral insufficiency, or coronary artery disease conditions that are further compromised by the loss of vascular tone.

Interactions

A number of drug interactions have been noted for guanethidine. Patients taking guanethidine are supersensitive to administered catecholamines. Patients become less responsive to guanethidine when an indirect-acting adrenergic drug (e.g., amphetamine, ephedrine) or a tricyclic antidepressant drug is taken. The indirect-acting adrenergic drugs release stored norepinephrine from neurons, an action that overcomes the effect of guanethidine to block release of norepinephrine. Tricyclic antidepressants block the uptake of guanethidine into the neuron so that guanethidine cannot reach its site of action.

guanadrel

Guanadrel (Hylorel) has actions similar to those of guanethidine but with more rapid onset of action and shorter duration of action. The side affects of guanadrel are similar to those of guanethidine but less severe.

reserpine and Related Drugs

Reserpine (Serpasil), Deserpidine (Harmonyl), and rauwolfia serpentina (Raudixin, others) and related drugs are often called rauwolfia alkaloids because reserpine was originally isolated from the *Rauwolfia serpentina* bush of India. Reserpine was originally used as an antipsychotic drug but has been replaced by the phenothiazine tranquilizers for this use. Reserpine is effective in lowering blood pressure because it depletes stores of norepinephrine from neurons both in the CNS and the peripheral nervous system. The central action produces sedation and tranquilization. The reported incidence of depression with reserpine has varied from 27% to 40%. Occasionally, patients who take reserpine will become severely depressed to the point of attempting suicide. More commonly, patients complain of a lethargic feeling, an increased appetite, and increased dreaming. Nightmares are sometimes a complaint.

Other side effects of reserpine can be related to the decreased sympathetic tone, such as vasodilation that results in a flushed, warm feeling and nasal congestion. Some side effects of reserpine can be related to the predominant parasympathetic tone when sympathetic tone is depressed: salivation, stomach cramps, and diarrhea. Because reserpine augments gastric acid secretion through the increased parasympathetic tone, it should not be used in patients with a peptic ulcer.

THERAPEUTIC AGENTS: VASODILATORS FOR TREATING CHRONIC HYPERTENSION

Vasodilators that are used to treat chronic hypertension are presented in the following sections: Angiotensin-Converting Enzyme Inhibitors, Angiotensin II Receptor Blockers, Calcium Channel Blockers, and Other Vasodilators.

Angiotensin-Converting Enzyme Inhibitors

General Characteristics

Mechanism of Action

Angiotensin II is a potent vasoconstrictor. As seen in Figure 13-1, angiotensin II is formed from angiotensin I by ACE. When this enzyme is inhibited, the amount of angiotensin II formed decreases. **Angiotensin-converting enzyme (ACE) inhibitors** therefore decrease the amount of the potent vasoconstrictor, angiotensin II. The ACE inhibitors also block the degradation of bradykinin and thus increase the amounts of this important vasodilator peptide. The net effect of ACE inhibitors is to decrease peripheral vascular resistance. This action makes the ACE inhibitors useful in treating congestive heart failure and hypertension.

Pharmacokinetics

ACE inhibitors are effective orally. Except for captopril and lisinopril, the ACE inhibitors are prodrugs and must be hydrolyzed in the body to active forms. Excretion tends to be predominantly renal.

Uses

ACE inhibitors are used alone or with a diuretic in the treatment of mild to severe hypertension. Because ACE inhibitors increase renal blood flow without changing the glomerular filtration rate, ACE inhibitors are the preferred antihypertensive therapy for patients with diabetic nephropathy or renal scleroderma.

ACE inhibitors have played a major role in reducing death from congestive heart failure. Studies have demonstrated a decrease in deaths by about 30% in patients with congestive heart failure when treated with enalapril. In patients with mild congestive heart failure, the development of severe heart failure was reduced by 37% in patients treated with captopril. Captopril, enalapril, and lisinopril have been approved for treatment of congestive heart failure in combination with digitalis and diuretics or in cases unresponsive to other therapies.

Adverse Reactions and Contraindications

ACE inhibitors are well tolerated and have little if any adverse effects on the CNS function or on carbohydrate or lipid metabolism. Dizziness, a skin rash, swelling, and an increase in serum potassium levels (hyperkalemia) have been reported. Some patients develop a cough during therapy that begins as a tickling sensation and progresses to a dry, nonproductive persistent cough that becomes worse at night. The cough disappears when the drug is withdrawn.

Patients with a history of angioedema, impaired renal function, or a renal transplant, or patients who are receiving renal dialysis or have renal artery stenosis should not be given ACE inhibitors. ACE inhibitors can cause fetal and neonatal problems and should not be administered to pregnant women. There is evidence for some ACE inhibitors that they are excreted in breast milk, so these drugs should not be taken by nursing mothers.

Interactions

Drug interactions have been reported for the ACE inhibitors. Foods or drugs high in potassium may contribute to hyperkalemia. The hypotensive effect of ACE inhibitors is enhanced by diuretics, alcohol, and beta-blockers. Patients who are sodium or water depleted through diuretic therapy should begin taking ACE inhibitors at about half the regular dose. Non-steroidal antiinflammatory drugs (NSAIDs), especially indomethacin, may antagonize the antihypertensive effect of the ACE inhibitors and cause sodium retention leading to edema.

Specific Angiotensin-Converting Enzyme Inhibitors

In addition to the drugs listed next, perindopril (Aceon) and spirapril (Renormax) are expected to join the list of ACE inhibitors on the market.

benazepril

Benazepril (Lotensin) is rapidly absorbed and metabolized by the liver. However, benazepril is also highly protein bound, and the main metabolite, benazeprilat, is also active, so the duration of action is 24 hours.

captopril

Captopril (Capoten) is rapidly absorbed after oral administration and is effective within 1 hour. About half of the drug is excreted unchanged in the urine, and there is no active metabolite. In addition to the treatment of hypertension, captopril is also used for treating congestive heart failure in combination with a diuretic and digoxin, for treating renovascular hypertension, for treating diabetic nephropathy, and for treating patients who have had a heart attack accompanied by dysfunction of the left ventricle.

▼ enalapril

Enalapril (Vasotec) is a prodrug designed to be absorbed orally. On absorption, enalapril is deesterified to the active drug, enalaprilat, which, like captopril, is an inhibitor of ACE. However, patients with liver disease may be unable to activate enalapril.

Enalapril is also used for treating congestive heart failure in combination with a diuretic and digoxin. Enalapril has been shown to reduce the onset of congestive heart failure in patients who have left ventricular dysfunction.

Enalaprilat injection (Vasotec injection) is the active form of enalapril in a dosage form suitable for treatment in a hypertensive emergency.

fosinopril

Fosinopril (Monopril) is slowly absorbed orally and metabolized by the liver and gastric mucosa to an active metabolite, fosinoprilat. Because the metabolite has a long duration of action, the drug's duration of action is about 24 hours.

lisinopril

Lisinopril (Prinivil, Zestril) is poorly absorbed, is not protein bound, and is not metabolized by the liver. Lisinopril is excreted in the urine unchanged. The duration of action is about 24 hours. The dosage must be greatly reduced for patients with impaired renal function. Lisinopril is also used for treating congestive heart failure in combination with a diuretic and digoxin.

moexipril

Moexipril (Univasc) is incompletely absorbed, and the rate of absorption is decreased by food. Moexipril is rapidly converted to moexiprilat, the active metabolite. Excretion is primarily in the feces. The duration of action is about 12 hours. The dosage must be reduced for patients with impaired renal function.

quinapril

Quinapril (Accupril) is well absorbed and metabolized by the liver and gastric mucosa to an active metabolite, quinaprilat, which is highly protein bound. The duration of action is about 24 hours.

Quinapril is also used for treating congestive heart failure in combination with a diuretic and digoxin.

ramipril

Ramipril (Altace) is rapidly absorbed and metabolized by the liver to ramiprilat, which has about six times the activity of ramipril itself. The duration of action is about 24 hours.

trandolapril

Trandolapril (Mavik) is a new long-acting ACE inhibitor similar to lisinopril and enalapril.

Angiotensin II Receptor Blockers

Angiotensin II receptor blockers are a new class of antihypertensive agents coming into clinical use. Angiotensin receptor blockers act to prevent the action of angiotensin II and therefore have a more selective mechanism of action. In addition to the losartan (Cozaar), irbesartan (Avapro), and valsartan (Diovan) covered in the following sections, cardesartan (Atacand) and eprosartan (Teveten) are expected to join the list of angiotensin II receptor blockers on the market.

▼ losartan

Mechanism of Action

Losartan (Cozaar) is a specific receptor antagonist for angiotensin II. Losartan blocks the vasoconstrictor and aldosterone-secreting effects of angiotensin II by inhibiting the binding of angiotensin II to its receptor (see Figure 13-1). The vasodilation resulting from losartan is like that of the ACE inhibitors.

Uses

Losartan is an alternative to an ACE inhibitor in the treatment of hypertension. Because losartan is a relatively new drug, its role relative to the ACE inhibitors in the treatment of hypertension remains to be tested. Diuretics increase the hypotensive effects of angiotensin II antagonists.

Pharmacokinetics

Losartan is administered orally but is extensively metabolized by the liver. The major metabolite is much more potent than the parent compound and has a half-life of 6 to 9 hours. Excretion is in both the feces and urine.

Adverse Reactions and Contraindications

The most common side effect of losartan is dizziness, especially after the first dose. The dry cough sometimes seen with ACE inhibitors is uncommon with losartan. Occasionally, headache, back pain, diarrhea, fatigue, and nasal congestion are reported. Rarely, angioedema with swelling in the face, mouth, hands, or feet occurs. Like the ACE inhibitors, losartan may cause birth defects and should not be taken during pregnancy. Patients with severe congestive heart failure or renal artery stenosis should not be treated with angiotensin II antagonists. These patients are especially susceptible to changes in the renin-angiotensin-aldosterone system and may experience oliguria, azotemia, acute renal failure, and death.

Interactions

The hypotensive action of losartan is aggravated by fluid loss caused by hot weather, exercise, or vomiting. Alcohol has vasodilatory activity and if ingested while taking losartan may cause increased dizziness or fainting.

irbesartan and valsartan

Irbesartan (Avapro) and valsartan (Diovan) are new drugs that like losartan are specific receptor antagonists for angiotensin II. High potassium levels may occur if a potassium supplement is given with valsartan. Occasionally, allergy, stomach irritation, dizziness, too low a blood pressure, or alterations in taste have been reported.

Calcium Channel Blockers

General Characteristics

Mechanism of Action

Calcium channel blockers decrease the entry of calcium into smooth muscle and thereby lower vascular tone, an action that reduces peripheral resistance and blood pressure. This reduction in blood pressure can produce a reflex increase in heart rate. Cardiac function is also depressed because of reduced intracellular calcium. Each of the various calcium channel blockers differs in its relative effect on vascular and cardiac tissue. In general, calcium channel blockers are useful for patients with coexisting angina (see Chapter 15).

Pharmacokinetics

Calcium channel blockers are generally well absorbed, and most have reduced bioavailability because the drug is extensively metabolized by the liver on absorption. Most of these agents are protein bound in the blood. Excretion of the drug or its metabolites is in the urine and feces.

Uses

Calcium channel blockers have rapidly become important in the treatment of various cardiovascular diseases. These drugs are effective in the treatment of angina, arrhythmias, and hypertension. In the treatment of hypertension, calcium channel blockers are especially effective in low-renin hypertension. Elderly and African-American patients have a better response to calcium channel blockers as the first drug to treat hypertension than to other antihypertensive drugs used alone. The addition of an ACE inhibitor, methyldopa, or beta-blocker enhances the antihypertensive response.

In general, calcium channel blockers are safe for patients with asthma, hyperlipidemia, diabetes, and renal dysfunction. They do not alter lipid values, uric acid, or electrolytes. They also do not alter exercise tolerance.

Adverse Reactions and Contraindications

Calcium channel blockers are well tolerated by various age and ethnic groups, and side effects are generally mild. Older adults may be more sensitive to the effects of these drugs than younger groups are. Headaches, dizziness, and edema are complaints in 20% or fewer of patients. A hypotensive response is more likely in older adults. Calcium channel blockers have not been tested in pregnant women. Adverse fetal effects have been found in animal studies when very large doses were given. Some of the calcium channel blockers have been found in breast milk.

Concern has been raised that calcium channel blockers may increase the rate of heart attacks or death. The fast-acting form of nifedipine at high dosages has been specifically implicated by recent studies as increasing mortality. Specifically, the fast-acting (immediate release) formulations of the dihydropyridine subclass of calcium channel blockers are implicated. Drugs in this subclass include amlodipine, felodipine, isradipine, nicardipine, nifedipine, and nimodipine. Studies are under way to determine how safe calcium channel blockers are.

Calcium channel blockers should be used with caution in patients with bradycardia or heart failure. These drugs do not improve and may worsen cardiac hemodynamics. Calcium channel blockers must also be used with caution in patients renal or hepatic failure, conditions which affect the metabolism and excretion of these drugs.

Some patients develop an allergic reaction to calcium channel blockers.

Interactions

Calcium channel blockers depress the atrioventricular (AV) nodal conduction that may lead to heart block. Beta-adrenergic blockers act synergistically with calcium channel blockers to depress both AV conduction and cardiac contractility. The digitalis glycosides act in an additive manner with the calcium channel blockers to depress AV conduction. Careful assessment should be used when combining calcium channel blockers with any other drugs that affect cardiac rhythm or contractility, especially disopyramide, flecainide, procainamide, quinidine, and hypokalemic medications.

Specific Calcium Channel Blockers

In addition to the drugs listed next, perindopril (Aceon) and spirapril (Renormax) are expected to join the list of ACE inhibitors on the market.

▼ amlodipine

Amlodipine (Norvasc) is used to treat angina and hypertension. It is relatively selective as a vasodilator, producing both peripheral arterial vasodilation and coronary dilation, making it a good antianginal agent. Reflex tachycardia is minimal. Amlodipine is absorbed slowly and has a prolonged effect, reaching steady plasma levels only after 7 to 10 days of therapy. The drug is highly protein bound. It is slowly metabolized in the liver and metabolites are excreted in the urine.

diltiazem

Diltiazem (Cardizem) depresses both the sinoatrial (SA) and AV nodes but produces little negative inotropic effect (decrease in the strength of the heartbeat). It is effective in dilating coronary vessels, making it a good antianginal agent. Diltiazem is well absorbed orally and extensively metabolized. The onset of action is 30 to 60 minutes for the tablet form and 2 to 3 hours for the extended-release capsule form. The duration of action is 4 to 8 hours for the tablet form, 12 hours for the sustained-release capsule form, and 24 hours for the controlled-dose capsule form. Diltiazem is extensively metabolized, and metabolites are excreted in the urine and feces.

felodipine

Felodipine (Plendil) is a potent peripheral vasodilator that does not depress the SA or AV node. With its use there tends to be a reflex increase in heart rate in response to the vasodilation. The drug is well absorbed but extensively metabolized by the liver after absorption. Felodipine is effective in 2 to 5 hours and has a duration of action of 24 hours. Metabolites are excreted in the urine.

isradipine

Isradipine (DynaCirc) is a potent vasodilator that does not depress the SA or AV node. With its use there tends to be a reflex increase in heart rate in response to the vasodilation. Isradipine is used primarily as an antihypertensive agent. It is effective in 2 to 3 hours and has a duration of action over 12 hours. Isradipine is extensively metabolized, and metabolites are excreted in the urine and feces.

nicardipine

Nicardipine (Cardene) is more selective for vascular smooth muscle than for cardiac muscle. This means that nicardipine is a potent vasodilator and also dilates the coronary vessels with little or no depression of conductivity. It is used both as an antihypertensive agent and an antianginal agent. Nicardipine is well absorbed and rapid acting; it has duration of action of about 8 hours. It is extensively metabolized, and metabolites are excreted in the urine and feces.

nifedipine

Nifedipine (Procardia, Adalat) is similar to nicardipine in being more selective for smooth muscle than for cardiac muscle. It has no real effect on the AV node and so does not directly depress the heart rate. It is used both as an antihypertensive agent and an antianginal agent. Nifedipine is rapidly absorbed with an onset of action of 20 minutes and a duration of action of 4 to 8 hours. Extended-release forms are available with longer durations. The drug is readily metabolized, and metabolites are excreted in the urine and feces.

nisoldipine

Nisoldipine (Sular) is a new calcium channel blocker for the treatment of hypertension. It is chemically related to nifedipine. Nisoldipine is available as an extended-release preparation for once-a-day administration. Nisoldipine is metabolized by the liver, and doses should be lowered for people with liver disease or the elderly. Gingival hyperplasia is a potential side effect, so meticulous dental hygiene should be encouraged.

verapamil

Verapamil (Calan, Isoptin) depresses the SA and AV nodes, an action that makes it a useful antiarrhythmic drug (see Chapter 19). A slowing of the heart rate (bradycardia) is common. Verapamil is used as both an antihypertensive agent and an antianginal agent. It is well absorbed. The onset of action is 4 to 12 hours, and the duration of action is 8 to 10 hours. Extended-release forms have a 24-hour duration of action. Verapamil is readily metabolized, and metabolites are excreted in the urine and feces.

Other Vasodilators

hydralazine

Hydralazine (Apresoline) acts directly on arteriolar smooth muscle to cause relaxation. The mechanism is unknown. The drop in arterial blood pressure is great enough to activate the baroreceptors of the aorta. This activation causes a reflex stimulation of the heart that increases cardiac output and partially compensates for the fall in blood pressure (reflex tachycardia). Hydralazine also causes sodium retention. Because hydralazine causes reflex stimulation of the heart and increases sodium retention, it is most effective in reducing hypertension when added to a diuretic to counteract the sodium retention and a beta-blocker (propranolol, nadolol, or metoprolol) to block the reflex stimulation of the heart.

Side effects common to hydralazine include headache, palpitation, loss of appetite, nausea, vomiting, and diarrhea. In the absence of a beta-antagonist, hydralazine can cause angina in susceptible individuals as a result of the reflex stimulation of the heart. Hydralazine is not a good drug for a patient with angina, coronary artery disease, or CHF because of the indirect cardiac effects.

An occasional effect of long-term therapy with hydralazine at high dosages is the appearance of a lupuslike syndrome. Lupus erythematosus is an autoimmune disease with symptoms of fever, joint pain, chest pain, edema, and circulating antibodies to DNA. The syndrome induced by hydralazine is similar, but it is reversed when the drug is discontinued. The appearance of lupuslike symptoms is rare when smaller doses of hydralazine are used in combination with diuretic and sympathetic blocking drug. Patients receiving hydralazine therapy are monitored for the appearance of the anti-DNA antibodies.

minoxidil

Minoxidil (Loniten) is a direct-acting vasodilator like hydralazine, but it is more potent. This drug must be given with a diuretic to control fluid retention and a beta-receptor blocker to prevent reflex tachycardia. A side effect of minoxidil is excessive hairiness, which may develop after a few weeks of treatment. Some patients experience transient nausea, headaches, or fatigue when treatment is started.

THERAPEUTIC AGENTS: CENTRALLY ACTING ANTIHYPERTENSIVE DRUGS

Clonidine, guanabenz, guanfacine, and methyldopa exert their antihypertensive activity through actions in the CNS.

Specific Drugs

▼ clonidine

Mechanism of Action

Clonidine (Catapres) has an antihypertensive effect that results from its action in the CNS. It activates alpha$_2$-receptors in the vasomotor center of the medulla, an action that inhibits activity of the sympathetic nervous system. Heart rate and cardiac output are decreased and account for the reduction in blood pressure.

Pharmacokinetics

Clonidine is well absorbed and becomes effective within 1 hour when taken orally. A transdermal system is also available for administering clonidine that requires 2 to 3 days before an effect is seen. More than half the drug is excreted unchanged in the urine. Patients with impaired renal function may require smaller doses or less frequent administration.

Uses

Clonidine is commonly used with a diuretic in antihypertensive therapy. New therapeutic uses for clonidine have been developed. Clonidine is used in the prophylaxis of vascular headaches and to treat the vasomotor symptoms of menopause. The symptoms of opioid withdrawal and nicotine withdrawal can often be controlled by clonidine. Gilles de la Tourette's syndrome, a condition of severe and multiple tics, is alleviated by clonidine therapy.

Adverse Reactions and Contraindications

Common side effects of clonidine therapy include drowsiness, dry mouth, and constipation. Sudden discontinuance can be dangerous. After discontinuing therapeutic doses for 12 to 48 hours, many patients experience symptoms of a sympathetic rebound: restlessness, insomnia, tremors, increased salivation, and increased heart rate (tachycardia). If clonidine is not reinstated, headaches, abdominal pain, and nausea follow. The most severe reaction is a hypertensive crisis that is best treated in the hospital with a combination of alpha-blocking and beta-blocking drugs: phentolamine and propranolol. To avoid these withdrawal problems, clonidine doses are gradually reduced over a week or more.

Interactions

The hypotensive action of clonidine may be decreased by antidepressants or appetite suppressants. If beta-blockers are taken concurrently, they should be discontinued gradually before clonidine is discontinued. If clonidine is discontinued while the patient is still taking a beta-blocker, this situation increases the risk of a clonidine-withdrawal hypertensive crisis.

guanabenz

Guanabenz (Wytensin) has a mechanism of action similar to that of clonidine; it inhibits sympathetic activity by activating alpha-receptors in the CNS. Guanabenz has a long duration of action, 12 to 24 hours, and may require only once-a-day dosage. It is metabolized and excreted in the urine.

The most common side effects are drowsiness, dry mouth, dizziness, weakness, and headache. Withdrawal rebound hypertension can occur if guanabenz is discontinued abruptly.

guanfacine

Guanfacine (Tenex), like clonidine and guanabenz, appears to act in the CNS. By stimulating central alpha-adrenergic receptors, there is a decreased sympathetic outflow and a lowering of blood pressure. Guanfacine has a long duration of action, about 24 hours, and can be taken once a day. It is well absorbed and is metabolized in the liver. The most common side effects are drowsiness, dry mouth, depression, and confusion.

methyldopa

Mechanism of Action

Methyldopa (Aldomet) is taken into sympathetic neurons and metabolized to methylnorepinephrine. Methylnorepinephrine is stored in granules and released on stimulation of the neuron. Methylnorepinephrine is called a false transmitter because it takes the place of norepinephrine. The antihypertensive effect of methylnorepinephrine is that it activates alpha$_2$-receptors in the vasomotor center of the medulla. This activation results in the inhibition of sympathetic nervous system. In addition to decreasing sympathetic tone, methyldopa metabolites produce a tranquilizing effect on behavior.

Pharmacokinetics

Methyldopa is administered orally two to four times daily. An injectable form of methyldopate is available for IV administration in a hypertensive crisis. However, methyldopate is relatively slow acting and does not act immediately to lower blood pressure. Methyldopa and its sulfated metabolite are excreted in the urine.

Uses

Methyldopa is used to treat moderate to severe hypertension, including that complicated by renal diseases. Methyldopa appears to be safe for the fetus when taken in the last trimester. An injectable form, methyldopate, is used in the treatment of hypertensive crisis. Because methyldopate has a slow onset of action, it is not the sole initial therapy for a hypertensive crisis.

Adverse Reactions and Contraindications

Side effects common to methyldopa are related largely to the decrease in central sympathetic activity. Drowsiness is common at the beginning of treatment. Unpleasant sedation, depressed mood, and nightmares are occasional complaints. Tiredness and fatigue may be noted. Peripheral effects include a slow heart rate (bradycardia), diarrhea, dry mouth, and occasional ejaculatory failure in men.

Interactions

Occasionally, methyldopa causes a false-positive Coombs' test. A positive Coombs' test indicates hemolytic anemia, but it is rare for the patient taking methyldopa to have hemolytic anemia despite the positive test. Methyldopa may also cause a mild alteration of liver function tests. Methyldopa is therefore not a drug to use for patients who already have impaired liver function because the drug will interfere with evaluating the course of the disease. This alteration of liver tests ordinarily occurs during the first 6 weeks of therapy and is reversed by discontinuing methyldopa.

Sympathomimetic drugs decrease the hypotensive effect of methyldopa and may themselves give exaggerated vasopressor responses. Methyldopa may cause hyperexcitability in patients receiving monoamine oxidase inhibitors.

THERAPEUTIC AGENTS: DRUGS USED IN HYPERTENSIVE EMERGENCIES

A **hypertensive emergency** cannot be simply defined. The blood pressure may be severely elevated or only moderately elevated. The important feature is that there is impending end-organ damage, usually of the brain, heart, or eyes. Unstable neurologic symptoms that suggest damage to the brain include headache, restlessness, confusion, and even convulsions. Hemorrhaging may be apparent in the eye.

Certain antihypertensive drugs discussed earlier in this chapter are available as IV formulations for the treatment of hypertensive crises. These drugs include enalaprilat, hydralazine, labetalol, methyldopa, and phentolamine. These drugs appear in Table 13-2. Additional drugs currently used to treat hypertensive emergencies by rapidly lowering blood pressure are listed in Table 13-3.

Vasodilators

diazoxide

As a vasodilator, diazoxide (Hyperstat) acts directly to relax arteriolar smooth muscle. This action lowers blood pressure but does not affect the venous side of circulation. Diazoxide is therefore not useful for those conditions requiring the decreased venous return produced by trimethaphan.

The advantage of diazoxide treatment is that a bolus of the drug can be given intravenously over 30 seconds and will usually be effective in 5 minutes and remain effective for 2 to 12 hours. Blood pressure does not need to be continuously monitored as with trimethaphan treatment. The patient rarely becomes excessively hypotensive. Diazoxide causes retention of sodium and water, which must be treated with a diuretic. Diazoxide also causes hyperglycemia.

▼ nitroglycerin

Nitroglycerin (Nitro-Bid IV, Nitrostat IV, Tridil) acts directly to relax smooth muscle with a greater effect on the venous than the arterial circulation. The advantage of nitroglycerin is its immediate action; it must be continuously infused. Because nitroglycerin is absorbed by PVC plastic, special non-PVC infusion sets are used.

sodium nitroprusside

Sodium nitroprusside (Nipride) acts directly on the smooth muscle of both arterioles and venous vessels. The result is an immediate decrease in blood pressure with no increase in venous return. There are no notable side effects with short-term use of nitroprusside. Blood pressure must be constantly monitored, and the drug is administered by IV drip. Nitroprusside is unstable in light, so it should not be used more than 4 hours after it is dissolved. Side effects arise from the use of nitroprusside for several days. Some of it is metabolized to thiocyanate, which can produce ringing in the ears (tinnitus), blurred vision, and hypothyroidism.

Ganglionic Blocking Drug: trimethaphan

Trimethaphan (Arfonad) blocks the receptors for acetylcholine in the ganglia and is a ganglionic blocking drug. Ganglionic blocking drugs inhibit both sympathetic and parasympathetic activity and therefore have limited clinical use. Trimethaphan is used in treating some hypertensive emergencies, particularly surgery for an aortic dissecting aneurysm. Because this drug has a short duration of action, it is administered by continuous IV drip; during this time

Table 13-3 Drugs Used in Hypertensive Emergencies

Generic Name	Trade Name	Administration/Dosage	Comments
diazoxide	Hyperstat*	INTRAVENOUS: *Adults*—150 mg or 5 mg/kg body weight. *Children*—5 mg/kg body weight. Administered over 30 sec. May be repeated after 30 min. FDA pregnancy category C.	Direct-acting vasodilator. Acts rapidly (2-5 min) and lasts 2-12 hr. Increases venous return and cardiac output. Blood pressure fall is rarely excessive, so blood pressure monitoring is not critical.
fenoldopam	Corlopam	INTRAVENOUS: *Adults*—Infuse, beginning at dosage of 0.1 μg/kg/min. Dosage is increased by 0.05-0.1 μg/kg/min at 15-min intervals if necessary. Maximum: 1.6 μg/kg/min. FDA pregnancy category B.	New vasodilator for in-hospital short-term management of severe hypertension. Rapidly eliminated in urine. Dilates coronary, renal, mesenteric, and peripheral blood vessels. May produce reflex tachycardia if blood pressure lowered too quickly.
nitroglycerin	Nitro-Bid* Nitrol Nitrostat* Tridil*	INTRAVENOUS: *Adults*—Initially 5 μg/min; increase in 5-μg increments every 3-5 min until clinical response or 20 μg/min is reached. FDA pregnancy category C.	Direct-acting vasodilator. Doses are stated for non-PVC infusion sets. PVC may absorb nitroglycerin. IV nitroglycerin is also used to reduce cardiac load or as antianginal agent in emergency situation. Effective immediately.
sodium nitroprusside	Nipride* Nitropress	INTRAVENOUS: *Adults*—dissolve 50 mg in 500-1000 ml of 5% dextrose. Infuse 0.5-10 μg/kg/min. Solution must be protected from light and discarded after 4 hr. *Children*—1.4 μg/kg/min. FDA pregnancy category C.	Direct-acting vasodilator. Acts rapidly (1-2 min). Continuous infusion is necessary to maintain hypotensive effect. Decreased venous return occurs with no change in heart rate. Blood pressure must be carefully monitored and infusion rate adjusted to maintain desired level.
trimethaphan camsylate	Arfonad*	INTRAVENOUS: *Adults*—0.1% (1 mg/ml) infusion in 5% dextrose. Rate of infusion is begun at 0.5-1 mg/min and increased gradually until blood pressure falls by 20 mm Hg. After several minutes, rate is again increased until blood pressure reaches desired level. FDA pregnancy category D.	Rapidly acting drug blocks acetylcholine receptors in ganglia. Inhibits sympathetic and parasympathetic nervous systems and decreases venous return and cardiac output. Blood pressure must be carefully monitored because hypotensive effect is variable and unpredictable.

*Available in Canada and the United States.

blood pressure must be constantly monitored. Side effects result from the inhibition of both sympathetic and parasympathetic tone. Severe hypotension can result from the inhibition of sympathetic tone. IV drip is then discontinued until the blood pressure begins to rise again. Side effects from loss of parasympathetic tone include pupillary dilation, loss of accommodation, drying of mucous surfaces, constipation, and urinary retention.

The disadvantages of trimethaphan therapy are that blood pressure must be carefully monitored and that the loss of pupillary reflexes makes it difficult to monitor ongoing neurologic damage to the brain (when neurologic damage was the presenting set of symptoms). In addition, trimethaphan can be unpredictable in its effects; patients already taking antihypertensive medication or those with a reduced blood volume may be unusually sensitive to trimethaphan. Some patients do not respond readily to trimethaphan; others are initially responsive but become unresponsive later.

Trimethaphan decreases venous return of blood and lowers cardiac output. These actions are helpful when the patient has a condition such as a dissecting aortic aneurysm, hypertensive encephalopathy, acute left ventricular failure, or cerebral hemorrhage because the pressure is removed from the weakened tissue.

Nursing Process Overview

Antihypertensive Drugs

Assessment

Assess the blood pressure with the patient at rest. Check both arms. Some physicians order lying, sitting, and standing blood pressure measurements. Monitor weight, serum electrolytes, blood urea nitrogen, and measures of renal and cardiovascular function. Obtain a dietary history that focuses on sodium intake. Assess patterns of smoking and alcohol consumption.

Nursing Diagnoses
- Sexual dysfunction related to drug's side effect: impotence
- Noncompliance related to intolerable side effects
- Risk for orthostatic hypotension

Patient Outcomes
The patient will maintain blood pressure within normal range. The patient will not discontinue antihypertensive medication without consulting the health care provider. The patient will not experience intolerable side effects.

Planning/Implementation
Patients in hypertensive crisis may be admitted to the acute-care setting for cardiac monitoring and IV drug therapy. Otherwise, therapy may be started in the hospitalized or ambulatory patient. Monitor the blood pressure and other vital signs, intake and output, weight, serum electrolyte levels, blood glucose levels, and other laboratory data specific to the side effects of individual drugs. In preparation for discharge, teach the patient about prescribed drugs and other prescribed therapies: sodium restriction, weight loss, smoking cessation, limited alcohol intake, and regular exercise.

Evaluation
Ideally, therapy will lower the blood pressure to below 140/90 mm Hg without serious side effects. Ascertain that the patient can explain the hazards of untreated hypertension, how to take the prescribed medications safely, why additional drugs such as diuretics or potassium may be needed, what to do about anticipated side effects, how to follow any dietary restrictions, and when to call the physician. If necessary, teach the patient to record weight or blood pressure regularly. If the patient is interested, refer him or her to local smoking-cessation clinics.

Nursing Implications Summary

General Guidelines: Antihypertensives
Drug Administration/Nursing in the Community
➤ Encourage the patient to lose weight to reach a desirable body weight and to restrict dietary intake of sodium because these changes may reduce the need for antihypertensive drug therapy. Other lifestyle changes that may lessen the need for antihypertensive medication include stopping smoking, cutting back on caffeine intake, and exercising regularly.
➤ Regularly assess the patient thoroughly and thoughtfully. Poor compliance with drug therapy may result if the patient feels worse, or not better, while taking antihypertensives. The patient may feel reluctant to discuss side effects such as impotence and may discontinue a drug if this or other side effects occur. In addition, the cost of drug therapy, especially when two or more drugs are required, may be prohibitive.
➤ Reinforce the need to take these medications as directed and not to discontinue therapy abruptly or without consulting the physician.
➤ Work with the patient to develop a system for remembering to take medicines. Activities such as marking off a calendar when doses are taken or preparing a week of doses at one time may keep the patient more involved and help serve as a reminder.

Nursing Implications Summary—cont'd

➤ Instruct the patient about orthostatic hypotension, a common side effect of antihypertensive therapy (see Patient Problems box).

➤ Monitor blood pressure and pulse at least every 4 hours when a patient begins antihypertensive therapy, during periods of dosage adjustment, or when orthostatic hypotension is a problem. Assess the blood pressure with the patient lying, then sitting, then standing; check both arms. For selected patients, it may be necessary to instruct a family member to measure and record the blood pressure in the home.

➤ Supervise the ambulation of the hospitalized patient undergoing antihypertensive therapy to guard against injury in case the patient becomes dizzy or faint. Be especially alert with older adult patients, who are more sensitive to drug effects.

➤ Teach the patient to keep all health care providers informed of all drugs being used and to avoid over-the-counter medications unless approved by the physician. The incidence of hypotensive episodes is increased if the patient taking antihypertensives takes other drugs that also cause hypotension, including diuretics, CNS depressants, barbiturates, antihistamines, or alcohol.

➤ Monitor the daily weight of the hospitalized patient. Weigh the patient under standard conditions (same time, same scales, same amount of clothing). Observe for signs of fluid retention such as pitting edema (edema characterized by indentations that remain in the skin for seconds to minutes after pressure has been applied by the examiner's finger); dependent edema; and tight rings, shoes, and clothing. Auscultate the lungs to detect pulmonary rales. If possible, instruct the patient to monitor and record his or her weight at home. Report to the physician a weight gain in excess of 2 lb/day or 5 lb/wk. Record intake and output in the hospitalized patient. Refer the patient to a dietitian or teach the patient about dietary sodium (see Dietary Considerations box earlier in chapter).

➤ When a patient is taking a combination product containing two or more drugs, teach about each drug in the product and assess for side effects for each drug. For example, Apresazide contains hydralazine and hydrochlorothiazide; the drug Ser-Ap-Es contains hydralazine, hydrochlorothiazide, and reserpine.

➤ If a dose is missed, instruct the patient to take the dose as soon as it is remembered, unless within 2 hours of the next dose, and then to resume the usual dosing schedule. Emphasize that the patient should not double up for missed doses.

➤ Caution the patient to avoid driving or operating hazardous equipment if sedation or sleepiness occurs. Review the box in Chapter 23 on measures to help patients with dry mouth.

Intravenous Antihypertensive Therapy

➤ Monitor the patient's blood pressure and pulse every 3 to 5 minutes until stable, then every 15 to 30 minutes. Use an electronic infusion monitor and/or a microdrip infusion set to titrate the drug dosage more accurately. Monitor the electrocardiogram. Ensure that the patient remains in bed for up to 3 hours after drug administration. Keep the call bell within reach and the siderails up.

Beta-Blockers

Drug Administration

➤ See general guidelines for antihypertensives.

➤ Take the apical pulse for a full minute before administering a dose. If the pulse is less than 60 beats/min in an adult or less than 90 to 110 beats/min in a child, withhold the dose and notify the physician. Specific guidelines may vary with an individual patient or by physician preference. Monitor the blood pressure. Review the general guidelines. Monitor the general parameters of cardiovascular function, including intake, output, daily weight, and serum electrolyte. Because beta-blockers accumulate in the presence of renal failure, monitor the blood urea nitrogen levels. Treatment of overdose with beta-blockers is symptomatic.

➤ Bronchospasm occurs occasionally. Assess for signs of respiratory distress, auscultate lung sounds, and monitor respiratory rate.

➤ Assess the patient for signs of depression, including withdrawal, insomnia, anorexia, and lack of interest in personal appearance.

➤ If beta-blockers are being used for treatment of angina pectoris, see the Nursing Implications Summary in Chapter 15.

Intravenous atenolol

➤ May be given by direct IV push at a rate of 5 mg injected evenly over 5 minutes. May also be diluted in 10 to 50 ml of compatible solution and given as an infusion. Monitor blood pressure, pulse, and electrocardiogram.

Intravenous labetalol

➤ May be given by direct IV push at a rate of 20 mg or less over at least 2 minutes. May be further diluted to provide a constant infusion. For example, dilute 200 mg (40 ml) in 160 ml of diluent to form a concentration of 1 mg/ml. Compatible with most IV fluids, including D5W; NS; D5NS; D5 in 0.2%, 0.33%, or 0.45% NS; Ringer's injection; or lactated Ringer's injection. Use microdrip tubing and/or a volume- or rate-controlling device to titrate dosage precisely. Monitor blood pressure every 2 to 5 minutes until stable. During IV administration, keep the patient supine. After administration, monitor blood pressure every 15 to 30 minutes until stable; this may take up to 3 hours. There is Y-site incompatibility with cefoperazone, furosemide, nafcillin, and sodium bicarbonate. Mixing labetalol with other drugs in syringe or solution is not recommended.

Intravenous metoprolol

➤ May be given by direct IV push. Administer dose (5 mg) rapidly. May repeat every 2 minutes for a total of three doses. Monitor blood pressure, pulse, and electrocardiogram.

Intravenous propranolol

➤ Check dose carefully; IV dose is much smaller than oral dose. May be given undiluted or diluted in 5% dextrose

Continued

solution. Administer at a rate of 1 mg/min or more slowly. May also be diluted in 50 ml of NS for infusion. Monitor blood pressure, pulse, and electrocardiogram.

Nursing in the Community

➤ Emphasize the importance of taking these drugs as prescribed for optimal benefit. Caution the patient not to discontinue these drugs without consulting the physician and not to let prescriptions run out. Stress that several weeks of therapy may be needed to gain maximum effects. Orthostatic hypotension may be a problem (review the Patient Problems box). Because chest pain from exercises or exertion may be reduced by beta-blockers, patients may overdo physical activity. Caution patients to discuss the limits of exercise with their physician.

➤ Instruct the patient to take oral doses with meals or snacks to reduce gastric irritation. Instruct the patient to swallow extended-release forms whole without chewing, crushing, or breaking (unless the tablet is scored). Instruct the patient taking concentrated oral propranolol to measure the dose with the calibrated dropper provided, then to mix the dose with a small amount of liquid or food such as water, juice, soda, applesauce, or pudding. Tell the patient to take the dose immediately after preparing it and to eat all the mixture to ensure that the whole dose is consumed.

➤ Emphasize the following points to the patient. For missed doses of atenolol, betaxolol, bisoprolol, carteolol, labetalol, nadolol, penbutolol, sotalol, or extended-release metoprolol, oxprenolol, or propranolol: Take when remembered unless within 8 hours of next scheduled dose, then omit. For missed doses of other beta-blockers: Take when remembered unless within 4 hours of next scheduled dose, then omit. Do not double up for missed doses. Wear a medical identification tag or bracelet.

➤ Many side effects can occur with beta-blockers. Tell the patient to report any unexpected sign or symptom to the physician. Teach the patient to report signs of thrombocytopenia (unexplained bruising or bleeding) or of leukopenia (unexplained fever or sore throat). Teach diabetic patients that beta-blockers may mask the symptoms of hypoglycemia; these patients should monitor blood glucose levels carefully during periods of dosage adjustment or when starting or stopping the drug.

➤ Tell the patient that if drowsiness occurs, driving or operating hazardous equipment should be avoided until this effect wears off. Instruct the patient to notify the physician if drowsiness is severe or persistent.

➤ Pregnant and breast-feeding women should talk with their physicians before using beta-blocking drugs.

➤ Instruct patients to avoid allergy shots or allergy skin testing while using beta-blockers until discussing this with the physician.

Alpha₁-Blockers: doxasin, prazosin, and terazosin
Drug Administration/Nursing in the Community
➤ See general guidelines for antihypertensives.

➤ A "first-dose" reaction may occur within 30 to 90 minutes after the initial dose has been administered. Monitor blood pressure; anticipate that orthostatic hypotension and/or fainting may occur. Supervise the patient closely during the first 2 hours after the first dose. A first-dose reaction is more common in older adults or volume-depleted or sodium-restricted patients. It also may occur if the dosage is increased. To help minimize this reaction, the first dose is often limited to 1 mg; also the first dose can be given at bedtime, if possible.

➤ Nasal congestion or runny nose may be a problem. Inform the patient that this side effect may decrease with continued use of the prescribed drug. Caution the patient to avoid the use of over-the-counter medications to self-treat this annoying side effect.

➤ Caution the patient to avoid driving or operating hazardous equipment until the effects of these medications are known. Blurred vision, dizziness, and lethargy may be common.

➤ Before discharge, teach the patient how to monitor for fluid retention. If diuretics are also prescribed, explain the importance of taking all drugs as ordered for maximum effects.

➤ These drugs are especially prone to cause orthostatic hypotension, particularly when therapy is started and during periods of increasing dosage. See the Patient Problems box for a discussion of orthostatic hypotension. Instruct the patient to take the first dose and any increased doses at bedtime and to be especially careful when getting up at night during the first few days of therapy. Warn the family members about this side effect so that they will not be frightened and will know that they should make the patient lie down until he or she is no longer dizzy.

➤ When these drugs are used to treat benign prostatic hypertrophy, teach the patient that 2 to 6 weeks of therapy may be needed before symptoms improve. Point out that these drugs will treat symptoms associated with prostatic enlargement but will not shrink the prostate; surgery may still be needed in the future.

Alpha₁-, Alpha₂-Blockers: phenoxybenzamine and phentolamine
Drug Administration
Intravenous phentolamine
➤ Dilute 5 mg with 1 ml of sterile water; may be further diluted. Administer at a rate of 5 mg or less over 1 minute. Monitor blood pressure and pulse every 30 seconds, and monitor electrocardiogram. Do not leave the patient unattended until stable. Treat overdose with dopamine; do not use epinephrine.

➤ When the drug is used to treat extravasation, 5 to 10 mg of phentolamine is diluted in 10 ml of sodium chloride injection, and the area of extravasation is infiltrated with this solution with a small-bore needle. There may be other protocols in different agencies. Phentolamine may also be added to infusions of norepinephrine to prevent damage from extravasation.

Nursing Implications Summary—cont'd

Nursing in the Community

➤ See general guidelines for antihypertensives.

➤ Nasal congestion may be a problem. Inform the patient that this side effect may decrease with continued use of the prescribed drug. Caution the patient to avoid the use of over-the-counter medications to self-treat this annoying side effect.

➤ Tachycardia may be a problem. Teach the patient to take and record his or her resting pulse; increases of 20 beats/min or more above normal should be reported to the physician. Orthostatic hypotension may develop (see Patient Problems box).

➤ Phenoxybenzamine may cause dry mouth (see Patient Problems box in Chapter 23). Caution the patient to avoid driving or operating hazardous equipment if drowsiness, confusion, or unusual tiredness develop. Phenoxybenzamine may also cause sexual dysfunction. Question the patient tactfully about sexual problems; many patients are reluctant to discuss sexual difficulties. Sexual problems may prompt the patient to discontinue the medication. Provide emotional support as needed. Remind the patient not to discontinue the medication without notifying the physician.

➤ Intracavernosal injection of phentolamine and/or papaverine is discussed in the Nursing Implications Summary of Chapter 15.

Sympatholytic Drugs: guanethidine and guanadrel
Drug Administration/Nursing in the Community

➤ See general guidelines for antihypertensives.

➤ Diarrhea may be severe (see Chapter 24). The drugs may cause hypoglycemia. Instruct the diabetic patient to monitor blood glucose levels closely during the start of therapy and periods of dosage adjustment. Dry mouth may occur (see Patient Problems box in Chapter 23). Nasal congestion may be a problem. Caution the patient to avoid treatment with over-the-counter products without consulting the physician.

reserpine and Related Drugs
Drug Administration/Nursing in the Community

➤ See general guidelines for antihypertensives.

➤ Serious mental depression is a side effect. Assess the patient carefully for changes in mood or affect, anorexia, insomnia, impotence, withdrawal, and mood swings. Instruct the family to report the development of any change in the patient's personality.

➤ Instruct patient to take doses with meals or a snack to reduce gastric irritation.

➤ Monitor the patient's pulse. Tell the patient to notify the physician if noticeable changes in heart rate occur. Explain that several weeks of therapy may be necessary to see the full drug benefit.

➤ Nasal stuffiness may occur. Remind patients not to use over-the-counter medications without first checking with the physician. Dry mouth may also occur; see the Patient Problems box in Chapter 23 on dry mouth.

Vasodilators for Treating Chronic Hypertension: ACE Inhibitors
Drug Administration

➤ Monitor serum potassium levels.

Intravenous enalaprilat

➤ Check the dose; a single IV dose is much smaller than the oral dose. May be given undiluted; or dilute with up to 50 ml of a compatible IV solution (see manufacturer's guidelines). Administer the dose over at least 5 minutes. Monitor blood pressure and pulse. Keep the patient supine until the blood pressure is stable.

Nursing in the Community

➤ See general guidelines for antihypertensives.

➤ Caution the patient to avoid excessive amounts of foods high in potassium (see the Dietary Considerations box in Chapter 14 on potassium). Teach the patient to avoid salt substitutes unless approved by the physician because these often contain large amounts of potassium.

➤ Tell the patient to take captopril on an empty stomach, 1 hour before meals, unless instructed otherwise by the physician. Other ACE inhibitors may be taken on a full or empty stomach. If a dose is missed, it should be taken as soon as remembered, unless close to the time for the next dose. Tell the patient not to double up for missed doses. Instruct the patient to report the development of fever, sore throat, or signs of infection. Caution the patient to avoid driving or operating hazardous equipment if dizziness develops; instruct the patient to consult the physician if dizziness is severe.

➤ Caution the female patient taking an ACE inhibitor to notify the physician immediately if she becomes pregnant. These drugs may also pass into breast milk.

Angiotensin Receptor Blockers: irbesartan, losartan, and valsartan
Drug Administration/Nursing in the Community

➤ Instruct patient to take doses with or without food.

➤ Caution patient to avoid dehydration, which may aggravate hypotension, and to avoid alcohol for the same reason.

Calcium Channel Blockers

➤ See Nursing Implications Summary in Chapter 15.

hydralazine
Drug Administration

➤ Hydralazine may be administered intramuscularly or intravenously (direct IV). It is recommended that it not be mixed with infusion fluids. Administer intravenously at a rate of 10 mg over 1 minute.

Nursing in the Community

➤ See general guidelines for antihypertensives.

➤ Diarrhea may occur (see Chapter 24). Teach the patient to monitor weight and to assess for fluid retention. Tell the patient to notify the physician if lupuslike symptoms develop: blisters on the skin or rash, malaise, weakness, muscle pain, joint pain, sore throat, fever.

Continued

Nursing Implications Summary—cont'd

➤ Instruct the patient to report the development of tingling of fingers or numbness because this sensation may signal peripheral neuropathy; pyridoxine may be prescribed. Instruct the patient to take oral doses with food or a snack to reduce gastric irritation. Tell the patient to avoid driving or operating hazardous equipment if dizziness develops.

minoxidil
Nursing in the Community
➤ See general guidelines for antihypertensives.
➤ This drug may cause hypertrichosis (excessive hairiness) after several weeks of therapy. Instruct the patient to report this side effect. The hair can be shaved, bleached, or removed, depending on the location and severity. Caution the patient not to discontinue the medication without contacting the physician. The excessive hair growth may slowly disappear after several months of therapy.
➤ The side effect of hypertrichosis led to the development of topical minoxidil (Rogaine), used to stimulate hair growth in men who are balding. Instruct the patient to follow the instructions supplied by the manufacturer. Wash hair daily before applying solution, and dry scalp and hair thoroughly. Apply the prescribed amount, with the applicator supplied. Wash hands to remove any solution left on the hands. Do not use a hair dryer to dry the scalp after drug application. If topical minoxidil is used at night, wait at least 30 minutes after applying solution before going to bed. If a dose is missed, the patient should apply it as soon as it is remembered, unless it is close to the time for the next dose; the patient should not double up for missed doses. Tell the patient to report local side effects (e.g., itching, scalp burning, skin irritation) or systemic effects (e.g., dizziness, flushing, headache, tingling of hands or feet, weight gain).
➤ Instruct the patient to report the development of shortness of breath, increased heart rate, or changes in heart rhythm. Teach the patient to monitor resting pulse and to report increases of 20 beats/min or more above normal to the physician. Assess for distended jugular veins and pulmonary rales.

Centrally Acting Antihypertensive Drugs: clonidine, guanabenz, and guanfacine
Drug Administration/Nursing in the Community
➤ See general guidelines for antihypertensives.
➤ Dry mouth may occur (see the Patient Problems box in Chapter 23). Constipation may occur (see the Patient Problems box in Chapter 24). Caution the patient to avoid driving or operating hazardous equipment if drowsiness occurs.
➤ Emphasize to the patient the importance of not discontinuing these drugs abruptly. Teach the patient to have prescriptions refilled before the supply on hand runs out. Patients who may not comply with dosage schedules should not take these drugs. See discussion of withdrawal symptoms in text. If an oral dose is missed, instruct the patient to take it as soon as it is remembered, unless within 2 hours of the next dose. Teach

the patient not to double up for missed doses. If two or more doses are missed, the patient should notify the physician.
➤ Clonidine is available in a transdermal form. Review the instruction leaflet provided by manufacturer with the patient. Emphasize the following points. Do not cut or trim the patch. Remove the old patch. Apply the new patch to clean hairless area, but avoid areas of skin irritation or scars. Rotate sites. If the patch becomes loose or falls off, replace it with a fresh one; if it is only slightly loose, cover it with an adhesive overlay provided by the manufacturer. Replace the patch weekly. If a patch is overdue for replacement by 3 days or more, notify the physician; do not apply two patches at once. To discard the patch, fold it in half, sticky sides together. Discard the patch out of reach of children.

methyldopa
Drug Administration/Nursing in the Community
➤ See general guidelines for antihypertensives.
➤ Dry mouth may occur (see the Patient Problems box in Chapter 23). Diarrhea may occur. Depression is a side effect. Assess the patient carefully for changes in mood or affect; assess for anorexia, insomnia, impotence, withdrawal, and mood swings. Instruct the family to report the development of any change in the patient's personality.
➤ Nasal congestion may be a problem. Caution the patient to avoid treatment with over-the-counter products without consulting the physician.
➤ Methyldopa may alter liver function tests. Teach the patient to report the development of malaise, fever, right upper quadrant abdominal pain, or any change in the color or consistency of stools. Monitor liver function tests. Tell the patient that urine may darken if exposed to the air.
➤ The IV form is methyldopate hydrochloride. Dilute the dose in 100 to 200 ml of 5% dextrose in water. Administer dose as an infusion over 30 to 60 minutes. Avoid intramuscular or subcutaneous administration.

Drugs Used in Hypertensive Emergencies
Drug Administration
➤ Drug dosage may be titrated to the patient's blood pressure. Use microdrip tubing or an infusion monitor to regulate infusion. Do not leave the patient unattended until stable. Keep siderails up. Ideally the patient should be in an intensive care unit. Monitor electrocardiogram, blood pressure, pulse, respirations, acid-base balance, oxygenation via pulse oximetry, level of consciousness, intake, and output; it may be necessary to insert a Foley catheter. Do not mix these drugs with other drugs in an infusion or a syringe. Keep the patient and family informed of the patient's condition.

Intravenous diazoxide
➤ Administer dose quickly, undiluted (e.g., 150 mg over 10 to 30 seconds). Other regimens may be ordered. Because diazoxide is highly alkaline, avoid intramuscular or subcutaneous injection. Make certain that the IV line is patent

Nursing Implications Summary—cont'd

before administering, and inspect the insertion site for irritation or redness. If extravasation occurs, apply ice packs. Treat drug overdose or severe hypotension with dopamine. Monitor the patient's blood glucose level because the diazoxide may cause hyperglycemia; insulin may be necessary.

Intravenous nitroglycerin

➤ Before administration nitroglycerin injection must be diluted in D5W or 0.9% sodium chloride injection. Mix well. Use glass solution bottles and non-PVC infusion sets. See manufacturer's dilution instructions. Nitroglycerin is also available in premixed volumes and concentrations. Do not use filters. Use microdrip tubing or an infusion monitor to help regulate the dosage precisely. Monitor heart rate and blood pressure continuously.

Intravenous sodium nitroprusside

➤ Dilute as directed by the manufacturer. Do not use an IV filter. Do not use if highly discolored; may be used if faintly brownish in color. Cover prepared infusion with sleeve provided by manufacturer or aluminum foil to protect from light. It is not necessary to cover the drip chamber or the tubing. Titrate dosage based on physician guidelines and patient response; a typical dose is 3 g/kg of body weight per minutes (adults) or 1.4 g/kg/min (small children). Use microdrip tubing and an infusion pump, preferably a volumetric pump. Monitor blood pressure continuously. Monitor serum cyanide and thiocyanate concentrations with prolonged use.

➤ To treat overdose, discontinue nitroprusside and use cyanide antidote kit. Administer amyl nitrate (see Chapter 9) for 15 to 30 seconds every minute until a sodium nitrite solution for IV administration can be prepared. Administer a 3% sodium nitrite solution in a dose of 4 to 6 mg/kg over 2 to 4 minutes. After this solution has been administered, inject sodium thiosulfate intravenously, 150 to 200 mg/kg. Monitor the patient carefully. Signs of overdose can reappear for up to several hours, and sodium nitrite and sodium thiosulfate can be repeated at half the dose listed. Monitor thiocyanate levels if the drug is used longer than 72 hours. Use dopamine to correct hypotension.

Intravenous trimethaphan

➤ Dilute a 500-mg ampule in 500 ml D5W to produce a concentration of 1 mg trimethaphan per milliliter. Titrate the dosage based on physician guidelines and patient response; a typical initial dose is 0.5 to 1.0 mg/min. Use microdrip tubing and an infusion control device. Monitor the patient's response closely. If blood pressure does not drop with the patient in the supine position, try raising the head of the bed. Monitor the patient closely for signs of cerebral anoxia; note that the drug produces pupillary dilation, so this objective sign may be of little significance. To treat severe hypotension, use phenylephrine or try dopamine.

CHAPTER REVIEW

Application

1. Describe the renal mechanisms that control blood pressure.
2. Describe the cardiovascular mechanisms that control blood pressure.
3. Name the beta-blockers that the nurse might see used as antihypertensive drugs. How does blockade of the beta-receptors lower blood pressure? What are the side effects of these drugs? What are cardioselective beta-blockers? List three cardioselective beta-blockers.
4. How does the action of phenoxybenzamine differ from that of phentolamine?
5. How does the use of prazosin differ from that of phentolamine?
6. List which antihypertensives act by interfering with storage and/or release of norepinephrine.
7. List which antihypertensives act centrally to inhibit sympathetic activity.
8. How do ACE inhibitors work? What are their limiting side effects?
9. How do calcium channel blockers decrease hypertension?

10. List those antihypertensives used in the chronic treatment of hypertension that are direct-acting vasodilators.
11. Which drug is both an alpha- and a beta-adrenergic antagonist?
12. List three drugs used to control a hypertensive emergency. Specify the mechanism of action for each drug.
13. What is orthostatic hypotension? Which antihypertensive drugs are commonly associated with orthostatic hypotension as a side effect?
14. Which antihypertensive is associated with the synthesis of a false transmitter?
15. Describe reflex tachycardia. Which antihypertensive drugs does the nurse anticipate to cause reflex tachycardia?

Critical Thinking

1. Lifestyle modifications that may help lower blood pressure are described in this chapter. Describe at least five specific interventions a patient can use to help stop smoking.
2. For what situations might the nurse see phentolamine used as an antihypertensive drug? What is the mechanism of action?

Continued

3. Develop a teaching plan for a patient taking an ACE inhibitor.
4. Develop a teaching plan for a patient taking a calcium channel blocker.
5. What is a limiting side effect of reserpine? How can the nurse assess the patient for this side effect?
6. What education can the nurse provide about orthostatic hypotension as a side effect of antihypertensive drugs?
7. What reaction may occur with the sudden discontinuation of clonidine? What counsel can the nurse give?
8. Why is patient compliance with antihypertensive therapy often poor? What actions can the nurse take to increase compliance?

References

Chase S: Pharmacology in practice: antihypertensives . . . overview, *RN* 60(6):33-40, 1997.

Davis L, Stecy P: Pharmacologic management of cardiovascular problems in women, *J Nurse Midwife* 42(3):176-185, 1997.

Eaton LE, Buck EA, Catanzaro JE: The nurse's role in facilitating compliance in clients with hypertension. *Medsurg Nurs* 5(5):339-345, 359, 1996.

Joint National Committee on Prevention, Detection, Evaluation, and Treatment of High Blood Pressure. *Arch Intern Med* 157(21):2413-2446, 1997.

Kuncl N, Nelson KM: Antihypertensive drugs, *Nursing* 27(8):46-49, 1997.

Sadowski AV, Redeker NS: The hypertensive elder: a review for the primary care provider, *Nurse Pract* 21(5):99-100, 102, 105-12 passim, 1996.

Thomas SA, DeKeyser F: Blood pressure, *Annu Rev Nurs Res* 14:3-22, 1996.

Wood MH: Current considerations in patients with coexistent diabetes and hypertension, *Nurse Pract* 21(4):19-20, 27-28, 30-31, 1996.

Chapter

14

Diuretics

OBJECTIVES

After studying this chapter, you should be able to do the following:

- *Explain why increasing sodium excretion is a desirable action of diuretics.*
- *Identify the class of diuretics with the highest potency.*
- *Name the loop diuretics.*
- *Name conditions for which loop diuretics or thiazide diuretics are used.*
- *Develop a nursing care plan for a patient receiving a loop diuretic, thiazide diuretic, potassium-sparing diuretic, carbonic anhydrase inhibitor, or osmotic diuretic or a combination of two diuretics.*

CHAPTER OVERVIEW

Diuretics are drugs that increase urine flow. There are several mechanisms by which drugs can produce this effect, but the clinically important drugs of this class act on the kidneys. This chapter reviews pertinent renal physiology and discusses the mechanism of action and clinical properties of diuretic drugs.

THERAPEUTIC RATIONALE: MODIFYING SALT AND WATER EXCRETION

The kidneys regulate water and electrolyte balance in the body so that the extracellular fluid volume may be held constant, a function that can influence blood pressure and the action of several organs. **Diuretics** act at various renal sites to modify salt and water excretion. The mechanisms by which these drugs act can be understood by first recalling normal renal function and then considering how diuretics alter the normal processes.

The Function of Nephrons

Urine is produced by the thousands of **nephrons** that comprise the kidneys (Figure 14-1). Glomerular filtration is the first step in forming urine. Blood contacts a filtering surface in the glomerulus, where water and small molecules pass freely into the tubule, leaving behind most proteins and protein-bound small molecules. The rest of the nephron adjusts the salt and water content of tubular

fluid to achieve **homeostasis,** a balanced condition in which the body retains the salt and water required for proper function and eliminates the excess. To understand diuretic drugs, six ions or molecules must be considered: sodium (Na^+), chloride (Cl^-), potassium (K^+), water, bicarbonate (HCO_3^-), and organic ions.

Renal Transport Mechanisms

Membranes are composed of lipid, which water and water-soluble materials like ions do not easily pass through. Several specific renal mechanisms allow such transport and regulate it. The various transporters have been given names, based on their function. *Symporters* move two or three ions all in the same direction in a process called cotransport. For example, chloride ion might be cotransported with a sodium ion. *Antiporters* are exchangers, in that they move two ions in opposite directions. For example, a sodium ion might be taken into a cell in exchange for a hydrogen ion, which is pumped out. These transporters, along with adenosine triphosphatase (ATP)-dependent pumps such as Na^+-K^+-ATPase, are called

161

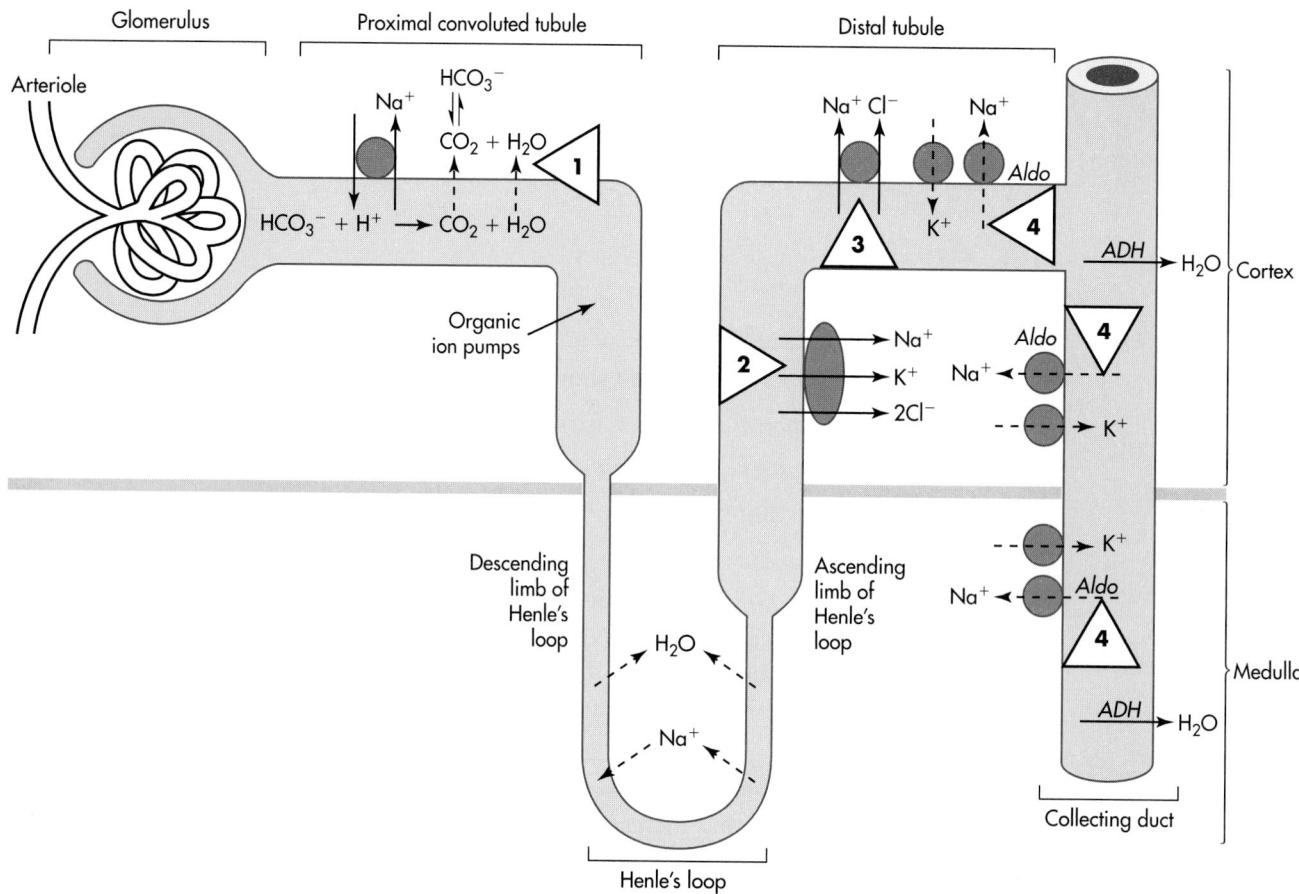

Figure 14-1 Sites of secretion and reabsorption of salt and water in nephron. Active (energy-requiring) processes are designated by solid arrows; passive transport is designated by broken arrows. Symporters, antiporters, and channels are shown as circles or ovals. The sites of major classes of diuretic agents are shown by the numbered triangles. *1*, carbonic anhydrase inhibitors; *2*, loop diuretics acting on the Na^+-K^+-$2Cl^-$ symporter; *3*, thiazide and thiazide-like drugs acting on the Na^+-Cl^- symporter; *4*, potassium-sparing diuretics acting on aldosterone-regulated sodium channels.

active transporters because they require cellular energy to drive them. With this energy these processes can cause an ion or molecule to move from an area of low concentration to an area of higher concentration, which is opposite to the movement that would be dictated by simple diffusion.

Passive transport includes not only simple diffusion but also processes that involve either channels or other carriers. These processes move ions or molecules from regions of higher concentration into areas of lower concentration, tending to lessen the concentration differences between the two sides of the membrane.

Sodium Ion Sites

Sodium ion freely enters tubular fluid from the glomerulus, so fluid entering the proximal convoluted tubule has the same sodium ion content as blood. The proximal convoluted tubule removes from the tubular fluid two thirds of the sodium ion that is presented to it. The pump mechanisms at this site include sodium symport with glucose, amino acids, or phosphate and sodium exchange with hydrogen ion. In

the ascending limb of Henle's loop, sodium ion is removed from tubular fluid by the Na^+-K^+-$2Cl^-$ symporter (see Figure 14-1). In the distal tubule, sodium ion is removed by a Na^+-Cl^- symporter and a Na^+-H^+ antiporter. At this point nearly 99% of the sodium that entered the tubular fluid from the glomerulus has been reabsorbed. Final adjustments to regulate sodium excretion occur in the collecting duct by way of sodium channels. Regulatory elements include the adrenal steroid aldosterone.

Chloride Ion Sites

Chloride ion is primarily removed from tubular fluid in the ascending limb of Henle's loop by the Na^+-K^+-$2Cl^-$ symporter (see Figure 14-1). Another important site is the Na^+-Cl^- symporter in the distal tubule.

Potassium Ion Sites

Potassium ion is not the primary ion involved in the action of any diuretic drug; diuretics are designed to alter sodium ion excretion patterns. Nevertheless, potassium

Table 14-1 Diuretic Effects on Tubular Transport of Ions

Drug	Excretion Increased				Excretion Blocked			
Loop diuretics	Na^+	K^+	Ca^+	Cl^-	Uric acid	Li^+	—	—
Thiazides and related drugs	Na^+	K^-	—	Cl^-	Uric acid	Li^+	Ca^+	—
Potassium-sparing diuretics	Na^+	—	Ca^+	—	Uric acid	Li^+	K^+, H^+	—
Carbonic anhydrase inhibitors	Na^+	K^-	Ca^+	—	Uric acid	—	—	Cl^-
Osmotic diuretics	$(Na^+)^*$	$(K^+)^*$	—	$(Cl^-)^*$	—	—	—	—

Li^+, Lithium ion; H^+, hydrogen ion.
*Large doses.
NOTE: The effects on ion transport shown are those commonly observed in humans during long-term therapy with normal clinical doses. With prolonged therapy, ions whose excretion is increased may become depleted from the body, whereas those whose excretion is blocked may accumulate. Lithium ion accumulation is clinically important only for those patients receiving lithium carbonate therapy for bipolar disorder. Uric acid accumulation is usually important only for those patients predisposed to gout.

excretion is altered by some of these agents, and the effects on some patients may be detrimental. Potassium ion is reabsorbed in the proximal tubule and ascending limb of Henle's loop. Secretion of potassium occurs in the distal tubule and collecting duct, where regulation of sodium ion secretion may secondarily affect potassium ion excretion (see Figure 14-1).

Water Sites

Water may be recovered from the tubule by diffusion in the proximal convoluted tubule and in the descending limb of Henle's loop. The ascending limb of Henle's loop is relatively impermeable to water. Final urine concentration is achieved primarily in the collecting duct. Removal of water at this site is regulated by antidiuretic hormone (ADH), which increases permeability of the tissue to water and thereby increases water retention.

Bicarbonate Sites

Bicarbonate, which is the main buffer in blood, freely enters tubular fluid from glomeruli and must be recovered for the body to maintain proper acid-base balance. Reabsorption of bicarbonate occurs in the proximal convoluted tubule and depends on the enzyme carbonic anhydrase. Carbonic anhydrase converts hydrogen ion and bicarbonate ion in tubular fluid to carbon dioxide and water. Carbon dioxide can freely pass into tubular epithelial cells and is reabsorbed, whereas bicarbonate ion stays in the tubule. The reabsorbed carbon dioxide is quickly reconverted to bicarbonate within renal cells and may reenter blood by way of a sodium-bicarbonate symporter.

Organic Ion Pumps

The kidneys rapidly secrete complex ions such as amino acids and other natural compounds. This secretion occurs in late portions of the proximal tubule. Many drugs, including several diuretics, enter tubular fluid by this mechanism, which is referred to as an organic anion pump. Because some diuretics work only from within the tubule, the action of the drug depends at least in part on the proper function of the organic ion pump.

Mechanism of Diuretic Action

The diuretics considered in this chapter achieve their effects mainly by increasing sodium ion excretion. Because water tends to follow sodium in the kidneys, it is excreted when sodium ion is excreted. The sites of action of the classes of diuretics are shown in Figure 14-1. Specific patterns of ion excretion produced by these drugs are summarized in Table 14-1, and mechanisms are discussed in detail in the following sections.

THERAPEUTIC AGENTS: DIURETICS

▼ Loop Diuretics: bumetanide, ethacrynic acid, furosemide, torsemide

Mechanism of Action

Bumetanide, ethacrynic acid, **furosemide,** and torsemide (Table 14-2) are called **loop diuretics** because the primary site of their diuretic action is in Henle's loop. These drugs inhibit the powerful Na^+-K^+-$2Cl^-$ symporter in the ascending limb of Henle's loop (see Figure 14-1). Therefore sodium chloride is retained in the tubule and excreted in urine, carrying water with it. The higher-than-normal delivery of sodium ion to the distal tubule and collecting duct promotes potassium and hydrogen ion excretion, which contributes nothing to the diuretic action but may produce serious side effects. Calcium ions are also excreted in higher-than-normal amounts in response to these drugs (see Table 14-1). At high dosages, furosemide may occasionally increase bicarbonate excretion, whereas other loop diuretics have little direct effect on such excretion.

Although all loop diuretics are similar in their mechanism of action, bumetanide is much more potent than other loop diuretics. For example, 1 mg of bumetanide given orally is as effective as approximately 40 mg of furosemide.

Pharmacokinetics

Loop diuretics are well absorbed from the gastrointestinal (GI) tract, producing a diuretic effect within 1 hour of administration. With intravenous (IV) doses, diuresis occurs within 5 to 10 minutes (see Table 14-2).

Table 14-2	**Loop Diuretics**				
Generic Name	Trade Name	Administration/Dosage	Diuretic Effect		
			Onset	Peak	Duration
bumetanide	Bumex	ORAL: *Adults*—0.5-2 mg each morning; if needed, a second dose may be given 4-5 hr later. Maximum daily dose: 10 mg. FDA pregnancy category C.	30-60 min	1-2 hr	4-6 hr
		INTRAVENOUS: *Adults*—0.5-1 mg for pulmonary edema; may repeat in 2 hr. Maximum daily dose: 10 mg.	5-10 min	15-30 min	3-4 hr
ethacrynic acid	Edecrin*	ORAL: *Adults*—50-100 mg initially; thereafter 50-200 mg daily. FDA pregnancy category B. *Children*—25 mg initially, increasing by 25 mg to maintain. Avoid in infants.	30 min	1-2 hr	6-8 hr
		INTRAVENEOUS: *Adults*—50 mg. Maximum daily dose: 100 mg. *Children*—1 mg/kg.	5-10 min	15-30 min	1-3 hr
furosemide	Lasix* Myrosemide Novosemide† Uritol†	ORAL: *Adults*—20-80 mg once or twice daily. Maximal daily dose: 600 mg. FDA pregnancy category C. *Children*—2 mg/kg initially, increasing by 1 or 2 mg/kg after 6-8 hr; maximum dose, 6 mg/kg.	20-60 min	1-2 hr	6-8 hr
		INTRAVENOUS: *Adults*—20-40 mg once or twice daily. *Children*—1 mg/kg initially, increasing by 1 mg/kg after 2 hr; maximum dose 6 mg/kg. Extend dosing interval in neonates.	5-10 min	15-30 min	1-3 hr
torsemide	Demadex	ORAL: *Adults*—5-20 mg once daily, adjusted as needed for therapeutic effect. Maximum daily dose: 200 mg, or 40 mg in hepatic cirrhosis. FDA pregnancy category B.	60 min	1-2 hr	6-8 hr
		INTRAVENOUS: *Adults*—5-20 mg once daily, adjusted as needed for therapeutic effect; not to exceed limits noted for oral.	5-10 min	1 hr	6-8 hr

*Available in Canada and the United States.
†Available in Canada only.

Ethacrynic acid should not be given by intramuscular (IM) or subcutaneous injection because the drug can cause severe pain and irritation at the injection site. Torsemide also is used parenterally only intravenously. Other loop diuretics can be given intramuscularly, but the IV route is preferred for parenteral administration.

Loop diuretics are bound to proteins in blood and in the protein-bound form are not available for glomerular filtration. These diuretics are secreted into tubules by the organic anion pump in the proximal tubule. Because diuresis is produced from within the tubule, the effectiveness of loop diuretics depends on their ability to enter tubules.

Excretion of loop diuretics is primarily renal, but some biotransformation to active and inactive products occurs. In moderate renal failure the half-life of torsemide is unchanged, but a relatively inactive metabolite accumulates.

Uses

Because loop diuretics promote the loss of excess salt and body water, they can control edematous states, such as those occurring in congestive heart failure, renal disease, and hepatic cirrhosis. Ethacrynic acid is also useful for lymphedema and ascites caused by malignancies or cirrhosis. Furosemide and torsemide are second-line drugs for hypertension. Bumetanide, ethacrynic acid, and furosemide can be used for hypercalcemia because these drugs promote calcium excretion.

Because loop diuretics cause rapid diuresis, rapid weight loss may occur as large volumes of fluid are lost, but this is not an accepted use of these agents (see Drug Abuse Alerts box).

Adverse Reactions and Contraindications

Electrolyte depletion, marked by weakness or lethargy, dizziness, leg cramps, anorexia, vomiting, and possibly mental confusion, may occur gradually. GI tract disturbances are also common with loop diuretics. Symptoms may include diarrhea, loss of appetite, and stomach pain or cramping. Ethacrynic acid causes GI tract disturbances more often than other loop diuretics, especially in patients receiving the drug continually for several months. A sudden, severe, watery diarrhea indicates that the drug should be withdrawn.

Orthostatic hypotension is common with these powerful diuretics. Patients who tend to rise quickly from a sitting or lying position must learn to move slowly to allow accommodation of blood pressure (see the box on p. 146). The most serious danger is risk of injury from falls.

Loop diuretics increase the loss of potassium and calcium ions, as well as sodium and chloride ions (see Table 14-1). Excessive potassium loss impairs proper functioning of the heart, skeletal muscle, kidneys, and other organs. Many physicians routinely prescribe a potassium replacement for their patients receiving loop diuretics for prolonged periods (see Dietary Considerations box). Loss of calcium may rarely

Diuretics

BACKGROUND

Diuretics may be abused by patients obsessed with weight loss. The acute weight loss produced by diuretics has been exploited by some diet clinics that may initiate the program with a diuretic so that dramatic weight loss will occur early; however, this weight loss is short-lived, and the earlier weight recurs with rehydration. Such acute weight loss is occasionally exploited in high school and college wrestling programs; the diuretics allow a wrestler to meet a weight limit at weigh-in, and the athlete usually attempts to rehydrate before wrestling. Diuretics may also be abused by patients, obsessed with excretory functions, who use the drugs to achieve large volumes of urine. Such patients, who may also abuse cathartics, often view this ritualistic drug taking as purification of the body.

PHARMACOLOGY

Diuretics promote an acute loss of body water and therefore cause an immediate drop in body weight. The amount of diuresis is related to the dose and strength of the drug used and also to the patient's water balance.

HEALTH HAZARDS

Long-term use of diuretics can cause severe electrolyte imbalances, especially if patients are not receiving careful counseling on dietary practices. If patients are receiving drugs from more than one physician or from unauthorized sources, follow-up care to monitor for the development of side effects may be lacking. The use of these drugs in weight control is unjustified, especially in healthy young athletes with no pre-existing edema.

DIETARY CONSIDERATIONS

Potassium Sources

Some drugs, especially the loop and thiazide diuretics, steroids, and amphotericin B, cause excessive loss of potassium, resulting in hypokalemia (low blood potassium levels). In mild cases hypokalemia may go unnoticed, but in severe cases it may contribute to toxicity from other drugs, as well as cardiac toxicity. Good dietary sources of potassium include the following:

■ Citrus fruits and juices
■ Bananas
■ Grape, cranberry, apple, pear, and apricot juices
■ Cereals
■ Leafy vegetables
■ Meat, fish, and fowl
■ Salt substitutes (read label)
■ Coffee, tea, and cola beverages
■ Nuts and peanut butter

Some sources of potassium may be contraindicated in persons who must also limit sodium intake. Licorice can cause potassium excretion and should be avoided by patients experiencing hypokalemia.

be sufficient to produce tetany. Most patients do not require calcium replacement, but serum calcium levels should be observed periodically. Uric acid excretion is partially blocked by loop diuretics. In susceptible patients gout may develop, but for most patients the increase in serum uric acid produces no symptoms.

Loop diuretics affect ion transport in several body organs other than the kidneys. Altered sodium and potassium transport may be associated with toxicity to certain cells in the inner ear. Transient or permanent deafness has been observed in patients receiving loop diuretics, especially those who receive high dosages or those who have reduced renal function in whom the drugs accumulate. Ototoxicity is more likely with ethacrynic acid than with other loop diuretics.

Loop diuretics impair glucose tolerance in some patients and rarely precipitate diabetes mellitus. Some patients experience sensitivity to sunlight while taking furosemide. Lupus erythematosus may be activated by ethacrynic acid and furosemide. Large doses of bumetanide may cause severe muscle pain (myalgia), chest pain, and premature ejaculation.

Loop diuretics should be used sparingly, if at all, in severe renal impairment. These drugs are less effective in anuric patients because the drugs fail to reach their site of action in the tubule. Loop diuretics also tend to accumulate in these patients, creating a greater risk of drug toxicity.

Toxicity

The loop diuretics are the most potent diuretics known. Their rapid, powerful action must be carefully monitored to avoid profound dehydration and salt depletion. Dehydration with reduction in blood volume can precipitate circulatory collapse. Vascular thromboses and emboli may be generated, especially in older adult patients (see Geriatric Considerations box).

Interactions

The potassium-depleting effect of loop diuretics makes these drugs dangerous for patients receiving digitalis. Lowered potassium content in tissues predisposes the heart to toxicity from cardiac glycosides, which may include fatal arrhythmias. Corticosteroids also deplete potassium and may add to the danger of electrolyte imbalance when given with loop diuretics.

Loop diuretics lower the renal clearance of lithium (see Table 14-1), a drug used to control manic cycles in manic-depressive psychosis. Under these conditions, lithium may accumulate and severe toxicity may occur. These drugs are ordinarily not given together.

Loop diuretics have an antihypertensive action that may be additive with that of other antihypertensive agents. Care

GERIATRIC CONSIDERATIONS

Diuretics

THE PROBLEM

Older adult patients are often more sensitive to the effects of diuretic drugs than are other adult patients. For example, loop diuretics and thiazides can cause excessive hypotension and severe electrolyte imbalances. Potassium-sparing diuretics more often cause hyperkalemia in older adults than in others.

SOLUTIONS

- Dosages of these drugs for older adults may be lower than for other adults.
- Blood pressure should be carefully monitored.
- Precautions should be taken against orthostatic hypotension.
- Electrolyte balance should be carefully monitored.
- Dietary counseling may be required to maintain potassium balance.

is required to prevent excessive hypotension when these drugs are used with antihypertensives.

The ototoxic effect of loop diuretics may be potentiated by aminoglycoside antibiotics (see Chapter 48), which are also ototoxic. This combination should be avoided because permanent deafness may result.

When given with loop diuretics, amphotericin B has the potential for increasing the risk of nephrotoxicity, ototoxicity, and hypokalemia.

Loop diuretics are strongly bound to serum proteins and may therefore displace other drugs from protein-binding sites. This action increases the concentration of the free, active form of the displaced drug. The anticoagulant warfarin is displaced in this way by loop diuretics. Higher concentrations of unbound warfarin produce greater anticoagulant effects and may produce toxicity.

Thiazide Diuretics

Mechanism of Action

Thiazide diuretics block sodium and chloride ion reabsorption in the distal tubule by inhibiting the Na^+-Cl^- symporter (see Figure 14-1). As a result potassium and hydrogen ion excretion is enhanced by thiazide diuretics, but this effect is not required for diuresis and is a mechanism that may lead to side effects. Thiazide diuretics also inhibit carbonic anhydrase in the proximal convoluted tubule, thereby elevating the excretion of bicarbonate ion and an additional increment of sodium ion. This effect is lost after a few days.

Pharmacokinetics

Thiazide diuretics are well absorbed from the GI tract and may take action in the kidney within 1 hour of ingestion. Peak diuretic action can occur from 2 to 6 hours after an oral

dose, depending on which thiazide preparation is used. Various preparations differ in timing and duration of diuretic effects (Table 14-3). In general, the longer-acting thiazide diuretics are highly bound to serum proteins. Their long duration of action is related to their slow elimination from these protein-binding sites.

Thiazide diuretics remain primarily in extracellular water in the body except for the drug concentrated in the kidneys. Thiazides are secreted into renal tubules by the organic anion pump. Most of the dose leaves the body by this route. Some drug is eliminated by the liver, which secretes these drugs into bile. Chlorothiazide may be administered intravenously. The onset of action is somewhat more rapid by this route, but the duration of effect is not greatly altered from that of oral doses. This preparation must never be administered intramuscularly or subcutaneously. Great care should be taken to prevent leakage of drug into tissues when it is given intravenously.

Uses

Thiazide diuretics are less potent than loop diuretics and are more suitable for use by outpatients. These drugs can control edema associated with heart or renal disease, as well as that caused by corticosteroid or estrogen therapy. The use of thiazide diuretics for hypertension is discussed in Chapter 13. **Hydrochlorothiazide** is one of the most widely used drugs of this class.

Adverse Reactions and Contraindications

Long-term use of thiazide diuretics can cause fluid and electrolyte imbalance, which may produce thirst, weakness, lethargy, restlessness, muscle cramps, and fatigue. The electrolyte imbalance most likely to occur is excessive potassium and chloride ion loss. The loss of these ions leads to metabolic alkalosis. Potassium supplements may be required to remedy this situation. Chloride loss alone is usually mild and does not require treatment.

Calcium excretion is blocked by thiazide diuretics, and increased serum calcium levels may result. The parathyroid glands may also be affected by long-term therapy with these diuretics. Uric acid excretion is also blocked, and the increased blood levels may precipitate an attack of gout in susceptible individuals.

Thiazide diuretics irritate the GI tract and may cause side effects ranging from simple nausea and vomiting to constipation, jaundice, and pancreatitis.

Thiazides may cause orthostatic hypotension. Chlorothiazide may lower the glomerular filtration rate when given intravenously. This action is not harmful to most patients, although patients with already reduced renal function may be adversely affected.

Thiazides are usually avoided in patients with severe impairment of renal function or anuria. Thiazides are less effective in these patients and may worsen renal function. Thiazides are also avoided in jaundiced infants because they

Table 14-3 Thiazide Diuretics and Agents with Similar Mechanisms

Generic Name	Trade Name	Administration/Dosage	Diuretic Effect		
			Onset	Peak	Duration
Thiazide Diuretics					
bendroflumethiazide	Naturetin*	ORAL: *Adults*—Initially, 2.5-20 mg once daily or divided dose; adjust dose by response. FDA pregnancy category C. *Children*—Maximum dosage 0.4 mg/kg/day in 1 or 2 doses; reduce dose for maintenance.	1-2 hr	4 hr	6-12 hr
benzthiazide	Exna	ORAL: *Adults*—25-100 mg once daily. FDA pregnancy category C. *Children*—0.9-3.9 mg/kg/day in 3 doses initially; dose reduced for maintenance.	2 hr	4-6 hr	12-18 hr
chlorothiazide	Diuril	ORAL: *Adults*—0.25-1 g once daily. FDA pregnancy category B. *Children*—10-20 mg/kg/day in 2 doses. *Infants <6 mo*—10-30 mg/kg/day in 2 doses.	2 hr	4 hr	6-12 hr
	Diuril (sodium)	INTRAVENOUS: *Adults*—500 mg twice daily.	15 min	30 min	6-12 hr
hydrochlorothiazide	Diuchlor-H† Esidrix HydroDiuril* Oretic Urozide†	ORAL: *Adults*—initially, 25-100 mg once daily or divided into 2 doses; maintenance, 25-100 mg/day. FDA pregnancy category B. *Children*—1-2 mg/kg/day in 2 doses. *Infants <6 mo*—Up to 3 mg/kg/day.	2 hr	4 hr	6-12 hr
hydroflumethiazide	Diucardin Saluron	ORAL: *Adults*—25-100 mg once daily or less frequently. FDA pregnancy category C. *Children*—1 mg/kg/day; adjust as needed for maintenance.	1-2 hr	3-4 hr	18-24 hr
methyclothiazide	Aquatensen Duretic† Enduron	ORAL: *Adults*—2.5-10 mg once daily FDA pregnancy category B. *Children*—0.05-0.2 mg/kg/day.	2 hr	6 hr	24 hr
polythiazide	Renese	ORAL: *Adults*—1-4 mg once daily or less frequently. *Children*—0.02-0.08 mg/kg/day.	2 hr	6 hr	36 hr
trichlormethiazide	Metahydrin Naqua Trichlorex	ORAL: *Adults*—1-4 mg once daily or less frequently. FDA pregnancy category C. *Children >6 mo*—0.07 mg/kg/day in single or divided dose.	2 hr	6 hr	24 hr
Nonthiazide Diuretics with Thiazide-Like Mechanisms					
chlorthalidone	Hygroton* Thalitone Uridon†	ORAL: *Adults*—25-100 mg after breakfast daily or less frequently. FDA pregnancy category B. *Children*—2 mg/kg once daily for 3 days/wk.	2 hr	2 hr	48-72 hr
indapamide	Lozide† Lozol	ORAL: *Adults*—2.5 mg/day; may be increased after few days to 5 mg/day. FDA pregnancy category B.	1-2 hr	2.3-3.5 hr	24-72 hr
metolazone	Mykrox Zaroxolyn*	ORAL: *Adults*—5-20 mg once daily for extended-release tablets. For prompt metolazone tablets (Mykrox), 0.5 mg once daily. FDA pregnancy category B.	1 hr	2 hr	12-24 hr
quinethazone	Hydromox	ORAL: *Adults*—50-200 mg once daily, or divided into 2 doses. Maximum daily dose: 200 mg.	2 hr	6 hr	18-24 hr

*Available in Canada and the United States.
†Available in Canada only.

may displace bilirubin from protein-binding sites, thereby increasing the risk of hyperbilirubinemia or kernicterus.

Toxicity

Thiazides affect the central nervous system (CNS). Mild symptoms include dizziness, headache, and paresthesia. At high concentrations, such as those found in drug overdose, mental lethargy may progress to coma, although heart function and respiration are not markedly depressed. Overdose requires stomach evacuation, with monitoring of electrolyte balance and renal function.

Interactions

The hypotensive activity of thiazide diuretics can potentiate the action of other antihypertensive agents, especially those that act at ganglionic or peripheral adrenergic sites (see Chapter 13). Thiazide diuretics are often included in fixed combinations that are marketed primarily as antihypertensives. Examples of these fixed combinations are shown in Table 14-4.

Thiazides cause loss of potassium, producing hypokalemia. Potassium loss is enhanced when thiazide diuretics are given with corticosteroids or adrenocorticotropic

Table 14-4   Fixed Combinations Including a Thiazide

Components	Trade Names	Use/Oral Adult Dose
Thiazide with ACE Inhibitor		
hydrochlorothiazide + captopril	Capozide	Antihypertensive; 1 tablet 2 or 3 times daily
hydrochlorothiazide + enalapril	Vaseretic	Antihypertensive; 1 tablet daily
hydrochlorothiazide + lisinopril	Prinzide, Zestoretic	Antihypertensive; 1 to 2 tablets once daily
Thiazide with Alpha-Blocker		
polythiazide + prazosin	Minizide	Antihypertensive; 1 capsule 2 or 3 times daily
Thiazide with Beta-Blocker		
bendroflumethiazide + nadolol	Corzide*	Antihypertensive; 1 tablet daily
chlorthalidone + atenolol	Tenoretic*	Antihypertensive; 1 or 2 tablets once daily
hydrochlorothiazide + bisoprolol	Ziac	Antihypertensive; 1 or 2 tablets once daily
hydrochlorothiazide + metoprolol	Lopressor HCT	Antihypertensive; 1 or 2 tablets daily
hydrochlorothiazide + pindolol	Viskazide†	Antihypertensive; 1 or 2 tablets once daily
hydrochlorothiazide + propranolol	Inderide LA	Antihypertensive; 1 capsule daily
hydrochlorothiazide + timolol	Timolide*	Antihypertensive; 1 tablet twice daily
Thiazide with Centrally Acting Antihypertensive		
chlorthalidone + clonidine	Combipres*	Antihypertensive; 1 to 2 tablets 2 to 4 times daily
chlorothiazide + methyldopa	Aldoclor, Supres†	Antihypertensive; 2 to 4 tablets daily
hydrochlorothiazide + methyldopa	Aldoril*, Dopazide†	Antihypertensive; 2 to 4 tablets daily
Thiazide with Potassium-Sparing Diuretics		
hydrochlorothiazide + amiloride	Moduretic, Moduret†	Diuretic or antihypertensive; 1 or 2 tablets daily
hydrochlorothiazide + spironolactone	Aldactazide*	Antihypertensive; 2 to 4 tablets daily Diuretic; 1 to 4 tablets daily
hydrochlorothiazide + triamterene	Dyazide†, Maxzide*	Diuretic or antihypertensive; 1 or 2 capsules or tablets daily
Thiazide with Rauwolfia		
chlorothiazide + reserpine	Diupres	Antihypertensive; 1 or 2 tablets 1 or 2 times daily
chlorthalidone + reserpine	Regroton	Antihypertensive; 1 to 2 tablets once daily
hydrochlorothiazide + deserpidine	Oreticyl	Antihypertensive; 1 tablet 2 times daily
hydrochlorothiazide + reserpine	Hydropres*, Mallopres	Antihypertensive; 1 tablet 1 to 4 times daily
methyclothiazide + deserpidine	Enduronyl, Dureticyl†	Antihypertensive; 1/2 to 1 tablet daily
methyclothiazide + reserpine	Diutensen-R	Antihypertensive; 1 to 4 tablets daily
polythiazide + reserpine	Renese-R	Antihypertensive; 1/2 to 2 tablets daily
trichlormethiazide + reserpine	Metatensin	Antihypertensive; 1 to 2 tablets daily
Thiazide with Vasodilator		
hydrochlorothiazide + hydralazine	Apresazide, Hydrazide	Antihypertensive; 1 capsule or tablet twice daily
Thiazide with Rauwolfia and Vasodilator		
hydrochlorothiazide + reserpine + hydralazine	Ser-Ap-Es*	Antihypertensive; 1 to 2 tablets 3 times daily

ACE, Angiotensin-converting enzyme.
*Available in Canada and the United States.
†Available in Canada only.

hormone (ACTH). Hypokalemia may make patients more sensitive to digitalis toxicity.

Thiazide diuretics often alter the requirement for insulin or other hypoglycemic agents. A diabetic patient who must receive one of the thiazides should be carefully observed during the first few days of thiazide therapy to prevent loss of diabetes control.

Lithium excretion is blocked by thiazides and other diuretics. The increased danger of lithium toxicity prevents the safe concurrent use of these drugs.

Cholestyramine and colestipol are solid resins used orally to treat hyperlipidemias (see Chapter 21). These agents can lower absorption of thiazide diuretics.

▼ Potassium-Sparing Diuretics: amiloride, spironolactone, and triamterene
Mechanism of Action

Potassium-sparing diuretics (Table 14-5) are rather weak diuretics that all reduce potassium loss in the kidneys, but two different mechanisms are involved. **Amiloride** and tri-

Table 14-5 Potassium-Sparing Diuretics

Generic Name	Trade Name	Administration/Dosage	Diuretic Effect		
			Onset	Peak	Duration
amiloride	Midamor*	ORAL: *Adults*—5-10 mg/day as a single dose. FDA pregnancy category B.	2 hr	6-10 hr	24 hr
spironolactone	Aldactone* Novospiroton†	ORAL: *Adults*—25-200 mg/day in divided doses. *Children*—1-3 mg/kg/day in divided doses.	Effects build over period of days		
triamterene	Dyrenium*	ORAL: *Adults*—25-100 mg/day; do not exceed 300 mg/day. FDA pregnancy category B. *Children*—2-4 mg/kg/day in divided doses.	2-4 hr (Maximal effect not seen for several days)		

*Available in Canada and the United States.
†Available in Canada only.

amterene inhibit sodium channels found in the distal tubule and collecting duct. The movement of sodium ion through these channels normally provokes excretion of potassium (see Figure 14-1). Inhibition of the sodium channels by amiloride and triamterene prevents this potassium loss and their action is relatively insensitive to the levels of aldosterone.

Spironolactone competitively blocks binding of the mineralocorticoid aldosterone to its intracellular receptor. Aldosterone bound to its receptor normally acts on the nucleus to induce proteins that activate sodium channels in the late distal tubule and collecting duct. Movement of sodium ion through these channels evokes excretion of potassium ions. By binding to the aldosterone receptor, spironolactone reduces sodium reabsorption and prevents potassium loss. Aldosterone is present in greater-than-normal amounts in edematous states resulting from congestive heart failure, nephrotic syndrome, and hepatic cirrhosis. Spironolactone is most effective when aldosterone is high.

Pharmacokinetics

Spironolactone, a steroid derivative, is not highly water soluble but is formulated using very fine particles to improve absorption from the GI tract. Peak therapeutic effects with spironolactone are observed several days after treatment begins (see Table 14-5). This delay is related to the mechanism of action of the drug and is not a result of delay in absorption or other pharmacokinetic properties of the drug. Spironolactone is extensively metabolized, much the same as the natural mineralocorticoids it chemically resembles. Metabolites of spironolactone appear in urine and in lesser quantities in bile.

Triamterene, although not a steroid like spironolactone, is also relatively insoluble in water. Intestinal absorption is somewhat variable but usually satisfactory. Elimination is by hepatic and renal mechanisms. The peak effect of triamterene is usually observed within a day.

Amiloride is more water soluble than triamterene or spironolactone and is excreted primarily renally. About 50%

of an oral dose is recovered unchanged in urine within 48 hours of administration.

Spironolactone is highly protein-bound in the blood, whereas triamterene is only moderately bound, and amiloride exists primarily as free drug.

Uses

Amiloride, spironolactone, and triamterene can be used to control edema in congestive heart failure, cirrhosis of the liver, and nephrotic syndrome. Spironolactone may lessen the effects of excessive aldosterone levels in patients with the endocrine disorder hyperaldosteronism. It may also be useful in treating hypertension and reversing potassium loss. Amiloride is also used in hypertension.

Adverse Reactions and Contraindications

Spironolactone, triamterene, and amiloride may cause dangerous increases in serum potassium levels. Patients with impaired renal function or high potassium intake are especially at risk. The earliest sign of hyperkalemia may be an irregular heartbeat. Fatal cardiac arrhythmias can occur.

Spironolactone can cause various endocrine alterations, since the drug chemically resembles not only mineralocorticoids but also androgens and progestins. Women may observe menstrual irregularities, hirsutism, and deepening of the voice. Men may observe gynecomastia (breast development) and have difficulty in achieving or maintaining erection. Symptoms in both sexes are usually reversed when the drug is discontinued.

Spironolactone produces tumors in rodents exposed to the drug for long periods; carcinomas have been reported in breasts of men and women taking this drug, but controlled trials have not been done to prove cause and effect. Nevertheless, the use of spironolactone should be restricted to cases in which the benefit clearly outweighs this risk. Spironolactone should not be used to control edema in pregnancy. If the drug is used by lactating women, breast-feeding should be discontinued because metabolites appear in breast milk.

CASE STUDY
Diuretics and Electrolyte Imbalance

Mr. Greene has been taking chlorothiazide (Diuril) for years as part of the treatment for mild congestive heart failure. But last month the physician changed his diuretic to spironolactone (Aldactone). Today he is in the office for a follow-up. His blood pressure is 130/88 mm Hg, and his weight is stable. He has trace edema on his lower extremities, and today complains of nausea and muscle weakness.

1. What is your main focus at this time for Mr. Greene? What additional assessments are needed?
2. Mr. Greene's serum potassium results indicate a level of 6.2 mEq/L. What, if any, treatment does this require?
3. Because of the change in diuretics, are there any dietary changes that are necessary for Mr. Greene?
4. Mr. Greene tells you that he does not cook his meals with salt, but does love to use a salt substitute with his meals. What do you need to tell him?

Triamterene and amiloride may produce a reversible azotemia revealed by an increased blood urea nitrogen (BUN) level. Triamterene has also been linked to blood dyscrasias and to photosensitivity. Skin rashes, GI tract disturbances (especially with spironolactone), dizziness, and fever have been observed in patients receiving potassium-sparing diuretics.

All potassium-sparing diuretics are contraindicated in patients with hyperkalemia.

Toxicity

Patients who overdose on potassium-sparing diuretics should have their stomachs evacuated. Electrolyte balance and renal function should be carefully monitored.

Interactions

Two potassium-sparing diuretics should not be administered concurrently, nor should these drugs be administered to a patient receiving potassium supplements or ingesting a diet high in potassium.

Use of potassium-sparing diuretics with antihypertensive agents may require reduction in doses of the latter drugs because spironolactone, triamterene, and amiloride may have additive antihypertensive effects with these agents. When spironolactone is combined with other diuretics, dosages may require reduction. Spironolactone can prevent distal tubular reabsorption of sodium, making diuretics that act upstream of this site in the nephron even more effective. Amiloride is less effective than spironolactone or triamterene when given in combination with hydrochlorothiazide.

Anticoagulant drugs are more potent when given with potassium-sparing diuretics, which may result in excessive anticoagulation and the risk of bleeding.

Lithium toxicity is increased by potassium-sparing diuretics because lithium excretion is blocked. Spironolactone increases the half-life of digoxin, leading to digoxin accumulation. Careful monitoring and dosage adjustment is required to keep digoxin blood levels in a safe range.

▼ Carbonic Anhydrase Inhibitors: acetazolamide, dichlorphenamide, and methazolamide

Mechanism of Action

Diuretics that inhibit renal **carbonic anhydrase** prevent secretion of hydrogen ion into tubular fluid and prevent reabsorption of carbon dioxide (Table 14-6). As a result, excretion of bicarbonate is rapidly increased and urine becomes alkaline. Carbonic anhydrase inhibitors have diuretic action because sodium ion accompanies the excreted bicarbonate. Bicarbonate excretion is much greater than sodium ion excretion, and these drugs are classified as weak diuretics. Moderate amounts of potassium and chloride ion are also lost in urine. When carbonic anhydrase inhibitors are given for long periods, metabolic acidosis may occur. Because metabolic acidosis prevents the diuretic action of these drugs, they are not suitable for long-term continuous administration as diuretics.

Pharmacokinetics

Carbonic anhydrase inhibitors are well absorbed from the GI tract. The most widely used drug of this class, **acetazolamide,** is concentrated in the kidneys, where tissue levels may be two to three times the plasma concentration within 30 minutes to 2 hours of an oral dose. Acetazolamide enters tubules by the organic anion pump. The drug also inhibits carbonic anhydrase in other tissues.

Acetazolamide is sometimes given on alternate days rather than continuously (see Table 14-6). This therapy is designed to prevent the kidneys from becoming resistant to the action of the drug (e.g., to prevent metabolic acidosis). During the day without the drug, acetazolamide is cleared from the body and renal function returns to its predrug condition. When the drug is readministered on the following day, it is as effective as when first given.

Uses

Carbonic anhydrase inhibitors are primarily used to treat glaucoma. In addition, acetazolamide is used for convulsive disorders and altitude sickness.

Adverse Reactions and Contraindications

Reactions to these drugs are uncommon, especially when they are used in intermittent or short-term therapy. Drug precipitation in urine has occurred, causing the formation of stones.

Carbonic anhydrase inhibitors act directly on the CNS, causing paresthesia, nervousness, sedation, lassitude, depression, headaches, vertigo, and other symptoms. Patients may complain of unusual tiredness or weakness. The conditions of patients already experiencing respiratory acidosis may

Table 14-6 Carbonic Anhydrase Inhibitors

Generic Name	Trade Name	Administration/Dosage	Clinical Effect		
			Onset	Peak	Duration
acetazolamide	Acetazolam† Diamox*	ORAL, INTRAVENOUS: *Adults*—250 mg 1-4 times daily; extended-release forms, 500 mg twice daily. FDA pregnancy category C. *Children*—4-30 mg/kg/day in divided doses.	About 1 hr (oral) IV: 2 min	2-4 hr (oral) IV: 15 min	6-12 hr (oral) IV: 4-5 hr
dichlorphenamide	Daranide	ORAL: *Adults*—initially 100-200 mg, then 100 mg every 12 hr until desired effect achieved; maintenance, 25-50 mg 1-3 times daily. FDA pregnancy category C.	0.5-1 hr	2-4 hr	6-12 hr
methazolamide	Neptazane*	ORAL: *Adults*—50-100 mg 2 or 3 times daily. FDA pregnancy category C.	2-4 hr	6-8 hr	10-18 hr

*Available in Canada and the United States.
†Available in Canada only.

worsen from these drugs, which tend to produce metabolic acidosis.

Carbonic anhydrase inhibitors cause a range of GI tract symptoms, including diarrhea, loss of appetite, nausea, vomiting, metallic taste, and weight loss.

Carbonic anhydrase inhibitors are usually avoided in patients at risk for electrolyte disturbances (e.g., adrenocortical insufficiency, hypokalemia, acidosis, hepatic disease, renal failure).

Toxicity

Renal function and acid-base balance must be carefully monitored in patients who have excessively high blood levels of carbonic anhydrase inhibitors.

Interactions

Carbonic anhydrase inhibitors produce more marked potassium excretion than sodium excretion. Potassium depletion is therefore likely to occur. This possibility is made even more likely by combining carbonic anhydrase inhibitors with corticosteroids or ACTH. Digitalis toxicity is increased in the presence of low serum potassium levels.

Excretion of amphetamines, anticholinergics, mecamylamine, and quinidine is slowed because carbonic anhydrase inhibitors alkalinize urine. Alkaline urine also blocks the effects of methenamine, which requires an acidic environment to be converted to formaldehyde, the active metabolite.

Osmotic Diuretics: mannitol and urea

Osmotic diuretics are nonelectrolytes that are filtered by the glomerulus but not significantly reabsorbed or metabolized. The high osmolality in tubules caused by the presence of these agents reduces reabsorption of water, which increases the production of urine. With a high urine output, sodium excretion is somewhat increased, with smaller increases in potassium, calcium, chloride, and bicarbonate excretion.

Osmotic diuresis may be used clinically to prevent permanent damage during acute renal failure. The usefulness of osmotic diuresis in these cases often depends on maintaining adequate urine volume without altering electrolyte balance. Osmotic diuretics also increase the osmolality of plasma, which allows reduction of osmotic pressure inside the eye and in cerebrospinal fluid.

The agents currently used as osmotic diuretics, mannitol and urea, are usually administered intravenously. Mannitol is the preferred agent.

Toxicity produced by these agents depends on how much drug is administered and how much the drug affects fluid balance. These drugs are retained within the extracellular space and can cause an acute expansion of extracellular fluid volume during IV administration. This volume expansion may be hazardous to a patient with reduced cardiac reserve.

Fluid and electrolyte imbalances may develop, especially if a degree of renal impairment exists. Under these circumstances the diuretics tend to accumulate in blood and may cause dangerous shifts in salt and water balance.

Pulmonary congestion, acidosis, thirst, blurred vision, convulsion, nausea and vomiting, diarrhea, tachycardia, fever, and angina-like pain may be noted occasionally. Local irritation with thrombophlebitis can also occur. Urea should not be used in patients with liver failure because the high levels of urea may place additional demands on liver function.

Nursing Process Overview

Diuretics

Assessment

Perform a total patient assessment, focusing on the presenting signs and symptoms and appropriate laboratory and other objective data that would help further define the nature of the patient's condition. Assess the patient's intake, output, weight, and blood pressure, and observe for signs of electrolyte imbalance, fluid retention, or dehydration.

Nursing Diagnoses

- Fluid volume deficit related to furosemide therapy as manifested by excessive urine output, decreased skin turgor, and orthostatic hypotension
- Potential complication: hypokalemia, or with potassium-sparing diuretics, hyperkalemia
- Risk for sleep pattern disturbance related to nocturia secondary to diuretic therapy

Patient Outcomes

The patient will have diuresis without drug-related side effects. The nurse will manage and minimize episodes of electrolyte imbalances. The patient will have drug dosage and dosing schedule adjusted to minimize sleep disturbance.

Planning/Implementation

Determine what actions are required to aid drug therapy. For example, dietary and fluid restrictions may be required to speed fluid removal and to prevent reaccumulation. Monitor fluid intake and output, serum electrolyte levels, BUN level, uric acid level, body weight, and blood pressure, and observe for the appearance of new signs or symptoms. Watch for side effects such as ototoxicity with ethacrynic acid.

Evaluation

Diuretic therapy is effective if excess fluid is lost and blood pressure is maintained and if abnormalities in electrolyte status or side effects do not result. For some patients, it is necessary to tolerate minor side effects to achieve required diuresis. Potassium depletion may be treated with potassium supplements. Teach the patient why the medication is necessary, what the major possible side effects are, and what symptoms should be reported to the physician. Discuss why additional medications such as potassium supplements may be needed. Teach selected patients to record daily weight, fluid intake and output, and blood pressure. If the physician has prescribed a restricted diet, verify that the patient understands how to choose menus within the limits of the diet plan. Be aware of the potential for abuse with these compounds (see Drug Abuse Alerts box).

Nursing Implications Summary

General Guidelines: Diuretics

➤ Carefully measure and record fluid intake and output. Report unexpected findings to the physician. For example, oliguria (scanty urine output) or anuria (no urine output) are unexpected after an increase in a diuretic dose. Patients who are at home are not usually required to measure intake and output, except in the case of severe kidney or heart disease, but encourage the patient to report abnormal output.

➤ Weigh the patient in the short-term care setting daily. Weigh the patient under standard conditions (e.g., at the same time [usually in the morning], after the patient has voided or the catheter bag has been emptied, but before breakfast). Use the same scale each day, and have the patient wear the same amount of clothing. If appropriate to their ability and resources, teach patients who are at home how to keep daily or weekly weight records. Instruct patients to report to the physician weight gains or losses greater than 2 lb/day or 5 lb/wk unless otherwise instructed by the physician.

➤ Monitor the blood pressure regularly. Although all patients receiving diuretic therapy would be expected to experience an initial drop in blood pressure, older adults, those receiving IV diuretics, and those also taking antihypertensives may experience a precipitous fall in blood pressure and in rare instances may go into shock. Other drugs that can cause hypotension, and can thus potentiate hypotension in patients receiving diuretics, include CNS depressants, barbiturates, narcotics, and antihypertensives. Initially, monitor the blood pressure with the patient in the standing, sitting, and lying positions and compare the measurements from each arm.

➤ Review with the patient the symptoms of orthostatic hypotension (see Patient Problems box in Chapter 13). Caution the patient to avoid the use of alcohol because it enhances hypotension.

➤ To monitor for fluid retention, measure the patient's abdominal girth or the circumference of one or both legs. To ensure accurate measurement, mark the patient's skin with small ink marks to indicate the correct placement of the tape measure from day to day.

➤ Check dependent areas daily for the presence of or change in the amount of pitting edema. In pitting edema an indentation or depressed area made by the examiner's finger remains visible in the skin for seconds to minutes after the pressure has been released. Dependent areas where this is more likely to occur include the sacral area and the feet and legs.

➤ Observe the patient for symptoms of dehydration, including thirst, decreased skin turgor, nausea, light-headedness, weakness, increased pulse, oliguria, decreased blood pressure, and elevated hemoglobin, hematocrit, and BUN levels.

➤ Assess the patient for electrolyte abnormalities, and monitor the serum levels of potassium, sodium, calcium, magnesium, and bicarbonate. The signs and symptoms of common electrolyte abnormalities are summarized in Table 17-1.

Nursing Implications Summary—cont'd

➤ Teach patients the importance of taking potassium supplements, if prescribed, and work with them to find a preparation they are willing to take (see Chapter 17). Many effervescent preparations are unpalatable. Enteric-coated tablets have been implicated in small bowel ulceration. Oral solutions are the preferred form of therapy, but they are often unpleasant tasting. Dilute these solutions in juice or milk to reduce the risk of gastric irritation and to make the taste tolerable. Instruct patients to take potassium with meals to reduce gastric irritation. Encourage hypokalemic patients to increase dietary intake of potassium-rich foods (see Dietary Considerations box).

➤ Caution the patient taking diuretics not to switch to salt substitutes without first consulting the physician. Salt substitutes contain a variety of electrolyte salts, and the exact proportions vary from product to product. A patient may inadvertently contribute to electrolyte abnormalities by using a salt substitute. For example, a patient taking a potassium-sparing diuretic may develop hyperkalemia if a salt substitute containing a high portion of potassium salts is used.

➤ Refer the patient as needed to the dietitian for instruction about special dietary restrictions, which may include sodium, calories, cholesterol, and other factors.

➤ Teach patients about their need for diuretic therapy, and review the anticipated side effects of the prescribed drugs. Poor compliance may stem from patient annoyance caused by frequent and excessive urination. Instruct patients to take once-daily diuretics in the morning and to take twice-daily diuretics in the morning and the last dose by 6 PM to avoid interrupting sleep to urinate.

➤ If diuretics are prescribed for hypertension, emphasize the importance of taking all drugs prescribed, even if the patient has no symptoms of hypertension. Teach patients that drug therapy for hypertension may be required for the rest of their lives. Emphasize the importance of continuing all therapies for hypertension that may be prescribed: weight loss, sodium restriction, stopping smoking, regular exercise, and medication.

➤ Dehydration and hypovolemia can contribute to thromboembolic disorders. Assess the patient for pain in the chest, calves, and pelvis that might indicate thromboembolism.

➤ For some patients intermittent therapy (every other day or M-W-F) will achieve the desired effects with fewer side effects.

➤ Teach the patient to take diuretics as ordered. If a dose is missed, it should be taken as soon as remembered, unless within a few hours of the next dose (this varies with the frequency of the dosing schedule), in which case it should be omitted and the regular dosing schedule resumed. Tell the patient not to double up for missed doses.

➤ Thirst is a common side effect (see Patient Problems box in Chapter 23 on dry mouth).

➤ Remind the patient to keep all health care providers informed of all drugs being taken.

Loop Diuretics
Drug Administration

➤ Review the general guidelines for patients receiving diuretics. Assess the patient for development of hyponatremia, hypocalcemia, hypokalemia, and hypochloremic alkalosis (see Table 17-1).

➤ Monitor serum electrolyte levels. Monitor blood glucose levels because these drugs may cause hyperglycemia.

➤ Review drug interactions, and counsel the patient as appropriate.

➤ Monitor serum uric acid levels, and assess the patient for signs of gout.

➤ Assess the patient for signs of ototoxicity, which include tinnitus (ringing in the ears), reduced hearing acuity, and vertigo.

➤ Question the patient about allergy to sulfonamides, thiazide diuretics, or any other loop diuretics before administering first doses. Observe for allergic response, including development of rashes.

➤ Teach patients taking the oral liquid form to measure doses with the calibrated dropper provided with the drug or to use a specially marked measuring spoon or medication cup to measure doses.

Intravenous bumetanide

➤ Bumetanide is usually given undiluted but may be mixed with 5% dextrose in water (D5W), normal saline, and lactated Ringer's solution.

➤ Administer dose evenly for a 2-minute period. After IV administration, monitor blood pressure every 15 to 30 minutes until stable, keep siderails up, and supervise ambulation.

Intravenous ethacrynic acid

➤ Ethacrynic acid may be given undiluted, or 50 mg may be diluted in 50 ml of D5W or 0.9% normal saline. Do not mix with other drugs. Do not administer if solution is discolored or contains particulate matter. Administer at a rate of 10 mg or less over a 1-minute period, or infuse total dose over 30 minutes. Check the infusion site carefully; thrombophlebitis is common, and extravasation causes pain and tissue irritation. After IV administration, monitor blood pressure every 15 to 30 minutes until stable, keep siderails up, and supervise ambulation.

Intravenous furosemide

➤ Furosemide may be given undiluted or added to D5W, normal saline, or lactated Ringer's injection. Inspect the solution before administering, and do not use it if it is yellow. Do not mix furosemide with other drugs.

➤ Administer at a rate of 40 mg evenly administered for a 1- to 2-minute period. If administered as an infusion, use an infusion control device and administer no faster than 4 mg/min. After IV administration, monitor blood pressure every 15 to 30 minutes until stable, keep siderails up, and supervise ambulation.

Intramuscular furosemide

➤ IM injection of furosemide may cause transient pain at the injection site.

Continued

Nursing Implications Summary—cont'd

Intravenous torsemide
➤ Torsemide may be given undiluted, at a rate of 1 dose evenly administered for a 2-minute period.

Nursing in the Community
➤ See the general guidelines for patients receiving diuretics.
➤ Potassium supplements are often prescribed concomitantly with loop diuretics. Emphasize the importance of taking potassium supplements as prescribed, refer to the dietitian as needed, and review good dietary sources of potassium. Instruct the patient that diarrhea, vomiting, and anorexia (loss of appetite), if prolonged or severe, may also cause hypokalemia and should be reported to the physician. Caution patients also taking a cardiac glycoside to be especially careful to avoid hypokalemia. Review other drug interactions with the patient, as appropriate.
➤ Caution diabetic patients to monitor blood glucose levels carefully because hyperglycemia may occur, requiring an adjustment in diet or dose of insulin. Instruct the patient to report signs of agranulocytosis (depressed production of white blood cells [leukopenia]), including unexplained fever, chills, sore throat, or enlarged lymph nodes. This is a rare but serious side effect of drug therapy (see Patient Problems box in Chapter 20).
➤ Instruct the patient to take oral preparations with meals or just after eating to reduce gastric irritation. Warn the patient in renal failure that bumetanide may cause myalgia. Tell the patient to report skin changes, rashes, nausea, vomiting, or any unexpected sign or symptom. For patients taking furosemide, review the Patient Problems box in Chapter 58 on photosensitivity.

Thiazide Diuretics
Drug Administration
➤ See the general guidelines for diuretic therapy. Thiazides may cause hypokalemia, hypochloremia, alkalosis, hyponatremia, and hypomagnesemia. Monitor the patient for these electrolyte abnormalities and monitor serum electrolyte levels (see Table 17-1).
➤ Monitor the patient's blood glucose levels because thiazide diuretics may cause hyperglycemia.
➤ Review drug interactions, and counsel the patient as appropriate.
➤ Monitor serum uric acid levels, and assess for signs of gout.
➤ Monitor the serum BUN levels and lipid levels.

Parenteral chlorothiazide
➤ Dilute each vial (0.5 g) with at least 18 ml of sterile water. Dilute further if desired with D5W or sodium chloride injection. Do not mix with other drugs or blood products. Administer at a rate of 0.5 g or less over a 5-minute period.
➤ Check the insertion site for signs of extravasation since the drug is extremely alkaline. Do not administer intramuscularly or subcutaneously. Thiazides can cause a paradoxical antidiuretic effect in patients who have diabetes insipidus (see Chapter 65).

Nursing in the Community
➤ See the general guidelines for diuretic therapy.
➤ Potassium supplements may be prescribed, but patients may be able to prevent hypokalemia by increasing their daily dietary intake of potassium-rich foods (see the Dietary Considerations box). If potassium supplements are prescribed, emphasize the importance of taking these as ordered. Instruct patients that diarrhea, vomiting, and anorexia, if prolonged or severe, can also cause hypokalemia and should be reported to the physician. Concomitant administration of adrenal corticosteroids may also predispose the patient to hypokalemia.
➤ Caution diabetic patients to monitor blood glucose levels carefully because hyperglycemia may occur, requiring an adjustment in diet or insulin dosage. Instruct patients to take oral doses with meals to reduce gastric irritation.
➤ Review the problem of photosensitivity (see the Patient Problems box in Chapter 58 on photosensitivity).

Potassium-Sparing Diuretics
Drug Administration
➤ See the general guidelines for diuretic therapy.
➤ Potassium-sparing diuretics may cause hyperkalemia or hyponatremia. Assess the patient for these electrolyte imbalances, and monitor serum electrolyte levels (see Table 17-1).
➤ Many combination products that contain both a potassium-depleting diuretic and a potassium-sparing diuretic are available. The combination is designed to promote diuresis while maintaining normal serum potassium levels. Patients receiving combination drugs are potentially at risk for side effects caused by any of the component drugs (see Table 14-4). Instruct the patient to report the development of any unexpected sign or symptom.
➤ Monitor BUN levels.

Nursing in the Community
➤ Patients should take doses with meals or a snack to reduce gastric irritation. Spironolactone tablets may be crushed and mixed in syrup or fluid of the patient's choice. The triamterene capsule may be opened and the contents mixed with food or fluid for patients who have difficulty swallowing. Check with the pharmacist.
➤ If a potassium-sparing diuretic has been newly prescribed or if a potassium-sparing diuretic is prescribed in addition to a potassium-depleting diuretic, emphasize the need to omit previous potassium supplements that may have been ordered; consult the physician. In addition, instruct the patient to limit intake of potassium-rich foods (see the Dietary Considerations box).
➤ Instruct the patient to avoid salt substitutes that contain potassium while taking potassium-sparing diuretics.
➤ Caution patients taking triamterene that photosensitivity may develop (see Patient Problems box in Chapter 58 on photosensitivity).
➤ Caution male patients taking spironolactone to notify the physician if gynecomastia develops.

Nursing Implications Summary—cont'd

Carbonic Anhydrase Inhibitors
Drug Administration
➤ Review the general guidelines for diuretic therapy.
➤ Monitor serum electrolyte levels, and assess the patient for electrolyte abnormalities, especially metabolic acidosis (see Table 17-1). Intermittent therapy may be used to limit the development of acidosis.
➤ Read the physician's orders carefully. Tablets and extended-release capsules are available. Review drug interactions, and counsel the patient as appropriate.
➤ Monitor serum uric acid and blood glucose levels.
➤ Monitor the patient for signs of kidney stone formation, such as renal colic (severe flank pain), hematuria (blood in the urine), and oliguria.

Intravenous acetazolamide
➤ Dilute each 500 mg of acetazolamide with at least 5 ml of sterile water for injection, and administer at a rate of 500 mg over at least a 1-minute period. The drug may be further diluted with standard IV fluids and administered over 4 to 8 hours. Avoid IM injection, which is very painful.

Nursing in the Community
➤ Review the guidelines for diuretic therapy.
➤ Instruct diabetic patients to monitor blood glucose levels; a change in diet or insulin dose may be required. Review expected effects and possible side effects. Instruct the patient to report any unexpected sign or symptom. Instruct the patient to avoid driving or operating hazardous equipment if drowsiness, dizziness, light-headedness, or visual changes occur and to notify the physician.
➤ A metallic taste in the mouth may occur. Sucking sugarless hard candy, chewing sugarless gum, brushing the teeth, or rinsing the mouth may help.
➤ Photosensitivity may occur (see Patient Problems box in Chapter 58 on photosensitivity).

Osmotic Diuretics
Drug Administration/Nursing in the Community
➤ See the general guidelines for diuretic therapy.
➤ Monitor serum electrolyte levels, and assess for electrolyte abnormalities (see Table 17-1). Assess the patient for signs of circulatory overload. Monitor vital signs for blood pressure, intake and output, and daily weight. Assess breath and heart sounds. Monitor the patient for signs of pulmonary congestion or congestive heart failure, including dyspnea, labored respiration, tachypnea, tachycardia, distended neck veins, rales, agitation, fluid retention, and weight gain.

➤ Osmotic diuretics are often given to patients with increased intracranial pressure. Assess level of consciousness, and monitor indicators of cerebral function, including blood pressure, pulse, intracranial pressure, and Glasgow Coma Scale or institutional equivalent.
➤ Determine the desired daily fluid balance with the physician. The infusion rate may be titrated to output. Diuresis may be copious, especially initially; a urinary catheter may be needed. If the urine output falls below 30 to 50 ml/hr, notify the physician.
➤ Oral fluids may not be permitted. Occasional ice chips may be permitted to help relieve thirst.
➤ If extravasation occurs, osmotic diuretics cause local skin and tissue damage. Before starting infusion, check that the IV line is secure and patent, with no signs of redness or infiltration, and that the rate of flow is not sluggish. Inspect infusion site regularly. If infiltration is suspected, discontinue infusion and restart in another site.

Intravenous mannitol
➤ Read the physician's order carefully. Mannitol is available in several concentrations. It is not necessary to dilute mannitol. Check ampule or bottle for crystallization, a common problem. If crystals are present, warm the container under running water until crystals dissolve. Cool to body temperature before administering. Use an in-line IV filter for 15%, 20%, and 25% solutions. Do not add to other IV solutions, medications, or blood products. The rate of administration is usually 1 to 2 g/kg for a 30- to 90-minute period but may vary.

Intravenous urea
➤ Urea must be diluted to make a 30% solution (30% solution equals 30 g of urea/100 ml or 300 mg/ml). Dilute with D5W or D10W or with 10% invert sugar in water; some manufacturers supply the diluent. Patients with hereditary fructose intolerance (aldolase deficiency) may have a severe reaction to the invert sugar solution if it is used as a diluent. Symptoms include hypoglycemia, nausea, vomiting, tremors, coma, and convulsions. Infuse at a rate of 4 ml/min (1200 mg/min) or slower. Use only fresh solutions, and discard any unused portions. Do not mix with blood or other drugs in the same syringe.
➤ These drugs are rarely used outside of the acute-care setting. Keep the patient and family informed of the patient's condition.

CHAPTER REVIEW

Application

1. What is a nephron?
2. What is the function of the glomerulus?
3. What is the difference between active transport and passive transport?
4. What is a symporter and how does it differ from an antiporter?
5. How is bicarbonate ion recovered from tubular fluid? Where does this occur?
6. What symporter is inhibited by loop diuretics?
7. What side effects are common with loop diuretics? Which of these is related to characteristics of the target symporter?
8. How does bumetanide differ from the other loop diuretics?
9. What symporter is inhibited by thiazide diuretics?
10. What side effects are characteristic of thiazide diuretics?
11. What are the two mechanisms by which potassium-sparing diuretics alter sodium excretion?
12. What side effects are associated with potassium-sparing diuretics?
13. How are carbonic anhydrase inhibitors used clinically?
14. What side effects are characteristic of carbonic anhydrase inhibitors?
15. What reactions occur with osmotic diuretics?

Critical Thinking

1. Develop a nursing care plan for a patient receiving one of the diuretics discussed in this chapter. How can you assess the drug's effectiveness? About what drug interactions should you instruct the patient?
2. Your older adult patient tells you the physician just began diuretic therapy, but the patient cannot remember the name of the drug. What should you warn the patient about?
3. An obese patient confides to you during weigh-in that she plans to join a weight loss program that starts off with pills that help you start losing weight quickly. What are some of the possible drugs that might be used this way? (See also Chapters 60 and 67.) What warnings should you give the patient?

References

Holcomb SS: Understanding the ins & outs of diuretic therapy, *Nursing* 27(2):34-40, 1997.

Morrison RT: Edema and principles of diuretic use, *Med Clin North Am* 81(3):689-704, 1997.

Perez A: Restoring electrolyte balance: hypokalemia, *RN* 58(12):33-36, 1995.

Suki WN: Use of diuretics in chronic renal failure, *Kidney Int Suppl* 59:S33-S35, 1997.

Valvo E, et al: Diuretics in hypertension, *Kidney Int Suppl* 59:S90-S96, 1997.

Antianginals and Other Vasodilators

OBJECTIVES

After studying this chapter, you should be able to do the following:

- *Describe drug therapy for angina pectoris, including differentiating among the nitrates, beta-blockers, and calcium channel blockers.*

- *Discuss the rationale for drug treatment of vasospastic disorders.*

- *Develop nursing care plans for patients receiving drugs from the following groups: nitrates, blockers, calcium channel blockers, vasodilators for vascular disease, and pentoxifylline.*

CHAPTER OVERVIEW

This chapter covers drugs used primarily to improve circulation: sympathomimetic drugs and selected vasodilators. Because beta-blockers and calcium channel blockers have gained widespread use in the treatment of angina, these drug classes are also discussed.

Vasodilators improve blood flow by increasing the size of the blood vessels. Vasodilation has been used in treating angina and peripheral vascular disease. Although some of the activity of vasodilators may be related to alpha- or beta-adrenergic receptors, most vasodilators work by a mechanism that was not understood until recently. As an understanding of these diseases progresses, the role of vasodilators is being reevaluated. Vasodilators used primarily as antihypertensive agents are discussed in Chapter 13.

THERAPEUTIC RATIONALE: ANGINA

Blood Circulation to the Heart

The heart has a very high requirement for oxygen and nutrients. These needs are met by the coronary circulation (Figure 15-1) because the heart muscle cannot use the blood pumped through its chambers. The right and left coronary arteries originate at the aorta as it leaves the heart. The left coronary artery divides into the circumflex branch and the anterior descending branch. The three major vessels of the heart are thus the right coronary artery, circumflex coronary branch of the left coronary artery, and the anterior descending branch of the left coronary artery. These vessels divide and subdivide to the capillaries that finally service the individual cardiac cells. Ordinarily, the heart receives an adequate supply of blood through these coronary vessels.

Angina Pectoris

Angina pectoris, which literally means a choking of the chest, is the result of a temporary insufficiency of oxygen to the heart. The heart has a large requirement for oxygen and

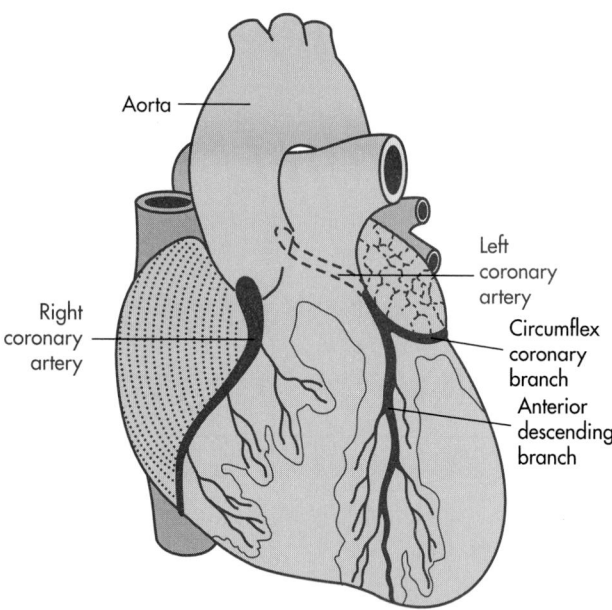

Figure 15-1 Coronary arteries. The three major coronary arteries are right coronary artery and two branches of left coronary artery; circumflex coronary branch and anterior descending branch. These arteries supply blood for heart muscle. Occlusion of one or more of these arteries can cause angina.

normally extracts maximum amounts of oxygen from the coronary circulation. The increased oxygen demands of the heart associated with increased work are normally met by increased coronary blood flow.

In about 1 of 50 American adults the coronary arteries become narrowed by fatty deposits that develop just underneath the inner lining of the vessel. This condition is called **coronary atherosclerosis.** The flow of blood in affected vessels is reduced, and the dependent heart muscle no longer receives an adequate blood supply. As the atherosclerosis worsens, the vascular system in the heart compensates by developing additional blood vessels (collateral circulation) to bypass the affected vessel. If a large enough area of the heart muscle does not receive sufficient oxygen, pain results.

Anginal pain is a sudden, severe, and pressing pain that begins behind the breast bone and radiates up to the left shoulder and arm. Often this pain initially may be a feeling of acute chest discomfort; it also may be felt in the neck, jaw, teeth, arms, or elbows, areas to which cardiac pain is physiologically referred. The pain gradually wears off when the person stops and rests. Drugs that increase the heart rate, decrease blood flow to the heart, or cause fluid retention may precipitate anginal episodes. Drugs shown to increase anginal attacks include bromocriptine, diazoxide, digitalis, dobutamine, dopamine, ergotamine, fluorouracil, hydralazine, indomethacin, minoxidil, nifedipine, prazosin, propranolol, and thyroid hormone.

Classic angina is often called stable angina or exertional angina. In classic angina the large coronary arteries are ob-

structed by atherosclerosis to the point that blood flow cannot increase to supply more oxygen required by increased work. Coronary atherosclerosis is the most common cause of angina.

Variant angina (Prinzmetal's angina) has a different origin than classic angina. Variant angina is caused by spasms of the large coronary arteries that result in obstruction of blood flow. These coronary spasms have no relationship to exercise and may occur at rest. Variant angina often has a daily rhythm, with episodes being more common in the morning. However, most patients with variant angina also have coronary atherosclerosis; in these patients anginal pain may also occur with exertion.

Unstable angina refers to angina that has a changing intensity. Pain comes at decreasing levels of exertion and often at rest. Patients who progress to unstable angina are the most likely to have a heart attack and should be medically reviewed immediately.

The treatment of angina depends on the recognition that the supply of oxygen to the heart does not meet the demand. On a long-term basis the demand for oxygen can be decreased by altering secondary factors that are known to adversely affect the heart. These factors include smoking, excess weight, hypertension, arrhythmias, anxiety, anemia, and lack of regular exercise. The major risk factors for the progression of atherosclerosis are cigarette smoking, hypertension, and high serum cholesterol levels. Evidence affirms that alteration of these risk factors in patients with angina related to coronary atherosclerosis prolongs life.

Coronary artery bypass surgery may be indicated when angina is severe because of coronary atherosclerosis. In this type of surgery one or more of the main coronary vessels is bypassed with a graft from the aorta to the lower end of the vessel. Replacement of vessels severely narrowed by atherosclerosis greatly improves coronary blood flow. About 70% of patients have no further angina, and another 20% have markedly reduced angina.

Percutaneous transluminal coronary angioplasty (PTCA) is a nonsurgical procedure for opening a coronary artery narrowed by atherosclerosis. A balloon catheter is inserted into the narrowed area. The balloon is inflated, and the vessel is widened. The PTCA procedure is most effective in patients with severe angina who have only one severely narrowed coronary artery. This is usually the left coronary artery servicing the more worked left ventricle.

THERAPEUTIC AGENTS: ANTIANGINAL DRUGS

Drug therapy for angina pectoris rests with three classes of drugs. The nitrates primarily offer acute relief of angina. The beta-blockers offer long-term relief in classic angina. The calcium channel blockers are especially effective in relieving the coronary spasms of variant angina. These three drug classes are discussed in detail in the following sections.

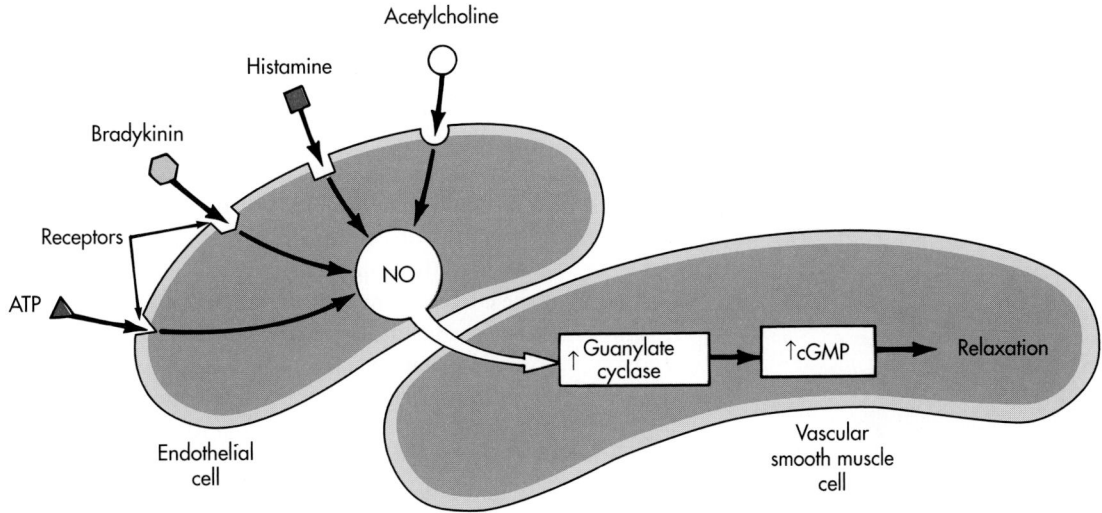

F i g u r e 15-2   Nitric oxide *(NO)* is a very potent vasodilator. Endothelial cell produces nitric oxide from argi-nine, an amino acid, in response to various substances such as acetylcholine, histamine, bradykinin, and adenosine triphosphate *(ATP)*. However, nitrates are also broken down to nitric oxide. Nitric oxide diffuses into vascular smooth muscle cells and stimulates enzyme, guanylate cyclase, which produces second-messenger cyclic guanosine monophosphate *(cGMP)*; cGMP activates intracellular events that result in vasodilation.

Nitrates

General Characteristics

Mechanism of Action

Nitric oxide is now recognized to be the endothelium-derived relaxing factor (EDRF) responsible for relaxation of vascular smooth muscle, resulting in vasodilation (Figure 15-2). Nitrates are broken down to nitric oxide. However, within cells, the endogenous source of nitric oxide is the amino acid arginine.

The nitrates were originally believed to dilate the coronary blood vessels, thereby increasing blood flow in the heart. It is now understood that most patients with angina have atherosclerosis of the coronary vessels and that atherosclerotic vessels cannot dilate. Furthermore, insufficient oxygen (ischemia) is itself a potent vasodilator; thus the coronary vessels are already dilated during an anginal attack. The nitrates act to dilate arterioles and veins in the periphery, thereby lowering blood pressure. The reduced blood pressure means that the work of the heart is greatly reduced. This reduced workload lowers the oxygen demand of the heart.

Pharmacokinetics

The organic nitrates, nitroglycerin, erythrityl tetranitrate, and isosorbide dinitrate, relieve anginal attacks within a few minutes when administered sublingually. Sublingual administration allows the drug to be distributed systemically without first going through liver. The organic nitrates are rapidly degraded by the liver, and therefore large doses are required for prophylactic use. Tolerance rapidly develops to organic

nitrates, reducing the duration of relief. Therefore organic nitrates are primarily used for acute relief of angina.

Uses

The nitrates, particularly nitroglycerin, are the mainstay of antianginal medication. The nitrates are most effectively used as needed to relieve an acute anginal attack. Patients who understand the factors that precipitate their own anginal attacks can take these medications prophylactically just before those activities.

Occasionally organic nitrates are administered orally in large doses to provide prophylactic treatment for angina.

Adverse Reactions and Contraindications

The side effects of sublingual nitrates result from the generalized vasodilation they produce. These side effects include flushing, headache, and dizziness. The flushing is a result of the vasodilation in the area of the neck and face. The headache is a result of the pressure imposed by dilated blood vessels in the brain. The incidence of headaches decreases 2 to 3 weeks after initial therapy. The dizziness is the result of the generalized hypotension. The patient should sit or lie down to avoid fainting after taking one of these drugs.

Nitrates should not be taken by patients with recent head trauma because of the increase in cerebrospinal fluid pressure. Patients for whom hypotension is a risk, especially after a myocardial infarction, should not take these drugs.

Toxicity

Severe hypotension is usually transitory. The legs should be elevated to aid venous return. Severe hypotension is

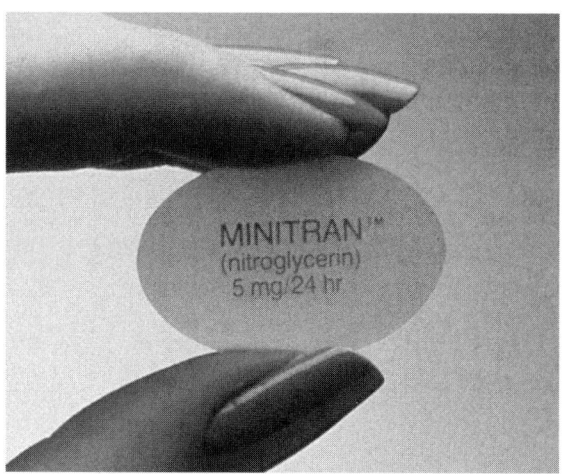

Figure 15-3 Minitran™ transdermal delivery system for controlled release of nitroglycerin for prevention of angina. *(Courtesy 3M Pharmaceuticals, St. Paul, MN.)*

accompanied by a reflex increase in heart rate, which increases the workload for the heart and makes the pain worse.

Interactions

The hypotensive effects of nitrates are enhanced by alcohol, beta-blockers, calcium channel blockers, and antidepressants. Patients taking drugs with anticholinergic action may have a dry mouth that delays dissolution of sublingual and buccal preparations.

Specific Nitrates

For summary information on specific nitrates, refer to Table 15-1.

▼ nitroglycerin

Nitroglycerin is considered the drug of choice for angina. When nitroglycerin is taken sublingually, its effect begins in 30 seconds, is maximal in 3 minutes, and lasts for about 10 minutes. A drawback to nitroglycerin is that it decomposes when exposed to light or heat. Nitroglycerin can also volatilize from the tablets, which therefore must be kept in airtight containers.

Several dosage forms for nitroglycerin are available. A variation of the sublingual form is nitroglycerin lingual aerosol, which allows the drug to be sprayed in a metered form on or under the tongue. The aerosol is a substitute for the sublingual tablets in the short-term relief of an anginal attack. Extended-release buccal forms are intended for prophylactic use. Extended-release capsules and tablets have up to 10 times the sublingual dose. These are swallowed and are effective for 8 to 12 hours. Nitroglycerin is very lipid soluble and probably enters the body from the gastrointestinal tract through the lymphatics rather than through the portal blood.

Nitroglycerin may also be administered through the skin. A measured amount of nitroglycerin ointment is spread on a nonhairy part of the body and held in place with plastic wrap taped over the area. This route of administration is said to produce relief for up to 3 hours. Nitroglycerin is also available impregnated in a polymer bonded to an adhesive bandage (Figure 15-3). This disk is applied to the skin, and nitroglycerin is absorbed through the skin (transdermally). It should be left in place for no more than 12 to 14 hours a day. If left on continually, the person will rapidly become tolerant to the drug (tachyphylaxis) and the patch will cease to be effective. The unit should be applied to a site free of hair, and the bandage should be placed at a new site each time to avoid irritation.

Nitroglycerin is administered intravenously in acute heart failure. Nitroglycerin can reduce the myocardial ischemia that results when the left side of the heart is failing. Because blood is not being pumped out effectively, pressure builds in the left ventricle. Pulmonary edema results because blood backs up in the lungs. Nitroglycerin is an effective dilator of the coronary arteries and therefore allows more oxygenated blood to reach the troubled heart muscle. The heart is able to perform better, and the symptoms of acute heart failure are relieved.

erythrityl tetranitrate

Erythrityl tetranitrate is the longest acting of the sublingual or chewable organic nitrates. This drug becomes effective in 5 minutes, and its effects last for 4 hours. This is a long duration compared with nitroglycerin or even isosorbide dinitrate, and therefore erythrityl tetranitrate is better for prophylactic use than for relief of acute attacks. Erythrityl tetranitrate is also available for oral administration.

isosorbide dinitrate

Isosorbide dinitrate is another organic nitrate that can be taken sublingually or chewed. It is effective in 2 to 5 minutes and can act for 1 to 2 hours.

pentaerythritol tetranitrate

Pentaerythritol tetranitrate has not been classified as possible effective as a prophylactic treatment of angina, but not for the treatment of acute attacks.

Beta-Blockers
General Characteristics

Beta-blockers decrease the oxygen requirements of the heart by reducing its workload. Blocking the beta$_1$-adrenergic receptors of the heart decreases the heart rate and the force of contraction, and a decrease in blood pressure follows. These actions also benefit coronary circulation by decreasing the resistance in the coronary circulation. However, beta-blockers are not vasodilators.

Mechanism of Action

There are two major subclasses of beta-receptors: beta$_1$ and beta$_2$. (For further discussion of beta-receptors, see Chapter 12.) The cardioselective beta-blockers are relatively

Table 15-1   Drugs Prescribed for the Relief of Angina Pectoris

Generic Name	Trade Name	Administration/Dosage	Comments
Nitrates and Nitrites			
erythrityl tetranitrate	Cardilate*	SUBLINGUAL, ORAL, OR BUCCAL: *Adults*—5-10 mg 3 times/day. If required, dose may be increased every 2-3 days up to 30 mg 3 times/day. Onset: 5 min for sublingual; 30 min for oral. Duration: 4 hr.	Prophylactic treatment prevents anginal attacks. Hypotension, headaches, and tolerance to nitrates are possible side effects.
isosorbide dinitrate	Iso-Bid Isordil* Isotrate Sorbitrate Others	SUBLINGUAL: *Adults*—2.5-5 mg. Chewable: 5-10 mg. Onset: 2-5 min. Duration: 1-2 hr. ORAL: *Adults*—5-30 mg 4 times/day. Timed-release forms: 40 mg 2-4 times/day. Onset: 15-30 min. Duration: 4-6 hr.	Drug relieves acute angina attacks. It is possibly effective prophylactically, especially if taken in anticipation of stressful situation. Hypotension is side effect limiting dose. It is possibly effective as prophylactic treatment to prevent anginal attacks. Headache can be severe. Tolerance to nitrates may develop.
isosorbide mononitrate	Monoket	ORAL (tablets): *Adults*—20 mg 2 times/day, 7 hr apart. ORAL (extended-release): *Adults*—30 or 60 mg once daily. May increase to 120 mg if needed. FDA pregnancy category C.	Drug is for prophylaxis and long-term treatment of angina caused by coronary artery disease.
nitroglycerin	Nitrostat	SUBLINGUAL: *Adults*—Tablets of 0.15-0.3 mg initially, up to 0.6 mg as required in individual. Individual dosages may be repeated at 5-min intervals, up to 3 tablets in 15 min. Peak action: 3 min. Duration: 10 min.	Drug is direct-acting vasodilator. It is drug of choice for angina pectoris. Patient takes at onset of acute anginal episodes or in anticipation of an episode, such as before exercise or sex. Storage containers should be kept cool to prevent disintegration and airtight to prevent volatilization.
	Nitrolingual*	SUBLINGUAL: *Adults*—1 or 2 metered doses (400 mg/dose) on or under tongue. Repeat at 5-min intervals for relief of anginal attack.	Sublingual spray should afford relief after total of 3 doses in 15 min.
	Klavikordal Nitrong* Nitronet Nitrong* Nitrogard Nitrogard SR†	ORAL (extended-release): *Adults*—2.5-6.5 mg every 8-12 hr. Onset: slow variable. Duration: 8-12 hr. BUCCAL: *Adults*—1 mg 3 times/day. May increase to 2 mg. Kept in mouth for several hours. May increase to 4 times/day or add extra for acute prophylaxis, but no more than every 2 hr.	Drug provides prophylactic administration of nitroglycerin. Effectiveness of this mode of therapy is not established.
nitroglycerin ointment, 2%	Nitro-Bid* Nitrol* Nitrong*	TOPICAL: *Adults*—Initially 1 inch is spread over area of skin. This is increased by 1/2-inch increments as required. Absorption is improved by covering area with plastic. Onset: 30-60 min. Duration: up to 3 hr.	Drug provides prophylactic administration of nitroglycerin. Excessive dose may cause violent headache. Area of administration will be irritated and should be rotated. On termination of treatment, area and frequency of administration should be reduced gradually over 4-6 wk to prevent withdrawal reactions.
	Nitrodisc Nitro-Dur* Transderm-Nitro*	TOPICAL: Apply to site free of hair for 12-14 hr/day. Do not apply to hands or feet. Change daily to new site.	Nitroglycerin is impregnated into polymer bound to adhesive bandages. Drug is absorbed through skin.
pentaerythritol tetranitrate	Peritrate* Pentylan Duotrate	ORAL: *Adults*—Initially 10-20 mg 4 times/day. If required, dosage may be adjusted up to 40 mg 4 times/day. Onset: 30 min. Duration: 4-5 hr. ORAL (sustained-release): *Adults*—30-80 mg twice day. Onset: 30-60 min. Duration: 12 hr.	Drug is possibly effective as prophylactic treatment for angina pectoris. Hypotension, headaches, and tolerance to nitrates are possible side effects. Tablets are taken 30 min before or 1 hr after meals and at bedtime. Drug is taken on empty stomach.
Beta-Adrenergic Blockers for Angina			
acebutolol	Monitan† Sectral*	ORAL: *Adults*—200 mg 2 times/day initially, then adjusted according to response.	Dosage should be reduced for patients with reduced liver or kidney function.
atenolol	Apo-Atenolol† Novo-Atenol† Tenormin*	ORAL: *Adults*—50-200 mg once daily.	Dose is given every other day to patients with severely impaired renal function.
carteolol	Cartrol	ORAL: *Adults*—Up to 10 mg/day.	Dosage interval is increased for patients with severely impaired renal function.
labetalol	Normodyne Trandate*	ORAL: *Adults*—150-300 mg 2 times/day.	Drug also has alpha₁-adrenergic blocking effects.

*Available in Canada and the United States.
†Available in Canada only.

Continued

Table 15-1   Drugs Prescribed for the Relief of Angina Pectoris—cont'd

Generic Name	Trade Name	Administration/Dosage	Comments
Beta-Adrenergic Blockers for Angina—cont'd			
metoprolol	Apo-Metoprolol† Betaloc† Lopressor* Novometoprol†	ORAL: *Adults*—50 mg 3 or 4 times/day. *For prophylaxis after myocardial infarction:* 100 mg 2 times/day.	Drug is readily metabolized by liver. Bioavailability is increased by food.
nadolol	Corgard* Syn-Nadolol†	ORAL: *Adults*—40-80 mg/day.	Drug is excreted unchanged in urine. Dosage interval is increased in patients with renal impairment.
penbutolol	Levatol	ORAL: *Adults*—20-40 mg once/day.	Drug is excreted unchanged in urine.
pindolol	Syn-Pindolol† Visken*	ORAL: *Adults*—10 mg 4 times/day.	Drug is well metabolized.
propranolol	Inderal*	ORAL: *Adults*—10-20 mg 3 or 4 times/day. Increase as required. Maintenance dose is usually 160-240 mg/day, in 4 doses.	Drug is well absorbed and extensively metabolized by liver.
sotalol	Betapace Sotacor†	ORAL: *Adults*—Initially 80 mg 2 times/day. Increase at weekly intervals as needed.	Drug is excreted unchanged in the urine. Dosage interval is increased in patients with renal impairment.
timolol	Apo-Timol† Blocadren* Novo-Timol†	ORAL: *Adults*—10-30 mg 2 times/day. *For prophylaxis for myocardial infarction:* 10 mg 2 times/day.	Drug is well absorbed and extensively metabolized by liver.
Calcium Channel Blockers for Angina			
amlodipine	Norvasc	ORAL: *Adults*—5-10 mg once daily.	Drug is a potent peripheral arteriolar vasodilator.
bepridil	Bepadin Vascor	ORAL: *Adults*—Initially 200 mg once daily. Increase after 10 days, if necessary, to 300 mg once daily. Maximum: 400 mg/day.	Drug also has significant cardiac effects: negative inotropy and bradycardia.
diltiazem	Cardizem SR*	ORAL: *Adults*—60 mg every 6 hr.	Drug is be taken before meals.
felodipine	Plendil* Renedil†	ORAL: *Adults*—10 mg once a day.	Geriatric patients may be more sensitive.
nicardipine	Cardene*	ORAL: *Adults*—20 mg 3 times/day, adjusted for need and tolerance.	Drug is potent peripheral vasodilator. Reflex increase in heart rate masks negative inotropy.
nifedipine	Adalat CC Adalat P.A.† Procardia XL	ORAL: *Adults*—30 or 60 mg once a day.	Procardia XL is a specially formulated system to release the drug in the intestine over 24 hr. Immediate release forms not recommended.
verapamil	Apo-Verap† Calan Isoptin* Novo-Veramil†	ORAL: *Adults*—240-480 mg/day in 3 or 4 divided doses.	Drug depresses sinoatrial and atrioventricular nodes and causes extensive first-pass metabolism. Half-life is increased in patients with cirrhosis, and dose should be lowered by 70%.

*Available in Canada and the United States.
†Available in Canada only.

selective for the beta$_1$-receptors. However, this selectivity is diminished at higher dosages. There is no evidence that any particular beta-blocker is better than another in the management of angina. Patients with asthma, diabetes, or peripheral vascular disease are better able to tolerate the selective beta$_1$-blockers. Beta$_1$-selective drugs include acebutolol, atenolol, and metoprolol. Non-selective drugs include nadolol, oxprenolol, pindolol, propranolol, sotalol, and timolol.

Pharmacokinetics

Beta-blockers are administered orally. The frequency of administration depends on the given drug. They are generally well absorbed and metabolized by the liver. Metabolites are generally excreted in the urine, although some metabolites are excreted in the feces through the biliary system.

Uses

Beta-blockers have become widely used in the management of classic angina. A beta-blocker is commonly prescribed as prophylactic therapy, and nitroglycerin is prescribed for acute anginal attacks. Long-term therapy reduces the frequency of anginal pain and decreases the requirements for nitroglycerin. The effective dose is highly individual for each patient. One index of dosage is the decrease in resting heart rate. In patients who have severe angina, enough medication may be given to lower the resting pulse to 50 to 60 beats/min. If gastrointestinal side effects such as nausea, cramping, or diarrhea occur, taking the drug with meals may lessen these symptoms.

Beta-blockers are widely used as antihypertensive agents. This use is discussed extensively in Chapter 13.

Another prophylactic use of beta-blockers is to prevent sudden death after a heart attack. Several studies have shown that administration of a beta-blocker after a heart attack reduces the incidence of sudden death by as much as 40%. In addition to reducing the workload of the heart, other actions of beta-blockers such as the antiarrhythmic and antiplatelet functions may be important.

Adverse Reactions and Contraindications

The most common side effects of beta-blockers are fatigue and mental lassitude. Depression, nightmares, and psychosis are more severe central nervous system (CNS) side effects sometimes seen. Peripheral vasoconstriction may cause cold hands or feet. Sexual dysfunction, including impotence, is a side effect, especially of propranolol and timolol. Beta-blockers are contraindicated for patients with severely impaired heart or circulatory function (e.g., congestive heart failure, heart block, severe sinus bradycardia, Raynaud's phenomenon). It is important to note that withdrawal of beta-blockers should be gradual. Sudden withdrawal can lead to unstable angina, a myocardial infarction, or even sudden death.

Adverse effects of beta-blockers include bronchospasm, hypoglycemia, and impairment of peripheral circulation. The bronchospasm arises from blockade of the beta$_2$-receptors of the bronchi. Beta-blockers mask symptoms of hypoglycemia such as an increase in heart rate and blood pressure. This makes it more difficult for diabetic patients to monitor their blood glucose. Dilation of peripheral blood vessels is mediated by beta$_2$-receptors. These adverse effects are less common with the beta$_1$-selective blockers.

Interactions

Beta-blockers inhibit glycogen breakdown, a process normally stimulated by epinephrine and norepinephrine. This interferes with the action of insulin and oral antidiabetic agents. Beta-blockers may exaggerate the hypotensive effects of other drugs such as calcium channel blockers, clonidine, diazoxide, guanabenz, and reserpine.

Specific Beta-Blockers

Many beta-blockers are now on the market. Those that have been specifically approved for use in the United States as antianginal agents are atenolol, metoprolol, nadolol, and propranolol. Additional beta-blockers used in the United States unofficially as antianginal drugs include acebutolol, carteolol, labetalol, penbutolol, pindolol, sotalol, and timolol. Atenolol, metoprolol, propranolol, and timolol have been approved for prophylaxis against myocardial reinfarction. Specific beta-blockers are listed in Table 15-1.

acebutolol

Acebutolol (Monitan, Sectral) is an intermediate-acting, cardioselective beta-blocker. The drug is metabolized by the liver and excreted both through the kidney and feces. Dosage should be reduced for patients with reduced liver or kidney function.

atenolol

Atenolol (Tenormin) is a long-acting, cardioselective beta-blocker. Poorly absorbed from the gastrointestinal tract, the drug is not metabolized but excreted unchanged in the urine. The time between doses must be increased in patients with impaired renal function.

carteolol

Carteolol (Cartrol) is a long-acting, nonselective beta-blocker. It is well absorbed and excreted largely unchanged in the urine. The dosage interval is increased for patients with impaired renal function.

labetalol

Labetalol (Normodyne, Trandate) is a long-acting, nonspecific beta-blocker that also has selective alpha$_1$-adrenergic blocking effects. It is well absorbed, metabolized by the liver, and excreted in the urine.

▼ metoprolol

Metoprolol (Betaloc, Lopressor) is a short-acting, cardioselective beta-blocker. It is well absorbed from the gastrointestinal tract and readily metabolized by the liver.

nadolol

Nadolol (Corgard) is a long-acting, nonselective beta-blocker. It is not well absorbed from the gastrointestinal tract, and up to one fourth of the dose may be excreted in the feces. Absorbed drug is excreted unchanged in the urine. The dosage interval is increased for patients with renal failure.

penbutolol

Penbutolol (Levatol) is a short-acting, nonselective beta-blocker. It is well absorbed and highly protein bound. The drug is excreted unchanged in the urine.

pindolol

Pindolol (Visken) is a short-acting, nonselective beta-blocker. It is well absorbed and metabolized by the liver.

propranolol

Propranolol (Inderal), a nonselective beta-blocker, is the oldest of the clinically used beta-blocking drugs. It is well absorbed orally, but it is readily metabolized by the liver.

sotalol

Sotalol (Betapace, Sotacor) is a nonselective beta-blocker. It is well absorbed and excreted primarily unchanged in the urine. The interval between doses must be increased for patients with impaired renal function.

timolol

Timolol (Apo-Timolol, Blocadren) is a short-acting nonselective beta-blocker. It is well absorbed from the gastrointestinal tract and metabolized by the liver.

Calcium Channel Blockers
General Characteristics

Calcium channel blockers, also called calcium antagonists or calcium entry blockers, are a class of drugs currently used in the treatment of angina, certain arrhythmias (see Chapter 19), and hypertension (see Chapter 13).

Mechanism of Action

Skeletal muscle has extensive stores of calcium in the sarcoplasmic reticulum, but both cardiac muscle and vascular smooth muscle lack these stores and must depend on the influx of extracellular calcium for the maintenance of contraction, or tone. The calcium channel blockers interfere with the initial influx of calcium through specific calcium channels on the cell surface.

At least four types of voltage-activated calcium channels have been described: L, T, N, and P. The L-type calcium channels are located on cardiac and smooth muscle and are the site of action of most calcium channel blockers. The T-type of calcium channel is associated mainly with the heart and especially in association with growth and remodeling of the heart and blood vessels.

Pharmacokinetics

Calcium channel blockers are administered orally for prophylactic treatment of angina. They are generally metabolized by the liver, with metabolites being excreted in the urine and sometimes the feces through biliary excretion.

Uses

Prophylactic Treatment of Angina. The calcium channel blockers decrease the oxygen requirements of the heart through several actions. They reduce peripheral vascular resistance by a systemic vasodilation. This means that the workload of the heart is decreased. Calcium channel blockers dilate the coronary vessels by inhibiting contractility of coronary smooth muscle. This action is especially important for relief from variant angina, in which coronary spasm prevents blood flow. However, it is becoming clear that there is a varying degree of coronary spasm even in classic angina. Patients with asthma, diabetes, and peripheral vascular disease who cannot tolerate beta-blockers can benefit from calcium channel blockers. The calcium channel blockers also reduce the cardiac contractility (negative inotropy), which decreases the oxygen requirement of the heart. These agents increase coronary blood flow through coronary vasodilation more selectively than they inhibit cardiac contractility. Without this selective preference, the calcium channel blockers would not be clinically useful because they would overly compromise cardiac function. The various drugs of this class differ in the degree of selectivity in coronary vasodilation versus decreased cardiac contractility.

Antihypertensive Therapy. The vasodilator effect of calcium channel blockers makes them useful antihypertensive agents. (See Chapter 13 for a complete discussion.)

Antiarrhythmic Therapy. Verapamil and diltiazem are used to treat supraventricular tachyarrhythmias.

Adverse Reactions and Contraindications

In general, the side effects of calcium channel blockers are mild. Headaches, light-headedness, and constipation are the most common ones. Some patients may feel unusually tired or weak. Side effects that require medical attention include difficulty in breathing, skin rash, heart rate less that 50 beats/min or an irregular or pounding heartbeat, or edema in the lower limbs.

Interactions

There are several important interactions of calcium channel blockers with other drugs. Beta-blockers and calcium channel blockers, if given concurrently, may cause cardiac problems, including a conduction block or arrhythmias and hypotension. Diltiazem and verapamil may inhibit the liver metabolism of several drugs, including carbamazepine, cyclosporine, quinidine, theophylline, and valproate. This may allow these drugs to reach toxic levels in the body. Digitalis glycosides may also accumulate in the presence of calcium channel blockers, resulting in excessive slowing of the heart or a heart block. Disopyramide depresses the force of the heartbeat (negative inotropic effect) and should not be administered within 48 hours of a calcium channel blocker.

Specific Calcium Channel Blockers

Seven calcium channel blockers are currently approved in the United States for use in the treatment of angina: amlodipine (Norvasc), bepridil (Vascor), diltiazem (Cardizem), nicardipine (Cardene), nifedipine (Aldalat, Procardia), and verapamil (Calan, Isoptin). Felodipine (Plendil, Renedil) and isradipine (DynaCirc) are also used as antianginals. Calcium channel blockers used in the treatment of hypertension are covered in Chapter 13.

bepridil

Bepridil (Vascor) is a nonselective calcium channel blocker that affects both cardiac and smooth muscle. It is used for the management of angina. It is rapidly absorbed. The 24-hour duration of action allows once-a-day dosage.

diltiazem

Diltiazem (Cardizem) produces cardiac effects similar to those produced by verapamil. The incidence of dizziness, headache, and hypotension is less with diltiazem than with nifedipine and verapamil.

Diltiazem is well absorbed orally and has a duration of action of 4 to 8 hours. Extended-release capsules are available. Diltiazem is extensively metabolized; metabolites are excreted in the urine (35%) and in the feces (65%).

▼ amlodipine, felodipine, isradipine, nicardipine, and nifedipine

Amlodipine (Norvasc), felodipine (Plendil), isradipine (DynaCirc), nicardipine (Cardene), and **nifedipine** (Adalat,

Procardia) are calcium channel blockers chemically related as dihydopyridines. Dihydopyridines are selective for vascular smooth muscle and are potent coronary and peripheral vasodilators. They act selectively at L-type calcium channels. The cardiodepressant effect of dihydropyridines is minor because they do not depress the sinoatrial or atrioventricular nodes and because reflex sympathetic activity caused by hypotension counteracts the negative inotropic effect. The hypotensive effect can be accompanied by a reflex tachycardia. If combined with a beta-blocker, these calcium channel blockers may produce excessive hypotension and rarely heart failure.

Dihydropyridines are well absorbed orally. Felodipine has a 24-hour duration of action and isradipine more than 12 hours. Nicardipine and nifedipine have a 4- to 8-hour duration of action, but nifedipine is available in extended-release forms for once-a-day dosage.

The side effects most commonly reported are related to peripheral vasodilation: headaches, hypotension, flushing, tingling in the extremities, and edema.

There are concerns that the immediate-release formulations of the dihydropyridines, especially nifedipine, nicardipine, and isradipine at high dosages, may increase mortality in cardiac disease. The physiologic basis is the reflex increase in sympathetic activity as a result of the marked hypotensive action of the of the dihydropyridines.

verapamil

Verapamil (Calan, Isoptin) depresses the atrioventricular node (negative chronotropism and negative dromotropism), an action that makes it a useful antiarrhythmic drug (see Chapter 19). A slowing of the heart rate (bradycardia) is common. Verapamil does not cause a pronounced decrease in blood pressure, and therefore reflex sympathetic activity to stimulate the heart is minimal. The slowing of the heart rate and the decrease in blood pressure reduce the oxygen requirements of the heart. Verapamil increases coronary blood flow, which increases the oxygen available to the heart.

Although verapamil is readily absorbed, it is rapidly metabolized by the liver. The tablet form must be taken three or four times a day, but extended-release tablets and capsules are available. Verapamil is generally well tolerated, with constipation being the most common side effect. Verapamil is contraindicated for patients with atrioventricular conduction disturbances or congestive heart failure.

Nursing Process Overview

Antianginal Drugs

Assessment

Patients with angina pectoris have a primary single complaint: chest pain. Obtain a thorough patient assessment, focusing on the subjective and objective signs. Determine the pulse, respiration, blood pressure, and level of conscious-ness. Question about the onset and duration of the pain, and ask about previous similar episodes and treatments. Obtain an electrocardiogram and appropriate laboratory work, including serum enzyme concentrations. When there is doubt about the cause of chest pain, the usual practice is to treat the patient as if a myocardial infarction has occurred.

Nursing Diagnoses
- Potential altered health maintenance related to insufficient knowledge about prescribed antianginal drugs
- Potential for injury related to orthostatic hypotension secondary to vasodilator therapy

Patient Outcomes
The patient will be able to use antianginal drugs as prescribed to treat or prevent attacks of angina. The patient will not experience side effects related to vasodilation or will demonstrate actions to lessen the problems with side effects, such as sitting down before using sublingual nitroglycerin. The patient will be able to explain any lifestyle changes prescribed.

Planning/Implementation
Administer drugs as ordered. Assess for further chest pain, monitor for drug side effects, and begin teaching the patient about the drugs in anticipation of the patient's discharge to home. Work with the patient and family to identify stresses that may precipitate angina attacks, and plan possible ways to decrease these stresses. Instruct the patient about other prescribed therapies: losing weight, stopping smoking, controlling blood pressure, and exercising regularly. Refer the patient as needed to the dietitian, the local heart association, or the visiting nurse association.

Evaluation
The drugs used to treat angina are successful if the pain is relieved and the patient experiences no side effects resulting from drug therapy. The drugs do not halt the progression of disease. Before the patient is discharged to home, determine that the patient can explain when and how to take the medications prescribed, can describe the drug side effects and how to treat them, and can explain what to do if drug therapy does not relieve the symptoms, how to correctly store the medication, and how to test for its continued effectiveness.

THERAPEUTIC RATIONALE: PERIPHERAL VASCULAR DISEASE

Vasospastic Disorders

Blood flow to the arms and legs, particularly the hands and feet, can be limited by peripheral vascular disease. Basically, the blood vessels may be narrowed by arteriosclerosis or by spasm of the vessels (vasospasm). If the vessel narrowing is a result of arteriosclerosis, vasodilator drugs are of little value. Vasodilator drugs may worsen the condition because vessels narrowed by arteriosclerosis do not dilate; adjacent vessels dilate and shunt the blood away from the occluded area. Blood flow in the occluded vessel therefore is reduced, not increased, by vasodilator drugs. On the other hand, if the narrowing of the vessel is a result of vasospasm, drugs are of benefit.

Raynaud's disease is the classic vasospastic disease in which primarily the fingers and toes are affected. In Raynaud's disease the blood vessels of the digits are readily thrown into spasm by cold or emotion and turn blue or white. Warming restores blood flow. Mild cases are best treated by having the patient dress warmly and avoid unnecessary cold exposure. Severe cases may be treated with a calcium channel blocker, usually nifedipine or diltiazem. Reserpine has also been used. Reserpine depresses sympathetic tone by depleting stored norepinephrine in the neurons. Other drugs that may bring relief include prazosin, methyldopa, guanethidine, and phenoxybenzamine. These drugs and their side effects are discussed fully in Chapter 13.

Impaired Cerebral Blood Flow

Vasodilators are sometimes prescribed to improve blood flow in the brain, particularly in older adult patients with arteriosclerosis of cerebral vessels who have had strokes or show signs of mental impairment. The problem is cerebral ischemia (insufficient oxygen to areas of the brain). Controlled medical trials are showing that this drug therapy is of little value. There is some medical opinion that vasodilator drugs may make the situation worse by shunting blood away from the unreactive, damaged vessels to areas with adequate blood flow already, as described for peripheral vascular insufficiency resulting from arteriosclerosis. Cyclandelate, ergoloid mesylates, and papaverine are sometimes prescribed to improve cerebral blood flow. There is no evidence that these drugs alter the progression of cerebral arteriosclerosis. They may improve some symptoms on a short-term basis.

THERAPEUTIC AGENTS: PERIPHERAL VASODILATORS

Unfortunately, a large number of "vasodilator" drugs advertised for treating peripheral vascular spasm are of doubtful clinical value. These drugs include cyclandelate, isoxsuprine, nicotinyl alcohol, nylidrin, and papaverine. However, the calcium channel blocker nimodipine has been shown effective in treating the neurologic problems associated with subarachnoid hemorrhage.

Specific Vasodilators

For summary information on specific vasodilators, refer to Table 15-2.

cyclandelate

Cyclandelate (Cyclospasmol) acts directly on vascular smooth muscle to cause relaxation. In the laboratory cyclandelate is a more effective vasodilator than papaverine,

ALTERNATIVE THERAPIES

Vasodilation

GINKGO
The drug consists of the dried leaves of *Ginkgo biloba* L. The active constituents of ginkgo include flavones, bioflavonoids, and diterpene lactones unique to ginkgo, such as ginkgolides A, B, C, and M. Of these, ginkgolide B is considered the most active. Most of the available information on the effects of ginkgo are based on studies of a specific, standardized extract of ginkgo leaf.

Ginkgo leaf extract exerts a vasodilatory effect on the vasculature and has been shown to enhance peripheral circulation in several conditions (e.g., varicose vessels, chronic cerebral insufficiency, short-term memory loss). Although these and other results are promising, more research is clearly warranted (*Br J Clin Pharm* 34:352-358, 1992).

The most common side effect reported for ginkgo extract are mild gastrointestinal disturbances. Rare side effects include headache, dizziness, and vertigo.

but the clinical effectiveness of cyclandelate is considered doubtful. Side effects include belching and heartburn, flushing, headache, weakness, and an increased heart rate.

ergoloid mesylates

Ergoloid mesylates (Hydergine) produce vasodilation in contrast to the ergot alkaloids, which produce vasoconstriction (see Chapter 71). Ergoloid mesylates are of definite value in treating brain disease secondary to hypertension, but the benefit is related to the fall in blood pressure. These alkaloids act centrally to reduce vascular tone and slow heart rate. They act peripherally to block alpha-adrenergic receptors. These alkaloids are available in a sublingual dosage form. Sublingual irritation, nausea, and gastrointestinal tract upset are the side effects. The dihydrogenated ergot alkaloids can markedly reduce heart rate through their central effect of lowering sympathetic tone.

isoxsuprine

Isoxsuprine (Vasodilan, Vasoprine) was originally thought to stimulate beta-receptors, but its vasodilating action is not blocked by drugs that are antagonists of the beta-receptors. Clinical tests have not demonstrated any usefulness for isoxsuprine. Side effects include flushing, hypotension, dizziness, an increased heart rate, and occasionally a rash.

nicotinyl alcohol

Nicotinyl alcohol (Ronigen, Rycotin) has been used as a vasodilator but without good evidence of clinical effectiveness. This drug causes a pronounced flushing, postural (orthostatic) hypotension, and gastrointestinal tract upset. It can also cause a rash.

Table 15-2 Vasodilator Drugs

Generic Name	Trade Name	Administration/Dosage	Comments
cyclandelate	Cyclospasmol†	ORAL: *Adults*—300-400 mg 4 times/day. Can be decreased gradually to 100-200 mg 4 times/day.	Direct vasodilator for use in vasospastic disorders may cause gastrointestinal tract disturbances.
ergoloid mesylates	Hydergine*	SUBLINGUAL, ORAL: *Adults*—1 mg 3 times/day.	Drug can cause marked bradycardia. It relieves symptoms in hypertensive brain disease by lowering blood pressure.
isoxsuprine	Vasodilan*	ORAL: *Adults*—10-20 mg 3-4 times/day. INTRAMUSCULAR: *Adults*—5-10 mg 2-3 times/day.	Drug is a direct-acting vasodilator with no proven use.
nicotinyl alcohol	Roniacol†	ORAL: *Adults*—50-100 mg 3 times/day. ORAL (timed-release): *Adults*—300-400 mg every 12 hr.	Drug is a direct vasodilator that causes pronounced blushing. Gastrointestinal tract disturbances, tingling sensation, and rashes are side effects. Use has not been proved effective for any vasospastic disorders.
nimodipine	Nimotop*	ORAL: *Adults*—60 mg every 4 hr, beginning within 4 days after subarachnoid hemorrhage and continuing for 21 days.	Calcium channel blocker treats cerebral vasospasm after subarachnoid hemorrhage.
nylidrin hydrochloride	Arlidin* PMS Nylidrin†	ORAL: *Adults*—3-12 mg 3-4 times/day.	Drug stimulates beta-adrenergic receptors and directly dilates vessels. It may cause dizziness, tachycardia, and hypotension.
papaverine hydrochloride	Many trade names	ORAL: *Adults*—100-300 mg 3-5 times/day. ORAL (timed-release): *Adults*—150 mg every 12 hr. Can give up to 150 mg every 8 hr or 300 mg every 12 hr. INTRAVENOUS: *Adults*—30-120 mg over 1-2 min. INTRAMUSCULAR: *Adults*—30-120 mg.	Drug depresses heart. It directly relaxes smooth muscle, particularly of large blood vessels. Use is to relieve smooth muscle spasm in vascular disease or colic. Its effectiveness has not been proved.
pentoxifylline	Trental*	ORAL: *Adults*—400 mg 3 times/day with meals.	Drug is not a vasodilator. It reduces blood viscosity and improves red blood cell flexibility to improve blood flow.

*Available in Canada and the United States.
†Available in Canada only.

nimodipine

Nimodipine (Nimotop) is a calcium channel blocker approved to treat cerebral vasospasm after a subarachnoid hemorrhage. This action alleviates the cerebral ischemia that can follow a stroke and, by maintaining blood flow, protects the brain from deterioration. This use of a calcium channel blocker is seen as the beginning of a new therapeutic approach for the treatment of various neurologic disorders. Calcium channel blockers for neurologic use cross the blood-brain barrier.

nylidrin

Nylidrin (Arlidin) is the classic example of a drug that stimulates blood flow in muscle. The rationale is to stimulate the beta-receptors of the blood vessels to produce vasodilation. However, blood vessels of the muscle, not the skin, have beta-receptors, so the approach is of little value in vasospastic disorders of the digits. The beta-blocker propranolol does not entirely reverse this stimulation, so nylidrin is believed to also act directly on smooth muscle. Side effects attributed to nylidrin include trembling, nervousness, weakness, dizziness, palpitations, and nausea and vomiting.

papaverine

Papaverine (various trade names) relaxes smooth muscle. In large doses papaverine also depresses cardiac muscle, slowing conduction and prolonging the refractory period.

Papaverine has long been used as a smooth muscle relaxant for ischemia of the brain, periphery, or heart. As with the other vasodilator drugs, there is little good evidence that papaverine improves peripheral vascular circulation. Side effects of papaverine can include flushing of the face, malaise, gastrointestinal tract upset, and headache. Other reported side effects include excess perspiration, loss of appetite, increased heart rate, and increased depth of respiration. Rarely, a hypersensitivity reaction involving the liver is seen. Symptoms of the liver damage may include jaundice, eosinophilia, and altered results of liver function tests.

Blood Viscosity–Reducing Drug: pentoxifylline

Pentoxifylline (Trental) is a different type of drug for the treatment of peripheral vascular disease. Pentoxifylline increases the flexibility of red blood cells and reduces blood viscosity. These actions improve blood flow through narrowed vessels. Pentoxifylline may improve the walking distance for some patients with intermittent claudication.

Side effects are rare but include dizziness, headache, nausea, and vomiting. Drug interactions include the potentiation of antihypertensive drugs. Smoking may interfere with the therapeutic action of pentoxifylline because nicotine constricts blood vessels. Toxic symptoms of pentoxifylline include excitement and seizures.

Nursing Process Overview

Vasodilator Therapy in Peripheral Vascular Disease

Assessment

Assess the patient, and obtain a history about onset and course of vascular disease. Assess the blood pressure and pulses, including peripheral pulses. Assess for altered sensation, poor healing of injuries on the feet, cool extremities, or symptoms of altered cerebral blood flow. Perform a mental status examination.

Nursing Diagnoses

- Potential for injury related to orthostatic hypotension associated with drug therapy
- Alteration in comfort: headache related to vasodilator therapy
- Alteration in comfort: nausea related to drug therapy

Patient Outcomes

The patient will be able to explain how to take prescribed medications correctly. The patient will demonstrate actions to minimize injury from side effects, such as sitting down when dizziness develops. The patient will be able to describe drug side effects and explain that some side effects will diminish with continued drug use. The patient will not discontinue medications without consulting the physician.

Planning/Implementation

Monitor the presenting signs and symptoms, especially blood pressure and pulses, and look for drug side effects. Instruct the patient about prescribed medications and begin teaching the patient about prevention of trauma to areas with decreased perfusion. Instruct the patient about other prescribed therapies: an exercise program, weight loss, and restriction of certain activities.

Evaluation

It is difficult to measure the effectiveness of these drugs. Before the patients discharge, determine that the patient can explain when and how to take the ordered medications, the side effects that might occur, and the situations that would require notification of the physician.

Nursing Implications Summary

Antianginal Drugs

Drug Administration

➤ In patients with chest pain, assess blood pressure and pulse; auscultate lungs and heart; assess intensity, duration, location, and quality of pain; assess response to medication; check for presence of diaphoresis, precipitating factors, electrocardiographic changes, or subjective and objective degree of patient distress; and obtain patient history. Chest pain in the person with a history of angina pectoris may have other causes.

➤ In the hospital it is often customary to keep a small supply of sublingual nitroglycerin tablets at the bedside of patients with a history of angina pectoris. Instruct patients to use as needed but to notify the nurse when tablets are used. Record the frequency of use, as well as a patient assessment, in the nurses' notes. Count and replenish the tablets each shift.

Nursing in the Community

➤ Encourage the patient to make all recommended lifestyle changes, including losing weight to reach desirable body weight, lowering cholesterol levels, ceasing smoking, and engaging in a regular exercise program after approval by the physician. Assist the patient and family in identifying activities that trigger anginal attacks such as eating a heavy meal, engaging in strenuous physical activities, lifting heavy objects, being exposed to cold weather, and having sex. Work with the patient to develop ways to decrease the frequency of attacks or to decrease the likelihood that activities will cause anginal pain to develop.

➤ Encourage the patient to notify the physician if the frequency, intensity, duration, location of pain, or response to antianginal drugs changes. Instruct the patient to avoid the use of alcohol because it potentiates the hypotensive effects of the nitrates and nitrites. Remind the patient to keep all health care providers informed of all drugs being used because diuretics, antihypertensives, CNS depressants, narcotics, and sedatives may potentiate the hypotensive effects of the antianginal drugs. Encourage the patient to maintain regular contact with the primary health care provider and not to stop drug therapy without medical consultation.

➤ If a headache regularly occurs when antianginal drugs are taken, it may indicate too high a dosage. For some patients it may be necessary to use mild analgesics with antianginal therapy; consult the physician.

Nitrates

Drug Administration

Intravenous nitroglycerin

➤ Consult the manufacturer's literature for specific instructions about dilution, dosage, and administration. Use a microdrip infusion set and a volume control or rate-controlling device to prevent overdosage and to accurately titrate the dose. Nitroglycerin migrates into plastic tubing. Dilutions should be prepared and kept in glass bottles. Use nonpolyvinyl chloride tubing. Monitor the blood pressure, heart rate, electrocardiographic changes, and pulmonary capillary wedge pressure (PCWP). Use intravenous

Nursing Implications Summary—cont'd

nitroglycerin only in settings where drugs and experienced personnel to treat cardiovascular emergencies are available.

Buccal Extended-Release Forms

➤ For buccal extended-release tablets, place the dose between the cheek and upper gum or between the upper lip and gum and allow it to dissolve over 5 hours. When eating or drinking, place the dose between the upper lip and gum. If the patient wears dentures, place the tablet between the cheek and gum. Tell the patient not to use chewing tobacco while using this form. Replace the tablet if it is accidentally swallowed. Tell the patient not to go to sleep with a tablet still in the mouth. Sublingual erythrityl tetranitrate, isosorbide dinitrate, and nitroglycerin tablets may also be administered buccally.

Chewable Tablets

➤ For chewable tablets, instruct the patient to chew it well, then hold it in the mouth for at least 2 minutes before swallowing. Instruct the patient not to drink, smoke, eat, or chew tobacco while using this form.

Extended-Release Capsules and Tablets

➤ Instruct the patient to swallow extended-release capsules whole, without chewing, crushing, or breaking.

Lingual Aerosol Forms

➤ Review the patient instruction leaflet supplied by the manufacturer. To use, remove the cover. Do not shake the container. Hold the container upright, close to the patients mouth. Spray 1 or 2 sprays (as prescribed by the physician) under the tongue. Close the mouth. Avoid swallowing for 1 or 2 minutes. This drug may be used like nitroglycerin tablets: when an attack of angina occurs, the patient should administer a dose as prescribed. If no relief is obtained in 5 minutes, the patient should repeat the dose. If there is no relief in another 5 minutes, the patient should repeat the dose. If no relief occurs after a total of 3 doses in 15 minutes, the patient should seek medical attention or notify the physician. The prescription may be modified for individual patient needs and by physician preference.

Topical Transdermal Forms

➤ Review the patient instruction leaflet supplied by the manufacturer. Do not trim or cut the adhesive patch. Remove the previous patch before applying a new patch. Rotate sites to avoid skin irritation. Apply the patch to an area that is clean and dry, with little or no hair. Avoid scratches, scars, or existing skin irritation. If the patch loosens or falls off, replace it with a new one. Side effects are the same as for other antianginal drugs in this group. Transdermal forms should not be used to treat an acute attack of angina. Tolerance to this therapy may be lessened if the patches are not used continuously; some physicians may prescribe a patch-free period each day (e.g., during the night).

Topical Ointments

➤ Review the patient instruction leaflet supplied by the manufacturer. Remove the ointment from a previous dose before applying a fresh dose. Measure the prescribed amount of ointment, using the measuring paper supplied by the manufacturer. Gently spread the ointment over a small area of about the same size each time with the measuring paper or small applicator (not the fingertips). Do not massage the ointment into the skin. Apply to areas with little or no hair. Avoid scratches and scars. Rotate sites to avoid skin irritation. Cover the area with plastic kitchen wrap or other dressing only if ordered by the physician. If a dressing is prescribed, it should be used each time the drug is used. If a dose is missed, apply it as soon as remembered, unless it is within 2 hours of the next dose, then follow the usual dosing schedule. Do not use more ointment than ordered and do not double up for missed doses.

Nursing in the Community

➤ If syncope (fainting), dizziness, or hypotension occurs with nitrate or nitrite use, instruct the patient to lie down before taking the prescribed dose of medication. Ascertain that the patient can correctly use sublingual drug forms before the patients discharge. This may be a new dosage form for the patient. In addition, teach the family how to place a dose under the patient's tongue in the event the patient cannot do it. Tell the patient not to eat, drink, chew tobacco, or smoke while the dose is dissolving.

➤ Review the standard instructions with the patient and family for antianginal agents used to relieve an attack of angina. When chest pain develops, the patient should sit down, then use one tablet, letting it dissolve under the tongue or in the cheek, or chew a chewable tablet. If relief is not obtained, the patient should repeat the dose in 5 minutes and again in another 5 minutes if needed, for a total of 3 tablets. If the pain persists after 3 tablets, the patient should notify the physician or seek medical help. These guidelines may be individualized based on the patient, the patient's condition, and the physician's preference.

➤ Instruct the patient to take oral nitrates with meals or a snack to reduce gastric irritation. Review the ordered drugs carefully with the patient, as well as exactly how and when to take the prescribed drugs, because many dosages and drug forms are available for these drugs.

➤ Storage instructions for these drugs include keeping drugs out of the reach of children and not storing in the bathroom or near the kitchen sink or other damp areas. Check expiration dates and replace drugs as needed. For sublingual nitroglycerin, follow the previous instructions and keep tablets in the original glass container. Once the bottle is opened, remove the cotton and do not replace it. Replace the cap tightly and quickly each time the bottle is opened. Do not put other medicines in the same bottle with the nitroglycerin. When pouring a dose (a tablet), pour one or more tablets into the lid of the bottle, take the dose out, and return remaining tablets to the bottle. Avoid replacing tablets from the palm of the hand into the bottle. Instruct the patient to obtain a small glass bottle from the pharmacist for carrying a small number of pills. Do not carry the small bottle too

Continued

Nursing Implications Summary—cont'd

close to the body because body warmth may cause the pills to lose their strength.

➤ To prevent an attack of angina, instruct patients to take the prescribed drug before engaging in the activity expected to produce anginal pain. For sublingual or chewable forms, this may be 5 to 10 minutes before engaging in such activities; for extended-release forms, patients may need to take the antianginal drug several hours before the activity. For specific patient needs, consult the physician.

➤ If doses are missed, instruct patients to take the dose as soon as remembered, unless within 2 hours of the next dose (extended-release forms or isosorbide dinitrate). Do not double up for missed doses.

Beta-Blockers
➤ See Nursing Implications Summary in Chapter 13.

Calcium Channel Blockers
Drug Administration
➤ Assess the patient with complaints of chest pain for intensity, duration, location, and quality of pain; response to medications; presence of diaphoresis; vital signs, blood pressure, and electrocardiographic changes; precipitating factors; patient history; auscultation of heart and lung sounds; and other subjective complaints. Chest pain in the patient with a history of angina pectoris may be due to other causes also.

➤ In patients taking calcium channel blockers, monitor the blood pressure, pulse, intake and output, and weight. Signs of fluid retention are peripheral edema and subjective complaints of tight shoes and rings. Signs of heart failure include dyspnea on exertion, distended jugular veins, orthopnea, or moist rales on pulmonary auscultation.

➤ If calcium channel blockers are prescribed for hypertension, see the general guidelines for patients receiving antihypertensives in Chapter 13.

bepridil
➤ Encourage the patient to take doses with meals or at bedtime if nausea is a problem.

nifedipine
➤ To administer sublingually or intrabuccally, puncture the fluid-filled capsule and squeeze the drug into the mouth. The patient may chew the capsule to break it and direct the contents to the cheek or under the tongue.

diltiazem
➤ Administer intravenous (IV) doses undiluted for at least 2 minutes in the adult. Monitor the electrocardiographic changes and the blood pressure. Diltiazem may also be diluted and administered as an infusion. See the manufacturers literature for various dilutions. Use microdrip tubing or an infusion control device to help maintain an even infusion. Monitor blood pressure, pulse, and electrocardiographic changes.

verapamil
➤ Administer IV doses undiluted over at least 2 minutes in the adult and 3 minutes in the older adult patient. Monitor the electrocardiographic changes and the blood pressure.

Nursing in the Community
➤ See the Patient Problems boxes for orthostatic hypotension (see Chapter 13) and constipation (see Chapter 24).

➤ If appropriate, teach the patient to take and record the pulse daily at home. Instruct the patient to report a change of 10 beats/min in the resting pulse or a pulse rate less than 50 beats/min. Appropriate candidates for such instruction may be those on multiple-drug regimens or those in whom control of side effects has been difficult. If appropriate, instruct the patient to monitor and record weight on a regular basis. Instruct patients to report a weight gain of greater than 2 lb/day or 5 lb/wk. Instruct the patient to report the development of tight rings, shoes, or clothing or signs of peripheral edema.

➤ Because of potential drug interactions with other medication, instruct the patient to keep all health care providers informed of all drugs being used. Instruct the patient to avoid the use of any over-the-counter preparations unless first cleared by the physician. In addition to using these drugs as prescribed, the patient may find additional relief by losing weight, stopping smoking, limiting caffeine intake, avoiding extremes of temperature, and becoming involved in a regular exercise program. The patient should consult the physician.

➤ Emphasize to the patient the importance of taking these drugs as prescribed and not discontinuing them without consultation with the physician. If a dose is missed, instruct the patient to take the missed dose as soon as remembered, but not within 2 hours of the next scheduled dose. Instruct the patient not to double up for missed doses.

➤ Headache may develop after a dose of medication is taken but will last only a short time. This side effect should gradually diminish with continued use of the drug. Instruct the patient to report any signs of liver problems such as right upper quadrant abdominal pain, jaundice, change in color or consistency of stools, fever, or malaise.

➤ The calcium channel blockers may cause tender gums or swelling or bleeding gums. Encourage the patient to have regular dental examinations. Review oral hygiene practices; encourage regular flossing and brushing. If gum problems develop, the patient should check with the physician or dentist.

➤ Instruct the patient to swallow extended-release capsules or tablets whole, without crushing or chewing. Instruct the patient using extended-release diltiazem capsules to check with the physician before changing brands of medication; the different brands should be given on different dosing schedules. Instruct the patient to take extended-release verapamil tablets whole, without chewing or crushing,

Nursing Implications Summary—cont'd

unless the physician has authorized breaking extended-release verapamil tablets in half.

Peripheral Vasodilators
Drug Administration
➤ Monitor the blood pressure and pulse when beginning therapy or when changing doses.

isoxsuprine
➤ Intramuscular (IM) doses of isoxsuprine may cause hypotension and tachycardia. Monitor the blood pressure and pulse.
➤ If isoxsuprine is used to prevent labor, monitor intensity, frequency, and duration of uterine contractions. Monitor fetal heart rate at regular intervals.

nimodipine
➤ See the nursing interventions for calcium channel blockers discussed earlier in this chapter. For patients who cannot swallow, withdraw the fluid from within the capsule and administer via a feeding tube, followed by 30 ml of 0.9% sodium chloride. To withdraw dose, puncture both ends of the capsule with an 18-gauge needle and withdraw fluid into a syringe.

papaverine
➤ Administer IV doses of papaverine undiluted at a rate of 30 mg or less over 2 minutes. IM injection is preferred. Monitor the electrocardiographic changes, pulse, respiration, and blood pressure during IV administration and for 1 hour afterward.

Nursing in the Community
➤ Instruct the patient to take doses with meals or antacids to diminish gastrointestinal tract symptoms. Review information about orthostatic hypotension with the patient (see Patient Problems box in Chapter 13). Hypotension may be potentiated in patients receiving vasodilators who are also receiving other drugs that can cause hypotension such as diuretics, antihypertensives, CNS depressants, narcotics, and sedatives. Instruct the patient to keep all health care providers informed of all medications being taken.
➤ Instruct the patient to avoid the use of alcohol because it potentiates the hypotensive effects of vasodilators. Instruct the patient to avoid smoking, which reduces peripheral blood flow.
➤ Instruct the patient to swallow timed-release formulations whole, without chewing or crushing. Encourage the patient to maintain desirable body weight to help decrease symptoms from peripheral vascular disease. Warn the patient that nicotinyl alcohol, pentoxifylline, or papaverine may produce pronounced flushing, which is not harmful. Caution the patient to avoid driving or operating hazardous equipment if side effects such as dizziness, weakness, drowsiness, or double vision occur.
➤ Encourage the patient to take peripheral vasodilators as prescribed. Regular long-term use may be necessary for full benefit to occur. Instruct the patient to take missed doses as soon as remembered, unless within 2 hours of the next dose. Do not double up for missed doses.
➤ Nylidrin may cause palpitations, especially if taken at bedtime. Work with the patient to develop a dosage schedule that avoids taking the last dose at bedtime.
➤ Papaverine or phentolamine may be used to produce erections in some impotent men. The patient should clean off the base of the penis with alcohol and inject the prescribed dose into the base of the penis as instructed by the physician. After injection, the patient should massage the penis and attempt intercourse within 2 hours. Teach the patient to consult the physician if the erection lasts more than 4 hours, the erection is painful, there is bleeding at the injection site that does not stop after pressure is applied, a lump develops where the medication was injected, or the penis is becoming curved.
➤ Instruct patients taking pentoxifylline to avoid the use of aspirin or aspirin-containing products while taking this drug. Assess patients for hypersensitivity or intolerance to methylxanthines before administering pentoxifylline. Methylxanthines include caffeine, theophylline, and theobromine (the active ingredients in coffee, tea, and chocolate). Pentoxifylline is contraindicated in persons with intolerance to methylxanthines.

CHAPTER REVIEW

Application

1. What is the origin of angina? Describe the differences between classic (exertional) angina, variant angina, and unstable angina.
2. How do the nitrates relieve angina?
3. How do the beta-blockers relieve angina? What are their side effects?
4. How do the calcium channel blockers relieve angina?
5. What are two causes of insufficient blood flow to the digits? Which cause is amenable to drug therapy? What role do vasodilators play?
6. List the seven drugs used as vasodilators for improving peripheral circulation. What are some of their common side effects?

Critical Thinking

1. How might the type of angina influence a teaching plan for a patient?
2. Outline the main teaching points for patients taking nitrates.
3. For which patients are the cardioselective beta-blockers especially indicated?
4. What would you include in the teaching plan for a patient taking a beta-blocker?
5. Why are calcium channel blockers especially effective for variant angina?
6. What would you teach a patient about the calcium channel blockers?

Drugs to Treat Hypotension and Shock

KEY TERMS

anaphylactic shock, p. 195
reflex bradycardia, p. 196
shock, p. 193
sympathomimetic drugs, p. 193

KEY DRUGS ▼

dopamine, p. 195
epinephrine, p. 195

OBJECTIVES

After studying this chapter, you should be able to do the following:

■ *Discuss the use of sympathomimetic amines in the treatment of shock.*

■ *Develop nursing care plans for patients receiving sympathomimetic amines.*

CHAPTER OVERVIEW

Shock is the result when too little blood flows through vital organs of the body. This chapter reviews the use of sympathomimetic drugs maintain blood pressure. Hypotension is low blood pressure.

THERAPEUTIC RATIONALE: SHOCK AND HYPOTENSION

Shock is a disruption of circulation. Often, the blood pressure is too low to force blood through vital tissues. Poor perfusion of the brain results in confusion or coma; poor perfusion of the kidney results in low urine output (less than 30 ml/hr); and poor perfusion of the skin makes the skin cold and clammy. In shock, the body has already activated the sympathetic nervous system to increase blood pressure. Fluid replacement or fluid addition is often the first choice in treating shock to overcome the decrease in the circulating volume caused by the constriction of the peripheral blood vessels. Selected use of direct-acting sympathomimetic amines is made in treating certain types of shock, raising blood pressure by increasing peripheral resistance (activation of alpha₁-adrenergic receptors) or by increasing cardiac output (activation of beta₁-adrenergic receptors).

Orthostatic hypotension is a decrease of 20 mm Hg in systolic or 10 mm Hg diastolic blood pressure for at least 3 minutes on rising to a standing position. Elderly persons often have a sluggish baroreflexor response that leads to hypotension on rising. However, the person can change from a lying to a standing position slowly so that blood pressure can adjust adequately. Orthostatic hypotension is a result of autonomic dysfunction. The cause may be primary but often is secondary to drugs such as those taken to control severe hypertension or from spinal anesthesia or secondary to nerve disorders caused by such diseases as diabetes or alcoholism.

THERAPEUTIC AGENTS: DIRECT-ACTING SYMPATHOMIMETIC DRUGS

As discussed in Chapter 12, the sympathetic nervous system plays a major role in controlling cardiovascular function. Stimulation of the alpha-adrenergic receptors of blood vessels causes vasoconstriction. On a systemic level, this vasoconstriction shows up as a higher blood pressure. Stimulation of the cardiac beta₁-receptors increases heart rate and force of contraction, resulting in an increased cardiac output. Stimulation of the beta₂-receptors, found primarily in the blood vessels of the skeletal muscle, causes vasodilation. Only in unusual circumstances, however, does systemic stimulation of the beta₂-receptors decrease blood pressure. The net change in cardiovascular function produced by direct-acting **sympathomimetic drugs** depends on the degree of activity at the three adrenergic receptor subtypes. For summary information on sympathomimetic drugs, refer to Table 16-1.

Table 16-1 Sympathomimetic Drugs Used to Treat Hypotension and Shock

Generic Name	Trade Name	Administration/Dosage	Comments
dobutamine hydrochloride	Dobutrex*	INTRAVENOUS: *Adults*—2.5-10 μg/kg/min. A 12.5-25 mg/ml solution is made and used. Onset: 1-2 min. Duration: 5 min.	Stimulates cardiac contractility in cardiogenic shock.
dopamine hydrochloride	Intropin*	INTRAVENOUS: *Adults*—1 ampule (40 mg of chloride salt in 5 ml) is diluted in 250 ml (800 μg/ml) or 500 ml (400 μg/ml) of solution. Initial intravenous infusion is 2-5 μg/kg/min. Onset: 5 min. Duration: 10 min. FDA pregnancy category C.	Maintains renal blood flow in shock with mild cardiac stimulation.
ephedrine	Generic	INTRAMUSCULAR, SUBCUTANEOUS: *Adults*—25 or 50 mg. FDA pregnancy category C. INTRAVENOUS, SUBCUTANEOUS: *Children*—0.75 mg/kg body weight or 25 mg/m² body surface.	Maintains blood pressure during spinal or general anesthesia.
epinephrine hydrochloride	Adrenalin chloride*	INTRAVENOUS: *Adults*—*For vasopressor response*: Infuse 1 μg/min. May increase dose to 2-10 μg/min for desired response. Onset: minutes. Duration: 1-4 hr. FDA pregnancy category C.	Treats anaphylactic shock. Higher doses are used to treat cardiac arrest.
isoproterenol hydrochloride	Isuprel hydrochloride*	INTRAVENOUS: *Adults*—1-2 mg (5-10 ml) diluted in D5W and infused at rate of 2-10 μg/min. Onset: minutes. Duration: 10 min. FDA pregnancy category C.	Stimulates cardiac contractility.
levarterenol (norepinephrine) bitartrate	Levophed bitartrate*	INTRAVENOUS: *Adults*—2-8 ml of 0.2% solution in 500 ml D5W and given by continuous infusion for desired response. Onset: immediate. Duration: minutes. FDA pregnancy category C.	Maintains blood pressure in life-threatening situations.
mephentermine sulfate	Wyamine sulfate	INTRAVENOUS: *Adults*—1 g is diluted in 1 L D5W and given by continuous infusion to maintain pressure. Onset: immediate. Duration: 15-30 min. FDA pregnancy category C.	Maintains arterial blood pressure during spinal, epidural, or general anesthesia.
metaraminol bitartrate	Aramine	INTRAVENOUS: *Adults*—*For hypotension*: 15-100 mg (base) in 500 ml NS or D5W given by continuous infusion to maintain pressure. Onset: 1-2 min. Duration: 20-60 min. FDA pregnancy category C.	Maintains blood pressure during spinal, epidural, or general anesthesia.
methoxamine hydrochloride	Vasoxyl*	INTRAMUSCULAR, INTRAVENOUS: *Adults*—5-20 mg in a single intramuscular dose or 3-5 mg intravenously (slow IV). Onset: 1-2 min (IV), 10 min (IM). Duration: 5-15 min (IV), 60-90 min (IM). FDA pregnancy category C.	Maintains blood pressure during spinal and general anesthesia. Controls hypotension after ganglionic blockade.
midodrine	ProAmatine	ORAL: *Adults*—10 mg 3 times/day in about 4-hr intervals during the day. Duration 4-6 hr. FDA pregnancy category C.	New drug to treat orthostatic hypotension.
phenylephrine hydrochloride	Neo-Synephrine hydrochloride*	INTRAMUSCULAR, SUBCUTANEOUS, INTRAVENOUS: *Adults*—2-5 mg intramuscularly or subcutaneously, repeated every 10-15 min if necessary; 0.2 mg given intravenously or 10 mg in 500 ml D5W infused slowly. Onset: very rapid. Duration: 5-20 min (IV), 45-60 min (IM,SC). FDA pregnancy category C.	Maintains blood pressure during general and spinal anesthesia.

*Available in Canada and the United States.
†Available in Canada only.

dobutamine

Mechanisms of Action

At low dosages, dobutamine (Dobutrex), like dopamine, will selectively increase the contractility of the heart without increasing the heart rate. Dobutamine neither stimulates the dopamine receptors of the kidney blood vessels nor releases norepinephrine. At high dosages, dobutamine does increase heart rate and conduction velocity (beta$_1$-adrenergic receptor) and stimulates beta$_2$-adrenergic receptors.

Pharmacokinetics

Dobutamine has a plasma half-life of about 2 minutes and must be administered by continuous intravenous (IV) infusion. Dobutamine is rapidly metabolized to inactive compounds in the liver.

Uses

Dobutamine improves cardiac output in patients with congestive heart failure with little effect on heart rate or systolic blood pressure.

Adverse Reactions and Contraindications

Increased heart rate and blood pressure are the most common side effects and can be reversed by lowering the infusion rate. Palpitations, shortness of breath, angina, nausea, and headache are less common side effects of dobutamine.

Dobutamine is contraindicated for patients in whom the increased force of contraction would be dangerous, as in idiopathic hypertrophic subaortic stenosis.

Interactions

Drugs that may sensitize the heart to the inotropic effects of dobutamine include hydrocarbon inhalation anesthetics and the reserpine antihypertensives. Dobutamine may block the effectiveness of the beta-blockers and several other antihypertensive agents: guanadrel, guanethidine, and nitroprusside.

▼ dopamine

Mechanism of Action

Dopamine (Dopastat, Intropin) is a naturally occurring catecholamine capable of acting at alpha- and beta-adrenergic receptors, as well as at its own specific dopaminergic receptors. Appropriate doses of this catecholamine can be selected such that cardiac output is increased while heart rate and mean blood pressure remain unchanged. The unusual and highly desirable property of dopamine is that renal blood flow is directly stimulated at these same doses. Renal function may therefore be maintained in patients being treated for shock as long as supportive therapy maintains adequate blood volume.

Pharmacokinetics

Dopamine must be administered by constant IV infusion. Dopamine is rapidly taken up and stored or destroyed by tissues. The infusion rate must be meticulously adjusted to achieve the desired therapeutic results.

Uses

Dopamine is the most widely used sympathomimetic amine for treating shock. The action of dopamine may be controlled by the rate of infusion. Dopamine is used primarily as a renal vasodilator to prevent renal failure in shock and secondarily to increase cardiac output. At low dosages (0.5 to 2 μg/kg/min), dopamine acts exclusively on dopamine receptors in the renal arterioles to cause vasodilation. At higher dosages (1 to 10 μg/kg/min), dopamine acts at cardiac beta$_1$-receptors to stimulate cardiac contractility. The beta$_1$-receptors controlling heart rate and the alpha-receptors controlling blood pressure are not activated. At dosages higher than these, dopamine causes the release of norepinephrine, thereby increasing heart rate and blood pressure.

Adverse Reactions and Contraindications

Dopamine can cause tachycardia (fast heart rate), palpitation, nausea and vomiting, angina, headache, hypertension, and vasoconstriction. A reduction or discontinuance of dopamine infusion is usually sufficient to reverse side effects because dopamine has such a short plasma half-life. Leakage of dopamine around the infusion site must be avoided, but if extravasation does occur, the alpha-adrenergic receptor antagonist phentolamine should be infused into the area to reverse vasoconstriction. Untreated extravasation can cause tissue death and sloughing.

Like the other sympathomimetic amines, dopamine is contraindicated for patients predisposed to cardiac arrhythmias.

Interactions

Dopamine is not stable in alkaline solutions and should not be made up in a sodium bicarbonate solution. Patients medicated with a monoamine oxidase inhibitor require only 10% of the usual dose of dopamine. Tricyclic antidepressants potentiate the hypertensive action of dopamine. Dopamine should not be administered to women in labor receiving an oxytocic drug because a severe persistent hypertension may be produced. Patients receiving one of the general anesthetics that sensitize the heart to catecholamines may develop arrhythmias if dopamine is administered. Because dopamine dilates renal arteries, the action of diuretic drugs is potentiated.

▼ epinephrine

Mechanism of Action

Epinephrine is a potent agonist of the beta$_1$-receptors of the heart, increasing heart rate and force of contraction. This cardiac stimulation is achieved with an increase in the oxygen demand of the heart, which may not be tolerable in cardiac disease. Epinephrine also stimulates alpha-receptors to cause vasoconstriction, particularly of the vessels in the skin, mucosa, kidney, and visceral organs. Epinephrine also stimulates beta$_2$-receptors, which alter blood flow because the receptors mediate vasodilation in the blood vessels in skeletal muscle. The overall response to IV administration of epinephrine is a marked increase in heart rate and force of contraction with little or no increase in blood pressure.

Pharmacokinetics

Epinephrine is not active when given orally because it is rapidly inactivated by the gastric mucosa. Epinephrine is administered intramuscularly or subcutaneously. Epinephrine may be inhaled from a nebulizer for relief of bronchospasm. IV administration of epinephrine must be done very slowly and cannot be done using one of the epinephrine suspensions. Intracardiac injection of epinephrine is a last step in attempting cardiac resuscitation when other measures have failed.

Epinephrine is rapidly degraded by monoamine oxidase and catechol *O*-methyltransferase of the liver and kidney. Epinephrine is unstable in alkaline solutions and when exposed to light or air. Pink or brown solutions should not be used.

Uses

Epinephrine, administered as soon as possible, is the drug of choice for treating **anaphylactic shock**. Anaphylactic shock is the result of massive histamine release caused by an allergic reaction and must be promptly treated. Histamine causes profound vasodilation and bronchial constriction. Epinephrine opposes the actions of histamine: epinephrine produces vasoconstriction, raising the blood pressure, and relaxes the bronchioles, restoring breathing. Epinephrine quickly reverses the edema of the larynx and the bronchospasm of anaphylactic shock.

Epinephrine is used to stimulate cardiac function when resuscitating a patient from cardiac arrest.

Epinephrine may be administered systemically or by inhalation for relief of bronchospasm resulting from asthma or allergic reactions. Because epinephrine causes vasoconstriction, it is applied topically as a hemostatic agent. Epinephrine injection prolongs the action of local anesthetics by slowing their systemic absorption.

Adverse Reactions and Contraindications

Fear and anxiety are side effects of epinephrine arising from stimulation of the central nervous system. Other side effects include a throbbing headache, dizziness, and pallor caused by vasoconstriction. Stimulation of skeletal muscle causes tremor and weakness, and stimulation of the heart causes palpitation. These effects are usually transient. Hyperthyroid and hypertensive patients are prone to an exaggerated hypertensive response to epinephrine. Cerebral hemorrhage and cardiac arrhythmias are serious reactions to epinephrine.

Epinephrine is contraindicated for patients receiving a general anesthetic that sensitizes the heart to catecholamines. Neither patients with narrow-angle glaucoma nor women in labor should receive epinephrine. Epinephrine must be used with extreme care in patients with cardiac arrhythmias, cardiovascular disease, hypertension, or hyperthyroidism. The hyperglycemic, hypoinsulinemic effects of epinephrine will interrupt control of diabetes mellitus.

Interactions

Epinephrine should not be administered simultaneously with isoproterenol because the combination can cause cardiac arrhythmias. Cardiac effects of epinephrine are also potentiated by tricyclic antidepressants, antihistamines, thyroxine, digitalis, and mercurial diuretics. A hypertensive response to epinephrine may be seen in patients receiving a monoamine oxidase inhibitor or oxytocin.

isoproterenol
Mechanism of Action

Isoproterenol (Isuprel) is a synthetic catecholamine that stimulates beta$_1$- and beta$_2$-adrenergic receptors but has little activity on alpha-adrenergic receptors. Isoproterenol will therefore stimulate heart rate and cardiac output. At sufficient dosages of isoproterenol, blood pressure will fall because activation of the beta$_2$-receptors of the blood vessels in skeletal muscle will shunt blood to the muscles and lower peripheral resistance. Smooth muscle, particularly the bronchial and gastrointestinal tract smooth muscle, is relaxed by isoproterenol. Isoproterenol is effective in treating bronchospasm when administered by inhalation.

Pharmacokinetics

Isoproterenol is not very effective orally. Absorption from a sublingual site is unreliable. Isoproterenol may be given effectively subcutaneously, intramuscularly, or intravenously. The catechol *O*-methyltransferase of the liver and other tissues is the major enzyme for degrading isoproterenol.

Uses

The principal use of isoproterenol is as a bronchodilator (see Chapter 28). Isoproterenol is rarely used as a cardiac stimulant in heart block and in cardiogenic shock secondary to a myocardial infarction or septicemia.

Adverse Reactions and Contraindications

Side effects of isoproterenol include palpitation, tachycardia (fast heart rate), headache, and flushing of the face. Sweating and mild tremors, nervousness, dizziness, and nausea may be experienced. Patients taking digitalis or otherwise disposed toward cardiac arrhythmias should not receive isoproterenol.

Interactions

Isoproterenol should not be administered with epinephrine because together they can induce severe cardiac arrhythmias.

levarterenol (norepinephrine)
Mechanism of Action

Levarterenol (Levophed), or norepinephrine, the neurotransmitter of the sympathetic nervous system, is a potent agonist of the alpha$_1$- and beta$_1$-adrenergic receptors when administered as the drug levarterenol. Levarterenol has relatively little effect on the beta$_2$-adrenergic receptors.

Levarterenol produces a potent peripheral vasoconstriction and inotropic response. Blood flow is shifted from the skin and visceral and renal vessels (where blood vessels are constricted) to the heart and brain (where blood vessels do not have alpha-receptors). On administration, levarterenol initially raises blood pressure dramatically. The increase is quickly great enough to stimulate the baroreceptors in the aorta, thereby triggering reflex stimulation of the vagus nerve, a physiologic process called **reflex bradycardia** (slow heart rate), which results because stimulation of the vagus nerve releases acetylcholine. Acetylcholine, however, slows the heart, and vagal stimulation from administration of acetylcholine counteracts the direct stimulation of the heart by levarterenol. The net result of administering levarterenol is therefore an increase in blood pressure with a modest and variable change in heart rate but very strong contractions of the heart.

Pharmacokinetics

Levarterenol is ineffective when taken orally, being rapidly degraded in the stomach. This drug is administered intravenously, and if it does infiltrate the infusion site, the alpha-adrenergic receptor antagonist phentolamine must be infiltrated in the area to counteract the profound vasoconstriction that may lead to tissue ischemia.

Levarterenol is rapidly inactivated by the liver. Like native norepinephrine, levarterenol is taken up and stored in sympathetic neurons identical to the native norepinephrine.

Uses

Levarterenol is used to restore blood pressure in acute hypotensive states but only after blood volume has been restored. In the absence of adequate blood volume, tissue perfusion is inadequate after vasoconstriction by levarterenol despite increased blood pressure. Kidney perfusion in particular is poor. Levarterenol provides a temporary treatment when the brain or heart is compromised in shock. Levarterenol may be used immediately after cardiac arrest has been terminated to restore and maintain blood pressure.

Adverse Reactions and Contraindications

Anxiety and a slow, forceful heartbeat are common side effects from administration of levarterenol. Some patients may develop a transient hypertension that is evidenced by a severe headache.

Levarterenol is contraindicated for patients who have vascular thrombosis because the resulting vasoconstriction could cause tissue death. Levarterenol should not be used to raise blood pressure in patients anesthetized with a drug that sensitizes the heart to catecholamine-induced arrhythmias (see Chapter 36).

Interactions

Administration of levarterenol to a patient taking an antidepressant drug (either a monoamine oxidase inhibitor or a tricyclic antidepressant) may cause a severe hypertensive response because antidepressant drugs interfere with the degradation and reuptake, respectively, of norepinephrine. A persistent hypertensive response may be elicited if levarterenol is administered after an oxytocic drug during labor.

methoxamine

Methoxamine (Vasoxyl) acts selectively to stimulate alpha-adrenergic receptors. Methoxamine, which is administered intravenously or intramuscularly, increases blood pressure for 60 to 90 minutes. This vasopressor action is used to treat the hypotension of anesthesia during surgery, primarily for spinal anesthesia when the patient is conscious and aware of the unpleasant effects of hypotension. The increased blood pressure in a patient with normal blood pressure will cause a reflex slowing of the heart rate (reflex bradycardia). Use of this action is made in terminating episodes of paroxysmal supraventricular tachycardia.

Side effects of methoxamine include sustained hypertension with a severe headache. Goose flesh (pilomotor erection), desire to urinate, and vomiting are occasional side effects.

Like the other sympathomimetic vasopressors, methoxamine should be used with caution in patients with heart disease or hypertension and is potentiated in patients receiving oxytocic drugs, monoamine oxidase inhibitors, tricyclic antidepressants, or general anesthetics of the type that sensitizes the heart to catecholamines.

midodrine

Midodrine (ProAmatine), a new drug, is a selective peripheral alpha$_1$-adrenergic agonist. It acts by increasing vascular tone and thereby elevating blood pressure. Midodrine is used for the treatment of orthostatic hypotension that cannot be controlled by such measures as support stockings, fluid expansion, or lifestyle changes. Midodrine is a prodrug and the active metabolite is desglymidodrine. It is given orally and is effective for 2 to 3 hours. Elimination is primarily in the urine.

Common side effects include burning, itching, or prickling of the scalp; chills, goosebumps; and urinary frequency, retention, or urgency. About 15% of patients experience supine hypertension, experienced as blurred vision, cardiac awareness, headache, and pounding in the ears. Patients with diabetes, visual problems, urinary retention problems, and renal dysfunction are at risk for hypertensive responses. Patients who should not be given midodrine include those who have severe cardiac disease, persistent hypertension, thyrotoxicosis, impaired renal function, or urinary retention. These conditions can worsen with midodrine.

Midodrine should not be given in combination with digitalis, sodium-retaining corticosteroids, or other vasoconstricting medications such as phenylephrine, phenylpropanolamine, and pseudoephedrine. Midodrine can block the excretion of drugs that are eliminated by active renal tubular excretion, causing elevated blood concentrations and potential toxic effects. This includes such drugs as cimetidine, flecainide, metformin, procainamide, quinidine, ranitidine, and triamterene.

phenylephrine

Phenylephrine (Isophrin, Neo-Synephrine) acts selectively to stimulate alpha-adrenergic receptors. The effect of phenylephrine is shorter in duration (20 to 50 minutes) than that of methoxamine, but otherwise the description of methoxamine and its uses, side effects, and drug interactions can be applied to phenylephrine.

Phenylephrine is used mainly as a nasal decongestant (see Chapter 30); it is also used to dilate the pupil (see Chapter 74). These actions result from stimulation of alpha-adrenergic receptors.

THERAPEUTIC AGENTS: INDIRECT-ACTING SYMPATHOMIMETIC DRUGS

Indirect-acting sympathomimetic drugs cause the release of norepinephrine from sympathetic neurons. The norepinephrine so released accounts for the activity of the drug. Like methoxamine, the selective alpha-adrenergic receptor agonist, the indirect-acting sympathomimetic amines are used primarily in treating the hypotension of spinal anesthesia. During spinal anesthesia, the sympathetic ganglia lying near the spinal cord may be affected, thereby disrupting sympathetic control of blood pressure. This is usually not to a degree that is life-threatening, but the sensation is unpleasant to the conscious patient. The indirect-acting sympathomimetic amines act directly on the postganglionic nerve terminals to release norepinephrine and restore blood pressure.

ephedrine

Mechanism of Action

Ephedrine is the prototype of the indirect-acting sympathomimetic amines, although ephedrine can be shown to have direct sympathomimetic actions at alpha- and beta-adrenergic receptors. Ephedrine, which has been isolated from several plants, has been used in Chinese medicine for 2000 years.

Pharmacokinetics

Ephedrine is active for 4 to 6 hours when administered orally, subcutaneously, intramuscularly, or intravenously.

Uses

The major use of ephedrine is as a bronchodilator (see Chapter 28). Ephedrine is occasionally used as a vasopressor to correct hypotension during spinal anesthesia. The vasopressor response to ephedrine is primarily a result of cardiac stimulation, increasing blood pressure through an increase in cardiac output.

Adverse Reactions and Contraindications

Ephedrine is a potent stimulant of the central nervous system, and this stimulation is the major side effect. Insomnia, agitation, euphoria, and confusion may be noted. Delirium and hallucinations can occur at high dosages. As with other sympathomimetic drugs, headache, palpitation, nausea and vomiting, and difficulty in voiding may be side effects. Repeated administration of ephedrine decreases the effectiveness of the drug. This rapidly developing tolerance (tachyphylaxis) results from the depletion of stored nor-epinephrine.

Ephedrine should be used cautiously in patients with hypertension, hyperthyroidism, diabetes mellitus, or (in males) prostate obstruction.

Interactions

The vasopressor response to ephedrine is potentiated by monoamine oxidase inhibitors, tricyclic antidepressants, and oxytocic drugs. Cardiac arrhythmias may be precipitated by ephedrine in the presence of digitalis or one of the general anesthetics that sensitize the heart to catecholamines.

metaraminol

Mechanism of Action

Metaraminol (Aramine) has both direct alpha-adrenergic agonist activity and an indirect sympathomimetic activity. Metaraminol can deplete norepinephrine stores on repeated administration to cause tachyphylaxis.

Pharmacokinetics

Metaraminol is administered intravenously, intramuscularly, or subcutaneously, with the onset of action being 1 to 2 minutes, 10 minutes, and 15 to 20 minutes, respectively. The activity persists for 20 to 60 minutes. Larger doses are administered by IV infusion, and care must be taken to avoid leakage of the drug at the infusion site. Metaraminol produces a rise in diastolic and systolic blood pressure, but heart rate is usually decreased as a result of reflex bradycardia. The force of contraction of the heart is increased.

Uses

Metaraminol is used clinically only to treat certain acute hypotensive states, as in spinal anesthesia.

Adverse Reactions and Contraindications

Metaraminol does not have any pronounced central nervous system effects. Otherwise side effects, contraindications, and drug interactions are identical to those described for ephedrine.

mephentermine

Mechanism of Action

Mephentermine (Wyamine) is an indirect-acting sympathomimetic drug. The major effect of mephentermine is an increased blood pressure resulting from increased cardiac output and peripheral vasoconstriction.

Pharmacokinetics

The effects of mephentermine persist for 30 to 60 minutes after subcutaneous administration and continue for up to 4 hours after intramuscular administration. Mephentermine can also be administered as a single IV dose. Mephentermine does not cause the tissue irritation characteristic of most vasopressor drugs.

Uses

Mephentermine is used to treat hypotension secondary to ganglionic blockade or to spinal anesthesia.

Adverse Reactions and Contraindications

Side effects of mephentermine are minimal and include drowsiness, weeping, incoherence, and occasionally, convulsions. Contraindications and drug interactions are those described for other vasopressor drugs.

Nursing Process Overview

Sympathomimetic Drugs

Assessment

Sympathomimetics treat shock, which can be caused by trauma, blood loss, burns, sepsis, cardiac failure (cardiogenic shock), anaphylaxis, and extreme reactions to some drugs. The patient in shock may appear pale, with clammy skin. The blood pressure is usually low or may even be absent; the pulse rate may be increased and thready. If alert, the patient may complain of fear of impending doom and may be anxious. The respiratory rate may be increased. Perform a rapid assessment, including the pulse, respirations, blood pressure, and level of consciousness. Examine for obvious causes of the shock. Monitor appropriate laboratory work: arterial blood gas concentrations, serum electrolyte concentrations, hematocrit and hemoglobin values, and serum glucose.

Nursing Diagnoses

Nursing diagnoses include the following:

- Risk for decreased cardiac output
- Risk for arrhythmias
- Risk for hypovolemic shock
- Risk for electrolyte imbalances
- Risk for septicemia
- Risk for renal insufficiency

Depending on the clinical picture of the patient, one or more of these risks may exist.

Patient Outcomes

The nurse will manage and minimize the complications associated with the potential complications identified for the patient. The patient will achieve and maintain a satisfactory blood pressure without experiencing permanent effects caused by the potential complication.

Planning/Implementation

Administer ordered vasopressors to increase and maintain the blood pressure; use an infusion control device and/or a microdrip infusion set. Monitor the vital signs frequently, continuously or as often as every 5 minutes. Administer ordered replacement fluids and blood. Monitor intake and output; insert a Foley catheter if necessary. Monitor the level of consciousness. Use a cardiac monitor to assess the patient's condition. Have available emergency care equipment, such as a suction machine and resuscitation equipment. Remain with the patient and stay calm. Continue to assess for changes in patient status and drug side effects. Keep the patient and family informed of what is being done.

Evaluation

Drugs to treat shock are successful if the blood pressure is maintained to provide adequate tissue perfusion. Few vasopressors are used in self-management situations; most are used only in the acute-care setting for the patient in shock. Epinephrine may be prescribed for patients with a history of previous serious allergic response. Before discharge, the patient should be able to explain when epinephrine should be used and how to use it, to demonstrate the correct administration technique, and to explain the side effects that result from the medication; the patient also should know when to seek emergency assistance.

Nursing Implications Summary

General Guidelines: Sympathomimetic Drugs
Drug Administration

➤ If possible, obtain medication history before administering these drugs to alert you to possible dosage adjustments that will be required.

➤ Use a microdrip IV administration and/or an electronic IV monitor or regulator to accurately control the rate of fluid and drug administration. Monitor the blood pressure and pulse continuously, or at least every 2 to 5 minutes until the blood pressure and rate of drug administration are stable, then every 15 minutes. Monitor the cardiac output, pulmonary artery pressure, pulmonary capillary wedge pressure (PCWP), central venous pressure (CVP), or other available indicators of hemodynamic response. Monitor the electrocardiographic changes. Monitor intake and output; monitor urinary output every 30 to 60 minutes. Dosage may be titrated to a combination of predetermined blood pressure, pulse, and urinary output. Monitor serum electrolytes. Do not leave the patient unattended. Monitor peripheral pulses and assess color and temperature of peripheral sites.

➤ Read drug labels carefully because some drug forms are not indicated for IV administration. Do not administer any drug intravenously if sediment or discoloration is visible. Do not mix sympathomimetic drugs with other drugs in a syringe or in IV solutions. If in doubt, consult the pharmacist. Observe the patient for development of hypertensive crisis. If it does occur, slow or stop vasopressor drugs, notify physician, and administer specific drug antidotes or phentolamine, an adrenergic blocking drug, as ordered.

➤ Avoid extravasation of these drugs. All sympathomimetic drugs cause vasoconstriction, which can lead to tissue necrosis or sloughing. Administer these drugs through a central venous catheter if possible. In the event of extravasation, infiltrate the site with a solution of 5 to 10 mg of phentolamine diluted in 10 to 15 ml of normal saline solution. Use a syringe with a fine hypodermic needle.

➤ Many of these preparations contain bisulfites, which can cause an allergic reaction in susceptible individuals. Although uncommon in the general population, this reaction may be seen more often in persons with a history of asthma. Symptoms include dizziness; feeling faint; bluish discoloration of the skin; skin rash or hives; swelling of the face, eyelids, or lips; and difficulty breathing. If possible, obtain a history of allergy or previous health problems preceding drug administration. Observe all patients for unexpected drug reactions. Keep the patient and family informed of the patient's condition. Provide calm reassurance. Note that shock produces a sense of impending doom and a feeling of

Continued

Nursing Implications Summary—cont'd

anxiety. Administration of adrenergic medication may also produce a tachycardia and palpitations, which contribute to a sense of anxiety.

➤ In many agencies, printed tables listing standard dilutions and rates of administration for these drugs are available in intensive care units. The manufacturer's insert provides detailed instructions about various dilutions and compatible IV fluids. Some of these drugs are available premixed (prediluted) and ready for infusion. Read labels carefully. Calculate dosages and dilutions carefully.

dobutamine
Drug Administration
➤ Dilute the concentrate for injection to a volume of at least 50 ml with a compatible IV solution before administration. The final concentration should be no greater than 5000 μg/ml (5 mg/ml). Solutions that are slightly pink in color may still be used. After mixing with IV solution, use within 24 hours.

dopamine
Drug Administration
➤ Dilute the concentrate for injection before infusion. Follow dilution guidelines for the agency. One protocol states "add 5 ml of concentrate containing 40 mg dopamine per ml (total of 200 mg of dopamine) to 500 ml of compatible IV solution to obtain a final concentration of 400 μg/ml." Also available prediluted at various concentrations in 250 ml or 500 ml of D5W.

ephedrine
Drug Administration
➤ Use IV ephedrine only if an immediate response is needed. May be given undiluted. Administer at a rate of 10 mg or less over 1 minute.

epinephrine
Drug Administration
➤ For anaphylactic shock, the usual dose of epinephrine is 0.1 to 1 ml (0.1 to 1 mg) of 1:1000 solution given subcutaneously.

➤ Read labels carefully; not all forms may be administered IV. For direct IV administration, epinephrine is available prediluted in syringes in a concentration of 1:10,000, or this concentration can be made by diluting 1 ml of 1:1000 solution to at least 10 ml with normal saline. For direct IV administration, use at a rate of 1 mg or less over 1 minute or longer. Follow each dose with 20 ml of IV flush to ensure that the entire dose has reached the patient. For infusion, the solution may be further diluted in 250 to 500 ml of 5% dextrose in water (D5W) and titrated to patient response.

➤ Epinephrine may be administered via the endotracheal route. Avoid administering epinephrine and isoproterenol simultaneously because they are both cardiac stimulants.

➤ Monitor the blood glucose because epinephrine causes hyperglycemia.

isoproterenol
Drug Administration
➤ For direct IV administration, administer each 1 ml of a 1:50,000 solution over 1 minute (1 ml of 20 μg/ml or 1 ml of 0.02 mg/ml). Follow dose with 20 ml of IV normal saline flush to insure patient receives entire dose.

➤ For infusion, dilute 1 mg (5 ml of 200 μg/ml or 0.2 mg/ml) of a 1:5000 solution in 250 ml of D5W. This makes a concentration of 4 μg/ml or a 1:250,000 solution. Other concentrations may be used. Titrate dose to patient response.

levarterenol (norepinephrine)
Drug Administration
➤ Dilute with D5W injection, with or without normal saline, before use. In the usual dilution, add 4 mg of drug to 1000 ml of D5W injection for a concentration of 4 μg/ml, or add 4 mg of drug to 250 ml of D5W injection for a concentration of 16 μg/ml.

mephentermine
Drug Administration
➤ Administer mephentermine undiluted at a rate of 30 mg or less over 1 minute. It may also be diluted by adding 600 mg to 500 ml of diluent to make a dilution of 1 mg/ml. Titrate infusion to patient response.

metaraminol
Drug Administration
➤ Administer a single dose up to 5 mg undiluted, at a rate of 5 mg over 1 minute. Metaraminol may also be diluted with D5W for injection or normal saline for injection. See manufacturer's directions for further guidelines. Titrate to patient response.

methoxamine
Drug Administration
➤ Administer methoxamine undiluted at a rate of 5 mg or less over at least 1 minute. For infusion, add 40 mg of methoxamine to 250 ml of D5W and titrate the rate to patient response.

midodrine
Drug Administration/Nursing in the Community
➤ Review dosing schedule. Supine hypertension is a potential problem. Usually, take first dose upon rising, second dose with the midday meal, and the third dose in the late afternoon or early evening, but no later than 6 PM. Administer doses at 4-hour intervals, although 3-hour intervals may be needed for some patients. Do not space doses closer than 3-hour intervals. Do not administer after the evening meal. Do not administer within 4 hours of bedtime. Do not

Nursing Implications Summary–cont'd

administer dose if patient plans to be supine shortly after taking dose.

➤ Monitor blood pressure when patient is supine. Check with physician before administering dose if supine systolic blood pressure exceeds 180 mm Hg.

➤ Instruct patient to avoid taking other medications unless approved by the physician.

➤ For missed doses, instruct patient to take missed dose as soon as remembered, unless almost time for next dose. Do not double up for missed doses. As noted, do not take doses after 6 PM or at bedtime.

➤ Emphasize the importance of and other prescribed therapies such as support stockings and maintaining fluid balance.

phenylephrine
Drug Administration

➤ For direct IV administration, dilute 1 mg (1 ml) with 9 ml of sterile water for injection (0.1 mg equals 1 ml); administer over 20 to 30 seconds for paroxysmal supraventricular tachycardia or over at least 1 minute for other conditions. For infusion, dilute 10 mg in 500 ml of diluent (makes a dilution of 20 mg/ml), and titrate to patient response.

CHAPTER REVIEW

Application

1. List the direct-acting sympathomimetic drugs. What is their receptor selectivity and what physiologic actions result?
2. List the indirect-acting sympathomimetic drugs. What is their receptor selectivity and what physiologic actions result?
3. What are symptoms of anaphylactic shock?
4. Which drug would the nurse expect to see used as a renal vasodilator?
5. Which drug is used as a selective stimulant of cardiac contractility?

Critical Thinking

1. Which drug would the nurse expect to see used to treat anaphylactic shock? What is the usual dosage range and how is it administered?
2. Develop a teaching plan for the patient discharged to home with a "bee sting" kit containing epinephrine.
3. Why are sympathomimetic drugs sometimes administered during spinal anesthesia?
4. Develop a table that compares and contrasts the drugs listed on Table 16-1. Some factors to compare include site of action, side effects, and advantages and disadvantages.

References

Harwood S: Action stat: anaphylaxis, *Nursing* 27(2):33, 1997.

Jerrard DA: ED management of insect stings, *Am J Emerg Med* 14(4):429-433, 1996.

Kellett PB: Latex allergy: a review, *J Emerg Nurs* 23(1):27-36, 1997.

Tuite PK: Recognition and management of shock in the pediatric patient, *Crit Care Nurs Q* 20(1):52-61, 1997.

Fluids and Electrolytes

OBJECTIVES

After studying this chapter, you should be able to do the following:

- *Explain what forces control the movement of water between body compartments.*
- *Describe the causes and signs of dehydration, and suggest fluids to reverse dehydration.*
- *Describe the causes and signs of fluid excess, and suggest ways to control it.*
- *Describe appropriate nursing actions in response to common problems encountered with intravenous fluids.*

CHAPTER OVERVIEW

Fluids and electrolyte solutions are used to reestablish proper salt and water balance. Because these solutions are used to return the body to homeostasis, they may be thought of as drugs. This chapter reviews the general classes of fluids and solutions that are commonly used in clinical practice. A full discussion of the clinical indications for these solutions is outside the scope of a pharmacology text, but the most important physiologic and clinical factors in the use of these solutions are covered.

THERAPEUTIC RATIONALE: FLUID OR ELECTROLYTE IMBALANCE

Regulation of Salt and Water Balance

Fluid Compartments

Water comprises 50 to 60% of an average person's weight. Although water passes easily through most tissues, certain physical and permeability barriers allow the body to be divided into compartments in which water content may be independently regulated. For example, a 70-kg man would contain 42 L of water, of which 28 L are inside cells (Figure 17-1). This water, along with its dissolved solutes, is called **intracellular fluid**. **Interstitial fluid** bathes the outside of cells and allows them to excrete waste products and receive nutrients. Plasma constitutes an important separate

fluid compartment similar to interstitial fluid, but it is more accessible to manipulation and testing. Extracellular fluid (ECF) primarily includes interstitial fluid and plasma but also other fluids such as lymph and cerebrospinal fluid.

Composition of Body Fluids

The fluid compartments in the body differ in the concentration of important ions and other solutes. In plasma the major solute is sodium chloride (Figure 17-2). The primary buffers maintaining the pH of blood at 7.4 are bicarbonate (HCO_3^{-1}, 27 mEq/L) and protein (16 mEq/L). Interstitial fluid is similar to plasma except that the protein content is much reduced.

Inside the cell, high concentrations of protein and potassium are found, but the sodium ion concentration is much lower. Phosphate is the major buffer for intracellular fluid.

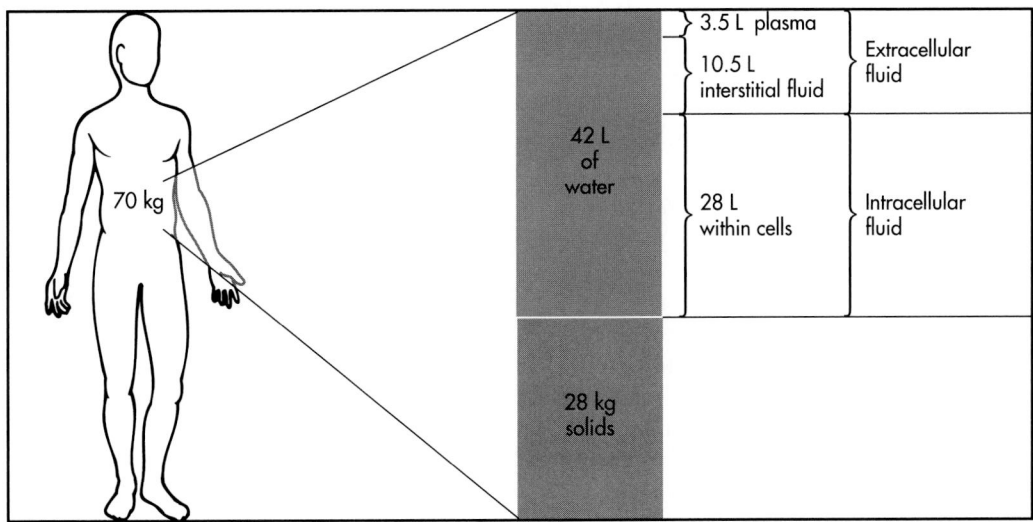

Figure 17-1   Distribution of water in men. In women, about 50% of body weight is found as water, but proportion of intracellular to extracellular fluid is same as for men.

Figure 17-2   Movement of water and solutes between body compartments. *Double-headed arrows* represent simple diffusion; *straight arrows* indicate pressure-regulated processes. *Arrows passing through or in contact with circles* represent active transport of solutes.

Phosphate is shown in Figure 17-2 as PO_4^{-3} but is actually present as a mixture of HPO_3^{-2} and $H_2PO_3^{-1}$. Magnesium ion, an important component of critical enzyme systems, is also a significant constituent of intracellular fluid.

Movement of Fluid and Electrolytes between Compartments

Water moves freely through the vascular walls separating plasma from interstitial fluid and through the cell membranes separating intracellular fluid from interstitial fluid. However, movement of ions and other solutes is rigidly con-

trolled so that optimum concentration differences are maintained between compartments. The concentrations of these solutes influence the disposition of water among the compartments. To understand the distribution of water and the various solutes, certain concepts from chemistry and physiology must be recalled.

Osmosis describes the movement of water across a semipermeable membrane (a membrane that selectively limits passage of some chemicals). For example, a cell membrane is semipermeable. The direction of movement is determined by the concentration of solutes in the water on either side of the membrane. Water moves toward the solution having the higher concentration. Osmosis reduces the difference in concentration of the solutions on either side of a semipermeable membrane.

The movement of water by osmosis across semipermeable membranes creates osmotic pressure. For example, if a glucose solution is enclosed in a synthetic membrane that allows water but not glucose to pass through the membrane and the sealed sac is submerged in pure water, two things will happen. Water will enter the sac at a greater rate than it leaves the sac. As water enters the solution-filled sac, pressure inside the sac increases and opposes the entry of more water. The pressure required to completely prevent the net movement of water into the sac is a measure of the osmotic pressure of the solution.

The osmotic properties of a solution relate to the concentration of solute, but the number of particles (ions, atoms, or molecules) is important, not the mass of the solute. For example, a 0.5 molar solution of glucose contains 90 g/L of glucose and has a potential osmotic pressure of 9650 mm Hg. In contrast, a 0.5 molar solution of sodium chloride contains 29 g/L of sodium chloride and has a potential osmotic pressure of 19,300 mm Hg. The greater potential osmotic pressure of the sodium chloride solution results from the ionization of sodium chloride to release two particles for every molecule of salt, a sodium ion and a chloride ion. Glucose does not ionize, and each molecule of the glucose remains a single particle.

Osmolarity of the ECF is determined mainly by the concentration of sodium chloride. Solutions that have the same osmolarity as plasma are called **isotonic**. Isotonic solutions include 5% dextrose and 0.9% sodium chloride solutions. Hypertonic solutions have an osmolarity above that of plasma (greater than 310 mOsm/L); hypotonic solutions have lower osmolarity than plasma.

Oncotic pressure regulates the movement of water between plasma and interstitial fluid. This pressure is generated by the difference in protein concentration between plasma and interstitial fluid. Although most solutes in plasma pass freely through pores of the vascular walls that separate plasma from interstitial fluid, proteins cannot leave plasma by that route. Proteins retained in plasma act like other solutes to promote the movement of water from interstitial fluid toward plasma.

Without a balancing force, oncotic pressure tends to dilute the protein in plasma and increase pressure in the plasma compartment. Oncotic pressure is balanced by **hydrostatic pressure** generated by the force of contraction of the heart. In arterioles where blood pressure is high, hydrostatic pressure exceeds oncotic pressure. In the arteriolar side of capillaries, water, along with dissolved nutrients and other solutes, moves from plasma into the interstitial fluid, where it is available to cells. Pressure on the venous side of the capillaries is lower and is not sufficient to fully block the movement of water. Oncotic pressure thus predominates on the venous side of capillaries, allowing water, solutes, and waste products to move back into plasma and be carried away.

Diffusion describes the movement of solutes across semipermeable membranes. The direction of movement is toward the less concentrated solution. As with osmosis, this process lowers the difference in concentration between the two solutions. Free diffusion of most ions and solutes takes place between plasma and interstitial fluid, but the cell membrane is not normally permeable to most solutes found in ECF. Sensitive control of uptake and release of solutes is maintained by active transport systems on the cell membrane. For example, the high intracellular concentration of potassium is maintained by Na^+-K^+-ATPase, an active transport system that hydrolyzes a molecule of adenosine triphosphate (ATP) to exchange three sodium ions for two potassium ions. Other active transport systems maintain the high intracellular concentrations of phosphate and magnesium ion.

Clinical Indications for Fluid Therapy

Loss of Extracellular Fluid Volume

Several clinical conditions can cause water and solutes to be lost from ECF. For example, sudden hemorrhage, prolonged vomiting, excessive diarrhea, or plasma loss through large

---

 PEDIATRIC CONSIDERATIONS

Diarrhea in Infants

THE PROBLEM
In most cases diarrhea is mild and self-limiting, but infants and young children may be thrown into dangerous states of dehydration and electrolyte imbalance if diarrhea is severe or prolonged. Hypotension and coma can arise when fluid losses equal 5% of body weight; losses of 10% can cause shock, and death ensues at higher losses.

ASSOCIATED OR CONTRIBUTING FACTORS
In underdeveloped nations diarrhea is a significant cause of mortality in infants and children, with death resulting from dehydration and electrolyte imbalance. Poor sanitation may expose children and adults to infectious agents that cause diarrhea. Even if the diarrhea is caused by bacterial contamination of food or water, treatment is often successful if salt and water balance are maintained. Intravenous replacement of fluids is expensive, unavailable to many people, and unnecessary in the majority of cases. Aggressive oral replacement with properly balanced solutions is first-line treatment.

SOLUTIONS
- Oral rehydration therapy (ORT) should begin early in the course of the disease.
- In the United States preparations are available under the trade names Lytren, Pedialyte, Rehydralyte, and Resol.
- In Canada, Lytren and Pedialyte are available.
- In other countries the World Health Organization (WHO) Diarrheal Disease Control Program supplies ORS-bicarbonate or ORS-citrate in premeasured packets that are mixed with 1 L of potable water before use.

areas of burned skin may cause fluid and salt loss, but the fluid remaining in the extracellular compartment may for a time stay essentially normal in composition. If the fluid loss is excessive and uncompensated, the patient may enter hypovolemic shock, in which the blood volume becomes so depleted that organ perfusion is compromised. The symptoms of this condition include lowered blood pressure, increased heart rate, rapid respiration, restlessness, pale and clammy skin, and decreased urine output. Without adequate perfusion the kidneys may fail completely. Hypovolemic shock is potentially life-threatening and requires rapid replacement of fluid and electrolytes.

In certain conditions, ECF volume may be decreased primarily by water loss. For example, patients who fail to take in adequate water may suffer dehydration. This condition is common in older adults who may have inefficient thirst centers in the brain. Unconscious patients lose between 1000 and 1700 ml of water in insensible perspiration, breath, and urine each day; this water must be replaced daily to avoid dehydration. In certain circumstances watery diarrhea and high-volume renal failure may cause loss of water in excess of salt loss (see Pediatric Considerations box). All these circumstances may require replacement of lost volume and restoration of the proper proportion of solutes in the ECF.

Fluid deficiency requiring therapy is associated with weight loss in excess of 5% of normal body weight, dry lips and eyes, decreased blood pressure, and depressed central nervous system (CNS) activity. Skin turgor is also diminished.

Fluid Excess

In certain conditions ECF volume is expanded to a degree that may impair cardiovascular functioning, in part by increasing venous pressure. Fluid excess may arise from conditions impairing the body's ability to eliminate fluid such as heart failure or renal impairment. Alternatively, fluid excess can arise from the improper administration of intravenous (IV) fluids. The main route for elimination of excess fluid is through the kidneys. Treatment aims to prevent further overload and, if necessary, to assist the kidneys by pharma-

cologic means. For example, digitalis given to strengthen contraction of the heart in heart failure improves perfusion of the kidneys and assists in mobilizing and eliminating excess fluid. Diuretics also enhance urine production.

Signs of fluid excess include swelling and edema, bounding pulse, distension of the jugular vein, difficult or noisy breathing, and warm, moist skin.

Electrolyte Imbalances

The proper concentrations of ions and solutes in the extracellular compartment can be disrupted by diseases or medical interventions (Table 17-1).

Sodium Ion. Sodium is the major determinant of osmolarity in plasma and interstitial fluid. **Hypernatremia** (excessive sodium ion concentration in plasma) can arise when a patient loses water but retains salt. Alternatively, hypernatremia may arise when excessive sodium has been administered with fluids or medications. In hypernatremia, water moves from cells into the ECF in an attempt to reduce the sodium ion concentration and restore equal osmolarity between the fluid compartments. **Hyponatremia** (plasma sodium concentrations less than 130 mEq/L) arises most commonly in patients who are losing water and electrolytes but are receiving water without adequate electrolyte replacement. In an extreme case this condition is called water intoxication. The low sodium ion concentration of the ECF causes water to move into cells in an attempt to restore equal osmolarity between the two compartments.

Potassium Ion. **Hyperkalemia** (excessive potassium ion concentration in plasma) causes less osmotic disturbance than a sodium ion imbalance, but potassium ion imbalances can be life-threatening because cardiac function may be impaired. Potassium-induced cardiac dysfunction appears in the electrocardiogram (ECG) as depressed ST segments, widened QRS complexes, and peaked T waves. Hyperkalemia may result from massive tissue injury when large numbers of cells die, releasing their high intracellular concentrations of

Table 17-1	**Common Electrolyte Imbalances**		
Solute	Normal Concentration in Plasma	Signs of Deficiency	Signs of Excess
Sodium ion	136-145 mEq/L	Anorexia, nausea, vomiting; increased intracranial pressure; oliguria leading to anuria	Dry sticky membranes; fever; weakness and disorientation; oliguria
Potassium ion	3.5-5 mEq/L	Muscle weakness; diminished tendon reflexes; paralytic ileus; cardiac arrhythmia	Nausea and vomiting; muscle weakness; electrocardiographic changes
Bicarbonate ion	24-31 mEq/L (pH 7.35-7.45)	Metabolic acidosis (pH <7.35); weakness; deep, rapid breathing (Kussmaul); stupor or unconsciousness	Metabolic alkalosis (pH >7.45); hypertonicity of muscles; depressed respirations; tetany
Calcium ion	4.7-5.6 mEq/L	Tetany; prolonged QT interval on electrocardiogram	Weakness, fatigue, thirst; nausea, anorexia, muscle cramping
Magnesium ion	1.3-2.3 mEq/L	Flushing, hypertension; neuromuscular irritability	Nausea, vomiting; diarrhea, colic

potassium into the ECF. Renal failure may also cause retention of potassium, as may the potassium-sparing diuretics discussed in Chapter 14.

Hypokalemia (low potassium ion concentration in the plasma) can be caused by the use of loop diuretics or the thiazides (see Chapter 14). Poor nutrition or poor gastrointestinal (GI) tract absorption may also cause hypokalemia. Vomiting depletes the body of potassium, along with fluid and other salts. Replacement of potassium is necessary to restore normal function, but the replacement should be spread out over several days to avoid excessive cardiac stress.

Hydrogen Ion and Bicarbonate Ion. The balance of these ions regulates the pH of plasma and interstitial fluid. An increase of hydrogen ion over bicarbonate ion lowers the pH of ECF, causing acidosis. An increase of bicarbonate ion over hydrogen ion causes a rise in pH of the ECF, or alkalosis. Acid-base imbalances arise from respiratory or metabolic causes. **Respiratory acidosis** arises when pulmonary ventilation is impaired. Without adequate ventilation the carbon dioxide concentration in blood rises. In blood, carbon dioxide becomes carbonic acid, which lowers blood pH. Pneumonia or pulmonary obstructive disease can produce respiratory acidosis. Therapy is aimed at the underlying disease. **Metabolic acidosis** arises when excess acid is produced, as in diabetic acidosis, lactic acidosis, starvation, and certain types of poisoning.

Respiratory alkalosis can be induced by hyperventilation, through which excessive amounts of carbon dioxide are lost. **Metabolic alkalosis** arises when excess hydrogen ion is lost, as in prolonged vomiting or nasogastric suctioning. Respiratory alkalosis seldom requires IV therapy, but metabolic alkalosis is often treated with isotonic saline. During metabolic alkalosis, bicarbonate excretion becomes limited by the progressive depletion of sodium. Administering isotonic saline allows the kidneys to sacrifice the sodium required to accompany excreted bicarbonate. With this assistance the kidneys usually reestablish acid-base balance.

THERAPEUTIC AGENTS: FLUID AND ELECTROLYTE SOLUTIONS

Hydrating Solutions

Conditions such as hemorrhage or shock, in which plasma volume is suddenly reduced, require replacement of fluid as initial therapy. Replacement of lost fluid volume allows maintenance of kidney function, preventing further development of dangerous electrolyte imbalances. Perfusion of other vital organs is also maintained by this strategy.

▼ Sodium Chloride in Water

Isotonic saline (Table 17-2) replaces ECF volume and treats sodium depletion and metabolic alkalosis. Dangers associated with its use include circulatory overload and hypernatremia. Metabolic acidosis may arise when excess chloride ion in blood promotes bicarbonate ion loss in the kidneys.

Hypokalemia may arise as excess sodium ion forces potassium ion excretion by the kidneys. Hypertonic saline solutions should be used in small volumes and administered carefully to correct severe hyponatremia. Use of sodium chloride solutions that contain preservative requires special precautions (see Pediatric Considerations box on benzyl alcohol).

Ringer's Solution and Lactated Ringer's Solution

Ringer's solution and lactated Ringer's solution are used to replace fluid, sodium, and other electrolytes (see Table 17-2). Often called balanced or maintenance solutions, these preparations are appropriate to replace volume if renal function is normal. The potassium found in these solutions cannot be eliminated and may accumulate to dangerous levels if renal function is impaired. Therefore renal function must be established before these fluids are administered.

Ringer's solution is appropriate replacement therapy for patients who have lost fluid and electrolytes through the GI tract, for burn patients, for postoperative patients, and for patients with dehydration or sodium depletion. Lactated Ringer's solution is most appropriate for patients who, along with other electrolyte imbalances, have acidosis. The lactate in this solution, converted to bicarbonate by the liver, provides stronger basic cations in the blood than simple inorganic salt solutions and elevates blood pH.

▼ Dextrose in Water

Dextrose, or glucose, in an isotonic solution (5%) is appropriate for most situations in which rehydration is needed. In addition to fluid, the solution supplies about 170 cal/L or 560 kJ/L. Electrolytes are not supplied in this solution. Hypertonic glucose solutions are given slowly to avoid tissue damage. These hypertonic solutions may be used to shift fluid from the interstitial space into the plasma. Isotonic dextrose solutions may be infused through peripheral veins to hydrate patients and to replace sodium loss, but hypertonic dextrose solutions should be infused through a central vein to avoid excessive irritation. Five percent dextrose in 0.45% saline may be used to shift fluid from plasma into the interstitial space, which may cause difficulty for patients with cardiac, renal, or liver disease who also have edema and poor venous return.

Dextrose solutions may have other components added for infusion, but not all additives are compatible. For example, dextrose solutions are never used in the same IV line with whole blood because the glucose causes hemolysis (rupture of red blood cells). The pharmacist or a standard reference such as *The Handbook on Injectable Drugs* (LA Trissel, Amer. Soc. of Health-system Pharmacists, Inc, 9th ed, 1996) can provide information about compatibilities of IV fluids.

Solutions to Correct Specific Electrolyte Imbalances

Calcium salts are used by IV infusion to correct acute hypocalcemia and to supply calcium for parenteral nutrition. Calcium salts have also been used to stimulate cardiac function, to treat hyperkalemia, to treat magnesium intoxi-

Table 17-2 Electrolyte Replacement Solutions

Principal Electrolyte	Intravenous Dosage	Comments
Bicarbonate		
Sodium bicarbonate in water (4.2%, 5%, 7.5%, 8.4%)	Individualized to reverse acidosis; usual dose 2-5 mEq/kg given in 4- to 8-hr infusion.	May be diluted; 1 L of 1.4% sodium bicarbonate contains 167 mEq/L of sodium ion.
Calcium		
Calcium acetate (0.5 mEq Ca^{++}/ml) Calcium chloride (1.36 mEq Ca^{++}/ml) Calcium gluceptate (0.9 mEq Ca^{++}/ml) Calcium gluconate (0.47 mEq Ca^{++}/ml)	Rate of infusion should not exceed 1.8 mEq Ca^{++} per minute.	Dosage based on calcium content of preparation.
Magnesium		
Magnesium sulfate (10%, 12.5%, 20%, 50%)	Infuse 10% solution at <1.5 ml/min.	10% solution is nearly isotonic.
Potassium		
KCl in water (0.1, 0.2, 0.3, 0.4, 1.5, or 2 mEq K$^+$/ml) KCl in 5% dextrose (10, 20, 30, or 40 mEq K$^+$/L) KCl in 0.9% saline (20 or 40 mEq K$^+$/L)	Dilute before use to 0.04 mEq/ml; infuse at 20 mEq/hr; higher rates occasionally are used for emergencies.	Solutions as supplied are hypertonic. Monitor ECG when infusion rates exceed 20 mEq/hr.
Sodium		
NaCl in water (0.45%, 0.9%, 3%, 5%) NaCl concentrate (2.5 or 4 mEq Na$^+$/L) NaCl in 2.5%, 5% or 10% dextrose (0.11%, 0.2%, 0.225%, 0.3%, 0.33%, 0.45%, or 0.9% in NaCl) NaCl in 5% dextrose with KCl (0.2%, 0.225%, 0.33%, 0.45%, or 0.9% NaCl with 0.075%, 0.15%, 0.224%, or 0.3% KCl)	Isotonic (0.9%) or hypotonic (0.45%) infused at 90-125 ml/hr or higher for initial therapy; 3% saline infused at <80 ml/hr; 5% saline infused at <50 ml/hr.	Isotonic saline supplies 154 mEq/L Na$^+$ and 154 mEq/L of Cl$^-$. NaCl concentrate used for mixing with other IV solutions. Monitor for potassium overload when using NaCl in dextrose with KCl.
Multiple Electrolytes		
Ringer's solution (0.86% NaCl, 0.03% KCl, 0.033% CaCl$_2$)	Common infusion rate is 90-125 ml/hr.	Balanced salt solution supplies, in mEq/L, the following ions: Na$^+$ 147, K$^+$ 4, Ca^{++} 4.5, Cl$^-$ 156.
Lactated Ringer's solution (0.6% NaCl, 0.03% KCl, 0.02% CaCl$_2$, 0.31% Na lactate)	Common infusion rate is 90-125 ml/hr.	Balanced salt solution supplies, in mEq/L, the following ions: Na$^+$ 130, K$^+$ 4, Ca^{++} 3, Cl$^-$ 109.
Electrolytes in 5% dextrose (Electrolyte No. 48, No. 75, Ionosol Isolyte, Normosol, Plasma-lyte)	Refer to specific information supplied with individual preparation.	Complex mixtures are used in special circumstances to correct massive electrolyte imbalances.

ECG, Electrocardiogram.

cation, and to replace calcium in patients receiving large volumes of citrated blood.

Magnesium sulfate is used to correct severe magnesium deficiencies and to control seizures in pregnancy (eclampsia). The 10% solution is nearly isotonic and may be used intravenously, but the 50% solution is strongly hypertonic and is used intramuscularly. Magnesium sulfate may be added to parenteral nutrition solutions for maintenance.

Potassium chloride may be added to IV fluids to replace potassium lost from the GI tract or through the kidneys. Replacement must be undertaken carefully to avoid causing hyperkalemia and its dangerous side effects. Dosage is calculated based on the estimated loss for the individual patient.

Plasma Expanders

In hemorrhage or hypovolemic shock, rapid filling of the plasma compartment may be a lifesaving measure. This

 PEDIATRIC CONSIDERATIONS

Benzyl Alcohol

THE PROBLEM
Benzyl alcohol is a bacteriostatic agent commonly used in solutions of sodium chloride and other drugs. Neonates are especially sensitive to this agent, and deaths have occurred when solutions containing benzyl alcohol were used in this age group.

SOLUTIONS
- Avoid administration of bacteriostatic saline (with benzyl alcohol) to newborns.
- Do not dilute drug with bacteriostatic saline if the drug is to be used in newborns.
- With newborns, do not flush intravenous lines with bacteriostatic saline.

volume replacement may be accomplished in several ways (Table 17-3), depending on the patient's needs.

Whole blood can be used in patients who have lost more than 20% of their blood volume. Crossmatching to test for blood group compatibility is required, although O-negative blood can be used until crossmatched blood is available. Whole blood replaces fluid, electrolytes, and oxygen-carrying capacity lost through hemorrhage. Before use, whole blood must be tested for evidence of viruses, including hepatitis and human immunodeficiency virus (HIV).

Plasma is a natural cell-free fluid that performs all the functions of whole blood except for oxygen transport. Crossmatching is not required.

Human albumin and plasma protein fractions expand plasma volume by increasing the plasma protein concentration. The resulting increase in plasma oncotic pressure causes water to move from the interstitial space into the plasma compartment. The albumin preparation contains appreciable amounts of sodium that may cause problems for certain patients with cardiovascular disease.

Dextran and hetastarch are complex carbohydrate molecules too large to pass out of the capillaries or vascular walls. Therefore these compounds are restricted to the vascular space. They generate osmotic forces that cause water to enter the blood vessels, thereby expanding plasma volume.

Intravenous Hyperalimentation

Patients unable to take oral foods and fluids require maintenance with IV nutrients. Dextrose solutions supply some calories, but only about 3 L of fluid can be administered daily without overloading the circulatory system. Therefore about 500 calories can be supplied each day from isotonic dextrose solutions. For longer-term therapy, more calories from different sources are required. Total parenteral nutrition (TPN) is now possible using synthetic amino acids, dextrose, and fat emulsions (Table 17-4).

Hypertonic dextrose is required for TPN. Solutions for administration are prepared from 50% or 60% dextrose stock solutions, but as they are administered the concentration of dextrose is only 25% to 30%. This hypertonic solution must be administered via a large central vein in which blood flow is sufficient to dilute the strong glucose solution and prevent tissue damage. A 10% dextrose solution is hypertonic but can be given peripherally without damage to veins.

Amino acids are used in TPN to prevent negative nitrogen balance and breakdown of protein in the body. Pure amino acid solutions, rather than protein hydrolysates, are preferred. At 3.5% concentrations the amino acid solutions offer about 140 cal/L and a variety of electrolytes. Extra potassium is often required by patients receiving amino acid solutions because potassium is depleted by amino acid metabolism.

Fat emulsions may be administered intravenously during TPN to prevent essential fatty acid deficiency. Because fats have a high caloric content, these preparations may supply a significant proportion (up to 60%) of the daily caloric requirement.

Vitamin and mineral supplements may need to be added to the TPN fluids. A variety of these preparations exist, allowing individual design of the nutrition program (see Dietary Considerations box).

Table 17-3   Blood, Blood Components, and Blood Substitutes

Preparation	Trade Names	Dosage/Administration	Comments
Whole blood		One unit: 340 ± 45 ml blood + 63 ml CPD (citrate-phosphate-dextrose) or CPDA-1 (citrate-phosphate-dextrose-adenine); give IV through 170-μm filter.	Used in patients who have lost more than 20% of blood volume; acts as volume expander; maintains oxygen transport.
Plasma		Monitored by clinical response to IV infusion.	Used as volume expander; does not support oxygen transport.
Albumin, human (5%, 25%)	Albuminar Albutein Buminate Plasbumin	Doses individualized, but normally <250 g/48 hr. FDA pregnancy category C.	Used to expand plasma volume. Preparations contain significant amounts of Na^+, which may be dangerous for certain patients.
Plasma protein fraction	Plasmanate Plasma Plex Plasmatein Protenate	*Adults*—250-500 ml of 5% solution infused at 5-8 ml/min, adjusted as necessary. FDA pregnancy category C. *Children*—22-33 ml/kg infused at 5-10 ml/min.	Used for hypovolemic shock in adults, to correct dehydration in children. Preparation contains 83% albumin, <17% globulin, <1% gamma globulin.
Dextrans in 5% dextrose or 0.9% saline	Dextran 40 Dextran 70 Dextran 75	Infusion rates may be rapid initially, but total daily dose should not exceed 10 ml/kg. FDA pregnancy category C.	Used for shock. Effects of Dextran 40 last 2-4 hr, but other dextrans are longer acting.
Hetastarch (6% in 0.9% NaCl)	Hespan	Rates of infusion normally <20 ml/kg/day. FDA pregnancy category C.	Used as plasma volume expander in shock or hypovolemia.

DIETARY CONSIDERATIONS

Vitamins

Vitamins are among the essential nutrients. If the patient's diet is varied and plentiful, vitamin deficiencies are rare. Digestive disorders and certain drugs can interfere with vitamin absorption. Good sources of major vitamins are listed in the following examples.

vitamin A (Retinol)
Liver, kidney, fish liver oils, cream, butter, whole milk, whole-milk cheese, fortified margarine, skim milk, skim-milk products, and dark green and deep yellow fruits and vegetables (all contain a precursor of vitamin A)

vitamin D
Exposure to sunlight, fortified milk, liver, egg yolk, butter, cream, fish, and liver oils

vitamin E
Widely distributed in foods, especially wheat germ and vegetable oils

vitamin K
Fruits and leafy vegetables, cereals, dairy products, meat, and tomatoes

vitamin C (ascorbic acid)
Citrus fruits, other fruits, and vegetables

B-COMPLEX VITAMINS

thiamine
Organ meats, legumes, nuts, whole or enriched grain products, wheat germ, and brewer's yeast

riboflavin
Milk and milk products, organ meats, eggs, leafy green vegetables, and whole or enriched grain products

niacin
Meats, legumes, nuts, peanut butter, and whole-grain and enriched-grain products. Tryptophan, a niacin precursor, is also found in protein foods of animal origin

pantothenic acid
Liver, kidney, salmon, eggs, legumes and peanuts, whole grains, milk, fruits, vegetables, molasses, and yeast

biotin
Organ meats, egg yolk, legumes, nuts, and mushrooms

folic acid
Leafy green vegetables, orange juice, liver, peanuts, legumes, whole-grain products, and wheat germ

vitamin B_{12}
Animal protein products only (meat, milk, fish and shellfish, eggs, and cheeses)

pyridoxine
Meat, fish, egg yolks, legumes and nuts, potatoes, whole grains, wheat germ, yeast, prunes and raisins, and bananas

---

Table 17-4 Fluids Used as Caloric Agents

Preparation	Trade Names	Dosage/Administration	Comments
Amino acids, crystalline	Aminosyn BranchAmin FreAmine HepatAmine NephrAmine Novamine ProcalAmine RenAmine Travasol TrophAmine	*Adults*—1 g/kg body weight per day, as needed to prevent protein breakdown and negative nitrogen balance. A 3.5% solution is nearly isotonic and may be administered via a peripheral vein. FDA pregnancy category C.	Solutions contain various mixtures of essential and nonessential amino acids, as well as appreciable amounts of sodium and other electrolytes. TrophAmine and Aminosyn contain taurine, an amino acid required by neonates.
Dextrose (2.5% to 11.5%)		Administer by peripheral IV line; can mix for TPN.	Adult requirement for dextrose is about 150 g/day.
Dextrose (5% to 38%)		Higher concentrations usually diluted or mixed before use.	Terminate infusion gradually to avoid rebound hypoglycemia.
Dextrose (40% to 70%)		Usually admixed with amino acids or other fluids; give by freely flowing central venous line.	Carefully maintain aseptic conditions; catheters remain in place for prolonged periods.
Fat emulsions (10% or 20%)	Intralipid Liposyn II Liposyn III Soyacal	*Adults*—IV by peripheral vein: 1 ml/min for 10% or 0.5 ml/min for 20% over 30 min as needed to supply calories (20% contains 2000 cal/L). *Infants, children*— Infuse at lower rates than for adults. Dosage for adults or children should not exceed 2.5 g fat/kg body weight daily.	Soybean oil stabilized with egg yolk phospholipids with glycerol to adjust isotonicity. Lipids should not supply more than 60% of total calories. Liposyn II contains both safflower and soybean oil, giving more linoleic acid but less linolenic acid than other preparations.

IV, Intravenous; *TPN*, total parenteral nutrition.

Nursing Process Overview

Fluids and Electrolytes

Assessment

Observe the patient for edema, especially in dependent areas; check skin turgor; auscultate breath and heart sounds; and monitor the vital signs, weight, and fluid intake and output. Observe the patient for specific electrolyte level imbalances. Observe for signs of nutritional deficiency, remembering that weight and intake measures alone are poor indicators. Monitor appropriate laboratory values, including serum electrolytes, blood urea nitrogen (BUN), and blood gas levels. If the patient is receiving IV fluids or nutrition, observe the administration setup, starting at the level of the patient. Check the insertion site; observe for signs of infiltration or infection; and check the placement and patency of the tubing, the rate of flow, and the amount of fluid remaining.

Nursing Diagnoses

- Risk for electrolyte imbalances
- Risk for negative nitrogen balance
- Risk for septicemia
- Risk for fluid volume excess related to excessive IV fluid intake

Patient Outcomes

The nurse will manage and minimize problems related to the potential complications listed previously. The patient will exhibit no edema from excessive fluid intake.

Planning/Implementation

The decision to initiate, terminate, or change the fluid and electrolyte therapy depends on the ongoing and cumulative database gathered during assessment. Keep the patient informed about the goals of therapy. Enlist the help of the patient and family in monitoring the IV line, and encourage them to report any unexpected subjective or objective finding. Continue to monitor the parameters identified previously. Observe patients for the desired and undesired effects of therapy. Label all IV fluids and medications carefully, monitor their rate of flow and their effects, and record carefully.

Evaluation

Therapy with fluids and electrolytes is effective if desired goals have been achieved without harmful consequences to the patient. If an oral electrolyte replacement is prescribed, review with the patient and family how the medication is administered, work with the patient to find an acceptable dosage form, review the need to continue the medication as desired, review side effects, and discuss situations that should cause the patient to call the physician or nurse (e.g., signs of electrolyte overload). Instruct the patient to measure fluid intake and output or weight at home. If the patient is to continue hyperalimentation at home, instruct the patient and family about the desired goals of therapy and review the technical tasks associated with the therapy (how to care for the insertion site, how to change the bottle, and what to do if the infusion line fails to function). Refer patients to social service and a visiting nurse agency as needed or discuss the patient's needs with the case manager.

Nursing Implications Summary

General Guidelines: Care of Patient Receiving IV Fluids

➤ Maintain vigilance whenever working with IV fluids or drugs because the administration of any substance directly into the vascular system can cause serious and rapid consequences.

➤ Inspect the patient receiving IV fluids at least hourly. Assess for correct infusion rate; inspect the bag or bottle, tubing, monitoring devices, and area surrounding the insertion site. Assess for signs of fluid overload and observe for any of the common problems associated with IV fluid therapy. See Table 17-5 for a summary of common IV problems and suggested nursing actions.

➤ Monitor skin turgor, intake and output, and weight; inspect dependent areas for edema; monitor vital signs; auscultate heart and lung sounds; and monitor central venous pressure and pulmonary capillary wedge pressure if available.

➤ Be familiar with agency or institutional policies and procedures regarding IV administration. Policies may specify who may start IV administrations, who may add electrolyte solutions or drugs to infusions, and what the procedures are for

routinely changing the tubing or insertion site or for redressing central line insertion sites.

➤ Use measures to prevent complications of IV administration, in addition to assessing for their development and subsequent treatment. For example, cleanse insertion sites thoroughly before initiating IV therapy, and wear sterile gloves when starting the IV line. Cleanse injection ports well with an alcohol or povidone-iodine solution before puncturing them. Use a Luer-Lok type of connection to prevent accidental pulling apart of IV tubing. Choose insertion sites where catheters are less likely to be dislodged by patient movement, and tape catheters securely. Wear gloves when discontinuing IV catheterization.

➤ Become familiar with the IV equipment used in the agency. Read the package inserts and attend in-service programs about new equipment.

➤ Check infusion rates carefully. If you have difficulty calculating IV drip rates, check calculations with another nurse. If a drip rate seems excessively fast or slow, discuss this with

Nursing Implications Summary—cont'd

another nurse. Some agencies require that two nurses check the infusion rate for infants and small children. See Chapter 6 for information about calculating IV rates of infusion.

➤ Inspect IV solutions carefully before using. Do not use solutions that are discolored, are leaking, or contain particulate matter.

➤ Choose a needle or catheter, administration set, and tubing length appropriate for the patient and the drug. For example, the larger the diameter of the needle or catheter, the

faster the fluid will infuse, but the larger the diameter, the more difficult it is to insert the needle or catheter into the chosen vein and the greater the risk of phlebitis. The higher the fluid reservoir (bag or bottle) is above the patient, the faster the rate of infusion; generally, the reservoir should be about 36 inches above the insertion site. The viscosity of the fluid influences the rate of flow; for example, blood infuses more slowly than normal saline or 5% dextrose solutions. The greater the length of tubing from the fluid reservoir to

Continued

Table 17-5   Intravenous Infusion: Problems, Signs and Symptoms, and Suggested Nursing Actions

Problem	Signs and Symptoms	Nursing Actions
Pain during infusion	Patient discomfort	Slow rate of infusion because some drugs are irritating to veins. Warm IV fluids to room temperature before hanging. Rule out phlebitis (below).
Occluded infusion	Decreased rate of infusion or no infusion Backup of blood into tubing Possible discomfort	Check to see that clamp is open or electronic device is turned on. Inspect tubing for kinks. Remove dressing over insertion site (using aseptic technique); check for kinks, remove old dressing, and retape insertion site. If fluid level in bag or bottle is low, raise level of bag or bottle or replace it with full bag or bottle. With some infusion devices (e.g., Port-A-Cath) or with multilumen central catheters, use thrombolytics such as urokinase to dissolve clots occluding IV flow; follow agency policies. If all else fails, restart IV.
Extravasation (leaking of fluid or drug into tissue surrounding vein, caused by tear in vein)	Decreased rate of infusion or no infusion Patient discomfort Puffiness, edema of extremity or insertion site Coolness distal to insertion site No blood return when bag or bottle is lowered below level of insertion site	Assess pulse. Elevate extremity. Discontinue IV and restart line at another site. Apply ice or warm soaks (follow agency procedure). If drug is known to be caustic (e.g., mechlorethamine), carry out any specific measures, including infiltration of area with steroids or drug antidote; consult physician or agency policies.
Phlebitis (irritation or inflammation of the vein)	Patient discomfort; site may be tender to touch Red streak coursing arm Site is warm to touch Possible edema Palpable cord along vein	Slow rate of infusion, while doing further assessment. If phlebitis is confirmed, discontinue IV and restart line at another site. Apply warm soaks (follow agency procedure). To prevent recurrence, consider one or more of the following: slowing IV rate, using a smaller-diameter catheter, adding an in-line filter, or diluting medication in a larger volume.
Septicemia (systemic infection)	Fever, chills, malaise Symptoms of shock, hypotension Normal appearance of IV insertion site Headache, nausea, vomiting	Notify physician. Monitor vital signs. Rule out other causes (respiratory tract infection, urinary tract infection, wound infection). Discontinue IV line, culture catheter tip and fluid (or as agency procedure directs), and restart IV line at another site.
Fluid overload	Noisy, rapid respiration, rales Distended neck veins Increased pulse rate or blood pressure Distress Puffiness, edema of dependent areas Weight gain	Slow infusion rate to keep line open. Raise of head of bed. Notify physician. Remain calm to reassure patient.
Embolism	Shortness of breath Chest and shoulder pain Unequal breath sounds Cyanosis Hypotension, weak pulse Loss of consciousness	Stop infusion. Place patient on left side, in Trendelenburg's position. Notify physician. Remain with patient, taking vital signs.

IV, Intravenous.

Nursing Implications Summary—cont'd

the patient, the slower the rate of flow. Choose a tubing long enough to allow safe movement by the patient but short enough to ensure that the tubing will not get tangled in the siderails or significantly restrict flow. Finally, choose an administration set appropriate to the ordered rate of flow. For example, if the rate of flow is 150 ml/hr, the drip rate on a minidrip set that delivers 60 gtt/ml would be 150 gtt/min, almost too fast to count. That same rate of administration with a set that delivers 10 gtt/ml would be 25 gtt/ml, an easy rate to count. Use a minidrip set for infants or small children, when a keep open or slow rate is in use, or when drug dose is measured according to patient response such as when an IV drug (e.g., dopamine) is adjusted based on the patient's blood pressure.

➤ Use volume control devices to limit the volume a patient could receive in a specified time. The nurse fills the volume control device with a specified volume of fluid and adjusts the flow rate. The patient can receive only the volume contained in the device until it is refilled. For example, consider an infant requiring IV fluids. Even if a 500-ml reservoir bag were hung instead of a 1000-ml bag, the danger of fluid overload would be significant if all 500 ml were to infuse rapidly. The nurse could fill the volume control device with the amount ordered for 1 hour (e.g., 30 ml for this patient) and adjust the flow rate. Even if all of the fluid in the device would infuse rapidly, the danger of fluid overload would be much less than with 500 ml. Volume control devices permit the addition of medications to the fluid in the chamber.

➤ IV pumps and controllers are widely used today. These electronic devices help maintain a constant rate of flow. Because they contain alarms, they warn the nurse when a problem occurs. The IV pump delivers the IV fluid with pressure, whereas the IV controller adjusts the rate of fluids infusing via gravity. Become familiar with devices used at your site. Electronic devices do not replace careful patient assessment and nursing care but can assist in managing IV therapy.

➤ The use of in-line IV filters for all medications and solutions is not universally accepted. Nevertheless, many agencies require them. Familiarize yourself with the advantages of the filters in use in your agency. For example, some filters remove only particulate matter, and some do not have air eliminating capability. The 0.22-mm filter can remove particulate matter, fungi, bacteria, and air but cannot filter TPN solutions because it is too small. Tubing for blood administration is equipped with a filter. Fat emulsions cannot be filtered.

➤ Label all fluid reservoirs as directed by agency procedure. A common way is to place a length of adhesive tape along the side of the bag or bottle next to the volume markers on the container. The correct fluid level per hour is marked on the tape. For example, if 1000 ml of fluid is started at 8 AM and the fluid is to infuse at 100 ml/hr, there should be 900 ml remaining at 9 AM and 800 ml at 10 AM. Thus any nurse on duty can determine at a glance whether the infusion is running at the correct rate. If you discover that an infusion is "behind," do not try to catch up by doubling or increasing the rate for the next hour or two. Assess the situation and, if necessary, restart the infusion at another site. If the solution is infusing too rapidly, slow the rate and assess the patient for signs of fluid overload (see Table 17-5). If the extra volume infused was minimal and the patient's condition is satisfactory, resume the prescribed rate. If the volume is excessive or signs of fluid overload are present, maintain the IV at the keep open rate and notify the physician.

➤ Label all IV solutions carefully, especially when additives such as potassium, vitamins, heparin, insulin, and other drugs have been included. Record the administration of all IV solutions carefully. See Chapter 5 for additional information about IV administration.

Oral and Intravenous potassium
Drug Administration

➤ Potassium chloride (KCl) is the most commonly administered electrolyte added to IV fluids. (Most sodium chloride administered is supplied by manufacturers in commonly used concentrations; potassium chloride is more often added by the nurse or pharmacy.) Ascertain that the patient has adequate kidney function before administering IV potassium. Always dilute potassium chloride before administering it intravenously. Carefully check the dose before adding it. Carefully label containers to which potassium has been added.

➤ Monitor the patient's ECG changes and serum potassium level. See Table 17-1 for signs of common electrolyte imbalances. The classic ECG changes seen with low potassium (hypokalemia) include ST-segment depression, flattened T waves, presence of U waves, and ventricular arrhythmias. The classic ECG changes with high potassium (hyperkalemia) include tall thin T waves, prolonged PR interval, ST depression, widened QRS complex, and loss of P waves.

➤ Carefully check the rate of administration of IV potassium. The usual dosage is 20 to 60 mEq/24 hr. If needed, IV potassium may be given at a rate of 10 to 15 mEq/hr of a solution containing 40 mEq/L unless the patient is severely potassium depleted.

➤ To treat hyperkalemia, discontinue potassium replacements (IV or oral) and limit potassium-rich foods (see Dietary Considerations box in Chapter 14). Emergency treatment includes IV sodium bicarbonate, calcium gluconate (if not contraindicated by existing cardiac conditions), and IV glucose and insulin (which help shift potassium into the cell). Dialysis may also be used.

➤ Subacute hyperkalemia is treated with cation exchange resins such as sodium polystyrene sulfonate (e.g., Kayexalate, SPS suspension), which exchanges sodium for potassium in the intestine. The effect is not evident for several hours to 1 day after administration. The resin is given orally, via nasogastric tube, or as a retention enema. Adverse effects include hypokalemia, hypocalcemia, anorexia, nausea, vomiting, and constipation. Monitor electrolyte levels. When the

Nursing Implications Summary—cont'd

resin is given orally or via nasogastric tube, constipation is common, so a mild laxative may be administered concurrently. For oral administration, dilute the drug in water, syrup, fruit juice, or soft drink.

➤ Monitor potassium levels carefully in patients with cardiac conditions because hypokalemia potentiates the effects of cardiac glycosides. Do not administer potassium to patients receiving potassium-sparing diuretics (see Chapter 14).

Nursing in the Community

➤ Review with patients the importance of taking potassium preparations as ordered. Some patients will be able to maintain potassium levels through dietary intake of potassium-rich foods (see Dietary Considerations box in Chapter 14).

➤ Work with patients to find an acceptable form of potassium. Oral preparations are often unpalatable or difficult to swallow. Enteric-coated tablets have been implicated in small bowel ulceration. Effervescent preparations are often unpalatable, and patients soon stop taking them. Oral solutions work well but often have a bitter, salty taste.

➤ Dilute oral solutions in juice or milk if acceptable to the patient. Avoid tomato juice if the patient is on a low-sodium diet.

➤ Dissolve the soluble powders, granules, or tablets in at least 4 ounces of juice or water; avoid tomato juice if the patient is on a low-sodium diet. Allow fizzing to stop before the patient drinks the dose.

➤ Extended-release tablets and capsules should be swallowed whole without being chewed or crushed. A few tablets may be crushed or broken and a few capsules may be opened, but most should not be; check with the pharmacist.

➤ Instruct patients to take potassium with meals to reduce gastric irritation.

➤ Instruct patients to take missed doses if remembered within 2 hours of when scheduled, otherwise omit the missed dose and resume regular dosing schedule. Do not double up for missed doses.

➤ Instruct patients to avoid salt substitutes and low-sodium foods or milk unless this is first discussed with the physician.

magnesium sulfate

Drug Administration/Nursing in the Community

➤ Magnesium sulfate is administered orally to promote defecation (see Chapter 24) and parenterally to treat or prevent hypomagnesemia. It is also available as an anticonvulsant, especially in pregnancy-induced hypertension (PIH).

➤ See Table 17-1 for signs of magnesium imbalances. If magnesium imbalance is suspected, monitor the serum magnesium level.

➤ Intramuscular (IM) administration of magnesium is painful. Use large muscle masses and rotate sites. Inject the drug slowly.

➤ The goal in treating PIH is to obtain a serum level that inhibits seizures but does not cause respiratory or cardiac paralysis. Several dosage regimens are followed for this purpose; most are initiated with a loading dose, followed by a maintenance dose. Assess the deep tendon reflexes, respiratory rate, ECG changes, and urinary output. If reflexes diminish or cease, if the respiratory rate decreases, or if the urinary output falls below 30 to 100 ml/hr, the dose of magnesium sulfate may require reduction. ECG changes caused by increasing magnesium levels include prolonged PQ interval and widened QRS complex. Monitor vital signs, intake and output, and serum magnesium levels. Monitor fetal heart sounds. In severe cases, monitor maternal ECG changes and attach a fetal monitor to assess infant status. Newborns of mothers who received magnesium sulfate should be monitored for several hours after delivery for signs of hypermagnesemia (see Table 17-1).

➤ Administer the 10% solution (1 g/10 ml or 8 mEq/10 ml) at a rate of 1.5 ml/min. Dilute the 50% solution to a 20% solution or less before IV administration.

➤ Have available equipment for resuscitation in settings where parenteral magnesium sulfate is administered. Have available calcium gluconate and calcium gluceptate as specific antidotes for magnesium overdose.

sodium bicarbonate

Drug Administration/Nursing in the Community

➤ Sodium bicarbonate is given orally to neutralize gastric acid (see Chapter 26) and to alkalinize urine.

➤ During resuscitation efforts, administer sodium bicarbonate via direct IV push to help correct metabolic acidosis. It is usually included in the emergency drug box or on the resuscitation cart, packaged in labeled, filled syringes.

➤ For general IV administration the drug is diluted and administered at a rate of 2 to 5 mEq/kg over 4 to 8 hours. Signs of overdose are metabolic alkalosis and hypernatremia (see Table 17-1). Monitor serum electrolyte and arterial blood gas levels.

calcium

Drug Administration/Nursing in the Community

➤ Oral calcium compounds are used as antacids (see Chapter 26). Read the physician's orders carefully.

➤ IV calcium compounds include calcium acetate, calcium gluconate, calcium chloride, and calcium gluceptate. When possible, warm drug to body temperature before administering. The IV route is preferred in infants, but scalp veins should be avoided because extravasation may cause tissue necrosis. Monitor ECG changes during IV administration. Keep patient recumbent for 30 minutes after IV administration; monitor blood pressure and serum calcium levels.

➤ If IV administration is not possible, calcium gluceptate, calcium gluconate, or a combination of calcium glycerophosphate and calcium lactate may be administered intramuscularly. (Do not give calcium chloride intramuscularly.) Use large muscle masses and rotate injection sites. If more than 5 ml is to be administered intramuscularly to an adult,

Continued

Nursing Implications Summary—cont'd

divide the dose in half and administer via two injections. With children, determine whether the dose should be divided.

➤ Severe hypocalcemia may manifest as tetany; Chvostek's sign and Trousseau's sign may be positive (see a text on physical assessment). Pad the siderails. Have resuscitation equipment readily available.

➤ For patients taking oral calcium supplements, review foods that are rich in calcium (see Dietary Considerations box in Chapter 68). Hypercalcemia is also discussed in Chapter 68.

Blood, Plasma, Albumin, and Plasma Protein Fraction
Drug Administration

➤ Review the general guidelines for care of patients receiving IV fluids and other replacement solutions.

➤ Whole blood is administered via a blood infusion tubing set, which usually contains an in-line filter. The infusion is established, usually with normal saline in the primary line; solutions with dextrose may hemolyze blood and solutions containing calcium, as in lactated Ringer's solution, may clot the blood. The blood is piggybacked to the primary solution via the second port in the set. This method helps prevent the blood from clotting; it also helps maintain a patent IV access line, even if infusion of the blood must be stopped, as might happen with an allergic reaction.

➤ Monitor hematocrit and hemoglobin levels, intake and output, and vital signs.

➤ Before beginning the transfusion, carefully check the patient's identification bracelet and the label on the container of blood. Blood type incompatibility is potentially fatal; death can occur after infusion of as little as 50 to 100 ml of an incorrect blood type. Most institutions provide specific, detailed procedures to ensure that blood is carefully checked beforehand. Signs and symptoms of a transfusion reaction include flushing, nausea, hypotension, increased pulse rate, difficulty breathing, tightness in the chest, chills, fever, headache, substernal chest pain, vomiting, and sense of impending doom. In addition, hematologic changes may occur, including disseminated intravascular coagulation (DIC), thrombocytopenia, and spontaneous bleeding. If the patient is anesthetized or unconscious, this reaction may be difficult to recognize.

➤ After starting a transfusion, remain with the patient for 10 to 15 minutes, monitoring and recording vital signs. Thoroughly investigate any unanticipated occurrence; stop the infusion, but maintain a patent IV access line by restarting the priming solution, and notify the physician. Hypersensitivity reactions include rashes, itching, and the symptoms of a transfusion reaction noted earlier. Minor reactions can often be treated with antihistamines or corticosteroids, but occasionally emergency life support measures, including epinephrine, are required. Know beforehand where emergency drugs and equipment are kept.

➤ Febrile reactions usually begin within the first 15 minutes of infusion but may not begin until 1 to 2 hours later. They are characterized by fever (39.4° to 40°C [103° to 104°F]), chills, headache, and malaise. Stop the infusion, notify the physician, and investigate the cause.

➤ Do not mix any medications with blood. If it is necessary to administer an IV medication via the same IV access line, stop the blood infusion, flush the line with saline, inject the medication, flush the line again with saline, and resume the blood infusion. Blood cells are large, so a large-diameter needle or catheter should be used.

➤ Circulatory overload is more common when whole blood is administered, when the patient is an older adult or an infant, or when the patient has cardiac disease. Monitor vital signs and cardiac and lung sounds, and observe for respiratory difficulty and cough.

➤ When fluid overload is a concern or large volumes must be transfused, whole blood components may be prescribed, such as packed red cells, platelets, cryoprecipitated factor VIII (for patients with hemophilia), and fibrinogen. These products are smaller in volume than whole blood but are generally administered the same way.

➤ Complete administration of a unit of whole blood within 2 to 4 hours; after this time, the blood may clot. (In extreme emergencies, pressure applied to the bag will afford delivery within 10 minutes or less.)

➤ Blood products deteriorate rapidly if not stored properly and used promptly. Do not thaw frozen products until they are to be used. Do not procure blood from the blood bank until the patient is ready for the infusion. Do not leave blood products in the patient care unit. Check and observe expiration dates of all blood products. Plasma, albumin, and plasma protein fraction are derived from blood, and the same general guidelines apply.

dextran
Drug Administration

➤ Monitor weight, blood pressure, pulse, and intake and output. Assess for signs of fluid overload (see Table 17-5). Monitor hematocrit, hemoglobin, serum electrolytes, serum protein, and serum protein electrophoresis levels. Assess patients for bleeding. Assess for dehydration because dextran promotes tissue dehydration.

➤ Notify physician if urine output falls below 30 ml/hr.

➤ Monitor patients for signs of allergic reaction. If blood must also be administered, flush tubing thoroughly between blood and dextran infusion because dextran coagulates blood in tubing.

➤ Use only clear solutions. If crystallization has occurred, heat bottle in warm water until crystals dissolve before administering. If drawing blood for laboratory tests, note on the requisition that dextran is being administered; this is important because dextran may cause falsely high serum glucose levels and alterations in other blood tests.

Nursing Implications Summary—cont'd

Hetastarch
Drug Administration
➤ Monitor for allergic reactions. Monitor vital signs. Monitor hematocrit, hemoglobin, plasma proteins, and platelet levels. Assess patients for signs of bleeding.

➤ Flush tubing with saline or change tubing before administering blood.

Total Parenteral Nutrition
Drug Administration/Nursing in the Community
➤ Review the general guidelines for care of patients receiving IV fluids.

➤ TPN, or hyperalimentation, must be administered via a central infusion line for solutions more concentrated than 10% dextrose. The central line is placed by the physician using aseptic technique, as described in Chapter 5.

➤ Follow aseptic technique when manipulating the TPN infusion. These fluids provide favorable conditions for growth of harmful bacteria. It is essential to prevent infection. Follow agency procedures for maintenance of TPN. Procedures usually specify how often to dress the insertion site, what method to use for dressing, what agent to use to clean injection sites (e.g., povidone-iodine or alcohol), and how often to change tubing.

➤ Monitor vital signs and assess for fluid overload (see Table 17-5). Monitor the patient's temperature every 4 hours in the hospital. Instruct the patient at home to notify the physician if fever develops.

➤ Hypertonic dextrose, amino acids, and fat emulsions are the mainstay of TPN therapy. The rate of flow, additives (vitamins, minerals, and electrolytes), and their concentrations must be ordered specifically by the physician. Most agencies have devised a protocol for monitoring the patient, including the frequency of blood work such as serum electrolyte levels, albumin levels, BUN levels, liver function studies, and blood glucose levels; the frequency of vitamin and mineral infusions; the procedures for culturing the catheter tip and fluid if infection develops; and the frequency of weighing the patient.

➤ Do not add medications to the solution or administer medications via the TPN line unless specifically permitted by agency protocol or the pharmacist. Usually, if other IV medications are needed, a separate peripheral IV line must be started and maintained.

➤ Maintain the infusion at a steady rate; usually an electronic monitoring device is used. Erratic infusion rates may cause fluctuations in blood glucose levels, which induces hyperglycemia and hypoglycemia. If the infusion stops or must be discontinued abruptly, standing orders (at most facilities) are to begin a peripheral infusion of 10% dextrose to prevent hypoglycemia. When the need for TPN therapy has resolved, gradually slow the rate of infusion to prevent hypoglycemia.

➤ Assess the patient for appearance of dry, flaky skin; hair loss; and rashes. These signs may indicate essential fatty acid or zinc deficiency.

➤ Prepare TPN solutions in a laminar flow hood, where risk of contamination is low.

➤ Some patients are suitable candidates for TPN administration at home. Assess learning needs with the patient and family. Provide reassurance. Ascertain that the patient and family are able to manipulate the equipment. Refer the patient to a social services agency and to a community-based nursing care service.

Amino Acid Infusions
Drug Administration
➤ Review the general guidelines for TPN. Assess for common side effects (nausea, vomiting, flushing, and a sensation of warmth). Less common side effects are chills, headache, abdominal pain, dizziness, rashes, hyperglycemia, and glycosuria.

➤ Monitor intake and output; serum electrolyte, magnesium, blood ammonia, phosphate, serum protein, cholesterol, and BUN levels; liver function studies; and blood glucose levels. Observe for signs of essential fatty acid deficiency (hair loss and dry, flaky skin).

➤ Vitamins, electrolytes, trace elements, heparin, and insulin may be administered via the same IV line, but other medications should not be. Do not premix these drugs with amino acid infusions; administer via a Y-connector.

➤ Use an IV filter. Infuse at a rate not exceeding 4 mg/kg/hr of nitrogen. Infuse at a steady rate; use an electronic infusion monitor if available.

Fat Emulsions
Drug Administration/Nursing in the Community
➤ Assess for history of allergy to eggs, legumes, soybeans, or previous fat emulsion before use.

➤ See general guidelines for IV therapy. Administer fat emulsions via a central or peripheral IV line. Read the manufacturer's information supplied with the bottle of fat emulsion. Fat emulsion should comprise no more than 60% of the total daily caloric intake. Inspect before using. If the emulsion has cracked (the oil separated from the other products), it should not be used. Do not shake the emulsion.

➤ Assess for side effects including thrombophlebitis, vomiting, chest pain, back pain, and allergic reactions. Begin the infusion slowly (e.g., 1 ml/min) and observe the patient. If no untoward effect has occurred after 15 to 30 minutes, increase the rate of infusion to the desired rate. Monitor serum triglyceride levels. Fat emulsions can cause hyperlipidemia, which should clear between infusions; if not, withhold the next dose and notify the physician.

➤ Do not filter a fat emulsion. If it is piggybacked into a line incorporating a filter, the fat emulsion must be inserted below the level of the filter (closer to the patient).

Continued

Nursing Implications Summary—cont'd

Vitamins

Drug Administration/Nursing in the Community

➤ Water-soluble vitamins may be given intravenously, whereas fat-soluble vitamins are administered via IM injection. Vitamins should be given parenterally when oral intake and di-

gestion are compromised. Patients with vitamin deficiencies who are able to eat and digest food should be counseled to increase their dietary intake of vitamin-rich foods (see Dietary Considerations box earlier in this chapter).

CHAPTER REVIEW

Application

1. What are the three main fluid compartments of the body?
2. What are the major buffers of plasma?
3. What is the major difference in composition between plasma and interstitial fluid?
4. What is osmosis?
5. What solute primarily determines the osmotic strength of plasma?
6. What is oncotic pressure?
7. Does the protein content of plasma cause water to move into or out of blood vessels?
8. What is hydrostatic pressure?
9. Does hydrostatic pressure cause water to move into or out of blood vessels?
10. What are signs of fluid overload?
11. What are the uses of isotonic saline?
12. What dangers are associated with saline administration?
13. What is the primary use for isotonic dextrose?
14. Dextrose solutions must not be mixed with whole blood for administration. Why?
15. What organ system must be functioning before potassium replacement is begun?

Critical Thinking

1. How are cells able to maintain high intracellular concentrations of potassium, phosphate, and magnesium?

2. What are signs of dehydration or fluid deficit? Give examples of patients who are at high risk for dehydration.
3. What can cause fluid excess or overload? Give examples of patients who are at high risk for fluid overload.
4. What is hypernatremia? hyponatremia? How would you assess for these?
5. What is hyperkalemia? hypokalemia? How would you assess for these?
6. What is respiratory acidosis? How does it differ from metabolic acidosis? How would you assess for these?
7. What is respiratory alkalosis? How does it differ from metabolic alkalosis? How would you assess for these?
8. Compare and contrast isotonic saline, Ringer's solution, and lactated Ringer's solution.
9. Why do solutions of large-molecular-weight proteins or carbohydrates expand plasma volume?
10. What special precautions for administration are necessary with hypertonic dextrose for parenteral nutrition?
11. What additional supplement may be required by patients receiving amino acid solutions for parenteral nutrition?
12. What is the primary advantage of fat emulsions in parenteral nutrition? What are some nursing care precautions in administering fat emulsions?
13. What teaching points are necessary for patients and families administering TPN in the home?

References

Bove LA: Restoring electrolyte balance: calcium & phosphorous. *RN* 59(3):47-52, 1996.

Bove LA: Restoring electrolyte balance: sodium & chloride. *RN* 59(1):25-29, 1996.

Carroll P: Analyzing the chem 7. *RN* 60(11):32-37, 1997.

Perez A: Electrolytes: restoring the balance: hyperkalemia. *RN* 58(11):32-37, 1995.

Perez A: Restoring electrolyte balance: hypokalemia. *RN* 58(12): 33-36, 1995.

Chapter 18

Drugs to Control Congestive Heart Failure

OBJECTIVES

After studying this chapter, you should be able to do the following:

■ *Explain why congestive heart failure produces symptoms of edema, shortness of breath, and rapid heart rate (tachycardia).*

■ *Explain how angiotensin-converting enzyme (ACE) inhibitors and other vasodilators might slow the progression of heart failure and improve survival.*

■ *Explain how cardiac glycosides relieve symptoms of congestive heart failure.*

■ *Explain how beta-adrenergic agents and diuretics relieve symptoms of congestive heart failure.*

■ *Develop a nursing care plan for a patient receiving a cardiac glycoside.*

CHAPTER OVERVIEW

Congestive heart failure leads to symptoms caused by the failure of the heart to adequately pump the blood delivered to it. The condition cannot be cured, but many medications can improve the situation by acting directly on the heart or by acting at other sites to interrupt the disease process.

THERAPEUTIC RATIONALE: CONGESTIVE HEART FAILURE

Cardiac Structure and Function

To understand the action of drugs on the heart, it is important to know how its tissues act together to produce the integrated function of the whole organ. The pumping action of the heart depends on an appropriately timed contraction of adequate force to deliver blood from the left ventricle into the arteries. The ability to pump blood into the arteries depends on the strength of ventricular contraction and the resistance against which the heart works (**afterload**). Afterload is determined by blood volume and pressure. **Contractility** refers to the strength of the muscular contraction of the heart. **Inotropic** refers to factors affecting the strength of

cardiac contraction. A positive inotropic response increases cardiac contractility, but a negative inotropic response decreases contractility.

Heart rate (the number of beats or ventricular contractions per minute) is normally the same as the rate of sinoatrial (SA) node firing because the impulse to beat normally originates at the SA node, a specialized group of cells in the right atrium (Figure 18-1). This impulse will not pass directly between the atria and ventricles because they are insulated from each other by a ring of nonconductive tissue. Another group of specialized fibers, the atrioventricular (AV) node, transmits the impulse to beat to the ventricles. The rate at which the impulse passes through the AV node causes an important delay that allows adequate filling of the ventricles. This rate of transmission of the impulse through the AV node is called the *conduction velocity*.

217

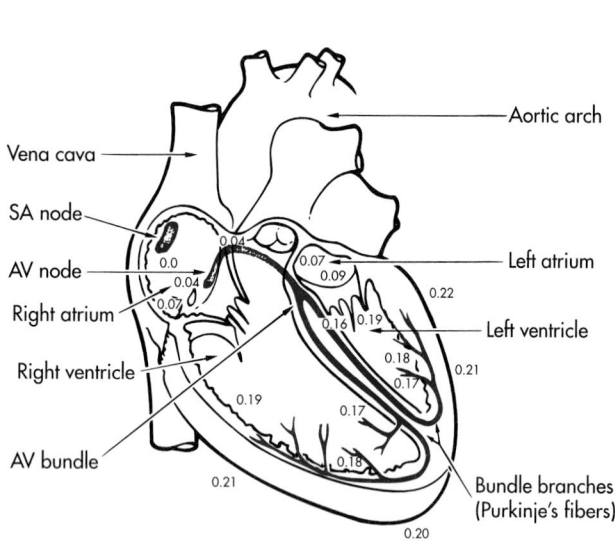

Figure 18-1 Transmission of action potentials through heart. Initiation of heartbeat occurs at sinoatrial (SA) node, and action potential is transmitted throughout atria before passing through atrioventricular (AV) node to ventricles. Numerals designate seconds it takes for impulse to travel from SA node to anatomic site designated by numeral. All parts of atria have received impulse with 0.09 seconds, but transmission to ventricles is delayed during its passage through AV node so that ventricles do not begin to contract until 0.16 seconds after SA node firing. Delay allows atria to contract and fill ventricles before ventricles begin to contract to force blood from heart.

Figure 18-2 Autonomic innervation of heart.

The heart is innervated by sympathetic and parasympathetic branches of the autonomic nervous system (Figure 18-2). The parasympathetic vagus nerve acts mainly in the nodes. Stimulation of the vagus nerve releases acetylcholine, which makes the cells less excitable. In the SA node, these actions decrease the rate of firing, which reduces heart rate. Stimulation of the vagus nerve also decreases conduction velocity through the AV node. Slowing conduction velocity increases the time between contraction of atria and ventricles and therefore slows heart rate.

Sympathetic nerve fibers innervate both atria and ventricles. Stimulation of sympathetic nerves releases norepinephrine, which activates beta$_1$-adrenergic receptors of the heart. Activation of the beta$_1$-receptors in conducting tissue of the heart increases heart rate and conduction velocity. Stimulation of the beta$_1$-adrenergic receptors in the ventricular muscle increases the force of contraction (positive inotropic response).

Alterations of Myocardial Output

Frank-Starling Law

The volume of blood that the heart delivers to the arteries varies with stress, exertion, and other factors. How the heart regulates its output to meet these variable demands is described by the **Frank-Starling law**. This principle of physiol-

ogy states that the force of muscular contraction is directly related to the stretch of the muscle; the more a muscle is stretched, within mechanical limits, the stronger its subsequent contraction. This principle applied to the heart means that when the ventricles are filled with larger-than-normal volumes of blood, they contract with greater-than-normal force to deliver their entire contents to the arteries. Blood does not normally accumulate in the veins, and all the blood coming into the heart is pumped out. If cardiac muscle fibers are stretched beyond their mechanical limits, however, the strength of contraction decreases and cardiac output falls.

Sympathetic Nervous System Stimulation

Stimulation of the sympathetic nervous system also increases the rate of cardiac contraction, which is a second mechanism for increasing output. The peak efficiency of the heart under these conditions is reached at about 150 to 175 beats/min. Faster rates result in incomplete filling of the ventricles and reduce the overall efficiency of the pump.

Cardiac Hypertrophy

If the heart is subjected to chronic demands for increased output, it may enlarge. This condition is called myocardial **hypertrophy** and may be a normal response to chronic stress. For example, long-distance runners and tennis players may have enlarged hearts. In other cases the enlargement of the heart may signal a pathologic process. For example, in chronic heart failure, myocardial output gradually falls below the required level, resulting from the failure of the myocardium as a pump. As output falls, normal regulatory mechanisms come into effect. Cardiac hypertrophy may occur as the body seeks to increase the efficiency of the pump. Sympathetic stimulation may also be increased to raise heart rate and hence output. In many cases, in the absence of acute demands on the heart, these mechanisms enable a weakened heart to maintain sufficient output. Patients may have few symptoms but on examination may have an enlarged heart and high heart rate.

Congestive Heart Failure

If the regulatory mechanisms fail and cardiac output falls below venous return, **congestive heart failure** results. The symptoms arise directly from insufficient cardiac output and indirectly from the body's attempts to adapt to lowered cardiac output. Blood pooled in the veins increases venous pressure. Excessive venous pressure stretches cardiac muscle fibers beyond their limit, and as predicted by the Frank-Starling law, the strength of contraction falls further. Chronic activation of the sympathetic nervous system causes systemic vasoconstriction, which contributes to the congestive symptoms and also limits renal blood flow. Reduced blood flow to the kidneys triggers sodium and water retention, which further worsens congestive symptoms. Moreover, the changes in renal perfusion cause the release of renin, which starts the cascade that leads to production of the potent vasoconstrictor angiotensin II (see Chapter 66). Angiotensin II stimulates the release of aldosterone, which further increases sodium and water retention, and the release of norepinephrine, which contributes to vasoconstriction. These effects increase the filling pressure caused by venous tone (preload) and the pressure against which the heart works as it forces blood into the arteries (afterload), further impairing cardiac output. Edema of the lungs and periphery develops as fluid leaks into tissues from the capillaries. The typical patient in congestive heart failure is therefore short of breath and has a rapid pulse resulting from sympathetic stimulation of the heart, obvious swelling of the hands and feet, and an enlarged heart.

Congestive heart failure may be divided into two broad categories. **Systolic heart failure** is the most common form of congestive heart failure and arises from weakness of the heart muscle. This weakness may be caused by ischemic coronary artery disease, chronic hypertension, chronic alcohol abuse, and a variety of less common conditions such as infections or exposure to toxins. This form of heart failure is termed systolic because in this state, ventricular filling pressure is normal but during systole the ventricles fail to deliver normal output to the arteries.

A less common form of heart failure is termed **diastolic heart failure**. This conditions arises when the ventricles are stiff and fail to fill adequately during diastole. To compensate, left ventricular filling pressures may go up, which helps adequately fill the left ventricle but also causes pulmonary venous hypertension. The most common cause of this type of heart failure is aging.

The drugs discussed in the next section relieve the symptoms of congestive heart failure by acting directly on the heart or by reducing some of the harmful adaptive mechanisms triggered by reduced cardiac output. Because many of the symptoms of congestive heart failure are caused by activation of the renin-angiotensin system and by overactivity of the sympathetic nervous system, agents that reduce these harmful adaptive mechanisms may produce dramatic improvement in function, as well as prolongation of life.

THERAPEUTIC AGENTS: DRUGS TO TREAT CONGESTIVE HEART FAILURE

▼ Agents to Counter Systemic Responses to Reduced Cardiac Output: Angiotensin-Converting Enzyme Inhibitors: captopril, enalapril, and lisinopril

Mechanism of Action

Angiotensin-converting enzyme (ACE) inhibitors block production of the potent vasoconstrictor angiotensin II and thus prevent many of the harmful adaptations that lead to symptoms of congestive heart failure and to mortality. Therapy with these drugs produces vasodilation, which reduces systemic and pulmonary vascular resistance. As a result, cardiac output improves but the workload of the heart declines, making the organ more efficient. In addition, therapy with ACE inhibitors prevents increased collagen deposition and fibrosis in the heart, factors that contribute to cardiac hypertrophy during heart failure. ACE inhibitors may also improve coronary artery blood flow by effects upon bradykinin.

Pharmacokinetics

Captopril, **enalapril,** and lisinopril are the three ACE inhibitors used for congestive heart failure (Table 18-1). All three drugs are oral agents, with captopril being the most efficiently absorbed and lisinopril the least efficiently absorbed; food affects absorption of captopril but not the other two agents. The onset of action is about 1 hour for each of these drugs, which corresponds to the peak effect for captopril, but the peak effects of enalapril and lisinopril occur at about 6 hours. The duration of action for captopril is 6 to 12 hours, but is 24 hours for enalapril and lisinopril. Captopril and enalapril are metabolized in the liver, but lisinopril is not. Enalapril is a prodrug and is converted to the active metabolite enalaprilat. Elimination of all three drugs is primarily renal, but for enalapril there is significant fecal elimination.

Uses

ACE inhibitors were originally introduced as antihypertensive agents (see Chapter 13), but are now also considered first-line drugs for systolic congestive heart failure and left ventricular dysfunction. Several large clinical trials have confirmed that ACE inhibitors not only improve cardiac function in these patients, and hence quality of life, but also reduce mortality from systolic congestive heart failure. Because these drugs block the harmful adaptions to lowered cardiac output, the ACE inhibitors can and should be used early in the process to slow development of congestive heart failure. There are no adequate clinical trials to evaluate the

Table 18-1 Summary of Agents Used in Congestive Heart Failure to Counter Systemic Responses to Reduced Cardiac Output

Generic Name	Trade Name	Administration/Dosage	Comments
Angiotensin-Converting Enzyme Inhibitors			
captopril	Capoten*	ORAL: *Adults*—6.25 mg initially; then 12.5 mg 2 or 3 times daily; may increase gradually to 50 mg three times daily.	See Chapter 13, Table 13-2 for full listing.
enalapril	Vasotec*	ORAL: *Adults*—2.5 mg 1 or 2 times daily; may increase to 20 mg daily in 1 or 2 doses.	See Chapter 13, Table 13-2 for full listing. Most clinical trials with ACE inhibitors for heart failure used this drug.
lisinopril	Prinivil*	ORAL: *Adults*—2.5-5 mg daily; may increase to 20 mg daily.	See Chapter 13, Table 13-2 for full listing.
Diuretics			
bumetanide	Bumex	ORAL: *Adults*—Maximum daily dose 10 mg.	See Chapter 14, Table 14-2 for full listing.
furosemide	Lasix*	ORAL: *Adults*—20-80 mg once or twice daily.	See Chapter 14, Table 14-2 for full listing.
torsemide	Demadex	ORAL: *Adults*—Maximum daily dose 200 mg.	See Chapter 14, Table 14-2 for full listing.
Nitrate Vasodilators			
isosorbide dinitrate	Isonate	ORAL: *Adults*—5-20 mg every 6 hr.	Used with hydralazine.
hydralazine	Apresolline*	ORAL: *Adults*—Initially up to 37.5 mg every 6 hr; gradually increased to 75 mg every 6 hr if needed.	Used with Isosorbide dinitrate.
Adrenergic Receptor Blocker			
carvedilol	Coreg	ORAL: *Adults*—3.125 mg twice daily; may double dose in 2 wk if tolerated. FDA pregnancy category C.	See Chapter 13, Table 13-2 for full listing. Dosage must start very low and be increased gradually to prevent sudden cardiac decompensation.

*Available in Canada and the United States.

effects of ACE inhibitors in diastolic congestive heart failure, but preliminary evidence suggests ACE inhibitors may be used to control myocardial fibrosis and left ventricular hypertrophy in these patients.

Adverse Reactions and Contraindications

Captopril, enalapril, and lisinopril have all been associated with renal impairment, which may include proteinuria. Hepatotoxicity has also been reported with these three drugs. The most common side effect is usually hypotension. Sodium depletion or volume depletion worsens this reaction. Another common side effect is a continuing dry cough that may be especially troublesome at night.

Because of the risk of induction of angioedema with ACE inhibitors, these drugs are usually avoided in patients with a history of angioedema. The drugs may also be avoided in patients with renal impairment, hyperkalemia, or sodium depletion.

Toxicity

The main effect of overdoses is severe hypotension. Thus treatment consists of expanding plasma volume to correct hypotension. Captopril, enalapril, and lisinopril may be removed by hemodialysis.

Interactions

Potassium-containing supplements, low-salt milk, or salt-substitutes that contain high amounts of potassium may lead to hyperkalemia when combined with ACE inhibitors.

Diuretics or other hypotensive agents may worsen hypotensive reactions to ACE inhibitors.

Agents to Counter Systemic Responses to Reduced Cardiac Output: Diuretics

Diuretics control the pulmonary edema that accompanies severe systolic congestive heart failure. Therapeutic guidelines suggest that diuretics be added if ACE inhibitors alone do not control volume overload or other cardiovascular symptoms. Commonly used agents include furosemide, bumetanide, and torsemide (see Table 18-1); other diuretics may also be effective (see Chapter 14).

In addition to relieving pulmonary edema, a side effect of congestive heart failure, diuretics may directly improve cardiac function in some patients. In end-stage congestive heart failure, venous pressure is elevated sufficiently to cause heart muscle fibers to stretch excessively during filling of the chambers. Diuretics lower the pressure forcing blood into the heart chambers. As a result, the muscle fibers are not so abnormally stretched; they are then able to contract with greater power. Therefore contractility of the heart muscle is improved. The major consideration limiting the use of diuretics in congestive heart failure is the risk of causing electrolyte or fluid imbalances, which may be especially dangerous to patients in heart failure. Volume depletion or excessive dehydration must be avoided. Patients receiving digitalis should be carefully observed to prevent complications because diuretics tend to alter potassium concentration in the blood (see Chapter 14).

Agents to Counter Systemic Responses to Reduced Cardiac Output: Vasodilators

Vasodilators reverse the persistent vasoconstriction in late chronic congestive heart failure resulting from long-term compensatory sympathetic nervous system stimulation. Sympathetic nervous system stimulation may drive a failing heart, but it constricts peripheral blood vessels, thereby reducing cardiac output and increasing the workload of the heart. Vasodilators reduce afterload, the resistance against which the left ventricle must force blood. Cardiac output is thus increased, and workload is reduced.

Several classes of vasodilators are used in congestive heart failure. Nitroprusside can be used for short-term IV therapy in severely ill patients. More commonly hydralazine and isosorbide are used in combination as oral therapy (see Chapter 15). This combination has been shown to improve survival, although the effects were not as great as with the ACE inhibitors, which in addition to being vasodilators also have other beneficial effects in heart failure.

Agents to Counter Systemic Responses to Reduced Cardiac Output: Adrenergic Receptor Blockers

Beta-adrenergic receptor blockers could in theory reduce the effects of overstimulation of the sympathetic nervous system seen in late stage congestive heart failure, but the negative inotropic effects of the drugs make them inappropriate. Third-generation beta-adrenergic blockers include the drug carvedilol, which is a nonselective agent that blocks beta-receptors as well as alpha-receptors. The effect on alpha-receptors makes the drug a vasodilator. This unique combination of actions led to a clinical trial in which carvedilol was shown to reduce risk of hospitalization in chronic heart failure and also to reduce risk of mortality from the disease, presumably by preventing arrhythmias arising from excess sympathetic stimulation.

Inotropic Agents: Cardiac Glycosides

▼ digoxin and digitoxin

Mechanism of Action

Digoxin and digitoxin are **cardiac glycosides** that inhibit Na^+-K^+-ATPase and promote accumulation within heart cells of the calcium needed for contraction. These actions directly increase contractility, which increases cardiac output, improves blood flow to the kidneys and periphery, reduces venous pressure, and allows excess fluid to be excreted as edema clears. The diuretic effect of cardiac glycosides results from these actions on the heart.

Pharmacokinetics

The use of cardiac glycosides often requires **loading doses** because of the long half-lives of the drugs. With repeated equal doses of any drug, the plateau of drug concentration in blood is achieved after about four elimination half-times (see Chapter 1). For cardiac glycosides, with half-lives of 2 to 7 days, the desired therapeutic concentration would not be achieved for weeks after therapy starts. To avoid such long delays, cardiac glycosides may be given first in a loading dose designed to raise the concentration in blood rapidly to the therapeutic range. After the loading dose or doses, a smaller dose is given on a regular schedule. This smaller dose, the maintenance dose, holds the concentration of drug in the therapeutic range; adjustments may be needed if the patient's condition changes.

Digoxin, the most commonly used cardiac glycoside, is usually given orally in a dose that produces and maintains a therapeutic plasma level of 0.8 to 1.6 ng/ml (Table 18-2). Loading doses range from 0.75 to 1.25 mg/day. The half-life of digoxin is 32 to 48 hours; thus the maintenance dose must replace the 37% of the total body store of drug that is lost every day, primarily through renal excretion. Maintenance doses range from 0.05 to 0.5 mg/day, depending on the drug form used.

Digitoxin is used less often because of its very long half-life. The therapeutic level in plasma is 14 to 26 ng/ml. Loading doses range from 0.4 to 1.2 mg/day. Because the half-life of digitoxin is 5 to 7 days, about 10% of the total body store of drug is excreted each day, primarily by hepatic mechanisms; the daily dose compensates for this loss. Maintenance doses range from 0.05 to 0.3 mg/day. Toxicity may persist for days after digitoxin is stopped because the drug is so slowly removed from the system.

Uses

Digoxin is avoided in diastolic congestive heart failure but is used to treat systolic congestive heart failure because it directly improves the strength of the heart muscle, elevating cardiac output. Numerous clinical trials have attempted to assess the outcome of digoxin therapy in congestive heart failure. Most studies suggest that optimal effects are seen when digoxin is combined with diuretics, vasodilators, or ACE inhibitors. The most clear-cut effect of digoxin is an improvement in exercise tolerance and hemodynamics; there is no documented improvement in long-term survival with digoxin.

Adverse Reactions and Contraindications

There is such a small difference between the therapeutic dose and toxic doses that most patients taking cardiac glycosides experience drug-related difficulties. The symptoms may be neurologic, visual, cardiac, or psychiatric. They tend to be vague and easily confused with those of congestive heart failure. Anorexia, nausea, and vomiting also occur.

The neurologic or central nervous system (CNS) effects of cardiac glycosides cause many of the characteristic side effects, such as weakness, fatigue, and fainting. Visual disturbances such as dimness of vision, double vision, blind spots, flashing lights, or altered color vision also occur. Psychiatric disturbances range from mood alterations to psychoses or hallucinations.

Patients receiving cardiac glycosides must be checked often for the appearance of extra heartbeats or other arrhythmias. It is routine practice in many hospitals to omit the dose if the heart rate is less than 60 beats/min. Although bradycardia is the most common sign of digitalis-induced arrhythmias,

Table 18-2 Summary of Inotropic Agents Used in Congestive Heart Failure

Generic Name	Trade Name	Administration/Dosage	Comments
digitoxin	Crystodigin Digitaline†	ORAL: *Adults*—Rapid loading: 0.6 mg, then 0.4 mg in 4-6 hr, followed by 0.2 mg 4-6 hr later. Slow loading: 0.2 mg twice daily for 4 days. Maintenance doses: 0.05-0.3 mg daily. FDA pregnancy category C.	Dosage forms are inconvenient for children; digoxin is preferred. Half-life is 5-7 days, with a duration of action of 14 days.
digoxin	Lanoxin*	ORAL (Tablets): *Adults*—Rapid loading: 0.75-1.25 mg divided into 2 or more doses given at 6- to 8-hr intervals. Maintenance dose (also used for slow loading): 0.125-0.5 mg daily. FDA pregnancy category C. *Children* (elixir)—Loading doses below should be divided and given every 6-8 hr. Premature to 1-mo-old infants—0.2-0.035 mg/kg. Infants-2 yr—0.035-0.06 mg/kg. 2-5 yr: 0.03-0.04 mg/kg. 5-10 yr—0.02-0.035 mg/kg. Older than 10 yr—usual adult dose (tablets). Maintenance dose for children: 20%-30% of loading dose.	Bioavailability of digoxin from tablet is variable and may be as low as 60%. Half-life is 32-48 hr, with a duration of action of 2-6 days.
	Lanoxicaps	ORAL (capsules) and INTRAVENOUS: *Adults*—Rapid loading: 0.4-0.6 mg, then 0.1-0.3 mg 2 or 3 more times at 4- to 6-hr intervals. Maintenance dose (also used for slow loading): 0.05-0.35 mg daily. *Children*—Divide loading doses below into portions given every 6 hr. Premature infants: 0.015-0.025 mg/kg. Newborns: 0.02-0.03 mg/kg. Infants-2 yr: 0.03-0.05 mg/kg. 2-5 yr: 0.025-0.035 mg/kg. 5-10 yr: 0.015-0.03 mg/kg. Over 10 yr: 0.008-0.012 mg/kg. Maintenance dose for premature infants: 20% to 30% of oral loading dose; for other children: 25%-30% of oral loading dose, divided for children under 10 yr.	Oral absorption from solution in soft gelatin capsule is nearly 100%.
amrinone	Inocor*	INTRAVENOUS: *Adults*—initially 0.75 mg/kg body weight given slowly over 2-3 min. Repeat after 30 min if needed. Maintenance: 0.005-0.01 mg/kg/min, according to clinical response. FDA pregnancy category C.	Patients with atrial flutter may require pretreatment with digitalis to prevent ventricular arrhythmia and with fluid to maintain adequate cardiac filling.
milrinone	Primacor	INTRAVENOUS: *Adults*—Initially 0.05 mg/kg body weight given slowly over 10 min. Maintenance: 0.375-0.75 µg/kg/min. FDA pregnancy category C.	Same precautions as amrinone. Milrinone is used primarily in patients who receive digitalis and diuretics.

*Available in Canada and the United States.
†Available in Canada only.

other changes in heart rate are possible. Therefore any change in heart rate or rhythm should be noted and reported.

Cardiac glycosides are avoided in patients with any sign of prior toxicity with one of the drugs or in ventricular fibrillation. Risk of arrhythmias may be increased by hyperkalemia, myxedema, pulmonary disease, or cardiac disease. Risks also rise in the elderly (see Geriatric Considerations box).

Toxicity

The toxic reactions caused by cardiac glycosides are dose related (see Chapter 1). Bradycardia (slow heart rate) may be an early sign of rising blood concentrations of cardiac glycosides, but as concentrations continue to rise, other arrhythmias appear; tachycardia and ultimately ventricular fibrillation and death may occur. Blood levels of cardiac glycosides are routinely monitored to aid in diagnosing drug toxicity.

With digoxin or digitoxin overdose, patients may continue to be at risk during the lengthy period required to eliminate these long-acting agents. If arrhythmias or hyperkalemia becomes life-threatening, digoxin immune Fab (Table 18-3) can be used to rapidly neutralize free drug. Arrhythmias and electrolyte imbalance can be reversed within 30 minutes. The inotropic effect of cardiac glycosides persists for several hours longer.

Accidental poisoning of children with cardiac glycosides can occur. Patients who are around small children should be warned of the danger their medicine poses to curious toddlers.

Interactions

Toxicity of cardiac glycosides may be increased by other drugs. For example, potassium-depleting diuretics such as thiazides or loop diuretics (see Chapter 14) may predispose a patient to cardiac toxicity because a low intracellular potassium level increases the likelihood of arrhythmias.

Inotropic Agents: Beta$_1$-Agonists

Stimulation of the beta$_1$ class of adrenergic receptors in the heart directly increases cardiac contractility by increasing cyclic adenosine monophosphate (cAMP) in heart muscle. An increase in cAMP can also be achieved by blocking phosphodiesterase, the enzyme that degrades cAMP. Drugs with these actions may be of value in treating symptoms of acute or chronic congestive heart failure.

Dobutamine (see Chapter 16) directly stimulates myocardial beta$_1$-receptors but has little effect on beta$_2$-receptors and alpha-receptors, which predominate in blood vessels. Dobutamine does not activate dopamine receptors in renal vasculature. The drug has little tendency to increase heart rate or elevate blood pressure. These properties make it an

GERIATRIC CONSIDERATIONS

Cardiac Glycosides

THE PROBLEM

Older adult patients receiving cardiac glycosides may have diminished renal or hepatic function and a decreased volume of distribution for cardiac glycosides. They are also more prone to electrolyte imbalances, including hypokalemia, which can increase drug toxicity. Appetite suppression caused by digoxin can aggravate the problem of poor nutrition in frail older adult patients.

SOLUTIONS

- Adjust dosages carefully to avoid toxicity. Maintenance dosages may be lower in older adult patients than in younger adults.
- Watch carefully for signs of electrolyte imbalance.
- Instruct the patient about appropriate dietary practices that minimize risk of electrolyte imbalances.
- Do not assume that complaints of fatigue, weakness, mood alterations, or other signs of toxicity are a normal part of aging or of heart disease, and observe patients carefully.

attractive agent for increasing cardiac output in severely ill patients. A disadvantage of dobutamine is that it must be given intravenously.

Dopamine (see Chapter 16) directly stimulates myocardial beta$_1$-receptors but also causes indirect stimulation at this site by releasing norepinephrine from nerve terminals in the heart. Dopamine also stimulates alpha-receptors in blood vessels and dopamine receptors in renal vasculature. Low dosages increase renal blood flow, thus promoting diuresis. Higher dosages directly stimulate the heart. Vasoconstriction caused by alpha-receptor stimulation appears with the highest dosages. Because dopamine can limit cardiac output by these actions in peripheral vessels, it is usually selected only for patients in congestive heart failure complicated by hypotension. Like dobutamine, dopamine must be administered intravenously and has a very short duration of action.

Despite positive effects in congestive heart failure, the beta$_1$-agonists dobutamine and dopamine also increase the risk of arrhythmias and mortality in these patients.

Inotropic Agents: amrinone and milrinone

Amrinone and milrinone inhibit phosphodiesterase, causing an increase in cellular concentrations of cAMP; thus the drugs increase the same second messenger that is elevated by stimulation of beta-adrenergic receptors (see Chapter 12). These drugs also have activity as vasodilators in the periphery.

Amrinone and milrinone are used for short-term intravenous (IV) treatment of congestive heart failure when

CASE STUDY
Polypharmacy and the Elderly

Mrs. Craine is an 83-year-old woman who has recently moved in with her son; previously she lived in another state. Today her son brought her in to the clinic because she seemed somewhat confused, "more unsteady on her feet" and was having "a hard time getting around the new house." Mrs. Craine has a history of mild congestive heart failure and arthritis and tells the nurse that she has been "borrowing" her son's sleeping pills because she has had problems falling asleep in her "new bedroom."

When asked about her medications, she tells you that she takes a "heart pill," an aspirin each day to "thin my blood," an "arthritis pill," and a "pain pill" when needed. Her son is able to remember the names digoxin and Darvon, but not the arthritis pill. He states that the arthritis medicine was given to her by a new rheumatologist just before she left her home and she has not yet been seen by his family doctor here in town. Laboratory work reveals a digoxin level of 1.0 ng/ml and a potassium level of 3.6 mEq/L. Mrs. Craine states that she is able to remember to take her pills "most of the time" and wants to remain as independent as possible even though she is now living with her son.

1. Why is polypharmacy a common problem with elderly clients?
2. Could any of the medications cited have contributed to her confusion or unsteadiness? How?
3. Describe strategies to prevent polypharmacy in the future.
4. Do the laboratory values show normal levels? What can be done to help Mrs. Craine remember to take her medications?

Table 18-3   Treatment of Cardiac Glycoside Overdose

Generic Name	Trade Name	Administration/Dosing
digoxin immune Fab	Digibind	INTRADERMAL: *Adults*—0.1 ml of 0.1 mg/ml solution. Inspect for redness and wheal 20 min later. Do not administer full dose if reaction is positive. FDA pregnancy category C. INTRAVENOUS: *Adults*—Give amount equimolar to total amount of digoxin or digitoxin in body. Digoxin immune Fab in a dose of 40 mg binds approximately 0.6 mg of drug. Consult package insert for aid in calculating dosage.

response to other agents has been poor. The drugs rapidly increase cardiac output and are usually given to patients also receiving diuretics and digitalis. Despite positive effects on cardiac function, both these drugs increase the risk of sudden death from cardiac arrhythmias.

Nursing Process Overview

Drugs to Control Congestive Heart Failure

Assessment

Obtain baseline assessment data, including the vital signs and blood pressure, weight, fluid intake and output, serum electrolyte and blood urea nitrogen (BUN) levels, electrocardiographic (ECG) changes, and other laboratory data. Auscultate heart and lungs and assess for the presence and location of edema. Obtain any subjective history of recent dysfunction such as dyspnea on exertion, shortness of breath, inability to perform activities of daily living, and orthopnea (needing to sleep with the head supported or elevated on several pillows).

Nursing Diagnoses

- Risk for health maintenance related to insufficient knowledge of cardiac drug therapy
- Risk for electrolyte imbalance or hypokalemia

Patient Outcomes

The patient will be able to manage adding drugs for congestive heart failure to the daily routine, that is, will take the drug reg-

ularly at approximately the same time, with few if any side effects. The nurse will manage and minimize episodes of electrolyte imbalance.

Planning/Implementation

Monitor the weight, fluid intake and output, ECG changes, serum electrolyte levels, blood pressure, and other parameters of cardiovascular function. Auscultate the heart and lungs.

Evaluation

Before discharge, make sure the patient can explain why and how to take all prescribed medication, what interrelations may exist (e.g., the need to take potassium supplements if certain diuretics and drugs for congestive heart failure are prescribed together), how to plan meals within prescribed dietary limitations, what side effects are anticipated, and what situations require consultation with a physician. If appropriate, the patient should be able to measure pulse, correctly record weight or pulse, and state what decisions should be made based on assessment of these data.

Nursing Implications Summary

Drugs to Control Congestive Heart Failure
Drug Administration

➤ Observe the patient carefully. Desired effects of therapy include a decrease in pulse rate; slower, less labored respirations; diuresis accompanied by weight loss; less coughing; less distended neck veins; and better tolerance of exertion. At the same time assess for signs and symptoms of drug toxicity. Sometimes in the elderly these are mistakenly attributed to the aging process or to general chronic disease but are in fact signs of drug toxicity. These signs and symptoms include abdominal discomfort, weakness, fatigue, confusion, restlessness, anorexia, nausea, vomiting, and mood changes.

➤ Monitor the vital signs, including blood pressure.

ACE Inhibitors

➤ The ACE inhibitors are discussed in Chapter 13.
➤ Monitor blood pressure. Monitor the signs and symptoms of congestive heart failure. Assess for persistent cough.

Diuretics

➤ Diuretics are discussed in Chapter 14.
➤ Monitor blood pressure. Monitor signs and symptoms of congestive heart failure. Assess for signs of electrolyte disturbance and monitor serum electrolytes (see Table 17-1).

➤ Assess for signs of dehydration: hypotension, poor skin turgor, confusion, and decreased urinary output.

Vasodilators

➤ Vasodilators are discussed in Chapter 15.
➤ Monitor blood pressure. Monitor signs and symptoms of congestive heart failure.

Cardiac Glycosides

➤ Monitor blood pressure. Monitor signs and symptoms of congestive heart failure.
➤ Take the apical pulse for a full minute before administering a cardiac glycoside. A slowing of the pulse rate is to be expected, and this alone does not warrant withholding the dose. However, a marked change in the apical pulse rate, accompanied by changes in rhythm or changes on ECG, warrants withholding the dose until consultation with the physician. Guidelines may vary according to institution or physician.
➤ Monitor serum electrolyte levels, especially potassium, calcium, and magnesium. Digitalis toxicity is aggravated in hypokalemia, and hyperkalemia and hypercalcemia may contribute to digitalis-induced arrhythmias. Signs of electrolyte imbalances are noted in Table 17-1. Recall that vomiting, chronic diarrhea, nasogastric suctioning, and alkalosis con-

Nursing Implications Summary—cont'd

tribute to hypokalemia, as can administration of potassium-depleting diuretics, long-term steroid therapy, amphotericin B, and long-term glucose therapy.

➤ Monitor serum drug levels when available. Withhold the drug and notify the physician if the serum drug level is higher than the therapeutic range.

➤ Monitor intake and output, daily weight, vital signs, and heart and lung sounds. Assess for dependent edema in the sacral area and feet and ankles. Assess for jugular venous distension. Use data from central venous or arterial lines if available. Monitor ECG changes; the cardiac glycosides can cause PR interval prolongation, ST-segment sagging, AV blockage, and other arrhythmias.

➤ Read the physician's orders and drug labels carefully; do not confuse digoxin with digitoxin.

Intravenous digoxin

➤ Monitor the apical pulse and check serum electrolyte and drug levels before administering IV digoxin. It may be administered undiluted or diluted in 4 ml of sterile water, normal saline, lactated Ringer's solution, or 5% dextrose in water (D5W); use diluted solution as soon as prepared. Administer each dose evenly over at least 5 minutes. If possible, monitor ECG changes during IV administration.

Nursing in the Community

➤ Review with the patient the expected benefits and possible side effects of drug therapy. Review in detail the signs of drug toxicity, especially if the patient is an older adult because older adults are more sensitive to the effects of cardiac glycosides.

➤ Discuss the importance of maintaining an adequate potassium level with cardiac glycosides. Review sources of dietary potassium (see Dietary Considerations box in Chapter 14). Many of the drugs used to treat congestive heart failure may contribute to electrolyte disturbance (e.g., diuretics), whereas other drugs are more toxic in the presence of abnormal electrolyte levels (cardiac glycosides). This may be confusing to patients.

➤ Patients with heart disease may need instruction about sodium-restricted, weight-reduction, and low-cholesterol diets; refer such patients to a dietitian as needed.

➤ Review all medications the patient is taking, and emphasize the importance of taking them as prescribed. The patient may be taking diuretics, potassium replacements, and antihypertensives.

➤ If appropriate for their abilities, resources, and medical conditions, instruct patients to monitor and record the apical pulse regularly. It may also be appropriate to instruct patients to measure and record weight regularly. Instruct patients to report weight gain greater than 2 lb/day (1 kg/day) or 5 lb/wk (2 kg/wk) to the physician.

➤ Assess the patient's diet. Doses of cardiac glycosides should not be taken at the same time as large amounts of fiber because the fiber may interfere with absorption of the glycoside.

➤ Instruct the patient to take cardiac glycosides with meals or snacks to lessen gastric irritation. The liquid form may be dispensed with a calibrated dropper; instruct the patient to measure doses with this dropper.

➤ There are many drug interactions with the cardiac glycosides. Remind patients to keep all health care providers informed of all drugs being taken, and to avoid over-the-counter medications unless first approved by the physician.

➤ For maintenance therapy, cardiac glycosides are usually taken once a day. For missed doses, instruct the patient to take the dose as soon as remembered on the day it was missed if within 12 hours of the usual time the dose is taken. Instruct the patient not to double up for missed doses and to take only one dose a day unless otherwise directed by the physician.

➤ Remind the patient to keep cardiac glycosides out of the reach of children, to keep all health care providers informed of all drugs being taken, and not to self-medicate with over-the-counter drugs without consulting the physician.

➤ Suggest that patients wear a medical identification tag or bracelet indicating that they are taking cardiac glycosides.

amrinone and milrinone
Drug Administration

➤ Review the information about cardiac glycosides.

➤ Monitor the platelet count; dosage of amrinone may need to be reduced in the presence of thrombocytopenia. Monitor serum electrolytes. Assess for orthopnea, dyspnea, and fatigue. Monitor blood pressure.

➤ Amrinone: Follow the dosage charts supplied by the manufacturer. Dose may be given as a bolus; administer over 2 to 3 minutes. It may be administered into fluids containing dextrose but should not be diluted with solutions containing dextrose. If given as an infusion, use microdrip tubing or an infusion monitor.

➤ Milrinone: Follow the dosage charts supplied by the manufacturer. Dose may be given as a bolus; administer a single dose over 10 minutes. It may be diluted for infusion with normal saline, 0.45% saline, or D5W. Also available prediluted in D5W for infusion. For infusion, use microdrip tubing or an infusion monitor.

➤ Monitor the ECG changes and other data available from central venous or arterial lines.

➤ Amrinone and milrinone are incompatible with furosemide. A precipitate will form if the two drugs mix in the same tubing.

➤ These drugs are used only in the acute-care setting. Keep the patient and family informed of the patient's condition.

digoxin immune Fab
Drug Administration

➤ Review the manufacturer's insert for the latest guidelines.

➤ Skin testing may be prescribed before the full dose is given (see manufacturer's guidelines). Be prepared to treat an anaphylactic reaction. Patients who are allergic to digoxin immune Fab should not be given the full dose unless absolutely

Continued

Nursing Implications Summary—cont'd

necessary. Have personnel, equipment, and drugs for resuscitation available.

➤ Prepare ordered dose and administer over 15 to 30 minutes, using IV tubing with a 0.22-micron filter unless cardiac arrest is imminent. Digoxin immune Fab may be given as a bolus in that situation. Monitor the ECG changes and data from central venous and arterial lines as available.

➤ Monitor temperature and blood pressure. Have readily available drugs, equipment, and personnel to treat acute allergic reactions.

➤ Monitor serum level of cardiac glycosides and serum electrolyte levels.

➤ Keep the patient and family informed of the patient's condition.

CHAPTER REVIEW

Application

1. Why is it important that the atria and ventricles not contract simultaneously?
2. Where does the impulse to beat originate in a healthy heart?
3. What structure transmits the impulse to beat from the atria to the ventricles?
4. How does systolic congestive heart failure differ from diastolic congestive heart failure?
5. What is the effect of parasympathetic stimulation on the heart?
6. What is the effect of sympathetic stimulation on the heart?
7. How does the Frank-Starling law apply to the heart?
8. What physiologic effect on the heart is shared by digoxin and beta$_1$-agonists?
9. What is the purpose of the loading dose at the beginning of therapy with cardiac glycosides?
10. Do cardiac glycosides have a high or a low therapeutic index?

Critical Thinking

1. What symptoms are typical of congestive heart failure? How would you assess for these?
2. What toxicity is common with cardiac glycoside therapy? What should you assess while monitoring for this toxicity?
3. Why are pulse rates measured before administering each prescribed dose of cardiac glycosides? What parameters should you use in assessing pulse rate data?
4. What inotropic drugs other than cardiac glycosides are used in congestive heart failure? What is the basis for their action in congestive heart failure?
5. Why are ACE inhibitors useful in congestive heart failure?
6. Diuretics relieve pulmonary congestion in congestive heart failure. How should you assess for this?

References

Bales AC, Sorrentino MJ: Causes of congestive heart failure, *Postgrad Med* 101(1):44-62, 1997.

Garg R, et al: The effect of digoxin on mortality and morbidity in patients with heart failure, *N Engl J Med* 336(8):525-533, 1997.

Packer M: Effects of beta-adrenergic blockade on survival of patients with chronic heart failure, *Am J Cardiol* 80(11A):46L-54L, 1997.

Schwabauer NJ: Retarding progression of heart failure: nursing actions, *DCCN* 15(6):307-317, 1996.

Sorrentino MJ: Drug therapy for congestive heart failure, *Postgrad Med* 101(1):83-96, 1997.

Spencer KT, Lang RM: Diastolic heart failure, *Postgrad Med* 101(1):63-82, 1997.

Chapter 19

Drugs to Control Cardiac Arrhythmias

OBJECTIVES

After studying this chapter, you should be able to do the following:

- *Explain how normal heart rhythm is maintained.*
- *Describe the four classes of antiarrhythmic agents.*
- *Explain how each class of antiarrhythmics suppresses arrhythmias.*
- *Discuss the cardiotoxicity of antiarrhythmic drugs.*
- *Develop a nursing care plan for a patient receiving an antiarrhythmic.*

CHAPTER OVERVIEW

Cardiac **arrhythmias** are defined as any change from the normal rate or pattern of heartbeat. Heart rates that are too slow (**bradycardia**), too fast (**tachycardia**), or irregular are included in this classification. Arrhythmias are also called dysrhythmias. The impulse to beat normally starts in the sinoatrial (SA) node; it spreads through the atria, causing them to contract, then passes through the atrioventricular (AV) node and enters the ventricles, causing contraction of that tissue (see Chapter 18). The electrical activity that allows this communication is discussed first in this chapter, followed by a description of classes of antiarrhythmic agents and individual drugs.

THERAPEUTIC RATIONALE: CARDIAC ARRHYTHMIAS

Electrophysiology of the Heart

Action Potentials

An action potential describes changes in electrical potential between a cell and its environment over time. Typical action potentials for three types of cardiac tissue are shown in Figure 19-1. Atrial and ventricular patterns are similar. Both begin with a rapid depolarization, marked by 0 on the curves, which is caused by a rapid rush of sodium ions into the cell. The inside of the cell therefore becomes more positive as the electrical potential shifts from about -90 mV to about $+20$ mV. This shift triggers a brief opening of channels that move potassium ions out of the cell; therefore the electrical potential starts to become more negative. This phase is marked by 1 on the curve. During the plateau period (phase 2, see Figure 19-1) sodium ions and calcium ions slowly enter the cell, and potassium ions leave. Over time, sodium and calcium ions stop flowing in, but potassium ions continue to flow out (phase 3). During this phase the electrical potential continues to become more negative. In the final phase of the action potential, sodium ions flow out of the cell in exchange for potassium ions, which enter the cell. At the end of this cycle, the cell has returned to the resting potential of about -90 mV and has regained the ability to generate another normal action potential. From the

227

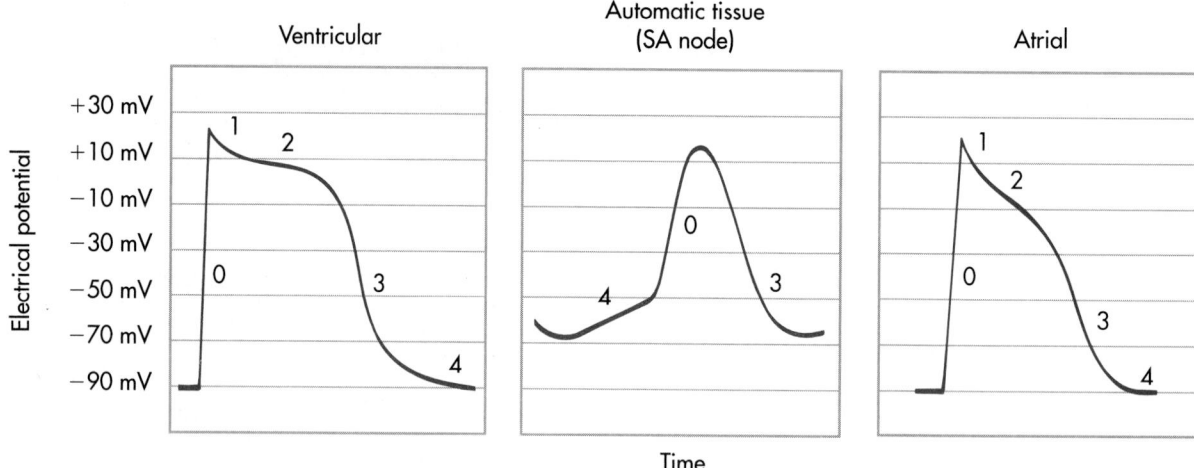

Figure 19-1   Typical action potential for three types of cardiac tissues. Action potentials are determined in laboratory in tissues from experimental animals.

beginning of phase 0 until sometime during the middle of phase 3, atrial or ventricular cells cannot be stimulated to beat again. This span of time is called the **refractory period.**

Automaticity of Normal Sinoatrial Nodal Cells

The action potential for the SA nodal tissue differs from that of atrial and ventricular cells. Most important in terms of cardiac physiology is the gradual depolarization that occurs during phase 4 (see Figure 19-1). This ability to gradually shift from a potential of about −70 mV to −50 or −40 mV triggers the start of the action potential (phase 0) in SA nodal cells. This process is called **automaticity:** the cells need no externally applied stimulus to initiate an action potential.

Electrocardiogram

In the clinical setting, information about the function of a patient's heart is gained from electrocardiographic (ECG) tracings (Figure 19-2). These ECG tracings are related to action potentials in various parts of the heart. The change in potential marked in Figure 19-2 as P (the P wave) is produced by the initial depolarization of atrial cells (phase 0 of the action potential). Very shortly after this wave of depolarization, the atrium contracts to complete filling of the ventricles. The waves marked Q, R, and S (QRS complex) result from depolarization of the ventricles. Repolarization of the atria occurs at this time but is masked by large changes produced by the ventricles. Ventricular contraction occurs between the QRS complex and the midpoint of the T wave. The T wave is generated by repolarization (phase 1 through 3 of the action potential) of the ventricles.

Mechanisms Producing Arrhythmias

Arrhythmias occur because of disorders in pacing of the heartbeat and/or disorders in conducting the impulse to beat through cardiac tissues. Disorders in cardiac pacing are often related to changes in automaticity of the heart. For example, the normal pacemaker in the SA node may become overstimulated by the sympathetic nervous system. Catecholamine neurotransmitters for this branch of the nervous system increase automaticity of the SA node. As a result, phase 4 on the action potential curve is steepened and shortened, phase 0 is triggered more often, and the heart beats more rapidly. In contrast, if the vagus nerve is predominant and sympathetic stimulation is removed, heart rate decreases. This action occurs because acetylcholine from the vagus nerve decreases the automaticity of the SA node.

Sinus bradycardia (slow atrial rate) is usually of minor importance and is not treated unless it is associated with reduced cardiac output. Sinus tachycardia (rapid atrial rate) may likewise be harmless unless the ventricular rate is also abnormally increased. Many physicians do not give antiarrhythmic drugs to patients with rapid atrial rates and no other symptoms. Sinus tachycardia may be produced in healthy persons by anxiety; ingestion of coffee, tea, or other caffeinated products; ingestion of alcoholic beverages; or smoking. Sympathomimetics, anticholinergics, or phenothiazines may also induce transient sinus tachycardia.

Disorders of conduction arise from various causes. For example, it is now known that hearts occasionally have a physical connection between the atria and ventricles that allows the conduction of an impulse to the ventricles not only through the AV node but also through this accessory path-

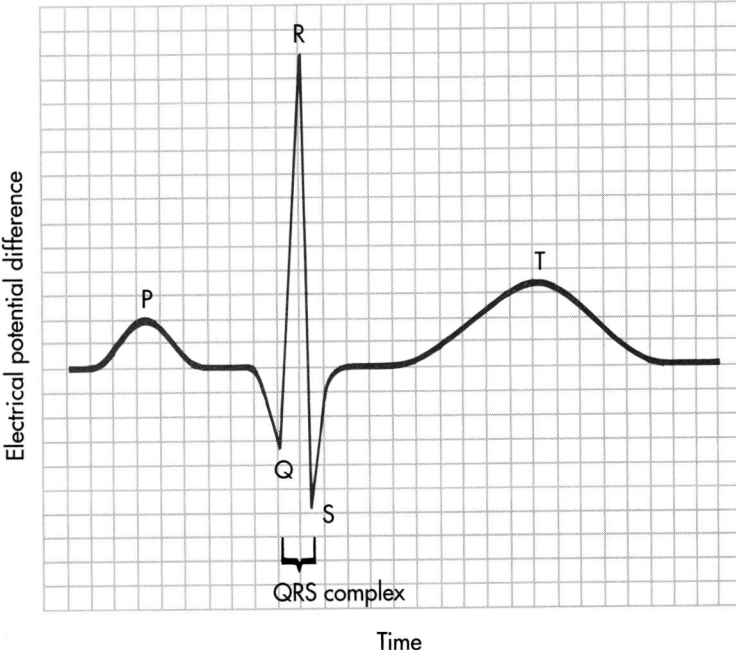

Figure 19-2 ECG tracing showing pattern typical of normal heart function.

way. This anatomic abnormality gives rise to an arrhythmia because the impulse passes rapidly through the accessory pathway but slowly through the AV node; thus, the impulse from the node may arrive at the accessory pathway just at the end of the refractory period of those rapidly conducting cells. A wave of depolarization may then pass from the ventricles through this pathway back into the atria, which may trigger a premature beat. An example of this type of anatomically defined arrhythmia is called the Wolff-Parkinson-White syndrome. A similar situation may exist without an anatomically defined separate pathway, especially if a section of tissue has been damaged by ischemia (oxygen deprivation), such as occurs with a myocardial infarction. The damaged area not only may fail to contract but also may fail to conduct an action potential properly. The key to understanding these arrhythmias is to recognize that two pathways exist for the impulse to travel to a distant site, and that one of the pathways is slower than the other, which allows the impulse to reenter the more rapidly conducting pathway and move back toward the source of the original impulse. This phenomenon is called **reentry** and is thought to be responsible not only for the Wolff-Parkinson-White syndrome but also for many cases of **atrial flutter** (a very rapid, rhythmic pattern), atrial **fibrillation** (a disorganized pattern that fails to produce a productive contraction), atrial tachycardia, paroxysmal supraventricular tachycardia (a rapid rhythm that begins abruptly with a premature atrial or junctional beat), and ventricular tachycardia.

The causes of many arrhythmias are not well understood. For example, **premature ventricular contractions (PVCs)** occur occasionally even in healthy persons. The ECG pattern

shows a normal QRS complex following a P wave (see Figure 19-2), plus an abnormal QRS complex that is isolated from a P wave. If PVCs are rare, they are ordinarily not treated unless the patient is recuperating from a myocardial infarction. Abstaining from coffee, tea, caffeine, and cigarettes may control the condition.

A recent innovation in controlling arrhythmias involves surgical ablation of the point of origin of a stable arrhythmia. Ablation may involve surgical interruption of tissue forming accessory pathways between the atria and ventricles or it may involve the use of high energy radiowaves delivered by means of a catheter to a site that has been mapped and shown to be the source of the arrhythmia. These surgical techniques are often curative. Drug therapy is usually less ambitious, being intended only to bring an acute arrhythmia under control. Long-term therapy with antiarrhythmic drugs does not necessarily improve mortality and is often associated with risks of secondary arrhythmias from the drugs themselves.

THERAPEUTIC AGENTS: DRUGS TO TREAT CARDIAC ARRHYTHMIAS

The classification system described in Table 19-1 is based on effects of the drugs on the action potential (see Figure 19-1). The classification system, although useful, is imperfect in that the effects of drugs within a category are now known to differ in some ways. Table 19-2 lists the major antiarrhythmic drugs by class, along with a summary of the overall effects of each drug on the various channels, receptors, and pumps that are important for regulating cardiac function.

Table 19-1 Classification of Antiarrhythmics with Indications for Use

Class	Drugs	Effect on Action Potential	Indications for Use
I-A	disopyramide procainamide quinidine	Depress phase 0; may prolong action potential duration	Ventricular arrhythmias; supraventricular arrhythmias (quinidine, procainamide)
I-B	lidocaine mexiletine tocainide	Depress phase 0 without involving autonomic nervous system	Ventricular arrhythmias
I-C	flecainide propafenone	Depress phase 0 markedly; profound slowing of conduction	Ventricular arrhythmias, life-threatening
II	esmolol	Depress phase 4 depolarization	Supraventricular and other tachyarrhythmias
III	amiodarone bretylium	Prolong phase 3 repolarization	Ventricular arrhythmias
IV	diltiazem verapamil	Depress phase 4 depolarization; lengthen phase 1 and 2	Supraventricular tachyarrhythmias

This summary, which is called the Sicilian gambit, came from the report of the Task Force of the Working Group on Antiarrhythmias of the European Society of Cardiology; it represents an attempt to further rationalize selection and use of antiarrhythmics.

The Sicilian gambit makes it clear that antiarrhythmics have many actions. For example, propranolol and esmolol block beta-adrenergic receptors (see Chapters 12 and 13); in the heart this action slows the rate at the SA node and slows conduction through the AV node. The effect at both sites is to slow heart rate. Anticholinergic drugs, such as atropine, may produce the opposite effect by blocking the muscarinic receptors by which the heart responds to vagal nerve stimulation. Calcium channel blocking drugs such as verapamil and diltiazem primarily change the responses of cells highly dependent on the so-called slow calcium current (e.g., AV nodal cells or cells in ischemic regions of muscle). Local anesthetics, such as lidocaine and related drugs, change the sodium ion influx that causes phase 0 of the action potential.

Table 19-3 gives an alphabetic listing of drugs used to control arrhythmias. In the following presentation the drugs are grouped according to mechanistic class.

CLASS I-A ANTIARRHYTHMIC DRUGS

Class I-A antiarrhythmic drugs block sodium channels, thus lowering automaticity. These drugs also prolong action potential duration because they block potassium channels (see Table 19-2). The effective refractory period is therefore prolonged in atria and ventricles, making the tissue less electrically responsive. Class I-A antiarrhythmics are indicated for treatment of ventricular tachycardia; quinidine and procainamide may also be used to treat atrial tachycardia or fibrillation.

disopyramide
Mechanism of Action
Disopyramide slows conduction and prolongs the effective refractory period in atrial and ventricular tissues, but it has little effect on the AV node or the His-Purkinje system.

Pharmacokinetics
Disopyramide is rapidly and almost completely absorbed orally. Biotransformation in liver produces metabolites with antimuscarinic and antiarrhythmic activities. About half of each dose is eliminated unchanged in urine. Dosages may be adjusted, based on renal function. Serum concentrations of disopyramide are not a reliable guide for adjusting dosage because of large patient-to-patient variation in protein binding.

Adverse Reactions and Contraindications
Difficulty in urination, an antimuscarinic effect, is experienced by 10% to 20% of treated patients. Up to 10% of patients have hypotension (dizziness or fainting), altered heart rhythm, or fluid retention (congestive heart failure). Dry mouth, another antimuscarinic effect, is very common but not dangerous.

Disopyramide is avoided in patients with AV block because of the risk of complete heart block. Disopyramide also worsens cardiogenic shock and is avoided in patients with this condition.

Toxicity
Overdose causes widening of the QRS complex and the QT interval of the ECG tracing. Cardiac arrhythmias may ensue. Apnea, loss of spontaneous respirations, and coma precede death by cardiovascular collapse.

Interactions
Disopyramide may worsen conduction in patients who have received other arrhythmics. Disopyramide is avoided for 48 hours before and 24 hours after a dose of verapamil; deaths from conduction blockade have occurred. Disopyramide may provoke arrhythmias in patients receiving pimozide.

Table 19-2   Antiarrhythmic Drug Summary Based on the "Sicilian Gambit"

Drug	Class*	Na† Fast	Na† Med	Na† Slow	Ca	K	Alpha	Beta	M2	P	Pumps Na⁺-K⁺-ATPase
lidocaine	I-B	★									
mexiletine	I-B	★									
tocainide	I-B	★									
moricizine	I-A	●									
procainamide	I-A		●			•					
disopyramide	I-A		●			•			★		
quinidine	I-A		●			•	★		★		
propafenone	I-C		●					★			
flecainide	I-C			●		★					
bepridil	IV	★			●	•					
verapamil	IV	★			●		•				
diltiazem	IV				•						
bretylium	III					●	◪	◪			
sotalol	III					●		●			
amiodarone	III	★			★	●	•	•			
nadolol	II							●			
propranolol	II	★						●			
adenosine										□	
atropine									●		
digoxin									□		●

*Class refers to the system described in Table 19-1.
†Sodium channel blockers have fast, medium, or slow onset and decline; the slow blockers prolong the QRS most markedly.
Na, Sodium channels; *Ca,* calcium channels; *K,* potassium channels; *alpha,* alpha-adrenergic receptors; *beta,* beta-adrenergic receptors; *M2,* muscarinic type 2 receptors; *P,* purinergic receptors;
★, blocker, low potency; •, blocker, moderate potency; ●, blocker, high potency; □, agonist; ◪, agonist/antagonist.

▼ procainamide

Mechanism of Action

Procainamide blocks sodium channels and, to a lesser degree, potassium channels. These blockades decrease cell excitability, conduction velocity, and automaticity, while prolonging the effective refractory period. These actions make procainamide effective against a variety of reentrant arrhythmias.

Pharmacokinetics

Procainamide reaches peak concentrations in serum (4 to 8 μg/ml) within 3 hours of an oral dose or within 30 minutes of an intramuscular dose. The active metabolite, *N*-acetylprocainamide (NAPA), is formed by the liver. The half-life of the parent drug in serum is 3 hours, and about half the drug dose is eliminated unchanged in urine; NAPA is cleared more slowly and can accumulate to toxic levels in renal failure.

Adverse Reactions and Contraindications

The most striking adverse effect with long-term use of procainamide is a syndrome resembling lupus erythematosus, with symptoms such as arthritis, arthralgia, myalgia, fever, and pericarditis. Procainamide also commonly causes gastrointestinal disturbances such as loss of appetite, diarrhea, and stomach pain.

Procainamide worsens torsades de pointes and is avoided in patients with this arrhythmia. Quinidine is avoided in digitalis toxicity or intraventricular conduction defects because the drug further slows conduction. Procainamide is avoided in AV block because of the risk of complete heart block.

Toxicity

Direct toxicity from procainamide usually changes conduction, especially in AV nodal tissue and conducting fibers of the ventricles. These direct toxic effects occur when blood levels exceed 12 μg/ml. Because normal therapeutic concentrations range from about 4 to 8 μg/ml, this drug, like other antiarrhythmic agents, has a narrow safety margin. Procainamide widens the QRS complex on ECG tracings.

Interactions

When used with other antiarrhythmics or pimozide, procainamide may cause increased heart-related side effects. Antihypertensives may produce hypotension if used with procainamide, especially in the elderly (see Geriatrics Considerations box). Antimyasthenic agents are antagonized by procainamide, but neuromuscular blocking agents are enhanced.

Table 19-3 Drugs Used to Control Cardiac Arrhythmias

Generic Name	Trade Name	Administration/Dosage	Comments
adenosine	Adenocard	INTRAVENOUS: *Adults*—6 mg given over 1-2 sec. If not effective, 12 mg may be given 1-2 min later. FDA pregnancy category C.	Extremely short half-life, thus side effects are usually self-limiting.
amiodarone	Cordarone*	ORAL: *Adults*—0.8-1.6 g daily in divided doses; reduce when control is adequate or side effects occur to 600-800 mg daily for 1 mo; maintain with lowest effective dose. FDA pregnancy category D. *Children*—10 mg/kg body weight or 800 mg/1.72 m² daily until control is adequate or side effects occur; reduce to 5 mg/kg or 400 mg/1.72 m² for several weeks; maintain with lowest effective dose.	Very long duration of action (weeks or months) and very slow onset (2 days-2 mo). Persists in body for months after drug is discontinued.
atropine		INTRAVENOUS: *Adults*—0.4-1 mg every 1-2 hr as needed, up to a maximum of 2 mg. FDA pregnancy category C. *Children*—0.01-0.03 mg/kg body weight.	Rapidly effective; excreted by the kidney within 12 hr of administration.
bretylium	Bretylol Bretylate†	INTRAMUSCULAR: *Adults*—5-10 mg/kg repeated in 1-2 hr, then every 6-8 hr. FDA pregnancy category C. INTRAVENOUS: *Adults*—5-10 mg/kg given over 8 min; for maintenance, infuse at 1-2 mg/min.	Excreted unchanged by the kidneys.
digoxin	Lanoxin*	ORAL: *Adults*—tablets or elixir, 0.375-0.625 mg repeated at 6-8 hr; maintain with 0.125-0.5 mg daily. Capsules, 0.4 to 0.6 mg once; maintain with 0.05 to 0.35 mg divided into 2 doses. FDA pregnancy category C. *Children*—Doses are individualized for age and body weight.	Effective serum level 1-2 ng/ml and toxic at 3 ng/ml. Bioavailability with capsules is higher so that 0.1 mg dose is equivalent to 0.125 mg in tablets.
disopyramide	Norpace* Rythmodan†	ORAL: *Adults*—300 mg loading dose. Maintenance with extended-release forms, 300 mg every 12 hr. FDA pregnancy category C. *Children*—6-30 mg/kg body weight daily divided into 4 doses. Avoid extended-release forms.	A 300-mg loading dose (regular capsules) takes effect in 0.5-3.5 hr.
esmolol	Brevibloc	INTRAVENOUS: *Adults*—0.5 mg/kg body weight in 1 min, then 0.05 mg/kg/min for 4 min. Increase maintenance dose as necessary up to 0.2 mg/kg/min. FDA pregnancy category C. *Children*—0.05 mg/kg body weight/min, titrated up to 0.3 mg/kg/min as needed.	This very short-acting drug must be given by continuous infusion. May be used up to 48 hr.
flecainide	Tambocor*	ORAL: *Adults*—50-100 mg every 12 hr, increasing in increments of 50 mg twice daily every 4 days as needed. Maximum daily dose, 400 mg. FDA pregnancy category C.	Toxicity increases at plasma concentrations above 0.7-1 μg/ml.
lidocaine	Xylocaine HCl* (for continuous IV infusion) Xylocard†	INTRAVENOUS: *Adults*—0.02-0.05 mg/kg at a rate of 1-4 mg/min, up to 300 mg in any 1-hr period. FDA pregnancy category B. *Children*—Continuous infusion, 20-50 μg/kg body weight/min.	Effective serum level 1-5 μg/ml; serum half-life 15-20 min; metabolized in liver.
mexiletine	Mexitil*	ORAL: *Adults*—200 mg every 8 hr; adjust up or down by 50-100 mg/dose every 2-3 days. Doses not to exceed 1200 mg daily. FDA pregnancy category C.	Effective plasma concentrations are 0.5-2 μg/ml, but toxicity may occur even at these levels.
moricizine	Ethmozine	ORAL: *Adults*—200-300 mg every 8 hr, not to exceed 900 mg daily. FDA pregnancy category B.	New ventricular arrhythmias may be fatal.
procainamide	Procan* Promine Pronestyl*	ORAL: *Adults*—6.25 mg/kg body weight every 3 hr. FDA pregnancy category C. *Children*—12.5 mg/kg every 6 hr. INTRAMUSCULAR: *Adults*—6.25 mg/kg every 3-6 hr. INTRAVENOUS: *Adults*—Initially 20 mg/min; maintain with 2-6 mg/min.	Effective serum level 4-8 μg/ml; serum half-life about 3 hr.
procainamide extended release	Procan SR* Pronestyl-SR*	ORAL: *Adults*—12.5 mg/kg every 6 hr.	For maintenance only.
propafenone	Rhythmol*	ORAL: *Adults*—Initially 150 mg every 8 hr, increasing gradually to a maximum of 225 mg every 8 hr. FDA pregnancy category C.	Plasma concentrations vary widely among patients.
quinidine gluconate	Duraquin Quinaglute* Quinalan Quinate†	ORAL: *Adults*—325-650 mg every 6-12 hr. FDA pregnancy category C. INTRAMUSCULAR: *Adults*—Initially 600 mg; 200-400 mg every 2-6 hr. INTRAVENOUS: *Adults*—20 mg/min.	More slowly absorbed than quinidine sulfate; intravenous doses require electrocardiographic and blood pressure monitoring.

*Available in Canada and the United States.
†Available in Canada only.

Table 19-3   Drugs Used to Control Cardiac Arrhythmias—cont'd

Generic Name	Trade Name	Administration/Dosage	Comments
quinidine polygalacturonate	Cardioquin*	ORAL: *Adults*—275 mg every 3-12 hr. *Children*—8.25 mg/kg 5 times daily.	Less gastrointestinal irritation than other forms of quinidine.
quinidine sulfate	Cin-Quin Quinora	ORAL: *Adults*—200-300 mg 3 or 4 times daily. *Children*—6 mg/kg 5 times daily.	Effective serum level 3-6 μg/ml.
tocainide	Tonocard*	ORAL: *Adults*—400 mg every 8 hr, adjusted as necessary; maintenance 400-600 mg every 8 hr. FDA pregnancy category C.	Bioavailability is high and is unaffected by food.
verapamil	Calan Isoptin*	ORAL: *Adults*—80-120 mg every 8 hr. FDA pregnancy category C. *Children*—4-8 mg/kg daily in divided doses. INTRAVENOUS: *Adults*—Initially 5-10 mg over 2-5 min, repeated if necessary at 30 min. *Children*—0.1-0.3 mg/kg over 2 min, repeated if necessary at 30 min.	Monitor electrocardiogram and blood pressure continuously with intravenous doses.

 GERIATRIC CONSIDERATIONS

Antiarrhythmics

THE PROBLEM

Older adults often respond differently to antiarrhythmic agents than do younger adults. Procainamide and tocainide are more likely to cause dizziness or hypotension in older persons. Amiodarone is more likely to cause ataxia or other neurologic problems in older adults. Older adults are more sensitive to the antimuscarinic effects (dry mouth, urinary retention) of disopyramide. Clearance of drugs like verapamil, flecainide, or the beta-adrenergic blockers is lower, and these drugs may accumulate. Especially with flecainide, higher serum levels may lead to development of dangerous drug-induced arrhythmias. Older persons may be more susceptible to hypothermia if they take beta-adrenergic blockers.

SOLUTIONS

- Lidocaine doses and rates of administration should be cut in half for patients older than 65 years.
- Blood pressure should be carefully monitored.
- Be alert to signs of neurologic toxicity and ataxia.
- Help patients develop strategies to avoid injury from falls if ataxia or dizziness is a problem.
- Watch for signs of urinary retention.
- Watch for hypothermia in older adult patients receiving beta-adrenergic drugs.

quinidine

Mechanism of Action

Quinidine blocks sodium and potassium channels, giving it an action similar to procainamide. In addition, quinidine also has atropine-like actions that block the effect of the vagus nerve on the heart, and blocks alpha-adrenergic receptors, which promotes vasodilation.

Pharmacokinetics

Quinidine preparations are best absorbed when taken with water on an empty stomach but may be taken with milk or food if needed to curb gastrointestinal irritation. Quinidine polygalacturonate may be less irritating to the gastrointestinal tract than other forms of quinidine. The half-life of quinidine is about 6 hours. Quinidine is metabolized in liver, but up to 50% of a dose may be excreted unchanged in urine; the drug may accumulate in patients in renal failure.

Adverse Reactions and Contraindications

The anticholinergic effects of quinidine may oppose its other actions. These dual effects have caused serious complications in treating atrial fibrillation. Although the direct effects of quinidine might be expected to slow atrial rates, the first observed effect may be an anticholinergic action that speeds conduction through the AV node, with the result that ventricular rates soar dangerously high before quinidine can slow atrial rates. Quinidine is avoided in AV block because of the risk of complete heart block.

The most serious noncardiac reactions to quinidine are allergic responses and cardiovascular toxicity. When the drug is given intravenously, hypotension may result because quinidine is a vasodilator. Quinidine also produces cinchonism, with symptoms of blurred vision, dizziness, headache, and ringing in the ears.

Quinidine also commonly causes loss of appetite, diarrhea, and stomach pain.

Toxicity

At doses producing blood levels above 8 μg/ml, quinidine may induce ventricular arrhythmias, including ectopic beats, tachycardia, and fibrillation. Quinidine causes a dose-dependent widening of the QRS complex. This effect can be used to monitor its therapeutic activity and to track the risk of toxicity.

Interactions

Quinidine serum levels rise when the urine becomes alkaline, as renal reabsorption of drug is enhanced; therefore urinary alkalinizers such as antacids, citrates, and carbonic anhydrase inhibitors must be used with care. Other arrhythmic agents, phenothiazines, rauwolfia alkaloids, and pimozide may have additive cardiac effects with quinidine. Actions of anticoagulants and neuromuscular blockers are enhanced by quinidine.

CLASS I-B ANTIARRHYTHMIC DRUGS

Class I-B antiarrhythmic drugs depress phase 0 of the action potential (see Figure 19-1), decreasing excitability and automaticity. They have little effect on the refractory period. Class I-B antiarrhythmic agents are indicated for ventricular arrhythmias, including those caused by myocardial infarction, cardiac surgery, cardiac catheterization, and digitalis toxicity.

▼ lidocaine

Mechanism of Action

Lidocaine is a local anesthetic (see Chapter 35), as well as an antiarrhythmic agent. The mechanism for both actions is rapid blockade of sodium channels.

Pharmacokinetics

More than 90% of a dose of lidocaine is rapidly destroyed in the liver. Therefore the drug is used primarily as a continuous infusion designed to produce therapeutic levels of 1.5 to 5 μg/ml in plasma.

Adverse Reactions and Contraindications

Lidocaine may cause anxiety, dizziness, drowsiness, nervousness, numbness, or the sensation of heat or cold. Reactions seldom persist after the infusion is discontinued because the half-life of lidocaine is so short.

Lidocaine may worsen Adams-Stokes syndrome or severe heart block.

Toxicity

Lidocaine causes central nervous system (CNS) reactions, ranging from muscle twitching and drowsiness to paresthesia, respiratory depression, convulsions, and coma. These reactions may be dose dependent. At serum lidocaine concentrations of 6 to 8 μg/ml, blurred vision, double vision, nausea, ringing in ears, tremors, twitching, and vomiting may occur. When serum concentrations exceed 8 μg/ml, patients may experience bradycardia, difficulty breathing, dizziness, fainting, and seizures. Toxic reactions to lidocaine are more common in patients with reduced hepatic function because the drug may accumulate in these patients.

Interactions

In administering lidocaine, it is important to remember that the drug has two separate clinical uses and is packaged differently for each. When intended for use as a local anesthetic, lidocaine is often packaged in solution with epinephrine (e.g., Xylocaine or other trade names with epinephrine). When used with the local anesthetic, epinephrine acts as a vasoconstrictor to reduce local blood flow and prolong the action of the anesthetic. If lidocaine with epinephrine were inadvertently used to treat a cardiac arrhythmia, the epinephrine might trigger a severe arrhythmia by stimulating automaticity of the heart. Lidocaine intended for use in cardiac emergencies is labeled "Xylocaine preservative-free" or "lidocaine for continuous intravenous (IV) infusion."

mexiletine

Mechanism of Action

Mexiletine is an oral antiarrhythmic drug with a mechanism of action similar to parenteral lidocaine. Both drugs have local anesthetic properties. Mexiletine also has anticonvulsant actions.

Pharmacokinetics

Mexiletine is well absorbed from the GI tract, making oral administration practical and effective. The onset of effect is within 2 hours. Elimination is primarily by hepatic metabolism; the half-life of the drug in the blood may be doubled in severe hepatic disease but only slightly increased in renal impairment.

Adverse Reactions and Contraindications

Side effects of mexiletine increase when plasma concentrations exceed 2 μg/ml. New ventricular arrhythmias, including premature ventricular contractions and torsades de pointes, may arise. Heartburn, nausea, and vomiting usually occur within 2 hours of administration. CNS effects include dizziness, trembling, nervousness, and unsteady gait.

Mexiletine is avoided in arrhythmias that respond to other drugs or are not life-threatening. It is also avoided in AV blockade or cardiogenic shock, which could be worsened by actions of the drug.

Toxicity

Overdose can cause death from respiratory failure and asystole. Acidifying the urine speeds excretion of mexiletine and may therefore help bring plasma concentrations back into a safe range.

Interactions

Mexiletine may decrease the metabolism of theophylline, increasing the risk of CNS toxicity. Mexiletine may worsen cardiac function if it is combined with beta-adrenergic agents.

tocainide

Mechanism of Action

Tocainide, like lidocaine, is a local anesthetic. Its action in the heart is similar to that of lidocaine.

Pharmacokinetics

Tocainide is completely absorbed orally, with or without food. The onset of action is within 2 hours, and the half-life is about 15 hours. Hepatic metabolism and renal excretion contribute equally to elimination.

Adverse Reactions and Contraindications

The most common side effects include dizziness, loss of appetite, and nausea. Blisters, peeling skin, or skin rashes may signal a rare but dangerous allergic reaction that can culminate in Stevens-Johnson syndrome. After several weeks of therapy, pulmonary damage can occur, with coughing and shortness of breath. Allergic reactions or pulmonary damage can be fatal.

Tocainide is avoided in AV blockade or in patients allergic to amide-type local anesthetics.

Toxicity

Shaking and trembling are early signs of toxicity. Overdoses may cause respiratory depression or seizures.

Interactions

Tocainide may increase risk of arrhythmias if combined with other antiarrhythmic drugs. It may also increase the risk of worsening contractility if combined with beta-adrenergic blocking agents.

moricizine
Mechanism of Action

In addition to blocking sodium channels, moricizine also has potent local anesthetic activity and membrane-stabilizing activity. The AV node and the His-Purkinje system are most sensitive to moricizine. Conduction through these tissues is slowed considerably, but there is little effect on the SA node. Moricizine is used only short-term to suppress life-threatening arrhythmias.

Pharmacokinetics

Moricizine is extensively biotransformed by the liver and has a half-life of about 2 hours. The drug is well absorbed orally but is subject to first-pass effects (see Chapter 1) that lower absolute bioavailability to about 38%. The onset of action is usually within 2 hours.

Adverse Reactions and Contraindications

Moricizine, like other antiarrhythmics, can induce new arrhythmias in some patients. Patients receiving the drug in controlled trials experienced more new or exacerbated ventricular arrhythmias than did patients receiving placebo. Other patients developed signs of congestive heart failure, AV block, or sinus arrest. Dizziness and other CNS effects may also be observed with long-term administration.

Moricizine is avoided in patients with AV block or right bundle branch block because risk of total heart block is substantial.

Toxicity

Overdoses of moricizine have been fatal, producing cardiotoxicity, coma, and respiratory failure. Most side effects are dose related and worsen as doses exceed the normal therapeutic range.

Interactions

Moricizine may hasten the metabolism of theophylline. If the drugs must be used together, theophylline concentrations should be monitored in blood and dosages should be adjusted accordingly to maintain effective control of pulmonary disease. Cimetidine slows clearance of moricizine.

CLASS I-C ANTIARRHYTHMIC DRUGS

Class I-C antiarrhythmic drugs markedly depress phase 0 of the action potential (see Figure 19-1) and profoundly slow conduction, especially in conductive fibers. They have little effect on the refractory period. Two members of this class, encainide and flecainide, were included in a large clinical trial that was designed to test the effectiveness of drugs in patients with asymptomatic, non-life-threatening ventricular arrhythmias who had a recent myocardial infarction. The Cardiac Arrhythmias Suppression Trial (CAST) showed both drugs more than doubled the risk for mortality or cardiac arrest (7.7%) over placebo (3%). As a result, encainide was withdrawn from the market and the remaining Class I-C drugs are indicated only for control of life-threatening ventricular arrhythmias.

flecainide
Mechanism of Action

Flecainide may have greater effects in ischemic than in normal cardiac tissue. It also has local anesthetic action and may decrease contractility of the heart.

Pharmacokinetics

Flecainide is nearly completely absorbed orally, with or without food. The major route of elimination is hepatic metabolism. The long half-life of approximately 20 hours may be increased by renal failure, hepatic failure, and congestive heart failure.

Adverse Reactions and Contraindications

Blurred vision and dizziness are common side effects. Trembling, chest pain, and arrhythmias can also occur. Flecainide is avoided when AV block or right bundle branch block exists because the risk of complete heart block is increased.

Toxicity

Flecainide has been associated with development of new and potentially fatal arrhythmias, especially when plasma concentrations exceed 1 μg/ml. Ventricular arrhythmias, congestive heart failure, and AV block are most common.

Interactions

Flecainide should not be used with other antiarrhythmic agents because such combinations may lead to fatal arrhythmias.

propafenone
Mechanism of Action

Propafenone primarily affects ventricular conductive tissue (His-Purkinje system), slowing conduction markedly. The drug also has a weak beta-adrenergic blocking effect and a strong local anesthetic action. Propafenone has a negative inotropic effect that increases the risk for congestive heart failure.

Pharmacokinetics

Propafenone is well absorbed orally, but a first-pass effect (see Chapter 1) reduces absolute bioavailability to 10% or less. The liver converts propafenone to several products, some of which are also active antiarrhythmics. Elimination is mostly by renal mechanisms. The half-life of the drug is 2 to 10 hours in most patients, but up to 10% of the population metabolizes propafenone much more slowly. For slow metabolizers the half-life is 10 to 32 hours. Steady-state concentrations of the drug are achieved after 4 or 5 days, but the steady-state plasma concentrations vary widely as a result of variations in metabolism.

Adverse Reactions and Contraindications

Propafenone, like other antiarrhythmics, can induce new arrhythmias in some patients. About 5% of patients receiving the drug in controlled trials experienced new or exacerbated ventricular arrhythmias. Other patients developed signs of congestive heart failure, AV block, or sinus bradycardia. Dizziness and other CNS effects may also be observed with long-term use. Many patients also report a change in their sense of taste.

Propafenone is avoided when AV block or right bundle branch block exists because the risk of complete heart block is increased.

Toxicity

The side effects (e.g., ventricular tachyarrhythmias) of propafenone are dose related; at high dosages, dangerous new arrhythmias, heart block, and severe congestive heart failure may appear.

Interactions

Propafenone interferes with metabolism or elimination of digoxin and warfarin and can significantly increase serum concentrations of these drugs. Dosages may need to be reduced and serum concentrations must be monitored when propafenone is also being given.

CLASS II ANTIARRHYTHMIC DRUGS

Class II antiarrhythmic drugs are beta-adrenergic receptor blockers (see Chapter 13) that depress phase 4 depolarization of the action potential (see Figure 19-1). Beta-adrenergic blockers are used for arrhythmias driven by excessive sympathetic stimulation. Trials have shown that beta-adrenergic receptor blockers reduce mortality after myocardial infarction. Nadolol and propranolol were included in European trials and therefore appear in Table 19-2. In the United States, acebutolol, a relatively cardioselective blocker of beta$_1$-receptors, has been used. Sotalol is also a beta-blocker that is an effective antiarrhythmic; it is included with class III drugs in Table 19-2 because of its additional strong inhibition of potassium channels. Esmolol is the only beta-blocker that is used in the United States primarily as an antiarrhythmic agent.

esmolol

Mechanism of Action

Esmolol is a relatively cardioselective blocker of beta$_1$-receptors, with little sympathomimetic or membrane-stabilizing activity.

Pharmacokinetics

Esmolol is used intravenously. It distributes to tissues within 2 minutes, and achieves therapeutic effects within 5 minutes. Effects last only 10 to 20 minutes after the infusion is stopped. The drug is rapidly destroyed by esterases in red blood cells.

Uses

Esmolol is intended for rapid, short-term control of ventricular rates in atrial flutter or fibrillation. It is primarily an emergency medication for perioperative or postoperative use.

Adverse Reactions and Contraindications

Hypotension is common in patients receiving esmolol, causing dizziness and sweating in up to 12% of patients. Reduced peripheral circulation and difficulty breathing may also occur. Esmolol is especially dangerous in patients with heart failure that has been compensated by increased sympathetic stimulation of the heart. Blockade of these sympathetic influences may produce bradycardia or heart arrest, especially if partial AV block already exists. Therefore esmolol should be avoided in cardiac failure, cardiogenic shock, AV block, and sinus bradycardia.

Toxicity

Overdose may cause slow or irregular heartbeat, dizziness, fainting, difficulty breathing, blue fingernail beds, or seizures. Treatment of overdose may include specific antiarrhythmics to control cardiac symptoms, a beta$_2$-agonist to halt bronchospasm, and glucagon to control bradycardia and hypotension.

Interactions

Esmolol should not be used with sympathomimetics because the effects of both drugs will be lost. Esmolol also blocks the therapeutic effects of aminophylline and theophylline. Risk of hypertension is increased with monoamine oxidase inhibitors. Esmolol masks signs of hypoglycemia, which can increase risks to patients receiving insulin or oral antidiabetic medications.

CLASS III ANTIARRHYTHMIC DRUGS

Class III antiarrhythmics primarily prolong phase 3, the repolarization phase, of the action potential (see Figure 19-1), thereby lengthening the duration of refractoriness. All the class III drugs strongly inhibit potassium channels (see Table 19-2). The drugs differ significantly in other actions.

amiodarone

Mechanism of Action

Amiodarone has many actions on cardiac tissues (see Table 19-2), which result in prolonging the refractory period and reducing automaticity. Amiodarone also may depress contractility and may cause vasodilation. The complex actions and long persistence in the body have caused amiodarone to be used only for prophylaxis or therapy for life-threatening ventricular arrhythmias when other drugs fail.

Pharmacokinetics

Oral absorption is variable, and most patients absorb less than half the administered dose. Amiodarone is highly lipid soluble and concentrates in adipose tissue, as well as other sites. As a result antiarrhythmic activity is not seen for days or even months. The duration of action is also greatly prolonged. Amiodarone may be detectable in plasma up to 9 months after its use has been discontinued.

Adverse Reactions and Contraindications

Sinus bradycardia is common, and arrest or heart block may occur. New arrhythmias occur in up to 5% of patients. Up to 15% of patients develop significant pulmonary toxicity, which may be fatal. Neurotoxicity, signaled by weakness, numbness, or ataxia, occurs in up to 40% of patients. Sensitivity to sun, ocular toxicity, and hypothyroidism also occur. Reversal of side effects may take months after therapy ends.

Amiodarone should be avoided in AV block because the drug may worsen blockade. Amiodarone is also avoided in conditions that produce bradycardia because the drug may lower SA node automaticity and create additional bradycardia that is resistant to atropine.

Toxicity

Overdose may result in hypotension, cardiovascular distress, and bradycardia. Because the drug has such a long duration of action, the patient may require monitoring or treatment for weeks after the use of amiodarone is discontinued.

Interactions

Amiodarone significantly increases serum concentrations of digoxin, digitoxin, and phenytoin, which increases the risk of toxicity. Amiodarone inhibits metabolism of coumarin anticoagulants, increasing their concentrations in plasma and thus increasing risk of bleeding. Amiodarone is likely to have additive cardiac effects with other antiarrhythmic agents, which may increase risk of cardiac toxicity.

bretylium

Mechanism of Action

Bretylium blocks potassium channels and hence increases action potential duration and prolongs the refractory period. It does not directly suppress automaticity or conduction velocity. Bretylium accumulates in sympathetic neurons and causes an initial release of norepinephrine that may stimulate contractility, heart rate, and automaticity, but ultimately the drug produces adrenergic blockade by preventing norepinephrine release.

Pharmacokinetics

Bretylium is administered by IV or intramuscular injection. The onset is usually within 20 minutes by either route, and the duration of action is 6 to 8 hours. Most of the drug is excreted by the kidneys.

Uses

Bretylium is used primarily for life-threatening ventricular tachycardia, especially episodes refractory to lidocaine or cardioversion, and for ventricular fibrillation.

Adverse Reactions and Contraindications

Major reactions to bretylium are precipitation of anginal attacks, bradycardia, and hypotension. Bretylium does not alter the ECG tracings. There are no specific contraindications to the use of bretylium.

Toxicity

Initial hypertension may be followed by marked hypotension.

Interactions

The early release of norepinephrine caused by bretylium may increase risk of toxicity with digoxin or digitoxin.

CLASS IV ANTIARRHYTHMIC DRUGS

Class IV antiarrhythmic drugs primarily depress phase 4 depolarization and lengthen phase 1 and 2 repolarization. The heart rate may slow significantly. These actions arise primarily from the calcium channel blockade produced by the drugs.

diltiazem and verapamil

Mechanism of Action

Calcium channel blockers are used primarily as antianginal or antihypertensive agents (see Chapters 13 and 15). Some of these agents are also useful antiarrhythmics because the slow calcium ion current blocked by these drugs is important for the activity of the AV node. Thus, the major antiarrhythmic effect of these drugs is a delay in conduction through the AV node, with a subsequent reduction of heart rate. These actions are shared by bepridil, diltiazem, and verapamil, but only the last two are currently used in the United States for this indication. Verapamil and diltiazem are used to control supraventricular arrhythmias.

Pharmacokinetics

Verapamil and diltiazem are well absorbed orally but are rapidly metabolized by the liver. This first-pass phenomenon significantly reduces bioavailability (see Chapter 1). Verapamil or diltiazem may be given intravenously when the oral route is inappropriate.

Adverse Reactions and Contraindications

Side effects related to cardiovascular function include hypotension, peripheral edema, congestive heart failure, and pulmonary edema.

Contraindications include AV block, SA node impairment, bradycardia, heart failure, cardiogenic shock, and hypotension. The drugs should also be avoided after myocardial infarction because they increase the risk of cardiac failure.

Toxicity

Acute overdose may produce bradycardia, progressing to hypotension and asystole. Treatment is symptomatic.

Interactions

Verapamil and diltiazem can increase serum concentrations of digoxin, which can lead to toxicity. Neither verapamil nor diltiazem should be given to patients receiving disopyramide or flecainide because the lower contractility produced by calcium channel blockers is additive with that produced by disopyramide or flecainide. The result can be dangerous cardiac failure.

UNCLASSIFIED ANTIARRHYTHMIC DRUGS

▼ adenosine

Adenosine is a naturally occurring metabolite that acts as an autocoid. Receptors for adenosine exist on the outer surface of many cells in the body, including cells in blood vessels and organs such as the brain, heart, and kidneys. Large doses of adenosine given by rapid IV injection are effective in terminating supraventricular tachycardia and returning the heart to normal sinus rhythm. Adenosine slows conduction in the SA and AV nodes and can interrupt reentry. In addition, adenosine may impair ventricular function, but because the drug has a half-life of about 10 seconds, this undesired action is considered minor and transient for most patients. The antiarrhythmic effect persists after the drug has been metabolized and removed.

atropine

Atropine, a blocker of muscarinic cholinergic receptors (see Chapter 11), may also be used to treat certain arrhythmias.

Its action as an antiarrhythmic drug depends on its ability to reduce the effects of vagal nerve stimulation, primarily on the SA node. Because stimulation of the vagus nerve slows heart rate, atropine increases heart rate by blocking that effect. Because it also speeds conduction through the AV node, atropine may lessen heart block in certain cases.

digoxin

Digoxin is primarily a cardiotonic agent (see Chapter 18), but in addition to the ability to strengthen contraction of the heart muscle, it also increases vagal tone at the AV node. Through this action and direct effects on nodal tissue, cardiac glycosides slow conduction through the AV node. This action is sought when digoxin is used to treat atrial flutter and fibrillation. By lowering conduction of impulses through the AV node, digoxin protects the ventricles from overstimulation. The short-term therapeutic goal is not to slow the atrial rate but to produce a partial heart block that allows fewer impulses from the atria to stimulate the ventricles to beat. The patient's condition may therefore be maintained with rapid atrial rates but with ventricular rates from 60 to 80 beats/min. Many patients spontaneously convert to normal sinus rhythm after a few days of treatment.

As with other antiarrhythmic drugs, higher concentrations of cardiac glycosides may also cause arrhythmias of various types, most characteristically bradycardia and PVCs. Bradycardia may be a sign of impending heart block (no impulse passes through the AV node to the ventricles). PVCs arise because cardiac glycosides increase the spontaneous rate of ventricular depolarization (phase 4 of the action potential). The first step in controlling these reactions is to discontinue the cardiac glycoside. If the arrhythmia is not severe, no further therapy may be required. However, cardiac glycosides are relatively long- acting drugs, and treating the arrhythmia while the cardiac glycoside is being eliminated from the system may be necessary (see Table 18-1). Potassium levels should be assessed in these patients because a low potassium level increases the sensitivity of the heart to digoxin and may predispose it to arrhythmias. Potassium supplements may be given if required.

Nursing Process Overview

Antiarrhythmic Therapy

Assessment

Antiarrhythmic therapy is used in patients with cardiac arrhythmias. An arrhythmia is diagnosed by use of the ECG tracings, although the patient may complain of missed beats, fluttering in the chest, pounding in the chest, or irregular heart rates or patterns. Perform a thorough cardiovascular assessment, and question the patient about previous cardiac problems.

Nursing Diagnoses
- Risk for arrhythmias
- Risk for activity intolerance related to insufficient knowledge of adaptive techniques needed related to impaired cardiac function

Patient Outcomes

The nurse will manage and minimize complications associated with arrhythmias. The patient will identify factors that increase cardiac workload, will identify modifications needed in activities of daily living, and will modify activities to maintain pulse, blood pressure, and respirations in normal range.

Planning/Implementation

Treatment may take place in the coronary care unit or in the outpatient care setting if the arrhythmia is less serious. Perform periodic or continuous ECG monitoring as needed. Monitor vital signs and blood pressure, weight, fluid intake and output, serum electrolyte levels, and laboratory work appropriate for the drug prescribed. Observe the general physical condition of the patient and watch for the appearance of side effects.

Evaluation

Before discharge, determine that the patient can explain interactions among prescribed drugs, plan meals within prescribed dietary restriction, state how to manage persistent side effects, describe side effects and the signs and symptoms of toxicity, and understand when to notify the physician.

Nursing Implications Summary

General Guidelines: Antiarrhythmic Therapy
Drug Administration
➤ Monitor vital signs and blood pressure. Although a change in the heart rate is often a desired outcome of therapy, a heart rate less than 60 beats/min or greater than 120 beats/min in an adult should be avoided.
➤ Establish specific guidelines for each patient in consultation with the physician.
➤ Monitor the ECG patterns continuously in the short-term care setting and periodically thereafter.
➤ Monitor other indicators of cardiovascular functioning as appropriate, including blood pressure, pulse, intake and output, weight, and heart and lung sounds. Assess for edema, especially in dependent areas, and jugular venous distension. Assess for activity tolerance with daily activities. Monitor other available data: central venous pressure and pulmonary capillary wedge pressure.
➤ Monitor the blood urea nitrogen (BUN) level, liver function studies, and serum drug levels if available.
➤ For IV administration, use microdrip tubing and/or an electronic infusion monitor. Usually, monitor the ECG during IV administration. Monitor the blood pressure and pulse. Keep the patient in the supine position after IV doses until vital signs are stable. Keep siderails up. Have available emergency equipment and drugs to treat toxicity or to resuscitate the patient.

Nursing in the Community
➤ Instruct the patient about the desired effects and common side effects of prescribed drugs. Emphasize that it is important to report the development of any unexpected sign or symptom. Point out that drugs or doses may require changing or adjustment if unusual side effects develop and that the patient should not hesitate to contact the health care provider with any questions.
➤ Review with the patient the importance of taking medications as ordered. Antiarrhythmic drugs are most effective when taken regularly, with doses spread evenly throughout the 24-hour day, as prescribed. If a dose is missed, the patient should not double up for it. Refer the patient as appropriate to community-based nursing care agencies.
➤ Instruct the patient not to discontinue antiarrhythmic medications without first consulting the physician.
➤ Stress the importance of concomitant therapies, if ordered, including modifying diet; losing weight; restricting sodium; using potassium replacements, diuretics, and antihypertensives; limiting caffeine intake; stopping smoking; and exercising regularly. Emphasize the importance of returning for follow-up visits as scheduled to monitor drug effectiveness.
➤ Assess the need for patients to monitor weight, pulse, blood pressure, or other parameters in the home. Consider the patient's medical condition, prescribed medication, ability, and resources when making this decision.
➤ Suggest that the patient carry a medical identification tag or bracelet indicating that antiarrhythmics are being used. Remind the patient to keep all health care providers, including dentists, informed of all drugs being used.
➤ Instruct the patient to avoid drinking alcoholic beverages unless approved by the physician.
➤ Remind the patient to keep all medications out of the reach of children.
➤ Digoxin is discussed in Chapter 18. Beta-adrenergic receptor blockers are discussed in Chapter 13. Calcium channel blockers are discussed in Chapter 15. Phenytoin is discussed in Chapter 61.

disopyramide
Drug Administration
➤ See the general guidelines for antiarrhythmic therapy.
➤ Assess for urinary retention. Monitor intake and output, question the patient about hesitancy or difficulty voiding, and palpate the bladder.
➤ Monitor blood glucose because disopyramide can cause hypoglycemia. Moderate to excessive alcohol intake may contribute to development of hypoglycemia.

Nursing in the Community
➤ See the general guidelines for antiarrhythmic therapy.
➤ Instruct the patient to take a missed dose as soon as remembered, unless within 4 hours of the next scheduled dose, then omit the missed dose and resume the regular dosing schedule.
➤ Disopyramide may cause the patient to sweat less. Instruct the patient to avoid becoming overheated or exercising excessively during hot weather.
➤ Instruct the patient to avoid driving or operating hazardous equipment if dizziness, light-headedness, or blurred vision develop.
➤ Emphasize to diabetic patients that it is important to monitor blood glucose carefully at the start of therapy and during

Continued

Nursing Implications Summary—cont'd

periods of dosage adjustment. A change in diet or insulin may be required; check with the physician. Review with the patient the signs of hypoglycemia, including fast heart rate, cold sweats, headache, hunger, nausea, nervousness, shakiness, unsteady walk, and anxious feeling. Instruct the patient to eat or drink a food containing sugar if any of these symptoms develop and to notify the physician.

➤ Instruct patients taking extended-release capsules or tablets to swallow the dose whole, without chewing, crushing, or breaking the medication.

➤ See the Patient Problems boxes on dry mouth (see Chapter 23), orthostatic hypotension (see Chapter 13), and constipation (see Chapter 24). Instruct the patient to report any difficulty urinating.

procainamide
Drug Administration
➤ See the general guidelines for antiarrhythmic therapy.

➤ Monitor antinuclear antibody (ANA) test and complete blood count. Monitor plasma procainamide levels and NAPA concentrations if available.

Intravenous Administration
➤ For direct IV injection, dilute each 100 mg with 5 to 10 ml of D5W. Administer at a rate of 20 mg/min. For infusion, add 1 g to 500 ml D5W for a dilution of 2 mg/ml; other dilutions may be used. Use microdrip tubing and/or an infusion control device, and infuse at a rate of 2 to 6 mg/min.

Nursing in the Community
➤ See the general guidelines for antiarrhythmic therapy.

➤ Doses are best taken on an empty stomach with a full (8 ounce) glass of water 1 hour before or 2 hours after meals. Instruct the patient to take doses consistently with meals or on an empty stomach. However, if GI symptoms are severe, instruct the patient to take doses with meals.

➤ Instruct patients taking extended-release formulations to swallow the medication whole without crushing or breaking it.

➤ Instruct the patient to report the development of arthritis, polyarthralgia, pleuritic pain, myalgia, skin lesions, fever, or any other new sign or symptom.

➤ Caution the patient to avoid driving or operating hazardous equipment if dizziness develops and to notify the physician if dizziness occurs.

➤ Instruct the patient to take a missed dose as soon as remembered if within 2 hours of when the dose was scheduled (4 hours for sustained-release preparations); otherwise the patient should omit the missed dose and resume the regular dosage schedule.

➤ Caution the patient that the matrix from extended-release tablets may be seen in the stool and that this situation is normal.

quinidine
Drug Administration
➤ See the general guidelines for antiarrhythmic therapy.

➤ Read medication labels carefully; do not confuse quinidine with quinine.

➤ Monitor liver function tests, blood count, platelet count, serum electrolyte levels, and prothrombin time. Monitor serum quinidine levels if available, and when daily doses exceed 2 g.

➤ A test dose may be ordered before the full dose is given to test for possible idiosyncrasy to quinidine.

➤ Assess for rash or skin changes.

➤ IM injections may be painful and may increase serum creatine phosphokinase (creatine phosphokinase [CPK] or creatine kinase [CK]) levels.

Intravenous Administration
➤ Dilute 800 mg (10 ml) in at least 40 ml of 5% dextrose in water (D5W). Do not add to IV solutions or mix with other drugs in a syringe. Administer at a rate of 1 ml (16 mg)/min. Use microdrip tubing and/or and IV monitor. Monitor ECG changes and blood pressure.

➤ IV quinidine may be used in treatment of life-threatening malaria; see Chapter 53.

Nursing in the Community
➤ See the general guidelines for antiarrhythmic therapy.

➤ Instruct the patient to take doses with full (8 ounce) glass of water on an empty stomach, 1 hour before or 2 hours after meals. If gastric irritation develops, instruct the patient to take doses with meals. Encourage the patient to take all doses the same way, either with or without food and to notify the physician if diarrhea develops.

➤ Remind patients taking extended-release tablets to swallow the tablet whole without breaking, chewing, or crushing it.

➤ Review with the patient the symptoms of cinchonism such as ringing in the ears, headache, nausea, or changes in vision. Instruct the patient to notify the physician if these occur; rarely patients may experience these symptoms after one or two doses.

➤ Warn the patient to avoid driving or operating hazardous equipment if visual changes occur and to notify the physician if these symptoms occur.

➤ Patients may develop a bitter taste in the mouth. There is little that can be done for this, but caution the patient not to discontinue the drug without consulting with the physician.

➤ Review with the patient the Patient Problems box in Chapter 55 on bleeding tendencies.

➤ Instruct the patients to report the development of any unexpected sign or symptom.

➤ Instruct the patient to take a missed dose as soon as remembered if within 2 hours of when scheduled; otherwise the patient should omit the missed dose and resume the regular dosing schedule.

lidocaine
Drug Administration
➤ See the general guidelines for antiarrhythmic therapy.

➤ Lidocaine is rarely used outside of the acute-care setting.

Nursing Implications Summary—cont'd

Keep the patient and family informed of the patient's condition.

➤ Assess for the side effects noted in the text. Instruct the patient to report any subjective changes. Monitor blood pressure, ECG, serum electrolytes, and serum lidocaine concentrations.

Intravenous Administration

➤ Read drug labels carefully. Use lidocaine labeled "preservative-free" or "lidocaine for continuous IV infusion." Lidocaine with epinephrine is not used as an antiarrhythmic. Label must state "for IV use." Bolus doses may be given undiluted at a rate of 25 to 50 mg/min; too rapid administration may cause seizures. For continuous infusion, dilute per agency protocol or consult manufacturer's literature. Premixed forms are available. Use microdrip tubing and/or an infusion control device, and adjust dose to patient response.

Nursing in the Community

➤ This drug is not used in the home care setting.

mexiletene

Drug Administration

➤ See the general guidelines for antiarrhythmic therapy.

➤ Monitor aspartate aminotransferase (AST, serum glutamic-oxaloacetic transaminase [SGOT]) white blood cell count, white blood cell differential, platelet count, and serum mexiletine concentrations if available.

➤ Assess the patient for ataxia, slurred speech, ringing in the ears, trembling, and development of CNS side effects.

Nursing in the Community

➤ See the Patient Problems boxes in Chapter 54 on bleeding tendencies and depressed white blood cell production. Instruct the patient to report the development of these rare but serious side effects.

➤ Caution the patient to avoid driving or operating hazardous equipment if dizziness or blurred vision develops and to notify the physician if these symptoms occur.

➤ Remind the patient to take doses with meals or a snack to lessen gastric irritation.

➤ Instruct the patient to take a missed dose as soon as remembered if within 4 hours of when the dose was due; otherwise the patient should omit the missed dose and resume the regular dosing schedule.

tocainide

Drug Administration

➤ See the general guidelines for antiarrhythmic therapy.

➤ Assess regularly for skin changes or rashes. Auscultate breath sounds and assess respiratory rate. Assess for tremor.

Nursing in the Community

➤ See the general guidelines for antiarrhythmic therapy.

➤ Instruct the patient to take doses with food or milk to lessen gastric irritation.

➤ Explain that the patient should notify the physician immediately if rashes, skin changes, peeling or scaling of skin, blisters on skin or mouth, cough, or shortness of breath develops.

➤ Caution the patient to avoid driving or operating hazardous equipment if dizziness, light-headedness, confusion, or visual changes develop; instruct the patient to notify the physician if these symptoms occur.

➤ Instruct the patient to take missed dose as soon as remembered if within 4 hours of when scheduled; otherwise the patient should omit the missed dose and resume the regular dosage schedule.

➤ See the Patient Problems box in Chapter 54 on bleeding tendencies.

moricizine

Drug Administration/Nursing in the Community

➤ See the general guidelines for antiarrhythmic therapy.

➤ Assess patient for diarrhea, dry mouth, stomach pain, insomnia, excessive fatigue, or weakness.

➤ Caution the patient to avoid driving or operating hazardous equipment if dizziness develops. Instruct the patient to notify the physician if dizziness develops.

➤ Instruct the patient to take a missed dose as soon as remembered if within 4 hours of when the dose was due; otherwise omit the missed dose and resume the regular dosing schedule.

flecainide

Drug Administration/Nursing in the Community

➤ See the general guidelines for antiarrhythmic therapy.

➤ Monitor complete blood count (CBC) and plasma flecainide levels if available.

➤ Caution the patient to avoid driving or operating hazardous equipment if dizziness or visual changes develop and to notify the physician if these symptoms occur.

➤ Instruct the patient to take a missed dose as soon as remembered if within 6 hours of when scheduled; otherwise the patient should omit the missed dose and resume the regular dosing schedule.

➤ Instruct the patient to notify the physician if jaundice, trembling, depression, anxiety, skin rash, or chest pain develops.

propafenone

Drug Administration/Nursing in the Community

➤ See the general guidelines for antiarrhythmic therapy.

➤ Caution the patient to avoid driving or operating hazardous equipment if dizziness, blurred vision, or light-headedness develop and to notify the physician if these symptoms occur.

➤ Review the Patient Problems boxes in Chapters 23 and 24 on dry mouth and constipation, respectively.

➤ Some patients develop a metallic taste in the mouth. If the patient is unable to tolerate this side effect, consult the physician. Remind the patient not to discontinue medication without consulting the physician. Monitor weight.

➤ Instruct the patient to take a missed dose as soon as remembered if within 4 hours of the scheduled time; otherwise the

Continued

Nursing Implications Summary—cont'd

patient should omit the missed dose and resume the regular dosage schedule.

esmolol
Drug Administration/Nursing in the Community
➤ See the general guidelines for antiarrhythmic therapy.
➤ Esmolol is rarely used outside of the short-term care setting. Keep the patient and family informed of the patient's condition.
Intravenous Administration
➤ Be alert to the physician's order and the strength of esmolol vial. Fatal overdoses have resulted from incorrect administration of the concentrated solution for the loading or bolus dose.
➤ Esmolol may be given undiluted for the loading dose; use only the 10 mg/ml concentration. Administer the dose as ordered (there may be one dose for the first minute, followed by a lower dose for 4 minutes).
➤ For infusion, see manufacturer's instructions. Aseptically withdraw 20 ml from a 500-ml bottle of compatible IV solution, then add 5 g esmolol to the remaining 480 ml to make a concentration of 10 mg/ml. Use microdrip tubing or an infusion control device to prevent overdose and keep administration rate steady. Monitor ECG changes and blood pressure.
➤ Monitor the patient for signs of toxicity described in the text.

amiodarone
Drug Administration
➤ See the general guidelines for antiarrhythmic therapy.
➤ Assess breath sounds, presence of cough, shortness of breath, and respiratory rate for signs of pulmonary toxicity. Questions patient about blurred vision or the presence of blue-green halos around lights, dry eyes, sensitivity to light. Assess for signs of hyperthyroidism (nervousness, sensitivity to heat, sweating, weight loss, trouble sleeping) or hypothyroidism (coldness, dry puffy skin, excessive fatigue, weight gain).
➤ Assess visual acuity at the start of therapy.
➤ Monitor laboratory work: alanine aminotransferase (ALT [SGPT]), alkaline phosphatase, and aspartate aminotransferase (AST [SGOT]).
Nursing in the Community
➤ See the general guidelines for antiarrhythmic therapy. Review the common side effects. Instruct the patient to report the development of respiratory difficulties, weakness, numbness, or ataxia.
➤ Review the Patient Problems box in Chapter 58 on photosensitivity. Patients receiving amiodarone who develop photosensitivity may be sensitive to sunlight coming through windows or through thin clothing. Photosensitivity may persist for up to several months after the drug is discontinued.
➤ Instruct the patient to report subjective visual or eye changes. Encourage patients who wear glasses to continue periodic ophthalmic examinations.

➤ Warn the patient that the skin may turn bluish gray but the discoloration should fade when therapy is discontinued. Instruct the patient to notify the physician if skin color begins to change.
➤ Review the Patient Problems box in Chapter 24 on constipation.
➤ Some patients develop a metallic taste in the mouth. If the patient is unable to tolerate this side effect, consult the physician. Remind the patient not to discontinue medication without consulting the physician. Monitor weight.
➤ Instruct the patient not to take a missed dose and not to double the next one but to go back to the regular dosing schedule. If two or more doses are missed, the patient should contact the physician.

bretylium
Drug Administration
➤ See the general guidelines for antiarrhythmic therapy.
Intramuscular Administration
➤ Administer in large muscle masses. Record and rotate injection sites. Do not dilute. Do not administer more than 5 ml into a single injection site; if a larger volume is ordered, divide the dose into two equal volumes for injection into two sites.
Intravenous Administration
➤ Bretylium may be given undiluted, one dose over 1 minute or less, for life-threatening ventricular arrhythmias.
➤ For intermittent infusion, dilute drug in at least 50 ml of diluent or use commercially prepared diluted solutions. Administer dose over 10 to 30 minutes. Too rapid an infusion may contribute to nausea and vomiting.
➤ For constant infusion, use microdrip tubing and/or an infusion control device.
➤ Monitor continuous ECG recording and blood pressure. Nausea and vomiting may occur with rapid IV administration.
➤ Bretylium is rarely used outside of the acute-care setting. Keep the patient and family informed of the patient's condition.

diltiazem and verapamil
Drug Administration/Nursing in the Community
➤ See the general guidelines for antiarrhythmic therapy.
➤ For additional information about diltiazem and verapamil, see Chapter 15.

adenosine
Drug Administration/Nursing in the Community
➤ See the general guidelines for antiarrhythmic therapy.
Intravenous Administration
➤ Read drug labels carefully. Do not confuse adenosine with adenosine phosphate. Inspect solution; use only clear solution, with no particulate matter.
➤ Adenosine may be given undiluted and should be given in an injection site as close to the IV insertion site as possible.

Nursing Implications Summary—cont'd

Administer as a rapid bolus over 1 to 2 seconds. Follow with a rapid normal saline flush (±50 ml) if given via IV line.

➤ For pharmacologic stress testing, dose is diluted and administered over 6 minutes.

➤ Monitor ECG changes and blood pressure.

➤ A variety of side effects have been reported but usually last less than 1 minute. These include chest pressure or pain, hyperventilation, hypotension, metallic taste in the mouth, neck or back pain, tight throat, nausea, and premature atrial contractions (PACs) or PVCs. Notify the physician of side effects that last longer than 1 minute. Because side effects are short lived, overdose is rarely a problem; however, xanthines are competitive antagonists that may be used if necessary.

➤ Adenosine is rarely used outside of the acute-care setting. Keep patient and family informed of the patient's condition.

atropine
Drug Administration/Nursing in the Community

➤ See the general guidelines for antiarrhythmic therapy, and review the patient care implications for anticholinergic drugs at the end of Chapter 23.

➤ See the Patient Problems boxes in Chapters 23 and 24 on dry mouth and constipation, respectively.

Intravenous Administration

➤ Atropine may be given undiluted or diluted in at least 10 ml of sterile water. Do not add to infusing fluids or drugs. Administer at a rate of 1 mg or less over 1 minute.

digoxin

➤ See the general guidelines for antiarrhythmic therapy. Digoxin is discussed in Chapter 18.

CHAPTER REVIEW

Application

1. What is an action potential?
2. What tissues in the heart are normally automatic?
3. What is the normal pacemaker of the heart?
4. What is the effect of vagus nerve stimulation on the heart?
5. What is the effect of sympathetic stimulation on the heart?
6. What is the refractory period?
7. What is reentry?
8. What is the mechanism of action of quinidine and procainamide?
9. What secondary action do both quinidine and procainamide share?
10. What is the mechanism of action of disopyramide?
11. Flecainide is reserved for what clinical indication? Why?
12. What is the antiarrhythmic effect shared by propranolol and esmolol?
13. What is the mechanism of action of amiodarone?
14. What are the uses of amiodarone?
15. What is the mechanism of action of bretylium as an antiarrhythmic agent?
16. What is the mechanism of action of verapamil as an antiarrhythmic agent?

Critical Thinking

1. Describe how the waves on an ECG tracing are related to electrical activity of different portions of the heart.
2. How may an ECG tracing help monitor a patient for toxicity caused by quinidine or procainamide?
3. What are the classes of antiarrhythmic drugs? On what is the classification based? How would you include this information in teaching plans?
4. How could you use the Sicilian gambit (see Table 19-2) to help you look for side effects of particular drugs?
5. How do the toxic effects of quinidine and procainamide differ? How would you assess the patient for them?
6. How does the use of lidocaine differ from that of mexiletine and tocainide?

References

Chase S, Cerrato PL: Pharmacology in practice: antiarrhythmics, *RN* 60(5):41-49, 1997.

Davenport J, Morton PG: Identifying nonischemic causes of life-threatening arrhythmias, *Am J Nurs* 97(11):50-55, 1997.

Hayes DD: Bradycardia: keeping the current flowing, *Nursing* 27(6):50-55, 1997.

Lazzara D: Dealing confidently with deadly arrhythmias, *Nursing* 28(1):41-45, 1998.

Rosen MR: Consequences of the Sicilian gambit. *Eur Heart J* 16(suppl G):32-36, 1995.

Strimike CL, Wojcik JM: Stopping atrial fibrillation with Ibutilide, *Am J Nurs* 98(1):32-34, 1998.

20

Agents Affecting Blood Coagulation

KEY TERMS

anticoagulant drugs, p. 246
antiplatelet drugs, p. 246
blood coagulation, p. 244
embolus, p. 244
hemophilia, p. 257
hemostatic drugs, p. 254
thrombocytes, p. 250
thrombus, p. 244

KEY DRUGS ▼

alteplase, p. 253
aspirin, p. 251
desmopressin, p. 257
heparin, p. 246

OBJECTIVES

After studying this chapter, you should be able to do the following:

- *Discuss the groups of drugs used in anticoagulation.*
- *Develop a nursing care plan for patients receiving an anticoagulant.*
- *Identify the antidotes for hemorrhage caused by drug overdose.*
- *Describe the use of antiplatelet therapy, thrombolytic therapy, and hemostatic therapy.*
- *Differentiate between treatments for hemophilia.*
- *Develop nursing care plans, including teaching points, for patients receiving drugs affecting blood coagulation.*

CHAPTER OVERVIEW

Blood can quickly produce plugs and clots when blood loss is threatened. This chapter describes blood coagulation and drugs and agents used to control it. Anticoagulants interfere with the process of coagulation. Antiplatelet drugs inhibit the aggregation of blood platelets and play a prophylactic role against heart attacks and strokes. Thrombolytic drugs degrade blood clots and can limit the damage of a heart attack. Hemostatic agents aid in promoting blood coagulation.

THERAPEUTIC RATIONALE: ANTICOAGULATION

Steps in Blood Coagulation

The process of **blood coagulation** is diagrammed in Figure 20-1. The initial step can be in the intrinsic pathway with the activation of the blood component factor XII (the Hageman factor) by contact with exposed collagen or an event in the extrinsic pathway (e.g., the release of tissue factor by damaged tissue). Either pathway results in the activation of factor X. Factor Xa (activated factor X) forms a complex with platelet phospholipids, calcium, and factor V. This complex, which is sometimes called thromboplastin, catalyzes the conversion of prothrombin (factor II) to thrombin. Thrombin then catalyzes the conversion of fibrinogen to

fibrin. After cross-linking of fibrin by factor XIIIa, fibrin becomes insoluble, forming a mesh that is the blood clot, also called a **thrombus.**

Blood clots in the arterial system are initially composed largely of platelets with a fibrin mesh (white thrombus). Blood clots in the venous system have only a few platelet aggregates and are composed largely of fibrin with trapped red blood cells (red thrombus). A thrombus in the arterial or venous system may dislodge, becoming an **embolus.** Venous emboli often lodge in the small arteries of the pulmonary circulation, thereby markedly blocking the oxygenating capacity of the lungs and increasing the blood pressure in the pulmonary system, a life-threatening situation. Thrombi form in veins in which blood flow is low, favoring the accumulation of activated clotting factors. Patients at risk for

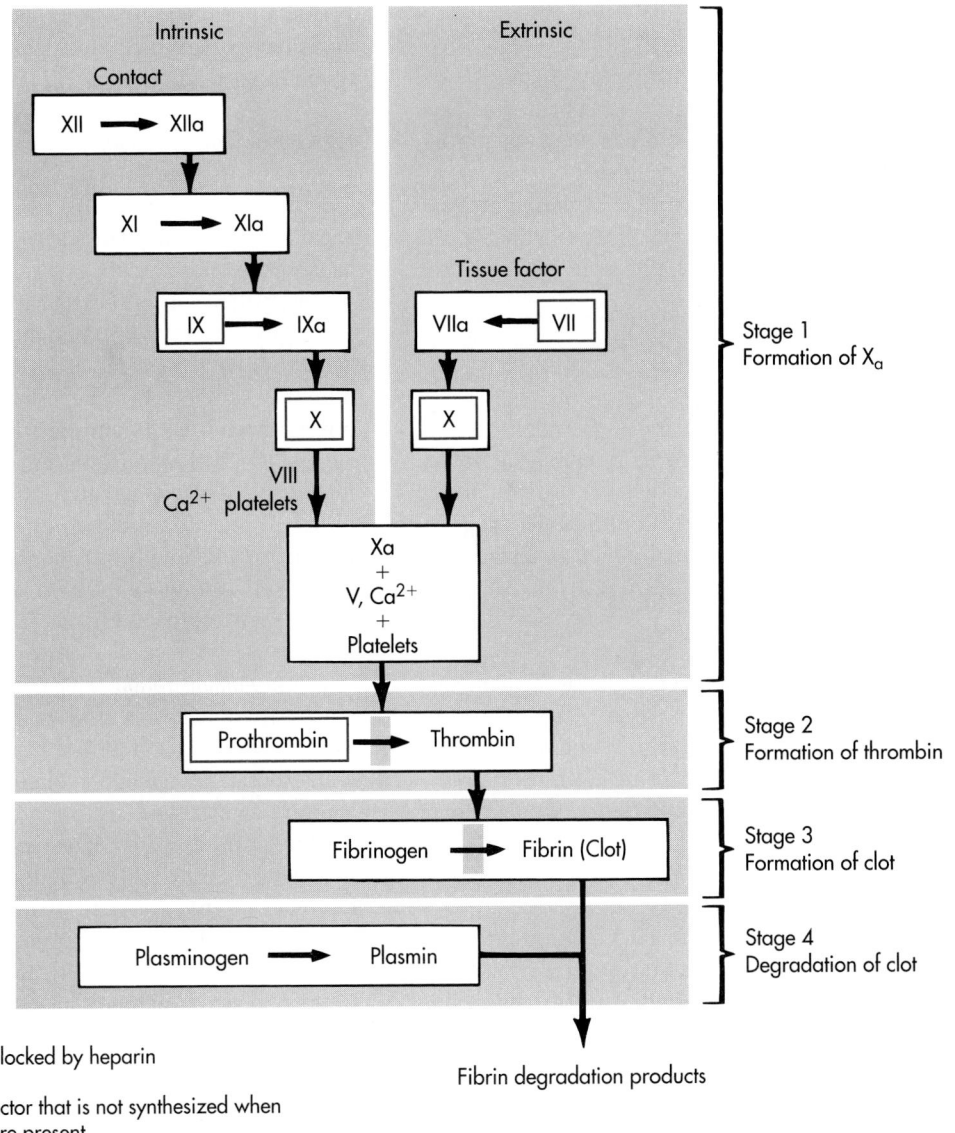

Indicates the step is blocked by heparin

Indicates a clotting factor that is not synthesized when
oral anticoagulants are present

Figure 20-1   Stages of blood coagulation. Actions of drug classes include four stages: *Stage 1,* Antiplatelet
drugs inhibit platelet aggregation in intrinsic pathway. Citrate and EDTA, which chelate calcium, prevent formation of factor Xa. Oral anticoagulants prevent synthesis of factors VII, IX, and X, which are necessary for stage 1. Local hemostatic
agents provide contact to activate intrinsic pathway. Not shown is the native inhibitor of anticoagulation, antithrombin III,
which acts in stage 1 to inhibit the activity of factor Xa and in stage 2 to inhibit the conversion of prothrombin to thrombin. Heparin and the low-molecular-weight heparins enhance the activity of antithrombin III by directly binding with antithrombin III. In stage 1, the heparin/antithrombin III complex inhibits factor Xa. *Stage 2,* Oral anticoagulants prevent
synthesis of prothrombin. *Stage 3,* The heparin/antithrombin III complex blocks thrombin (factor IIa) activity. Low-molecular-weight heparins are relatively ineffective activating antithrombin III to block thrombin. *Stage 4,* Aminocaproic acid
inhibits activation of plasminogen and thus inhibits clot degradation. Aprotinin inhibits plasmin. By contrast alteplase,
anistreplase, streptokinase, and urokinase activate plasminogen to promote clot digestion.

experiencing venous thrombosis include those immobilized
as a result of trauma or surgery and those with a history of
thromboembolism.

Role of Calcium in Blood Coagulation

Calcium is a cofactor for each of the steps through the
activation of prothrombin. The removal of calcium prevents the coagulation of blood. Citrate and ethylenediaminetetraacetic acid (EDTA) are compounds that complex calcium, making calcium unavailable for blood coagulation. When blood is drawn for testing or storage, citrate or EDTA may be used to keep the blood from clotting
in the container. Because calcium is essential for many
biochemical events, anticoagulants that complex calcium
can be used only in storage containers (in vitro), not in a
patient (in vivo).

Mechanisms for Anticoagulant and Antiplatelet Drugs

Anticoagulant drugs interfere with any of the steps depicted in Figure 20-1, leading to the formation of fibrin. Blood coagulation is often referred to as a cascade phenomenon because the process becomes magnified at every step. Each activated factor is a catalyst leading to the formation of many molecules of the next activated factor. The earlier in the process that a step can be blocked, the more efficient is the inhibition of blood coagulation.

THERAPEUTIC AGENTS: ANTICOAGULANT AND ANTIPLATELET DRUGS

Anticoagulant drugs prevent clot formation; they do not affect existing clots. They can be classified into two groups: the drug heparin and oral anticoagulants. **Antiplatelet drugs** inhibit the aggregation of platelets and inhibit coagulation in the arterial system.

▼ heparin

Heparin (Calciparine, Liquaemin) is an anticoagulant that can be either administered to the patient (Table 20-1) or added to a storage container. Heparin is a naturally occurring glycosaminoglycan extracted from pig intestines and bovine lungs. As extracted, heparin consists of polymers of varying molecular weights.

Mechanism of Action

Heparin forms a complex with a plasma protein, antithrombin III. Antithrombin III neutralizes factor Xa, the factor activating the conversion of prothrombin to thrombin. Antithrombin III can also directly neutralize thrombin. When heparin complexes with antithrombin III, both of these actions of antithrombin III are greatly enhanced. However, the inhibition of factor Xa, rather than the inhibition of thrombin, appears to be primarily responsible for the effective anticoagulant action of heparin at low dosages.

Heparin is also an antiplatelet drug. In vitro, heparin stimulates platelet aggregation. In vivo, however, heparin appears to coat the endothelial lining of the vessels. Because heparin is a highly negatively charged polymer, it adds a negative charge to the endothelium that keeps platelets from attaching and forming a thrombus.

Pharmacokinetics

Heparin is administered intravenously or by deep subcutaneous injection. Heparin is not administered intramuscularly because it can lead to painful hematomas. Heparin is active within minutes and has a plasma half-life of 1 to 2 hours. Small doses of heparin are taken up by mast cells. Large doses are excreted in the urine.

Uses

The clinical uses of heparin differ in dose and route of administration. It achieves anticoagulation (in large doses), prevents postoperative thromboembolism (in small doses), and prevents coagulation of laboratory samples and stored blood in vitro.

High-Dose Administration. Heparin is used in the hospital to prevent the further growth of venous thrombi. Large doses (35 to 100 U/kg) must be administered intravenously to achieve this anticoagulation. Heparin cannot be taken orally because it is not absorbed and causes a painful hematoma if administered intramuscularly. Heparin may be given as an intravenous (IV) injection, achieving immediate anticoagulation, with the same or lesser dose repeated every 4 to 6 hours. Blood levels of heparin decrease by half every $1\frac{1}{2}$ hours. Intermittent IV administration results in virtual incoagulability after administration and is associated with a higher risk of bleeding than continuous IV infusion. Thus an initial IV injection followed by continuous infusion at approximately 1000 U/hr is commonly given. An IV drip must be carefully monitored if used to deliver heparin, or overdosing may result; an infusion monitor is usually used.

Low-Dose Administration. Heparin may also be given subcutaneously to achieve a slow, continual administration over 8 to 12 hours. Low-dose heparin is used for patients older than 40 years of age undergoing thoracoabdominal surgery who are at increased risk for thrombosis. (Heparin is not used in brain, spinal cord, or eye surgery, in which even minor hemorrhage could be catastrophic. It is not effective in hip replacement surgery.) Heparin is administered subcutaneously (5000 U) 2 hours before thoracoabdominal surgery, and then 5000 U is administered every 8 to 12 hours until the patient is walking. This regimen can reduce the incidence of deep leg vein thrombosis by 50% in thoracoabdominal surgical patients without significantly affecting their bleeding or clotting times. The effectiveness of this therapy results from heparin activating antithrombin III, which rapidly inactivates newly formed factor Xa. After antithrombin III has inactivated factor Xa, the heparin can dissociate from this inactive complex and act again to cause further inactivation.

In Vitro Use. Heparin prevents the coagulation of blood after it leaves the body. Tubing used to shunt blood can be pretreated with heparin to prevent clotting. The negative charge of the heparin coating on the wall of the tubing that prevents platelet adherence is probably the effective anticoagulant mechanism. Heparin is also added to containers used for blood collection. For transfusions, 4 to 6 U of heparin per milliliter of blood is used. For laboratory samples, 7 to 15 U of heparin per milliliter of blood is used.

Adverse Reactions and Contraindications

Heparin is a natural compound, extracted from animal lungs or intestines. Some patients become allergic to heparin. The usual symptoms of heparin hypersensitivity are chills, fever, and urticaria, but other allergic reactions such as asthma,

Table 20-1 Anticoagulant Drugs

Generic Name	Trade Name	Administration/Dosage	Comments
heparin and Related Compounds			
heparin	Calciparine* Calcilean† Liquaemin Hepalean†	INTRAVENOUS: *Adults—Intermittent*—10,000 U then 5000- 10,000 U every 4-6 hr. *Continuous*—20,000-40,000 U daily in 1000 ml. SUBCUTANEOUS: *Adults*—5000 U 2 hr before surgery, then every 8-12 hr until ambulatory. FDA pregnancy category C.	High dosage is for therapeutic anticoagulation. Low dosage is for prophylaxis of postoperative thromboembolism.
ardeparin	Normiflo	SUBCUTANEOUS: *Adults*—50 anti-factor Xa units/kg body weight every 12 hr after knee replacement surgery. Begin the evening of the day of surgery or the next morning, continue for up to 14 days or until patient is ambulatory. FDA pregnancy category C.	Prophylaxis of postoperative thromboembolism. Use deep intrafat injection. Do not mix with other injections or infusions.
dalteparin	Fragmin	SUBCUTANEOUS: *Adults*—2500 IU. Begin 1-2 hr before abdominal surgery, then repeat once a day every evening for 5-10 days until the patient is mobile. FDA pregnancy category C.	Prophylaxis of postoperative embolism. Also used with hemodialysis.
danaparoid	Orgaran	SUBCUTANEOUS: *Adults*—750 antifactor Xa units/kg body weight every 12 hr after knee replacement surgery. Begin 1-4 hr before surgery and no later than 2 hr after surgery. Continue until the risk of deep venous thrombosis has diminished (7-10 days) or up to 14 days. FDA pregnancy category C.	Store ampules between 2° and 30° C (35.6° and 86° F).
enoxaprin	Lovenox*	SUBCUTANEOUS: 30 mg twice a day for 7-10 days.	Prophylaxis for postsurgical thrombosis; administer within 24 hr of surgery. Risk of epidural or spinal hematomas with concurrent use with spinal/epidural anesthesia. Hematomas can cause neurologic injury, including long-term or permanent paralysis.
Oral Anticoagulants			
anisindione	Miradon	ORAL: *Adults*—300 mg on day 1; 200 mg on day 2; 100 mg on day 3; 25-250 mg daily for maintenance.	Half-life is 3-5 days. Peak effect occurs in 2-3 days. Anticoagulant effect persists 1-3 days after discontinuance. Dermatitis is a side effect. Drug imparts orange color to alkaline urine.
dicumarol (bishydroxy-coumarin)	Generic	ORAL: *Adults*—200-300 mg on day 1; 25-200 mg daily for maintenance.	Dicumarol is prototype oral anticoagulant. Half-life is 1-2 days. Peak effect occurs in 1-4 days. Anticoagulant effect persists 2-10 days after discontinuance. This coumarin is poorly and erratically absorbed.
warfarin	Coumadin* Panwarfin Sofarin Warfilone†	ORAL, INTRAMUSCULAR, INTRAVENOUS: *Adults*—10-15 mg daily until prothrombin time is in therapeutic range; 2-10 mg daily for maintenance. Loading dose of 40-60 mg (20-30 mg in older adult patients) may be given initially.	Half-life is 2 days. Peak effect occurs in 1-3 days. Anticoagulant effect persists 4-5 days after discontinuance.

*Available in Canada and the United States.
†Available in Canada only.

rhinitis, lacrimation, and anaphylaxis have been reported. In some patients heparin has caused thrombocytopenia; thus the platelet count should be measured daily after therapy.

Toxicity

The major side effect of heparin is hemorrhage. Because the half-life of intravenously administered heparin is only 1½ hours, discontinuing heparin therapy is usually sufficient to reverse a hemorrhagic episode. If hemorrhaging must be stopped immediately, protamine sulfate may be given by slow IV infusion. Protamine sulfate is a highly positively charged molecule that complexes the negatively charged heparin. It is an anticoagulant and has a longer half-life than

heparin. Protamine sulfate may persist and cause bleeding after heparin is eliminated. One milligram of protamine sulfate neutralizes 100 U of heparin. No more than 50 mg of protamine sulfate should be administered in 10 minutes.

Heparin can also bind to platelets, causing platelet aggregation and leading to thrombocytopenia. This heparin-induced platelet aggregation can result in a paradoxical thromboembolism that is seen in fewer than 5% of patients receiving heparin. Lepirudin (Refludan) is a new drug for the treatment of heparin-induced thromboembolism. Lepirudin binds specifically to thrombin to prevent clot formation. Lepirudin is a recombinant form of hirudin. Hirudin is a family of polypeptides released by medicinal leeches to

RESEARCH HIGHLIGHTS

Patency of 24-Gauge Peripheral Intermittent Infusion Devices: A Comparison of Heparin and Saline Flush Solutions

—Mudge B, Forcier D, Slattery MJ: Pediatr Nurs 24(2):142-145, 149, 1998.

PURPOSE

Maintaining patency of peripheral intermittent infusion devices (PIIDs) is important for facilitating administration of medications and fluids to patients, preventing the discomfort of repeated device reinsertions, and limiting costs associated with use of new equipment and nursing care to reinsert devices. Many studies comparing the efficacy of saline with heparinized saline as a flush solution have been done, with varying results. Little research has been done on the small-bore, 24-gauge PIIDs used with neonates and infants. This study was designed to compare the two flush solutions in 24-gauge PIIDs.

METHODS

A prospective, nonrandomized, sequential, blinded design was used. The two flush solutions were heparin sodium 10 units in 0.9% sodium chloride per 1 ml (group 1) and 0.9% sodium chloride per 1 ml (group 2). The sample consisted of 134 24-gauge catheters in 61 patients. Ages of children ranged from newborn to 2 years. Chi-square analysis indicated no significant difference between the two groups for factors such as age (less than 30 days versus more than 30 days), catheter placement site, irritating substances infused, and whether the catheter was started as a continuous infusion before converting to a PIID. The mean admission weight of the heparin group was significantly greater than that of the saline group, but weight was not found to be correlated with catheter duration.

RESULTS

Catheters flushed with heparin solution had a median duration of 42 hours (range 5.9 to 116.5 hours), whereas catheters flushed with normal saline had a median duration of 35 hours (range 4 to 125 hours). Catheters flushed with heparin solution lasted significantly longer than catheters flushed with normal saline alone (X^2 stratified $= 5.43$, $p = 0.2$). In addition, 52% ($n = 29$) of the catheters flushed with the heparin solution were removed because of problems, compared to 71% ($n = 55$) of the catheters flushed with saline, and this was also statistically significant ($X^2 = 4.89$, $p = 0.27$).

IMPLICATIONS

In this study, catheters flushed with a heparin solution lasted longer than catheters flushed with saline alone, and there were fewer problems requiring catheter removal in the heparin flush group. Heparinized saline is more costly as a flush solution than normal saline alone. However, reinsertion of catheters causes patient distress and, in the case of pediatric patients, also causes distress to their parents. This study suggests that a single solution for flushing PIIDs may not apply across all patient age groups and all catheter sizes.

CRITICAL THINKING: How can a researcher quantify the costs of nursing care involved in a procedure (e.g., restarting an infusion)? How can a researcher decide if in-house pharmacy prepared heparinized flush solution is cheaper or more expensive than commercially prepared heparinized flush solution?

---

prevent thrombosis. Medicinal leeches are used to prevent thrombosis in the fine vessels of reattached digits.

Low-Molecular-Weight Heparins: General Characteristics

Specific low-molecular-weight heparins include ardeparin (Normiflo), dalteparin (Fragmin), danaparoid (Orgaran), and enoxaparin (Lovenox).

Mechanism of Action

Heparin is a naturally occurring glycosaminoglycan extracted from pig intestines and bovine lungs. As extracted, heparin consists of polymers of varying molecular weights. Heparin acts by complexing with antithrombin III. Recently it has been found that the low-molecular-weight fraction of heparin is as effective as heparin in forming a complex with antithrombin III to inhibit the activation of factor Xa. However, this complex is not an effective inhibitor of thrombin directly. Low-molecular-weight heparin will have a minimal effect on in vitro clotting tests.

Pharmacokinetics

Low-molecular-weight heparins are administered by subcutaneous injection. They are characterized by a high degree of bioavailability and a peak plasma concentration in 3 to 5 hours. They are active for about 24 hours and are eliminated in the urine. Patients with renal impairment will need to have the dosage interval modified.

Uses

Low-molecular-weight heparins have been approved for the prophylactic treatment of pulmonary thromboembolism and deep vein thrombosis. They are used prophylactically in knee and hip replacement surgery.

Adverse Reactions, Contraindications, and Interactions

Injection of low-molecular-weight heparins may be accompanied by pain at the injection site and nausea. Because these anticoagulants have only a small effect on routine coagulation tests, these tests cannot be used to monitor anticoagulant activity. Coadministration of oral anticoagulants or platelet aggregation inhibitors will increase the risk of bleeding.

Low-molecular-weight heparins are not suitable for patients with blood abnormalities, stroke, or ulcers, or those who are undergoing brain, spinal, or eye surgery. Patients sensitive to heparin, pork products or sulfites may have an allergic response to low-molecular-weight heparins. There is a risk of epidural or spinal hematomas with concurrent use of the low-molecular-weight heparins and spinal or epidural anesthesia or spinal puncture. These hematomas may cause neurologic injury, including paralysis. The risk of hematomas in increased by the use of indwelling epidural catheters; the concurrent use of nonsteroidal antiinflammatory drugs (NSAIDs), platelet inhibitors, or other anticoagulants; or by repeated epidural or spinal puncture.

Oral Anticoagulants: General Characteristics

Only three oral anticoagulant drugs are currently in use: dicumarol, warfarin, and anisindione. Dicumarol and warfarin belong to the coumarin drug class and are often referred to as coumarins.

Coumarins are well tolerated but have two very distinctive features. One is that they bind very tightly to plasma proteins from which they are only slowly released, thereby greatly prolonging their action. The second is that coumarins have a large number of interactions with other drugs that calls for careful monitoring of any drugs the patient is taking.

The third oral anticoagulant is anisindione, which belongs to the indandione drug class. Indandiones can cause a number of side effects and are not widely used.

Mechanism of Action

Clotting factors II (prothrombin), VII, IX, and X are synthesized in the liver, with vitamin K as a necessary cofactor. If vitamin K is deficient, these clotting factors are synthesized in a functionally inactive state, impairing blood coagulation. The coumarins and the indandiones interfere with the regeneration of active vitamin K in the liver and thereby produce vitamin K deficiency. Because the synthesis of functional clotting factors II, VII, IX, and X is inhibited, the anticoagulant effect does not appear until preexisting factors II, VII, IX, and X are removed by normal degradation. This takes 1 day or longer. Factor II, prothrombin, is the longest lived of these clotting factors, and 24 hours are required to deplete half the existing prothrombin. A one-stage prothrombin test often determines whether the dose of oral anticoagulants is appropriate. Therapeutic doses of the oral anticoagulants increase the prothrombin time (PT) by 1.5 to 2.5 times the baseline values. Anticoagulant therapy must be individualized for each patient (see Table 20-1).

Pharmacokinetics

Warfarin is the most widely used coumarin. It is the only coumarin that can be administered intramuscularly or intravenously. Warfarin is well absorbed orally. Its peak effect

CASE STUDY
Oral Anticoagulants

Mr. Holmberg is a 48-year-old social worker who has been treated for deep vein thrombosis in his left leg. He experienced pain and swelling of the left lower leg over several days. He was in the hospital for 2 weeks on strict bed rest while receiving intravenous heparin. Before his discharge, he was switched to oral warfarin. His prothrombin times showed adequate levels of anticoagulation at the time of discharge.

At his 2-week checkup, the blood prothrombin times show a decrease in anticoagulation. Mr. Holmberg says he has taken the medication every day at the same time and is not taking any other medications. He says he has been "taking it easy" and working to harvest his wife's kale and collards crop before the winter weather sets in. He has been drinking Ensure and taking multivitamins "to improve my health."

1. What could be interfering with the anticoagulant effect of the warfarin?
2. Mr. Holmberg asks you whether he should resume the Bufferin he has taken for minor arthritis pain and whether he can take "a few drinks" to relax at night. What is your answer?
3. What other safety measures do you review with Mr. Holmberg?
4. Warfarin is highly bound to protein. If Mr. Holmberg takes another highly protein-bound drug that displaces the warfarin from the albumin, what will be the effect on the coagulation?

occurs 36 to 72 hours after administration, and the duration of action is 4 to 5 days.

Dicumarol is longer acting than warfarin. The peak action is 3 to 5 days after administration, and the duration of action is up to 10 days. Dicumarol is not well absorbed and causes flatulence and diarrhea.

Anisindione is well absorbed orally. The onset of action is 2 to 3 days, and duration of action after discontinuing therapy is 1 to 3 days.

Protein binding is important to the pharmacokinetics of coumarins. The coumarins stay in the body a long time because they are bound tightly to plasma albumin. This tight binding has several consequences. Only a small amount of the total drug in the body is free to diffuse to the site of action in the liver. The liver also degrades the coumarin to inactive forms that are then excreted in the urine so that only a small amount of the total coumarin is available for degradation. Other drugs can displace coumarins from albumin. This displacement dramatically increases the effective concentration of coumarin. For example, if only 1% of the total coumarin is not bound and displacement causes another 1% to be free, the concentration of free coumarin drug has doubled. The albumin-bound coumarin acts as a reservoir for the drug. After administration is discontinued, several days are required for the drug to dissociate from the albumin and to be degraded by the liver.

Uses

The major indication for the oral anticoagulants is the prophylaxis or treatment for a deep venous or pulmonary thrombus. However, low-dose heparin administered during surgery has significantly reduced the risk of thrombus formation. The oral coumarins were widely used as prophylaxis against myocardial reinfarction, a use never well substantiated by controlled studies. Recently, the number of available oral anticoagulants has dropped to two coumarins (warfarin and dicumarol) and one indandione (anisindione). Anticoagulants that are vitamin K antagonists do not prevent coagulation of blood after it is drawn because the clotting factors are already synthesized and present.

Adverse Reactions and Contraindications

The principal side effect of oral anticoagulant therapy is hemorrhage, commonly first seen as bleeding of the gingiva. Other signs of overdose include blood in the urine or stools, causing them to turn red, orange, smoky, or black. The drug can be discontinued temporarily when minor hemorrhaging occurs. When hemorrhaging is severe, fresh or frozen plasma may be transfused to replace clotting factors immediately. Less severe hemorrhage can be treated by administering 10 mg (up to 50 mg) of vitamin K_1 phytonadione. This adds excess vitamin K to overcome the block caused by the coumarins. Clotting factors are then again synthesized by the liver, returning the PT to normal in about 24 hours. Side effects other than hemorrhaging are rare.

Anisindione more commonly causes other side effects, including rashes, depression of the bone marrow, hepatitis, and renal damage.

Interactions

Drug interactions are not prominent with anisindione. However, drug interactions are especially numerous with the coumarins dicumarol and warfarin. Many drugs alter the effectiveness of dicumarol and warfarin. No drug should be added to or deleted from a therapeutic regimen that includes a coumarin without considering drug interactions and appropriately modifying dosages.

The anticoagulant action of both heparin and coumarins is enhanced by drugs that decrease platelet adhesion (e.g., aspirin, clofibrate, dextran, dipyridamole, hydroxychloroquine, ibuprofen, indomethacin, phenylbutazone). The anticoagulant action of coumarins is enhanced by drugs that inhibit coumarin degradation, such as clofibrate, disulfiram, metronidazole, oxyphenbutazone, phenylbutazone, and trimethoprim; drugs that displace bound anticoagulant, such as chloral hydrate, oxyphenbutazone, and phenylbutazone; and drugs that interact by unknown mechanisms, such as anabolic steroids, cimetidine, D-thyroxine,

glucagon, quinidine, and sulfinpyrazone. The anticoagulant action of coumarins is diminished by drugs that accelerate coumarin degradation, such as barbiturates, ethchlorvynol, glutethimide, griseofulvin, and rifampin; drugs that decrease gastrointestinal (GI) tract absorption of coumarins, such as cholestyramine; and drugs that interact by unknown mechanisms, such as 6-mercaptopurine. Dicumarol enhances the action of phenytoin. This list summarizes the major drug interactions but is not exhaustive.

Antiplatelet Drugs: General Characteristics

Mechanism of Action

Platelets (**thrombocytes**) are the small cell fragments in blood derived from giant bone marrow cells called megakaryocytes. Ordinarily, platelets do not stick to each other or to the endothelial lining of the blood vessels. When there is a break in the endothelial lining, however, platelets readily attach to the collagen in the exposed tissue. This attachment causes the platelets to aggregate, rapidly forming a plug that stops the bleeding and aids in the formation of a thrombus. This aggregation of platelets in the presence of abnormal surfaces is the initial step in the normal repair system for the blood vessels. Drugs that interfere with this process are termed antiplatelet or antithrombic drugs (Table 20-2).

The search for antiplatelet drugs began in the late 1970s. It was discovered that when the platelets adhere to a surface, they synthesize thromboxane A_2, a substance related to the prostaglandins. Thromboxane A_2 is a potent stimulus for the further aggregation of platelets and thereby accelerates the formation of the platelet plug. Because aspirin was found to block the synthesis of thromboxane A_2, this action explained the antiplatelet action of aspirin.

Currently attention is directed at agents that prevent the binding of platelets to fibrinogen, the step that results in an aggregated plug. The platelet receptor binding fibrinogen is called glycoprotein IIb/IIIa (GP IIb/IIIa). Several factors, including thromboxane A_2 and adenosine diphosphate (ADP), are involved in activating this receptor. Aspirin, dipyridamole, clopidogrel (Plavix), and ticlopidine (Ticlid) interfere with this activation. Newer drugs, including abciximab (ReoPro), eptifibatide (Integril), and tirofiban (Aggrastat), block the GPIIb/IIIa receptor directly.

Uses

The role of platelet aggregation as the initial step leading to blood coagulation is well established. In particular, the blood clots forming in the arterial system, as opposed to the venous system, are highly linked to conditions promoting platelet aggregation. Patients at risk for developing arterial clots are those who have already had a myocardial infarction (MI) or a stroke. Another established clinical use of antiplatelet drugs is for heart valve prostheses, disorders, and shunts.

Table 20-2 Antiplatelet Drugs

Generic Name	Trade Name	Administration/Dosage	Comments
abciximab	ReoPro	INTRAVENOUS: *Adults*—Intially, 250 μg/kg body weight administered 10-60 min before start of percutaneous transluminal coronary angioplasty (PTCA). Maintenance: 10 μg/min for 12 hr.	Prophylaxis to prevent clots or thrombus during PTCA.
aspirin	Various	ORAL: *Adults—After transient ischemic attack:* 325 mg with each meal and at bedtime or 650 mg twice a day. *Prosthetic heart valve:* 325 mg with each meal. *Atrioventricular shunt or fistula:* 160 mg with each meal and at bedtime. *Graft patency:* 325 mg after each meal. *Prevention of myocardial infarction (MI) or sudden death in patient with unstable angina:* 325 mg with each meal and at bedtime. *Prevention of recurrent MI or coronary death post-MI:* 325-1300 mg/day.	Prophylaxis to prevent platelet aggregation in transient ischemic attacks, strokes, MIs, thromboembolism after hip surgery; may be combined with dipyramidole to reduce risk of thrombosis or occlusion of bypass grafts.
clopidolgrel bisulfate	Plavix	ORAL: *Adults*—75 mg/day.	Prophylaxis for stroke and MI.
dipyridamole	Persantine* Apo-Dypridamole†	ORAL: *Adults*—75-100 mg 4 times/day. FDA pregnancy category B.	Taken to prevent thrombi formation with prosthetic heart valve or to maintain graft patency. Taken with warfarin for prosthetic heart valve. May also be taken with aspirin for prosthetic heart valve or graft patency.
eptifibatide	Integril	*For prevention of acute coronary thrombosis:* INTRAVENOUS: 180 μg/kg body weight over 1-2 min, followed by 2 μg/kg body weight/min until surgery or discharge, for up to 72 hr.	Adjunct to aspirin and heparin in preventing coronary thrombosis in patients at high risk. Also used in patients undergoing procedures with cardiac catheters.
ticlopidine	Ticlid*	ORAL: *Adults*—250 mg 2 times/day with food.	Prophylaxis for stroke.
tirofiban	Aggrastat	INTRAVENOUS INFUSION: 0.4 μg/kg body weight/min for 30 min, then 0.1 μg/kg body weight/min for 48-108 hr.	Adjunct to aspirin and heparin in preventing coronary thrombosis in patients at high risk. Also used in patients undergoing procedures with cardiac catheters.

*Available in Canada and the United States.
†Available in Canada only.

Specific Antiplatelet Agents

abciximab

Abciximab (ReoPro) is a chimeric human-mouse monoclonal antibody fragment. It binds to a platelet receptor (GP IIb/IIIa) and prevents that receptor from binding fibrin. This action inhibits thrombus formation. Abciximab is used with heparin and aspirin to prevent complications in patients undergoing angioplasty who are at high risk for vessel closure. The temporary oxygen deprivation to the treated vessel can precipitate thrombus formation without treatment.

▼ aspirin

Aspirin is the most widely studied antiplatelet drug. It provides effective prophylactic treatment for the following:

- Patients who have experienced a transient ischemic attack (TIA, a ministroke) have a decreased incidence of further TIAs, strokes, or death. This is a dramatic effect in men but probably not in women. Sulfinpyrazone and dipyridamole were not effective.

- Patients who have had an MI or who have stable or unstable angina have a decreased incidence of subsequent heart attacks. These results are from studies in men and may not apply to women.

Primary prevention of heart attacks has been demonstrated. Large scale studies in both men and women have shown that taking 325 mg aspirin (1 adult tablet) or less per day is effective in preventing an MI, especially in those individuals over 50 years old who have risk factors for atherosclerotic cardiovascular disease (e.g., high blood pressure, high cholesterol levels, smoking).

The dosage of aspirin may be important to its effectiveness in preventing thrombus formation. A low dosage of aspirin (80 to 180 mg/day) inhibits the synthesis of thromboxane A_2 by the platelets. A higher dosage of aspirin (1000 mg/day) also inhibits the synthesis of prostacyclin (prostaglandin I_2) by the epithelial lining of the blood vessel. Prostacyclin inhibits the aggregation of platelets, an action directly opposite that of thromboxane A_2. Prostacyclin therefore prevents the formation of a platelet plug. For this reason, a high dosage of aspirin may be less effective than the low dosage in preventing the formation of a thrombus. However, for prophylaxis following a TIA, only high dosages have been found effective.

clopidogrel

Clopidogrel (Plavix) is a new drug that is an alternative to aspirin for lowering the risk of heart attacks or strokes for patients who have already had one or who have peripheral artery disease. The main side effects are rash and diarrhea.

dipyridamole

Dipyridamole (Persantine) combined with warfarin is used for patients with artificial heart valves. It has not been shown effective as prophylaxis in preventing heart attacks or strokes.

eptifibatide

Eptifibatide (Integril) is a new platelet inhibitor. Like abciximab, epifibatide binds to a platelet receptor (GP IIb/IIIa) and prevents that receptor from binding fibrin. This action inhibits thrombus formation. Epifibatide is given as an adjunct to aspirin and heparin to hospitalized patients at high risk for MI or patients undergoing a cardiac catheterization procedure. An initial dose is administered intravenously, followed by a continuous IV infusion. Significant inhibition of platelet function has been observed 1 hour after administration. Normalization of bleeding times has occurred 15 minutes after discontinuation of infusion; recovery of platelet function has occurred at 4 hours. Plasma protein binding is approximately 25%. Clearance is predominantly renal, with no evidence of metabolism in the circulation or liver.

ticlopidine

Ticlopidine (Ticlid) is a new drug approved as prophylactic therapy for strokes. It inhibits platelet aggregation irreversibly. The onset of action is about 2 days, and the inhibition of platelet aggregation persists for 1 to 2 weeks. Ticlopidine is somewhat more effective than aspirin but also causes more adverse effects. The most common adverse effects include nausea, vomiting, cramps, and diarrhea. Occasionally a rash or urticaria develops during the first month of therapy. The most serious side effects include bleeding complications, agranulocytosis, leukopenia, and thrombocytopenia.

tirofiban

Tirofiban (Aggrastat) is a new platelet inhibitor. Like abciximab, tirofiban binds to a platelet receptor (GP IIb/IIIa) and prevents that receptor from binding fibrin. This action inhibits thrombus formation. Tirofiban is given as an adjunct to aspirin and heparin to hospitalized patients at high risk for MI or patients undergoing a cardiac catheterization procedure. An initial dose is administered intravenously, followed by a continuous IV infusion. Platelet aggregation is inhibited as early as 5 minutes after initiation of IV administration; bleeding times return to normal 3 to 4 hours after discontinuation of an IV infusion.

Nursing Process Overview

Anticoagulant and Antiplatelet Drugs

Assessment

Anticoagulation prevents clot formation; it does not dissolve existing clots. Obtain a history of problems with clots. Assess the patient's mental status, vital signs, and ability to perform activities of daily living. Assess the general physical condition of the patient, including bruising or easy bleeding. Monitor blood coagulation studies, including PT, partial thromboplastin time (PTT), platelet count, and clotting times. Document the presence of any bleeding.

Nursing Diagnoses

- Risk for hemorrhage
- Risk for altered health maintenance related to insufficient knowledge of the implication of anticoagulant or antiplatelet therapy

Patient Outcomes

The patient will not have a TIA, stroke, thromboembolism, or other vascular problem while taking one or more of these drugs as prescribed. The patient will not have side effects caused by any of these drugs.

Planning/Implementation

Assess for bleeding from any site and check stools for occult blood. Evaluate any symptoms signaling possible thrombus formation such as chest or leg pain or any symptom of internal bleeding such as headache. Monitor blood coagulation studies carefully. Use an infusion monitoring device for infusions of heparin and check dosages carefully. Keep antidotes readily available for the drugs being used.

Evaluation

Before discharge, determine that the patient can explain why the drug is needed, how to take or administer the drug, what signs and symptoms of bleeding should be reported, how to avoid injury and bruising, what side effects may be related to the drug but do not involve bleeding, and which additional side effects require notification of the physician. Finally, verify that the patient can state which other drugs, such as aspirin, to avoid while taking anticoagulants.

THERAPEUTIC RATIONALE: THROMBOLYTIC THERAPY

As shown in Figure 20-1, the plasma contains the enzyme plasmin, which degrades the fibrin network of a clot into small, soluble fragments. Plasmin normally exists in an inactive form, plasminogen. Plasminogen is activated to plasmin by various factors in the plasma, primarily tissue plasminogen activator (TPA), which originates in the blood vessel wall. Plasminogen and TPA bind to fibrin, and TPA converts

Table 20-3 **Thrombolytic Drugs**

Generic Name	Trade Name	Administration/Dosage	Comments
alteplase, recombinant	Activase Activase rt-PA†	INTRAVENOUS: *Adults*—Initially, bolus of 6-10 mg over 1-2 min, followed by infusion of 60 mg for 1 hr and 20 mg for next 2 hr. For patients weighing <65 kg, total dose is 1.25 mg/kg.	Monitor for arrhythmias, reocclusion.
anistreplase (APSAC)	Eminase*	INTRAVENOUS: *Adults*—30 U injected over 2-5 min.	Monitor for bleeding.
reteplase	Retavase	INTRAVENOUS: *Adults*—10 U over not more than 2 min followed in 30 min by another 10 U.	Monitor for bleeding.
streptokinase	Kabikinase* Streptase*	INTRAVENOUS: *Adults*—Loading dose of 250,000 IU infused over 30 min, then infusion of 100,000 IU/hr. Dosage is continued for 24-72 hr for pulmonary embolism and for 72 hr for deep vein embolism. *For coronary thrombosis:* INTRAVENOUS: *Adults*—1.5 million IU, administered within 1 hr. INTRAARTERIAL (via coronary artery catheter)—20,000 IU initially, followed by 2000 IU/min for 1 hr.	Monitor thrombin times every 12 hr. Allergic reactions are common (15% of patients); usually of milder variety (itching, flushing, nausea, headache). Treat with antihistamines.
urokinase	Abbokinase* Open-Cath*	INTRAVENOUS: *Adults*—Loading dose of 4400 IU/kg infused over 10 min by infusion, then 4400 IU/kg for 12 hr. FDA pregnancy category B.	Isolated from human urine. Not as allergenic as streptokinase.

*Available in Canada and the United States.

plasminogen to plasmin and plasmin digests fibrin. Degradation products of fibrin act as anticoagulants, thereby limiting further clot formation.

Although the steps in coagulation occur very rapidly, the dissolution of a blood clot may take several days. Drugs to speed the clot dissolution process are widely used. The treatment of choice for an acute MI has become the injection of a clot-dissolving drug as quickly as possible, which prevents the myocardial ischemia that leads to tissue death. Patients can leave the hospital after 3 days instead of 10 and may not require prolonged recovery at home. The drugs available are alteplase, streptokinase, anistreplase, and urokinase (Table 20-3). Thrombolytic therapy is also used in acute pulmonary embolism, deep vein thrombosis, and peripheral arterial occlusion. This therapy helps locally clear atrioventricular (AV) shunts in patients receiving long-term renal dialysis; however, clotting often recurs.

THERAPEUTIC AGENTS: THROMBOLYTIC DRUGS

Thrombolytic agents are used to dissolve thrombi. They are administered after a heart attack to prevent prolonged myocardial ischemia and are also used to treat pulmonary emboli and deep vein thrombosis. The thrombolytic agents are proteins and must be infused. Except for anistreplase, they are relatively short-acting (30 minutes or less). Bleeding or its complications are potential side effects of thrombolytic drugs.

Contraindications for the use of thrombolytic drugs include those conditions for which such therapy might severely compromise the patient: surgery or organ biopsy within 10 days, serious gastrointestinal bleeding within 3 months, uncontrolled hypertension, an active bleeding or hemorrhagic disorder, history of cerebrovascular bleeding or neoplasm, or presence of an aneurysm.

▼ alteplase recombinant

Alteplase (Activase) is a naturally occurring product produced by recombinant DNA technology. Alteplase is an enzyme that binds to fibrin, is activated, and catalyzes conversion of plasminogen to plasmin. Plasmin is the enzyme that degrades fibrin, dissolving a thrombus (clot). Alteplase is most effective if administered within 6 hours of a heart attack because it is effective in promoting thrombus reduction in 2 hours. Alteplase also treats pulmonary thromboembolism. Alteplase has recently been approved as an acute treatment for strokes, but only within the first 3 hours after onset of the stroke. A computed tomographic scan of the brain is necessary to rule out evidence of recent major infarction, edema, or possible hemorrhage. Unbound alteplase is rapidly cleared by the liver.

anistreplase

Anistreplase (APSAC [anisoylated plasminogen-streptokinase activator complex], Eminase) is a complex of streptokinase and human plasminogen. The human plasminogen has been modified with a blocking group so that it is not readily activated. The injected complex binds to the fibrin of a clot, and the plasminogen slowly loses its blocking group and is activated by streptokinase. This happens at a controlled rate and at the fibrin network of the clot. Anistreplase treats acute MI and is active for about 6 hours.

reteplase

Reteplase (Retavase) is a variant of plasminogen activator produced by recombinant DNA technology. Reteplase has fewer amino acids than does alteplase. Reteplase does not bind as tightly to fibrin nor does it compete with native plasminogen for binding to fibrin. As a result, native plasminogen is activated, while reteplase can diffuse more freely through the clot. Reteplase has a half-life of 11 to 19 minutes and is excreted in the urine. It is administered as a bolus by IV injection, followed by a second bolus 30 minutes later.

streptokinase

Streptokinase (Streptase) is isolated from group C beta-hemolytic streptococci; it acts by forming a complex with plasminogen to activate it. Streptokinase is antigenic and may cause allergic reactions. The cost of streptokinase treatment is about one-tenth that of alteplase or anistreplase and appears to be as effective in treating coronary thrombosis. Streptokinase also treats pulmonary thromboembolism and clears arterial cannulas and IV catheters.

urokinase

Urokinase (Abbokinase) is isolated from human urine; it is an enzyme that cleaves plasminogen to plasmin. Urokinase treats thromboembolisms but not coronary thrombosis. Urokinase also clears arterial cannulas and IV catheters.

Nursing Process Overview

Thrombolytic Drugs
Thrombolytic drugs have revolutionized the treatment of myocardial infarction and other problems caused by clots. They promote the digestion of fibrin, thereby dissolving the clot.

Assessment
Anticoagulant therapy prevents clots, and thrombolytic therapy dissolves clots. Both alter the normal coagulation mechanism to cause anticoagulation. Obtain a history of the presenting problem. Assess vital signs and blood pressure. Assess mental status and neurologic status. Assess the size and location of the clot and the signs and symptoms caused by the clot. Assess for a recent patient history of streptococcal infection or previous exposure to thrombolytic agents because this would influence the choice of agents.

Nursing Diagnoses
- Risk for arrhythmias (reperfusion arrhythmias)
- Risk for hemorrhage/excessive bleeding

Patient Outcomes
The nurse will manage and minimize arrhythmic episodes or hemorrhage. The clot will be successfully lysed, and the patient will experience no lasting side effects from the clot or the medications used to lyse it.

Planning/Implementation
Use systemic thrombolytic drugs only in short-term care settings. Monitor patients for signs of clot dissolution and hemorrhage.

Monitor the usual tests for blood coagulation and check the hematocrit level daily because it may drop even when bleeding is not present. Use an infusion monitoring device for infusions. Have available appropriate drugs to control bleeding, such as aminocaproic acid.

Evaluation
If effective, a thrombolytic drug dissolves the existing clot without causing hemorrhage. Patients are not discharged while still receiving systemic thrombolytic therapy.

THERAPEUTIC RATIONALE: CONTROL OF EXCESSIVE BLEEDING WITH HEMOSTATIC DRUGS

Hemostatic drugs are systemic or local agents used to control excessive bleeding. Specialized biologic hemostatics are used to control bleeding episodes in individuals with hemophilia (Table 20-4).

THERAPEUTIC AGENTS: SYSTEMIC HEMOSTATIC DRUGS

aminocaproic acid

Aminocaproic acid (Amicar) inhibits the activation of plasminogen to the active enzyme plasmin. The lack of plasmin inhibits dissolution of blood clots. Aminocaproic acid is used when it is desirable to protect blood clots, such in as surgery on the prostate, after a ruptured cerebral aneurysm, or for patients with hemophilia after a tooth extraction.

Aminocaproic acid can be given orally or intravenously. It is rapidly excreted in the urine. Side effects are transient and minor and include nausea, cramps, dizziness, headache, ringing in the ear, and stuffy nose. When IV therapy is used, aminocaproic acid can irritate the veins and give rise to thrombophlebitis. This effect may be minimized by diluting the drug before use and by carefully placing the needle.

aprotinin

Aprotinin (Trasylol) inhibits the degradation of certain enzymes. The activation of plasminogen to plasmin involves limited proteolysis, and aprotinin inhibits this activation. The major use of aprotinin is during open heart surgery to reduce bleeding from cardiopulmonary bypass with heparin. Because about 1 in 200 patients have an anaphylactic reaction to aprotinin, a small test dose is administered first.

tranexamic acid

Tranexamic acid (Cyklokapron), like aminocaproic acid, inhibits the activation of plasminogen to the active enzyme plasmin. Tranexamic acid also directly inhibits plasmin. As an antifibrinolytic agent, it is 5 to 10 times more potent than aminocaproic acid. The major indication for the drug is in patients with hemophilia undergoing dental surgery.

Table 20-4 Hemostatic Agents

Generic Name	Trade Name	Administration/Dosage	Comments
Systemic Hemostatic Agents			
aminocaproic acid	Amicar*	ORAL, INTRAVENOUS: *Adults*—5-6 g initially orally or by slow IV infusion, then 1 g hourly or 6 g every 6 hr. Maximum in 24 hr is 30 g. Reduced dosage is used with low renal output or renal disease. *Children*—100 mg/kg body weight every 6 hr for 6 days.	Prevents activation of plasminogen (fibrinolysis) so that blood clots are not broken down. Used in special surgical situations.
aprotinin	Traysylol*	INTRAVENOUS: *Adults*—Test dose: 10,000 KIU; initial dose: 1 million KIU; maintenance dose: 250,000 KIU/hr; "pump prime" dose added to priming fluid: 1 million KIU. The high-dose regimen doubles all except the test dose.	Prophylaxis for hemorrhage associated with coronary bypass graft surgery.
phytonadione (vitamin K₁)	AquaMEPHYTON Konakion* Mephyton	ORAL, INTRAMUSCULAR, SUBCUTANEOUS: *Adults and children*—2.5-25 mg. INTRAMUSCULAR, SUBCUTANEOUS, INTRAVENOUS: *Newborns*—0.5-1 mg immediately after birth. Alternatively, mother is given 1-5 mg 12-24 hr before delivery.	Intravenous route can be dangerous. Use only in emergencies for oral anticoagulant overdose, and dilute so that no more than 1 mg is given per minute. Subcutaneous and intramuscular injection may be painful.
menadiol sodium diphosphate (vitamin K₄)	Synkayvite	ORAL, INTRAMUSCULAR, SUBCUTANEOUS, INTRAVENOUS: *Adults*—5-15 mg once or twice daily. *Children*—5-10 mg once or twice daily.	Used to correct secondary hypoprothrombinemia. Converted to menadione (vitamin K₃) in body.
tranexamic acid	Cyklokapron*	ORAL: *Adults and children*—25 mg/kg 3 or 4 times/day before surgery and 2-8 days after surgery. INTRAVENOUS: *Adults and children*—10 mg/kg before surgery, administered with factor VIII or IX, and 10 mg/kg 3 or 4 times daily for 2-8 days after surgery. FDA pregnancy category B.	Indicated use is for patients with hemophilia who are undergoing dental surgery.
Local Hemostatic Agents			
absorbable gelatin sponge	Gelfoam	Blocks and cones of various sizes. Also sterile (surgical) and nonsterile (dental) powder.	Used to control bleeding in wound or at operative site.
absorbable gelatin film	Gelfilm	Thin film strips.	Used to repair membranes in neural, thoracic, and ocular surgery.
oxidized cellulose	Oxycel*	Type of gauze pads or strips. Also as sponges 2 × 1 × 1 inch.	Used to control hemorrhage and absorb blood. May be left in wound. Not for packing around bone fractures or to be left on skin.
oxidized regenerated cellulose	Surgicel	Knitted fabric strips.	Used like oxidized cellulose, but may be left on skin.
microfibrillar collagen hemostat	Avitene	Sterile powder. 1 g should cover 50 × 50 cm (20 × 20 inches) to control light bleeding.	Used to control bleeding in wound or at operative site. May be used on skin. Discard unused material because it cannot be resterilized.
thrombin	Fibrindex Thrombin, topical	Sterile powder. Packaged by units. May be dissolved in sterile saline solution and applied in absorbable gelatin sponge.	Used to control bleeding in wound or at operative site. Discard unused material because it cannot be resterilized and solution is unstable.
Replacement Therapy for Hemophilia			
antihemophilic factor (AHF)—human	Hemofil M* Koate-HP Others	INTRAVENOUS: *Adults and children*—Usually single dose of 15-20 U/kg given at rate of 10-15 ml/min maintains activities sufficient for clotting.	There are four different methods of purifying factor VIII from plasma.
cryoprecipitated antihemophilic factor-human		INTRAVENOUS: *Adults and children*—Usually single dose of 15-20 U/kg given at rate of 10-15 ml/min maintains activities sufficient for clotting.	This product is prepared by hospital blood bank. Thaw in water bath at 37° C (98.6° F); keep at room temperature and use within 3 hr.
antihemophilic factor—porcine	Hyate: C	INTRAVENOUS: *Adults and children*—Initially, 100-150 U/kg. If this is insufficient, second larger dose should then be given, followed by third dose if necessary.	This product is purified freeze-dried concentrate of AHF from pig. It can be used for patients who have developed antibodies to human product.
antihemophilic factor—recombinant	Helixate Kogenate* others	INTRAVENOUS: *Adults and children*—Usually single dose of 15-20 U/kg given at rate of 10-15 ml/min maintains activities sufficient for clotting.	Product is made synthetically through recombinant technology rather than extracted from blood.
antithrombin III	ATnativ Thrombate III	INTRAVENOUS: *Adults and children*—Initially, 50-100 U/min is administered over 5-10 min. Final dosage is determined by level of deficiency, response, and weight of patient.	Anticoagulant to treat thromboembolism associated with hereditary antithrombin III deficiency. It is prepared from human plasma to be free of human immunodeficiency virus and hepatitis B and is heat treated.

*Available in Canada and the United States.
†Available in Canada only.

Continued

Table 20-4   Hemostatic Agents—cont'd

Generic Name	Trade Name	Administration/Dosage	Comments
desmopressin	DDAVP* Octostim† Stimate	INTRAVENOUS: *Adults and children*—0.3 μg/kg is infused slowly over 15-30 min. Dosage should not be repeated within 24 hr.	This synthetic analogue of arginine vasopressin is used for short-term hemostatic control in patients with mild or moderate factor VIII deficiency and in those with type I von Willebrand's disease.
factor IX complex human	Bebulin VH* Konyne-80 Profilnin, heat treated	INTRAVENOUS: *Adults and children*—For non-life-threatening bleeding in patients with hemophilia who have factor VIII inhibitors, 75 U/kg is initial dose, repeated in 8-12 hr if necessary.	Factor IX complex treats bleeding associated with Christmas disease or deficiency of one or more of the other factors in this preparation (factors II, VII, and X).
coagulation Factor IX (recombinant)	BeneFix*	INTRAVENOUS: *Adults and children*—For non-life-threatening bleeding in patients with hemophilia who have factor VIII inhibitors, 75 U/kg is initial dose, repeated in 8-12 hr if necessary.	Product is made synthetically by recombinant technology. Prophylaxis for hemophilia B; control of perisurgical hemostasis.

*Available in Canada and the United States.
†Available in Canada only.

Patients receiving tranexamic acid should be monitored for signs of thromboembolic complications. If they are to receive the drug for more than a few days, they should also receive an ophthalmologic examination; animal studies have indicated that high dosages of the drug can cause focal areas of retinal degeneration. More common side effects are GI tract upsets, including diarrhea, nausea, and vomiting. Tranexamic acid is eliminated largely unchanged in the urine.

vitamin K

Vitamin K is a fat-soluble vitamin required for the synthesis of clotting factors II, VII, IX, and X in the liver. Vitamin K is contained in many foods. Humans cannot synthesize vitamin K, but bacteria in the GI tract can synthesize vitamin K for absorption by the host. Conditions that can produce vitamin K deficiency include the following:

- Long-term IV feeding
- Debilitation resulting from poor diet
- Prolonged oral antibiotic therapy
- Malabsorption syndrome
- Acute diarrhea in infants
- Biliary disease

In addition, the oral anticoagulant drugs produce a relative vitamin K deficiency by inhibiting the reactivation of vitamin K.

Vitamin K is available as vitamin K_1 (phytonadione) and vitamin K_4 (menadiol) for replacement therapy, but only phytonadione is effective as an antidote for severe bleeding episodes caused by an overdose of one of the oral anticoagulants. Vitamin K is safest when taken orally. IV injection must be made slowly with a dilute solution and even then may cause a severe reaction. Reactions to IV injection include flushing, a heavy feeling on the chest, sweating, vascular collapse, and an anaphylactic reaction. Intramuscular

(IM) and subcutaneous administration may cause pain and bleeding at the injection site.

In infants and anyone with a deficiency of the enzyme glucose-6-phosphate dehydrogenase, menadiol can produce hemolysis but phytonadione does not. These vitamins do not promote clotting in a patient with liver disease or a hereditary deficiency of one of the vitamin K–dependent clotting factors.

THERAPEUTIC AGENTS: LOCAL ABSORBABLE HEMOSTATIC DRUGS

Local absorbable hemostatics provide a surface that promotes platelet adhesion and thereby promotes blood clotting where the agent is applied (see Table 20-4).

absorbable gelatin sponge: Gelfoam

Gelfoam is a sterile absorbable gelatin sponge that is moistened with sterile saline solution and applied to bleeding capillary beds that cannot be readily sutured. It is absorbed in 4 to 6 weeks.

absorbable gelatin film: Gelfilm

Gelfilm is a thin, sterile absorbable gelatin film used in neurologic, thoracic, and ocular surgery to repair membrane surfaces. Reabsorption may take from 1 week to 6 months, depending on the size and site of the film.

oxidized cellulose

Oxidized cellulose (Oxycel) and oxidized regenerated cellulose (Surgicel) are used much like the absorbable gelatin sponge. They interfere with bone regeneration and therefore cannot be packed around fractures. Oxycel retards formation of new skin and cannot be used as a surface dressing. Small implants are reabsorbed in 1 week, but large ones may require 6 weeks for reabsorption.

microfibrillar collagen hemostat

Microfibrillar collagen hemostat (Avitene) is a water-insoluble powder that is applied to a bleeding surface to activate natural clotting. The collagen is absorbed in 7 weeks. Microfibrillar collagen is used during surgery to control bleeding in capillary beds, liver, and skin graft sites. It does not interfere with the healing of skin or bone. Microfibrillar collagen must be kept dry and cannot be resterilized after the container is opened.

thrombin, thromboplastin, human fibrin foam

Thrombin is an activated clotting factor (see Figure 20-1). Thrombin is applied topically only as a sterile protein powder to bleeding surfaces. It must be kept cold and dry until use or it becomes inactive. Thrombin can be applied topically as a solution; however, it is important to note that it must not be injected.

Like thrombin, thromboplastin and human fibrin foam are naturally occurring clotting factors that can be applied topically to reduce bleeding. They are especially used in dental surgery.

THERAPEUTIC AGENTS: HEMOSTATIC DRUGS FOR REPLACEMENT THERAPY FOR HEMOPHILIA

Hemophilia is an inherited disorder in which there is a deficiency of one of the factors necessary for coagulation of the blood. Hemophilia A, or classic hemophilia, is a deficiency of factor VIII, which is important in the activation of factor X. Hemophilia A is inherited as an X-linked recessive disorder and is seen almost exclusively in boys and men. Hemophilia B, or Christmas disease, is an inherited X-linked recessive disorder characterized by a deficiency of factor IX. Von Willebrand's disease is a non–sex-linked (autosomal) codominant disorder in which von Willebrand's factor is decreased or abnormal. Von Willebrand's factor is important for the adhesion of platelets to the blood vessels and as a carrier for factor VIII.

antihemophilic factor

There are several methods of isolating factor VIII from human plasma. A unit of antihemophilic factor (AHF) may represent a pool from as many as 25,000 donors because of the viral inactivation steps now needed. (It is estimated that 80% of patients with severe hemophilia are infected with human immunodeficiency virus [HIV] because of contaminated supplies of antihemophilic factor from the early 1980s.) Cryoprecipitated AHFs are made from the plasma of one unit of whole blood. This product may be kept frozen for about 1 year.

Factor VIII, produced by recombinant DNA technology, is currently being tested clinically. Availability of factor VIII from a source other than the blood supply would eliminate the risk of blood-transmitted diseases such as HIV and hepatitis.

antithrombin III, human

A deficiency of antithrombin III is seen in several thousand Americans and results in an increased risk of thromboembolic diseases and venous thrombosis, especially after surgery and obstetric procedures. Antithrombin III (AT-III) is now prepared from plasma tested and treated to exclude viruses.

▼ desmopressin

Desmopressin (DDAVP, Stimate) temporarily increases the concentrations of factor VIII and von Willebrand's factor. This action controls mild to moderate bleeding in patients with mild hemophilia A or classic von Willebrand's disease (type I). Desmopressin is a synthetic analogue of the pituitary hormone vasopressin.

Adverse reactions to desmopressin may be seen in patients who have certain blood disorders that predispose them to reactions. Therefore desmopressin should not be used for patients with type IIB of von Willebrand's disease and should be used with caution for patients with coronary artery disease, hypertension, or atherosclerosis or for older adult patients.

factor IX complex, human

Factor IX is derived from human plasma and used to treat bleeding episodes in hemophilia B or factor IX deficiency (Christmas disease). Patients receiving factor IX may experience transient fever, chills, itching, nausea, vomiting, headache, flushing, or tingling. Slow administration can reduce these reactions. Patients, particularly those undergoing surgery, may experience thromboembolic complications.

PATIENT PROBLEMS

Agranulocytosis

Agranulocytosis, also called malignant neutropenia, is characterized by very low granulocyte levels. It can develop during the course of some diseases but is most often caused by drug toxicity or hypersensitivity. Although rare, it is potentially fatal if not recognized. Symptoms include the following:

- High fever and chills
- Sore throat
- Ulcers or sores in the mouth and pharynx and difficulty swallowing
- Weakness, severe fatigue
- Cough or hoarseness, lower back or side pain, painful or difficult urination

Laboratory work indicates leukopenia (low white blood cell count) with extremely low polymorphonuclear (PMN) cell count of 0% to 2%.

Treatment involves discontinuing the suspected causative drug, placing the patient in protective isolation or protecting the patient from infection, treating any existing infection, and providing supportive care.

Nursing Process Overview

Hemostatic Drugs

Assessment

Assess the type, location, and amount of bleeding; the symptoms related to the bleeding, such as pain, swelling, and level of consciousness; appropriate blood coagulation tests such as PTT, PT, clotting time, platelet count, and hematocrit; and general physical condition of the patient.

Nursing Diagnoses

- Altered health maintenance related to insufficient knowledge of how to manage injectable antihemophilic agent

Patient Outcomes

The patient will become adept at preparing and administering the prescribed injectable agent, will use it appropriately, and will experience less severe bleeding episodes.

Planning/Implementation

Observe the patient for signs that bleeding is stopping and for side effects of the drugs. Overdose with the systemic hemostatic agents is possible; ensure that the patient receives the correct dose. Monitor the appropriate coagulation studies and the hematocrit.

Evaluation

The goal of therapy with hemostatic agents is to stop bleeding without causing side effects resulting from the drug therapy. Many hemostatic agents are discussed in this section. Some are used only in the hospital setting, whereas others would be prescribed for short-term or long-term management by the patient.

Nursing Implications Summary

General Guidelines: Patient Receiving Anticoagulants
Drug Administration

➤ Inspect the patient twice daily for the appearance of bruising and bleeding.

➤ Check the patient's stool for guaiac or blood.

➤ Monitor vital signs at regular intervals. Be alert for signs of hemorrhage such as hypotension, rapid pulse, pale color, or weakness. In pregnant women hemorrhage occurs most often in the third trimester or immediate postpartum period.

➤ Avoid the use of restraints. If necessary to use them, pad the extremities well and remove the restraints frequently to inspect the area.

➤ Handle the patient carefully to avoid bruising.

➤ Have experienced personnel perform venipuncture. Apply pressure to the venipuncture site for 10 minutes after blood is drawn to help prevent bruising.

Nursing in the Community

➤ Instruct the patient to notify the physician if nosebleeds, bleeding gums, blood in stool or urine, unexplained or severe bruising, severe headache, or stiff neck occurs.

➤ Suggest that patients wear a medical identification tag or bracelet indicating they are taking anticoagulants.

➤ Instruct the patient to keep all health care providers, including dentists and oral surgeons, informed of anticoagulant use.

➤ Tell the patient to avoid using razors with blades and to use electric shavers instead.

➤ Instruct the patient not to take any medications (except those prescribed) without checking with the physician. This precaution applies especially to aspirin or over-the-counter drugs that might contain aspirin.

➤ Emphasize to the patient that it is important to brush teeth with a soft-bristle brush if bleeding from gums is prolonged and to avoid flossing. Remind the patient to use water-spray oral care devices on low settings only.

➤ Instruct the patient not to walk barefoot.

➤ Caution the patient to avoid rough contact activities or sports while taking anticoagulants.

ANTICOAGULANT AND ANTIPLATELET DRUGS
heparin
Drug Administration

➤ Review the general guidelines for the patient receiving anticoagulants.

➤ It is recommended that patients with a history of allergies or asthma receive a test dose of 1000 U before a full dose.

➤ Monitor blood work before administering doses, especially with high-dose heparin (more than 15,000 U/24 hr). Some agencies have protocols for monitoring blood work in patients receiving heparin. Monitor activated PTT (aPTT); the goal of anticoagulation therapy is 1.5 to 2.5 times the control in seconds. Other tests that may be monitored include the Lee-White Whole Blood Clotting Time (WBCT) (desired level is $2\frac{1}{2}$ to 3 times the control value in minutes) and the activated clotting time (ACT; the desired level is 2 to 3 times the control value in seconds). Blood specimens for these tests are usually obtained shortly ($\frac{1}{2}$ hour) before an ordered dose is to be administered with intermittent therapy. If laboratory work indicates anticoagulation above the desired range, notify the physician before administering the dose. There will be little or no change in coagulation studies when low-dose heparin is used. With constant infusion, blood will

Nursing Implications Summary—cont'd

be drawn 1½ to 2 hours after the infusion is begun, and again every 4 hours until stable, then at least daily. Notify the physician immediately if laboratory work indicates anticoagulation above the desired range.

➤ Monitor platelet count and hematocrit.

➤ If the patient is receiving heparin and an oral anticoagulant, monitor laboratory work appropriate to both drugs.

➤ For mild heparin overdose, the physician may simply discontinue heparin until the laboratory findings return to the therapeutic range. Keep protamine sulfate available for treatment of severe overdose (see discussion of toxicity earlier in this chapter). Transfusion of whole blood or plasma may also be ordered for severe overdose; the transfusion dilutes the heparin in the patient's body but does not neutralize it.

➤ Read medication labels carefully. Several strengths of heparin are available. Check calculations carefully; some institutions require that two nurses check doses of heparin before administration.

➤ Place a note above the patient's bed (or as is customary in the institution) stating that the patient is receiving heparin therapy so that laboratory personnel will use care to avoid excessive bleeding after venipuncture.

➤ Avoid IM injections in patients receiving high-dose heparin.

Subcutaneous Administration, Intermittent Doses

➤ Any subcutaneous site may be used (see Chapter 5), but the abdomen is preferred because it contains few muscles and bruising is less of a cosmetic problem. Avoid using the arms.

➤ Keep a record of sites used and rotate sites, even if the abdomen is used for all doses. Avoid the area 2 inches around the umbilicus and any abdominal scars.

➤ Use careful technique to avoid bruising, but be aware that bruising may occur with even the best technique. Avoid areas that are already bruised. Use a concentrated heparin solution because the smaller volume is less likely to cause bruising.

➤ After drawing up the dose, change needles. Pinch the skin and create a subcutaneous "pocket." After careful assessment to avoid injection into a muscle, inject dose into the pocket with a ⅝- to ½-inch 25- to 28-gauge needle at a 45- to 90-degree angle. Do not aspirate the needle before injecting the drug. Do not rub the area after injecting the drug.

Continuous IV Infusion of heparin

➤ Use microdrip tubing and/or an electronic infusion monitoring device, or a mechanical syringe pump.

➤ Prepackaged dilutions of heparin suitable for constant infusion are available, or they may be prepared by the pharmacy. Read medication labels carefully.

➤ Many drugs are incompatible with heparin. If other IV drugs must be administered, establish a second IV infusion line for these medications, or flush the tubing containing heparin with normal saline before and after administering other medications. Heparin blood levels will be erratic if the heparin infusion is interrupted frequently or for long periods.

Intermittent IV heparin via heparin Well or Other Infusion Access Devices

➤ Insert the heparin well (heparin lock) into the vein with an accepted venipuncture technique and secure the well in place.

➤ Prime the well with a small amount (1 to 2 ml) of heparin of the same strength that will be used for anticoagulation.

➤ Inject each dose of heparin into the heparin well. The injected dose displaces the heparin remaining in the well each time a dose is given, so flushing the well after the dose is administered is not necessary. Follow agency procedures if different from those listed.

Other IV Medications via heparin Well or heparin-Primed Infusion Access Devices

➤ Insert the heparin well or other venous access device into the vein with an accepted venipuncture technique, and secure the well in place.

➤ Prime the heparin well with 1 ml of a solution of normal saline containing 10 or 100 U of heparin per milliliter (as agency policy dictates). Implanted ports may require up to 5 ml; consult the manufacturer's literature. These solutions are available in prepackaged syringes and multiple-dose vials or can be prepared by the nurse or pharmacist. Some institutions use only normal saline for flushing.

➤ Each time a dose of medication is given, flush the heparin well with 1 to 2 ml of saline (unless there is only saline in the heparin well); administer the prescribed medications via IV push or infusion; flush the well again with 1 to 2 ml of normal saline; finally, flush with 1 ml of the dilute heparin solution. Follow agency procedures if different from those listed.

➤ Check for patency and correct location of the heparin well before administering heparin or other medications. Assess for pain, tenderness, swelling, or redness. It should be possible to gently aspirate blood from the heparin well. It should be possible to smoothly but slowly inject drugs via the well with no patient discomfort or resistance. If in doubt that the heparin well is patent and in the vein, remove it and insert another one elsewhere.

Nursing in the Community

➤ See the general guidelines for the patient receiving anticoagulants.

➤ If heparin is prescribed for home management, instruct the patient in the necessary techniques involved (subcutaneous injection or injection via implanted ports, heparin well, or catheter, and safe disposal of syringes). Provide positive reinforcement and encouragement. Supervise return demonstrations. Refer the patient to a community-based nursing care agency.

➤ Inform the patient that a variety of side effects may occur and that the physician should be notified immediately if any of the following develop: fast or irregular breathing, shortness of breath, tightness in the chest, skin rash, hives, itching, frequent or persistent erection, or fever. Other side effects include alopecia (hair loss), burning sensation of the feet,

Continued

myalgia, and bone pain. Encourage the patient to notify the physician of any unusual sign or symptom.

➤ Instruct the patient to take a missed dose as soon as remembered, unless almost time for the next dose, and then omit the missed dose and resume the regular dosing schedule; do not double up for missed doses because it may cause bleeding. Suggest that the patient keep a record of drug doses and times administered and take the record to the physician at each visit.

➤ Emphasize the importance of returning for follow-up visits to monitor blood work.

Low-Molecular-Weight Heparins
Drug Administration

➤ Review the general guidelines for the patient receiving anticoagulants.

➤ Monitor baseline blood work before administering the first dose: aPTT, PT, thrombin time, hemoglobin, hematocrit, and platelet count. Low-molecular-weight heparins should not alter these test results.

➤ For mild overdose, the physician may simply discontinue the drug until the laboratory findings return to the therapeutic range. Keep protamine sulfate available for treatment of severe overdose.

➤ Place a note above the patient's bed (or as is customary in the institution) that the patient is receiving low-molecular-weight heparin therapy so that laboratory personnel will use care to avoid excessive bleeding after venipuncture.

Subcutaneous Administration, Intermittent Doses

➤ Any subcutaneous site may be used (see Chapter 5), but the abdomen is preferred because it contains few muscles and bruising is less of a cosmetic problem. Avoid using the arms.

➤ Keep a record of sites used and rotate sites, even if the abdomen is used for all doses. Avoid the area 2 inches around the umbilicus and any abdominal scars.

➤ After drawing up the dose, change needles. Pinch the skin and create a subcutaneous "pocket." After careful assessment to avoid injection into a muscle, inject the dose into the pocket with a $^5/_8$- to $^1/_2$-inch, 25- to 28-gauge needle at a 45- to 90-degree angle. Do not aspirate the needle before injecting the drug. Do not rub the area after injecting the drug.

Nursing in the Community

➤ See the general guidelines for the patient receiving anticoagulants.

➤ If a low-molecular-weight heparin is prescribed for home management, instruct the patient in the necessary techniques involved for subcutaneous injection and safe disposal of syringes. Provide positive reinforcement and encouragement. Supervise return demonstrations. Refer patients to a community-based nursing care agency.

➤ Inform the patient that a variety of side effects may occur and that the physician should be notified immediately if any of the following develops: shortness of breath, tightness in the chest, and fast or irregular heartbeat. Other side effects include increased menstrual bleeding, nausea, and vomiting.

Encourage the patient to notify the physician of any unusual sign or symptom.

➤ Instruct the patient to take a missed dose as soon as remembered, unless within 4 hours of the next dose, and then omit the missed dose and resume the regular dosing schedule; do not double up for missed doses.

➤ Emphasize the importance of returning for follow-up visits to monitor blood work.

protamine sulfate
Drug Administration

➤ The dose of protamine sulfate is based on the amount of heparin or low-molecular-weight heparin administered during the preceding 3 to 4 hours. Protamine sulfate injection USP may be given undiluted. Administer intravenously at a rate of 5 mg or less over 1 minute. Do not exceed 50 mg in 10 minutes. The solution may be further diluted for infusion in 5% dextrose in water (D5W) or normal saline.

➤ Monitor vital signs; protamine sulfate may cause hypotension.

➤ Warn the patient that flushing and a feeling of warmth may occur.

➤ Patients receiving protamine zinc insulin may be sensitized to protamine and may experience a severe reaction.

➤ Keep available appropriate drugs and equipment to treat anaphylactic shock.

➤ Continue to assess the patient and monitor blood work because the effects of heparin or low-molecular-weight heparin may persist longer than the protamine, necessitating additional doses of protamine. Monitor the aPTT, ACT, and thrombin time (TT). These tests may not be useful with overdose of a low-molecular-weight heparin.

➤ Protamine sulfate is rarely used outside of a hospital setting. Keep the patient and family informed regarding the patient's condition.

Oral Anticoagulant Drugs: Coumarins and Indandiones
Drug Administration

➤ See the general guidelines for the patient receiving anticoagulants.

➤ Monitor the PT. A guideline for the desired therapeutic range is 1.3 to 1.5 times the control value, unless there is an especially high risk of thromboembolism, when the therapeutic range may be 1.5 to 2 times the control value. In recent years the World Health Organization instituted a standardized system based on the International Normalized Ratio (INR). PT values of 1.3 to 1.5 times the control value are equivalent to INR values of 2 to 3 times the control value; PT values of 1.5 to 2 times the control value are equivalent to INR values of 3 to 4.5 times the control value. The specific desired therapeutic range for PT or INR varies with the patient's medical problem and should be prescribed by the physician. Laboratory work will be done before the first dose is administered and daily until the patient's condition is stable. Check laboratory results before administering each dose.

Nursing Implications Summary—cont'd

If laboratory results indicate excessive anticoagulation, withhold the dose and contact the physician.

➤ If the patient is receiving heparin and an oral anticoagulant, monitor the appropriate blood work for both drugs.

➤ Monitor the white blood cell differential and platelet count.

➤ For mild overdose, the physician will withhold the anticoagulant until the blood results return to the therapeutic range. Keep phytonadione available to treat severe overdose with the oral anticoagulants.

➤ Pregnant women requiring anticoagulants are usually treated with heparin because the oral agents cross the placenta and may cause birth defects. Anticoagulation is usually discontinued at about the 37th week of pregnancy in anticipation of labor and delivery.

Parenteral Administration of warfarin

➤ Reconstitute by adding 2 ml of sterile water for injection to the vial containing 50 mg of warfarin. May be given intramuscularly or intravenously. Administer IV doses at a rate of 25 mg/min direct IV push. Do not mix with IV fluids.

Nursing in the Community

➤ See the general guidelines for the patient receiving anticoagulants.

➤ Inform the patient that anisindione may turn alkaline urine orange, which may be mistaken for blood. If in doubt, the patient should consult the physician.

➤ Rare side effects may develop in patients taking oral anticoagulants. Emphasize the importance of notifying the physician if unexpected signs or symptoms develop.

➤ Instruct patients to avoid drinking alcoholic beverages while taking anticoagulants.

➤ Instruct the patient to take a missed dose as soon as remembered if it is during the same day, otherwise omit the missed dose and resume the regular dosing schedule; do not double up for missed doses because doing so may contribute to bleeding.

➤ Emphasize the importance of returning for follow-up visits to monitor laboratory studies.

➤ Anticoagulant drugs act by creating a vitamin K deficiency (see text). Instruct patients not to change their diet significantly while taking an oral anticoagulant; they should not begin a weight-reduction diet, begin nutritional or vitamin supplements, or otherwise change their diet without consulting with the physician because the dose of anticoagulant may require alteration. Encourage patients to maintain a well-balanced diet and not to make changes in the amount of vitamin K in the diet. Sources of vitamin K are listed in the Dietary Considerations box in Chapter 17 on vitamins. Also instruct patients to notify physician if persistent GI tract upset, fever, or diarrhea develops.

abciximab

Drug Administration

➤ May be given undiluted for bolus injection. For infusion, dilute 4.5 ml (9 mg) with 250 ml normal saline or D5W to make a dilution of 36 μg/ml. Administer at a rate of 17 ml/hr to deliver 10 μg/min. Administer through an in-line, nonpyrogenic, low protein binding 0.2- or 0.22-micron filter, and use an infusion control device.

➤ Monitor the complete blood count (CBC), ACT, aPTT, PT, and platelet count.

➤ Assess potential bleeding sites regularly: catheter insertion sites, arterial and venous puncture sites, cutdown sites, needle puncture sites. Be alert for GI, genitourinary (GU), retroperitoneal, or intracranial bleeding.

➤ Monitor vital signs and blood pressure. Perform neurologic check at least hourly. In addition to bleeding and/or hypotension, hypersensitivity or anaphylaxis may occur at any time. Have readily available drugs, equipment, and personnel to treat an acute allergic reaction.

➤ See manufacturer's literature for recommended technique of femoral artery sheath placement. While the femoral sheath is in place, keep patient on strict bed rest with the head of the bed at less than a 30-degree elevation. Check distal pulses regularly.

➤ Use care in handling patient to avoid bruising or bleeding. Avoid arterial or venous puncture and IM injections. Apply steady pressure over invaded sites for 30 minutes, then apply pressure dressing.

➤ Review with patients the potential for bleeding. Instruct the patient to report any signs of bleeding or oozing. This drug is used in the acute-care unit.

➤ Keep family informed of patient's condition.

aspirin

➤ For a detailed discussion of aspirin, see Chapter 31.

dipyridamole

Drug Administration

➤ Dipyridamole may also be used for some diagnostic studies such as myocardial perfusion imaging.

➤ For IV administration, dilute the dose in sufficient 0.45% or 0.9% sodium chloride injection or D5W to make a volume of 20 to 50 ml. The dose is determined by the patient's weight. Administer at a rate of 142 μg/kg/min for 4 minutes. Monitor vital signs, especially blood pressure, and electrocardiographic changes.

➤ Have IV aminophylline and nitroglycerin readily available to treat adverse effects.

Nursing in the Community

➤ Instruct the patient to take doses with a full glass (8 ounces) of water. It is best to take doses on an empty stomach, 1 hour before or 2 hours after meals. However, if gastric irritation is a problem, instruct the patient to take doses with meals, milk, or a snack.

➤ Dipyridamole may be prescribed with aspirin or another anticoagulant. Review with the patient the importance of taking both drugs as ordered and not increasing the dose of either drug without consulting the physician.

Continued

Nursing Implications Summary—cont'd

➤ Remind the patient to keep all health care providers informed of all drugs being taken. Instruct the patient not to take aspirin or any blood thinner (anticoagulant) unless prescribed by the same physician who prescribed the dipyridamole.

➤ Instruct the patient to avoid over-the-counter medications, especially aspirin-containing products, unless approved by the physician.

➤ Tell the patient to space doses evenly throughout the day. Instruct the patient to take a missed dose as soon as remembered, unless within 4 hours of the next dose, then omit the missed dose and resume the regular dosing schedule; do not double up for missed doses.

➤ Instruct the patient to notify the physician if bruising, bleeding gums, nosebleeds, or bleeding in the stool occurs. Also notify the physician if skin rash or itching, tightness in the chest, or chest pain develops.

ticlopidine
Nursing in the Community
➤ Instruct the patient to take doses with meals or snack.

➤ Emphasize the importance of returning for scheduled follow-up visits. It is especially important during the first 3 months of therapy to monitor for side effects.

➤ Remind the patient to keep all health care providers informed of all medications being used. Ticlopidine may increase the risk of bleeding from surgery or dental procedures, so the drug may need to be stopped for 1 to 2 weeks before scheduled procedures.

➤ Notify the physician if bleeding, unexplained or excessive bruising, blood in urine or stool, black tarry stools, severe headache, bleeding gums, excessively heavy menstrual periods, or nosebleeds develop.

➤ Review the signs of agranulocytosis with the patient (see Patient Problems box earlier in this chapter).

➤ Advise the patient to check with the physician before discharge regarding any possible restrictions in activities while taking ticlopidine.

THROMBOLYTIC DRUGS
Drug Administration
➤ Monitor vital signs and temperature. Be alert to signs of hemorrhage such as hypotension, rapid pulse, or other signs of shock. Monitor mental status and neurologic status. Assess for nosebleeds, bleeding gums, blood in urine, stool, vomitus, or bleeding at IV sites; notify physician. Heparin may also be prescribed, which puts the patient at even greater risk for hemorrhage.

➤ Assess the patient systematically. Many other side effects have been reported, including nausea, vomiting, rash, fever, muscle aches, and dyspnea. Sometimes it is difficult to distinguish drug side effects from symptoms of the underlying medical condition.

➤ Monitor laboratory work, including CBC, TT, aPTT, PT, creatine phosphokinase (CPK), fibrinogen level, and platelet count.

➤ Monitor continuous electrocardiogram (ECG). Reperfusion arrhythmias occur frequently.

➤ Check stools daily for presence of blood.

➤ Use caution in handling and moving the patient to avoid excessive bleeding or bruising. Do not restrain the patient.

➤ If arterial puncture is necessary, apply pressure to the puncture site for 30 minutes after the procedure and use pressure dressings. Check the site regularly for signs of bleeding.

➤ For continuous infusion, use microdrip tubing and an electronic infusion monitoring device. Use a separate infusion line from the one being used for other medications.

➤ Do not administer IM injections to patients receiving these drugs.

➤ Avoid venipuncture unless absolutely necessary. Apply pressure to the site for at least 15 minutes after venipuncture. Label the bed (or as agency custom dictates) so that personnel from the laboratory use appropriate technique to minimize bleeding after venipuncture.

➤ Anaphylaxis has been reported. Keep available appropriate drugs and equipment to treat acute allergic reactions.

➤ For systemic infusion these drugs are used only in short-term care settings. Keep the patient and family informed of the patient's condition.

➤ For arteriovenous cannula occlusion clearance, try to clear the cannula by using a heparinized saline solution. If that is not successful, wait until the effects of the heparin have diminished. Inject the thrombolytic agent into the cannula, and then clamp cannula for 2 hours. Assess the patient for side effects during that period. After 2 hours, aspirate the contents of the affected cannula; then flush the cannula with saline.

➤ For IV catheter obstruction clearance, see the manufacturer's literature supplied with urokinase.

Intravenous alteplase
➤ Dilute as directed by the manufacturer. There are separate directions for the 50- and 100-mg vials. Use the diluent provided to make a concentration of 1 mg/ml. IV alteplase may be given undiluted or further diluted with an equal volume of 0.9% sodium chloride injection or 5% dextrose injection to make a concentration of 0.5 mg/ml. No other diluents should be used.

Intravenous anistreplase
➤ Assess for history of allergic response to streptokinase or anistreplase or previous administration of either of these drugs within the past 12 months.

➤ Have available appropriate drugs, equipment, and personnel to treat acute allergic reactions.

➤ Reconstitute anistreplase as directed by the manufacturer. Roll vial to mix powder and diluent; avoid shaking because foaming may occur. There is no preservative. Use each vial

Nursing Implications Summary—cont'd

for 1 dose then discard vial. Administer the dose within 30 minutes of reconstitution. Administer the dose over 2 to 5 minutes; 4 to 5 minutes is the usual time.

Intravenous reteplase
➤ Reconstitute as directed by the manufacturer.
➤ Use reconstituted solution within 4 hours.

Intravenous streptokinase
➤ Assess the patient for history of allergic response to streptokinase or anistreplase or previous administration of either of these drugs within the past 12 months.
➤ Have available appropriate drugs, equipment, and personnel to treat acute allergic reactions.
➤ Reconstitute as directed by the manufacturer.

Intravenous urokinase
➤ Reconstitute as directed by the manufacturer. When mixing, roll vial; avoid shaking.
➤ For clearing occluded IV catheters, see the manufacturer's insert. Before disconnecting a central venous catheter, instruct the patient to exhale and hold breath until the catheter is disconnected and reconnected to the tubing or syringe. Avoid excessive pressure when injecting the dose. Because catheters may be occluded by material that will not be dissolved by the injected thrombolytic, urokinase may not be successful in clearing obstruction. Be careful not to force precipitate substance into the circulation.

SYSTEMIC HEMOSTATIC DRUGS
aminocaproic acid and tranexamic acid
Drug Administration
➤ Aminocaproic acid and tranexamic acid may be used to treat overdose with fibrinolytic drugs.

Intravenous aminocaproic acid
➤ Dilute the 250 mg/ml concentration with sterile water for injection, normal saline, D5NS, D5W, or lactated Ringer's injection. See the manufacturer's directions. Do not dilute with sterile water for injection if it is to be used for subarachnoid hemorrhage.
➤ Administer at a rate of 5 g or less over 1 hour, followed by 1 g/hr. Use an infusion control device. Too rapid infusion or insufficient dilution may cause hypotension, bradycardia, or arrhythmias.
➤ Because aminocaproic acid can cause clot formation, be alert to signs of possible thrombosis such as pain in extremities, one extremity cooler than the other, loss of pulse in an extremity, shortness of breath, chest pain, slurred speech, changes in vision, and Homans' sign. When aminocaproic acid is used after urologic surgery, the bladder should be free of clots before aminocaproic acid is administered or the drug may accumulate in the clots, preventing them from dissolving. This situation could lead to bladder obstruction, manifested by decreased urination and eventually bladder pain.
➤ Monitor vital signs.

Intravenous tranexamic acid
➤ Dilute a single dose to at least 50 ml with normal saline, D5NS, D5W, Ringer's solution, amino acids, or dextran. Heparin may be added to the solution if needed. Do not mix tranexamic acid with penicillin or blood. Administer a dose over at least 1 minute. Monitor blood pressure. Too rapid administration may cause hypotension.
➤ Because tranexamic acid can cause clot formation, be alert to signs of possible thrombosis, such as pain in extremities, one extremity cooler than the other, loss of pulse in an extremity, shortness of breath, chest pain, slurred speech, changes in vision, and Homans' sign.
➤ Other routes of administration being investigated include using diluted tranexamic acid as a bladder irrigant, applying the drug topically to the nasal mucosa as a spray, and soaking gauze that is then packed into the nasal cavity. See the manufacturer's insert.

Nursing in the Community
➤ Review the goals of therapy with the patient. Therapy is usually short term, but side effects may develop. Review the symptoms of clot development described under IV forms, previously. The development of clots is rare, but instruct the patient to notify the physician if any of the symptoms develop. Encourage the patient to notify the physician if any unexpected sign or symptom develops.
➤ Instruct the patient to take a missed dose of aminocaproic acid as soon as remembered, unless almost time for next dose, then omit the missed dose and resume the regular dosing schedule; do not double up for missed doses.
➤ Instruct the patient to take a missed dose of tranexamic acid as soon as remembered then space remaining doses evenly through the rest of the day; do not double up for missed doses; contact the physician with questions.
➤ For long-term use of tranexamic acid, the physician may recommend regular ophthalmic examinations to check for side effects.

aprotinin
Drug Administration
➤ Review patient's record for previous exposure to aprotinin and possible allergic reaction. Administer a test dose to assess for possible allergic reaction at least 10 minutes before the loading dose. Administer a test dose of 1 ml (10,000 KIU).
➤ Administer all IV doses through a central venous line. Do not administer any other medications through the same IV line as aprotinin.
➤ Monitor vital signs. Have available equipment, drugs, and personnel to treat acute allergic reactions.

phytonadione
Drug Administration
➤ Assess for history of allergy before administering. Monitor vital signs and blood pressure. Remain with the patient for 5 to 10 minutes after administration. Have available

Continued

appropriate drugs, equipment, and personnel to treat an acute allergic response.

➤ IM injection is painful, and the injection site may be tender. Use large muscle masses. Record and rotate injection sites.

➤ Monitor the PT.

➤ Read labels carefully. Konakion is for IM injection only. AquaMEPHYTON may be given intramuscularly, intravenously, or subcutaneously.

Intravenous phytonadione

➤ Dilute with sodium chloride injection, 5% dextrose injection, or D5NS. Diluents containing benzyl alcohol should not be used in neonates or infants. Administer diluted solution at a rate of 1 mg or less over 1 minute. The IM route is preferred. Solution is light sensitive; prepare dose just before administration.

menadiol
Drug Administration

➤ Assess for glucose-6-phosphate dehydrogenase deficiency before administering; if present, do not administer.

➤ IM injection is painful, and the injection site may be tender. Use large muscle masses. Record and rotate injection sites.

➤ Monitor the PT.

Intravenous menadiol

➤ May be given undiluted or added to most infusion solutions. Administer undiluted dose over at least 1 minute.

Nursing in the Community for phytonadione or menadiol

➤ Review with the patient the expected benefits of therapy.

➤ Dietary deficiency of vitamin K is rare in adults. For dietary sources of vitamin K, see the Dietary Considerations box in Chapter 17 on vitamins.

➤ Instruct the patient to take a missed dose as soon as remembered, unless almost time for next dose, and then omit the missed dose and resume the regular dosing schedule; do not double up for missed doses. Encourage the patient to keep a record of missed doses and to inform the physician of these omissions on the next visit.

➤ Emphasize to the patient the importance of follow-up visits to monitor drug effectiveness.

➤ Remind the patient to keep all health care providers, including dentists, informed of all drugs being used.

HEMOSTATIC DRUGS FOR REPLACEMENT THERAPY FOR HEMOPHILIA
antihemophilic factor and cryoprecipitated antihemophilic factor
Drug Administration

➤ Monitor vital signs and remain with the patient for 5 to 10 minutes after beginning drug administration to watch for allergic reaction. Symptoms include fast or irregular breathing, tightness in the chest, swelling of eyelids, skin rash, hives or itching, and hypotension. If allergic reaction occurs, discontinue use of the remaining AHF, but keep the IV line patent. Notify the physician.

➤ Monitor plasma factor VIII and antibodies to factor VIII periodically.

➤ For the dry form, bring the concentrate and diluent to room temperature. Use plastic disposable syringe and filter needle to prepare dose. Reconstitute with the diluent provided by the manufacturer, adding diluent to the vial by directing the stream against the side of the vial to prevent foaming. Do not shake the vial. Administer within 1 to 3 hours after reconstitution (see the manufacturer's instructions with the preparation being used).

➤ Cryoprecipitated AHF is handled like all blood products (see Chapter 17). Thaw in a water bath at 30° to 37° C (86° to 98.6° F) for up to 15 minutes.

➤ Administer through a separate IV line; do not mix with other IV fluids or medications (except for 0.9% sodium chloride with cryoprecipitated form).

Nursing in the Community

➤ Some patients may be candidates to learn how to administer AHF at home. Review the directions for reconstitution. Have the patient give return demonstration. In addition to teaching how to reconstitute and administer a dose, demonstrate the appropriate disposal technique for used syringes, needles, and equipment. Review the side effects.

➤ Patients recently diagnosed with hemophilia should be immunized against hepatitis A and B; consult the physician.

➤ Instruct patients with hemophilia to wear a medical identification tag or bracelet indicating their condition and treatment.

➤ Instruct the patient to contact the physician for missed doses. If unable to contact the physician, instruct the patient to take a missed dose as soon as remembered, unless almost time for next dose, then omit the missed dose and resume the regular dosing schedule; do not double up for missed doses.

antithrombin III
Drug Administration

➤ Review the manufacturer's instructions provided with the preparation. Reconstitute as directed. Roll the vial to mix. Do not shake the vial because foaming may occur.

➤ Administer ATnativ at a rate of 50 IU of less over 1 minute; do not exceed 100 IU/minute. Administer a single dose of Thrombate III over 10 to 20 minutes.

desmopressin
Drug Administration

➤ Desmopressin is also discussed in Chapter 65.

➤ For treatment of hemophilia A and von Willebrand's disease, dilute a single dose in 10 ml of normal saline for children weighing less than 10 kg and in 50 ml for children weighing more than 10 kg and adults. Administer a dose over 15 to 30 minutes.

➤ Monitor blood pressure and pulse. Other side effects include headache, nausea, flushing, abdominal cramps, and pain at the injection site.

Nursing Implications Summary—cont'd

➤ Desmopressin has an antidiuretic effect. Monitor intake and output. Caution the patient to limit fluid intake.

➤ Monitor blood work such as factor VIII coagulant, factor VIII antigen, and ristocetin cofactor, depending on diagnosis.

factor IX complex
Drug Administration
➤ Review the manufacturer's instructions provided with the preparation. Reconstitute as directed. Roll the vial to mix. Do not shake the vial because foaming may occur. Use plastic syringes and filter needles.

➤ Administer at a rate of 2 to 3 ml/min or 100 U/min, although it may vary according to patient's condition. Do not exceed 10 ml/min. Slow the infusion rate if chills, fever, flushing, headache, tingling, or pain at the injection site develops. Monitor blood pressure and pulse.

➤ Administer through a separate line; do not mix with other drugs or IV fluids.

Nursing in the Community
➤ Some patients may be candidates to learn how to administer factor IX at home. Review the directions for reconstitution, and have the patient give a return demonstration. In addition to teaching how to reconstitute and administer dose, demonstrate the appropriate disposal technique for used syringes, needles, and equipment. Review the side effects.

➤ Patients recently diagnosed with hemophilia should be immunized against hepatitis A and B; consult the physician.

➤ Instruct patients with hemophilia to wear a medical identification tag or bracelet indicating their condition and treatment.

➤ For missed doses, instruct the patient to notify the physician as soon as possible.

CHAPTER REVIEW

Application

1. Describe the major steps in blood coagulation.
2. What are the groups of anticoagulants you see in clinical practice? What is the mechanism of action of each group?
3. Which anticoagulants would you expect to see in test tubes when blood is drawn for storage or testing?
4. How does protein binding affect the pharmacodynamics of the coumarins?
5. What are the therapeutic limitations of the indandiones?
6. How do platelets initiate clot formation?
7. What drugs might you see prescribed to inhibit platelet aggregation?
8. What roles do thromboxane A$_2$ and prostacyclin play in platelet aggregation?
9. What is the action of thrombolytic drugs? Name the thrombolytic drugs.
10. What is the mechanism of action of aminocaproic acid? of vitamin K? When would these drugs be used?
11. List the agents used as local hemostatics. What is their mechanism of action?

Critical Thinking

1. Differentiate between nursing care activities required to administer heparin in high-dose and low-dose therapy.
2. Compare and contrast how protamine sulfate and vitamin K function as antidotes for drug-induced hemorrhage.
3. Compare and contrast heparin with warfarin; consider action, side effects, ease of administration, and contraindications.
4. How do the actions of thromboxane$_2$ and prostacyclin influence the dose of aspirin used to prevent thrombus formation?
5. Compare and contrast the four thrombolytics. Call the pharmacy and include cost in your discussion.
6. Compare and contrast hemophilia A, hemophilia B, and von Willebrand's disease.
7. What drugs are used to treat hemophilia? What are the nursing care implications of these drugs?

References

Braimah J, et al: Nursing care of acute stroke patients after receiving rt-PA therapy, *J Neurosci Nurs* 29(6):373-377, 382-383, 1997.

Falter HJ: Deep vein thrombosis in pregnancy and the puerperium: a comprehensive review, *J Vasc Nurs* 15(2):58-62, 1997.

Fritz DL, Chung DJ, Merli GJ: Understanding hypercoagulability, *Nursing* 27(1):32a-32b, 32f, 32h, 1997.

Gibbar-Clements T, Shirrell D, Free C: PT and APTT: Seeing beyond the numbers, *Nursing* 27(7):49-51, 1997.

Gregory S, Stockman L: Reducing the risks from postprocedure anticoagulation therapy, *Nursing* 27(8):32cc1-2, 32cc4-5, 1997.

Kongable GL: Code stroke: Using t-PA to prevent ischemic brain injury, *Am J Nurs* 97(11):16BB,16DD-16FF, 16HH, 1997.

Lechner DL: A standardized weight-based heparin protocol: improving clinical outcomes, *Nurs Manage* 28(4):29-32, 1997.

Majors DS: Medication review. Thrombolytic therapy with urokinase, *ANNA J* 23(6):627-629, 1996.

Rapp K, et al: Code stroke: Rapid transport, triage and treatment using rt-PA therapy, *J Neurosci Nurs* 29(6):361-366, 1997.

Selig PM: Pearls for practice. Management of anticoagulation therapy with the International Normalized Ratio, *J Am Acad Nurse Pract* 8(2):77-80, 1996.

Sparks KS: Are you up to date on weight-based heparin dosing? *Am J Nurs* 96(4):Nurse Pract Extra Ed: 33-37, 1996.

Drugs to Lower Blood Lipid Levels

OBJECTIVES

After studying this chapter, you should be able to do the following:

- *Differentiate between the two main types of lipids in the blood and the four major classes of lipoprotein.*
- *State the normal blood level of cholesterol.*
- *Discuss the four types of lipoproteins.*
- *Develop a teaching plan for a patient who needs to decrease cholesterol intake.*
- *Develop a nursing care plan for a patient who is taking one of the drugs discussed in this chapter.*

CHAPTER OVERVIEW

Atherosclerosis is the gradual blocking of arteries by a buildup of plaque. This clogging of the arteries is the major factor behind heart attacks, strokes, and peripheral vascular disease. Lipids, particularly cholesterol, are a major component of atherosclerotic plaques. The association of high blood levels of cholesterol with atherosclerosis has led to preventive measures to control cholesterol. This chapter reviews the current pharmacologic approaches to controlling blood cholesterol.

THERAPEUTIC RATIONALE: ATHEROSCLEROSIS AND CORONARY HEART DISEASE

Origin of Blood Lipids and Their Role in Atherosclerosis

The **lipids** in the blood are triglyceride and cholesterol. **Triglyceride** is an energy source for muscle and is stored in fat. **Cholesterol** is a fatlike substance that is present in cell membranes and is a precursor of bile acids and steroid hormones. Triglycerides and cholesterol are bound to special proteins to form soluble lipoprotein.

The major classes of **lipoprotein** are chylomicrons, very-low-density lipoprotein (VLDL), low-density lipoprotein (LDL), and high-density lipoprotein (HDL). Chylomicrons and VLDLs are largely composed of triglycerides; they transport triglycerides to tissues for metabolic use or storage. LDLs and HDLs transport cholesterol. The role and composition of lipoprotein are summarized in Figure 21-1.

Chylomicrons

Chylomicrons are very large lipoproteins that contain about 90% triglyceride by weight. After a meal the ingested fat is processed by the intestine into chylomicrons, which are transported through the lymphatic system to the plasma.

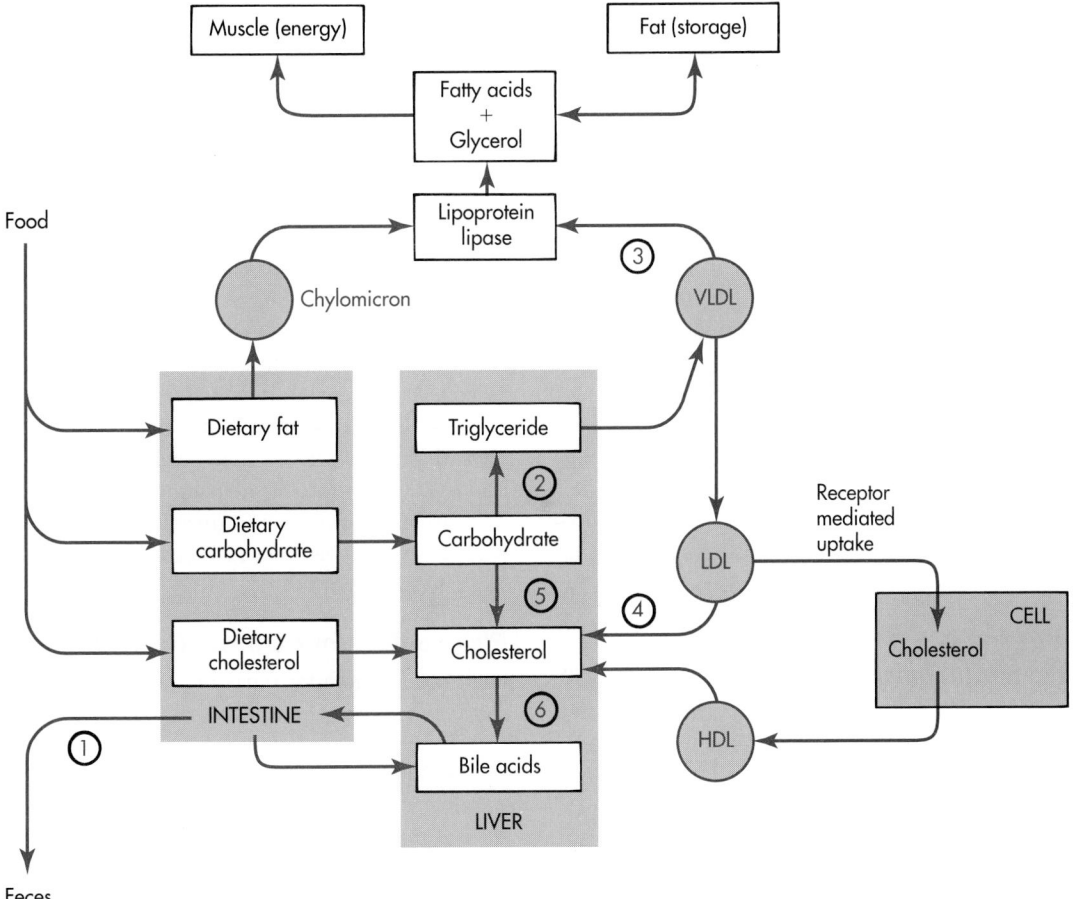

Figure 21-1   Diagram of origin and fate of lipids. Drug actions that lower excessive plasma concentrations of lipids include *(1)* bile acid resins lower cholesterol by increasing excretion of bile acids; *(2)* fibric acid derivatives and nicotinic acid lower triglycerides by inhibiting hepatic triglyceride synthesis; *(3)* clofibrate lowers VLDL, inhibiting its release and activating lipoprotein lipase; *(4)* statins lower cholesterol by stimulating LDL uptake; *(5)* statins inhibit cholesterol synthesis; and *(6)* clofibrate increases cholesterol excretion into bile.

Chylomicrons are normally found in the blood only during the 8 to 12 hours after a meal. Because chylomicrons represent dietary fat, patients who are evaluated for triglyceride abnormalities should not eat for 12 to 16 hours before a blood sample is drawn.

Very-Low-Density Lipoproteins

VLDLs are 60% triglyceride by weight. This triglyceride pool is synthesized by the liver from carbohydrate sources for export as fuel to other tissues. Triglycerides cannot be transported directly into cells for use. Tissues that require triglycerides, particularly muscle and fat tissues, secrete an enzyme called lipoprotein lipase, which breaks down the triglycerides to fatty acids and glycerol, compounds that can be taken into the cells.

Low-Density Lipoproteins

LDLs ("bad cholesterol") are only 5% triglyceride but are 50% cholesterol by weight. About 60% to 70% of the total

serum cholesterol in a fasting serum sample is found in LDLs. When triglyceride values are less than 400 mg/dl, the calculation for LDL cholesterol is made from the following formula:

LDL cholesterol =
Total cholesterol − HDL cholesterol − (triglyceride/5)

The desirable level of LDL is less than 130 mg/dl. LDLs are the remains of the VLDLs after removal of triglycerides and some protein. When cells need cholesterol, they synthesize receptors for LDL. LDLs bind to these receptors and are taken into the cell by pinocytosis and degraded. Most cells can synthesize cholesterol, but this synthesis is turned off when the cholesterol from LDL is used. When the cell has sufficient cholesterol, it stops making LDL receptors.

High-Density Lipoproteins

HDLs ("good cholesterol") are 50% protein, 20% cholesterol, and 5% triglyceride by weight. Only about 20% of the total plasma cholesterol is found in HDL. The HDLs remove excess cholesterol from peripheral tissues. HDLs can also remove cholesterol from cells and can inhibit the uptake of LDL by cells. Recent studies indicate that persons with high concentrations of HDLs (more than 65 mg/dl) have a lower incidence of atherosclerosis and the related problems of heart disease and strokes. Higher HDL levels can be promoted by exercise, weight reduction, and smoking cessation. On the other hand, individuals with a very low HDL level (less than 35 mg/dl) have an increased risk for atherosclerosis even if the LDL level is in the "normal" range.

Degradation of Cholesterol

The liver degrades cholesterol to bile acids, which are excreted into the small intestine. Bile acids emulsify lipids to aid in fat absorption. Some bile acids are absorbed into the portal vein for transport back to the liver. This circulation between the liver and small intestine is called **enterohepatic circulation.**

Atherosclerosis and Blood Cholesterol
Role of LDLs in Atherosclerosis

Research has focused on the role of LDLs in **atherosclerosis** because the concentration of LDLs reflects the total cholesterol concentration. Increased total plasma cholesterol concentration is linked to increased incidence of atherosclerosis. When there is injury to the epithelial cells of arteries or when the amount of circulating LDLs becomes high, the receptor mechanism controlling LDL uptake no longer operates properly, and the cell becomes overwhelmed with cholesterol. This situation is believed to be an origin of atherosclerotic plaques.

Atherosclerotic Plaques

Platelets may also initiate atherosclerosis. Aggregated platelets release factors that stimulate smooth muscle growth. This stimulation of growth heals the minute breaks in the normal blood vessel. When the epithelial cells are overloaded with cholesterol and aggregated platelets stimulate an overgrowth of smooth muscle cells, an atherosclerotic plaque is formed. The outcome of atherosclerosis is the narrowing of an artery so that the blood flow is reduced and may not be sufficient to maintain tissue function (Figure 21-2).

Reduced blood flow also favors the formation of a clot that may completely obstruct flow. A stroke may result when the cerebral arteries are involved, or a myocardial infarction may result when the coronary arteries are involved. When the legs are affected, limbs may be lost to gangrene. Renovascular hypertension is associated with atherosclerosis.

Recent studies suggest that about 10% to 20% of atherosclerotic lesions are unstable plaques that may rupture and lead to 80% or more of such clinical events as sudden death, myocardial infarction, or worsening angina. These unstable plaques seem to be those depleted or regressed by aggressive diet and drug therapy.

Risk Factors for Coronary Heart Disease

High blood cholesterol has been shown to be a major risk factor for coronary heart disease. The classification of total cholesterol levels is as follows:

<200 mg/dl	Desirable total blood cholesterol
200-239 mg/dl	Borderline high total blood cholesterol
>240 mg/dl	High total blood cholesterol

Epidemiologic studies support a direct relationship between the level of total serum cholesterol and the rate of coronary heart disease. Migration studies show that within one generation of moving, a population adopts both the blood cholesterol levels and the coronary heart disease rate of the new country. The risk for death from coronary heart disease in men rises fivefold over the range of blood cholesterol levels. In recent years studies have examined the outcome of lowering high blood cholesterol levels in individu-

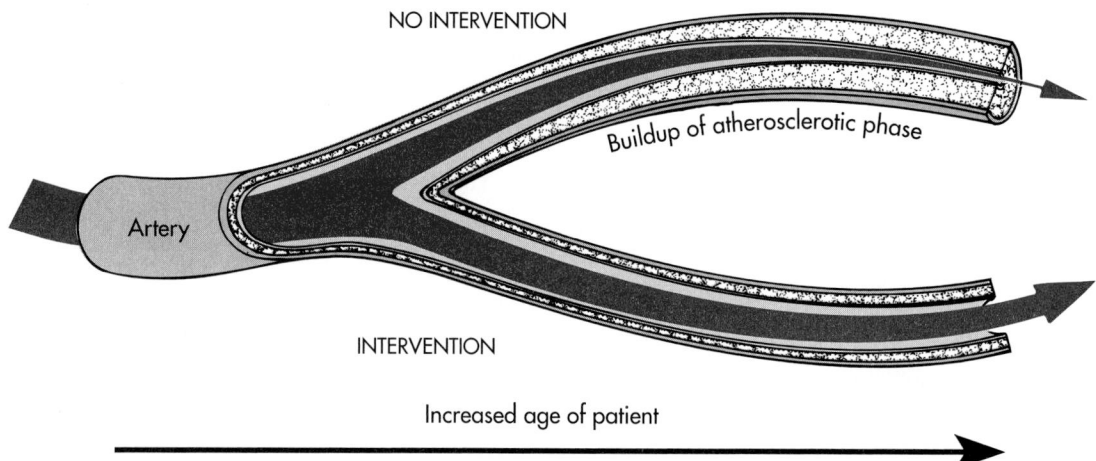

F i g u r e 21-2   Diagram of increasing blockage of artery caused by atherosclerotic plaque. Buildup of plaque is shown as time-dependent phenomenon. Intervention, through diet, exercise, or drugs, can slow buildup. Recent studies have shown that some interventions can reverse atherosclerosis.

als with established coronary heart disease. Lowering cholesterol levels reduces rates of recurrent coronary heart disease events along with a strong trend toward decreased total mortality rates.

The emphasis today for preventing coronary heart disease is twofold: first, to identify individuals at high risk who will benefit from intensive intervention efforts (Box 21-1) and, second, to promote lower blood cholesterol levels in the whole population by encouraging changes in dietary habits (see Dietary Considerations box) and physical activity levels.

Genetic Factors in Atherosclerosis

The fact that atherosclerosis runs in families has prompted searches for the genetic factors underlying unusually high blood lipid levels. Hypercholesterolemia in its severest form

---

Box 21-1   Risk Factors Identified for Coronary Heart Disease

- Age: Men older than 45 years; women older than 55 years or those who have undergone premature menopause without estrogen replacement therapy
- Family history of premature coronary heart disease (myocardial infarction or sudden death before 55 years of age in a male first-degree relative or 65 years of age in a female first-degree relative)
- Current cigarette smoking
- Hypertension
- Low high-density lipoprotein (HDL) cholesterol (<35 mg/dl)
- Diabetes mellitus

There is one protective (negative risk) factor:
- High HDL cholesterol ≥60 mg/dl

An individual with two or more risk factors should be given dietary consultation and drug therapy if needed to achieve and keep cholesterol levels in the desirable range.

DIETARY CONSIDERATIONS

Reducing Cholesterol

Dietary changes to lower serum cholesterol levels usually involve decreasing cholesterol intake, lowering the intake of saturated fat, and increasing the intake of polyunsaturated fat. As with all major dietary prescriptions, refer patients to a dietitian for more extensive teaching and explanation if necessary.

FOODS ALLOWED

Meat
Lean, well-trimmed meat; poultry, fish (not shrimp), and veal preferred, with occasional ham, pork, lamb, beef

Eggs and Other Meat Alternatives
Egg white only, no-cholesterol egg substitutes, legumes, soy protein, peanut butter, nuts (e.g., walnuts, pecans, almonds)

Milk and Cheese
Skim milk and skim milk products, buttermilk, low-fat cheese, cottage cheese, yogurt containing up to 1% milkfat, sherbet

Vegetables and Fruits
Fresh, canned, frozen, or dried fruits or vegetables; juices; vegetables prepared without animal fat; vegetarian baked beans

Fat
Vegetable oils, soft margarine listing allowed liquid oil as first ingredient, mayonnaise, salad dressings not containing sour cream or cheese

Breads and Cereals
Cooked and dry cereal; rice; flour; pasta; breads made with minimum of saturated fat; white, whole-wheat, rye, pumpernickel, raisin, Italian, and French breads; English muffins; hard rolls; matzo; pretzels; saltines; homemade breads made without whole milk, egg yolk, or saturated shortening

Soup
Bouillon; clear broths; fat-free vegetable soup and pot liquor; cream soups made with skim milk and allowed fat; packaged dehydrated soup

Desserts and Sweets
Angel food cake; fruit ices; sherbet (1%-2% fat); gelatin desserts; meringues; homemade pastries made with allowed fat, skim milk, and egg white; pure sugar candies; jam; jelly; honey; syrup made without fat; molasses; sugar

Miscellaneous
Coffee, tea, caffeine-free coffee, carbonated beverages, relishes, fat-free barbecue sauce, catsup, chili sauce, spices, herbs, extracts, lemon juice, vinegar

FOODS TO AVOID OR LIMIT
- Fatty meat, regular ground beef, bacon, sausage, luncheon meat, fried meat, meat in gravy, shrimp, organ meats, fish roe
- Egg yolk, canned pork and beans, cashews, macadamia nuts
- Whole milk and milk products, malted milk and milkshakes, cream (sweet and sour), ice cream and ice milk, nondairy substitutes for cream, whipped toppings containing coconut or palm oil, cheese made from cream or whole milk
- Buttered, creamed, or fried vegetables; pork and beans, avocado (use sparingly)
- Other margarines, including low-calorie; butter, hydrogenated vegetable shortening, bacon, lard, meat drippings, salt pork, suet, cream; coconut, palm, and peanut oils; gravies (unless made with allowed fat and skim milk)
- Egg noodles; egg bread; commercial biscuits, muffins, donuts, pancakes, waffles, and butter rolls; mixes for preceding; corn chips, potato chips, and other deep-fried snacks; cheese crackers
- All other soups
- Commercial pies, cakes, mixes; desserts and candy containing nonallowed fat, egg yolk, and whole milk; chocolate; coconut

is caused by mutations in the gene responsible for producing a functional LDL receptor. Without a functional LDL receptor, LDLs cannot be taken into cells and cholesterol cannot be used. Instead, cholesterol remains circulating while bound to LDLs. Individuals monozygous for this trait are 1 in 1 million and have severe atherosclerosis by their twenties. Far more common (1 in 500) are individuals who are heterozygous for a defective LDL receptor but still have about 50% of the normal number of LDL receptors. These individuals show premature atherosclerosis. Most cases of hypercholesterolemia have no specific genetic abnormality, however. Multiple genetic and environmental factors are being identified.

High levels of total cholesterol combined with elevated levels of triglycerides are designated as combined **hyperlipidemia** and reflect elevated LDL and VLDL levels. This condition is commonly found to run in families, although specific genetic factors have not been determined and in fact may be multiple. Combined hyperlipidemia is also caused by obesity, diabetes mellitus, and nephrotic syndrome.

Dietary Modification and Physical Activity

Dietary modification, weight reduction in overweight individuals, and increased physical activity are important lifestyle modifications for lowering blood cholesterol levels. Weight reduction may be important in itself or through its beneficial effect in reducing hypertension or moderating diabetes mellitus. Physical activity increases HDL cholesterol.

Diet modification is always the first therapeutic intervention (see Dietary Considerations box). A trial of at least 6 months can determine whether diet modification alone is sufficient to lower blood cholesterol without addition of drug therapy. The goal of a step I diet is to reduce saturated fat intake to less than 10% of calories, total fat to 30% or less of total calories, and cholesterol to less than 300 mg/day. The goal of a step II diet is to reduce saturated fat to less than 7% of total calories, total fat to 30% or less of total calories, and cholesterol to less than 200 mg/day.

THERAPEUTIC AGENTS: DRUGS TO LOWER BLOOD CHOLESTEROL

Drugs that are used to reduce blood lipid concentrations are listed in Table 21-1. The major drugs used include the 3-hydroxy-3-methylglutaryl coenzyme A (HMG-CoA) reductase inhibitors ("statins"), the bile acid sequestrants, and nicotinic acid. Other drugs include the fibric acid derivatives and estrogens. Treatment decisions are based on the LDL level rather than total cholesterol. Box 21-2 outlines treatment decisions for adding these drugs to dietary therapy. The treatment decision is influenced by the presence of coronary heart disease or its risk factors.

▼ HMG-CoA Reductase Inhibitors (Statins)

Recent clinical trials have shown dramatic reductions in myocardial infarctions and death when patients with established coronary heart disease were treated aggressively with diet and simvastatin or pravastatin to lower elevated cholesterol levels. **Simvastatin** (Zocor) and pravastatin (Pravachol) are two of the HMG-CoA reductase inhibitors—

Box 21-2   Treatment Decisions Based on LDL Cholesterol and Coronary Heart Disease (CHD)

Dietary Therapy

	Initiation Level	LDL Goal
Without CHD and with fewer than two risk factors	≥160 mg/dl	<160 mg/dl
Without CHD and with two or more risk factors	≥130 mg/dl	<130 mg/dl
With CHD	>100 mg/dl	≤100 mg/dl

Drug Therapy

	Consideration Level	LDL Goal
Without CHD and with fewer than two risk factors	≥190 mg/dl	<160 mg/dl
Without CHD and with two or more risk factors	≥160 mg/dl	<130 mg/dl
With CHD	>130 mg/dl	≤100 mg/dl

Drug Selection

	Single Drug	Combination Drug
1) Elevated LDL cholesterol and triglycerides <200 mg/dl	Bile-acid sequestrant (BAS)	BAS + Statin
	HMG-CoA reductase inhibitor (statin)	Statin + NA*
	Nicotinic acid (NA)	NA + BAS
2) Elevated LDL cholesterol and triglycerides 200-400 mg/dl	Nicotinic acid	NA + Statin*
	HMG-CoA reductase inhibitor	Statin + Gem†
		NA + BAS
	Gemfibrozil (GEM)	NA + Gem

From Second Report of the Expert Panel on Detection, Evaluation, and Treatment of High Blood Cholesterol in Adults, National Institutes of Health Publication No. 93-3095, September, 1993, US Department of Health and Human Services, Public Health Service.
*Possible increased risk of myopathy and hepatitis.
†Increased risk of myopathy. Must be used with caution.

commonly called statins—currently available. Others include atorvastatin (Lipitor), cerivastatin (Baycol), fluvastatin (Lescol), and lovastatin (Mevacor).

Mechanism of Action

The HMG-CoA reductase inhibitors block an early step in the synthesis of cholesterol by the liver. This inhibition in cholesterol production leads cells, especially in the liver, to increase the number of LDL receptors. The increased number of receptors causes LDL to be removed from the serum, lowering LDL cholesterol 20% to 60%, whereas HDL cholesterol increases 5% to 15%. Triglycerides are lowered by 10% to 40%.

Pharmacokinetics

The statins are taken as a single dose in the evening. Lovastatin should be taken with a meal to maximize absorption, but the other drugs may be taken with a meal or on an empty stomach. Atorvastatin, lovastatin, and simvastatin are metabolized to active metabolites, whereas cerivastatin, fluvastatin, and pravastatin are active as administered. The LDL reduction stabilizes after 4 to 6 weeks of therapy, at which time the drug and dose can be evaluated.

The statins are metabolized by the liver and excretion is primarily fecal. The duration of action persists 4 to 6 weeks after therapy is discontinued.

Table 21-1 Drugs to Lower Blood Cholesterol

Generic Name	Trade Name	Administration/Dosage	Comments
HMG-CoA Reductase Inhibitors (Statins)			
atorvastatin	Lipitor	ORAL: *Adults*—10 mg once a day. May increase at 2- to 4-wk intervals up to 80 mg daily. FDA pregnancy category X.	New drug.
cerivastatin	Baycol	ORAL: *Adults*—0.3 mg once a day in the evening. FDA pregnancy category X.	New drug.
fluvastatin	Lescol	ORAL: *Adults*—20 mg once a day in the evening. May increase to 40 mg if needed. FDA pregnancy category X.	New drug.
lovastatin	Mevacor*	ORAL: *Adults*—20 mg once a day with the evening meal. May adjust at 4-wk intervals. Maintenance: 20-80 mg/day, as a single dose or in divided doses, with meals. FDA pregnancy category X.	First statin available. Should be taken with meals. Combined therapy with cholestyramine resin shown to reduce progression of atherosclerosis in bypass grafts.
pravastatin	Pravachol*	ORAL: *Adults*—10-20 mg once a day at bedtime. May adjust at 4-wk intervals. Maintenance: 10-40 mg/day, as a single dose at bedtime. FDA pregnancy category X.	Shown to decrease new heart attacks in patients who had survived one, even when cholesterol levels were not elevated.
simvastatin	Zocor*	ORAL: *Adults*—5-10 mg once a day in the evening. May adjust at 4-wk intervals. Maintenance: 5-40 mg/day, as a single dose in the evening. FDA pregnancy category X.	Scandinavian Simvastatin Survival Study showed 34% reduction in coronary events, 42% reduction in coronary heart disease mortality.
Bile Acid Sequestrants			
cholestyramine	Questran*	ORAL: *Adults and children*—4 g 1 or 2 times a day before meals. Maintenance: 8-24 g in 2-6 doses.	Valuable for isolated elevations of LDL cholesterol. Stays in the intestine removing bile acids and thereby increasing cholesterol degradation by the liver.
colestipol	Colestid*	ORAL: *Adults*—15-30 mg/day before meals in 2-4 divided doses.	Valuable for isolated elevations of LDL cholesterol. Stays in the intestine removing bile acids and thereby increasing cholesterol degradation by the liver.
Fibric Acid Derivatives			
clofibrate	Abitrate Atromid-S* Claripex† Novofibrate†	ORAL: *Adults*—1.5-2 g/day in 2-4 divided doses. FDA pregnancy category C.	Inhibits triglyceride synthesis in the liver and inhibits the breakdown of triglycerides in fat tissue. Triglycerides are lowered; HDL concentration may be increased.
fenofibrate	Tricor	ORAL: *Adults*—Initially 1 capsule (67 mg) per day, taken with a meal. May increase at 4- to 8-wk intervals if necessary, depending on triglyceride measurements. Maximum daily dose: 201 mg.	Inhibits tryglyceride synthesis in the liver and inhibits the breakdown of tryglycerides in fat tissue. Tryglycerides are lowered; HDL concentration may be increased.
gemfibrozil	Lopid*	ORAL: *Adults*—1.2 g/day in 2 divided doses 30 min before morning and evening meals. FDA pregnancy category C.	Inhibits triglyceride synthesis in the liver and inhibits the breakdown of triglycerides in fat tissue. Triglycerides are lowered; HDL concentration may be increased.
Other Agent			
nicotinic acid	Niacor Novo-Niacin†	ORAL: *Adults*—1 g 3 times/day. May increase by 500 mg/day every 2-4 wk as needed.	Reduce VLDL production by the liver. Useful in most lipid and lipoprotein abnormalities.

LDL, Low-density lipoprotein; *HDL*, high-density lipoprotein; *VLDL*, very-low-density lipoprotein.
*Available in Canada and the United States.
†Available in Canada only.

Uses

Statins are used to treat hypercholesterolemia caused by elevated LDL. At therapeutic doses they reduce, but do not completely block, synthesis of cholesterol. As a result, liver cells produce more LDL receptors to capture LDL from the plasma, thereby clearing excess LDL from the blood. A long-term study of patients taking simvastatin showed that those with both high blood cholesterol and heart disease cut their risk of dying by about 30% over 5 years. This patient population tends to be older. The long-term safety among middle-aged adults is unknown, but as the clinical experience continues, few safety concerns have emerged.

Adverse Reactions, Contraindications, and Toxicity

Statins are well tolerated. Unlike the fibric acids, they do not increase the risk of gallstones. The most common side effects include dyspepsia, flatulence, constipation, and abdominal pain or cramps. High dosages occasionally increase hepatic transaminase levels. An uncommon severe side effect is myopathy with muscle aches, soreness, weakness, and elevated creatine kinase values.

These drugs are contraindicated in patients with allergies or active liver disease. Because they block synthesis of cholesterol, a key compound for growth and maintenance, they pose potential harm to the fetus and should not be used during pregnancy or by nursing mothers.

Interactions

Concurrent administration of cyclosporine, gemfibrozil, or niacin with a statin is associated with an increased risk for muscle damage (rhabdomyolysis) and acute renal failure. Creatine kinase values may also be higher. Simvastatin given with digoxin will cause a slight increase in digoxin levels.

▼ Bile Acid Sequestrants

Cholestyramine (Questran) and colestipol (Colestid) are the bile acid sequestrants used to treat high LDL cholesterol levels. They have been shown in prevention trials to reduce the risk for coronary heart disease while having a long-term safety record.

Mechanism of Action

The bile acids sequestrants are resins that are not absorbed systemically. In the intestine they bind bile acids, which are then excreted, interrupting the enterohepatic circulation of bile acids. This action causes the liver to convert more cholesterol to bile acids. With hepatic cholesterol lowered, more LDL receptors are formed on cells, and LDL removal is enhanced. The overall result is a lowering of LDL cholesterol levels.

Pharmacokinetics

Bile acid sequestrants are powders mixed with water or fruit juice. They are taken in one or two doses daily with meals. Alternatively, they may be given in one large dose after the evening meal in order not to absorb other drugs that must be taken earlier in the day. A lowering of LDL cholesterol is usually seen within 2 weeks of beginning therapy. Cholestyramine and colestipol are not absorbed and are excreted in the feces.

Uses

Cholestyramine and colestipol are especially effective in lowering LDL cholesterol levels. A 15% to 30% reduction is commonly seen. Because of their safety and proven effectiveness, these drugs are the first to be prescribed when diet therapy alone is not sufficient and the patient is younger and has moderate hypercholesterolemia (men younger than 45 years and women younger than 55 years, LDL cholesterol 160 to 220 mg/dl). These drugs are also effective in combination of the HMG-CoA reductase inhibitors in treating patients with severe hypercholesterolemia.

Adverse Reactions and Contraindications

Gastrointestinal (GI) symptoms are the major side effects of the bile acid sequestrants. Symptoms include constipation, bloating, epigastric fullness, nausea, and flatulence. Serum triglyceride levels may increase in some patients as a result of increased hepatic VLDL production. Therefore bile acid sequestrants are not recommended for patients with triglyceride levels of about 200 mg/dl.

Interactions

Bile acid sequestrants may bind other drugs and prevent their absorption. Other drugs should be taken at least 1 hour before or 4 hours after cholestyramine or colestipol. In particular, decreased absorption of digitoxin, warfarin, thyroxine, thiazide diuretics, and beta-blockers has been shown. It may be advisable to administer some drugs early in the day and to administer cholestyramine or colestipol with the evening meal.

▼ Fibric Acid Derivatives

Gemfibrozil (Lopid), clofibrate (Abitrate, Atromid-S, Claripex, Novofibrate), and fenofibrate (Tricor) are the fibric acid derivatives available in the United States. Gemfibrozil is more commonly used. It is not recommended as a single agent for lowering cholesterol; it is added to treatment with nicotinic acid or a statin.

Mechanism of Action

Fibric acid derivatives primarily lower triglycerides. They act in a complex manner to increase lipoprotein lipase activity, thereby enhancing catabolism of VLDLs and LDLs and reducing triglyceride levels. They also decrease the synthesis of VLDL triglycerides and partially inhibit the synthesis of cholesterol and bile acids to increase the secretion of cholesterol in bile.

Pharmacokinetics

Clofibrate, fenofibrate, and gemfibrozil are administered orally and are well absorbed from the GI tract. They are given in two daily doses 30 minutes before breakfast and dinner. Gemfibrozil is metabolized by the liver. Clofibrate and fenofibrate are also metabolized in the GI tract to an active form, clofibric acid and fenofibric acid. The drugs and metabolites are excreted in the urine.

A measurable onset of action is seen in 2 to 5 days with continuous administration. The peak effect is seen in 3 weeks for clofibrate and in 4 weeks to several months for gemfibrozil. VLDL levels will return to pretreatment values about 3 weeks after therapy is discontinued.

Uses

Clofibrate and gemfibrozil reduce triglycerides by 20% to 50% and increase HDLs by 10% to 15%. The primary use of clofibrate is to treat severe hyperlipidemia in persons with a significant risk of coronary artery disease or at risk for pancreatitis. Gemfibrozil is added to therapy with nicotinic acid or a statin for primary prevention of coronary heart disease in those with elevated LDLs, high triglycerides, and low HDLs. Gemfibrozil is also used to treat severe hyperlipidemia.

Adverse Reactions, Contraindications, and Toxicity

The fibric acid derivatives are generally well tolerated. The most common side effects are GI complaints. Patients with impaired renal or hepatic function may require a reduced dose. This drug class increases the likelihood of developing cholesterol gallstones.

A large trial by the World Health Organization found an increase in overall mortality associated with clofibrate therapy that may be associated with gallstone disease. The Helsinki Heart Study did not find an increased overall mortality associated with gemfibrozil. Clofibrate is not recommended for use during pregnancy because it crosses the placenta. Clofibrate is also excreted in breast milk and should therefore not be taken by nursing mothers. Gemfibrozil may significantly increase LDL values in patients with type IV hyperlipidemia (relatively normal cholesterol but elevated triglycerides) and therefore is not recommended.

ALTERNATIVE THERAPIES

Antihyperlipidemic

GARLIC

Garlic consists of the dried or fresh bulbs of *Alliium sativum* L. of the lily family. The main components of the volatile oil in garlic are sulfur compounds, especially allicin, which is considered to be the most important. Allicin is formed enzymatically when the bulb is crushed or bruised. Allicin is also responsible for the characteristic odor of garlic.

Garlic is considered antibacterial, antifungal, antithrombotic, antihypertensive, and antihyperlipidemic, among others. Of these, the antihyperlipidemic properties of garlic have been the most substantiated. The daily dose is equivalent to 400 to 1200 mg of dried garlic powder, or 2 to 5 g of the fresh bulb, which is equivalent to 2 to 5 mg of allicin. At these doses, garlic may cause discomfort.

Interactions

Fibric acid derivatives can significantly increase the anticoagulant effect of coumarin and indanedione anticoagulants. Clofibrate displaces several drugs from albumin, including coumarins, phenytoin, and tolbutamide. The concurrent use of a statin with gemfibrozil is associated with an increased risk for myopathy, leading to elevated creatine kinase levels and myoglobinuria.

▼ nicotinic acid (Niacin)

Mechanism of Action

Nicotinic acid is a vitamin B_3 (niacin) for which the minimum daily requirement (MDR) is 20 mg. At dosages 10 to 20 times higher than the MDR, niacin is a vasodilator. At dosages 100 to 200 times higher than the MDR, niacin depresses the synthesis of VLDLs by the liver and thereby reduces LDLs. Serum total and LDL cholesterol are lowered by 10% to 25%, triglyceride levels are lowered by 20% to 50%, and HDL cholesterol levels are raised by 15% to 35%.

Pharmacokinetics

Nicotinic acid is readily absorbed from the GI tract and has a short half-life; it is readily excreted unchanged in the urine. A reduction in triglyceride concentration is seen in a few hours, but a reduction in cholesterol concentration is seen only after several days. To reduce side effects, patients are commonly started at 125 mg twice a day and gradually increased to 1.5 to 3 g per day as needed. In addition to being available in tablets, nicotinic acid is also available in extended-release capsules.

Uses

Nicotinic acid is effective in treating most hyperlipidemias. Nicotinic acid or a bile acid sequestrant is the initial medication recommended to lower LDL cholesterol when dietary and other lifestyle modifications have not been effective. LDL cholesterol is usually lowered by 10% to 25%, triglycerides are lowered by 20% to 50%, and HDL cholesterol is usually raised by 15% to 35%.

Adverse Reactions, Contraindications, and Toxicity

The high dosages of nicotinic acid needed as an antilipemic agent produce troublesome side effects in most patients, and only a few patients can tolerate continued use of nicotinic acid. Most patients experience marked flushing because of its vasodilator action. Itching and GI upset are also common side effects. Tolerance to these symptoms may develop; thus the dosage is usually low at first and increased gradually to avoid severe reactions. Niacin can cause or aggravate peptic ulcer, glucose intolerance (diabetes), and high plasma uric acid (gout). Chronic liver disease is a contraindication for use of nicotinic acid. An extended-release form of nicotinic acid is available but is associated with a greater prevalence of hepatotoxicity.

Conjugated Estrogens

Conjugated estrogens have been shown to decrease the risk for coronary heart disease in postmenopausal women by about 50%. The levels of LDL are decreased by 15%, and the levels of HDL are increased by 15%. Triglycerides are also increased. Estrogen may be given alone if the woman has had a hysterectomy. However, women with a uterus should also receive a progestin either cyclically or continuously to reduce the risk of endometrial cancer (see Chapter 70). Although there is concern that estrogen administration may increase the risk for breast cancer, this association has not been substantiated in clinical trials to date. The National Institutes of Health is addressing this concern in the Women's Health Initiative. Estrogen also protects postmenopausal women against osteoporosis. Estrogen given to men not only causes feminization but also increases the incidence of heart attacks.

Nursing Process Overview

Blood Lipid Levels

Assessment

Baseline assessment should include a general physical assessment and weight, serum cholesterol and triglyceride levels, blood pressure, and dietary history. Be sure to include exercise and smoking patterns in the assessment.

Nursing Diagnoses

- Altered health maintenance related to insufficient knowledge of effects of tobacco use
- Altered nutrition: more than body requirements related to lack of knowledge of nutritional needs and exercise
- Altered bowel elimination: diarrhea related to antilipemic therapy
- Health-seeking behaviors: low cholesterol diet, available smoking cessation clinics, or age-appropriate exercise programs

Patient Outcomes

The patient will lose weight to ideal body weight by limiting fat and caloric intake and adhering to a low-fat, low-cholesterol diet. The patient will achieve a lower serum cholesterol level through dietary modification, exercise, and the use of medications, with no intolerable side effects caused by the medications. The patient will stop smoking.

Planning/Implementation

These drugs have few side effects in usual doses. Evaluate new signs or symptoms. Discharge planning should include instruction by the dietitian, particularly if the type of hyperlipidemia can be better treated by dietary restriction or weight loss.

Evaluation

By discharge, ascertain that the patient can explain why and how to take the prescribed drug, when to take it in relation to meals, what anticipated side effects to expect and what to do about them, which symptoms should be reported immediately to the physician, and how to plan meals within prescribed dietary restrictions.

Nursing Implications Summary

General Guidelines: Drugs to Lower Blood Lipid Levels
Nursing in the Community

➤ Many of the drugs cause GI side effects. Forewarn the patient about this. Provide emotional support as needed. Instruct the patient about the importance of taking the drug as prescribed for best effect.

➤ Review the Patient Problems box in Chapter 24 on constipation.

➤ Tell the patient to report persistent or severe diarrhea to the physician.

➤ Teach the patient about necessary changes in diet to lower fat, carbohydrate, and cholesterol intake, as needed; see the Dietary Considerations box on cholesterol earlier in this chapter. Refer the patient to the dietitian as needed. Teach the patients that these drugs must be taken for weeks to months before their full benefit can be seen. If the drugs prove to be beneficial, they may then be prescribed on a long-term basis.

➤ Remind the patient not to discontinue taking the drug without consulting the physician. Doses of other medications may be prescribed based on their effect when the patient is taking the prescribed antilipemic agent. Discontinuing the antilipemic therapy may result in incorrect doses of other drugs being taken. Because antilipemic agents may interfere with absorption of other prescribed drugs, remind the patient to keep all health care providers informed of all drugs being taken.

➤ Emphasize the importance of all prescribed activities, including drug therapy, smoking cessation, exercise, and diet modification in lowering cholesterol and reducing the risk of heart and vascular disease.

Nursing Implications Summary—cont'd

➤ For missed doses, instruct the patient to take the missed dose as soon as remembered unless almost time for the next dose, then omit missed dose and resume regular dosing schedule. Do not double up for missed doses.

➤ It may be appropriate to screen children for the presence of familial hyperlipidemias; if necessary, place them on therapeutic diets to lower lipid levels.

HMG-CoA Reductase Inhibitors (Statins)
Nursing in the Community

➤ Review the general guidelines.

➤ GI discomfort may occur, and a variety of other side effects have been reported. Instruct the patient to report the development of any unexpected sign or symptom.

➤ Instruct the patient to notify the physician immediately if pregnancy is suspected.

➤ For pravastatin and simvastatin, instruct the patient to take doses in the evening or at bedtime. For lovastatin, instruct the patient take doses with the evening meal if ordered once a day, or if ordered more than once a day, to take each dose with a meal or snack.

Bile Acid Sequestrants: cholestyramine and colestipol
Drug Administration

➤ Monitor intake and output, weight, urinalysis, and vital signs. Assess the patient for skin changes and rashes.

➤ Schedule drug administration times to allow as much time as possible between cholestyramine or colestipol and other drugs taken orally. At minimum, other drugs should be taken 1 hour before or 4 hours after cholestyramine or colestipol.

Nursing in the Community

➤ Review the general guidelines.

➤ GI side effects are the most common. Instruct the patient to report the development of any unexpected sign or symptom.

➤ Review all the drugs the patient is taking. Plan a dosing schedule to allow as much time as possible to elapse between the administration of the antilipemic and other medications.

➤ Instruct the patient not to take the powder in dry form. Always mix it with fluid or food or fruit with a high fluid content such as applesauce, crushed pineapple, or thin soups, or with milk in hot or regular breakfast cereals. Fill a glass with 2 ounces of chosen fluid. Put the correct dose of medication on top of the fluid and mix thoroughly. Add an additional 2 to 4 ounces of fluid and again mix thoroughly. Instruct the patient to drink the mixture while the drug is still suspended. The drug will not dissolve in the fluid. Add a little more of the selected beverage to rinse the glass, and drink this also. If a carbonated beverage is chosen, use a large glass to prevent spillover because the mixture will foam up. To prevent swallowing air, especially if a carbonated beverage is chosen, drink the mixture slowly. Take doses before meals and at bedtime as ordered.

➤ Because these drugs interfere with absorption of fat-soluble vitamins, supplemental vitamins may be necessary; consult the physician.

➤ If these drugs are used to treat the pruritus of biliary stasis, the pruritus may reappear if the drug is discontinued.

Fibric Acid Derivative: clofibrate
Nursing in the Community

➤ See the general guidelines.

➤ Nausea and diarrhea are the most common side effects, but others occasionally occur. Tell the patient to report the development of any unexpected sign or symptom. Impotence and decreased libido have occurred; the patient may be reluctant to mention these effects. Assess the patient carefully for sexual side effects. Provide emotional support. It may be possible to change the dose or the drug; consult the physician.

➤ Instruct the patient to notify the physician if pregnancy occurs. Do not take this drug when breast-feeding.

➤ Instruct the patient to take doses with meals to lessen gastric irritation. Nausea may diminish with continued use of the drug.

Fibric Acid Derivative: gemfibrozil
Nursing in the Community

➤ Review the general guidelines.

➤ Instruct the patient to take doses 30 minutes before breakfast and the evening meal.

➤ GI upset is the most common side effect, but others occasionally occur. Tell the patient to report the development of any unexpected sign or symptom.

nicotinic acid (Niacin)
Nursing in the Community

➤ Review the general guidelines.

➤ Most patients experience flushing of the face and neck after taking the high dosage needed for the antilipemic effect. This effect usually diminishes with continued use of the drug. Starting with low dosages and gradually increasing them may also help reduce flushing and pruritus. Flushing may be ameliorated by taking one regular (300 mg) aspirin tablet 30 minutes before the niacin dose (check with physician). GI discomfort may occur, and a variety of other side effects have been reported. Instruct the patient to report the development of any unexpected sign or symptom. Taking doses with meals or milk may reduce GI irritation.

➤ For information about dietary sources of niacin, see the Dietary Considerations box in Chapter 17 on vitamins.

➤ Instruct the patient to swallow extended-release forms whole, without chewing or crushing. Scored tablets may be broken in half. Contents of capsules may be poured into a small amount of food and swallowed but should not be chewed.

➤ Caution diabetic patients to monitor blood glucose levels carefully during periods of dosage adjustment while taking niacin.

➤ Parenteral forms: Niacin may be added to total parenteral nutrition solutions. Intravenous and intramuscular forms are also available to treat deficiency. Administer intravenous doses slowly. See manufacturer's literature for information about dilution and rate of administration.

CHAPTER REVIEW

Application

1. List the four categories of lipoprotein and describe the role of each.
2. What is hyperlipidemia? What causes it?
3. Name drugs and their mechanism of action for lowering triglyceride levels.

Critical Thinking

1. Compare and contrast the bile acid sequestrants, fibric acid derivatives, and HMG-CoA reductase inhibitors. Consider actions, side effects, and potential for patient compliance. Call the pharmacy and find the cost for a 30-day supply of each drug.
2. Develop a teaching plan for the patient who needs to decrease dietary intake of cholesterol.
3. Consider the risk factors identified for coronary heart disease (see Box 21-1). Which ones can you help the patient lower the risk for heart disease?

Reference

Carson MA: The impact of a relaxation technique on the lipid profile, *Nurs Res* 45(5):271-276, 1996.

Drugs to Treat Anemia

OBJECTIVES

After studying this chapter, you should be able to do the following:

- *Explain the role of iron in normal body functioning.*
- *Develop a nursing care plan for the patient receiving iron therapy.*
- *Describe the treatment of iron toxicity.*
- *Explain the treatment of pernicious anemia and develop a nursing care plan for patients who receive vitamin B_{12}.*
- *Outline dietary sources of iron, folic acid, and vitamin B_{12}.*
- *Explain the use of epoetin alfa and develop a nursing care plan for patients receiving it.*

CHAPTER OVERVIEW

This chapter discusses iron, vitamin B_{12}, folic acid, and related agents used to treat anemia. These agents are most commonly associated with anemia of nutritional origin. They play a major role in the production of new red blood cells—the process of hematopoiesis.

Erythropoietin, a growth factor produced by the kidney, promotes the production of red blood cells. Erythropoietin is a product produced with recombinant DNA technology.

THERAPEUTIC RATIONALE: ANEMIA

Iron, vitamin B_{12}, and folic acid are essential for the production of new blood cells. A deficiency results in anemia.

Iron Deficiency Anemia

Iron is available in many foods (see Dietary Considerations box). The absorption of iron from food is regulated. Iron is taken up by active transport into the mucosal cells of the duodenum and upper jejunum in the small intestine. These cells contain the protein ferritin that binds the iron. When ferritin is saturated with iron, further absorption of iron is limited. It remains in the mucosal cells unless transferred to the plasma protein transferrin. Iron not transferred within 5 days is lost in the feces when the mucosal cell is sloughed. Iron bound to transferrin is carried in the plasma and transferred to the proteins ferritin and hemosiderin, which act

as storage forms of iron within the liver, spleen, and bone marrow.

When the intake of iron is inadequate to meet the demand, iron is first taken from the iron stores in hemosiderin and ferritin. Absorption of iron from the gastrointestinal (GI) tract can increase twofold when the ferritin within the mucosal cells is no longer saturated with iron. When iron stores are exhausted and the intake of iron is still inadequate, the newly made red blood cells are small (microcytic) and do not have much color (hypochromic) because there is not enough iron to make an adequate amount of hemoglobin to fill the cells. **Iron deficiency anemia** is therefore a microcytic hypochromic anemia.

Megaloblastic Macrocytic Anemia

Both vitamin B_{12} and folic acid are required for a key reaction in the synthesis of thymidylate, a component of DNA.

Whereas folic acid is the immediate cofactor in this synthesis, vitamin B_{12} regenerates the active form of folic acid. Deficiency of folic acid or vitamin B_{12} results in the release of too few red blood cells. Those red blood cells that are released are large and immature because of the deficiency of DNA synthesis required for cell division and maturation. This condition is a **megaloblastic macrocytic anemia,** or immature large cell anemia. Other tissue cells that turn over rapidly and require active DNA synthesis include some white and mucosal cells of the GI tract. A deficiency in white cell counts and GI upset can appear in vitamin B_{12} or folic acid deficiency.

Vitamin B₁₂ and Pernicious Anemia

Vitamin B_{12} is unique because it requires a special binding protein for transport into the intestinal cells. This binding protein is called **intrinsic factor,** which is produced and released by the parietal cells of the stomach. (Parietal cells also release hydrochloric acid.) **Pernicious anemia** is the relative or complete lack of intrinsic factor so that vitamin B_{12} is no longer absorbed. The body has a large store of vitamin B_{12}, 4 to 5 mg, and a deficiency will not occur for 2 to 5 years after intrinsic factor is no longer released. Stomach atrophy is a normal part of the aging process, and pernicious anemia appears more commonly in patients older than 50 years of age than in younger patients. Any condition that damages the stomach can also cause pernicious anemia.

Anemia Related to Kidney Failure

Chronic renal failure is associated with underproduction of red blood cells. This happens because the kidney is the major producer of the growth factor erythropoietin, which is critical to the production of red blood cells. When the kidneys fail, erythropoietin is not produced in sufficient quantity to maintain adequate red blood cell production in the bone marrow.

 DIETARY CONSIDERATIONS

Iron

Inadequate iron intake contributes to iron deficiency anemia, the most common nutritional deficiency in the United States. Good dietary sources of iron include the following:

- Red meats
- Legumes and nuts
- Whole grains
- Molasses
- Dried fruits
- Organ meats
- Green leafy vegetables
- Enriched bread and cereal
- Brewer's yeast
- Oysters

THERAPEUTIC AGENTS: DRUGS TO TREAT ANEMIA

▼ iron

Mechanism of Action

Iron is an essential component of several key proteins that carry or use oxygen. More than 70% of body iron is part of hemoglobin, the protein of red blood cells that transports oxygen to tissues and carbon dioxide away from tissues. The red color of blood is caused by the iron-oxygen complex in the heme portion of hemoglobin. Iron is also part of several of the electron transport enzymes of the mitochondria responsible for the oxidation-reduction reactions essential to functioning cells.

Pharmacokinetics and Uses

Recycling of the Body's Iron. Given the importance of iron, it is not surprising that the body uses iron efficiently. The total iron content of a 70-kg man is about 4 g, yet iron is reused so efficiently that less than 1 mg of iron is lost daily. Not only is the iron of the red blood cell reused after cell degradation, but 10% to 35% of the iron is in a storage form for use when required. Iron is lost only as body cells are lost through shedding of cells from the GI tract, skin, fingernails, and hair and in fluids such as bile, urine, and sweat.

Iron deficiency anemia commonly results from blood loss or rapid growth. This condition is reflected in the varying requirements for dietary iron. The average American diet contains about 6 mg of iron per 1000 calories, and only 10% of dietary iron is actually absorbed, although up to 20% may be

---

CASE STUDY
Anemia and Pregnancy

Emily and Tom stay after the Prepared Childbirth class this evening to ask you, the RN educator, some questions. Emily is 25 and in the seventh month of her first pregnancy. She says that she has been feeling "so tired and listless" all the time and that she can barely gather enough energy to attend the evening classes. You suspect iron deficiency anemia, and instruct her to call her obstetrician in the morning to check her blood count. The next afternoon she calls you, upset, because the doctor told her that she has anemia. "Isn't that a fatal disease?" she asks.

1. What do you tell Emily about iron deficiency anemia in pregnancy? What is the daily requirement of iron for a pregnant woman?
2. Which form of oral iron preparation contains the largest amount of iron per gram of iron salt consumed?
3. What foods are good dietary sources of iron? Are there any foods that enhance or inhibit the absorption of dietary iron?
4. What patient teaching should be included for Emily?

absorbed in iron-deficient individuals. Adult men and post-menopausal women have the lowest daily requirement for dietary iron (5 to 10 mg). Menstruating women have a higher daily requirement, depending on the amount of blood loss during menstruation (7 to 20 mg). Pregnant women have the highest daily requirement (20 to 58 mg) because of the added demand of the placenta and developing fetus. Children and adolescents have a higher requirement per unit weight (4 to 20 mg total) than adults because of their rapid growth.

Administration of iron. Iron for replacement therapy is most commonly given orally as a **ferrous salt**. Iron preparations are listed in Table 22-1. Ferrous sulfate is the standard for

Table 22-1 Drugs to Treat Nutritional Anemias

Generic Name	Trade Name	Administration/Dosage	Comments
Iron Salts for Iron Deficiency Anemia			
ferrous fumarate (33% elemental iron)	Femiron Fumerin Palafer† Various others	Replacement therapy requires 90-300 mg of elemental iron daily in divided doses before meals if tolerated or with meals.	Timed-release or enteric-coated forms ARE considered less effective because of poor iron absorption beyond duodenum.
ferrous gluconate (11.6% elemental iron)	Fergon Fertinic† Various others	See above.	See above.
ferrous sulfate (20% elemental iron)	Feosol Fer-In-Sol* Fero-Gradumet Various others	See above.	See above.
iron-dextran injection	DexFerrum DexIron†	INTRAVENOUS: *Adults and children*—No more than 100 mg daily, no faster than 50 mg (1 ml)/min of undiluted solution, or dilute in 500-1000 ml normal saline solution and administer by drip over 10 hr. FDA pregnancy category C.	Reserved for use in severe iron deficiency anemia when oral iron is contraindicated (gastrointestinal disease) or unsuccessful. Serious toxic effects, including anaphylaxis, may accompany parenteral administration and are more common with IM than with IV administration.
iron-polysaccharide complex	Hytinic Niferex	See above.	Not well absorbed. May be milder to stomach than other formulations.
Antidote for Iron Toxicity			
deferoxamine mesylate	Desferal*	INTRAMUSCULAR: Initially 90 mg/kg followed by 45 mg every 4-12 hr; not to exceed 6 g/day. INTRAVENOUS: In face of cardiovascular collapse; as IM but infused at 15 mg/kg/hr. Not to exceed 6 g in 24 hr.	A specific chelator for iron. To manage acute iron intoxication. Will turn urine pink to red. Can be administered long term to manage secondary hemochromatosis.
Vitamin B$_{12}$ (Cyanocobalamin) for Pernicious Anemia			
hydroxocobalamin	Alphamin Various others	As for cyanocobalamin.	Like cyanocobalamin. Somewhat longer acting.
vitamin B$_{12}$ (cyanocobalamin)	Anacobin† Cobex Rubramin PC Various others	INTRAMUSCULAR: 100 μg daily for 6-7 days, then 100 μg every other day for 7 doses; maintenance: 100-200 μg monthly.	For pernicious anemia, only IM injection effective. Oral forms taken for dietary deficiency. RDA is 2 μg daily for healthy adults.
Folic Acid for Anemia			
folic acid	Apo-Folic† Folvite*	ANY ROUTE: *Adults and children*—1 mg daily.	Solutions of sodium salt used for parenteral administration. RDA is 400 μg for healthy adults.
leucovorin calcium	Wellcovorin Generic	For megaloblastic anemia, 1 mg daily. To counter folic acid antagonists, give in amounts equal to weight of antagonist.	Metabolically active form of folic acid. Expense does not justify use for anemia, but protects normal tissue when given with methotrexate (antineoplastic drug) or pyrimethamine (antimalarial drug).
Hormone for Anemia			
epoetin alfa, recombinant	Epogen Eprex† Procrit	INTRAVENOUS, SUBCUTANEOUS: *Adults and children*—Initially, 50-100 units/kg 3 times weekly. Dosage is adjusted to reach hematocrit of 30%-33%.	Epoetin is protein hormone, erythropoietin, produced by recombinant DNA technology. Used to treat anemia of chronic renal failure.

*Available in Canada and the United States.
†Available in Canada only.

these preparations. The usual daily dose of iron in iron deficiency anemia is 50 to 100 mg. The amount of iron per tablet depends on the ferrous salt used. A 300-mg tablet of ferrous sulfate contains 60 mg of iron and 240 mg of sulfate; a 300-mg tablet of ferrous gluconate contains 37 mg of iron and 263 mg of gluconate; and a 300-mg tablet of ferrous fumarate contains 99 mg of iron and 201 mg of fumarate.

Iron in the ferrous form is absorbed most readily in the presence of acid. Therefore optimum absorption occurs when a tablet of ferrous sulfate or other soluble ferrous salt is taken before meals. However, iron is also highly irritating to the GI tract; many patients cannot tolerate iron tablets taken on an empty stomach and have to take iron with meals. Enteric forms are not satisfactory because they generally dissolve past the duodenum, where there is little capacity for the absorption of iron. Infants and children given iron-supplemented formula or vitamins may develop acute diarrhea from the GI irritation.

Patients with iron deficiency anemia respond to iron therapy in the first 2 days with increased energy and appetite. Because this is too soon to correct the hemoglobin deficiency, the response may be caused by restoration of the cellular enzymes containing iron. After 1 week there is an increase in the number of reticulocytes (immature red blood cells) and the rate of hemoglobin synthesis. Although the microcytic anemia of iron deficiency is eliminated after a few weeks of therapy, at least 6 months of therapy is necessary to restore iron storage sites.

Iron may also be given parenterally as iron dextran when oral administration is not possible. Slow intravenous (IV) injection is preferred. If administered by deep intramuscular (IM) injection, the "Z-track" injection technique is used to avoid discoloration of the injection site. An anaphylactic response is more common after IM than after IV injection.

Adverse Reactions and Contraindications

Iron taken orally can cause GI discomfort. Infants are especially sensitive to the iron in infant formulas and vitamins. Liquid dosage forms can stain the teeth. More seriously, iron can occasionally cause an allergic reaction with skin rash or hives and trouble breathing. This reaction is more common after parenteral administration. Iron is contraindicated for persons with hemochromatosis or hemosiderosis and for those with hemolytic anemia or thalassemia.

Toxicity

Acute Toxicity. Acute toxicity from iron is uncommon in adults and is primarily seen in young children. The population most likely to take iron tablets includes pregnant women who may also have small children. Many iron tablets are brightly colored and look like candy, leading young children to swallow many tablets at once. The child often experiences acute nausea and vomiting 30 to 60 minutes after ingesting the tablets. Treatment is gastric lavage with sodium phosphate or sodium bicarbonate to remove undissolved tablets, to create an alkaline environment that re-

tards absorption, and to complex the ferrous iron into insoluble salts.

Within a few hours of ingestion, metabolic acidosis is common and cardiovascular collapse can occur. If supportive treatment carries the child through these stages, the next stage originates from tissue injury. The high concentration of iron overloads the uptake capacity of the mucosal cells so that a high concentration of free ferrous iron enters the portal circulation. Signs of extensive damage to the liver and kidney are evident in children who die of iron toxicity after 24 hours.

deferoxamine. To avoid damage from high plasma concentrations of iron, a specific antidote, deferoxamine mesylate (Desferal), is given as soon as possible and concurrently with lavage and supportive measures. Deferoxamine is given intravenously or intravenously and combines with iron in the plasma to form a water-soluble complex that is excreted in urine (67%) and in bile (33%). This complex gives a pink to red color to urine, which shows elevated concentrations of iron in the plasma. The free deferoxamine imparts no color to urine.

Chronic Toxicity. Because the body has no mechanisms to remove excess iron, excess intake can cause iron overload, called **hemosiderosis** (after the storage protein for iron). Chronic iron overload can occur in patients treated with parenteral iron who receive frequent blood transfusions because each milliliter of blood contains 0.5 mg of iron. Some patients have a genetic tendency to store excess iron; this genetic disorder is called **hemochromatosis**. Iron overload traditionally imparts a bronze color to the skin of the face, neck, upper chest, genitalia, hands, and forearms. The pancreas is especially sensitive to damage, and diabetes mellitus can result. Liver damage is seen on biopsy but is generally not serious unless superimposed on liver disease. Patients with iron overload generally die of heart failure. Treatment for iron overload is weekly bleeding (phlebotomy).

Interactions

Absorption of iron salts is increased with ingestion of large doses of ascorbic acid (vitamin C). Cereal and eggs decrease absorption, as do antacids, particularly magnesium trisilicate, and tetracyclines because all these bind to iron and prevent its uptake by the mucosal cells in the small intestine.

vitamin B$_{12}$
Mechanism of Action

Vitamin B$_{12}$ is required for the synthesis of thymidylate, a component of DNA. Deficiency of vitamin B$_{12}$, like folic acid, affects the maturation of red blood cells and results in a megaloblastic macrocytic anemia. In addition, vitamin B$_{12}$ is required for maintenance of the myelin sheath of nerves.

Pharmacokinetics

A diet that includes animal protein, eggs, and dairy products contains adequate vitamin B$_{12}$. The usual American diet contains 5 to 15 mg of vitamin B$_{12}$, although the minimum daily requirement is only 1 to 2 mg. Only strict vegetarians may develop dietary vitamin B$_{12}$ deficiency over several years. Vitamin B$_{12}$ bound to intrinsic factor is absorbed in the distal ileum, the part of the small intestine just ahead of the large intestine, and this absorption requires a slightly alkaline pH. Conditions in which the distal ileum is damaged or removed or in which the pancreas fails to secrete sufficient bicarbonate to keep the intestine at a slightly alkaline pH slow absorption of vitamin B$_{12}$. After absorption, vitamin B$_{12}$ is carried to storage sites. Some vitamin B$_{12}$ is excreted in the bile but is later reabsorbed.

The IM injection of vitamin B$_{12}$ to bypass the intestine for systemic absorption is the treatment for pernicious anemia. Initial therapy is administered daily for about 1 week, then monthly throughout life. Oral vitamin B$_{12}$ is indicated only for the rare dietary deficiency of vitamin B$_{12}$ when there is an adequate amount of intrinsic factor released.

Uses

Vitamin B$_{12}$ is indicated for the treatment of pernicious anemia. Neurologic damage may result from deficiency of vitamin B$_{12}$. This damage arises because vitamin B$_{12}$ is a cofactor for an enzymatic step necessary for producing the myelin sheath of nerves. A common initial neurologic symptom of vitamin B$_{12}$ deficiency is a tingling sensation of the extremities (paresthesia) from neurologic damage. Neurologic damage becomes irreversible if vitamin B$_{12}$ deficiency persists.

Vitamin B$_{12}$ injections have been given indiscriminately to older adult patients as a general tonic, which it is not. Vitamin B$_{12}$ injections are also not of therapeutic value for general neurologic disorders, psychiatric disorders, general malnutrition, or loss of appetite.

Adverse Reactions, Contraindications, and Toxicity

Vitamin B$_{12}$ injections are virtually free of side effects. Patients who receive vitamin B$_{12}$ injections for pernicious anemia must understand that injections must be continued for the rest of their lives to avoid irreversible neurologic damage.

Interactions

Folic acid taken in large doses will overcome the block in DNA synthesis caused by the deficiency of vitamin B$_{12}$. Folic acid will thereby cure the anemia, but folic acid cannot affect the vitamin B$_{12}$–dependent reaction necessary for myelin synthesis. If folic acid is taken indiscriminately, the anemia of vitamin B$_{12}$ deficiency will never appear, but neurologic damage may proceed until it is irreversible.

▼ folic acid

Mechanism of Action

Like vitamin B$_{12}$, **folic acid** is required for the synthesis of thymidylate, a component of DNA. Deficiency of folic acid, like vitamin B$_{12}$, affects the maturation of red blood cells and results in a megaloblastic macrocytic anemia.

Pharmacokinetics

Folic acid is found in most meats, fresh vegetables, and fresh fruits, but it is destroyed when these foods are cooked for longer than 15 minutes. Folic acid preparations are listed in Table 22-1. The minimum daily requirement is 50 μg, and the average American diet contains 200 to 300 μg. Unlike vitamin B$_{12}$, stores of folic acid are not large and can be depleted in a few weeks when the diet is deficient in folic acid. It is readily absorbed in the intestine and administered orally. Individuals with poor diets and chronic alcoholics may be deficient in folic acid.

Uses and Interactions

Pregnant women and nursing mothers have increased requirements for folic acid, and this agent is commonly given as a routine supplement to these women. Studies have shown that 400μg folic acid taken daily during pregnancy reduces the incidence of neurologic defects in newborn infants.

Methotrexate, antineoplastic drugs, and pyrimethamine (an antimalarial drug) are folic acid antagonists. When these drugs are used, folinic acid (leucovorin), the metabolically active form of folic acid, can be given to protect normal tissues from folic acid deficiency. Other drugs that interfere with the use of folic acid include phenytoin, oral contraceptives, glucocorticoids, and aspirin.

Adverse Reactions, Contraindications, and Toxicity

Folic acid is nontoxic. The greatest danger associated with the indiscriminate ingestion of folic acid is that it may correct the anemia of pernicious anemia but leave the neurologic damage untreated.

▼ epoetin alfa
Mechanism of Action

Epoetin alfa (Epogen and Eprex, Procrit) is the human hormone erythropoietin, manufactured by recombinant DNA technology, that stimulates the production of red blood cells.

Pharmacokinetics

Epoetin alfa is a protein and must be administered intravenously or subcutaneously. It is commonly administered three times a week. The effect is seen in 1 to 2 weeks. The dosage should not be adjusted for 8 weeks, and it should not be changed more often than every 4 weeks. The dosage should be discontinued gradually by lowering the dose by 25 units/kg body weight every 4 weeks.

Uses

Epoetin counteracts the anemia associated with chronic renal failure. This effect eliminates the need for transfusion of red blood cells and greatly improves the patient's quality of life. Patients should be evaluated to ensure that they have adequate iron stores to support red blood cell production. Epoetin is being evaluated for treatment of anemia resulting in a number of other conditions, including azathioprine (AZT) treatment and cancer.

Adverse Reactions, Contraindications, and Toxicity

Side effects of epoetin are minimal. Occasional headaches and joint pain are reported. About one third of patients have elevated blood pressure that may require drug therapy. However, renal function does not worsen. Epoetin should not be administered to individuals with uncontrolled hypertension.

Abuse of epoetin has been reported among athletes in high-endurance sports, especially cyclists. The increased production of red blood cells enhances athletic performance by increasing the blood's ability to carry oxygen. The increased number of red blood cells makes the blood more viscous, and this viscosity is enhanced by the dehydration of performance. Death from heart blockage was reported in one young athlete who was taking epoetin.

Nursing Process Overview

Iron Therapy

Assessment

Patients who require iron therapy may have fatigue, pallor, and lethargy. Folic acid and vitamin B_{12} deficiency are usually diagnosed from blood studies but may be seen in patients with iron deficiency anemia. Assess vital signs, weight, and diet history; blood studies, including hemoglobin level, peripheral blood smear, and reticulocyte count; and any neurologic symptoms such as tingling in the fingers or toes.

Nursing Diagnoses

- Altered bowel elimination: constipation related to iron therapy
- Fatigue related to anemia

Patient Outcomes

The patient will display increased energy and less pallor as anemia is treated. The patient will state that his or her energy level is better.

Planning/Implementation

At usual dosages, few side effects occur with these drugs. If the source of anemia is diet related, provide dietary instruction about iron-rich foods. If pernicious anemia is diagnosed, instruct the patient about the need for continued treatment.

Evaluation

Determine that the patient can explain what kind of anemia is present, what the goals of drug therapy are, how to take the prescribed medications correctly, what anticipated side effects are and what to do about them, and which symptoms can be expected to improve and which will not. (The neurologic damage in pernicious anemia may be permanent.) Verify that the patient can identify dietary sources of needed iron or folic acid.

Nursing Implications Summary

General Guidelines: Patient Receiving Iron Therapy

Drug Administration

➤ Do not administer parenteral and oral iron preparations concurrently because this combination increases the incidence of toxic reactions.

➤ Parenteral doses of iron may cause anaphylactic reactions. Before giving the first dose of IM or IV iron dextran, administer a test dose of 25 mg. Monitor the vital signs. Wait at least 1 hour before administering the remaining dose. Have available appropriate equipment, drugs, and personnel to treat anaphylactic reactions. Other reactions may include febrile reactions, arthralgias, myalgia, headache, transitory paresthesias, nausea, shivering, and rash.

➤ Monitor hemoglobin and hematocrit.

Intramuscular iron dextran

➤ Use large muscle masses, preferably the buttocks. The drug may stain the skin, which is cosmetically unacceptable on the

thigh. Consult the physician when administering this drug to small children and infants. Draw up the prescribed dose. Put a fresh needle on the syringe. Use the Z-track method of administration (see Chapter 5).

Intravenous iron dextran

➤ Read the vial carefully; use preparations labeled "for IV use." The drug may be given undiluted or diluted in 50 to 250 ml normal saline solution. Administer a test dose over at least 5 minutes. Administer other doses at a rate of 50 mg/min. Flush the IV line with normal saline solution before and after administering dose. Keep the patient in a supine position for 30 minutes after IV doses; monitor vital signs and blood pressure.

Nursing in the Community

➤ Review the dietary sources of iron with the patient (see the Dietary Considerations box earlier in this chapter on iron). Remind the patient to keep all medications out of the reach

Nursing Implications Summary—cont'd

of children. Instruct the family to have ipecac available when iron preparations are in use but always to call the poison control center or emergency department before using ipecac to induce vomiting. Tell the patient to notify the physician immediately if overdose with iron is suspected.

➤ Instruct the patient to take liquid iron preparations through a straw to avoid staining the teeth. Teach the patient to dilute the preparation well with water or fruit juice and to rinse the mouth thoroughly after taking the dose. If doses must be administered with a dropper, place dose in the back of the mouth and follow with water or juice. Advise the patient to brush teeth with baking soda or hydrogen peroxide 3% to remove stains.

➤ Ideally, instruct the patient to take the iron preparation on an empty stomach, 1 hour before or 2 hours after meals, although this may cause significant GI upset. Teach the patient to take doses with a full glass (240 ml) of fluid for an adult or one half glass (120 ml) of fluid for children. Teach the patient to take drug with meals or snack to reduce gastric irritation. Take iron 2 hours after or 1 hour before eating cheese, yogurt, eggs, milk, spinach, tea, coffee, whole-grain breads and cereals, or bran. Do not take iron at the same time as antacids or calcium supplements; space doses of these 1 to 2 hours apart. Ascorbic acid (vitamin C) increases the absorption of iron; some patients may wish to take the iron with orange or other citrus juice.

➤ Inform the patient that regular use of iron will cause the feces to turn dark green or black and to become more tarry in consistency. Patients who have no change in stool should notify the physician. If there is doubt about whether the cause of a change in color or consistency in stools is caused by blood or ingestion of iron, test the stool for the presence of blood.

➤ Most patients experience constipation while taking iron preparations; some experience diarrhea (see the Patient Problems box in Chapter 24 on constipation). If diarrhea is severe or persistent, notify the physician. To decrease gastric irritation, suggest that the patient take smaller but more frequent doses of iron (check with the physician).

deferoxamine mesylate
Drug Administration
➤ See Chapter 9.
➤ Deferoxamine may be administered via IM, IV, or subcutaneous (SC) injection, usually by subcutaneous pump. IM or SC injection may cause swelling, irritation, pain, and itching at the injection site.
➤ Deferoxamine has been associated with allergic reactions, including anaphylactic reactions. Monitor vital signs. Have equipment and drugs available to treat acute allergic reactions.

Intravenous Deferoxamine
➤ Dilute as directed in the manufacturer's literature. Administer at a rate not exceeding 15 mg/kg/hr. Monitor the blood

pressure and vital signs. Treatment of acute iron overdose should be done in the acute-care setting.

vitamin B₁₂
Drug Administration
➤ Administer parenteral doses via the IM route only.
➤ Allergic reactions have been reported. Monitor vital signs and blood pressure. Have available drugs and equipment to treat acute allergic responses.

Nursing in the Community
➤ Teach patients with pernicious anemia about their disease. It may be difficult for them to understand why the vitamin B₁₂ cannot be taken orally and why it must be continued for life.
➤ Review dietary sources of vitamin B₁₂ (see the Dietary Considerations box in Chapter 17 on vitamins) with patients in whom vitamin B₁₂ deficiency is due to dietary causes. Strict vegetarians may require vitamin supplements that contain vitamin B₁₂.
➤ Instruct patients to limit the consumption of alcohol while taking vitamin B₁₂.

folic acid
Drug Administration
➤ In addition to the more common oral administration, folic acid may be given by the IM, IV, or SC route.
➤ IV folic acid may be given undiluted or added to most IV solutions and given as an infusion. For direct IV administration, administer at a rate not to exceed 5 mg/min.
➤ Allergic reactions, although rare, have been reported. Monitor vital signs after parenteral administration. Have drugs and equipment available to treat acute allergic reactions.

Nursing in the Community
➤ Review the dietary sources of folic acid (see the Dietary Considerations box in Chapter 17 on vitamins).
➤ Warn the patient that self-treatment with large doses of vitamins is unwise and may mask some health problems. Large doses of vitamins should be taken only under the direction of a physician.

leucovorin
Drug Administration/Nursing in the Community
➤ Leucovorin is the calcium salt of folinic acid, a metabolite of folic acid. It is not affected by folic acid antagonists. Read the physician's orders carefully. The drug may be given orally, intramuscularly, or intravenously. Parenteral administration is usually used when the drug is given to counteract some of the toxic effects of the folic acid antagonists, especially some cancer chemotherapy drugs (called leucovorin rescue) (see Chapter 55). It may also be used in combination with fluorouracil in treatment of advanced colorectal cancer.

Parenteral Administration
➤ Reconstitute as directed on the vial. For total doses less than 10 mg/m², dilute with bacteriostatic water that contains benzyl alcohol as a preservative for injection. For doses greater

Continued

Nursing Implications Summary—cont'd

than 10 mg/m², use sterile water without a preservative. Further dilute in 100 to 500 ml of common IV fluid. Administer dilute volume at a rate not exceeding 160 mg/min because of the calcium content. Monitor vital signs.

➤ For leucovorin rescue/folinic acid rescue, several protocols may be used. The dose is based on the dose of methotrexate and the body surface area of the patient. Monitor the serum creatinine level.

➤ Review with the patient and family the reason leucovorin is being used. Instruct them to report the development of any unexpected sign or symptom.

epoetin alfa
Drug Administration

➤ This drug may be given undiluted as an IV bolus. Read the accompanying literature. Do not shake the vial. Prepare only 1 dose per single-dose vial. Discard the multiple-dose vial after 21 days. The multiple-dose vial contains benzyl alcohol as a preservative. Because of this, do not use the multiple-dose vial to prepare doses for neonates.

➤ Administer the dose over at least 1 minute. For dialysis patients, it may be administered via the venous line at the end of dialysis. This agent may also be administered intravenously or subcutaneously in patients not receiving dialysis. Monitor blood pressure, and report increases to the physician.

➤ Dose and length of therapy are based on patient response. Monitor the complete blood cell count with differential, platelet count, hematocrit, blood urea nitrogen, uric acid, serum creatinine, phosphorus, serum electrolytes, and serum uric acid.

➤ Assess patients for chest pain, edema, rash, hives, bone pain, muscle weakness, diarrhea, vomiting. Some patients develop flulike symptoms 1 to 2 hours after drug administration; the symptoms may last up to 12 hours. Monitor vital signs and blood pressure.

Nursing in the Community

➤ Although usually given by a nurse, this drug may be prescribed for self-administration at home by some patients. Teach the patient how to administer and have the patient give a return demonstration of the injection technique.

➤ This drug may cause seizures, especially during the first 90 days. This side effect is rare, but caution the patient to avoid driving or operating hazardous equipment during this period until the effects of the medication are known.

➤ Review the reasons for epoetin therapy. Instruct the patient to report the development of any new sign or symptom. Emphasize the importance of returning for scheduled follow-up visits and taking doses as ordered, even if the patient is feeling better. Emphasize the importance of prescribed therapies, including other medications and special dietary restrictions.

CHAPTER REVIEW

Application

1. What is the role of iron?
2. Describe factors governing the absorption of iron.
3. What are the symptoms of iron toxicity?
4. How does deferoxamine function as an antidote for iron toxicity?
5. What is pernicious anemia?
6. Why does vitamin B₁₂ have to be injected intramuscularly to treat pernicious anemia?
7. What role do vitamin B₁₂ and folic acid play in red blood cell maturation?

8. Why is folic acid contraindicated for treatment of pernicious anemia?
9. Why is chronic renal failure associated with underproduction of red blood cells?

Critical Thinking

1. Why is iron poisoning so dangerous in young children?
2. What are important teaching points about epoetin alfa?
3. How would you respond to a student athlete colleague who wants to know about epoetin to increase athletic endurance?

Drugs Affecting Motility: Cholinergic Stimulants and Anticholinergics/Antispasmodics

OBJECTIVES

After studying this chapter, you should be able to do the following:

- *Discuss the use of drugs that alter gastrointestinal tone and motility.*

- *Develop a nursing care plan for patients receiving the following drugs or drug groups: bethanechol, cisapride, metoclopramide, neostigmine, belladonna alkaloids, atropine and related drugs, and antispasmodics.*

- *Develop a teaching plan for patients who have xerostomia.*

CHAPTER OVERVIEW

Motility of the gastrointestinal (GI) system is controlled at two levels (Figure 23-1). The higher level of control is through the autonomic nervous system. The cholinergic nervous system stimulates GI activity. The local control of smooth muscle tone is modulated by two major nerve plexuses that provide the intrinsic control and use acetylcholine as the neurotransmitter. These two intrinsic nerve plexuses are the myenteric plexus, located between the longitudinal and circular layers of the intestinal smooth muscle, and the submucous nerve plexus, located in the submucosal region. These local nerve complexes not only respond to local events but are subject to regulation by the autonomic nervous system. The release of acetylcholine from the cholinergic neurons to the ganglia of the intrinsic nerve plexuses is controlled by dopaminergic presynaptic receptors.

Drugs that mimic acetylcholine or stimulate its release promote GI motility. Drugs that antagonize acetylcholine or its release inhibit GI motility.

THERAPEUTIC RATIONALE: GASTRIC HYPOMOTILITY

Gastric hypomotility is characterized by delayed emptying of liquid and solid contents. This condition can arise after surgery or result from conditions such as gastroesophageal reflux disease, diabetic gastroparesis, or gastric stasis. Atonic conditions of the intestine include intestinal atony, pseudoobstruction, and adynamic colon. Symptoms may include nausea, vomiting, heartburn, and indigestion.

THERAPEUTIC AGENTS: GASTROINTESTINAL STIMULANTS

Drugs used to treat an atonic GI tract act directly or indirectly to stimulate the muscarinic receptors of the intrinsic nervous system that control motility in the intestine. The cholinomimetic drugs bethanechol and neostigmine act at the level of the smooth muscle. Metoclopramide, a dopaminergic antagonist, acts at presynaptic dopamine receptors of the parasympathetic nervous system to promote

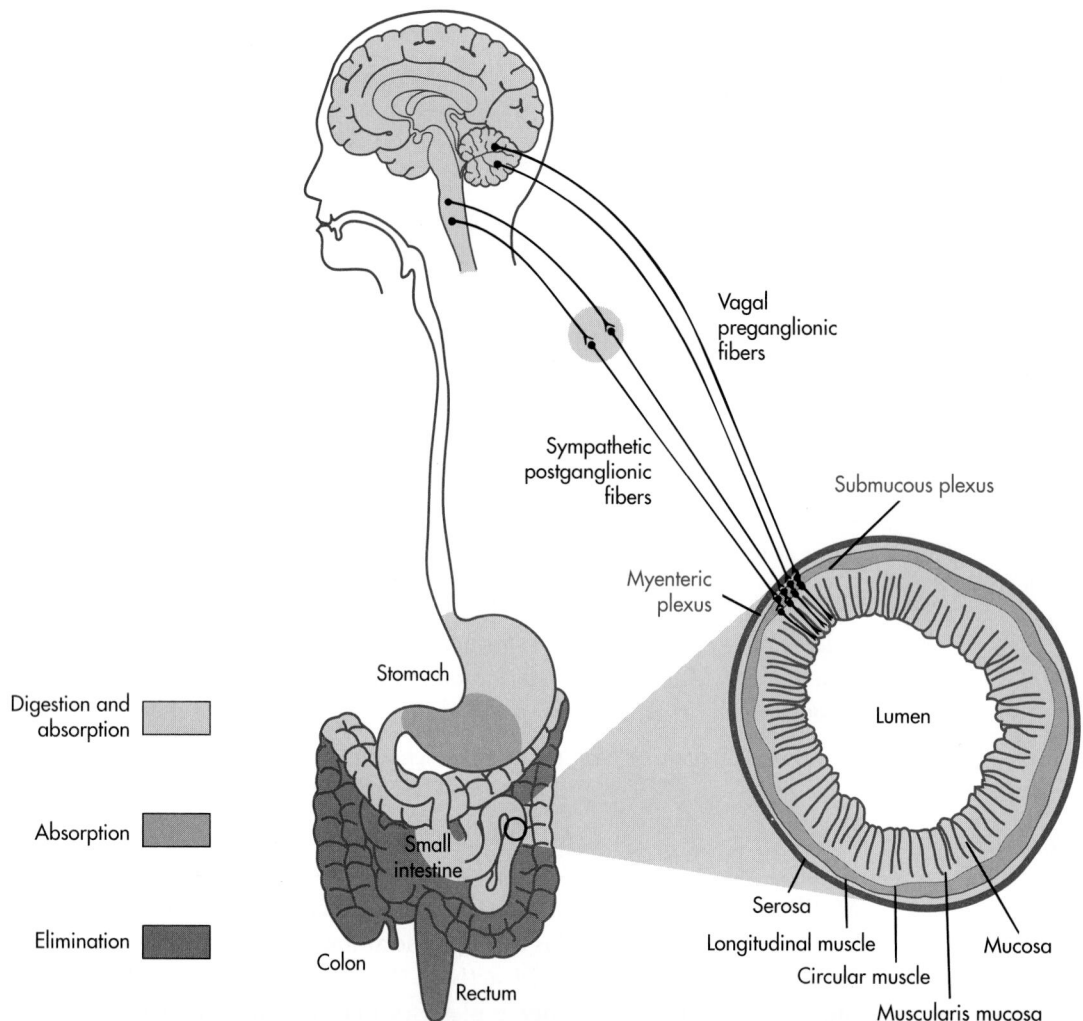

Figure 23-1   Overall functions of the gastrointestinal tract. Autonomic nervous system modulates longitudinal musculature of the small intestine. The small intestine also has a complex intrinsic autonomic system controlling circular musculature and secretion.

release of acetylcholine. Cisapride stimulates the release of acetylcholine by an action on the myenteric plexus. These drugs are listed in Table 23-1.

bethanechol

Mechanism of Action

Bethanechol (Urecholine) is the only direct-acting cholinomimetic drug with sufficient tissue specificity to be administered systemically. It directly stimulates muscarinic receptors in the intestinal smooth muscle.

Pharmacokinetics

Bethanechol may be administered orally or subcutaneously. Absorption is rapid and complete. The onset of action is 30 to 60 minutes with a half-life of 7 to 10 hours. Bethanechol is metabolized by the liver and excreted in the urine.

Uses

At therapeutic doses bethanechol is relatively specific for the urinary and GI tracts. The stimulation it produces is use-

ful for situations in which the bladder or intestine has lost its tone, such as after childbirth, surgery, or other abdominal trauma.

Adverse Reactions and Contraindications

Side effects of bethanechol are expected from muscarinic stimulation such as salivation, flushing of the skin, sweating, diarrhea, nausea and belching, and abdominal cramps. Because of these widespread side effects, the use of bethanechol has decreased with the introduction of newer agents.

Bethanechol should never be administered if there is any mechanical obstruction of the GI or urinary tract, such as stones or adhesions, because the hypermotility caused by the drug could lead to rupture of the tissue in the presence of an obstruction. Also, bethanechol is never administered intravenously or intramuscularly because the rate of absorption is so fast that toxic plasma concentrations of the drug are reached, resulting in possible heart block or a severe drop in blood pressure. Bethanechol may be administered subcutaneously if the oral route is not effective.

Table 23-1   Drugs to Increase Gastrointestinal Tone and Motility

Generic Name	Trade Name	Administration/Dosage	Comments
bethanechol chloride	Duvoid* Urabeth Urecholine*	ORAL: *Adults*—10-50 mg every 6-8 hr. SUBCUTANEOUS: *Adults*—2.5-5 mg every 6-8 hr; maximum, 10 mg/day. Never give intravenously or intramuscularly. Onset: 30 min. FDA pregnancy category C.	Direct-acting cholinomimetic that stimulates atonic bladder and gastrointestinal tract.
cisapride	Propulsid*	ORAL: *Adults—Prophylaxis for gastroesophageal reflux:* 10 mg 2 times/day, before breakfast and at bedtime or 20 mg at bedtime. *Treatment:* 5-10 mg every 6-8 hr, 15 min before meals and at bedtime. FDA pregnancy category C. *Children*—0.15-0.3 mg/kg body weight every 6-8 hr, before meals.	Serotonin antagonist; treats gastroesophageal reflux.
domperidone†	Motilium†	ORAL: *Adults*—10 mg 3 or 4 times/day before meals, bedtime. *Children*—0.3 mg/kg 3 or 4 times/day before meals, bedtime.	Dopamine antagonist that hastens gastric emptying in diabetic gastroparesis and after barium administration. Related to metoclopramide but does not cross blood-brain barrier.
metoclopramide	Apo-Metoclop† Clopra Emex† Maxeran† Octamide Reclomide Reglan*	INTRAVENOUS: *Adults—Peristaltic stimulant:* 10 mg injected over 1-2 min. *Children*—1 mg/kg body weight; may repeat 1 time after 60 min. ORAL: *Adults*—10 mg 30 min before each meal and at bedtime. FDA pregnancy category B. *Children 6-14 yr*—2.5-5.0 mg 3 times/day 30 min before meals. Onset: 1-3 min IV; 30-60 min orally.	Dopamine antagonist that hastens gastric emptying in diabetic gastroparesis and after barium administration. Antiemetic for chemotherapy.
neostigmine methylsulfate	Prostigmin*	SUBCUTANEOUS, INTRAMUSCULAR: *Adults*—0.25-0.5 mg every 3-4 hr to stimulate bladder or gastrointestinal tract. Onset: 10-20 min. FDA pregnancy category C.	Acetylcholinesterase inhibitor used postsurgically to stimulate atonic bladder and gastrointestinal tract.

*Available in Canada and the United States.
†Available in Canada only.

Interactions

Bethanechol interferes with anticholinergic or ganglionic blocking drugs. Bethanechol synergizes the action of cholinergic agents, especially cholinesterase inhibitors.

cisapride

Mechanism of Action

Cisapride (Propulsid) is a serotonin receptor antagonist that increases the release of acetylcholine from the myenteric plexus. This action increases several activities, including esophageal clearance, tone of the lower esophageal sphincter, gastric emptying, and propulsion in the small intestine and colon.

Pharmacokinetics

Cisapride is absorbed rapidly and completely after oral administration. The onset of action is 30 to 60 minutes with a half-life of 7 to 10 hours. Cisapride is metabolized by the liver and excreted in the urine and feces.

Uses

Cisapride is used to manage gastroesophageal reflux disease, diabetic gastroparesis, intestinal atony, and adynamic colon. Treatment may continue for 2 to 3 months, but tolerance will often develop, limiting effectiveness.

Adverse Reactions and Contraindications

The most common side effect is diarrhea, which is dose dependent. Abdominal cramping, nausea, headache, and fatigue are other side effects sometimes reported. Rarely, seizures have been reported in patients with a history of seizures.

Cisapride is contraindicated for patients with GI hemorrhage, mechanical obstruction, or perforation. Dosage should be reduced for patients with hepatic or renal insufficiency because of the reduced clearance of cisapride. Nursing mothers should not take the drug because small amounts appear in breast milk.

Interactions

The absorption of cimetidine and ranitidine is accelerated because of the increased gastric emptying. The sedative effects of benzodiazepines and alcohol are enhanced. **Anticholinergic drugs** antagonize the effect of cisapride.

▼ metoclopramide

Mechanism of Action

Metoclopramide (Reglan, others) is a dopamine antagonist that promotes the release of acetylcholine from the myenteric plexus. It stimulates motility of the upper GI tract without stimulating gastric, biliary, or pancreatic secretions. The tone and amplitude of gastric contractions are increased, as is peristalsis of the small intestine, so gastric emptying and intestinal transit times are increased.

Pharmacokinetics

Metoclopramide may be administered intramuscularly, intravenously, and orally. The onset of action is 10 to 15 minutes after intramuscular injection and 30 to 60 minutes after oral administration. The half-life is 4 to 6 hours. Metoclopramide crosses the blood-brain barrier and can produce effects in the central nervous system (CNS). The drug is excreted in the urine as unchanged drug and sulfate and glucuronide conjugates.

Uses

The gastrostimulatory action of metoclopramide is useful in treating diabetic gastroparesis, a condition in which stomach tone is lost and contents are not emptied readily into the intestine. Metoclopramide also facilitates intubation of the small intestine for biopsy and stimulates gastric emptying and intestinal transit of barium in radiologic examinations.

Metoclopramide is also effective as an antiemetic, probably through a CNS action in the chemoreceptor trigger zone and vomiting center. The antiemetic effect is especially helpful in controlling emesis that occurs during cancer chemotherapy, especially with cisplatin or cyclophosphamide (see Chapter 25).

Adverse Reactions and Contraindications

About 10% of patients experience the side effects of metoclopramide, including restlessness, drowsiness, fatigue, and lassitude. Metoclopramide is contraindicated in patients with mechanical obstruction, perforation, or possible hemorrhage of the GI tract. An increase in GI motility poses danger for such patients.

Interactions

Anticholinergic drugs and narcotic analgesics inhibit GI tone and thereby antagonize the action of metoclopramide. Sedation is intensified with the concurrent use of alcohol, tranquilizers, sleeping medications, and narcotic analgesics.

ADDITIONAL GASTROINTESTINAL STIMULANTS

domperidone

Domperidone (Motilium) is related to metoclopramide. It is similar to that drug except that domperidone does not cross the blood-brain barrier and is not effective as metoclopramide an antiemetic. Domperidone is available in Canada but not in the United States.

erythromycin

Erythromycin is an antibiotic with GI side effects (see Chapter 46). Recently the ability of erythromycin to stimulate GI motility has been shown directly. Erythromycin appears to stimulate the receptor for motilin, a GI hormone. Erythromycin is being used to improve gastric emptying and increase propulsion throughout the GI tract for such conditions as gastroparesis and intestinal hypomotility.

neostigmine

Neostigmine (Prostigmin) is a reversible acetylcholinesterase inhibitor prescribed for its muscarinic and neuromuscular effects (see Chapter 42). Neostigmine may be given subcutaneously or intramuscularly in place of bethanechol to restore bladder or intestinal tone after surgery. If urination does not occur within 1 hour, a catheter should be inserted.

Nursing Process Overview

Drugs to Increase Gastrointestinal Tone and Motility

Assessment

Drugs to increase GI tone and motility are used after trauma, after surgery to treat atonic intestines or bladder, and when barium is used for radiologic examination. They are also used to treat diabetic gastroparesis. Assess the patient to rule out any obstruction of the bladder or intestine. Also assess vital signs, check for the presence of bowel sounds, check intake and output, palpate the bladder for distension, and check the patency of urinary catheters.

Nursing Diagnoses

- Altered comfort related to abdominal cramps or diarrhea
- Diarrhea related to drug action or side effect

Patient Outcomes

The patient will have a bowel movement and return to usual defecation pattern. The patient having difficulty voiding will be able to void and will return to usual elimination pattern. The patient who has undergone a diagnostic test will expel the barium without difficulty.

Planning/Implementation

After administering bethanechol or neostigmine, remain at the patient's bedside for 15 minutes to observe for side effects. Side effects often occur with subcutaneous bethanechol. Have the antidote atropine readily available before bethanechol is administered. After the drug is administered, monitor vital signs and measure output. If side effects become serious, notify the physician or consider administering atropine (0.6 mg). If metoclopramide is administered intravenously, remain at the bedside; oral administration produces much slower effects.

Evaluation

These drugs are effective if they enhance the patient's ability to defecate or urinate. Some patients require only one or two doses, whereas other patients require continued use of these drugs. Before discharging a patient, assess the patient's knowledge of how to take the drug correctly, the anticipated effects, the possible side effects and what to do about them, and the symptoms requiring medical attention.

THERAPEUTIC RATIONALE: DECREASING GASTROINTESTINAL SECRETIONS, TONE, AND MOTILITY

Selected anticholinergic agents are used as preanesthetic medications to block salivation and respiratory tract secretions during surgery.

Irritable bowel syndrome, also called spastic colitis, is a common GI disorder characterized by hyperactivity of the colon. Abdominal pain coincides with hypermotility of the colon. Constipation or diarrhea are characteristic. Psychologic or emotional factors are also commonly associated with the irritable bowel syndrome. Some patients have had a previous bout of infectious diarrhea; others may have laxative abuse as a predisposing factor.

Behavioral and dietary therapy are the first treatments for irritable bowel syndrome. Anticholinergic drugs administered alone or with an antianxiety agent may be helpful.

THERAPEUTIC AGENTS: ATROPINE AND ANTISPASMODIC AGENTS

A number of **anticholinergic** and **antispasmodic drugs** have been developed to decrease GI tone and motility. Anticholinergic drugs (drugs that block muscarinic receptors) inhibit gastric acid secretion and depress GI motility. These drugs are listed in Table 23-2.

▼ atropine and Related Drugs

Atropine was originally derived from the plant Atropa belladonna, or deadly nightshade. Other belladonna alkaloids include hyoscyamine and scopolamine. Charged derivatives of atropine include homatropine and methscopolamine. These are listed in Table 23-2.

Mechanism of Action

Atropine is the prototypic anticholinergic agent, blocking acetylcholine at the muscarinic receptors. This action blocks the parasympathetic nervous system at various end organs (see Chapter 11).

Pharmacokinetics

Atropine may be administered orally, intramuscularly, subcutaneously, or intravenously. The duration of action is 4 to 6 hours. About 30% to 50% of the drug is excreted unchanged in the urine. See Table 23-2 for information on other atropine-like drugs.

Uses

Atropine and related drugs are used as anticholinergic agents for the treatment of irritable bowel syndrome and as a treatment adjunct for peptic ulcer. Atropine is also used as an antidote for the toxicity of cholinesterase inhibitors, including organophosphate pesticides, and for muscarinic mushroom poisoning.

Scopolamine is occasionally used as a preanesthetic medication to reduce salivation and respiratory secretions.

Atropine and related drugs are used in ophthalmology (see Chapter 73). Atropine is used to treat selected arrhythmias (see Chapter 19).

Adverse Reactions and Contraindications

Common side effects of anticholinergic drugs include dry mouth (**xerostomia**) (see Patient Problems box), photophobia from dilated pupils (mydriasis), blurred vision (cycloplegia), fast heart rate (tachycardia), constipation, and acute urinary retention. If patients do not have dry mouth (xerostomia), they are not getting a dose large enough to suppress acid secretion.

Children and elderly patients are more susceptible to the effects of atropine and other antispasmodic drugs.

Toxicity

Toxic doses of the uncharged anticholinergic drugs atropine (and its L-isomer, hyoscyamine) and oxyphencyclimine reach the CNS and produce CNS stimulation such as restlessness, tremor, irritability, delirium, and hallucinations. Infants and children are especially susceptible. Toxic doses of the charged anticholinergic drugs that do not reach the CNS cause ganglionic blockade (usually seen as orthostatic hypotension) or neuromuscular blockade. Death can result from respiratory arrest related to neuromuscular blockade.

In contrast to atropine, scopolamine produces sleepiness, sedation and amnesia at toxic levels, although scopolamine can produce hallucinations as well.

PATIENT PROBLEMS

Dry Mouth (Xerostomia)

THE PROBLEM
Some drugs produce an excessively dry mouth. This effect may cause discomfort, trauma to the mouth, bad breath, irritation from dentures, potential for the development of dental caries, and potential for injury to the oral mucosa.

SIGNS AND SYMPTOMS
Dry oral mucous membranes; bad breath; dry and sticky feeling mouth

MEASURES TO DECREASE PATIENT DISCOMFORT
- Perform thorough, regular oral hygiene, with teeth brushing.
- Rinse mouth with a pleasant tasting rinse or normal saline solution (dissolve 1 tsp of salt in 1 pint water).
- Sip water frequently.
- Suck on sugarless hard candy or chew sugarless gum.
- Avoid drying mouthwashes (those containing alcohol).
- Avoid lemon-glycerin swabs for oral hygiene.
- Keep lips moist with lip moisturizer.
- Keep environmental air moist with a humidifier.
- Consider using a commercially available saliva substitute.
- Have regular dental checkups.

Table 23-2	Drugs to Decrease Gastrointestinal Tone and Motility		
Generic Name	Trade Name	Administration/Dosage	Comments
Belladonna Alkaloids (Uncharged)			
atropine sulfate		ORAL, SUBCUTANEOUS: *Adults*—0.3-1.2 mg every 4-6 hr. FDA pregnancy category C. SUBCUTANEOUS: *Children*—0.01 mg/kg every 4-6 hr.	Anticholinergic also used as a urinary antispasmodic, for biliary tract disorders, and as a preanesthetic to reduce saliva.
belladonna tincture		ORAL: *Adults*—180-300 μg 3-4 times/day. FDA pregnancy category C. *Children*—0.03 ml/kg in 3 or 4 divided doses.	As above. Atropine is active ingredient. Administer 30-60 min before meals and at bedtime.
hyoscyamine sulfate	Anaspaz Cystospaz Gastrosed Levsin	ORAL: *Adults*—0.125-0.25 mg every 4-6 hr. *Children 2-10 yr*—½ adult dosage. *Children <2 yr*—¼ adult dosage. INTRAMUSCULAR, INTRAVENOUS, SUBCUTANEOUS: *Adults*—0.25-0.5 mg every 4-6 hr. FDA pregnancy category C.	As above. Atropine is active ingredient. Administer 30-60 min before meals and at bedtime.
scopolamine butylbromide	Buscopan†	ORAL: *Adults*—10-20 mg 3 or 4 times/day. INTRAMUSCULAR, INTRAVENOUS, SUBCUTANEOUS: *Adults*—10-20 mg 3 or 4 times/day. FDA pregnancy category C.	Anticholinergic also used as a urinary antispasmodic, for biliary tract disorders, and as a preanesthetic to reduce saliva. Also an antiemetic and antivertigo agent.
scopolamine hydrobromide	Generic	INTRAMUSCULAR, INTRAVENOUS, SUBCUTANEOUS: *Adults*—0.3-0.6 mg as single dose. FDA pregnancy category C.	As above.
Charged Derivatives of atropine			
homatropine methylbromide	Homapin	ORAL: *Adults*—5-10 mg 3 or 4 times/day. *Children*—3-6 mg every 6 hr. *Infants*—0.3 mg dissolved in water every 4 hr.	Anticholinergic.
methscopolamine bromide	Pamine	ORAL: *Adults*—2.5-5 mg every 6 hr. *Children*—0.2 mg/kg every 6 hr.	Anticholinergic. Administer 30 min before meals and at bedtime.
Synthetic Substitutes for atropine			
anisotropine methylbromide	Generic	ORAL: *Adults*—50 mg 3 times/day. Onset: 1 hr.	Anticholinergic.
clidinium bromide	Quarzan	ORAL: *Adults*—2.5-5 mg 3 or 4 times/day before meals and at bedtime. Reduce dosage to 2.5 mg 3 times/day before meals for older adult patients.	Anticholinergic. Administer before meals and at bedtime.
glycopyrrolate	Robinul*	ORAL: *Adults*—1-2 mg 3 times/day initially; then 1-2 mg 2 times/day for maintenance. Onset: 1 hr. INTRAMUSCULAR, SUBCUTANEOUS, INTRAVENOUS: *Adults*—0.1-0.2 mg every 4 hr. Onset: 10 min. FDA pregnancy category B.	Anticholinergic. Also given before surgery to block secretion of saliva and respiratory fluids. Antidiarrheal agent.
mepenzolate bromide	Cantil	ORAL: *Adults*—25 mg 4 times/day. Increase to 50 mg if necessary.	Anticholinergic.
methantheline bromide	Banthine	ORAL: *Adults*—50-100 mg every 6 hr initially; reduce by half for maintenance. *Children*—6 mg/kg/day in 4 doses. Onset: 30 min.	Anticholinergic.
propantheline bromide	Pro-Banthine* Propanthel†	ORAL: *Adults*—15 mg 3 times/day plus 30 mg at bedtime. FDA pregnancy category C. *Children*—1.5 mg/kg/day every 6 hr.	Anticholinergic. Also used to treat urinary incontinence and to prepare for duodenography. Administer 30 min before meals and at bedtime.
Antispasmodic Drugs			
dicyclomine hydrochloride	Antispas Bentyl Bentylol† Others	ORAL, INTRAMUSCULAR: *Adults*—10-20 mg 3 or 4 times/day. *Children*—10 mg 3 or 4 times/day. *Infants*—5 mg 3 or 4 times/day.	Antispasmodic.
pirenzepine†	Gastrozepin†	ORAL: *Adults*—50 mg 2 times/day. May be increased to 3 times/day if needed.	Antispasmodic.

*Available in Canada and the United States.
†Available in Canada only.

Interactions

Atropine and related drugs give additive anticholinergic effects with phenothiazines, amantadine, antiparkinson drugs, glutethimide, meperidine, tricyclic antidepressants, quinidine, disopyramide, and some antihistamines. Levodopa absorption is decreased, but digoxin absorption is increased. Antacids will decrease the absorption of anticholinergics when taken concurrently.

Synthetic Substitutes for atropine

A number of synthetic substitutes for atropine were developed as antiulcer medications: anisotropine, clidinium, glcopyrrolate, mepenzolate, and methantheline (see Table 23-2). They are no longer commonly used in the treatment of ulcers. Glycopyrrolate is used as preanesthetic medication to prevent or reduce salivation and respiratory tract secretions.

Antispasmodic Agents

In addition to atropine and related drugs, dicyclomine and pirenzepine have antispasmodic but not anticholinergic effects (see Table 23-2). These drugs relax the smooth muscle of the GI tract and are used to treat hyperactivity or spasm of the intestine. Their side effects are not as prominent as those reported for the anticholinergic drugs. Side effects reported include constipation or diarrhea, rash, euphoria, dizziness, drowsiness, headache, nausea, and weakness.

Nursing Process Overview

Drugs to Decrease Gastrointestinal Secretion, Tone, and Motility

Assessment
Assess the patient with attention to vital signs, any subjective complaints, frequency and character of stools, and presence of occult blood in the stool.

Nursing Diagnoses
- Colonic constipation related to drug side effects
- Altered oral mucous membranes related to dry mouth produced as a drug side effect

Patient Outcomes
The patient will have symptomatic relief of ulcer pain without constipation. The patient with irritable bowel disease will have less pain and decreased frequency of bowel movements. The patient who is nauseated will have relief of nausea without vomiting. The patient treated for poisoning will have reversal of the effects of the poisons.

Planning/Implementation
These drugs are used with dietary management and other therapies. Continue to monitor the patient's subjective complaints and vital signs and to assess the patient for side effects. Anticholinergic drugs and related compounds produce side effects if administered in effective dosages. Assist the patient in dealing with unpleasant side effects (e.g., sucking on hard candy for treatment of dry mouth). Monitor intake and output and assess for constipation. Watch for CNS effects such as restlessness, tremor, or irritability, which may indicate a need to reduce the drug dose.

Evaluation
These drugs are effective if the patient complains of fewer symptoms or the signs of ulcer disease disappear. Before discharge, the patient should be able to explain why and how to take the medications, which side effects will probably occur, how to treat these side effects, which symptoms warrant medical attention, and how to carry out related therapies such as dietary modification for treatment of ulcer disease.

Nursing Implications Summary

Cholinomimetics: bethanechol and neostigmine
Drug Administration
➤ Have atropine sulfate (0.5 to 1.0 mg for adults; 10 mg/kg for infants and children) on hand to counteract excessive cholinergic side effects when administering cholinomimetics subcutaneously.

➤ Check doses carefully. The oral dose of bethanechol may be as high as 50 mg, whereas the subcutaneous dose should not exceed 5 mg.

➤ Remain at the bedside of patients for the first 10 minutes after administering subcutaneous bethanechol to assess for side effects, and check periodically for the next hour.

➤ The physician may order a test dose of half or less of the usual dose to check for patient response. Monitor vital signs.

➤ Check the pulse before administering neostigmine. Notify the physician if the rate is less than 80 beats/min, and withhold the dose pending physician approval. For additional information about neostigmine, see Chapter 42.

Nursing in the Community
➤ Teach the patient to take oral doses of bethanechol on an empty stomach 1 hour before or 2 hours after eating.

➤ If a dose is missed, instruct the patient to take the missed dose if within 2 hours of the scheduled time. If close to the next dosing time, omit the missed dose and resume the usual dosing schedule. Do not double up for missed doses.

➤ See the Patient Problems box in Chapter 13 on orthostatic hypotension.

➤ Remind the patient to keep these and all medications out of the reach of children.

cisapride
Nursing in the Community
➤ Instruct the patient to take doses 15 minutes before meals and at bedtime with a beverage. Shake suspensions well before preparing dose.

Continued

Nursing Implications Summary—cont'd

➤ For missed doses, instruct the patient to take the missed dose as soon as remembered, unless almost time for the next dose, then omit missed dose and resume regular schedule.

➤ Avoid alcohol intake unless first approved by the physician

➤ Avoid driving or operating hazardous equipment if drowsiness occurs.

➤ Remind patients to keep all health care providers informed of all medications being taken. Concurrent use of cisapride with certain antibiotics or antifungal agents has resulted in cardiac arrhythmias.

metoclopramide
Drug Administration

➤ If dose does not exceed 10 mg, may administer undiluted intravenous (IV) doses over 2 minutes; too rapid administration may cause intense anxiety, restlessness, and then drowsiness. Dilute doses larger than 10 mg in at least 50 ml of solution and administer slowly, over at least 15 minutes. Give doses administered in conjunction with cancer chemotherapy 30 minutes before chemotherapy is begun. A second dose may be given in 2 hours and a third dose in 3 hours. Doses for this purpose may be as high as 2 mg/kg body weight. Other regimens may be used.

➤ Allergic reactions may occur. Treat overdose of extrapyramidal reactions with diphenhydramine.

Nursing in the Community

➤ Instruct the patient to take oral doses 30 minutes before meals; doses may also be taken at bedtime.

➤ Metoclopramide may produce extrapyramidal reactions (see Table 58-3). Instruct the patient to report any unusual side effects, especially protrusion of the tongue, puffing of the cheeks, chewing movements, and involuntary movements of any body parts. Although rare, these side effects occur more often in children and older adults.

➤ Caution the patient to avoid driving or operating hazardous equipment until the effects of the medication can be evaluated.

➤ Caution the patient to avoid alcohol intake while taking this drug, as well as any drug that may depress the CNS, such as sleeping medications, tranquilizers, narcotic analgesics, and other drugs that cause drowsiness.

➤ Agranulocytosis occurs rarely. Assess the patient for chills, fever, sore throat, and fatigue (see Patient Problems box in Chapter 20).

erythromycin

➤ Erythromycin is discussed in Chapter 46.

Anticholinergics and Antispasmodics
Drug Administration

➤ Use anticholinergics and antispasmodics cautiously in patients with prostatic hypertrophy, pyloric obstruction, obstruction of the bladder neck, or serious cardiac disease. Assess for preexisting glaucoma because anticholinergics may precipitate an attack of acute angle closure glaucoma.

➤ Assess for urinary retention, especially in older men with preexisting prostatic hypertrophy. Monitor intake and output. Instruct the patient to report inability to void, increasing difficulty in initiating urination, or a sensation of incomplete bladder emptying. Instruct the patient to void before taking each dose.

➤ Monitor the patient's pulse before administering doses. Withhold the dose if the resting pulse exceeds 90 to 100 beats/min in an adult. Administer anticholinergics with caution in patients with a history of heart disease characterized by tachycardia. Auscultate bowel sounds. Keep a record of bowel movements. Treat overdose with neostigmine.

➤ Administer intramuscular doses into a large muscle mass, such as the dorsogluteal site or rectus femoris muscle in adults or the vastus lateralis muscle in infants and small children. Use careful technique; aspirate before administering the dose to avoid inadvertent IV administration.

➤ Tincture of belladonna may be prescribed by number of drops. Dilute the dose in 15 to 30 ml of water before administering. If drowsiness or disorientation develops, supervise ambulation, keep siderails up, and use night lights.

➤ IV atropine: may be given undiluted at a rate of 1.0 mg or less over 1 minute. May also be diluted in up to 10 ml sterile water for injection, and administered slowly.

➤ IV hyoscyamine: May be given undiluted, at a rate of 1 dose over at least 1 minute.

➤ IV scopolamine: Dilute dose in at least 10 ml sterile water for injection. Administer at a rate of 0.6 mg or less over 1 minute.

➤ IV glycopyrrolate: May be given undiluted at a rate of 0.2 mg or less over 1 to 2 minutes.

Nursing in the Community

➤ Instruct the patient to take doses 30 minutes to 1 hour before meals and at bedtime unless a timed-release form is used. If antacids are also prescribed, take doses 30 minutes before or 2 hours after antacid doses.

➤ Inform the patient that constipation is a common side effect. Instruct the patient to increase the daily fluid intake to at least 3000 ml, to increase dietary intake of fruits and fiber, and to exercise regularly. Tell the patient to record bowel movements; if a bowel movement has not occurred in 3 days, instruct the patient to consult the physician. Teach the patient to avoid cathartics or laxatives unless instructed to use specific ones by the physician because they may be contraindicated in certain medical conditions that require anticholinergics. Remind the patient to avoid drugs for diarrhea while taking these drugs, unless approved by the physician.

➤ Caution the patient to avoid driving or operating hazardous equipment until the effects of the medication can be evaluated; drowsiness and blurred vision may occur. Encourage the patient to wear sunglasses and avoid bright sunlight if photophobia develops; keep room lights dim.

➤ Teach the patient to suck on sugarless hard candy or chew sugarless gum to relieve dry mouth. Refer the patient to the pharmacist for commercially available saliva substitutes (see Patient Problems box earlier in this chapter).

Nursing Implications Summary—cont'd

➤ Instruct the patient to be careful about undertaking strenuous activities on warm days because these drugs inhibit the body's ability to perspire. Tell the patient to take frequent rest periods to cool off. Inform the patient that atropine may produce a fever, especially in children.

➤ Because these drugs often produce side effects when taken in therapeutic doses, patient compliance may be poor. Provide emotional support as needed. Teach the patient the importance of taking drugs as prescribed. Reinforce the importance of keeping all drugs out of the reach of children. If combination products are prescribed, review the side effects of each drug with the patient.

➤ Review signs of overdose, including clumsiness, dizziness, severe drowsiness, slurred speech or confusion, shortness of breath, nervousness, restlessness, fast heartbeat, and warm, drug-flushed skin. If overdose is suspected, seek medical attention immediately.

➤ Patients using scopolamine should avoid the use of alcohol.

➤ Review the correct use of suppositories or transdermal patches if these drug forms are prescribed. Scopolamine transdermal patches are applied behind the ear; review the patient instruction sheet supplied by the manufacturer. Patients may experience photophobia while using the transdermal patch form, and this side effect may persist for several hours after removing it. When used for its antiemetic effect, apply patch at least 4 hours before effect is needed (U.S. brand: Transderm-Scop, or 12 hours in advance for Canadian brand (Transderm-V).

CHAPTER REVIEW

Application

1. How do cholinomimetic drugs act on the GI tract? Name two cholinomimetic drugs that are used for their activity on the GI tract.
2. How do the mechanisms of metoclopramide and cisapride differ from direct-acting cholinomimetic drugs?
3. What actions do anticholinergic drugs have on the GI tract?

Critical Thinking

1. What is the antidote for bethanechol? Under what circumstances should you consider administering the antidote? What symptoms would you see with excessive bethanechol dosage?
2. The drug atropine is classically given as a preoperative medication. What are the desired effects? For the patient using atropine regularly (long term), what are the side effects, and how would you suggest the patient manage them?

References

Shuster J: Adverse drug reaction. Anticholinergics and cavities, *Nursing* 27(1):71, 1997

Walizer EM, Ephraim PM, Rudy S: Double-blind cross-over controlled clinical trial of vegetable oil versus xerolube for xerostomia: an expanded study abstract, *ORL Head Neck Nurs* 14(1): 11-12, 1996.

Laxatives and Antidiarrheals

OBJECTIVES

After studying this chapter, you should be able to do the following:

- *Discuss the use of laxatives and antidiarrheals.*
- *Develop a nursing care plan for patients receiving laxatives or antidiarrheals.*
- *Develop a teaching plan for patients who have constipation or diarrhea.*

CHAPTER OVERVIEW

A normal bowel movement refers to whatever pattern of defecation results in readily passed feces for a given individual. Constipation arises when the frequency of bowel movements decreases and defecation yields hard stools that are difficult to pass (see Patients Problems box on constipation). Laxatives are agents used to promote or ease defecation. Diarrhea refers to frequent or fluid stools. Antidiarrheals are agents that suppress intestinal motility.

THERAPEUTIC RATIONALE: CONSTIPATION

The major muscular activity of the large intestine is a contraction of circular smooth muscle, which decreases the diameter to segment and knead the fecal mass without moving it along. About 8 L of fluid travel through the intestines of the average adult in 24 hours. Water ingested in food or drink accounts for about 2 L, and secretions (salivary, gastric, biliary, and pancreatic) account for about 6 L. Because only 100 to 200 ml of water is normally excreted daily in feces, the intestines are highly efficient in reabsorbing water and electrolytes.

About 2 L of water are removed from the fecal mass in the large intestine. Bulk in the large intestine stimulates stretch receptors to cause a reflex peristalsis, which moves the fecal mass forward. Usually three to four times daily, strong propulsive contractions occur spontaneously to move the fecal mass through the large intestine. The strongest movements usually occur after the first meal of the day, and the perception of the need to defecate follows the filling of the rectum. The relaxation of the external anal sphincter is a voluntary act, as are the straining movements to expel the feces. The pattern of defecation described implies that defecation is a regular morning event, but the timing of defecation is highly individual and may occur more or less frequently. **Constipation** results when the propulsive contractions of the large intestine fail to move the fecal mass sufficiently.

THERAPEUTIC AGENTS: LAXATIVES

Laxative, cathartic, and *purgative* describe agents that act on the large intestine (colon, bowel) to promote defecation, but these terms have evolved to represent different degrees of action. A laxative produces soft stools with a minimal incidence of abdominal cramping. A cathartic produces a soft to fluid stool and may also cause abdominal cramping. A purgative produces a watery stool and violent cramping to such an extent that shock and hemorrhaging may result. Purgatives are no longer used in medical practice, and only some cathartics, also called stimulant cathartics, are commonly used.

Table 24-1 lists the drugs used as laxatives. Traditionally, laxatives are classified as bulk-forming, stimulant (irritant) cathartic, saline (osmotic) cathartic, wetting agent (stool softener), and lubricant. Laxatives are indicated for patients with true constipation. Causes of constipation include poor

PATIENT PROBLEMS

Constipation

THE PROBLEM
The patient is not having bowel movements as often as necessary.

SIGNS AND SYMPTOMS
Abdominal discomfort; feeling a need to defecate but inability to do so; dry, firm, hard stools when bowel movements do occur; infrequent defecation (the meaning of *infrequent* may vary with each patient)

ASSOCIATED OR CONTRIBUTING FACTORS
Dehydration or inadequate fluid intake; constipating medications; misuse or overuse of antidiarrheal medications or improper use of cathartics, causing the patient to move from constipation to diarrhea; and immobility

MEASURES TO HELP ELIMINATE CONSTIPATION
- Keep a record of bowel movements to help verify the problem, and note any associated factors.
- Increase daily fluid intake to 2500 to 3000 ml.
- Increase dietary intake of fruit and fruit juices.
- Increase dietary intake of fiber (see Dietary Considerations box in this chapter).
- Increase level of exercise.
- Examine use of drugs causing diarrhea or constipation.
- Examine the use of foods that may contribute to constipation: cheese and sweets such as cake, pastries, and pudding.

ADDITIONAL NURSING CARE MEASURES
- Keep a record of bowel movements for all hospitalized, immobilized, or institutionalized patients because constipation is easier to prevent than to treat.
- Auscultate bowel sounds in patients complaining of constipation.

DIETARY CONSIDERATIONS

Fiber

Adequate amounts of dietary fiber may help prevent constipation and colon diseases, maintain blood glucose levels, and lower blood cholesterol levels. Good sources of dietary fiber include fruits and vegetables, especially raw, unpeeled, or with edible seeds, and whole grains and whole-grain products, such as bread, cereals, pastas, bran, oats, peas, beans, and lentils.

DRUG ABUSE ALERTS

Cathartics

BACKGROUND
Cathartics are subject to two types of abuse. Individuals may fixate on being regular. Individuals with eating disorders may use cathartic laxatives in excess to get rid of ingested food.

PHARMACOLOGY
Cathartics are laxatives that produce a soft to fluid stool in 6 to 12 hours. They directly stimulate the colon.

HEALTH HAZARDS
The colon becomes unresponsive when cathartics are used for more than 1 week. Persistent diarrhea may result, which in its most severe form causes dehydration and produces electrolyte imbalances. Therapy is supportive as the cathartic is discontinued.

---

bowel habits, narcotic analgesics, drugs with anticholinergic side effects, and intestinal muscle tone loss because of surgery, bed rest, or age. Laxatives are also indicated when straining is painful or risky, such as in women with episiotomies and patients with hemorrhoids, hernias, or aneurysms. Laxatives are also used to clean out the large intestine before surgery or examination. With the exception of mineral oil, laxatives act by providing a greater bulk to the fecal mass, primarily by keeping water in the large intestine. The large, hydrated fecal mass can fill the rectum to stimulate defecation, which is then accomplished with minimal irritation or strain.

Bulk-Forming Laxatives

Bulk-forming laxatives includes bran, **methylcellulose,** polycarbophil, and psyllium hydrophilic mucilloid. They act by retaining water so that the stool remains large and soft. Bulk-

forming laxatives provide what should be a part of good nutrition. It is generally believed that people in developed countries eat a diet containing too little fiber that favors the formation of small, hard stools. Including bran, whole grain products, and fibrous fruits and vegetables in the diet promotes the formation of large, soft stools that readily stimulate the large intestine and the rectum (see Dietary Considerations box).

In a patient who does not regularly use laxatives, bulk-forming laxatives are effective in 12 to 24 hours. Bulk-forming laxatives can also relieve a mild watery diarrhea by absorbing water to produce a soft stool. Psyllium hydrophilic mucilloid is often added to enteral feedings for patients receiving nutrition through feeding tubes.

Stimulant Cathartics

Stimulant (irritant) cathartics include bisacodyl, cascara, castor oil, glycerin, phenolphthalein, and senna. These drugs usually form a soft to fluid stool in 6 to 12 hours. Stimulant cathartics were believed to act only by directly stimulating the motility of the large intestine; however, newer research indicates that these drugs also inhibit the reabsorption of water in the large intestine.

Table 24-1   Drugs to Relieve Constipation

Generic Name	Trade Name	Administration/Dosage	Comments
Bulk-Forming Agents			
methylcellulose; carboxymethyl-cellulose	Citrucel Cologel	ORAL: *Adults*—4-6 g/day. *Children <6 yr*—1-1.5 g/day.	Nonprescription drug. Take with a full glass of water or more. Effective in 12 hr to 3 days.
polycarbophil	Fibercon Mitrolan†	ORAL: *Adults*—4-6 g/day. *Children 6-12 yr*—1.5-3 g/day. *Children 2-5 yr*—1-1.5 g/day.	Nonprescription drug. Take with a full glass of water or more. Effective in 12 hr to 3 days.
psyllium hydrophilic mucilloid	Fiberall Konsyl Metamucil* Modane Bulk Serutan	ORAL: *Adults*—1 round tsp (7 g) or 1 packet. Add to glass of water and drink rapidly and then follow with second glass of water. Repeat 1-2 times/day if necessary.	Nonprescription drug. Effective in 12 hr to 3 days.
Stimulant (Irritant) Cathartics			
bisacodyl	Bisco-Lax† Dulcolax Others	ORAL: *Adults*—10 mg. Up to 30 mg may be given to clear gastrointestinal tract. *Children >6 yr*—5 mg. RECTAL: *Adults and children >2 yr*—10 mg. *Children <2 yr*—5 mg.	Nonprescription drug. Initial response occurs in 6-12 hr. Patient should not take it within 60 min of milk or antacids. Rectal administration is effective in 15 min.
cascara sagrada	Generic	ORAL: *Adults*—200-400 mg of extract, 0.5-1.5 ml of fluid extract, or 5 ml of aromatic extract, or 325-mg tablet.	Nonprescription drug. It is one of mildest of stimulant cathartics. Action is more rapid if taken on an empty stomach.
castor oil	Generic	ORAL: *Adults*—15-60 ml. *Children >2 yr*—5-15 ml. *Children <2 yr*—1-5 ml.	Nonprescription drug. Castor oil is degraded to ricinoleic acid, which is an active drug.
castor oil, emulsified	Neoloid	ORAL: *Adults*—30-60 ml. *Children >2 yr*—7.5-30 ml. *Children <2 yr*—2.5-7.5 ml.	Nonprescription drug. This emulsion is mint flavored. It turns alkaline urine pink.
phenolphthalein	Ex-Lax* Others	ORAL: *Adults*—30-270 mg/day. *Children >6 yr*—30-60 mg/day. *Children 2-6 yr*—15-20 mg/day.	Nonprescription drug. It turns alkaline urine pink. The FDA has proposed a ban on phenolphthalein for over-the-counter drugs.
senna concentrate	Senexon Senna-Gen Others	ORAL: *Adults*—Twice daily give 1-2 tsp (granules), 2-3 tsp (syrup), or 2-4 tablets. *Children, pregnant or postpartum women, or geriatric patients*—½ adult dose. *Children 1 mo-1 yr*—1.25-2.5 ml (syrup). RECTAL: *Adults*—1 suppository. *Children >60 lb*—½ suppository.	Nonprescription drug. Not all preparations are recommended for children.
sennosides	Glysennid† Herbal Laxative	ORAL: *Adults*—12-24 mg at bedtime. *Children >10 yr*—Same as adult. *Children 6-10 yr*—12 mg at bedtime.	Nonprescription drug.
Osmotic Cathartics			
glycerin suppositories	Senokot	RECTAL: *Adults*—3 g. *Children <6 yr*—1-1.5 g.	Nonprescription drug. It is effective in 15-30 min.
lactulose	Chronulac* Constilac Others	ORAL: *Adults*—15-30 ml, increased to 60 ml/day if necessary (15 ml = 10 g).	Nonprescription drug. It works by osmotic effect in 1-3 days.
magnesium citrate	Citroma	ORAL: *Adults*—1 glassful (about 240 ml). *Children*—0.5 ml/kg body weight.	Nonprescription drug.
magnesium hydroxide	Phillips' Milk of Magnesia	ORAL: *Adults*—10-15 ml (concentrated) or 15-30 ml (regular). *Children*—0.5 ml (regular)/kg body weight.	Nonprescription drug.
magnesium sulfate	Epsom Salts	ORAL: *Adults*—15 g in glass of water. *Children*—0.25 g/kg.	Nonprescription drug.
potassium bitartrate and sodium bicarbonate	Coe-Two*	RECTAL: *Adults*—1-2 suppositories.	Nonprescription drug. Releases carbon dioxide to stimulate rectum.
sodium phosphates	Fleet Phospho-Soda Fleet Enema*	ORAL: *Adults*—20-40 ml in glass of cold water. *Children*—5-15 ml. RECTAL: *Adults*—Solution prepackaged: 26 g salts in 118 ml.	Nonprescription drug.
Wetting Agents (Stool Softeners)			
ducosate sodium (calcium, potassium forms also used)	Colace D-S-S Many others	ORAL: *Adults*—50-360 mg. *Children 6-12 yr*—40-120 mg. *Children 3-6 yr*—20-60 mg. *Children <3 yr*—10-40 mg.	Nonprescription drug.

*Available in Canada and the United States.
†Available in Canada only.

Table 24-1	**Drugs to Relieve Constipation—cont'd**		
Generic Name	Trade Name	Administration/Dosage	Comments
Lubricant mineral oil	Agoral, Plain Kondremul, Plain* Neo-Cultol Petrogalar, Plain	ORAL: *Adults*—15-30 ml at bedtime. *Children >6 yr*— 5-10 ml at bedtime.	Nonprescription drug. It eases strain of passing hard stools. It should not be used regularly because fat-soluble vitamins (A, D, E, and K) are not absorbed. Response occurs in 1-3 days.

Stimulant cathartics are the most abused laxatives (see Drug Abuse Alerts box). When a stimulant cathartic is used for more than 1 week, the large intestine loses its tone and becomes less responsive to any stimulation. Continued use of a stimulant cathartic can produce diarrhea severe enough to cause dehydration and to lower blood concentrations of sodium and potassium.

bisacodyl

Bisacodyl is a synthetic compound available in suppositories, enemas, and tablets. As a suppository, bisacodyl is effective in 15 to 60 minutes and as a tablet, in 6 hours. Because bisacodyl irritates the stomach, the tablet is coated to dissolve only in the intestine. This enteric-coated tablet should not be taken within 1 hour of ingestion of milk products or antacids, which neutralize stomach acid. Bisacodyl is often used to clear the large intestine for proctoscopic or colonoscopic examination.

cascara and senna

Cascara and senna are extracted from plants. Cascara is the milder and senna the more potent cathartic. They should not be used by breast-feeding mothers because these laxatives are excreted in the milk. Senna and cascara turn acid urine yellow-brown and alkaline urine red. These are often taken at bedtime to produce results the next morning.

castor oil

Castor oil is an old remedy for constipation and is still used medically. Castor oil is the most potent of the stimulant cathartics, producing a watery stool in 2 to 6 hours, which thoroughly removes gas and feces from the intestine. Castor oil has an unpleasant taste and is best disguised by chilling and administering with fruit juice.

phenolphthalein

Phenolphthalein has been found in many over-the-counter laxative preparations. However, the Food and Drug Administration (FDA) has proposed a ban on products containing phenolphthalein because of safety concerns. Animal studies have shown that tumors and genetic damage can arise from long-term, high-dose use.

Phenolphthalein enters the enterohepatic circulation and may be effective for several days. In alkaline urine, phenolphthalein is pink.

Osmotic Cathartics

glycerin

Glycerin is administered as a suppository. It acts by attracting water to increase bulk, which stimulates the rectum. Glycerin is effective in 15 to 60 minutes.

lactulose

Lactulose is a synthetic disaccharide that is not hydrolyzed by intestinal enzymes and is not absorbed. Instead, lactulose is degraded by bacteria in the colon to short-chain organic acids that are not absorbed and act as osmotic agents. The net effect is a moderate fluid accumulation in the colon and the formation of a soft stool. Lactulose may initially produce gas and cramps. Lactulose acts slowly and is often used for long-term treatment of chronic constipation. This agent has reduced the incidence of fecal impaction in older adults. However, older adult patients should have serum electrolyte levels monitored after treatment for more than 6 months. Lactulose also reduces the amount of ammonia in the blood and is sometimes used with liver dysfunction.

Saline Cathartics

Saline cathartics are poorly absorbed salts of magnesium or sodium such as magnesium carbonate, oxide, citrate, hydroxide, or sulfate and sodium phosphate. Concentrated solutions of these salts attract water osmotically into the lumen of the large intestine, and the resulting bulk stimulates peristalsis. Saline cathartics empty the bowel in 2 to 6 hours when administered orally. Sodium phosphates administered as rectal solutions are effective in 2 to 5 minutes. Patients with poor kidney function should not use saline cathartics because they cannot excrete the small fraction of the salt that is absorbed systemically.

The combination of potassium and sodium tartrate delivered rectally results in the release of a gas, carbon dioxide. The gas pushes against the intestinal wall, causing contractions that move the fecal mass. This enema is administered as a suppository and is effective in 5 to 30 minutes.

▼ Wetting Agents

Wetting agents, or stool softeners, are detergents that inhibit the absorption of water so that the fecal mass remains large and soft. This class of laxatives is indicated when the objective is to avoid straining to pass the stools. The most widely used agent is **docusate** (dioctyl sulfosuccinate). Another agent is poloxamer 188. Results may be seen in 1 to 2 days after the first dose, although in some individuals results take 3 to 5 days.

Lubricants

The only lubricant laxative still used is mineral oil, which is indigestible and acts to soften the feces, thus easing the strain of passing stools and lessening irritation to hemorrhoids. Long-term use of mineral oil interferes with the absorption of fat-soluble vitamins A, D, E, and K. It should not be taken within 2 hours of meals to avoid interference with the absorption of vitamins and nutrients. Mineral oil is often taken at bedtime because it requires 6 to 8 hours to produce results. It should not be taken while lying down because it can cause a lipid pneumonia if accidentally aspirated. Wetting agents are considered superior to mineral oil in softening the stools for easy passage.

Nursing Process Overview

Drugs to Relieve Constipation

Assessment

Assess vital signs, fluid intake and output, and presence of bowel sounds. Perform a digital rectal examination to determine the presence of impacted stool. Obtain a history of previous constipation and its treatment, the patient's perception of constipation, and any recent change in lifestyle, diet, or medications.

Nursing Diagnoses

- Diarrhea related to drug side effects
- Perceived constipation

Patient Outcomes

The patient will have relief of constipation and will learn how to avoid constipation in the future.

Planning/Implementation

The treatment of uncomplicated constipation is usually simple. If constipation is persistent, the physician must rule out serious causes such as cancer. Administer ordered medications and teach the patient about other factors that influence the frequency of stools such as diet, fluid intake, and exercise.

Evaluation

Drugs to relieve constipation are effective if they produce a bowel movement. Before a patient is discharged, verify that the patient can explain how to take the ordered medications and what the desired effects of the medications are.

THERAPEUTIC RATIONALE: DIARRHEA

Diarrhea has no precise definition but refers to bowel movements that are frequent (more than 3 per day), fluid (unformed stools), or large (more than 200 g/day). Acute diarrhea lasts for hours or days, whereas chronic diarrhea lasts for more than 3 to 4 weeks. A patient with chronic diarrhea must be thoroughly examined to establish a cause, which can then be specifically treated. Acute diarrhea rarely requires treatment beyond avoidance of food and maintenance of adequate liquid intake.

The primary treatment of diarrhea is replacement of lost fluids and electrolytes. Glucose is required for the intestinal absorption of water and electrolytes. Mild dehydration can be treated with carbonated drinks, which add glucose and bicarbonate, and broths or clear soups, which add sodium and chloride. Infants and older adults can become seriously dehydrated if adequate intake of glucose and salts is not maintained to replace the fluid and electrolytes lost. Commercially available drinks for replacement of glucose and electrolytes include Gatorade and Lytren. A similar drink can be made at home with ½ teaspoon of corn syrup or honey and a pinch of table salt added to 1 cup (8 ounces) of fruit juice (to provide potassium), alternating with a drink made by adding ¼ teaspoon of baking soda (sodium bicarbonate) to 1 cup (8 ounces) of water. A simpler drink is made with the following recipe: 1 teaspoon table salt, 1 teaspoon baking soda, and 4 teaspoons of sugar in a quart of boiled water. Because the latter recipe does not provide needed potassium, ½ teaspoon of potassium chloride should be added to a quart of the solution.

THERAPEUTIC AGENTS: ANTIDIARRHEALS

Table 24-2 lists the drugs used to treat diarrhea. There are two general categories of agents: the opioids and related drugs and the absorbent agents. In addition, the somatostatin analog octreotide is effective in treating diarrhea in selective cases.

Opioid-Related Drugs

The most effective nonspecific antidiarrheal agents are the opioids, which decrease the tone of the small and large intestines in a manner that slows the transit of material. The longitudinal contractions propelling the contents (peristalsis) are inhibited by the opioids, but the circular contractions, which cause the segmental activity that mixes the intestinal contents, are stimulated by the opioids. The treatment of diarrhea with opioids is nonspecific, and when diarrhea is caused by poisons, infections, or bacterial toxins, opioids can make the condition worse by delaying the elimination of these agents. Opioids that are used to control diarrhea include opium tincture, codeine, difenoxin, and diphenoxylate (Lomotil). The effective antidiarrheal dose is lower than that which can cause euphoria or analgesia. Toxic

RESEARCH HIGHLIGHTS

Do Rehabilitation Patients Continue Prescribed Bowel Medications after Discharge?

—*Graham C, Kunkle C:* Rehab Nursing *21(6):298-302, 1996.*

PURPOSE

Patients requiring inpatient rehabilitation often experience constipation, incontinence, and loss of independence in toileting. Bowel problems may result from neurogenic factors (e.g., stroke) and changes in diet, fluid intake, mobility, and medications. Bowel programs include bulk agents, stool softeners, stimulants, suppositories, and enemas. At home, patients may select from hundreds of over-the-counter medications. The purpose of this descriptive, exploratory study was to assess the use of bowel medications 1 month after discharge from a rehabilitation center.

METHODS

Subjects were patients who had been inpatients for at least 7 days, were taking an oral diet, and were not discharged to a hospital or an extended-care facility. Data were obtained from the medical record at time of discharge, and a telephone interview conducted 1 month later. All 114 eligible subjects agreed to participate at time of discharge, but only 102 could be included in the follow-up interview. Ages ranged from 19 to 88 years, and 59% were female. Of the 114, 89% took a regular texture diet and the others had diets modified for dysphagia.

RESULTS

At discharge, 66% of the 114 patients took bowel medications, but at 1 month, 42% of 102 took any bowel medication regularly, and 32% took the same medication, same dose as at time of discharge. The reasons patients changed bowel medications fell into two categories: physiology (e.g., 35 patients no longer needed any bowel medication) or personal choice (e.g., patient preferred another medication or family or friend advised a change). Individual situations varied widely: one patient's wife who had been taught to administer a suppository to her husband who had suffered a stroke stopped the medication at home and cleaned up an incontinent stool once or twice daily. Self-report of bowel movement frequency at home varied from every 1 to 2 days to once a week. More than half of the patients had a home health nurse, but no patient reported changing medications as a result of advice from the nurse.

IMPLICATIONS

Although medications for bowel management may be appropriate in the inpatient setting, it may also be that health care providers prescribe too many medications, if patients do not feel the need to continue them at home. Another possibility is that health care providers do not sufficiently question patients to learn what medications the patient prefers to use at home. Finally, some of these patients indicated lack of knowledge about normal bowel function.

CRITICAL THINKING: What bowel medications do you see routinely prescribed in your clinical setting? Are there nondrug therapies that could be used to help some of your patients? What are they?

Table 24-2 **Drugs to Control Diarrhea**

Generic Name	Trade Name	Administration/Dosage	Comments
Opioids and Related Drugs			
codeine phosphate; codeine sulfate	Generic	ORAL: *Adults and children >12 yr*—15-60 mg every 4-8 hr as needed. INTRAMUSCULAR: *Adults and children >12 yr*—15-30 mg every 2-4 hr.	Codeine phosphate and sulfate are schedule II drugs.
difenoxin with atropine	Motofen	ORAL: *Adults*—2 mg initially, then 1 mg after each loose stool or every 3-4 hr as needed. FDA pregnancy category C.	Difenoxin with atropine is schedule IV drug.
diphenoxylate hydrochloride with atropine	Lofene Lomotil* Others	ORAL: *Adults*—5 mg 3-4 times daily. FDA pregnancy category C. *Children 8-12 yr*—10 mg/day in 5 divided doses. *Children 5-8 yr*—8 mg/day in 4 divided doses. *Children 2-5 yr*—6 mg/day in 3 divided doses.	Diphenoxylate hydrochloride with atropine is schedule V drug.
loperamide	Imodium	ORAL: *Adults*—4 mg initially, then 2 mg with each diarrheal episode, up to 16 mg/day. FDA pregnancy category B.	Drug is also available as nonprescription drug.
opium tincture	Generic	ORAL: 0.6 ml 4 times/day. Maximum single dose is 1 ml. Maximum daily dose is 6 ml.	Opium tincture is schedule II drug.

*Available in Canada and the United States.
†Available in Canada only.

Continued

Table 24-2	**Drugs to Control Diarrhea—cont'd**		
Generic Name	Trade Name	Administration/Dosage	Comments
Absorbent Antidiarrheals			
bismuth subsalicylate	Pepto-Bismol	ORAL: *Adults—30 ml. Children 10-14 yr—20 ml. Children 6-10 yr—10 ml. Children 3-6 yr—5 ml.*	This nonprescription drug is effective for "traveler's" diarrhea. It may turn stools gray-black.
kaolin and pectin	Donnagel-MB† Kao-Spen Kapectolin	ORAL: (after each loose bowel movement): *Adults-60-120 ml. Children ≥12 yr—45-60 ml. Children 6-12 yr—30-60 ml. Children 3-6 yr—15-30 ml.*	Nonprescription drug. Should be used only as adjunct to fluid and diet therapy.
Somatostatin Analog			
octreotide	Sandostatin*	SUBCUTANEOUS: *Carcinoid tumor:* 100-600 μg/day in 2-4 doses. *VIPoma:* 200-300 μg/day in 2-4 doses. *AIDS:* 100-1800 μg daily in 2-4 doses.	This is a potent antidiarrheal used for selected conditions.

AIDS, Acquired immunodeficiency syndrome.
*Available in Canada and the United States.
†Available in Canada only.

RESEARCH HIGHLIGHTS

The Effect of Dietary Fiber in Tube-Fed Elderly Patients

—Bass DJ, Forman LP, Abrams SE, Hsueh AM: J Gerontol Nurs *22(10):37-44, 1996.*

PURPOSE

Diarrhea is a common problem with tube-fed patients. Reasons for this may include hyperosmolar formula, rapid administration, bacterial contamination of the formula, improper tube placement, and decreased dietary bulk. Other contributing factors in some patients may include concurrent broad-spectrum antibiotic use or hypoalbuminemia. One difficulty with adding dietary fiber to tube feedings has been finding a fiber form that was compatible with the diet being administered and that could be given via a tube without clogging the tube. The purpose of this study was to determine whether the addition of dietary fiber to tube feedings was associated with a decrease in number of loose stools. The definition of diarrhea for this study was any alteration of the bowel habit associated with loose and/or liquid stools sufficient to be noticed by the patient or nursing staff.

METHODS

A retrospective review of records of patients admitted over a 30-month period to a 10-bed continuing care facility was done. Subjects had to have required a tube feeding for at least 3 weeks; 50 charts met this criterion. There were 29 men and 21 women, ranging in age from 28 to 83 years; the median age was 71 years. Medical diagnoses included cerebrovascular accident, respiratory failure, closed head injury, pneumonia, and others. Formula type was coded as fiber-containing formula (FCF) or fiber-free formula (FFF); 35 patients received FCF and 15 re-

ceived FFF. All patients in the FCF group received a formula that provides 14 g of fiber/L.

RESULTS

The FCF group had a mean number of 3.0 liquid/loose stools over 21 days, and the FFF group experienced 12.9 ($p < -0.014$). The FCF group had a mean of 49.6 formed stools over the 21-day period, and the FFF group experienced 19.5 formed stools ($p < -0.001$). Age was not significantly correlated with the number of stools, and no correlation was found between stool outcome and antibiotic use. Most patients (72%) had a serum concentration of albumin below the normal limit of 3.5 g/dl. There was a weak, significant negative correlation between serum albumin and liquid/loose stools (Pearson's $r = -0.2903$).

IMPLICATIONS

In this study the use of a tube-feeding formula containing fiber was associated with patients having significantly more formed stools than with tube feedings without fiber.

CRITICAL THINKING: Review the contents of tube-feeding formulas available in your clinical agency. Is there a range of the amount of fiber available? Why might tube feedings containing fiber (or not containing fiber) be prescribed?

---

doses produce respiratory depression, which can be reversed with a narcotic antagonist.

codeine

Codeine can be given orally, or the drug can be administered intramuscularly.

diphenoxylate and difenoxin

Diphenoxylate (Lomotil) is an opioid that has a lower potential than codeine or opium tincture for causing drug dependence. Difenoxin (Motofen), an active metabolite of diphenoxylate, has about five times greater activity than diphenoxylate. These drugs are combined with atropine to diminish abdominal cramping while reducing the loss of water and electrolytes.

▼ loperamide

Loperamide (Imodium) depresses longitudinal and circular contractions of the intestinal smooth muscles and decreases the release of acetylcholine. Loperamide has a broader spectrum of actions on the intestine than the opioids. Loperamide is structurally related to diphenoxylate but has no effects on the central nervous system (CNS) and does not appear to produce physical dependence. Originally available as a schedule V drug, loperamide is now available over the counter. Loperamide is concentrated by the liver and excreted into the bile. Its use is contraindicated in liver disease.

opium tincture

Opium tincture is a 10% solution of opium containing 10 mg/ml morphine. The antidiarrheal dose of opium tincture is measured in drops (usually 6 to 20 drops), and such a dose does not usually produce euphoria or analgesia.

Absorbent Antidiarrheal Agents

In addition to opioids that depress intestinal motility, many agents have been used as antidiarrheal drugs in the belief that they absorb toxins and thus remove the cause of diarrhea. Of these, only bismuth salts have been proved effective.

bismuth salts

Bismuth subsalicylate (Pepto-Bismol) is effective in controlling traveler's diarrhea, apparently by binding the bacterial toxins. Bismuth causes the feces to become black, which does not indicate the presence of blood. Use is discouraged in infants or older adults because it may produce feces that cannot be expelled (impacted feces).

kaolin and pectin

Kaolin is hydrated aluminum silicate and is thought to adsorb bacteria and toxins. Pectin is a carbohydrate extracted from apples and citrus fruits. This combination has not been found to decrease diarrhea. If parasites are suspected as the cause of diarrhea, kaolin may interfere with stool analyses.

octreotide

Mechanism of Action

Octreotide (Sandostatin) is a synthetic analog of the hypothalamic hormone somatostatin. Like somatostatin, octreotide inhibits gastric acid and pepsinogen secretion, inhibits secretion of gastric hormones (gastrin, cholecystokinin, secretin, serotonin, vasoactive intestinal polypeptide, and motilin), inhibits intestinal fluid and bicarbonate secretion, and diminishes smooth muscle contractility.

Pharmacokinetics

Octreotide is a peptide that must be administered subcutaneously or intravenously. It is effective in 30 minutes and

---

CASE STUDY
Laxative Use and Abuse

Mrs. Lankford is at home recovering from left total knee replacement surgery. She is 78 years old and finds herself sitting more than she is used to since the surgery. She goes to physical therapy daily but finds that she is very tired afterward. She is able to fix cereal for breakfast and soup for lunch, and her daughter visits every evening to help with her dinner and her hygiene needs.

Today she has called the doctor's office to complain of constipation. She says that she has had no bowel movement this morning, and had a "small hard stool" yesterday. She states that she is constipated if she does not have "one big bowel movement each morning." She blames the pain medication, Vicodin, that she takes only at bedtime for causing her constipation. Upon questioning, she states she takes Surfak once daily, Citrucel daily, and a Dulcolax (bisacodyl) tablet at bedtime if she did not have a "good" bowel movement that morning. The Surfak was prescribed after her surgery, and the other medications she buys over the counter.

1. What has contributed to Mrs. Lankford's perception of constipation?
2. What is the difference in the actions of the Surfak, the Citrucel, and the Dulcolax? Does she need all three of them?
3. When should she take a stimulant laxative, if ever? What are the concerns about using these laxatives?
4. What nonpharmacologic means can she take to promote bowel elimination?

---

has a duration of action up to 12 hours. It is eliminated in the urine.

Uses

Octreotide is used to treat the symptoms of tumors of the gastrointestinal (GI) tract, especially of carcinoid tumors and vasoactive intestinal peptide tumors that are associated with a severe diarrhea. Octreotide can be effective in treating diarrhea that does not respond to other treatments, such a acquired immunodeficiency syndrome (AIDS)-related diarrhea.

Adverse Reactions and Contraindications

About 10% of patients will experience abdominal or stomach pain or discomfort. Octreotide can cause mild hypoglycemia or hyperglycemia because it alters the balance between insulin, glucagon, and growth hormone. Patients with diabetes, severe renal impairment, or gallbladder disease are at risk for complications when taking octreotide.

Interactions

The combination of octreotide and antidiabetic agents or the hormones glucagon, growth hormone, or insulin, can cause hypoglycemia or hyperglycemia.

Nursing Process Overview

Drugs to Control Diarrhea

Assessment

Assess patients, focusing on vital signs, intake and output of solids and liquids, presence and character of bowel sounds, and the character of diarrhea. Question patients about recent exposure to new water or dietary sources, infectious agents, international travel, and any medications taken recently. Appropriate laboratory studies include culturing a stool specimen and testing stools for ova, parasites, and occult blood.

Nursing Diagnoses

- Altered thought processes related to drowsiness produced as a drug side effect
- Colonic constipation related to drug side effects

Patient Outcomes

The patient will have no diarrhea and will return to normal bowel patterns.

Planning/Implementation

Diarrhea treatment aims to provide symptomatic relief and identify and treat the cause. Monitor vital signs and intake and output, and observe the frequency and character of bowel movements. Limit the diet to clear liquids. If the diarrhea results from milk intolerance or other dietary cause, refer the patient to a dietitian for instruction. Observe the patient for drug side effects, especially constipation and sedation. If diarrhea is severe, monitor serum electrolyte levels and provide replacement fluids as ordered (see Patient Problems box on diarrhea and Table 17-1).

Evaluation

Drugs to control diarrhea are effective if the frequency of bowel movements is decreased to the patient's normal range. Before discharge patients should be able to explain when and how to take the medication prescribed, symptoms that may indicate too high a dosage, and what to do if drugs do not relieve the symptoms.

PATIENT PROBLEMS

Diarrhea

THE PROBLEM

The patient is experiencing diarrhea: frequent loose or unformed stools.

SIGNS AND SYMPTOMS

Frequent urge to defecate; abdominal cramping or discomfort; dizziness; symptoms of dehydration (e.g., weight loss, poor skin turgor, confusion, dry mucous membranes); anal tenderness and irritation (severity will vary with the patient and the cause)

ASSOCIATED OR CONTRIBUTING FACTORS

Misuse or overuse of drugs to treat constipation; antibiotics or other drugs that may cause diarrhea; concurrent gastrointestinal (GI) pathologic condition; excessive intake of food items that are irritating to that individual; GI infection; exposure to contaminated water

MEASURES TO HELP TREAT DIARRHEA

- Initially, switch to a clear liquid diet.
- Add gelatin or carbonated drinks, but avoid diet and caffeine-containing forms, to add glucose and carbonate.
- Add broths and clear soups, which will add sodium and chloride.
- Add Gatorade, Lytren, or other commercially available replacement, or make a similar drink at home (see text).

- Avoid alcohol, caffeine, acidic fruit or juices, fried foods, milk and milk products, and raw fruits. Slowly add bland foods such as crackers, bread, and cooked cereals.
- Clean rectal area carefully after each bowel movement: wash with mild soap or just water, and dry thoroughly, or use a cleansing wipe. Consider sitz baths three or four times a day. For irritated skin, apply a thin layer of petroleum jelly around anus.
- Wash hands thoroughly with soap and water after each bowel movement or after changing infant's diaper. If it is suspected that the diarrhea may be infectious and it is possible to do so, have patient use bathroom facilities separate from others in the family. Dispose of contaminated diapers in closed container, away from kitchen and food preparation areas, or put into closed hamper. In the home, wash contaminated linens promptly; in the hospital, use infection control guidelines.
- Wash dishes and eating utensils of person with diarrhea thoroughly, with soap and hot water, or put into dishwasher. Do not let others in the family share dishes with patient if diarrhea might be contagious.

ADDITIONAL NURSING CARE MEASURES

- Monitor weight, blood pressure.
- Take diet history, if indicated.
- If contaminated well water is a possible source of microorganisms, have water tested.

Nursing Implications Summary

Drugs to Relieve Constipation

Drug Administration

➤ Keep a record of bowel movements on all institutionalized, immobilized, or incapacitated patients. Prevention and early detection and treatment of constipation are much easier and less time-consuming than treatment of severe constipation or impaction. Assess bowel sounds before administering any drug to relieve constipation. If bowel sounds are absent, withhold drug dose and notify the physician.

➤ Read medication orders and labels carefully. Many drugs have similar names. Be alert to the action of each component drug in combination products. For example, Colace contains the stool softener docusate sodium, whereas Peri-Colace contains docusate and casanthranol, a mild stimulant laxative.

➤ Physicians also sometimes prescribe bulk-forming agents to treat diarrhea, especially diarrhea associated with tube feedings. If the agent is to be given through a feeding tube, dilute the solution with sufficient fluid to prevent clogging of the tube and flush the tube with water after administration. Large-bore tubes are better suited to administer these agents.

➤ Castor oil does not mix with a water-based diluent. Add a small amount of baking soda (less than ¼ teaspoon) immediately before administering to cause the mixture to fizz, and the castor oil will be partially suspended in the juice for 1 or 2 minutes. Patients may find it easier to drink castor oil this way. In an institution, the routine use of baking soda for this purpose must be cleared by the pharmacy or physician.

➤ Monitor the serum electrolyte levels of patients receiving lactulose, especially older adult patients.

➤ Lactulose is also used to treat elevated serum ammonia levels.

Nursing in the Community

➤ Instruct the patient that a daily bowel movement is not necessary for normal bowel function. Review with parents the inadvisability of encouraging laxative dependence in small children. To help keep a regular bowel schedule, teach the patient to increase daily fluid intake to 2500 to 3000 ml. If necessary, suggest that the patient drink a full (8 ounce) glass of water before each meal and a full glass with each meal.

➤ Instruct the patient to increase daily dietary intake of bran in cereals and other foods such as fruits and vegetables, fruit juices, and foods known by the patient to be stimulating to defecation (e.g., hot chocolate, coffee). Encourage the patient to exercise regularly to promote bowel regularity.

➤ Remind the patient to use laxatives only as directed. Many laxatives are available without prescription. They may be misused or abused by patients who do not understand that increasing dependence on these drugs can develop with regular use.

➤ Review with the patient using laxatives in preparation for GI tract diagnostic procedures the importance of following the prescribed regimen. The major reason that many studies of the GI tract are poor in quality or must be repeated is that the preparation of the gut or colon was inadequate.

➤ Inform women who are pregnant or lactating that drugs to relieve constipation should be used only under the direction of a physician.

➤ Inform the patient that sudden or persistent changes in bowel habits should be thoroughly evaluated by a physician.

➤ Bulk-forming laxatives: Teach the patient to stir the prescribed dose into an 8-ounce glass of fluid and drink the mixture while the drug is still suspended in the liquid. For best results, follow the first glass with a second full glass of water. Never take these drugs dry since they can cause obstruction. Pills should be swallowed whole and not chewed. Under most circumstances, use these agents regularly, one to three times daily, to promote regular defecation.

➤ Remind the patient to take daily doses of stimulant (irritant) cathartics, but not castor oil, at bedtime to promote regular defecation in the morning. Take doses on an empty stomach for best result. Swallow enteric-coated preparations, such as bisacodyl, whole and do not chew them. The patient should not take bisacodyl preparations within 1 hour of drinking milk or taking antacids.

➤ Castor oil has an unpleasant taste; inquire whether the patient would like it mixed with fruit juice. Some patients prefer to take castor oil straight and then drink juice as a follow-up so that the taste of the juice is not ruined by the medication. Encourage the patient to chill the castor oil to help lessen the unpleasant taste and to take doses early in the day because results usually occur within 2 to 6 hours. Flavored forms of castor oil are available.

➤ Inform the patient that storing suppositories in the refrigerator will make them firmer and easier to insert.

➤ Note in Table 24-1 that many of these drugs change the color of urine. Warn the patient about these changes.

➤ Encourage the patient to chill magnesium citrate before drinking to make it more palatable. The patient should drink the entire prescribed amount at once for best results.

➤ Instruct patients adhering to a sodium-restricted diet to avoid saline cathartics.

➤ Saline cathartics are often used to eliminate parasites after anthelminthic therapy if the trophozoites are not destroyed.

➤ The patient should be warned that when mineral oil is used regularly there may be leakage of the oil or fecal material from the anus. Mineral oil stains clothing. Suggest that the patient wear a perianal pad or incontinence shield to protect clothing and sheets. Regular mineral oil use is associated with increased incidence of lipid pneumonia, especially in older adults. Encourage the patient to always sit upright or stand when taking this medication. For long-term treatment of constipation, drugs other than mineral oil are preferred. Warn the family not to use mineral oil or any oil-based substance to lubricate the nose or mouth of an immobilized patient because the patient may inadvertently aspirate small amounts. Instruct the patient not to take doses of mineral oil within 2 hours of meals because the mineral oil may interfere with absorption of fat-soluble vitamins

Continued

Nursing Implications Summary—cont'd

and other nutrients. Avoid mineral oil in children less than 6 years of age.

➤ Explain the action of fecal softeners to the patient. Many patients misunderstand their function and expect defecation to occur a few hours after taking a single dose. Inform the patient that best results are achieved by using fecal softeners daily as prescribed. The patient may take liquid forms in milk or fruit juice, if desired.

➤ Encourage the patient taking saline cathartics or lactulose to follow doses with an additional glass of water, if possible, to facilitate laxative action. If the laxative leaves an unpleasant taste in the mouth, the patient should drink a glass of fruit juice or carbonated beverage after the dose, rather than water.

➤ Caution diabetic patients to monitor blood glucose levels carefully when taking lactulose because the drug contains high concentrations of lactose and galactose. Warn patients taking lactulose that flatulence and abdominal cramps are common initially but will subside with continued therapy.

➤ Review with the patient how to administer suppositories or enemas if these routes of administration are prescribed.

Drugs to Control Diarrhea
Drug Administration

➤ Assess the patient with diarrhea for a history of recent travel, especially international travel; recent antibiotic use; recent cancer chemotherapy; and recent work with children in day-care centers or other settings where harmful microorganisms are easily spread.

➤ Monitor intake and output, daily weight, skin turgor, level of consciousness, blood pressure, and pulse. Monitor serum electrolyte level. See the Patient Problems box earlier in this chapter on diarrhea.

➤ Dilute opium tincture in 15 to 30 ml of water to ensure that the patient receives the entire dose.

➤ Codeine is discussed in greater detail in Chapter 32.

➤ Theoretically, addiction to diphenoxylate or difenoxin is possible. Overdose with this drug resembles an overdose with a narcotic analgesic and is treated in a similar manner (see Chapter 32).

➤ Diphenoxylate and difenoxin preparations contain a small amount of atropine. A single dose of these preparations causes few side effects from the atropine, but the accumulated dose after 1 or 2 days of treatment might cause problems. Review the side effects of and contraindications to atropine use (see Chapter 23).

Nursing in the Community

➤ Review side effects with the patient. Note that loperamide is now available over the counter, but caution the patient that side effects may be associated with excessive or long-term use.

➤ Encourage the patient to keep a record of bowel movements. After several days of treatment for diarrhea, the patient may become constipated.

➤ Many cases of diarrhea are self-limiting. Instruct the patient to consult the physician if diarrhea persists longer than 3 to 5 days, if prescribed antidiarrheal medications are not affording relief, if stools are especially foul smelling or contain flecks of blood or large amounts of mucus, if or the patient is unable to take in sufficient replacement fluids. Review with the patient the symptoms of hypokalemia such as muscle weakness, fatigue, anorexia, vomiting, drowsiness, irritability, and eventually coma and death. Review with the patient the symptoms of hypochloremia, including hypertonic muscles, tetany, and depressed respiration.

➤ Caution the patient to avoid drinking alcohol and to avoid driving or operating hazardous equipment if drowsiness develops. This effect may be dose related.

➤ Caution the patient to avoid the use of bismuth salts in infants or children who are recovering from the flu or chicken pox. If nausea and vomiting are present, the patient should check with the physician because these symptoms may indicate Reye's syndrome.

➤ Instruct patients taking bismuth subsalicylate to read the labels of other drugs they may be taking and to avoid other salicylate-containing drugs. Also, large amounts of bismuth salts may interfere with urine glucose tests. Instruct diabetic patients to be alert to this possibility.

 CHAPTER REVIEW

Application

1. List some teaching points about ways to prevent constipation without using medications.
2. What drugs might you use for the treatment of diarrhea? What is their mechanism of action?

Critical Thinking

1. List the five classes of laxatives. How do they differ in the time for a laxative effect to be produced and in the type of stool produced?
2. Why does the continued use of the stimulant (irritant) cathartics not help establish regular bowel habits?
3. What is diarrhea? Why do you need to monitor fluid and electrolyte replacement for the patient with diarrhea?

References

Abyad A, Mourad F: Constipation: common sense care of the older patient, *Geriatrics* 51(12):28-32, 34, 36, 1996.

Bass DJ, et al: The effect of dietary fiber in tube-fed elderly patients, *J Gerontol Nurs* 22(10):37-44, 1996.

Belknap D, Davidson LJ, Smith CR: Diarrhea with enteral feedings. The effects of psyllium hydrophilic mucilloid on diarrhea in enterally fed patients, *Heart Lung J Acute Crit Care* 26(3):229-237, 1997.

Benton JM, et al: Changing bowel hygiene practice successfully: a program to reduce laxative use in a chronic care hospital, *Geriatr Nurs* 18(1):12-17, 1997.

Bisanz A: Managing bowel elimination problems in patients with cancer, *Oncol Nurs Forum* 24(4):679-688, 1997.

Brucker MC, Faucher MA: Pharmacologic management of common gastrointestinal health problems in women, *J Nurse Midwife* 42(3):145-162, 1997.

Graham C, Kunkle C: Do rehabilitation patients continue prescribed bowel medications after discharge? *Rehabil Nurs* 21(6):298-302, 1996.

Ouellet LL, et al: Dietary fiber and laxatives in postop orthopedic patients, *Clin Nurs Res* 5(4):428-440, 1996.

Saphire LS, Doran B: International travel preparedness: a guideline for occupational health professionals, *AAOHN J* 44(3):123-128, 1996.

Young RJ: Pediatric constipation, *Gatroenterol Nurs* 19(3):88-95, 1996.

Antiemetics

OBJECTIVES

After studying this chapter, you should be able to do the following:

- *Discuss the use of antiemetic drugs.*
- *Develop a care plan for patients receiving one of the various antiemetic drugs.*

CHAPTER OVERVIEW

Nausea and vomiting are most commonly associated with motion sickness, anesthesia, radiation therapy, and cancer chemotherapy. A variety of agents with different mechanisms of action are effective against selected causes of nausea and vomiting.

THERAPEUTIC RATIONALE: VOMITING

Antiemetics are drugs to control vomiting. Vomiting (**emesis**) is an involuntary act of regurgitating the contents of the stomach and is coordinated by an area in the medulla called the vomiting center (Figure 25-1). **Nausea** is the unpleasant sensation that usually precedes vomiting. Input from three major neural sites can stimulate the vomiting center. The first input is controlled by the higher central nervous system (CNS) functions, with vomiting being secondary to emotion, pain, or disequilibrium (motion sickness). The second pathway arises from peripheral stimuli, with vomiting related to injury or disease of a body tissue or organ. In particular, irritation of the mucosa of the gastrointestinal (GI) tract or bowel or biliary distension stimulates the vomiting center by way of the autonomic neurons carrying information to the CNS (afferent neurons). A third pathway is from the **chemoreceptor trigger zone**, a medullary center sensitive to stimulation by circulating drugs and toxins.

Nausea and vomiting are not necessarily treated with drugs. For instance, because antiemetic drugs have caused fetal abnormalities in experimental animals, the recommended treatment for the nausea and vomiting of pregnancy is having patients sip water or tea and eat small meals.

Many drugs cause nausea and vomiting because they act directly on the chemoreceptor trigger zone. Examples of such drugs include levodopa, digitalis, opiates (narcotic analgesics), and aminophylline. The effective treatment is to lower the dosage of the offending drug or to increase the dosage slowly. Drugs may also irritate the gastric mucosa, thus causing a reflex stimulation of nausea and vomiting. Aspirin is an example of an irritant drug. To dilute the drug, patients should take it with a large volume of liquid or with a meal.

THERAPEUTIC AGENTS: ANTIEMETICS

Drugs used to prevent nausea and vomiting are listed by drug class in Table 25-1. These drugs include antagonists of serotonin, dopamine, histamine, and acetylcholine. Serotonin and dopamine play major roles as neurotransmitters in the emetic pathway. Acetylcholine and histamine play a minor role but are involved in transmission from the vestibular apparatus to the emetic center. Drugs for treating nausea and vomiting are most effective when administered before nausea and vomiting have begun rather than after.

The choice of an antiemetic is determined by the cause of the nausea and vomiting. The drugs effective in reducing the

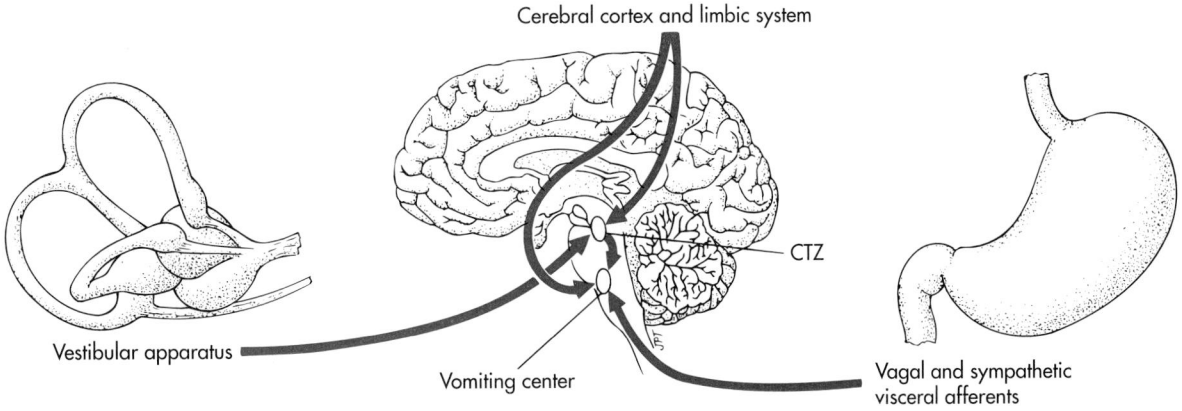

Figure 25-1 Vomiting action. Once stimulated, vomiting center acts on cranial nerves, spinal nerves to diaphragm, and abdominal muscles, which results in autonomic response of vomiting. *CTZ,* Chemoreceptor trigger zone. *(From Beare PG, Myers JL:* Adult health nursing, *ed 3, St Louis, 1998, Mosby.)*

Table 25-1   Drugs to Control Vomiting

Generic Name	Trade Name	Administration/Dosage	Comments
Antiserotonergic Antiemetics (HT₃ Antagonists)			
dolasetron	Anzemet	*Chemotherapy:* INTRAVENOUS, ORAL: *Adults and children ≥2 yr*—1.8 mg/kg, up to 100 mg as a single dose 30 min (IV) or 60 min (PO) before chemotherapy. FDA pregnancy category B. *Postoperative:* INTRAVENOUS: *Adults*—12.5 mg 15 min before cessation of anesthesia or when nausea begins postsurgically. *Children >2 yr*—0.35 mg/kg up to 12.5 mg as a single dose 15 min before cessation of anesthesia or when nausea begins postsurgically. ORAL: *Children >2 yr*—1.2 mg/kg, up to 100 mg as a single dose 2 hr before surgery.	Effective in controlling nausea and vomiting associated with emetogenic cancer chemotherapy, including cisplatin. Intravenous administration can be administered over 30 seconds or diluted up to 50 ml and infused over up to 15 min.
granisetron	Kytril	INTRAVENOUS: *Adults and children ≥2 yr*—10 µg/kg 30 min before chemotherapy, administered over 5 min. ORAL: *Adults*—1 mg up to 1 hr before chemotherapy with a second dose 12 hr later. FDA pregnancy category B.	Effective in controlling nausea and vomiting associated with emetogenic cancer chemotherapy, including cisplatin. Also used to control emesis associated with cancer radiation therapy.
ondansetron	Zofran*	*Chemotherapy:* INTRAVENOUS: *Adults and children 4-12 yr*—150 µg/kg 30 min before chemotherapy, administered over 15 min; administer 2 additional doses 4 and 8 hr later. ORAL: *Adults*—8 mg 30 min before chemotherapy, followed by additional doses every 12 hr for 1 or 2 days. *Children 4-12 yr*—4 mg 30 min before chemotherapy, followed by additional doses every 12 hr for 1 or 2 days. *Postoperative:* INTRAVENOUS: *Adults*—4 mg administered over 2-5 min just before induction of surgery or postoperatively. ORAL: *Adults*—16 mg 1 hr before surgery. FDA pregnancy category B.	Effective in controlling nausea and vomiting associated with emetogenic cancer chemotherapy, including cisplatin. Also used to control emesis associated with surgery and with cancer radiation therapy.
Antidopaminergic Drugs			
chlorpromazine hydrochloride	Largactil† Novo-Chlorpromazine† Thorazine Thor-Prom	RECTAL: *Adults*—50-100 mg every 6-8 hr. *Children*—1 mg/kg body weight every 6-8 hr. INTRAMUSCULAR: *Adults*—25 mg, then 25-50 mg every 3-4 hr to stop vomiting. *Children*—0.5 mg/kg body weight every 6-8 hr; maximum, 40 mg (up to 5 yr or 50 lb), 75 mg (5-12 yr or 50-100 lb) daily. ORAL: *Adults*—10-25 mg every 4-6 hr. *Children*—0.5 mg/kg body weight every 4-6 hr.	Effective for postoperative nausea and vomiting and that caused by toxins, radiation therapy, or chemotherapy. Nurse watches for hypotension with initial injection. Drug may cause considerable drowsiness.

*Available in Canada and the United States.
†Available in Canada only.

Continued

Table 25-1	Drugs to Control Vomiting—cont'd		
Generic Name	Trade Name	Administration/Dosage	Comments
haloperidol	Haldol*	INTRAMUSCULAR, ORAL: *Adults*—1, 2, or 5 mg every 12 hr as needed. FDA pregnancy category C.	Effective for postoperative nausea and vomiting and that caused by toxins, radiation therapy, or chemotherapy.
metoclopramide	Clopra Emext† Maxeran† Reclomide Reglan*	INTRAVENOUS: *Adults*—10-20 mg, administered over 2 min. *Children up to 6 yr*—0.1 mg/kg body weight. *Children 6-14 yr*—2.5-5 mg. ORAL: *Adults*—5-10 mg 3 times/day 15-30 min before meals. FDA pregnancy category B.	Acts centrally to block stimulation of chemoreceptor trigger zone and peripherally to enhance gastrointestinal tone. High-dose therapy is effective in reducing nausea and vomiting caused by cisplatin therapy or use in low dose with corticosteroid.
perphenazine	Trilafon*	ORAL: *Adults*—8-16 mg 2-4 times/day, up to 24 mg/day. INTRAMUSCULAR: *Adults*—5 mg/day.	Effective for postoperative nausea and vomiting and that caused by toxins, radiation therapy, or chemotherapy.
prochlorperazine	Compazine Prorazin† Stemetil†	RECTAL: *Adults*—25 mg 2 times/day. *Children ≤10 kg*— 0.4 mg/kg body weight daily divided into 3-4 doses.	Effective for postoperative nausea and vomiting and that caused by toxins, radiation therapy, or chemotherapy.
prochlorperazine edisylate	Compazine Compa-Z	DEEP INTRAMUSCULAR: *Adults*—5-10 mg every 3-4 hr; maximum, 40 mg/day. *Children ≥10 kg*—0.2 mg/kg body weight daily.	As above.
prochlorperazine maleate	Compazine Prorazin† Stemetil†	ORAL: *Adults*—5-10 mg every 3-4 hr; maximum, 40 mg/day. *Children >10 kg*—0.2 mg/kg body weight daily.	As above.
thiethylperazine malate (injection) or maleate (oral)	Norzine Torecon*	INTRAMUSCULAR: *Adults*—10 mg 1-3 times/day. ORAL: *Adults*—10 mg 1-3 times/day.	Effective for postoperative nausea and vomiting and that caused by toxins, radiation therapy, or chemotherapy.
triflupromazine hydrochloride	Vesprin	ORAL: *Adults*—25-30 mg/day. *Children*—0.2 mg/kg body weight divided into 3 doses; maximum daily dose, 10 mg. INTRAMUSCULAR: *Adults*—5-15 mg every 4 hr as needed; maximum daily dose, 60 mg. *Older adults*—2.5-15 mg/day. *Children*—0.2-0.25 mg/kg body weight; maximum daily dose, 10 mg.	Effective for postoperative nausea and vomiting and that caused by toxins, radiation therapy, or chemotherapy.
trimethobenzamide hydrochloride	Tigan*	INTRAMUSCULAR: *Adults*—200 mg 3-4 times/day. For preventing postoperative nausea and vomiting, give 1 dose before or during surgery and another 3 hr after surgery.	Drug relieves nausea and vomiting of radiation therapy, in immediate postoperative period, and in gastroenteritis.
Cannabinoids			
dronabinol	Marinol*	ORAL: *Adults*—5 mg/m² 1-3 hr before chemotherapy, then every 4-6 hr after chemotherapy, for a total of 4-6 doses/day.	Dronabinol is delta-9-tetrahydrocannabinol, major active ingredient in marijuana. It is particularly effective antiemetic when combined with phenothiazine. It is schedule II drug in the United States and N in Canada.
nabilone	Cesamet†	ORAL: *Adults*—1 or 2 mg the night before chemotherapy, then 1 or 2 mg 1-3 hr before chemotherapy. Continue 2-3 times/day for 48 hr past the last dose of chemotherapy.	Especially effective antiemetic for cisplatin chemotherapy. Controlled substance in Canada.
Miscellaneous Antiemetics			
dexamethasone sodium phosphate	Decadron Phosphate* Others	INTRAVENOUS: *Adults*—20 mg.	Effective against moderately emetogenic chemotherapy; enhances overall antiemetic effect of other drugs.
diphenidol hydrochloride	Vontrol*	ORAL: *Adults*—25-50 mg 4 times/day. *Children >6 mo and ≥12 kg*—5 mg/kg body weight daily divided into 4 doses.	Acts on vestibular apparatus to prevent vertigo after surgery on middle ear. It is effective for postoperative nausea and vomiting and that caused by toxins, radiation therapy, or chemotherapy.
Anticholinergic Drugs			
scopolamine	Transderm-Scop Transderm-V†	TOPICAL: *Adults*—1 adhesive unit is placed behind ear several hours before travel. Duration is 72 hr.	Sustained release protects most patients from motion sickness while greatly reducing anticholinergic side effects (blurred vision, sensitivity to light, dry mouth, and drowsiness).

*Available in Canada and the United States.
†Available in Canada only.

Table 25-1   Drugs to Control Vomiting—cont'd

Generic Name	Trade Name	Administration/Dosage	Comments
scopolamine hydrobromide	Bucospan†	ORAL, SUBCUTANEOUS: *Adults*—0.6-1.0 mg. *Children*—0.006 mg/kg body weight.	One of most effective drugs in preventing motion sickness, but side effects (dry mouth, drowsiness) limit its use.

Antihistaminic Drugs

Generic Name	Trade Name	Administration/Dosage	Comments
cyclizine hydrochloride; cyclizine lactate	Marezine Marzin†	ORAL: *Adults*—50 mg 30 min before traveling and 4-6 hr later; maximum, 300 mg/day. *Children 6-10 yr*—3 mg/kg body weight divided into 3 doses/day.	Effective for preventing motion sickness and vertigo.
dimenhydrinate	Dramamine* Gravol† Others	INTRAMUSCULAR: *Adults*—50 mg as needed. *Children*—5 mg/kg body weight divided into 4 doses/day; maximum, 300 mg/day. INTRAVENOUS: *Adults*—50 mg diluted in 10 mg saline solution, injected over 2 min. ORAL: *Adults*—50-100 mg every 4 hr. *Children*—5 mg/kg body weight divided into 4 doses; maximum, 150 mg/day. RECTAL: *Adults*—100 mg 1-2 times/day. FDA pregnancy category B.	Effective for preventing vertigo, motion sickness, and nausea and vomiting of pregnancy. It also causes drowsiness.
diphenhydramine hydrochloride	Benadryl* Others	DEEP INTRAMUSCULAR: *Adults*—10 mg increased to 20-50 mg every 2-3 hr if needed; maximum, 400 mg/day. *Children*—5 mg/kg body weight divided into 4 doses; maximum, 300 mg/day. INTRAVENOUS: *Adults*—Same as deep intramuscular. ORAL: *Adults*—50 mg 30 min before traveling, then 50 mg before each meal. FDA pregnancy category B. *Children*—5 mg/kg body weight divided into 4 doses; maximum, 300 mg/day.	Drug causes sedation. It is effective for preventing vertigo, motion sickness, and nausea and vomiting of pregnancy.
hydroxyzine hydrochloride	Atarax* Vistaject	INTRAMUSCULAR: *Adults*—25-100 mg. *Children*—1 mg/kg body weight.	Antianxiety drug is effective for preventing motion sickness and postoperative nausea and vomiting.
hydroxyzine pamoate	Vistaril	ORAL: *Adults*—25-100 mg 3-4 times/day. *Children >6 yr*—50-100 mg/day divided into 4 doses. *Children <6 yr*—50 mg/day divided into 4 doses.	As above.
meclizine hydrochloride	Antivert* D-Vert Others	ORAL: *Adults*—25-50 mg once daily, taken 60 min or longer before traveling; 25-100 mg/day in divided doses for vertigo or radiation sickness. FDA pregnancy category B.	Effective for preventing motion sickness, vertigo, and nausea and vomiting of radiation therapy. It is longer acting than most antihistamines.
promethazine hydrochloride	Phenazine Phenergan* Others	INTRAMUSCULAR, RECTAL: *Adults*—12.5-25 mg every 4 hr as needed. *Children <12 yr*—0.25-0.5 mg/kg every 4 hr as needed. ORAL: *Adults*—25 mg then 10-25 mg every 4-6 hr as needed. FDA pregnancy category C. *Children*—0.5 mg/kg every 4-6 hr as needed.	Effective for preventing motion sickness, vertigo, and postoperative nausea and vomiting.

*Available in Canada and the United States.
†Available in Canada only.

vomiting of chemotherapy and radiation therapy are the serotonin antagonists and the dopamine antagonists. These agents may also be used to prevent postsurgical nausea and vomiting. The cannabinoids (active ingredients in marijuana) dronabinol and nabilone are also used for cancer chemotherapy. For the severely emetic chemotherapeutic agents cisplatin, dacarbazine, and mechlorethamine, the serotonin receptor antagonists are the most effective antiemetic agents, especially when combined with the glucocorticoid dexamethasone. Motion sickness and vertigo are most effectively treated prophylactically with scopolamine or antihistamines. Diphenidol also acts on the aural vestibular apparatus to control nausea and vomiting.

Antiserotinergic Antiemetics

Mechanism of Action

Serotonin is the major neurotransmitter for emesis. A specific subtype of serotonin receptor, the 5-HT$_3$ receptor, is located on vagal nerve terminals in the stomach and small intestine and in the CNS in the chemoreceptor trigger zone and solitary tract nucleus. Serotonin antagonists block the action of serotonin at the 5-HT$_3$ receptor, preventing initiation of the signal for nausea and vomiting.

Pharmacokinetics

Serotonin antagonists are available in oral and intravenous formulations. They are administered before chemotherapy or surgery. Ondansetron is shorter acting and administered more often than granisetron. Dolasetron is the longest acting and requires only a single dose. These agents are metabolized by the liver.

Uses

The major use of serotonin antagonists is to prevent the nausea and vomiting in chemotherapy and surgery patients. Chemotherapeutic agents that are destructive to cells also release serotonin from the enterochromaffin cells in the GI tract, which sets off a severe emetic response. The serotonin antagonists block the action of serotonin at the 5-HT$_3$ receptors both in the GI tract and in the chemoreceptor trigger zone. Studies have demonstrated an efficacy of 60% to 90% in preventing significant nausea or vomiting following chemotherapy.

The serotonin antagonists may also be effective in preventing nausea and vomiting after radiation therapy for cancer or bone marrow transplantation.

Adverse Reactions, Contraindications, and Interactions

Serotonin antagonists have few side effects other than headaches occasionally or constipation or diarrhea. The major contraindication is a history of an allergic reaction to the drug. No significant drug interactions have been reported.

Specific Antiserotonergic Antiemetics

dolasetron

Dolasetron (Anzemet) is metabolized to hyodolasetron, an active metabolite. A single dose is effective in preventing nausea and vomiting. Dolasetron is administered intravenously 30 minutes before chemotherapy or 15 minutes before the cessation of anesthesia to prevent nausea and vomiting. Dolasetron may also be given orally 1 hour before chemotherapy or 2 hours before surgery.

▼ granisetron

Granisetron (Kytril) is administered intravenously over a 5-minute period 30 minutes before chemotherapy or radiation therapy. It can be administered into a Y-site with the following medications: cyclophosphamide, cytarabine, dacarbazine, dexamethasone, doxorubicin, fluorouracil, furosemide, ifosfamide, magnesium sulfate, methotrexate, and potassium chloride. When given orally, it is administered 1 hour before chemotherapy and repeated 12 hours later.

ondansetron

Ondansetron (Zofran) is administered intravenously over a 15-minute period 30 minutes before chemotherapy. Ondansetron is also administered over 2 to 5 minutes in a smaller dose just before surgery to prevent postoperative

---

RESEARCH HIGHLIGHTS

The Safety and Efficacy of Granisetron in Postoperative Vomiting in Pediatric Patients Undergoing Tonsillectomy

—Carnahan D, Dato K, Hartsuff J: J Am Assoc Nurs Anesthetists 65(2):154-159, 1997.

PURPOSE
Children undergoing tonsillectomy and adenoidectomy (T & A) often suffer from vomiting, and vomiting is the leading cause of prolonged hospital stay and unanticipated overnight stay. Severe vomiting may result in dehydration, bleeding, electrolyte imbalance, and aspiration. A newer group of drugs, the 5-hydroxytryptamine (5-HT$_3$) receptor antagonists, has been shown to be effective in preventing nausea and vomiting. Ondansetron, the first drug in the group, was short acting, so repeated doses were often required. A newer drug in the group, granisetron, has a longer duration of action. The purpose of this study was to evaluate the effectiveness of granisetron in preventing postoperative vomiting in pediatric patients having T & A.

METHODS
A random assignment, double-blinded prospective study design was used. Subjects were 54 children, ages 2 to 8, admitted for T & A. All met the initial health screening criteria. All subjects received drugs and monitoring routine for the surgery at the research institution. Experimental subjects received granisetron 10 μg/kg diluted in 20 ml of normal saline solution, and control subjects received 20 ml of normal saline IV over 2 minutes after induction and intubation. Episodes of vomiting were assessed and recorded after admission to the postanesthesia care unit. A

telephone interview with the patient's parent was conducted the day after surgery.

RESULTS
The incidence of vomiting in the control group was 69% in-hospital and 61.5% postdischarge. The incidence of vomiting in the granisetron group was 17.8% in-hospital and 14% postdischarge ($p \le -0.01$). The severity of vomiting was significantly reduced in the granisetron group also ($p \le -0.05$). None of the granisetron subjects vomited more than twice in the hospital, whereas in the placebo group, 15.3% vomited three to four times. The mean discharge time for the placebo group was 320.8 + 118.22 minutes, whereas for the granisetron group, it was 250.0 + 147.27 minutes ($p \le -0.05$). After discharge, one patient reported diarrhea, one complained of headache, and six reported an increase in appetite.

IMPLICATIONS
Decreasing postoperative vomiting in pediatric T & A patients reduces the risk of bleeding, dehydration, and aspiration, as well as general discomfort associated with vomiting, and distress of parents caring for their children. Shorter hospital stays save money and make the surgical experience less difficult for patient and family. Finally, a single dose of antiemetic is less costly than repeated doses of antiemetic medication.

nausea and vomiting. Ondansetron should not be mixed with solutions containing acyclovir, aminophylline, amphotericin B, ampicillin, ampicillin and sulbactam, amsacrine, cefoperazone, furosemide, ganciclovir, lorazepam, methylprednisolone, mezlocillin, perperacillin, or sargramostim.

When given orally, ondansetron is administered 30 minutes before chemotherapy and every 12 hours for 1 to 2 days.

Antidopaminergic Antiemetics

Mechanism of Action

Antidopaminergic antiemetics act at the chemoreceptor trigger zone. They are antagonists of dopamine, the major neurotransmitter of the chemoreceptor trigger zone. Most of these dopamine antagonists are drugs that are used as antipsychotic drugs (see Chapter 58).

Pharmacokinetics

In addition to oral administration, most of these drugs are available for intramuscular (IM) or intravenous (IV) injection. In general, the drug is metabolized by the liver and excreted in the urine.

Uses

Antidopaminergic drugs are effective in reducing vomiting from chemotherapy and radiation therapy of cancer. They also control postoperative vomiting, although they do not prevent motion sickness.

Adverse Reactions and Contraindications

Occasionally, extrapyramidal symptoms are seen with the antidopaminergics. Extrapyramidal symptoms are disorders of motor control associated with too little dopamine in a certain area of the brain. The side effects of the antidopaminergics are more fully discussed in Chapter 58.

Interactions

The major drug interaction of antiemetics is a synergistic depression with drugs depressing the CNS, particularly when respiratory depression is involved. For instance, vomiting that is related to alcohol intoxication or ingestion of narcotic analgesics can be relieved with an antidopaminergic, but the resultant respiratory depression makes this treatment undesirable.

Specific Antidopaminergic Antiemetics

▼ chlorpromazine

Chlorpromazine (Thorazine) is used to prevent nausea and vomiting associated with use of chemotherapeutic agents that are not highly emetic. Chlorpromazine causes considerable sedation and orthostatic hypotension, actions that limit its use.

haloperidol

Haloperidol (Haldol) is used to treat nausea and vomiting associated with use of opioids and surgery, radiation therapy, cancer chemotherapy, and GI tract disorders.

metoclopramide

Metoclopramide (Octamide PFS, Maxolon, Reglan) blocks both dopaminergic (D_2) receptors and serotonergic (HT_3) receptors. One action is stimulation of the GI system, which counteracts the loss of tone in vomiting. In addition, metoclopramide acts at the chemoreceptor trigger zone to prevent vomiting. Metoclopramide is effective in preventing severe chemotherapy-induced vomiting, especially when combined with dexamethasone.

perphenazine

Perphenazine (Trilafon) is effective in treating nausea and vomiting associated with surgery and use of opioids and radiation.

prochlorperazine

Prochlorperazine (Compazine) is widely used to prevent nausea and vomiting associated with use of mildly emetic chemotherapeutic agents, toxins, and radiation. Prochlorperazine does not produce the profound sedation associated with chlorpromazine. Hypotension is minimized by administering prochlorperazine in a slow IV infusion over 15 to 20 minutes.

thiethylperazine

Thiethylperazine (Torecan) is considered very effective to prevent postoperative nausea and vomiting. It is also effective in treating nausea and vomiting caused by the use of mildly emetogenic chemotherapeutic drugs, radiation, and toxins.

triflupromazine

Triflupromazine (Vesprin) is used primarily to prevent postoperative nausea and vomiting.

trimethobenzamide

Trimethobenzamide (Tigan) inhibits stimulation of the chemoreceptor trigger zone and prevents vomiting. It is believed to inhibit both dopamine and serotonin.

Other Antiemetic Drugs

dexamethasone

Dexamethasone (Decadron) is a long-acting glucocorticoid. Glucocorticoids have antiemetic properties. Although effective alone against moderate chemotherapy-induced nausea and vomiting, glucocorticoids greatly enhance the overall antiemetic effect of other antiemetic agents against severe chemotherapy-induced nausea and vomiting. Glucocorticoids are discussed more completely in Chapter 41.

diphenidol

Diphenidol (Vontrol) acts on the aural vestibular apparatus to prevent nausea associated with surgery on the middle and inner ear. It is also effective in treating postoperative nausea and vomiting as well as that associated with toxins, radiation therapy, and some chemotherapeutic agents.

dronabinol

Dronabinol (Marinol) is the major active substance in marijuana and appears to be an especially effective antiemetic when combined with a phenothiazine. Cannabinoids are new additions to antiemetic therapy for cancer chemotherapy (see Drug Abuse Alerts box). Patients who smoked marijuana before receiving cancer chemotherapy reported a decreased incidence of nausea and vomiting. Research revealed that the active ingredients, cannabinoids, appeared to depress the chemoreceptor trigger zone.

nabilone

Nabilone (Cesamet) is an active cannabinoid-like dronabinol that appears to be especially effective for relieving the nausea from low-dose cisplatin therapy. It is available in Canada but not in the United States.

▼ Anticholinergic Antiemetic: scopolamine

Mechanism of Action

Scopolamine is an anticholinergic agent. Its effectiveness in preventing motion sickness is attributed to blockade of muscarinic receptors in the vestibular system.

Pharmacokinetics

Scopolamine is well absorbed and readily crosses the blood-brain barrier. When administered orally, scopolamine causes significant anticholinergic side effects. For preventing motion sickness, a transdermal patch is preferred to decrease side effects. The patch is applied at least 4 hours in advance of travel and delivers scopolamine over 3 days. The patch should not be used by children because of their sensitivity to the anticholinergic effects. Administered orally, scopolamine is effective in 30 minutes and has a duration of action of 4 to 6 hours. It is metabolized by the liver and excreted in the urine.

Uses

Scopolamine is considered the most effective agent available for prophylactic treatment of motion sickness. Scopolamine is also administered as a preanesthetic agent to depress respiratory secretions and salivation.

Adverse Reactions and Contraindications

Anticholinergic effects of scopolamine include dry mouth, blurred vision, decreased sweating, urinary hesitancy, and constipation. Drowsiness, amnesia, and fatigue may also be experienced. Because vagal tone is depressed, patients with cardiac disease may experience an undesirable increase in heart rate. Children are sensitive to the anticholinergic effects, and with the reduced sweating, they may have significant fevers. Children and older adults are more sensitive to the effects of urinary retention, constipation, and disorientation. Men with prostatic hypertrophy are also likely to have difficulty with urination.

Lactation may be inhibited by scopolamine. Moreover, scopolamine is secreted in breast milk and should be avoided by nursing mothers because infants may be sensitive to the anticholinergic effects. Patients with glaucoma should be given scopolamine cautiously because of the increase in intraocular pressure resulting from the anticholinergic effect.

Interactions

Scopolamine causes additive anticholinergic effects with other agents having this activity. In particular, antiparkinsonian drugs, disopyramide, glutethimide, opioids, phenothiazines, tricyclic antidepressants, quinidine, and some antihistamines have significant anticholinergic activity.

Antihistaminic Antiemetics

Mechanism of Action

Selected antihistamines have been developed that help prevent motion sickness and vertigo. Stimulation of receptors in the labyrinth of the ear from which signals governing the sense of equilibrium arise is suppressed. A central anticholinergic action depresses the chemoreceptor trigger zone.

Pharmacokinetics

Most antihistamines are taken orally 30 minutes before travel and every 4 to 6 hours as needed. Metabolites are excreted in the urine within 24 hours.

Uses

Antihistamines are primarily effective for treating motion sickness and vertigo. Therapy is most effective when given prophylactically, 30 minutes before travel.

DRUG ABUSE ALERTS

Marijuana

BACKGROUND
Tetrahydrocannabinols are the active ingredients found in the marijuana plant. The leaves and tops of the marijuana plant are smoked or eaten. Users seek relaxation and feeling of heightened perception. However, the only medical use of cannabinols is for their antiemetic effect during cancer chemotherapy.

PHARMACOLOGY
Cannabinols impair memory and judgment and raise blood pressure. Characteristically, the user's eyes are bloodshot. When cannabinols are smoked, effects are felt after a few inhalations and reach a maximum about 20 minutes after the last inhalation. Intoxication includes euphoria, depersonalization, and uncontrollable laughter. Acute effects last about 3 hours.

HEALTH HAZARDS
Acute intoxication may impair judgment; thus the intoxicated individual should not drive or perform potentially dangerous tasks. Anxiety, paranoia, loss of concentration, slower movements, and time distortion are effects of overdose. Long-term health effects have not been clearly shown. Addiction is psychologic. There is no major withdrawal syndrome, although insomnia, hyperactivity, and decreased appetite have been reported.

Adverse Reactions and Contraindications

The most common side effects are drowsiness and dry mouth. Headache and jitters may also occur. Older adults tend to be more sensitive to the anticholinergic effects of dryness of mouth and urinary retention. Older adults are also more likely to become sedated, confused, or dizzy.

Antihistamines can worsen the symptoms of urinary retention, prostatic hypertrophy, bladder neck obstruction, and pyloroduodenal obstruction. Therapy for glaucoma may require alteration.

Interactions

Antihistamines cause additive depression with concurrent use of CNS depressants and alcohol. Anticholinergic effects are enhanced with concurrent administration of other drugs that have anticholinergic activity.

Specific Antihistaminic Antiemetics

cyclizine

Cyclizine (Marezine) is effective for motion sickness, vertigo, and symptoms of vestibular disorders.

dimenhydrinate

Dimenhydrinate (Dramamine) is effective in treating vertigo and motion sickness. It is also effective in treating nausea and vomiting during pregnancy. Dimenhydrinate can be administered intramuscularly, intravenously, orally, or rectally. Drowsiness is a common side effect.

▼ diphenhydramine

Diphenhydramine (Benadryl) has actions and uses similar to those of dimenhydrinate. When given intravenously, diphenhydramine is especially effective in treating dystonic reactions caused by dopaminergic blockers such as metoclopramide. Diphenhydramine causes drowsiness.

ALTERNATIVE THERAPIES

Gastrointestinal Disorder

GINGER

Ginger is the dried or fresh rhizome of *Zingiber officinale* Rosc. It is considered by some to be both an effective aid to digestion and a prophylaxis for motion sickness. Although the clinical literature in this regard is not extensive, at least one double-blind study (*Lancet* I:655-657, 1982) found that 940 mg of powered ginger was superior to 100 mg of dimenhydrinate or placebo in preventing nausea and vomiting in 36 subjects prone to motion sickness.

To date there are no reported side effects or toxicities associated with the doses usually taken to prevent motion sickness. This dose is two 500-mg capsules 30 minutes before travel, with one or two capsules every 4 hours as needed up to a total daily dose of 2 to 4 g. At this time, ginger should not be recommended for prevention of postsurgical nausea or the nausea of pregnancy.

---

hydroxyzine

Hydroxyzine (Atarax, Vistaril) is used for preventing motion sickness. Given intramuscularly, it also reduces postsurgical nausea and vomiting.

meclizine

Meclizine (Antivert, Bonine) has a slower onset (60 minutes) and longer duration (24 hours) than other antihistamines. It is especially useful in treating the nausea of vestibular disorders such as labyrinthitis and Meniere's disease. It is also used to prevent motion sickness.

promethazine

Promethazine (Phenergan) is a phenothiazine with pronounced antihistaminic activity in addition to strong central cholinergic blocking activity. It is effective in preventing both motion sickness and postoperative nausea.

Nursing Process Overview

Drugs to Treat Nausea and Vomiting

Assessment

Patients develop nausea with associated vomiting from a variety of causes. Assess the patient, focusing on the vital signs, character and quantity of any emesis, presence of bowel sounds, and intake and output. Perform a brief neurologic examination. Obtain a history of precipitating factors, exposure to recent infectious processes, and recent changes in diet or medications.

Nursing Diagnoses

- Altered thought processes related to drowsiness produced as a drug side effect
- Risk for injury related to impaired vision related to drug side effect (e.g., scopolamine)

Patient Outcomes

The patient will have relief of nausea, without vomiting.

Planning/Implementation

Antiemetics are used to relieve symptoms. Continue to monitor the vital signs and intake and output, and assess the subjective complaints of nausea and vomiting. Observe the patient for side effects, although these are usually not severe. CNS depression, hypotension, and dry mouth are often seen. Limit odors in the patient's environment, limit intake to clear liquids, and provide backrubs or cool washcloths to the forehead to aid comfort.

Evaluation

Success is measured by a reduction in the subjective complaint of nausea and by less vomiting. Before discharge, patients should be able to explain why and how to take the drug, the frequency of drug administration, the anticipated side effects of the medication, and what to do if nausea and vomiting are unrelieved by the medication.

Nursing Implications Summary

Antiemetics

Drug Administration

➤ Measure emesis as part of fluid intake and output.

➤ Use antiemetics with caution in children who may have Reye's syndrome. This syndrome is characterized by an abrupt onset of persistent severe vomiting, lethargy, irrational behavior, progressive encephalopathy, convulsions, coma, and death.

➤ Cannabinoids: Be alert to patient response to the cannabinoids; some patients may hesitate to use drugs derived from marijuana. Inform the patient that psychologic or physical dependence is unlikely at therapeutic dosages and with short-term use of these drugs. Because the gelatin capsule form of dronabinol contains sesame seed oil, check for allergy to this oil before administering the first dose.

➤ Avoid IM trimethobenzamide in children.

➤ Dolasetron mesylate injection may be administered orally, diluted in apple or apple-grape juice, and administered to children approximately 1 hour before cancer chemotherapy.

➤ IV dolasetron: May be given undiluted, at a rate of 100 mg/30 seconds, or may be further diluted in normal saline, D5W, D5/0.45% sodium chloride injection, D5LR, lactated Ringer's, or 10% mannitol injection and administered as an infusion, administered over 15 minutes. Administer approximately 30 minutes before cancer chemotherapy.

➤ IV granisetron: Dilute dose in 20 to 50 ml of D5W or 0.9% sodium chloride. Administer dose over 5 minutes, 30 minutes before chemotherapy or radiotherapy.

➤ IV ondansetron: Dilute dose in 50 ml of D5W or 0.9% sodium chloride. Administer dose over 15 minutes.

➤ IV dimenhydrinate: Dilute 50 mg of drug in 10 ml of 0.9% sodium chloride injection. Administer at 25 mg/min.

➤ IV diphenhydramine: May be given undiluted. Administer at a rate of 25 mg or less over 1 minute. May be administered more slowly, especially in children.

➤ IV promethazine: Dilute with normal saline to at least 25 mg/ml, preferably to 2.5 to 5 mg/ml. Administer at 25 mg/min. Slightly yellow solutions may be safely used; discard highly discolored solutions. Avoid spilling on hands because it may cause contact dermatitis.

➤ Other antihistamines are discussed in detail in Chapter 29. The antidopaminergic drugs are discussed in detail in Chapter 58. Scopolamine is also discussed in Chapter 23. Dexamethasone and other corticosteroids are discussed in Chapters 41 and 66.

Nursing in the Community

➤ Review the side effects of antiemetics with the patient. Warn the patient to use antiemetics only as prescribed and not to self-medicate with leftover doses. The use of these drugs in pregnant women is contraindicated unless the benefit outweighs the risk. Warn the patient to avoid drinking alcohol or operating hazardous equipment when taking antiemetics because sedation and drowsiness are common side effects. Caution the patient to avoid other drugs that may depress the CNS while using antiemetics. These drugs include alcohol, tranquilizers, sleeping medications, and narcotic analgesics.

➤ For treatment of motion sickness, suggest that the patient ride in the front seat of the car if possible, facing forward. Suggest that the patient take prophylactic drugs 1 to 2 hours before a trip rather than when nausea develops.

➤ For sustained-release transdermal drugs, emphasize the importance of reading the manufacturer's instructions. Instruct the patient to wash hands before and after applying the device. The disk is usually applied behind the ear, in front of the hairline. The patient should avoid cut or denuded skin and should replace the disk every 3 days or as directed by the physician. If the disk falls off, the patient should apply a new one. Instruct the patient to apply the disk 4 hours before a trip (Transderm-Scop) or 12 hours for the Canadian brand (Transderm-V).

➤ For dry mouth, suggest that the patient chew sugarless gum or suck sugarless hard candy. Provide frequent mouth care, but avoid drying, alcohol-containing mouthwashes and lemon and glycerin swabs. See the Patient Problems box in Chapter 23 on dry mouth. For the person who can have nothing by mouth (NPO) or who has vomited, provide frequent mouth care. Suggest that the patient suck ice chips; consult the physician for the NPO patient.

➤ Encourage the family to keep the environment free of odors and to keep food out of sight of the nauseated person. The patient should try clear liquids in small amounts before progressing to a more complete diet.

➤ If dry eyes are a problem, suggest that the patient regularly use artificial tears; consult the physician. Warn the patient that IM antiemetics often produce burning at the injection site. Remind the patient to keep these and all drugs out of the reach of children.

➤ Review the drug administration technique that the patient is to use at home. If the patient is to inject the medication intravenously or intramuscularly, have the patient give a return demonstration before discharge.

CHAPTER REVIEW

Application

1. What are the three major pathways that stimulate vomiting?

Critical Thinking

1. What are some nonpharmacologic treatments of nausea and vomiting you might recommend?

2. Differentiate between antihistamines vs. the antidopaminergic drugs for types of nausea and vomiting, actions, and effectiveness.

References

Carnahan D, Dato K, Hartsuff J: The safety and efficacy of granisetron in post-operative vomiting in pediatric patients undergoing tonsillectomy, *AANA J* 65(2):154-159, 1997.

Ferrara-Love R, Sekeres L, Bircher NG: Nonpharmacologic treatment of postoperative nausea, *J PeriAnesth Nurs* 11(6):378-383, 1996.

Fessele KS: Managing the multiple causes of nausea and vomiting in the patient with cancer, *Oncol Nurs Forum* 23(9):1409-1417, 1996.

Johnson MH, Moroney CE, Gay CF: Relieving nausea and vomiting in patients with cancer: a treatment algorithm, *Oncol Nurs Forum* 24(1):51-57, 1997.

Chapter

26

Drugs to Treat Acid Reflux and Ulcers

KEY TERMS

acid reflux, p. 316
H₂ antagonists, p. 318
hydrochloric acid, p. 317
peptic ulcer, p. 316
secretin, p. 317
ulcer, p. 316

KEY DRUGS ▼

cimetidine, p. 318
omeprazole, p. 321

OBJECTIVES

After studying this chapter, you should be able to do the following:

- *Discuss the use of drugs to treat ulcers.*
- *Develop a nursing care plan for patients receiving the following drugs or drug groups: antacids, histamine H₂-receptor antagonists, omeprazole, sucralfate, and misoprostol.*

CHAPTER OVERVIEW

A key component of stomach secretions is hydrochloric acid. Although hydrochloric acid is necessary for the proper digestion of food, reflux of the acid mass into the esophagus produces heartburn, which can damage the esophagus if severe and recurring. Ulcers can be another consequence of stomach acid. It is estimated that about 25 million Americans suffer each year from ulcers. Peptic ulcers occur when the mucosal defense system of the gastroduodenal tract fails to protect the tissue from erosive effects of acid and pepsin. The treatment of ulcers has changed dramatically in recent years with the introduction of H₂ antagonists and proton pump inhibitors that effectively suppress acid secretion. The demonstration that a bacterium, *Helicobacter pylori,* is a significant risk factor for ulcer formation has changed the treatment of ulcers.

THERAPEUTIC RATIONALE: ACID REFLUX AND ULCERS

Definitions

Acid reflux, or gastroesophageal reflux, occurs when stomach acid backs up into the esophagus. The result is "heartburn," a burning pain beginning in the pit of the stomach and moving upward toward the throat. Triggers of acid reflux include large meals and overeating, caffeine and nicotine, fatty or fried foods, alcohol, chocolate, and peppermint.

An **ulcer** is the loss of the skin or mucosal tissue that provides the protective layer of cells normally surrounding an organ. A **peptic ulcer** occurs in the esophagus, stomach, or duodenum after the mucosal barrier is destroyed, exposing the underlying tissue to stomach acid; as a result, the

anatomic structure of the stomach and the regulation of stomach secretions are affected. The common symptom is a gnawing or burning pain the upper abdomen, usually occurring between meals and early in the morning, that is relieved by food or antacids. Ulcers can also cause nausea, vomiting, and loss of appetite and weight.

The goal in treating an ulcer had been to depress or neutralize stomach acid, thereby allowing the ulcer to heal. The recognition that a bacterial cause underlies most ulcers has led to therapies that include eradication of the causative agent, *Helicobacter pylori.*

An esophageal ulcer results when there is reflux of stomach acid into the esophagus because of a defective esophageal sphincter. An ulcer in the duodenum results from overactive secretion of acid in the stomach so that stomach contents cannot be neutralized in the duodenum. The acidic contents then damage the duodenal mucosa. Stomach ulcers can result from the reflux of duodenal contents back into the stomach because of a faulty pyloric sphincter. The duodenal contents contain bile acids that disrupt the mucosal barrier normally protecting the stomach from acid and pepsin.

Control of Acid Secretion

Factors controlling the secretion of **hydrochloric acid** by the parietal cells of the stomach are diagrammed in Figure 26-1. The neurotransmitter acetylcholine (released from a branch of the vagus nerve), the hormone gastrin, and histamine stimulate the secretion of acid. Hydrochloric acid aids in the breakdown of connective tissue in food, activates pepsinogen to pepsin (which degrades protein), and kills any bacteria ingested in food. The acidic digest leaves the stomach to enter the duodenum. This movement of digested food lessens stomach distension and thereby removes a stimulus for the release of gastrin and for vagal activity. In response to acidity the duodenum releases **secretin,** a hormone that stimulates the release of bicarbonate and digestive enzymes from the pancreas. Secretin also depresses the release of hydrochloric acid by the parietal cells and depresses the motility of the stomach. The bicarbonate released by the pancreas neutralizes the acidity of the partially digested food entering the duodenum. This neutralization is also necessary for the digestive enzymes in the intestine to be active.

Risk Factors for Ulcers

Bacteria

Recent attention has focused on a bacterial cause of ulcers. The bacterium *H. pylori* accounts for 70% to 90% of all stomach and duodenal ulcers. This bacterium attaches to the mucus-secreting gastric epithelial cells that line the stomach and survives by breaking down urea to neutralize the acid in its microenvironment. This leads to the loss of mucus that protects the lining of the stomach and duodenum from acid. However, most persons infected with this organism do not develop an ulcer, so other risk factors also play a role. Evidence is accumulating that chronic *H. pylori* infection can also lead to acid hypersecretion and gastritis.

Eradication of *H. pylori* can be achieved with a combination therapy that includes suppression of acid production and antibiotics. When eradication therapy is used, the recurrence rate for ulcers drops to 5%. Previous therapies had a recurrence rate of 60% to 80%.

Drugs

Nonsteroidal antiinflammatory drugs (NSAIDs) inhibit prostaglandin synthesis. Because prostaglandins are important in maintaining the gastric mucosal system, use of NSAIDs is associated with upper gastrointestinal (GI) tract bleeding, and prolonged use can cause peptic ulcers. Older adults are especially sensitive to this effect. Corticosteroids

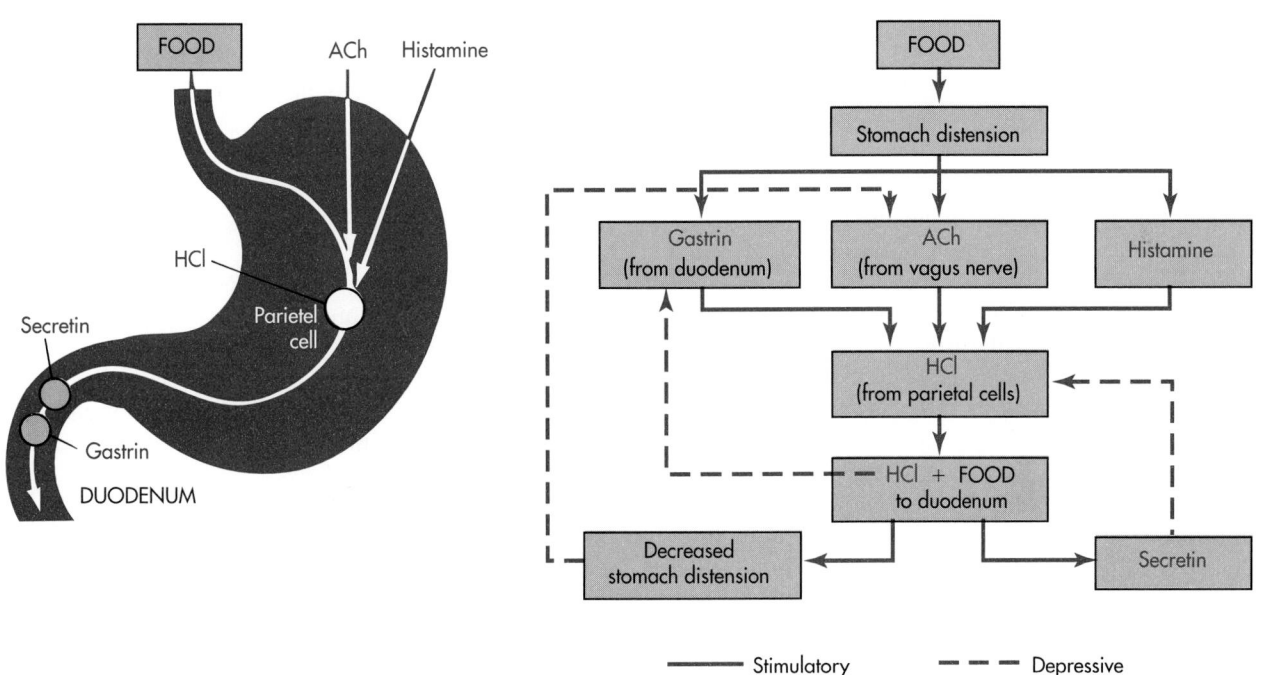

F i g u r e 26-1 Secretion of acid parietal cells of stomach is controlled by duodenally released hormone, gastrin; parasympathetic nervous system, via neurotransmitter acetylcholine *(ACh);* and histamine. Histamine is most effective stimulant of gastric acid secretion. Acid secretion is discontinued when food reaches duodenum, where hydrochloric acid *(HCl)* inhibits gastrin release and stimulates secretin release, and distension of stomach is lessened, decreasing vagal stimulation.

enhance the incidence of ulcer formation in patients, especially those also taking NSAIDs.

Other Factors

In the past, much attention was given to dietary and emotional factors. However, these are exacerbating factors and not causal factors for ulcers. Smoking is also an aggravating factor.

THERAPEUTIC RATIONALE: DRUGS TO TREAT ACID SECRETION AND ULCERS

Until recently, the control of acid secretion was the goal of ulcer treatment. Now control of acid secretion is just part of the treatment. Drugs to treat acid secretion are listed in Table 26-1. The introduction of H_2-receptor antagonists and proton pump inhibitors in the past decade dramatically improved the ability to control acid secretion and allow ulcer healing. Mucosal protective agents also aid ulcer healing. Antacids and anticholinergic drugs, once a mainstay of ulcer therapy, now play a minor role.

Histamine H_2-Receptor Antagonists

Mechanism of Action

The **H_2 antagonists** specifically block the H_2 receptors that control the basal and stimulated secretion of hydrochloric acid by the parietal cells (see Figure 26-1). (H_1 receptors are blocked by the antihistamines discussed in Chapter 29.) Gastrin and acetylcholine are believed to act through histamine to cause the release of hydrochloric acid because H_2 antagonists are so effective in decreasing acid secretion stimulated by pentagastrin (an active analog of gastrin) or bethanechol (an agonist of acetylcholine), as well as by food, insulin, and caffeine.

Pharmacokinetics

The H_2 antagonists are taken orally and absorbed rapidly. They are effective within an hour. Cimetidine has a duration of action of up to 6 hours, whereas other H_2 antagonists have a duration of up to 12 hours. They are partially metabolized by the liver and excreted in the urine. Patients with severe renal disease should receive reduced doses.

Uses

H_2 antagonists became available in 1995 as over-the-counter drugs for the prevention and relief of heartburn. Because H_2 antagonists dramatically decrease stomach acid, they alleviate many conditions in which stomach acid impedes therapy, including the following:

- Duodenal and gastric ulcers: H_2 antagonists are used in combination with other drugs in the treatment of ulcers.
- Zollinger-Ellison syndrome: A tumor secretes excessive gastrin that stimulates excessive acid production. H_2 antagonists depress this acid production.
- GI hemorrhage: Stomach acid intensifies inflammation of the stomach, worsening the hemorrhaging.

- Pancreatic insufficiency: Digestive enzymes must be administered orally. Without H_2 antagonists, stomach acid inactivates most of the administered enzymes.

Adverse Reactions and Contraindications

H_2 antagonists are remarkably free of general side effects. Central nervous system (CNS) effects include mental confusion, agitation, and hallucinations; these symptoms are reversible when the drug is discontinued. CNS effects are more common in patients with liver or renal disease.

Interactions

All H_2 antagonists decrease the gastric acidity that can alter the absorption of other drugs. The absorption of ketoconazole and itraconazole in particular is reduced unless it is taken at least 2 hours before the H_2 antagonist. The absorption of the H_2 antagonists is slowed by concurrent administration of antacids.

Cimetidine inhibits the liver cytochrome P-450 system that metabolizes many drugs. Some of the drugs whose metabolism is inhibited include warfarin, theophylline, and phenytoin. The doses of these drugs should be reduced. Cimetidine also inhibits the gastric metabolism of alcohol. The other H_2 antagonists do not affect drug metabolism.

Cimetidine given in large doses over a long time has a feminizing effect on men, producing gynecomastia, impotence, and loss of libido. These effects are not characteristic of the other H_2 antagonists.

Specific Histamine H_2-Receptor Antagonists
▼ cimetidine

Cimetidine (Tagamet) was the first histamine H_2-receptor antagonist released for commercial use. It has a shorter duration of action than the other H_2 antagonists. Cimetidine is also available without a prescription.

famotidine

Famotidine (Pepcid) can be taken once a day. Famotidine is also available without a prescription.

nizatidine

Nizatidine (Axid) can be taken once a day and is also available without a prescription.

ranitidine and ranitidine bismuth citrate

Ranitidine (Zantac) can be taken once a day and is also available without a prescription. Ranitidine bismuth citrate (Tritec) is a new formulation for the treatment of active duodenal ulcers associated with *H. pylori* when used with the antibiotic clarithromycin.

Acid (Proton) Pump Inhibitors
Mechanism of Action

Acid (or proton) pump inhibitors block the enzyme that "pumps" hydrogen ion (or proton) into the secretory side of the parietal cells of the stomach. This activity more

Table 26-1   Drugs to Treat Acid Secretion and Ulcers

Generic Name	Trade Name	Administration/Dosage	Comments
H₂-Receptor Antagonists			
cimetidine	Tagamet Apo-Cimetidine† Novocimetidine† Peptol†	*For heartburn, indigestion:* ORAL: *Adults*—200 mg with water as symptoms appear or prophylactically 1 hr before a meal. Take only once daily. *For ulcer therapy:* ORAL: *Adults*—300 mg with meals and at bedtime or 400 or 600 mg twice daily or 800 mg at bedtime. FDA pregnancy category B.	Nurse should administer with meals because food slows absorption and prolongs action of cimetidine. Nurse should administer at least 1 hr after antacids or metoclopramide, which reduces absorption of cimetidine if taken concurrently.
cimetidine hydrochloride	Tagamet* Hydroxide	INTRAVENOUS: *Adults*—1-4 mg/kg/hr or 300 mg diluted and infused over 15-20 min. INTRAMUSCULAR: *Adults*—300 mg every 6 hr. FDA pregnancy category B. ORAL, INTRAVENOUS: *Children*—20-40 mg/kg in divided doses.	Nurse should switch to oral doses when ulcer bleeding has stopped.
famotidine	Pepcid* Ulcidine†	*For heartburn, indigestion:* ORAL: *Adults*—10 mg as symptoms appear or prophylactically 1 hr before a meal. Take only once daily. *For ulcer therapy:* ORAL: *Adults*—40 mg/day at bedtime, or in 2 divided doses. INTRAVENOUS: *Adults*—20 mg every 12 hr. FDA pregnancy category B.	Famotidine acts longer than cimetidine.
nizatidine	Axid*	*For heartburn, indigestion:* ORAL: *Adults*—75 mg as symptoms appear or prophylactically 30-60 min before a meal. Take only once daily. *For ulcer therapy:* ORAL: *Adults*—300 mg/day at bedtime to heal ulcer, then 150 mg/day to prevent recurrence. FDA pregnancy category B.	Nizatidine acts longer than cimetidine.
ranitidine hydrochloride	Zantac* Apo-Ranitidine†	*For heartburn, indigestion:* ORAL: *Adults*—75 mg as symptoms appear or prophylactically 1 hr before a meal. Take only once daily. *For ulcer therapy:* ORAL: *Adults*—150 mg every 12 hr. INTRAMUSCULAR/SLOW INTRAVENOUS: *Adults*—50 mg every 6-8 hr. Maximum daily dose is 400 mg. FDA pregnancy category B.	Ranitidine hydrochloride acts longer than cimetidine.
ranitidine bismuth citrate	Tritec	ORAL: *Adults*—400 mg twice a day for 8 wk in combination with clarithromycin 500 mg 3 times/day for 2 wk. FDA pregnancy category B.	Bismuth salt formulated for eradicating *H. pylori*.
Acid Pump Inhibitors			
lansoprazole	Prevacid*	*For erosive esophagitis:* ORAL: *Adults*—30 mg/day, before eating, for 8-16 wk. *For ulcer:* ORAL: *Adults*—15-30 mg in the morning before eating, for 4 wk. *For hypersecretion:* ORAL: *Adults*—60 mg in the morning before eating. FDA pregnancy category B.	Delayed-release capsules. Also used in combination with clarithromycin and/or metronidazole, amoxicillin to eradicate *H. pylori*.
omeprazole	Losec† Prilosec	ORAL: *Adults*—20-40 mg once a day for 4-8 wk. FDA pregnancy category C.	Delayed-release capsules/tablets. Also used in combination with clarithromycin and/or metronidazole, amoxicillin to eradicate *H. pylori*.
pantoprozole†	Pantoloc†	*For erosive esophagitis:* ORAL: *Adults*—40 mg/day, before eating, for 4-8 wk. *For ulcer:* ORAL: *Adults*—40 mg, in the morning before eating, for 4-8 wk.	New drug.
Mucosal Protective Agents			
aluminum hydroxide gel	AlternaGEL Amphojel*	ORAL: *Adults*—5-30 ml up to 40 ml every 30 min if pain is severe.	Antacid. Aluminum hydroxide gel is constipating. Long-term use may cause hypophosphatemia. The drug complexes with tetracycline and can interfere with absorption of warfarin, digoxin, quinine, and quinidine.

*Available in Canada and the United States.
†Available in Canada only.

Continued

Table 26-1 Drugs to Treat Acid Secretion and Ulcers—cont'd

Generic Name	Trade Name	Administration/Dosage	Comments
aluminum carbonate gel	Basaljel*	ORAL: *Adults*—5-20 ml or 2 capsules every 2 hr up to 12 times/day.	Antacid. See aluminum hydroxide gel.
bismuth subsalicylate	Pepto-Bismol* Others	*For ulcers:* ORAL: *Adults*—525 mg (15-30 ml or 2 tablets) 3 times/day 1 hr before meals and at bedtime.	Used in combination therapy with antibiotics to eradicate *H. pylori*.
calcium carbonate	Dicarbosil Titralac Tums Others	ORAL: *Adults*—1-4 g 1 and 3 hr after meals and at bedtime. (Tablets should be chewed before swallowing.)	Antacid. Calcium carbonate is constipating. It can be used hourly to keep acid neutralized, but some patients become hypercalcemic.
magnesium carbonate magnesium hydroxide magnesium oxide magnesium phosphate magnesium trisilicate	Milk of Magnesia Others	ORAL: *Adults*—Check individual product label for information.	Antacid. These magnesium salts are laxatives and must be taken with aluminum or calcium antacid to maintain normal stool consistency.
misoprostol	Cytotec	ORAL: *Adults*—200 μg 4 times/day at meals and bedtime or 400 μg 2 times/day. FDA pregnancy category X.	Misoprostol protects against ulcers from nonsteroidal antiinflammatory drugs used for arthritis. It is also effective for healing peptic ulcers.
sucralfate	Carafate Sulcrate†	ORAL: *Adults*—1 g 4 times/day taken 1 hr before meals and 1 hr before bedtime.	If antacids are prescribed for pain relief, they should not be taken 30 min before or after sucralfate.
Antimicrobials Effective Against *H. pylori*			
amoxicillin	Amoxil* Trimox Others	ORAL: *Adults*—1 g 2 times/day.	Requires acid suppression with acid pump inhibitor or H_2 antagonist to be effective.
clarithromycin	Biaxin*	ORAL: *Adults*—500 mg 2 times/day.	Requires acid suppression with acid pump inhibitor or H_2 antagonist to be effective.
metronidazole	Flagyl* Prostat Novonidazol† Others	ORAL: *Adults*—250 mg 4 times/day or 500 mg 2 times/day.	Resistance develops rapidly. Best given with another antimicrobial, bismuth, and acid suppression with acid pump inhibitor or H_2 antagonist.
tetracycline	Achromycin* Novotetra† Sumycin Others	ORAL: *Adults*—500 mg 4 times/day.	Oxytetracycline may be substituted. Best given with another antimicrobial, bismuth, and acid suppression with acid pump inhibitor or H_2 antagonist.

*Available in Canada and the United States.
†Available in Canada only.

completely blocks stomach acid production than do the H_2-receptor antagonists.

Pharmacokinetics

The onset of action for these drugs is within 1 hour. The duration of action is prolonged; more than 39 hours for lansoprazole and 72 hours for omeprazole. Lansoprazole is metabolized by the liver into inactive metabolites that are excreted in the feces. Omeprazole is metabolized by the liver into inactive metabolites that are excreted in the urine.

Uses

Acid pump inhibitors are more potent that the H_2-receptor antagonists but are used for the same indications. They are effective in treating severe erosive esophagitis that has not responded to therapy with H_2-receptor antagonists. They also are used in the short-term treatment of active peptic ulcer disease, especially when combined with an antibiotic to eradicate *H. pylori*. Pathologic gastric hypersecretion disorders such as Zollinger-Ellison syndrome are treated with acid pump inhibitors.

Adverse Reactions and Contraindications

Acid pump inhibitors are very effective and have a few side effects with short-term therapy. The major concern for long-term therapy is the potential for leading to overproduction of gastrin, which can lead to gastric carcinoid tumors. At present this is a theoretical rather than an observed risk, but more experience with these drugs will be needed to assess safety with long-term use.

Interactions

Omeprazole inhibits the hepatic cytochrome P-450 system and can interfere with the metabolism of oral anticoagulants, diazepam, and phenytoin, leading to high blood levels of these drugs.

CASE STUDY

Gastrointestinal Tract Ulceration

Mr. Hanson is 47 years old and has been admitted to the hospital with the diagnosis of "acute GI bleeding." He has a history of peptic ulcer disease and has had abdominal pain and tarry stools for the past 3 weeks. He has been self-treating himself with Maalox several times a day. His history also reveals that he is a pack-a-day smoker and that he drinks alcohol approximately 6 days per week. His admission orders include famotidine (Pepcid) 20 mg IV every 12 hours.

1. Although the mechanisms of action of Maalox and famotidine differ, the therapeutic effects are the same. Explain.
2. Mr. Hanson asks the nurse, "Why isn't my doctor having me take the Maalox anymore?" What should the nurse consider in formulating a response?
3. Mr. Hanson has an endoscopy performed, which reveals a large duodenal ulcer that is not actively bleeding. Biopsies are performed, and his physician discontinues the famotidine and prescribed omeprazole (Prilosec) 20 mg PO twice daily. Mr. Hanson asks you how the omeprazole differs from the famotidine he was previously taking. Explain the difference.
4. What aspects of Mr. Hanson's lifestyle have placed him at risk for ulcer formation?
5. What is *Helicobacter pylori* and how would you expect Mr. Hanson's medication regime to change?
6. What medication teaching is important to cover with Mr. Hanson before his discharge?

Specific Proton Pump Inhibitors

lansoprazole

Lansoprazole (Prevacid) is available as a delayed-release capsule for once-a-day administration.

▼ omeprazole

Omeprazole (Prilosec) is available in delayed-release form for once-a-day administration. The Food and Drug Administration (FDA) has approved a combination therapy of omeprazole and the antibiotic clarithromycin (Biaxin) for the treatment of peptic ulcers.

pantoprazole

Pantoprazole (Pantoloc) is a new acid pump inhibitor available in enteric-coated tablets.

Mucosal Protective Agents

Antacids

Antacids are weak bases that can be ingested to neutralize the hydrochloric acid secreted by the stomach.

Sodium bicarbonate (baking soda) reacts with hydrochloric acid to yield water and carbon dioxide. Carbon dioxide is a gas that causes the frequent belching associated with the ingestion of sodium bicarbonate. Sodium bicarbonate is the only common antacid that is readily absorbed from the GI tract. Taken in excess, sodium bicarbonate also makes the blood slightly alkaline, thus making urine alkaline. Excess bicarbonate stimulates the stomach to secrete more acid (rebound hypersecretion). This hypersecretion can persist after the bicarbonate has been absorbed. For these reasons, sodium bicarbonate is not an antacid of choice when prolonged therapy is required.

Nonsystemic antacids include alkaline salts of aluminum, magnesium, and calcium, which neutralize acid but are not readily absorbed into the bloodstream. Aluminum and calcium salts tend to cause constipation, whereas magnesium salts tend to loosen the bowels. Therefore most antacids combine a magnesium salt or hydroxide and an aluminum or calcium salt or hydroxide. However, calcium carbonate has a greater potential for allowing acid rebound and leading to the formation of kidney stones. As an adjunct to ulcer therapy, 1444 mEq of acid neutralizing capacity taken 1 to 3 hours after meals and at bedtime gives adequate acid control and relieves the pain of ulcers.

Nonsystemic antacids are available as liquids or chewable tablets. The most common side effect is diarrhea or constipation, even with a combination antacid. The patient must then add more aluminum or calcium antacid to correct diarrhea or more magnesium antacid to correct constipation. Antacids can impede the absorption of drugs, notably tetracyclines (antibiotics), digoxin (a cardiac glycoside), and quinidine (a cardiac antiarrhythmic drug).

bismuth subsalicylate

Bismuth subsalicylate (Pepto-Bismol, others) is used in combination with one or more antimicrobials and to treat ulcers. Bismuth is toxic to *H. pylori* without the development of resistance. Because of its short half-life, bismuth subsalicylate should be taken four times a day. It can turn the tongue and stools black.

Bismuth has been added to the H₂ antagonist ranitidine as ranitidine bismuth citrate (Tritec). This combination of the bacteriocidal activity of bismuth with the suppression of acid secretion by ranitidine is approved for the treatment of ulcers.

misoprostol

Misoprostol (Cytotec) is an ester of prostaglandin E₁. Prostaglandin E₁ is normally synthesized in the stomach, where it blocks gastric acid secretion. NSAIDs, including aspirin, inhibit the synthesis of naturally occurring prostaglandin E₁ when they dissolve in the stomach. Therefore bleeding from gastric ulcers is a significant problem with long-term use of NSAIDs. Patients with arthritis who must take NSAIDs to relieve inflammation and pain are a major market for misoprostol. Misoprostol replaces the prostaglandin E₁ that is not produced in the stomach when NSAIDs are present. With the protection of misoprostol, excess acid secretion is blocked, and therefore stomach mucosa is protected. Misoprostol is also used to treat duodenal and peptic ulcers caused by NSAID use.

Minor effects such as diarrhea, mild nausea, abdominal discomfort, and dizziness are occasionally reported. Serious side effects are bleeding and abortion in pregnant women, an action expected of a prostaglandin E_1 analog. In one study there was bleeding in 50% of pregnant women and a 7% incidence of abortion. Therefore misoprostol is contraindicated for pregnant women and should be used cautiously by women of childbearing age.

sucralfate

Sucralfate (Carafate) is a complex of sulfated sucrose and aluminum hydroxide that is changed by stomach acid into viscous material that binds to proteins in ulcerated tissue. This action protects the ulcer from the destructive action of the digestive enzyme pepsin. Sucralfate is used in the initial treatment (first 1 to 2 months) of a duodenal ulcer. Sucralfate does not neutralize stomach acid or inhibit acid secretion. Sucralfate should be given alone 30 to 60 minutes before mealtime so that it can be activated by stomach acid and coat the ulcer. Sucralfate binds digoxin, tetracycline, warfarin, phenytoin, quinidine, and theophylline; thus these drugs should be taken at different times. Sucralfate also decreases the bioavailability of ciprofloxacin and norfloxacin.

Antimicrobial Therapy for *H. pylori*

The identification of *H. pylori* as the major causative agent for peptic ulcers has added antimicrobials as the key to effective treatment of ulcers. *H. pylori* infection is endemic worldwide. The highest infection rates are associated with food and water contamination. For instance, the infection rate is lowest in Australia at 20% and highest in west Africa at 90%. Although infection occurs during childhood, the individual may remain asymptomatic throughout life. For individuals with symptoms of an ulcer, the presence of *H. pylori* can be confirmed by serologic testing or by the urease breath assay. A 2-week therapy with two appropriate antimicrobial agents and acid suppression or bismuth leads to eradication of *H. pylori* in 80% of cases. Examples of some of the currently used combination therapies are listed (Box 26-1). In the future, a vaccine may be developed to prevent infection.

amoxicillin

Amoxicillin (Amoxil, Trimox, others) is concentrated in gastric secretions and can therefore achieve effective antimicrobial concentrations in the lumen. Because amoxicillin is not very active in an acid environment, suppression of acid secretion enhances antimicrobial activity. *H. pylori* does not become resistant to amoxicillin. Side effects of amoxicillin include diarrhea and yeast infections. See Chapter 44 for further information on amoxicillin.

clarithromycin

Clarithromycin (Biaxin) is active against *H. pylori*. It can replace metronidazole in treatment therapies for *H. pylori*.

Side effects include diarrhea, nausea, headache, and a bad taste in the mouth. Resistance can develop to clarithromycin. Clarithromycin is contraindicated for patients taking cisapride, an agent used in treating gastroesophageal reflux. The combination may cause cardiac arrhythmias. See Chapter 46 for further information on clarithromycin.

Two-drug combination therapies have been developed using clarithromycin as the sole antimicrobial. A combination therapy of clarithromycin and omeprazole has been approved by the FDA for treatment of ulcers and *H. pylori* infection. Clarithromycin is given at a dosage of 500 mg three times daily for 2 weeks. Omeprazole is given at a dosage of 40 mg once a day for 2 weeks followed by 2 weeks at 20 mg once daily. A second combination is ranitidine bismuth citrate and clarithromycin. Clarithromycin is given at a dosage of 500 mg three times daily for 2 weeks. Ranitidine bismuth citrate is given at a dosage of 400 mg twice daily for 4 weeks. The goal of two-drug combination therapies is to increase the compliance rate, which can be low with the more complicated triple and quadruple combination therapies.

metronidazole

Metronidazole (Flagyl, others) is selective against bacteria that grow under low oxygen. It is secreted in gastric secretions and is not affected by acidic conditions. Although *H. pylori* is sensitive to metronidazole, resistance rapidly develops. Side effects such as diarrhea, nausea, vomiting, and a

---

Box 26-1   Examples of Triple or Quadruple Combination Therapy for Eradication of *H. pylori*

1. Acid pump inhibitor twice daily
   plus
   clarithromycin twice daily
   plus
   metronidazole twice daily
   or
   amoxicillin twice daily

2. Acid pump inhibitor once daily
   or
   H₂ antagonist at bedtime
   plus
   bismuth subsalicylate four times daily
   plus
   metronidazole four times daily
   plus
   tetracycline four times daily

3. Acid pump inhibitor once daily
   or
   H₂ antagonist at bedtime
   plus
   amoxicillin three times daily
   plus
   clarithromycin three times daily
   plus (optional)
   bismuth subsalicylate four times daily

*These are examples and not exhaustive of therapeutic combinations for eradication of *H. pylori*. Combination 1 is given for 7 days; combinations 2 and 3 for 7-14 days.

metallic taste in the mouth are common. A disulfiram-like reaction can develop if someone drinks an alcoholic beverage while taking metronidazole. See Chapter 53 for further information on metronidazole.

tetracycline

Tetracycline is combined with bismuth and metronidazole to eradicate *H. pylori*. Like amoxicillin, tetracycline concentrates in the gastric mucosa; however, tetracycline is active in an acidic environment. In treating ulcers, tetracycline is taken with bismuth at meals to promote binding of tetracycline to bismuth, a combination that promotes activity against *H. pylori*. Side effects of tetracycline include diarrhea and photosensitivity. Tetracycline is not recommended for pregnant women or children less than 8 years old. See Chapter 47 for further information on tetracycline.

Nursing Process Overview

Drugs to Treat Ulcers

Assessment

Patients with suspected ulcer disease may have a variety of symptoms. Obtain a baseline patient assessment, focusing on the vital signs, level of consciousness, and character or quality of any emesis or stool, including the presence of occult blood. Monitor the patient's intake and output. Question the patient about relevant history, such as recent alcohol intake or previous ulcer disease. Monitor the hematocrit and hemoglobin levels.

Nursing Diagnoses

- Altered thought processes related to drug side effect (H$_2$ antagonists)
- Altered health maintenance related to complicated dosing regimens when patient is taking several drugs

Patient Outcomes

The patient will state there is relief of GI discomfort.

Planning/Implementation

The goal of treating an ulcer is to stop blood loss and to promote the healing of the ulcerated area. Monitor the patient's vital signs, intake and output, level of consciousness, and character of any emesis or stool. Monitor hematocrit, hemoglobin, and serum electrolyte levels. Prepare the patient for ordered diagnostic studies. Teach the patient about any ordered dietary restrictions.

Evaluation

Before discharge, the patient should be able to explain why the drugs have been ordered, how to take them correctly, how to treat side effects, which side effects require medical attention, and how to implement dietary or other restrictions prescribed by the physician.

Nursing Implications Summary

HISTAMINE RECEPTOR ANTAGONISTS

cimetidine

Drug Administration

➤ For direct intravenous (IV) injection, dilute 300 mg in at least 18 ml of normal saline (total volume is 20 ml). Administer at a rate of 300 mg or less over 5 minutes. For intermittent IV infusion, dilute 300 mg of drug in at least 50 ml of compatible IV solution. Do not add to continuously infusing fluids. Administer over 15 to 20 minutes. The solution may also be diluted and administered over 24 hours; use an infusion control device.

➤ Warn the patient that there may be discomfort associated with intramuscular administration.

➤ Read medication labels carefully. Prefilled syringes are intended for intramuscular use or for diluting for intermittent infusion. Prefilled syringes are not for direct IV injection. This drug is incompatible with many other drugs for infusion. Do not add other drugs to infusions of cimetidine.

➤ Administer once-daily doses before bedtime, twice-daily doses in the morning and at bedtime, and more frequent doses with meals and at bedtime. If antacids or metoclopramide are also ordered, they should be administered 1 hour before or after the cimetidine dose.

➤ Because cimetidine is metabolized by the liver and excreted through the kidney, the action of many drugs, including aminophylline, caffeine, anticoagulants, and some heart medications, may be potentiated when the patient is also receiving cimetidine. Assess the patient carefully for side effects and monitor appropriate laboratory tests carefully because dosages of other drugs may require adjustment.

➤ Monitor level of consciousness, blood pressure and pulse, intake and output, and complete blood count. Assess the patient for skin changes and gynecomastia. For Nursing in the Community, see below the Drug Administration section of the remaining histamine H$_2$-receptor antagonists.

famotidine, nizatidine, and ranitidine

Drug Administration

➤ Administer once-daily doses before bedtime, twice-daily doses in the morning and at bedtime, and more frequent

Continued

Nursing Implications Summary—cont'd

doses with meals and at bedtime. If antacids or metoclopramide are also ordered, they should be administered 1 hour before or after the histamine H$_2$-receptor antagonists.

➤ For direct IV use of famotidine, dilute 20 mg with 5 to 10 ml of compatible solution, and administer over at least 2 minutes. For intermittent infusion of famotidine, dilute 20 mg in 100 ml of compatible solution, and administer dose over 15 to 30 minutes.

➤ For direct IV use of ranitidine, dilute 50 mg with 20 ml of compatible IV solution, and administer over at least 5 minutes. For intermittent infusion of ranitidine, dilute 50 mg in 50 to 100 ml of compatible IV solution, and administer over 15 to 20 minutes. Also available as a premixed 0.5 mg/ml solution in 100 ml. The solution may also be diluted and administered over 24 hours; use an infusion control device.

➤ Be alert when administering ranitidine intravenously; too rapid administration has been associated with bradycardia, tachycardia, and premature ventricular contractions (PVCs).

➤ Monitor pulse and blood pressure. Monitor level of consciousness, blood pressure, and pulse; assess for constipation or diarrhea and monitor complete blood count and blood urea nitrogen.

Nursing in the Community

➤ Warn patients taking nonprescription strength of these drugs to take doses no longer than 2 weeks on a regular basis unless approved by the physician.

➤ Review with the patient the side effects associated with the prescribed drug and instruct the patient to report the development of these side effects to the physician. Review all prescribed medications with the patient, and help the patient develop a dosing schedule that is consistent with the therapy goals and possible drug interactions.

➤ Warn the patient to avoid alcohol and smoking while taking these drugs, especially after the final dose of the day. Emphasize the importance of all aspects of therapy, which may include modifying the diet, taking other drugs, and limiting caffeine intake. Warn the patient to avoid using over-the-counter preparations while taking histamine H$_2$-receptor antagonists.

➤ Teach patients using ranitidine effervescent granules or effervescent tablets to dissolve dose in 6 to 8 oz of water before drinking.

➤ Note: this Nursing in the Community information also applies to cimetidine.

lansoprazole and omeprazole
Nursing in the Community

➤ Instruct the patient to take lansoprazole and omeprazole capsules immediately before a meal, preferable in the morning. Omeprazole tablets may be taken on an empty stomach or with food. Instruct the patient to swallow capsules whole, not to break or chew them. Omeprazole may be taken with antacids if ordered.

➤ Instruct the patient to take missed doses as soon as remembered, unless almost time for the next dose, then omit missed dose. Do not double up for missed doses.

➤ Remind patients to keep all health care providers aware of all drugs being used.

MUCOSAL PROTECTIVE AGENTS
Antacids
Nursing in the Community

➤ Instruct the patient to avoid administering antacids with tetracyclines, digoxin, or quinidine. Review with the patient the complete list of medications, and schedule home drug administration that prevents the antacids from interfering with absorption of any other drugs. Try to schedule antacids for 30 minutes before or 1 hour after sucralfate; try to schedule histamine H$_2$-receptor antagonists 1 hour before or after antacids.

➤ Remind the patient to chew antacid tablets, not to swallow them whole.

➤ Instruct the patient to take a small amount of water after doses of antacid liquid to ensure that the antacid dose is carried to the stomach.

➤ Instruct the patient to alternate aluminum or calcium salts with magnesium salts to prevent diarrhea or constipation unless a specific antacid is ordered. Also instruct the patient to increase fluid intake to 2500 to 3000 ml/day and increase dietary intake of fruits and fiber to prevent constipation.

➤ Patients with renal failure should not increase fluid intake and may require concomitant stool softeners.

➤ Instruct the patient to read labels carefully. Antacids vary in their strength, acid-neutralizing ability, and sodium content, especially if other drugs are included in the formulation. Commonly included drugs are magaldrate, another antacid, and simethicone, an antigas drug.

➤ Instruct the patient taking aluminum carbonate, aluminum hydroxide, or calcium carbonate products for hyperphosphatemia not to substitute other antacids. Doses of antacids used to bind phosphates are often administered with meals. Refer the patient to a dietitian for instruction in following a low-phosphate diet if indicated.

➤ Antacids used to treat ulcers are often administered 1 and 3 hours after meals and at bedtime; review prescription orders with patients. Instruct the patient taking antacids to prevent kidney stones by increasing daily fluid intake to 3000 ml.

➤ Instruct the patient requiring sodium restriction for heart disease or other health problems to avoid antacids high in sodium; consult the physician or pharmacist. Low-sodium or sodium-free products include Alka-Mints, Equilet, Maalox tablets, magaldrate, and Mylanta. Products relatively high in sodium include Gaviscon-2 chewable tablets (36.8 mg) and Genaton Extra Strength tablets (35 mg). Instruct the patient to use antacids as prescribed and avoid frequent self-medication with over-the-counter products unless advised to do so by a physician.

Nursing Implications Summary—cont'd

bismuth subsalicylate
Nursing in the Community

➤ Caution the patient to avoid the use of bismuth salts in infants or children who are recovering from the flu or chicken pox. If nausea and vomiting are present, the patient should check with the physician because these symptoms may indicate Reye's syndrome.

➤ Instruct patients taking bismuth subsalicylate to read the labels of other drugs they may be taking and to avoid other salicylate-containing drugs. Also, large amounts of bismuth salts may interfere with urine glucose tests. Instruct diabetic patients to be alert to this possibility.

➤ Warn patients that this drug may cause discoloration of the tongue and that stools will turn black.

misoprostol
Drug Administration/Nursing in the Community

➤ Question female patients about possible pregnancy before administering first dose. Ensure that women of childbearing age are informed of the possible side effects of bleeding and abortion before administering first dose.

➤ Instruct the patient to report severe or persistent diarrhea. Instruct the patient to avoid concurrent use of magnesium-containing antacids; they may aggravate diarrhea. Encourage the patient to take misoprostol with or after meals and at bedtime for best effect. Instruct the patient to report any new sign or symptom.

sucralfate
Drug Administration/Nursing in the Community

➤ Instruct the patient to take antacids 30 minutes before or after sucralfate. For best effects, instruct the patient to take sucralfate with water on an empty stomach 1 hour before meals and at bedtime.

➤ Review with the patient the complete list of medications prescribed, and develop a dosing schedule that is suitable considering known drug interactions. The patient should take cimetidine, digoxin, phenytoin, tetracyclines, and fat-soluble vitamins at different times than sucralfate.

➤ Instruct the patient to keep a record of bowel movements. If constipation develops, instruct the patient to increase daily intake of fluids to 2500 to 3000 ml, increase level of activity, and increase dietary intake of fruit and fiber. If the patient is taking antacids, changing the brand of antacid may also help; consult the physician.

CHAPTER REVIEW

Application

1. What three factors stimulate the secretion of stomach acid?
2. How do ulcers arise? What does the location of the ulcer indicate?
3. What do antacids do?
4. Name the major side effects you might expect with the use of sodium bicarbonate, aluminum and calcium alkaline salts, and magnesium alkaline salts.

Critical Thinking

1. Why does cimetidine inhibit gastric acid secretion, whereas antihistamines used to treat hay fever do not?
2. Differentiate among lansoprazole and omeprazole, misoprostol, and sucralfate. Would two of these be ordered concurrently?

References

Aronson B: Update on peptic ulcer drugs, *Am J Nurs* 98(1):41-46, 1998.

Brozenec SA: Ulcer therapy update, *RN* 59(9):48-50, 52-54, 1996.

Cottrill MRB: *Helicobacter pylori*, *Prof Nurse* 12(1):46-48, 1996.

Heslin JM: Peptic ulcer disease: making a case against the prime suspect, *Nursing* 27(1):34-39, 1997.

Podolski JL: Recent advances in peptic ulcer disease: *Helicobacter pylori* infection and its treatment, *Gastroenterol Nurs* 19(4):128-136, 1996.

Turner LW, et al: Dietary management in the patient with chronic renal failure, *Am J Nurs* 97(9):16B, 16D, 16F, 16H, 1997.

Chapter 27

Drugs to Treat Gallbladder and Pancreatic Diseases

KEY TERMS

bile, p. 326

cholecystectomy, p. 326

cholelithiasis, p. 326

gallstones, p. 326

pancreatic enzymes, p. 329

KEY DRUGS ▼

chenodiol, p. 328

pancreatin, p. 329

OBJECTIVES

After studying this chapter, you should be able to do the following:

- *Discuss drugs used to dissolve gallstones and drugs for pancreatic enzyme replacement.*
- *Develop a plan of care for patients receiving one of the drugs discussed in this chapter.*

CHAPTER OVERVIEW

This chapter reviews drugs to aid in the dissolution of gallstones and agents to replace pancreatic enzymes.

THERAPEUTIC RATIONALE: GALLBLADDER DISEASES

The gallbladder is a small organ located beneath the right side of the liver (Figure 27-1). The liver produces **bile**, which is a yellow-brown watery fluid consisting of cholesterol, lipids, bile salts, and bilirubin. As much as 3 cups a day are produced, and up to 1 cup of concentrated bile is stored by the gallbladder. A duct connects the gallbladder with the small intestine. As food leaves the stomach and enters the small intestine, the gallbladder contracts and propels stored bile into the small intestine. Bile disperses the fat in food, and it is important for digestion of lipids in the small intestine. Normally, most of the bile is reabsorbed by the small intestine and returned to the liver.

Gallstones are composed principally of cholesterol and are believed to result when crystals form from bile supersaturated with cholesterol, compounded by poor motility of the gallbladder. Usually gallstones remain small, less than 2 cm in diameter. **Cholelithiasis** refers to the presence of gallstones, and most individuals with gallstones do not have symptoms for many years. When symptoms appear, they include brief episodes of biliary pain, sometimes mislabeled as colic.

About 1% to 10% of the U.S. adult population has gallstones. More than 1 million people are newly diagnosed each year. Risk factors for gallstones include age, female gender with multiple pregnancies, obesity, and rapid weight loss (Box 27-1). Most people with gallstones have no symptoms. Gallstones are most commonly detected from an abdominal x-ray examination, computed tomography (CT) scan, or abdominal ultrasound taken for an unrelated problem.

Diagnosis of gallstones is made with ultrasound. A gallstone attack usually gives rise to a steady, severe pain in the upper abdomen that last from 20 to 30 minutes up to several hours. The pain may also be felt in the back between the shoulder blades or in the right shoulder. Nausea and vomiting may also be present. Attacks may not occur often. A common complication of gallstones is that they lodge in the cystic duct, the channel connecting the gallbladder with the common bile duct, and cause cholecystitis, an inflammation of the gallbladder. A more serious problem is blockage of the common bile duct, obstructing the flow of bile from the liver, or even blockage of the flow of digestive fluids from the pancreas. Blockage of any of the ducts can cause severe damage to the gallbladder, liver, or pancreas.

THERAPEUTIC AGENTS: TREATMENT OF GALLSTONES

Removal of the gallbladder, **cholecystectomy**, is the most common method for treating gallstones, with more than 500,000 patients undergoing this surgery each year in the United States. Standard cholecystectomy, involving a 5- to

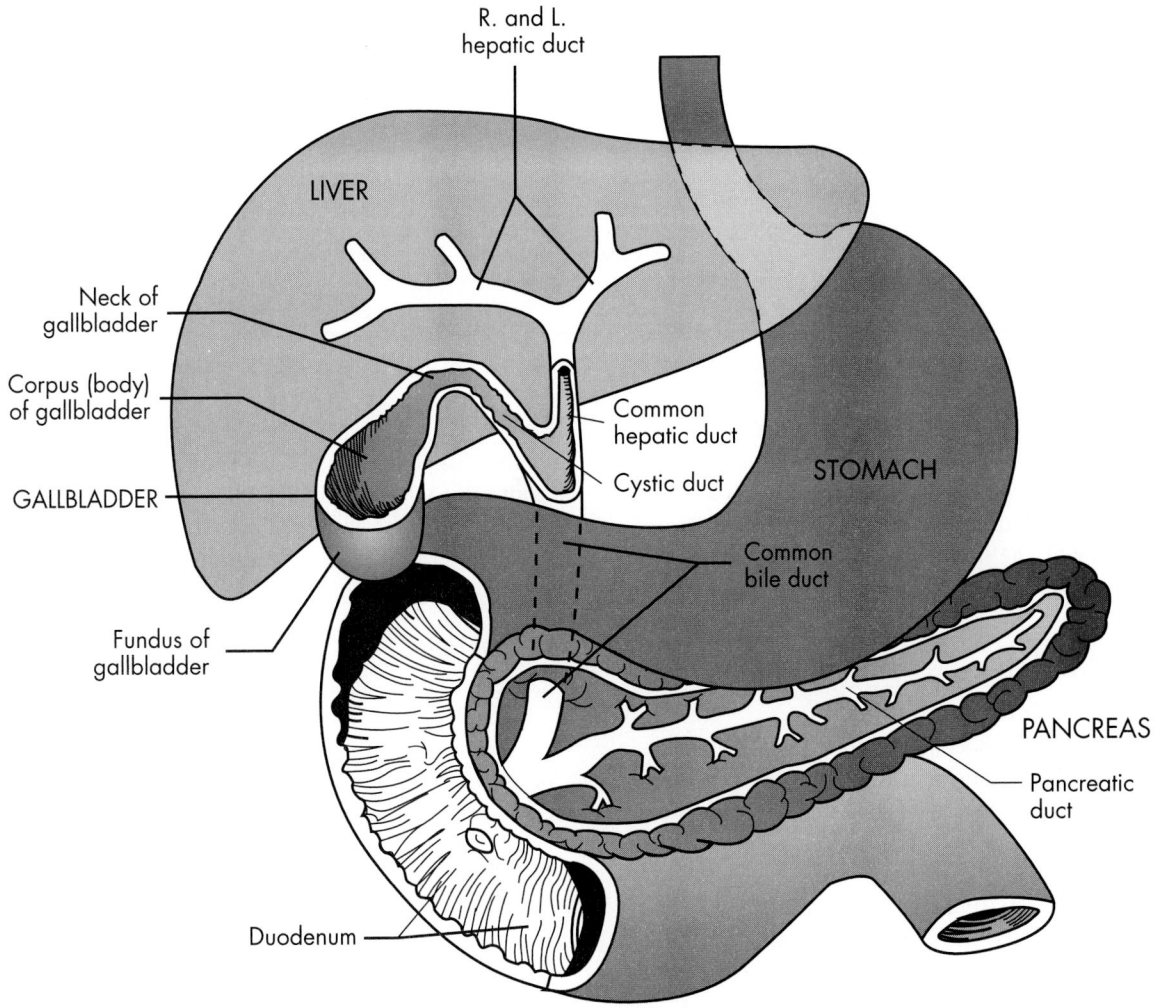

Figure 27-1 Bile is secreted by the liver and stored in the gallbladder. As food passes into the small intestine, the gallbladder contracts and sends stored bile into the cystic duct, which connects into the common bile duct. Bile salts enter the intestine, where they aid in digestion by dispersing lipids. Symptomatic gallstones are most commonly lodged in the cystic duct and less often in the common bile duct. The pancreas is a major source of digestive enzymes: amylase (carbohydrates), trypsin, chymotrypsin, and carboxypeptidase (proteins) and lipase (lipids), as well a bicarbonate to neutralize stomach acid. Pancreatic secretions enter the intestine at the lower end of the common bile duct. *R,* Right; *L,* left. (Courtesy Donald O'Connor)

Box 27-1 Risk Factors for Gallstones

Those most likely to develop gallstones are as follows:

- Women between 20 and 60 years of age (twice as likely as men to develop gallstones)
- Men and women over age 60 years
- Pregnant women or women who have used birth control pills or estrogen replacement therapy
- Native Americans (have the highest prevalence of gallstones in the United States)
- Mexican-American men and women of all ages
- Men and women who are overweight
- People who go on "crash" diets or who lose a lot of weight quickly

From National Institutes of Health Publication No. 95-2897, March 1993.

8-inch abdominal incision to remove the gallbladder, is being replaced by laparoscopic cholecystectomy. Laparoscopic surgery requires only small incisions to be made, avoiding damage to the abdominal muscles. Recovery from this surgery is in days rather than in weeks.

Although surgery is the treatment of choice for symptomatic gallstones, pharmacologic treatment is available for small stones that are predominantly cholesterol. These pharmacologic agents, chenodiol and ursodiol, are derived from bile acids naturally found in bile. They work slowly and must be taken daily for up to 2 years to dissolve gallstones. Specific agents to dissolve gallstones are listed in Table 27-1.

Two experimental procedures for treatment of gallstones are being explored. One treatment is methyl-tert-butyl-ether,

Table 27-1	**Drugs to Dissolve Gallstones**			
Generic Name	Trade Name	Administration/Dosage		Comments
chenodiol	Generic	ORAL: *Adults*—13-16 mg/kg body weight daily divided into 2 doses and taken with food or milk in the morning and at night. FDA pregnancy category X.		Gallstone dissolution may require 3 months to 2 years. Overweight patients are less responsive, may require higher dosage.
ursodiol	Actigall Ursofalk†	ORAL: *Adults*—8-10 mg/kg body weight daily divided into 2 or 3 doses and taken with meals. FDA pregnancy category B.		Gallstone dissolution may require 3 months to 2 years. Also used for cholestatic hepatic disease and gallstone prophylaxis.

†Available in Canada only.

a contact solvent that dissolves cholesterol when instilled into the gallbladder via a catheter. Another treatment is the use of extracorporeal shock-wave lithotripsy in which acoustic shock waves break the stones into smaller pieces. This treatment is followed by pharmacologic therapy to dissolve the stones.

▼ chenodiol

Mechanism of Action

Chenodiol (Chenix) reduces the saturation of cholesterol in bile by increasing the ratio of bile acids to cholesterol. This allows the gradual dissolution of cholesterol from gallstones.

Pharmacokinetics

Chenodiol is taken twice daily with meals. It is readily absorbed from the small intestine and enters the bile through enterohepatic circulation. The liver is also able to metabolize chenodiol into taurine and glycine conjugates that are excreted into the bile. Elimination is in the feces.

Uses

Pharmacologic therapy is used to treat uncomplicated gallstone disease in patients with a functioning gallbladder. The gallstone would be radiolucent indicating a predominant cholesterol content. The insoluble calcium-containing stones are not radiolucent. Dissolution of gallstones generally requires at least 3 months and may take 2 years of daily therapy. Response is monitored with oral cholecystograms or ultrasonograms performed every 6 to 9 months. If no response is seen in 18 months, therapy is discontinued. If a response is seen, therapy is continued until dissolution has been confirmed by two successive ultrasonograms.

Adverse Reactions and Contraindications

The major side effect of chenodiol is diarrhea. This is usually mild and transient; severe diarrhea may indicate an overdose of drug. Occasionally there is constipation, gas, or a frequent urge for bowel movement. These symptoms are most common in the first month of therapy and tend to decrease with time.

Chenodiol is contraindicated during pregnancy because animal studies have indicated damage to fetal organs. Pa-

tients with abnormalities of the bile duct or complications from gallstones are not candidates for pharmacologic therapy. Patients with impaired hepatic function may have further problems of impaired bile acid metabolism and should not receive chenodiol.

Interactions

Cholestyramine, antacids, and colestipol may bind chenodiol and prevent absorption of chenodiol. Clofibrate, estrogens, progestins, and neomycin depress the action of chenodiol because they tend to increase the concentration of cholesterol in the bile.

ursodiol

Mechanism of Action

Ursodiol (Actigall) is concentrated in bile and decreases biliary cholesterol saturation by suppressing hepatic synthesis and secretion of cholesterol. Ursodiol also increases bile flow.

Pharmacokinetics

Ursodiol is usually given orally three times a day with meals. It well absorbed from the intestine and is metabolized in the liver to its taurine and glycine conjugates. These are excreted into the bile. Elimination is through the feces.

Uses

Ursodiol has the same indication for the treatment of gallstones as chenodiol. Pharmacologic therapy is used to treat uncomplicated gallstone disease in patients with a functioning gallbladder. The gallstone would be radiolucent, indicating a predominant cholesterol content. The insoluble calcium-containing stones are not radiolucent. Dissolution of gallstones generally requires at least 3 months and may take 2 years of daily therapy. Response is monitored with oral cholecystograms or ultrasonograms performed every 6 to 9 months. If no response is seen in 18 months, therapy is discontinued. If a response is seen, therapy is continued until dissolution has been confirmed by two successive ultrasonograms.

Ursodiol is also used in the treatment of some chronic liver diseases because of its action to increase bile flow and to

Table 27-2 Agents for Pancreatic Enzyme Replacement

Generic Name	Trade Name	Administration/Dosage	Comments
pancreatin	Generic Creon	ORAL: *Adults*—4-18 g extract daily in divided doses with meals; extra dose with snacks.	Available as tablets and as enteric-coated microspheres (Creon). Each preparation differs, and dosage must be individualized.
pancrelipase	Cotazym* Ilozyme Ku-Zyme HP Pancrease* Protilase Viokase	ORAL: *Adults*—300-900 mg before each meal, 900 mg with meals, 600 mg within 1 hr after meals, and 300 mg with any food eaten between meals. *Children*—300-600 mg taken in the same manner as described for adults.	Available as tablets and as enteric-coated microspheres. Each preparation differs, and dosage must be individualized.

*Available in Canada and the United States.

reduce the detergent properties of bile salts. Ursodiol appears to have a protective effect on liver cells from the damaging activity of toxic bile salts, which increase in chronic liver disease.

Adverse Reactions and Contraindications

Ursodiol has few side effects. Diarrhea is occasionally experienced. Ursodiol does not have adverse effects on the fetus in animal studies and is not contraindicated in pregnancy. Patients with complications from gallstones are usually treated surgically because of the long response time to therapy with ursodiol.

Interactions

Cholestyramine, antacids, and colestipol may bind ursodiol and prevent its absorption. Clofibrate, estrogens, progestins, and neomycin depress the action of ursodiol because they tend to increase the concentration of cholesterol in the bile.

THERAPEUTIC RATIONALE: PANCREATIC DISEASES

Like the gallbladder, the pancreas secretes agents to aid in digestion into the small intestine. Pancreatic secretions enter the small intestine through the common bile duct via the pancreatic duct (see Figure 27-1). The pancreas secretes the enzymes lipase, amylase, trypsin, and chymotrypsin, which are important in the digestion of fat, carbohydrate, and protein. Bicarbonate is also secreted to neutralize stomach acid. Replacement of the **pancreatic enzymes** is required when pancreatic secretion is impaired by chronic pancreatitis, cystic fibrosis, removal of the pancreas, or obstruction of the pancreatic duct.

THERAPEUTIC AGENTS: PANCREATIC ENZYME REPLACEMENT

Therapy is directed at replacing enzymes (Table 27-2). A mixture containing pancreatin, pepsin, bile salts, hyoscyamine, atropine, scopolamine, and phenobarbital is marketed as Donnazyme. The use of such mixtures is questioned; each component should be prescribed as needed.

▼ pancreatin

Mechanism of Action

Pancreatin (generic; Creon for enteric-coated) is a combination of amylase, proteases, and lipases derived from hog pancreata. They supplement or replace these pancreatic enzymes.

Pharmacokinetics

Pancreatin tablets are taken with meals and with any snacks. The food helps buffer stomach acid. Pancreatin is also formulated into enteric microspheres to avoid degradation of the enzymes by stomach acid. Dosage is individualized by both the patient and the brand of preparation used. The enzymes are degraded in the intestine.

Uses

Replacement therapy is used for conditions that are characterized by a marked decrease in the secretion of pancreatic enzymes: chronic pancreatitis, benign or malignant pancreatic tumors, cystic fibrosis, and pancreatectomy. There is no rationale for replacement therapy as a digestive aid.

Adverse Reactions and Contraindications

The major complication of replacement therapy is diarrhea, nausea, abdominal cramps, or pain, especially when the preparation is taken in large doses. Children taking large doses may show elevated levels of uric acid in their blood and urine, but this does not seem to be significant. Individuals occasionally may show allergy to the animal protein in these preparations.

Interactions

A high-fiber diet may decrease the efficacy of pancreatin. Some patients with a high content of gastric acid may require the use of an H_2 antagonist or omeprazole to inhibit gastric acid secretion (see Chapter 26) to preserve activity of pancreatin.

pancrelipase

Pancrelipase (Cotazym, Ilozyme, Ku-Zyme HP, Viokase), like pancreatin, is derived from hog pancreata and contains lipase, proteases, and amylase. It is formulated both as tablets and enteric-coated microspheres. Its use and side effects are like those of pancreatin.

Nursing Process Overview

Drugs to Treat Gallbladder and Pancreatic Disease

Assessment

Assess vital signs and weight. For patients with gallstones, assess history of previous symptoms, treatments, and effectiveness of treatment. For patients requiring pancreatic enzymes, assess weight and characteristics of stool. If patients have cystic fibrosis or other conditions, assess the effects of these problems.

Nursing Diagnoses

- Diarrhea related to drug therapy

Patient Outcomes

The patient will have no further pain related to gallstones. For patients taking pancreatic enzymes, the patient will have more normal digestion with less fat in the stools. For all of the drugs in the chapter, the patient will not have diarrhea as a drug side effect.

Implementation

For the patient with gallstones, review the proper technique for taking the prescribed drug. Emphasize the importance of returning for follow-up visits to monitor the drug effectiveness. For patients taking pancreatic enzymes, review the reasons for drug therapy. Review the correct technique for taking the prescribed form. Encourage regular follow-up to monitor drug effectiveness.

Evaluation

Chenodiol and ursodiol are effective if the gallstones dissolve. In addition, the patient does not need surgery. Pancreatic enzymes are successful if digestion approximates normal, without severe or persistent diarrhea or gastrointestinal symptoms.

Nursing Implications Summary

chenodiol and ursodiol
Nursing in the Community

➤ Tell patients to take doses with food or milk.

➤ Emphasize the importance of taking the drug as ordered for the full course of therapy and returning for regular follow-up visits to monitor effectiveness, even if the patient feels better. Weeks to months of therapy may be needed to achieve dissolution of all gallstones. Emphasize the importance of concomitant therapies: dietary restrictions, weight loss, and medications.

➤ Instruct the patient to avoid taking aluminum-containing antacids while taking chenodiol.

➤ Instruct the patient to notify the physician if severe or persistent diarrhea, severe nausea and vomiting, severe abdominal pain, or right upper quadrant abdominal pain develop.

➤ Maintaining ideal or low body weight and eating a high-fiber diet may help in the prevention and treatment of gallstones. Check with physician and instruct patient in dietary changes as needed.

pancreatin
Nursing in the Community

➤ Emphasize the importance of taking the drug as ordered, and returning for regular follow-up visits to monitor effectiveness, even if the patient feels better. Emphasize the importance of concomitant therapies including dietary restrictions.

➤ Tell patients to take doses with meals or snacks, unless the physician directs otherwise. Swallow tablets quickly, without chewing, to avoid mouth irritation.

➤ Donnazyme contains a mixture of drugs; patients may experience side effects for each of the component drugs. Instruct the patient to avoid or limit the use of alcohol or drugs that depress the central nervous system. Example drugs to avoid include antihistamines, sedatives, sleeping medications, prescription drugs for pain, and muscle relaxants. Tell the patient to avoid driving or operating hazardous equipment if the medication causes drowsiness or blurred vision. See Chapter 23 for further information about atropine, hyoscyamine, and scopolamine, and Chapter 57 for additional information about phenobarbital.

pancrelipase
Nursing in the Community

➤ Tell patients to take doses with meals or snacks, unless the physician directs otherwise. Swallow tablets quickly, without chewing, to avoid mouth irritation.

➤ Teach patients taking the capsule containing enteric-coated spheres to swallow the capsule whole, without crushing or chewing. If the capsule cannot be swallowed, it can be opened and the contents sprinkled on a small amount of liquid or soft food such as gelatin or applesauce, and swallowed without chewing. Do not mix the contents with foods such as milk or ice cream.

Nursing Implications Summary—cont'd

➤ Tell patients taking the capsule containing powder to swallow the capsule whole, without crushing or chewing. There is also a powder form of the drug that does not come in a capsule. The contents of the capsule or the powder form can be mixed with a small amount of food or liquid. Be careful not to breathe in the drug powder because it may cause irritation to the nose, shortness of breath, or trouble breathing.

➤ Do not change brands of pancrelipase without checking with the physician.

➤ Emphasize the importance of taking the drug as ordered and returning for regular follow-up visits to monitor effectiveness, even if the patient feels better. Emphasize the importance of concomitant therapies, including dietary restrictions and other medications.

➤ If antacids are also prescribed, teach patients to avoid products containing calcium carbonate and/or magnesium hydroxide because these may interfere with the action of the pancrelipase.

CHAPTER REVIEW

Application

1. Explain the role of bile salts in digestion.
2. Describe the origin of gallstones. How are chenodiol and ursodiol thought to aid in the dissolution of gallstones?
3. Describe the action of pancreatic enzymes in digestion.

Critical Thinking

1. An abdominal x-ray film reveals gallstones. When would treatment be considered? What are the therapeutic options?
2. You are working with a family whose child has just be diagnosed with cystic fibrosis. How would you assess this child? Why is pancreatin used for this condition?

References

American College of Physicians: Guidelines for the treatment of gallstones, *Ann Intern Med* 119(7):620, 1993.

Gollan JL, et al: Gallstones and laparoscopic cholecystectomy, *NIH Consensus Statement Online* 10(3):1-20, 1992.

Poupon RE, Poupon R, Balkau B, the UDCA-PBC Study Group: Ursodiol for the long-term treatment of primary biliary cirrhosis, *N Engl J Med* 330:1342, 1994.

Ransohoff DF, Gracie WA: Treatment of gallstones, *Ann Intern Med* 119(7):606, 1993.

Drugs to Treat Asthma and Other Pulmonary Diseases

OBJECTIVES

After studying this chapter, you should be able to do the following:

- *Discuss the role of inhaled corticosteroids, nonselective and selective beta-adrenergic bronchodilators, xanthines, cromolyn, ketotifen, and ipratropium in treating asthma.*
- *Describe the alpha, beta$_1$, beta$_2$, and central nervous system (CNS) effects of sympathomimetic bronchodilators.*
- *Discuss the role of alpha$_1$-proteinase inhibitor in the treatment of chronic obstructive pulmonary disease.*
- *Discuss the role of surfactant in infants with respiratory distress syndrome.*
- *Develop a nursing care plan for patients receiving one or more of the groups of drugs discussed in this chapter.*

CHAPTER OVERVIEW

Asthma results from an allergic reaction in the airways leading to acute bronchospasm with difficulty in breathing. Recently, attention has focused on the inflammatory origins of asthma. Inhaled steroids and agents modifying mast cells decrease inflammation. A new class of drugs, the leukotriene modifiers, may prove to be effective agents in controlling asthma. Treatment previously focused on bronchodilators to dilate the constricted bronchioles and to relieve the wheezing, difficult breathing, and coughing that occur during an asthma attack. Theophylline and beta-adrenergic bronchodilators are still used as agents to relieve asthma. This chapter also introduces the new surfactant drugs used to prevent lung collapse in premature infants.

THERAPEUTIC RATIONALE: ASTHMA AND OBSTRUCTIVE LUNG DISEASES

Asthma

Asthma is an inflammatory disease characterized by an increased responsiveness of the trachea and bronchi to various stimuli and manifested by a widespread narrowing of the airways that changes in severity either spontaneously or as a result of therapy. Symptoms of asthma include shortness of breath, coughing, and wheezing. Episodes of these symptoms alternate with periods of no symptoms. An asthma attack involves not only constriction of the bronchioles but also edema of the bronchial mucosa and excess secretion of mucus, combining to restrict the caliber of the airway, as diagrammed in Figure 28-1. Asthma is classified as extrinsic asthma if an allergic response is the primary stimulus for

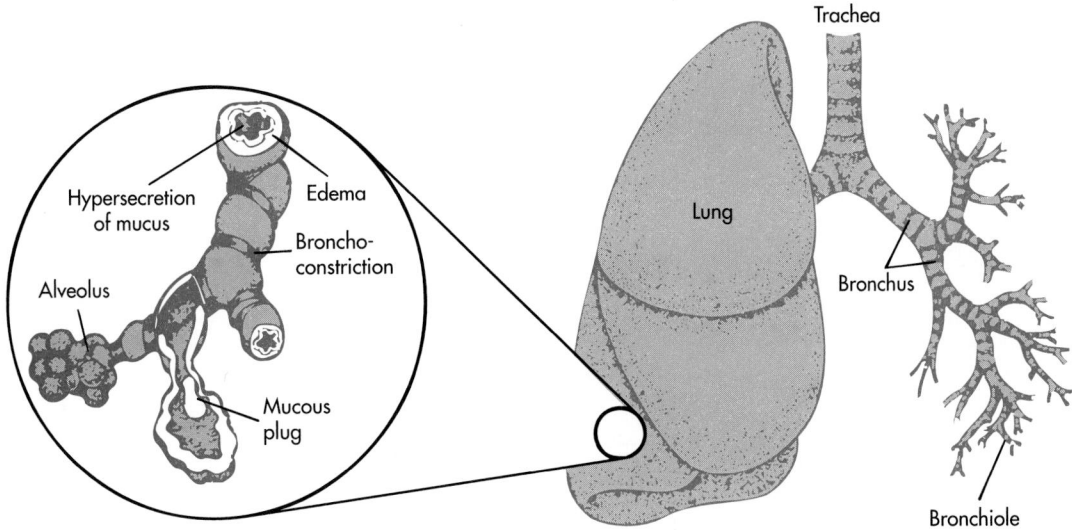

Figure 28-1   Factors restricting airway include hypersecretion of mucus, mucosal edema, and bronchoconstriction. Mucous plugs may form in alveoli.

bronchial constriction. When no such response can be identified, asthma is classified as intrinsic asthma.

Factors Triggering an Asthma Episode

About 15 million Americans, or 4% to 5% of the population, have asthma; about 5000 die of severe asthma attacks each year. Cases of asthma have doubled since 1980, with children and African-Americans groups disproportionately affected. Why some individuals become asthmatic is unknown. Asthma appears to be a disease of civilization. One current theory is that childhood infections, especially exposure to tuberculosis, paradoxically protect against asthma by altering the primary immune response. Those who are asthmatic have airways that become overly responsive to environmental factors. Some of the agents that trigger an asthma episode include the following:

- Allergens such as pollens, foods, dust, mold, feathers, or animal dander; key allergens are dust mites, animal dander from pets, cockroaches, and indoor mold
- Irritants in the air such as dirt, cigarette smoke, gases, and odors
- Respiratory infections such as colds, flu, sore throats, and bronchitis
- Too much exertion such as running upstairs too fast or carrying heavy loads
- Emotional stress such as excessive fear or excitement
- Very cold or windy weather or sudden changes in weather
- Some medications such as aspirin and related drugs and some drugs to treat glaucoma and high blood pressure

Because each person with asthma reacts differently, each should learn to identify individual triggers and either avoid the trigger or be prepared to take prophylactic medication.

Immune Mechanisms in Extrinsic Asthma

The airway inflammation of asthma involves an immunologic mechanism. The mast cells play a major role in precipitating the attack (Figure 28-2). In the lung, mast cells are primarily located in the epithelial layer and exposed to the surface. Immunoglobulin E (IgE) antibodies bind to mast cells; when an antigen appears, it binds to the IgE. The formation of the antigen-antibody complex causes the mast cells to degranulate, releasing several substances, including histamine and leukotrienes C and D.

The leukotrienes are potent bronchoconstrictors, chemically related to the prostaglandins. Recently, leukotriene modifiers have been approved for treatment of asthma. Histamine, also a bronchoconstrictor, also induces vasodilation and increased capillary permeability, which results in the mucosal edema characteristic of asthma. Antihistamines are not used for the treatment of asthma, however. They are used to treat allergic rhinitis (see Chapter 29).

Adrenergic Mechanisms in Controlling Bronchioles

There is little, if any, direct innervation of the bronchioles by the sympathetic nervous system. However, there is indirect involvement because sympathetic nerve terminals in pulmonary blood vessels release norepinephrine, which can act on the beta$_2$-receptors in the bronchioles. Norepinephrine is not a potent stimulant of beta$_2$-receptors. The beta$_2$-receptors are activated by epinephrine released from the adrenal medulla in response to stress.

As diagrammed in Figure 28-2, the beta-adrenergic system affects relaxation of bronchial smooth muscle and inhibits degranulation of the mast cells. Activation of the beta$_2$-receptor stimulates an enzyme, adenylate cyclase, to synthesize more cyclic adenosine monophosphate (cAMP), which is a second messenger for the beta$_2$-receptor (see

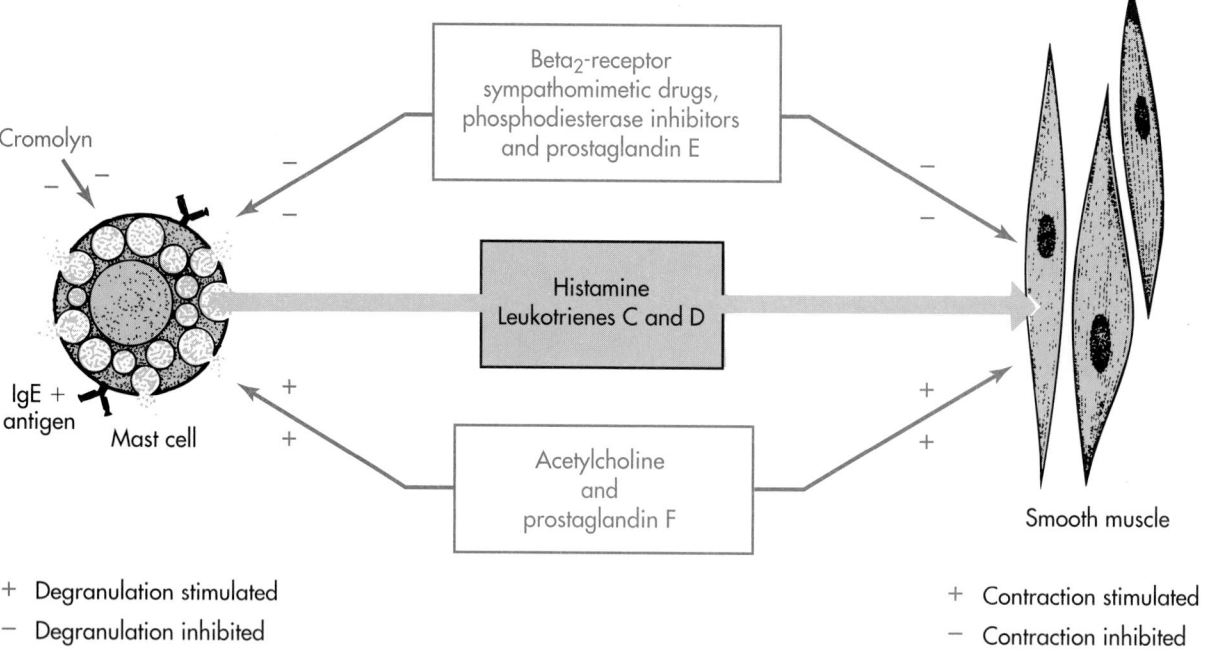

Figure 28-2   Histamine and leukotrienes C and D released from mast cells stimulate smooth muscle contraction to produce bronchoconstriction. Mast cell degranulation and smooth muscle contraction are stimulated by acetylcholine and prostaglandin F. Smooth muscle relaxation and inhibition of mast cell degranulation are promoted by beta$_2$-receptor agonists, phosphodiesterase inhibitors, and prostaglandin E.

Chapter 12); cAMP activates intracellular pathways, resulting in relaxation of smooth muscle, inhibition of mast cell degranulation, and stimulation of the ciliary apparatus to remove secretions more effectively.

Drugs that increase cAMP are **bronchodilators,** inhibitors of mast cell degranulation, and promoters of secretion flow in the bronchioles. These drugs include beta-adrenergic agonists, which stimulate the beta$_2$-receptor, and phosphodiesterase inhibitors, which inhibit the breakdown of cAMP. Xanthine compounds are used clinically as bronchodilators because they inhibit phosphodiesterase.

Cholinergic Mechanisms Controlling Bronchioles

Acetylcholine, the neurotransmitter of the parasympathetic nervous system, acts on muscarinic receptors to cause bronchoconstriction through the intracellular second messenger, cyclic guanosine monophosphate (cGMP). Mast cell degranulation is also promoted by agents that stimulate the formation of cGMP. Intrinsic asthma is believed to arise from direct stimulation of the enzyme guanylate cyclase, which synthesizes cGMP. Irritants such as noxious gases can stimulate guanylate cyclase. Asthmatic individuals respond to low dosages of inhaled methacholine, a cholinomimetic drug, with bronchospasm, whereas high dosages are required to induce bronchospasm in nonasthmatic individuals. Intrinsic asthma may therefore primarily involve a parasympathetic response, mediated by cGMP, to inhaled bronchial irritants. Blocking the muscarinic receptor with atropine or scopol-

amine causes bronchodilation. The atropine-like drug ipratropium is used for bronchodilation.

Other Airflow Obstructive Lung Diseases

Obstruction of airflow is a component of other pulmonary diseases. Chronic bronchitis and emphysema are referred to as **chronic obstructive pulmonary disease (COPD).** Patients with COPD commonly have some degree of reversible airflow obstruction. As with asthma, bronchodilators and corticosteroids play a major role in supportive therapy. In longstanding pulmonary disease, irreversible changes take place so that the elastic smooth muscle tissue is replaced with inelastic scar tissue. This can occur in the bronchioles in chronic bronchitis or in the alveoli in emphysema. These irreversible changes cannot be modified with drugs. The drug alpha$_1$-antitrypsin can slow these changes. However, because the early stages of chronic bronchitis and emphysema often involve reversible bronchospasm, ipratropium and bronchodilators can provide some relief.

About 60,000 to 70,000 American premature infants develop **respiratory distress syndrome** each year, with 6000 to 10,000 of those affected dying. In addition, about half of the 150,000 adult Americans who develop respiratory distress syndrome as a result of injuries or blood infections die. Respiratory distress syndrome, also called hyaline membrane disease, is caused by a collapse of the tiny air sacs of the lung related to a deficiency of surfactant. Surfactant is a lipoprotein material coating the air sacs in mature lungs, lowering

Table 28-1 **Drug Therapy for Asthma**

Type of Asthma	Controller Medications	Reliever Medications
Mild Intermittent Episodes of wheezing, coughing, or chest tightness twice a week or less Nighttime problems with breathing less than twice a month Often associated with exercise Few severe attacks	No daily medication needed	Short-acting inhaled bronchodilator, usually beta$_2$-agonist; inhaled beta$_2$-agonist or cromolyn before exercise or exposure to antigen; alternative: ipratropium
Mild Persistent Episodes of wheezing, coughing, or chest tightness more than twice a week but less than daily Nighttime problems with breathing more than twice a month Severe attacks that affect activity	Low daily dosage of inhaled corticosteroids; *or* Daily dosage of mast cell inhibitor (especially effective for children) *or* Daily dosage of sustained-release theophylline *or* Leukotriene modifier (patients 12 years and older)	Short-acting inhaled bronchodilator, usually beta$_2$-agonist; Alternatives: oral beta$_2$-agonist as needed up to 4 times/day; or ipratropium; or oral short-acting theophylline (if not on sustained release form)
Moderate Persistent Daily episodes of wheezing, coughing, or chest tightness Nighttime problems with breathing more than once a week Severe attacks that affect activity two or more times weekly	Medium daily dosage of inhaled corticosteroids *or* Small daily dosage of inhaled corticosteroid combined with long-acting agent such as salmeterol or sustained-release theophylline	Short-acting inhaled bronchodilator, usually beta$_2$-agonist; Alternative: oral beta$_2$-agonist as needed up to 4 times/day (children); ipratropium (if excessive tachycardia)
Severe Persistent Continual wheezing, coughing, or chest tightness and frequent nighttime breathing problems Limited physical activity because of breathing problems Frequent serious attacks	High daily dosages of inhaled corticosteroid, combined with long-acting agent such as salmeterol or sustained-release theophylline and oral doses of corticosteroid	Short-acting inhaled bronchodilator, usually beta$_2$-agonist; Alternative: oral beta$_2$-agonist as needed up to 4 times/day (children)

the surface tension, and thereby allowing ready inflation of the lungs. Synthetic surfactant preparations are available to treat respiratory distress syndrome.

THERAPEUTIC AGENTS: DRUGS TO TREAT ASTHMA

The 1997 Expert Panel report of the National Heart, Lung and Blood Institute emphasized that children or adults with three or more asthmatic episodes per week should receive daily treatment to reduce airway inflammation. As shown in Table 28-1, treatment guidelines are stratified for severity. Drug therapy is divided into *controller* medications and *reliever* medications. This is a shift in treatment guidelines, which previously emphasized symptomatic relief with bronchodilators.

Controller medications treat the underlying inflammatory condition. The goal is to prevent or decrease the severity of asthmatic episodes. These drugs are not appropriate to treat an acute asthmatic attack. Controller medications include inhaled corticosteroids, inhaled cromolyn or nedocromil, oral long-acting theophylline, leukotriene modifiers, and a long-acting inhaled beta$_2$-agonist or oral slow-release beta$_2$-agonist. Even mild asthma is treated with controller drugs if symptoms occur three times a week or more.

Reliever medications control asthmatic episodes. Reliever medications include short-acting inhaled beta$_2$-agonists, oral short-acting theophylline, and inhaled anticholinergic. If exercise precipitates an asthmatic attack or if exposure to antigens is anticipated, a beta$_2$-agonist or cromolyn might be taken.

Treatment of Special Populations

Infants and Young Children

Daily antiinflammatory treatment relies on cromolyn or nedocromil, drugs that have no side effects. If inhaled corticosteroids are needed, doses are kept to 400 to 800 μg/day. Systemic corticosteroids may be used to control moderate to severe symptoms associated with viral respiratory infections. Inhaled ipratropium and oral beta₂-agonists are used as reliever medications.

Pregnant Women

Most asthma medications do not pose a problem for the mother or fetus. However, oral corticosteroids are associated with an increased risk of preeclampsia.

Geriatric Patients

Older patients often have other medical conditions. Medications used to treat asthma may aggravate other conditions. Systemic and even inhaled corticosteroids increase the risk of osteoporosis, cataracts, and diabetes. Beta₂-agonists can cause tremor and tachycardia, aggravating heart conditions. Theophylline dosage may need to be decreased because of reduced clearance in older people. Medications that can make asthma worse include nonsteroidal antiinflammatory drugs taken for arthritis or nonselective beta-blocking agents taken for glaucoma or heart conditions.

Inhaled Corticosteroids

Corticosteroids are controller drugs for asthma. Drugs for asthma control are listed in Table 28-2. Asthma specialists now advocate the use of aerosol glucocorticoids over theophylline or beta-adrenergic agonists in the daily management of persistent asthma. Glucocorticoids available as aerosols include **beclomethasone** (Beclovent, Vanceril), budesonide (Pulmicort, Nebuamp), flunisolide (AeroBid, Bronalide), fluticasone (Flovent), and triamcinolone (Azmacort).

Mechanism of Action

Corticosteroids are potent antiinflammatory agents that, among other actions, inhibit the release of inflammation promoting cytokines from lymphocytes, macrophages, mast cells, fibroblasts, and eosinophils.

Pharmacokinetics

Aerosol corticosteroids have been developed that can be inhaled daily without producing adrenal suppression or Cushing's syndrome. As with other aerosol medications, the patient must be carefully instructed in the administration of the aerosol glucocorticoids (Figure 28-3). The aerosol cannot be used during an episode of acute bronchospasm because the powder causes further irritation and the bronchospasm prevents adequate inhalation. An oral glucocorticoid is indicated instead.

Beclomethasone is transformed in the lung to an active metabolite. The other corticosteroids are unchanged. Drug that reaches the plasma is rapidly degraded in the liver to inactive metabolites. Maximum improvement in pulmonary function may take 4 weeks. Reduction in airway responsiveness occurs over weeks to months. Unfortunately, many patients discontinue the medication when they feel better and lose the benefit.

Uses

Aerosolized corticosteroids are used as the mainstay of controller therapy for persistent asthma, especially in adults. Corticosteroids do not relieve acute bronchospasm or bronchitis not caused by asthma.

Figure 28-3 Inhaled drugs commonly used in asthma treatment include beta-adrenergic bronchodilators, cromolyn sodium, and aerosol glucocorticoids. Metered-dose inhaler **(A)** should not be put in mouth but held about two fingerwidths (1½ inch) in front of mouth. Alternatively, inhaler with spacer device **(B)** can be used. Patients should breathe deeply once before activating the inhaler and then continue breathing in for about 5 seconds. Patients should then hold the breath for 10 to 15 seconds before breathing out slowly. If second dose is needed, patients should wait 1 to 2 minutes before taking another dose.

Adverse Reactions, Contraindications, and Toxicity

Patients using these aerosols should gargle after use to prevent the drug trapped in the throat from being swallowed and absorbed systemically and to avoid a *Candida* infection (a fungal infection) in the mouth or throat. Bronchospasm or cough may be experienced. Systemic side effects are uncommon with inhaled corticosteroids. However, children may be at risk for retarded growth rate and depressed adrenal function when administered high aerosol dosages.

Inhaled Nonsteroidal Antiallergy Agents

Cromolyn (Intal) and nedocromil (Tilade) are controller drugs for persistent asthma, especially for children or for adults prone to exercise-induced asthma.

Table 28-2 Drugs for Asthma Control

Generic Name	Trade Name	Administration/Dosage	Comments
Corticosteroids			
beclomethasone dipropionate	Beclovent* Vanceril*	INHALATION (metered-dose inhaler): Each spray is 50 μg. *Adults*—2 inhalations 3-4 times/day. *Children 6-12 yr*—1-2 inhalations 3-4 times/day.	Inhaled corticosteroid. Patients transferring from oral corticosteroids to beclomethasone must be carefully monitored because adrenal function is impaired and may require months to begin functioning adequately.
budesonide†	Pulmicort Nebuamp†	INHALATION: *Adults and adolescents*—1-2 mg in 2-4 ml, administered via nebulization over 10-15 min 2 times/day. *Children 3 mo-12 yr*—½ adult dose.	Inhalation suspension not available in the United States.
flunisolide	AeroBid Bronalide†	INHALATION (metered-dose inhaler): Each inhalation is 250 μg. *Adults and children >4 yr*—2 inhalations 2 times/day.	Inhaled corticosteroid. See comments for beclomethasone.
fluticasone propionate	Flovent	INHALATION (metered-dose inhaler): 3 dose levels: 44, 110, 220 μg per inhalation. *Adults and children >12 yr*—2 inhalations 2 times/day.	Inhaled corticosteroid. See comments for beclomethasone.
triamcinolone	Azmacort*	INHALATION (metered-dose inhaler): Each inhalation is 100 μg. *Adults*—2 sprays 3 or 4 times/day, up to 12-16 sprays daily. *Children 6-12 yr*—1 or 2 sprays 3 or 4 times/day, up to 12 sprays daily for severe cases.	Inhaled corticosteroid. See comments for beclomethasone.
Inhaled Nonsteroidal Antiallergy Agents			
cromolyn sodium	Intal*	INHALATION: *Adults and children >5 yr*—20-mg capsule inhaled 4 times/day (Spinhaler); 2 inhalations 4 times/day (inhalation aerosol). FDA pregnancy category B.	Prophylactic drug used to inhibit mast cell degranulation. Cough or bronchospasm is occasionally experienced after inhaling dry powder.
nedocromil	Tilade*	INHALATION (metered-dose inhaler): *Adults and children >12 yr*—2 inhalations 4 times/day.	New prophylactic drug used to inhibit mast cell degranulation.
Leukotriene Modifiers			
montelukast	Singulair	ORAL: *Adults*—10 mg/day. *Children 6-14 yr*—5 mg/day.	New drug. Blocks receptor for leukotrienes. Prophylactic for asthma.
zafirlukast	Accolate	ORAL: *Adults and children >12 yr*—20 mg twice daily.	New drug. Blocks receptor for leukotrienes. Take 1 hr before or 2 hr after meals. Prophylactive for asthma.
zileuton	Zyflo	ORAL: *Adults and children >12 yr*—600 mg 4 times/day.	New drugs. Selective inhibitor of enzyme synthesizing leukotrienes. Prophylactic for asthma.
Other Drugs			
ipratropium	Atrovent*	INHALATION (metered-dose inhaler): Each dose is 18 μg. *Adults*—1-4 inhalations 4 times/day as necessary. FDA pregnancy category B.	Anticholinergic bronchodilator.
ketotifen†	Zaditen†	ORAL: *Children >3 yr*—1 mg 2 times daily with morning and evening meals.	Prophylactic for asthma in children.

*Available in Canada and the United States.
†Available in Canada only.

Mechanism of Action

Cromolyn and nedocromil inhibit mast cell degranulation and the release of bronchospastic agents caused by immunologic (antigen IgE) or nonimmunologic (exercise or hyperventilation) stimulation. They also inhibit the recruitment of inflammatory cells into the airway, and they inhibit late bronchoconstriction. These agents do not treat an ongoing asthma attack or prevent asthma attacks brought on by vagal reflexes rather than by mast cell degranulation. Cromolyn and nedocromil do not have bronchodilator or anti-inflammatory activity.

Pharmacokinetics

Cromolyn is available as a metered inhalation aerosol. Cromolyn can also be administered with a Spinhaler, a hand-held, hand-operated device that when activated, punctures a capsule, releasing a dry powder. This powder is dispersed by the air current from a small rotor blade and enters the lungs during deep inhalation. A solution for nebulization is also available. In addition, cromolyn is formulated for nasal administration (Nasalcrom and Rynacrom), as prophylaxis for allergic rhinitis, for ophthalmic administration (Opticrom and Vistacrom) for allergic conjunctivitis, and oral administration for food allergies. Cromolyn is rapidly excreted unchanged in the urine so that blood levels are negligible.

Nedocromil is available as a metered dose inhalation aerosol. It is effective when administered 30 minutes before exposure to an allergen or chemical or before exercise. The drug is rapidly excreted unchanged in the bile and urine.

Uses

Cromolyn and nedocromil are used prophylactically, especially in children, to treat asthma. No tolerance develops to the drug. They are used in place of glucocorticoids or to allow the gradual reduction in the dose of glucocorticoids. These agents are more effective in treating children than adults for asthma. They are effective in adults when taken before exercise or exposure to allergen to provide prophylaxis for 1 to 2 hours. Continued therapy increases control of symptoms.

Adverse Reactions, Contraindications, and Toxicity

Because cromolyn and nedocromil are rapidly excreted unchanged, they are practically nontoxic. The major side effect that can limit use is bronchospasm caused by the dry powder in sensitive individuals. Some individuals become allergic to cromolyn or nedocromil.

Leukotriene Modifiers

The newest class of drugs for control of persistent asthma are the leukotriene modifiers (see Table 28-2). The first drugs released are montelukast (Singulair), zafirlukast (Accolate), and zileuton (Zyflo).

Mechanism of Action

The cyclooxygenase pathway converts arachidonic acid to inflammatory mediators that include prostaglandins, thromboxanes, and leukotrienes. Zileuton selectively inhibits the path to leukotrienes. Montelukast and zafirlukast block receptors for leukotrienes at receptors in the smooth muscle of airways. The result is that the inflammatory action of leukotrienes is blocked.

Pharmacokinetics

Leukotriene modifiers are administered orally. The onset of action of zileuton is rapid, within 2 hours of administration. The action of montelukast or zafirlukast is apparent after 1 to 3 weeks of therapy. All three drugs are metabolized in the liver.

Uses

Leukotrienes are intended be taken prophylactically on an ongoing basis to control symptoms of persistent asthma. They are not for the treatment of acute asthma. They may replace inhaled corticosteroids, cromolyn, or nedocromil for the control of mild to moderate persistent asthma.

Adverse Reactions, Contraindications, Interactions, and Toxicity

Side effects are minimal. Because the leukotriene modifiers are metabolized by the hepatic cytochrome P-450 isoenzyme CYP3A4, there is the potential for elevated liver enzymes. Patients with liver disease or active alcoholism should not take these drugs. Leukotriene modifiers enhance the plasma concentration of the following drugs taken concurrently: beta-adrenergic blockers, theophylline, and warfarin.

Beta-Adrenergic Agonists

Beta-adrenergic agonists are reliever drugs for asthma. A number of beta-adrenergic agonists have been developed to treat asthma (Table 28-3). Most are available in metered aerosol canisters that deliver the drug in a spray taken by inhalation (see Figure 28-3). These are used to relieve acute episodes of asthma. Oral and parenteral forms are available of some beta-adrenergic agonists for use when the inhalation route is not possible. Salmeterol is a new long-acting beta-adrenergic agonist that is used only prophylactically.

Mechanism of Action

The most widely used beta-adrenergic bronchodilators are relatively specific beta$_2$-receptor agonists. The beta-receptors of the bronchial smooth muscle are beta$_2$-receptors, whereas cardiac beta-receptors are beta$_1$-receptors. The goal has been to develop drugs that are selective in stimulating only beta$_2$-receptors because stimulation of the heart is not desirable and can limit the use of the drug.

Pharmacokinetics

The route of administration and the onset and duration of action are important in selecting a beta-adrenergic bron-

Table 28-3 **Bronchodilators**

Generic Name	Trade Name	Administration/Dosage	Comments
Beta-Receptor Agonists			
albuterol	Proventil Ventolin	INHALATION: *Adults and children >12 yr*—1 or 2 inhalations from metered aerosol every 4-6 hr; 0.05-0.15 mg/kg body weight by nebulization over 5-15 min every 4-6 hr. ORAL: *Adults and children >12 yr*—2-6 mg 3 or 4 times/day. FDA pregnancy category C.	Relatively selective for beta$_2$-receptors (bronchial). May cause fine finger tremor. Injectable form available in Canada.
bitolterol	Tornalate	INHALATION: *Adults*—2 inhalations from metered aerosol every 8 hr for prophylaxis. To treat an attack, 1 inhalation followed by a second after 1-3 min; then 2 inhalations every 4 hr or 3 inhalations every 6 hr. Nebulizer dose is 1.5-3.5 mg delivered over 10-15 min, 3-4 times/day, not less than 4 hr apart. FDA pregnancy category C.	Selective for beta$_2$-receptors (bronchial).
ephedrine sulfate	Generic	ORAL: *Adults*—25-50 mg every 3-4 hr as needed. FDA pregnancy category C. *Children 6-12 yr*—6.25-12.5 mg every 4-6 hr. *Children 2-6 yr*—0.3-0.5 mg/kg every 4-6 hr. INTRAMUSCULAR, SUBCUTANEOUS: *Adults*—12.5-25 mg, up to 150 mg in 24 hr. *Children*—3 mg/kg body weight daily divided in 4-6 doses.	Oral or parenteral administration only. Central nervous system stimulation is a common side effect. Not selective for beta$_2$-receptors.
epinephrine (base) suspension	Sus-Phrine	INTRAMUSCULAR, SUBCUTANEOUS: *Adults*—For 1:200 solutions, 0.1-0.3 ml not more often than every 4 hr, maximum test dose, 0.1 ml. FDA pregnancy category C. *Children*—For 1:200 solutions, 0.005 ml/kg body weight not more than every 4 hr, maximum test dose, 0.15 ml.	Long-acting suspension. Effect may persist for 8-10 hr.
epinephrine epinephrine bitartrate	AsthmaHaler Mist Bronkaid Suspension Mist	INHALATION: Aerosol nebulizers metered to deliver 0.16-0.2 mg epinephrine with each inhalation. Repeat once after 1-2 min if necessary; allow 3 hr before next dose.	Overuse can cause serious adverse effects, leading to death. Reduce dosage if bronchial irritation or central nervous system stimulation arises. For symptomatic relief only.
epinephrine (racemic)	Vaponefrin* Asthma Nefrin (2-2.25% epinephrine)	INHALATION: *Adults and children >4 yr*—Hand-bulb nebulizer: 10 drops to provide 1-3 inhalations; jet nebulizer: 4-10 drops diluted and delivered over 15 min. Repeat after 3-4 hr if necessary.	Excessive use causes bronchial inflammation and stimulation of heart and central nervous system.
epinephrine hydrochloride	Adrenalin Chloride (1% epinephrine)	INHALATION: *Adults and children >4 yr*—Hand-bulb nebulizer: 10 drops to provide 1-3 inhalations. Repeat after 3-4 hr if necessary.	
ethylnorepinephrine	Bronkephrine	INTRAMUSCULAR, SUBCUTANEOUS: *Adults*—1-2 mg. FDA pregnancy category C. *Children*—0.2-1 mg.	A beta$_2$-selective bronchodilator.
fenoterol†	Berotec†	INHALATION: *Adults*—1 or 2 inhalations from metered aerosol every 6 hr as needed.	A beta$_2$-selective bronchodilator. Not available in the United States.
isoetharine hydrochloride isoetharine mesylate	Bronkosol Various others Bronkometer	INHALATION: Nebulized solution: 3-7 inhalations. FDA pregnancy category C. INHALATION: 1-4 inhalations from metered aerosol every 3-6 hr, maximum 12 inhalations daily.	A beta$_2$-selective drug. Phenylephrine is included to relieve congestion and prolong duration of action.
isoproterenol hydrochloride	Isuprel Glossets Various others	SUBLINGUAL: *Adults*—10 mg initially. No more than 15 mg 4 times/day or 20 mg 3 times/day. FDA pregnancy category C. *Children*—5-10 mg, not exceeding 30 mg/day. INTRAVENOUS: *Children only*—Initial infusion rate is 0.1 μg/kg/min. Increase by 0.1 μg/kg/min every 15 min until heart rate exceeds 180 beats per minute or clinical improvement is seen or infusion rate is 0.8 μg/kg/min.	Sublingual absorption is unreliable. Patients should not swallow saliva until tablet has completely disintegrated. This route of administration is used only in pediatric intensive care units for children in respiratory failure.
	Isuprel Mistometer*	INHALATION (solution for nebulization, 0.5% to 1%): *Adults*—1 or 2 deep inhalations, repeated no more than every 4 hr.	Excessive use has caused refractory bronchial obstruction and tolerance to drug. In some individuals inhalation precipitates a severe, prolonged asthma attack.
isoproterenol sulfate	Medihaler-Iso*	INHALATION: *Adults*—1 or 2 deep inhalations from metered aerosol repeated once or twice at 5- to 10-min intervals	Excessive use has caused refractory bronchial obstruction and tolerance

*Available in Canada and the United States.
†Available in Canada only.

Continued

Table 28-3 Bronchodilators—cont'd

Generic Name	Trade Name	Administration/Dosage	Comments
isoproterenol sulfate—cont'd		if necessary. Repeat after 4 hr. *Children*—5-15 deep inhalations of 1:200 aerosol repeated in 10-30 min if necessary.	to drug. In some individuals inhalation precipitates a severe, prolonged asthma attack.
metaproterenol sulfate	Alupent* Metaprel	ORAL: *Adults*—20 mg 3 or 4 times/day. FDA pregnancy category C. *Children 6-9 yr*—10 mg 3 or 4 times/day. *Children >9 yr or 60 lb*—20 mg 3 or 4 times/day.	Longer acting than isoproterenol. Patients are less likely to develop tolerance to metaproterenol than to isoproterenol.
	Alupent* Arm-a-Med Metaproterenol Dey-Lute Metaproterenol	INHALATION: *Adults and children 12 yr only*—2-3 inhalations from metered aerosol every 3-4 hr, not to exceed 12 inhalations daily.	
pirbuterol	Maxair Autohaler*	INHALATION: *Adults*—1 or 2 inhalations from metered aerosol every 4-6 hr as needed. FDA pregnancy category C.	A beta$_2$-selective bronchodilator.
procaterol	Pro-Air†	INHALATION: *Adults*—2 inhalations from metered aerosol 3 times/day.	A beta$_2$-selective bronchodilator.
salmeterol	Servent*	INHALATION: *Adults*—2 inhalations from metered aerosol morning and evening.	New long-acting beta$_2$-selective bronchodilator. Prophylactic use only for asthma.
terbutaline sulfate	Brethine	SUBCUTANEOUS: *Adults*—0.25 mg repeated in 15-30 min if necessary, with no more than 0.5 mg administered in any 4 hr period. FDA pregnancy category B. *Children*—0.01 mg/kg body weight to maximum of 0.25 mg.	Shakiness is the most common side effect.
	Bricanyl*	ORAL: *Adults*—initially 2.5 mg every 8 hr, increased to 5 mg every 8 hr 3 times/day over 2-4 wk. Dosage may be lowered to 2.5 mg if side effects are too disturbing. *Children 12 yr*—1.25-2.5 mg 3 times/day during waking hours.	Side effects are mild. Headache, nausea, and gastrointestinal upset are the most common.
	Brethaire Bricanyl Turbuhaler†	INHALATION: *Adults and children <12 yr*—2 inhalations from metered aerosol 1 min apart, every 4-6 hr.	
Xanthines aminophylline	Generic	*For acute asthma attack:* INTRAVENOUS: Solutions should be diluted to 25 mg/ml and injected no more rapidly than 25 mg/min to avoid circulatory collapse. Loading dose: 5.6 mg/kg over 30 min. Maintenance dose: No more than 0.9 mg/kg/hr by continuous infusion. Dosage is determined by age, cardiac and liver status, and smoking history.	85% theophylline, so 116 mg of aminophylline is equivalent to 100 mg theophylline. Watch for nausea, wakefulness, restlessness, and irritability as early symptoms of toxicity. Serious toxic effects of IV include delirium, convulsions, hyperthermia, and circulatory collapse.
	Truphylline	RECTAL: *Adults*—250-500 mg 1-3 times/day. FDA pregnancy category C. *Children*—5 mg/kg not more often than every 6 hr.	
	Generic	ORAL: *Adults*—500 mg for acute attack. Maintenance dose: 200-250 mg every 6-8 hr. *Children*—7.5 mg/kg for acute attack. Maintenance dose: 5 mg/kg every 6 hr.	
	Phyllocontin	ORAL (extended release): *Adults and children >6 yr*—300 mg/day initially, increasing gradually to 600 mg if needed.	
	Generic	INTRAMUSCULAR: *Adults*—250-500 mg.	
oxtriphylline	Apo-Oxtriphylline† Choledyl PMS-Oxtriphylline† Choledyl-SA*	ORAL: *Adults*—200 mg every 6 hr. *Children 2-12 yr*—100 mg/60 lb every 6 hr. ORAL (extended release): *Adults and children >6 yr*—Up to 1 g/day. FDA pregnancy category C.	64% theophylline, so 156 mg is equivalent to 100 mg theophylline. Oral solution formulation contains alcohol; not recommended for children. Syrup formulation available for young children.
theophylline	Many names, elixirs, syrups, tablets, capsules, timed-release preparation, and suppositories	ORAL: *Adults*—Initial dose: 3-5 mg/kg every 6 hr. *For maintenance: Adults*—100-200 mg every 6 hr. FDA pregnancy category C. *Children*—50-100 mg every 6 hr. RECTAL: *Adults*—250-500 mg every 8-12 hr. *Children*—10-12 mg/kg/24 hr. Administered no more than every 6 hr.	Headache, dizziness, nervousness, nausea, vomiting, and epigastric pain are most common side effects of oral administration. Therapeutic levels are 10-20 mg/ml serum.

*Available in Canada and the United States.
†Available in Canada only.

chodilator. Inhalation is a particularly effective route of administration for the bronchodilators because most are degraded if swallowed. Inhalation also places the drug near the site of action.

Many bronchodilators are available in metered aerosol form so that one inhalation delivers a given amount of a drug. The metered-dose inhaler (MDI) has emerged as the standard for aerosol therapy. The correct use of the inhaler is illustrated in Figure 28-3. Bronchodilators available as MDIs include albuterol, bitolterol, epinephrine, fenoterol, isoetharine, isoproterenol, metaproterenol, pirbuterol, procaterol, salmeterol, and terbutaline (see Table 28-3). If more than one inhalation is administered, patients should wait a minute or so between inhalations. Because only about 10% of the delivered drug is deposited in the lung, the likelihood of overdosing is small. However, recent studies indicate that overuse of inhalers (more than one incident per month) may be associated with an increased death rate.

Another inhalation technique is to put a solution of the drug into a nebulizer, which disperses the drug solution in tiny drops to be taken into the lungs by deep inhalation. Bronchodilators available in solutions for nebulization include albuterol, bitolterol, epinephrine, fenoterol, isoetharine, isoproterenol, and metaproterenol.

Albuterol, ephedrine, fenoterol, isoproterenol, metaproterenol, and terbutaline are available in oral forms. Although oral administration is convenient, especially for children, the patient is exposed to more side effects with oral administration than with aerosol administration.

Finally, albuterol, ephedrine, epinephrine, ethylnorepinephrine, isoproterenol, and terbutaline are available in parenteral formulations. These are generally reserved for relieving severe bronchospasm or conditions in which inhalation or oral administration is not possible.

Uses

Beta-adrenergic bronchodilators are now used as reliever drugs during acute attacks of asthma. They may also be used prophylactically for exercise-induced asthma or when exposure to antigens is anticipated, for instance, contact with animals or during periods when pollen counts are high.

Adverse Reactions and Contraindications

The older beta-adrenergic bronchodilators, ephedrine, epinephrine, and isoproterenol, are not selective for the beta$_2$-adrenergic receptor. They have a range of side effects resulting from their nonselective action. Side effects are related to stimulation of the heart and include palpitation, tachycardia, and arrhythmias. CNS activity can cause tremors, headache, nervousness, and hypotension. Beta$_1$-adrenergic activity promotes the breakdown of glycogen to glucose, which impairs control in patients with diabetes mellitus.

The newer beta-adrenergic bronchodilators are relatively selective for the beta$_2$-receptor, the adrenergic receptor mediating bronchodilation. Because of this selective action, these drugs are less likely to cause unwanted cardiac effects or breakdown of liver glycogen to glucose. Patients with hypertension, cardiac disease, or diabetes can better tolerate the selective beta-adrenergic bronchodilators. Occasionally, nervousness or restlessness are side effects.

Toxicity

Overdose with beta-adrenergic drugs can cause chest discomfort and pain with an irregular heartbeat and irregular blood pressure. Chills, fever, light-headedness, and dizziness may be experienced. Other symptoms of overdose include nervousness, restlessness, unusual anxiety, and trembling. Inhalation medication should be discontinued and supportive therapy given.

Interactions

Beta-adrenergic drugs are potentiated by drugs that have direct or indirect sympathomimetic activity, including monoamine oxidase inhibitors, tricyclic antidepressants, and other sympathomimetic agents. This interaction may aggravate cardiovascular conditions such as arrhythmias and hypertension. Thyroid hormones may also aggravate cardiovascular conditions when taken with beta-adrenergic drugs.

Selective Beta-Adrenergic Bronchodilators

The second generation of beta-adrenergic bronchodilators are relatively selective for the beta$_2$-receptor, the adrenergic receptor mediating bronchodilation. These drugs are available in metered aerosol inhalers for easy administration. Albuterol, fenoterol, metaproterenol, and terbutaline are also available in oral forms.

▼ albuterol

Albuterol (Proventil, Ventolin) is available in forms for oral and inhalation administration for treatment of acute asthma. The inhalation forms include a metered aerosol and a solution. The solution is administered by nebulizer or intermittent positive pressure breathing (IPPB). The onset of action is 5 to 15 minutes, and the duration of action 3 to 6 hours. For oral administration, albuterol is available as a syrup, tablets, or extended-release tablets. The onset of action is 15 to 30 minutes, and the duration of action is 8 hours. In Canada an injectable form is also available with a duration of action of 12 hours. Albuterol is metabolized by the liver to an inactive form and excreted in the urine.

bitolterol

Bitolterol (Tornalate) is available in metered aerosol form for treatment of acute asthma. The onset of action is 3 to 4 minutes, and the duration of action is 5 to 8 hours. Bitolterol is conjugated and excreted in the urine.

fenoterol

Fenoterol (Berotec) is available in metered aerosol form, as a solution, and as tablets for the treatment of acute asthma.

The onset of action for the inhaled drug is 5 minutes, with a duration of action of 3 to 6 hours. The oral form is effective in 30 to 60 minutes and has a duration of action of 6 to 8 hours. Although available in Canada, fenoterol is not available in the United States.

isoetharine

Isoetharine (Bronkometer, others) is available in metered aerosol form and as a solution for the treatment of acute asthma. The onset of action is 1 to 6 minutes, and the duration of action is 1 to 4 hours. Isoetharine is metabolized by the liver and excreted in the urine.

metaproterenol

Metaproterenol (Alupent, others) is available as a metered aerosol and as a solution for inhalation administration and as a syrup and tablet for oral administration. Metaproterenol is used for treatment of acute asthma. The aerosol form has an onset of action of 1 minute and a duration of action of 1 to 5 hours. The solution, administered by hand-bulb nebulizer or IPPB, has a slower onset of action (5 to 30 minutes) and a duration of action of 2 to 6 hours. Oral forms are effective in 15 to 30 minutes for up to 4 hours. Metaproterenol is metabolized by the liver and excreted in the urine.

pirbuterol

Pirbuterol (Maxair) is available as a metered aerosol for the treatment of acute asthma. The onset of action is 5 minutes, and the duration of action is 5 hours. Pirbuterol is conjugated and excreted in the urine.

procaterol

Procaterol (Pro-Air) is available as a metered aerosol for asthma but is available only in Canada. The onset of action is 5 minutes, and the duration of action is 6 to 8 hours.

salmeterol

Salmeterol (Servent) is a new long-acting beta$_2$-agonist that is used for prophylactic treatment of asthma, especially asthma or bronchiole constriction in the presence of chronic obstructive lung disease. Salmeterol is available as a metered aerosol. Onset of action is 10 to 20 minutes, with peak effect in 3 to 4 hours and a duration of action of 12 hours. Patients should be cautioned not to use salmeterol to relieve an acute asthma episode. Because the onset is so slow, patients have overmedicated with salmeterol, leading to exacerbation of heart problems and even death in older patients.

terbutaline

Terbutaline (Brethine, Bricanyl) is available as metered aerosol, tablets, and an injection for the treatment of acute asthma or for prophylaxis in chronic asthma. Inhaled terbutaline is effective in 5 to 30 minutes and has a duration of action of 3 to 6 hours. With oral administration, the onset of action is 1 to 2 hours, and the duration of action is 4 to 8 hours. When injected, onset of action is within 15 minutes,

and the duration of action is ½ to 4 hours. Terbutaline is metabolized by the liver and excreted in the urine.

Nonselective Beta-Adrenergic Bronchodilators

The older beta-adrenergic bronchodilators, ephedrine, epinephrine, and isoproterenol, are not selective for the beta$_2$-adrenergic receptor. They have a range of side effects resulting from their nonselective action. These drugs are listed in Table 28-3.

epinephrine

Epinephrine (Adrenalin, Asmolin, Medihaler-Epi, others) can be administered subcutaneously to relieve an acute asthmatic attack. The drug causes bronchodilation and vasoconstriction to relieve bronchial edema. Given subcutaneously, an aqueous suspension of epinephrine (Sus-Phrine) lasts 8 hours; the hydrochloride salt lasts only 3 hours. Epinephrine is also available in MDIs as an aerosol or in solution for use in a nebulizer.

ephedrine

Ephedrine (generic) acts like epinephrine but is effective orally. Ephedrine is a weaker bronchodilator than epinephrine and is of no use for an acute asthma attack. It is used as a prophylactic for patients with mild to moderate asthma. Several formulations combine ephedrine with theophylline and a sedative in a single pill.

Ephedrine releases stored norepinephrine from sympathetic neurons, an indirect sympathomimetic effect that explains the weak bronchodilator action. The major metabolite is phenylpropanolamine, an active alpha-adrenergic drug often used as a decongestant.

ethylnorepinephrine

Ethylnorepinephrine (Bronkephrine) acts on beta$_1$- and beta$_2$-adrenergic receptors. It also exerts some vasoconstrictive activity that reduces bronchial congestion. Ethylnorepinephrine is available only for subcutaneous or intramuscular (IM) administration.

isoproterenol

Isoproterenol (Isuprel Hydrochloride, Medihaler-Iso) was the first widely used adrenergic drug with selectivity for beta- rather than alpha-receptors. It is not selective for beta$_2$-receptors and therefore stimulates the heart. Isoproterenol is primarily given by inhalation and relieves bronchoconstriction for up to 2 hours. If swallowed, it is degraded in the gut wall. It is available as a sublingual tablet, but absorption is so erratic that this route is rarely used.

▼ theophylline and Related Xanthines

Theophylline and related drugs are listed in Table 28-3. Short-acting forms are used to treat acute asthma. Although theophylline is also used as a prophylactic drug for asthma, inhaled steroids are now preferred as prophylaxis for persistent asthma because of the side effects associated with theophylline. However, long-acting formulations of theophylline are effective and are considerably less expensive than other medications.

Mechanism of Action

Theophylline is the prototype of the xanthines used to treat asthma. Like beta-adrenergic agonists, theophylline acts by increasing cellular cAMP concentrations, which relaxes bronchial smooth muscle and inhibits mast cell degranulation. Theophylline and the other xanthines accomplish this by inhibiting the degradation of cAMP by the enzyme phosphodiesterase. This action complements that of the beta-agonists, and the two kinds of agents may be included in therapy when the effect of either drug alone is insufficient to control bronchospasm.

Pharmacokinetics

Theophylline can be given intravenously (as aminophylline) to control acute bronchospasm in status asthmaticus or orally to control the bronchospasm of mild, moderate, or severe asthma. Theophylline is not highly water soluble, and there are many formulations to improve the solubility. Studies have shown that theophylline tablets are well absorbed, with more than 96% of the drug appearing in the plasma within 2 hours. Aminophylline, the most common soluble form of theophylline, is the only form that can be administered intravenously.

Several soluble salts of theophylline are available, and dosage is determined by the theophylline content. The drug is also available in slow- and fast-release preparations, alcoholic or aqueous solutions, and suppositories. Only the suppository is erratically absorbed and therefore unreliable. Rectal solutions are well absorbed. Theophylline is combined with ephedrine and a sedative in several combination products for treating asthma. Most clinicians prefer to individualize doses of each ingredient to minimize side effects while maximizing therapeutic effects and therefore do not favor combination drugs. Theophylline is not effective when administered by inhalation. IM injections of theophylline are not used because they are painful.

Theophylline is metabolized by the liver into inactive compounds excreted in the urine. There is a wide variability among individuals as to the plasma half-life of theophylline. In normal, nonsmoking adults the plasma half-life is about 6 hours but can vary from 3 to 12 hours. In smokers and children the plasma half-life is shorter, whereas in older adult patients, premature infants, and patients with liver disease or congestive heart failure with pulmonary edema, the plasma half-life is prolonged.

Uses

Theophylline and related drugs are used for the prophylaxis and treatment of asthma. They relieve the shortness of breath, wheezing, and dyspnea of asthma. Stimulation of the medullary centers of respiration may occur, which is benefi-

cial if the asthmatic patient is hypoxic. Theophylline treats Cheyne-Stokes respiration, in which the medullary sensitivity to hypoxia is decreased. Theophylline stimulates respiration in newborns who do not breathe well.

Adverse Reactions, Contraindications, and Toxicity

The most common side effects of theophylline after oral administration are nausea and epigastric pain. Headache, dizziness, and nervousness are also common. The effectiveness of theophylline is determined by its plasma concentrations, and the therapeutic range is 10 to 20 μg/ml. Agitation, exaggerated reflexes, and mild muscle tremors (fasciculation) are often seen when plasma levels are 20 to 30 μg/ml. Seizures and cardiac arrhythmias may occur when plasma levels exceed 30 μg/ml but occasionally occur with plasma concentrations between 20 and 30 μg/ml.

Other actions of theophylline seen in the therapeutic dose range are dilation of blood vessels and mild diuresis resulting from the increased renal blood flow and glomerular filtration. Stomach acid secretion is increased, which may be a problem for a patient with an ulcer.

Interactions

Phenobarbital increases the metabolism of theophylline, so larger doses are required. The serum concentration of theophylline is increased by cimetidine, erythromycin, influenza virus vaccine, and troleandomycin. Sympathomimetic drugs enhance CNS stimulation. Theophylline decreases the effects of phenytoin, lithium, nondepolarizing muscle relaxants, and beta-blockers.

Cigarette or marijuana smoking induces hepatic metabolism of theophylline. Smokers may require a 50% to 100% increase in the dose of theophylline.

Other Agents for Asthma

For information related to drugs in this category, refer to Table 28-2.

Oral Glucocorticoids

Oral glucocorticoids (corticosteroids) treat asthmatic patients with severe symptoms that are not controlled by bronchodilator therapy. Initially, very large doses (up to 1 g of methylprednisolone) of a glucocorticoid may be administered for as long as 5 days to bring a severe asthma attack under control when intravenous (IV) aminophylline and sympathomimetics have proved inadequate. High dosages of glucocorticoids can be tolerated for short periods but cause many severe side effects when used on a long-term basis. Few patients with asthma require glucocorticoids even after an acute attack. The mechanisms by which these drugs act to alleviate asthma are unknown, but they potentiate the action of the bronchodilators. To minimize the long-term toxic effects of glucocorticoids, they are administered in small doses (20 mg) every other day. This schedule minimizes suppression of adrenal function and also avoids excessive use, which could cause Cushing's syndrome (characteristic of excessive glucocorticoid administration; see Chapter 66). Oral glucocorticoids are covered more thoroughly in Chapter 41.

ipratropium

Ipratropium bromide (Atrovent) is the first anticholinergic drug available to treat asthma and conditions such as chronic bronchitis and emphysema in which bronchoconstriction is present. Ipratropium is an adjunct to antiinflammatory and bronchodilator therapy in the treatment of asthma. Ipratropium opens narrowed breathing passages by blocking vagal nerve impulses that tighten the muscles in the walls of the bronchial tubes. Mucus secretion is also reduced. Ipratropium is administered by inhalation. The onset of action is 5 to 15 minutes, and the duration of action is 3 to 6 hours. The drug is primarily excreted unchanged in the feces. It has negligible cardiovascular effects. Atropine-like side effects are rare with inhalation administration.

ketotifen

Ketotifen (Zaditen) is an antihistamine with cromolyn-like activity. It can be taken orally and has a duration of action of 12 to 24 hours. This drug may be prophylactic for asthma and relief of the sneezing and eye irritation from allergies. Side effects include sedation, dizziness, nausea, headache, and dry mouth. Asthma and bronchospasm may be aggravated. Ketotifen is available in Canada but not in the United States.

THERAPEUTIC AGENT: DRUG TO TREAT CHRONIC OBSTRUCTIVE PULMONARY DISEASE

Alpha₁-Proteinase Inhibitor

Lung damage in COPD results from the destruction of elastin, a major structural protein of the lung. Elastin is destroyed when there is an imbalance between the lung pro-teinase, elastase, which breaks down elastin, and alpha₁-proteinase inhibitor (Prolastin) (also called alpha₁-antitrypsin), a protein that inhibits elastase. Smoking depresses alpha₁-proteinase inhibitor, which can account for the high association between smoking and COPD. Some people have a genetic defect that results in low levels of alpha₁-proteinase inhibitor (Table 28-4). alpha₁-Proteinase inhibitor (Prolastin) is available for replacement therapy in patients with a congenital deficiency of alpha₁-proteinase inhibitor. This drug is currently purified from human plasma and administered intravenously. The recommended dosage is 60 mg/kg body weight administered once weekly.

THERAPEUTIC AGENTS: DRUGS TO TREAT RESPIRATORY DISTRESS SYNDROME

Surfactant Preparations

Surfactant preparations that diminish the mortality from respiratory distress syndrome in infants (see Table 28-4) have become available recently. It is not clear whether it is preferable to give surfactant for prophylaxis or as treatment only. Dosing schedules are still being refined.

Beractant or surfactant TA (Survanta) is derived from cow's lungs. For high-risk infants weighing 600 to 1250 g, beractant is administered prophylactically in a single 100-mg dose immediately after birth. For infants with respiratory distress syndrome, 100-mg doses are given no more than every 6 hours, up to 4 doses. All doses are administered intratracheally.

The combination of colfosceril palmitate, cetyl alcohol, and tyloxapol (Exosurf) is a synthetic mixture. The colfoceril palmitate is the lipid and active ingredient. Cetyl alcohol is a spreading agent, and tyloxapol is a nonionic detergent that serves as a dispersing agent. For high-risk infants weighing less than 1350 g, 80 mg/kg is given shortly after birth and again at 12 and 24 hours. For infants with respiratory distress syndrome, two doses of 80 mg/kg are given at 12-hour intervals. All doses are administered intratracheally.

Table 28-4	**Miscellaneous Drugs for Pulmonary Conditions**		
Generic Name	Trade Name	Administration/Dosage	Comments
alpha₁-proteinase inhibitor, human	Prolastin*	INTRAVENOUS: *Adults*—60 mg/kg body weight, administered at rate of 0.08 ml/kg body weight/min, once a week.	For emphysema caused by a deficiency of alpha₁-antitrypsin.
beractant	Survanta*	INTRATRACHEAL: *Neonates*—100 mg immediately after birth. Doses may be repeated every 6 hr, up to 4 doses.	Pulmonary surfactant for respiratory distress syndrome of neonates.
colfosceril palmitate, cetyl alcohol, and tyloxapol	Exosurf Neonatal*	INTRATRACHEAL: *Neonates*—80 mg/kg just after birth and again at 12 and 24 hr for high-risk infants. For infants with respiratory distress syndrome, 2 doses of 80 mg/kg at 12-hr intervals.	Pulmonary surfactant for respiratory distress syndrome of neonates.

*Available in Canada and the United States.

Nursing Process Overview

Bronchodilators

Assessment

Perform a general assessment of the patient. The focus is often on the respiratory system. Check the vital signs, the amount and characteristics of secretions, and the level of fatigue; auscultate breathing sounds; determine arterial blood gas levels and vital capacity; and assess subjective complaints and patient's ability to perform and tolerate activities of daily living. Obtain relevant history regarding issues such as smoking, exposure to irritants, infection, and stress. Assess history of medications used and their effect.

Nursing Diagnoses

- Anxiety related to difficult breathing, air hunger, tachycardia, and drug side effects
- Possible complication: hypertension secondary to bronchodilator use

Patient Outcomes

The patient will state a subjective feeling of less anxiety. Pulse rate will be lower, and breathing will be subjectively easier. Hypertension will be diagnosed if it occurs, and appropriate measures to lower blood pressure will be developed by nurse and physician.

Planning/Implementation

Monitor vital signs; a short-term care unit may be appropriate for the patient in acute respiratory distress. Monitor fluid intake and output, level of consciousness, blood gas levels, vital capacity, and treatment of any infectious process. Use an infusion control device for IV drugs. Monitor serum xanthine levels and blood glucose level in patients receiving xanthine therapy.

Evaluation

Bronchodilators are successful if the patient's condition is subjectively and objectively improved. The vital capacity should increase, arterial blood gas levels should be closer to normal values, the respiratory rate should decrease, and the patient should appear to be in less respiratory distress. Subjectively, the patient should report easier breathing, less shortness of breath, less fatigue, and better tolerance for activities of daily living.

Before discharge, verify that the patient can explain which drugs are to be taken and how to take them correctly, what situations require notification of the physician because of exacerbation of the disease process or because of effects resulting from drug therapy, how to perform measures such as exercises for respiratory management, and how to use oxygen correctly. Determine that the patient can demonstrate correct use of any equipment such as IPPB machines or drug administration devices such as inhalers or nebulizers. Finally, check that the patient can explain which respiratory irritants should be avoided.

Nursing Implications Summary

GENERAL GUIDELINES: DRUGS TO TREAT ASTHMA AND OTHER PULMONARY DISEASES

Drug Administration

➤ Review the side effects discussed in the text and the information in Tables 28-1 to 28-3.

➤ Monitor pulse, blood pressure, and respiratory rate. Auscultate lung sounds. The frequency of monitoring varies with the drug, dosage, route of administration, and patient condition. During IV administration, monitor vital signs every 5 to 15 minutes until stable. With subcutaneous and inhalation administration, monitor every 15 minutes.

➤ Monitor all patients requiring bronchodilators but especially older adult patients and those with cardiovascular or hypertensive disease or diabetes mellitus.

➤ Patients with acute asthma may require admission to the intensive care unit. Characteristics of severe acute asthma include poor air exchange, diminished breath sounds, marked retraction of accessory muscles of respiration, obtunded mentation, cyanosis, confusion, signs of exhaustion, and forced expiratory volume less than 1 L. Monitor pulse oximetry, and obtain arterial blood gases if indicated. Administer oxygen. Establish an IV line to provide access for medications and to keep patient hydrated.

➤ Anxiety, insomnia, fear, and other emotional responses may aggravate bronchospasm and air hunger. Maintain a calm but efficient attitude in caring for patients. Do not leave patients unattended for long periods. Keep the call bell within easy reach.

➤ With subcutaneous or IM injection, perform aspiration before administering dose to avoid inadvertent IV administration.

➤ For continuous IV infusion, use an infusion control device and (usually) microdrip tubing. Monitor intake and output and vital signs.

➤ Monitor blood glucose levels of diabetic patients because bronchodilators may produce hyperglycemia.

Continued

Nursing Implications Summary—cont'd

Nursing in the Community

➤ After the acute respiratory distress episode is over, review with the patient the common side effects of the prescribed drugs.

➤ Many bronchodilators are dispensed with patient instruction leaflets; review the leaflets with the patient.

➤ Encourage patients with respiratory problems to stop smoking. Provide them with information about local resources available to help smokers quit.

➤ Before discharge, the patient should be able to describe or demonstrate the correct way to take ordered medication, including frequency, route of administration, and use of inhalation devices; and the patient should also know under what circumstances to return to the physician or emergency room if the drugs are not effective. Caution the patient to use these drugs only as prescribed and not to increase the dose or frequency unless directed to do so by the physician. Patients who find relief with MDIs may begin using them more often than prescribed. These drugs soon become ineffective, or patients will experience significant side effects.

➤ In consultation with the physician, develop a written plan for the patient and family that outlines the specific plan of action to manage an exacerbation.

➤ Warn diabetic patients to monitor blood glucose levels carefully, especially when changing doses of a bronchodilator.

➤ The patient should let sublingual tablets dissolve under the tongue. Instruct the patient not to swallow saliva until the tablet is completely dissolved.

➤ Instruct the patient to take oral doses with meals or snacks to lessen gastric irritation.

➤ Ensure that the patient can use the MDI correctly when using it for the first time. Review manufacturer's instruction sheet with the patient. Have the patient assemble the inhaler and shake the canister. The patient should exhale deeply, then put the mouthpiece into the mouth with the opening directed to the back of the throat. The patient should grasp the mouthpiece with the teeth and lips. The patient should inhale deeply while depressing the aerosol container or activating the spray mechanism. The patient should inhale for 5 to 10 seconds, then hold his or her breath as long as possible before exhaling. Instruct the patient to wait several minutes before taking a second dose (if prescribed). Remember to shake the canister again before administering the second dose. For children, it may be necessary to hold the nose shut. When finished, tell the patient to wash and dry the mouthpiece (see Figure 28-3).

➤ Special devices can help children use inhalation medications if they are having difficulty using the MDI; examples include the Inhal-Aid and InspirEase devices. The patient should consult the pharmacist.

➤ The nurse should periodically watch the patient use the MDI to verify that the patient is continuing to use the device correctly.

➤ When two drugs are ordered via inhalation, the patient should use the bronchodilator first, then take the second drug such as beclomethasone.

➤ Some patients experience drug or food induced asthma. The following are some triggers for some patients: sulfites, bisulfites, and metabisulfites found in food and other drugs; tartrazine dye (see Patient Problems box in Chapter 31 for tartrazine allergy); monosodium glutamate (MSG), commonly used in oriental cooking, but used in many prepared foods; and nonselective beta-blocking agents used to treat other health problems the patient may have. Angiotensin-converting enzyme inhibitors may be a trigger in a small number of patients.

➤ Some of the drugs used to treat asthma contain sulfites. If the patient is allergic to sulfites, instruct him or her to read carefully all literature provided with the prescriptions to see whether any contain sulfites and to work with the pharmacist to obtain sulfite-free brands.

➤ Strategies that may be helpful for exercise-induced bronchospasm include extending the warm-up period before exercising, choosing a less strenuous sport, avoiding exercise during periods of high air pollution, and using one or more medications prophylactically before exercising (consult physician for specific drugs and dose).

➤ To decrease exposure to common irritants, teach the patient to vacuum the home often, encase mattress and pillows with plastic, use high-energy particulate air filters (HEPA) for the heating/air conditioning system, use an air conditioner if possible, and keep the windows closed.

➤ If tachycardia is a problem, suggest that the patient limit caffeine intake.

➤ Instruct the patient to check the supply of drug on hand to avoid running out at inopportune times. To check the amount in a canister, drop the canister into water (without mouthpiece). Full containers sink to the bottom, and half-full containers float with part of the container out of the water. The empty container floats on its side, half submerged (see Figure 5-25). Consult the manufacturer's literature for additional information.

➤ Remind the patient to inform all health care providers of all drugs being taken. Remind the patient to avoid over-the-counter drugs unless first approved by the physician. Many decongestants and cold remedies contain products that duplicate the effects of the bronchodilators, causing increased side effects.

➤ Instruct the patient to keep these and all drugs out of the reach of children.

➤ No drugs should be used during pregnancy or lactation unless first approved by the physician.

Inhaled Glucocorticoids
Drug Administration/Nursing in the Community

➤ See Chapters 41 and 66 for a detailed discussion of systemic glucocorticoid therapy.

➤ Systemic side effects with inhaled forms are uncommon but may occur. These side effects include development of osteoporosis, easy bruising, and suppression of the hypothalamic-pituitary-adrenal axis.

Nursing Implications Summary—cont'd

➤ See the general guidelines for drugs to treat asthma for a discussion of the use of MDIs.

➤ For best effect, glucocorticoids should be used at evenly spaced intervals throughout the 24 hours as prescribed. Several weeks of therapy may be required to see full benefit of therapy.

➤ Glucocorticoids for inhalation are dispensed with an inhaler and a patient instruction leaflet. Review this leaflet with the patient.

➤ Glucocorticoids for inhalation are also available as powder or capsules containing powder. These forms require a special device that punctures the capsule or blister containing the powder and releases it into the inhaler. Review manufacturer's leaflet with the patient.

➤ Instruct the patient to gargle and rinse the mouth, but not to swallow the gargle liquid, after each use of the inhaler to help prevent fungal infections.

➤ Instruct patients to notify the physician if they experience unusual stress such as surgery or illness, have an asthma attack that does not respond to usual treatment, develop an infection of the mouth or throat, or their general physical condition worsens. Also, instruct patients taking glucocorticoids regularly to wear a medical identification tag or bracelet. Finally, instruct patients not to discontinue any medications prescribed for asthma without consulting with physician.

cromolyn and nedocromil
Nursing in the Community

➤ See the general guidelines for bronchodilator therapy for a discussion of MDIs. Unlike other drugs administered via inhalation, neither the cromolyn nor the nedocromil canister can be floated to estimate the number of doses remaining. Teach patients using this form to keep a record of doses used. There are about 112 or 200 inhalations per canister of cromolyn, depending on the size canister prescribed. The drug may also be administered with a Spinhaler or a Halermatic device or in a nebulizer; the drug is packaged with detailed instructions, which should be reviewed with the patient.

➤ About 56 or 122 inhalations are in a canister of nedocromil, depending on the size prescribed by the physician. Nedocromil is available only in aerosol canisters.

➤ Inform the patient of the importance of taking cromolyn or nedocromil as ordered, on a regular basis. Spreading doses out evenly throughout the day is more beneficial than erratic use. These drugs are useful for prophylactic treatment of asthma but will not control an acute attack of asthma. Several weeks of therapy may be required to see full benefit of therapy. Instruct patients to continue all concomitant therapy, even if they begin to feel better.

➤ See the Patient Problems box in Chapter 23 on dry mouth.

➤ For missed doses, instruct the patient to take dose as soon as remembered, then space remaining doses for that day evenly throughout that day.

➤ Side effects are rare, but encourage the patient to report unexpected signs or symptoms.

➤ There are also cromolyn capsules for oral administration, and cromolyn eye drops. All should be dispensed with patient instruction leaflets. Review these instructions with the patient.

Leukotriene Modifiers
Nursing in the Community

➤ Teach patients that these drugs are used to prevent attacks of asthma, not to treat acute attacks. For best effect, they need to be used regularly, as prescribed, even if the patient is feeling better. It may require several weeks of therapy for full effect to be realized.

➤ Do not discontinue other medications for asthma while taking a leukotriene modifier. Consult physician with questions.

➤ Take zafirlukast on an empty stomach, 1 hour before or 2 hours after a meal.

➤ Montelukast is available as a tablet and as a chewable tablet. Review the form prescribed with the patient.

➤ For missed doses, instruct the patient to take dose as soon as remembered, unless almost time for the next dose, then omit the missed dose and resume usual schedule. Do not double up for missed doses.

Beta-Adrenergic Bronchodilators
Nursing in the Community

➤ Review the general guidelines for drugs used for asthma. The first dose from an MDI may contain inadequate amounts of medication. When the canister is new or when it has not been used in a while, especially if stored in an upright position, the patient should activate the canister at least once, into the air, before using it again to administer the dose(s). Avoid getting the priming mist into the eyes.

➤ Caution patients to contact their physicians if the usual doses of medication are not controlling their asthma. Do not increase doses without medical advice. The need for increased medication may signal a worsening of the condition, and medical advice is needed.

➤ Instruct patients to keep a record of inhalations from each canister. Floating the canister in water provides only a rough estimate of the amount of medication remaining. Consult the pharmacist for information about the number of doses per canister prescribed, or consult manufacturer's literature.

➤ Review the Patient Problems boxes on dry mouth (Chapter 23) and orthostatic hypotension (Chapter 13).

➤ Beta-receptor agonists are available in a variety of dosage forms: oral solution, oral syrup, tablets, extended-release tablets, capsules, forms for injection, as well as aerosol, solution, and powder for inhalation. Review the patient's medications to verify that the patient is taking prescribed forms correctly.

➤ Isoproterenol may cause saliva to turn pinkish to red; this effect is harmless.

➤ Ephedrine may cause trouble sleeping. Instruct the patient to take the last dose of this drug several hours before bedtime.

Continued

Nursing Implications Summary—cont'd

➤ Sustained-release formulations should be swallowed whole, without chewing or crushing. If there is a question about a specific product, instruct the patient to consult the pharmacist.

epinephrine
Drug Administration

➤ Epinephrine hydrochloride (adrenalin chloride) is used via subcutaneous or IM injection to treat anaphylactic allergic reactions. The dose is 0.1 to 0.5 mg (0.1 to 0.5 ml) of 1:1000 injection.

➤ Epinephrine can be administered via endotracheal tube if the patient is intubated, at the same dosage used for IV injection.

➤ To use epinephrine inhalation solution, place about 10 drops of a 1% solution in the reservoir of the nebulizer.

➤ See the general guidelines for bronchodilator therapy. Monitor the pulse and blood pressure carefully.

➤ Sus-Phrine is a suspension. Rotate the vial between the hands to mix the suspension before preparing the dose, and administer immediately so that the drug does not settle out of suspension.

➤ See Chapter 16 for a discussion of use of epinephrine in shock.

XANTHINES TO TREAT ASTHMA
Drug Administration

➤ Review the general guidelines for drugs to treat asthma.

➤ Monitor the vital signs and blood pressure, and auscultate lung sounds. Hypotension may be pronounced. Supervise ambulation. Keep siderails up.

➤ Monitor serum theophylline levels, pulmonary function tests, and serum caffeine concentration if ordered.

➤ When using oral liquid forms of aminophylline or theophylline to treat neonatal apnea, use the less concentrated form (5 mg/ml) to reduce the possibility of error in measuring the small volumes needed of the more concentrated solution.

Intravenous aminophylline

➤ Read labels carefully; the label must state for IV use. Only the concentration of 25 mg/ml may be given undiluted, by direct IV push, at a rate of 20 mg/min. Usually, aminophylline is diluted in at least 100 to 200 ml of 5% dextrose in water and given as an infusion, based on serum levels or patient's response, 1 dose over 20 to 30 minutes. Even when diluted, do not administer at a rate faster than 20 mg/min. It is available prediluted. It is incompatible with many drugs, so do not administer it piggyback; start and maintain a separate IV for replacement fluids and other drugs.

Nursing in the Community

➤ Review the general guidelines for drugs to treat asthma.

➤ Instruct the patient to take oral doses on an empty stomach with a full glass (8 ounces) of water, 1 hour before meals or 2 hours after meals. Doses can also be taken with meals or

snack to lessen gastric irritation. Whichever way the patient takes the medication, it should be taken the same way each day to decrease fluctuations in serum levels.

➤ Inform the patient taking once-a-day doses to take the dose after fasting through the night and 1 hour before eating or in the evening with or without food, depending on the product. Encourage the patient to take the medication at the same time and in the same way each day.

➤ Instruct the patient to notify the physician if fever, diarrhea, or symptoms of the flu develop. Encourage the patient to return for follow-up visits to have blood work done to monitor serum drug levels.

➤ Review the Patient Problems box in Chapter 13 on orthostatic hypotension.

➤ Warn the patient to avoid driving or operating hazardous equipment if dizziness, light-headedness, or vertigo develop; if these symptoms occur, tell the patient to notify the physician.

➤ Instruct the patient to read drug prescriptions and labels carefully. Many xanthines are available in regular and sustained-release formulations; they cannot be interchanged on the same dosing schedule. See Chapter 5 for a discussion of sustained-release products. In addition, various brands are not interchangeable. Inform the patient not to switch brands or dosage forms without checking with physician.

➤ Inform patients who have difficulty swallowing extended-release capsules that the contents may be sprinkled on a small amount of food such as jam, jelly, or applesauce and swallowed without chewing.

➤ Instruct the patient to limit or avoid the use of coffee, tea, chocolate, and other methylxanthines because they may affect xanthine metabolism.

➤ Instruct the patient to avoid smoking cigarettes or marijuana, which may alter serum levels. Instruct the patient not to start or stop smoking without talking with the physician because the dose of xanthine may need to be adjusted.

OTHER AGENTS TO TREAT ASTHMA
ipratropium
Nursing in the Community

➤ See the general guidelines for drugs to treat asthma for a discussion of MDIs. Ipratropium is usually dispensed with a patient instruction leaflet; review the leaflet with the patient.

➤ Review the Patient Problems boxes on dry mouth (Chapter 23) and constipation (Chapter 24). See Chapter 23 for a detailed discussion of anticholinergics.

➤ Instruct patients to notify the physician if they do not have the usual response to ipratropium or if their condition worsens.

➤ Ipratropium is also prescribed in an inhalation solution form. If used concurrently with cromolyn inhalation solution, teach patients to use the preservative-free ipratropium inhalation solution.

➤ Ipratropium is also available as a nasal aerosol.

Nursing Implications Summary—cont'd

ketotifen

Nursing in the Community

➤ Inform the patient of the importance of taking this drug as ordered, on a regular basis. This drug is useful for prophylactic treatment of asthma.

➤ Instruct the patient to avoid driving or operating hazardous equipment if sedation or dizziness occur and to notify the physician.

➤ See the Patient Problems box in Chapter 23 on dry mouth.

DRUG TO TREAT CHRONIC OBSTRUCTIVE PULMONARY DISEASE

Alpha$_1$-Proteinase Inhibitor

Drug Administration

➤ Consult the manufacturer's literature for current guidelines.

➤ Store the drug in the refrigerator before reconstitution and at room temperature after reconstitution and administer within 3 hours. Use diluent supplied by the manufacturer to prepare the dilution. Diluted solution is approximately 20 mg/ml.

➤ Monitor vital signs. Administer intravenously at 0.08 ml/kg/min.

➤ Patients should be immunized against hepatitis B because the drug is prepared from pooled human plasma.

➤ Monitor serum alpha$_1$-proteinase inhibitor levels if available.

Nursing in the Community

➤ This drug is administered intravenously. If used by the patient for self-administration, teach the patient how to store drug and prepare doses, manage infusion, and dispose of contaminated needles, tubing, and equipment.

DRUGS TO TREAT RESPIRATORY DISTRESS SYNDROME

Surfactant Preparations

Drug Administration

➤ Protocols for administration of these agents are being developed and refined. Check the hospital protocol for guidelines. Administration may be restricted to the physician.

➤ Beractant suspension should be warmed before administration. Let stand at room temperature for 20 minutes, or warm in the hand for at least 8 minutes. Do not use artificial warming methods. For prophylactic doses, begin warming before infant's birth. Rotate vial to suspend or resuspend drug in diluent. Use each vial for a single dose. Discard unused suspension.

➤ Reconstitute colfosceril palmitate, cetyl alcohol, and tyloxapol with diluent provided by manufacturer. See manufacturer's instructions for preferred method. Reconstitute immediately before use because the product does not contain antibacterial preservatives.

➤ Dosage is based on weight. Inject drug intratracheally via an endotracheal tube. The manufacturer of Exosurf provides an endotracheal tube adapter to permit injection.

➤ Aspirate an infant's lungs before administration of surfactant; avoid suctioning if possible for at least 2 hours after administration of the drug and for as long as 6 hours, if tolerated by infant.

➤ To distribute the drug throughout the lungs, it may be necessary to gently rotate the infant's body from side to side.

➤ Monitor clinical appearance, pulse oximetry, partial pressure of oxygen (Po_2), carbon dioxide partial pressure (Pco_2), arterial blood gases, lung sounds, and cardiac monitoring.

➤ Keep the mother and family informed of the infant's condition.

CHAPTER REVIEW

Application

1. What three components restrict the airway in extrinsic asthma?

2. Which beta-adrenergic agonists used as bronchodilators are relatively specific for the beta$_2$-receptor?

3. What side effects are associated with bronchodilators?

4. How does cromolyn treat extrinsic asthma? What is its mechanism of action?

5. For what purpose are surfactant preparations used? How would you administer them?

Critical Thinking

1. Compare and contrast the mechanisms responsible for extrinsic and intrinsic asthma.

2. What is the mechanism of action of the bronchodilators (beta-adrenergic receptor agonists and theophylline)? List three beneficial responses attributed to this mechanism.

3. How do beclomethasone and other glucocorticoids treat extrinsic asthma? What is their mechanism of action?

4. How does alpha$_1$-proteinase inhibitor treat COPD? What are the nursing considerations in its administration?

References

Berg J, Dunbar-Jacob J, Sereika SM: An evaluation of a self-management program for adults with asthma, *Clin Nurs Res* 6(3):225-238, 1997.

Canales MAP: Asthma management: putting your patient on the team, *Nursing* 27(12):33-38, 1997.

Chiocca E, Russo L: Acute asthma attack, *Nursing* 27(7):43, 1997.

Eisenbeis C: Full partner in care, *Nursing* 26(1):48-51, 1996.

Gazarian PK: Teaching your patient to use a metered-dose inhaler: the direct route for asthma therapy, *Nursing* 27(10):52-54, 1997.

LeNoir MA: Bronchodilator therapy for asthma, *RT* 9(1):115-116, 118, 120-121, 1996.

Middleton AD: Managing asthma. It takes teamwork, *Am J Nurs* 97(1):39-43, 1997.

Rokosky JM: Misuse of metered-dose inhalers: helping patients get it right, *Home Healthc Nurse* 15(1):13-21, 23-24, 1997.

Roncolli MT: Asthma medications for children: guidelines for the primary care practitioner. *J Am Acad Nurse Pract* 8(5):243-255, 1996.

Antihistamines

OBJECTIVES

After studying this chapter, you should be able to do the following:

■ *Describe localized and generalized allergic responses.*

■ *Discuss the role of histamine in allergic responses.*

■ *Describe the common side effects of antihistamines, including the anticholinergic effects.*

■ *Develop a nursing care plan for a patient taking an antihistamine.*

CHAPTER OVERVIEW

Histamine is a naturally occurring amine that is formed from the amino acid histidine. Histamine is found in mast cells, which are numerous in the lung and skin, and basophils, the counterparts of mast cells in the blood. The histamine released from the mast cells causes many of the symptoms associated with allergic reactions. It is also found in the gastrointestinal (GI) tract, where histamine is a potent stimulant for the secretion of acid in the stomach. Histamine is also found in parts of the brain, where it is believed to be a neurotransmitter. At present, the role of histamine in the brain is speculative but may involve regulating the level of arousal. This chapter focuses on the role of histamine in allergic reactions and the drugs available to treat these reactions. The role of histamine in the stomach is discussed in Chapter 26.

THERAPEUTIC RATIONALE: ALLERGIES

Histamine Release and Metabolism

Histamine in mast cells and basophils is complexed with heparin and stored in granules. The typical allergic reaction such as hay fever or contact dermatitis involves the release of these granules in response to an antigen. Antibodies of the immunoglobulin E (IgE) class fix to the mast cells and basophils. When an antigen binds to the fixed IgE, the cells degranulate, releasing histamine, heparin, and other compounds, which alter capillary permeability and attract phagocytes to degrade the bound antigen. This process is illustrated in Figure 29-1.

In addition to antigen-induced degranulation, many drugs and venoms cause degranulation. These include drugs

and dyes that carry a positive charge, large molecules that occur in animal sera and dextran solutions, and venoms and enzymes that damage tissue.

Once histamine is released, it is metabolized to inactive compounds in 5 to 15 minutes. One of the degradative pathways is inhibited by aspirin so that histamine may persist. This is the mechanism for one type of aspirin sensitivity.

Allergic Responses Explained by the Action of Histamine

Local allergic responses involving histamine are as follows:

■ **Anaphylaxis:** Systemic; onset usually indicated by a generalized itching and tingling sensation and a feeling of apprehension; profound hypotension leading to shock may follow, and the bronchioles are constricted, causing a choking sensation

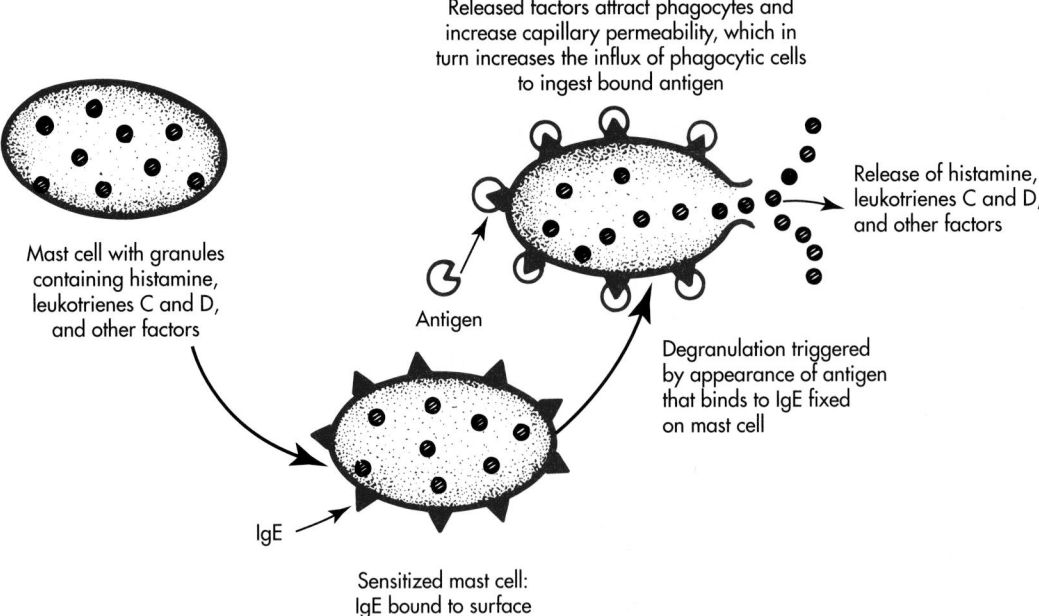

Figure 29-1 Immunologic mechanism underlying release of histamine from mast cells. Antibodies of immunoglobulin E *(IgE)* class are bound to surface of mast cells. Binding of antigen to IgE triggers degranulation of mast cell, releasing histamine and leukotrienes C and D. Histamine is responsible for many allergy and asthma symptoms.

- **Angioedema:** Swelling caused by plasma leakage and blood vessel dilation in the skin or mucous membranes ("giant hives")
- **Asthma:** Spasm of the bronchial smooth muscle
- **Eczema:** Inflamed areas of skin
- **Purpura:** Red spots on the skin caused by the leakage of blood from small vessels
- **Rhinitis:** Inflammation of the nasal mucous membranes that allows fluid to escape
- **Urticaria:** Hives, which are large wheals caused by leakage of plasma and are accompanied by severe itching

Two actions of histamine are prominent in explaining allergic responses. Histamine is a potent dilator of arterioles and renders the capillaries more permeable so that fluid and protein are lost into the extravascular space. This explains the bump that appears after an insect sting. Initially, a red spot reflects the dilation of the small blood vessels; as fluid leaks into the extravascular space, the bump, representing local edema, appears. Histamine also stimulates the contraction of smooth muscle, particularly the bronchial smooth muscle. When mast cells are degranulated in the lung, as in asthma, the airway is narrowed and patients have difficulty breathing.

Histamine released systemically causes anaphylaxis, characterized by a profound fall in blood pressure resulting from vasodilation and severe constriction of the bronchioles, making breathing difficult. The loss of fluid from circulation resulting from the increased capillary permeability causes the shock that develops in an untreated anaphylactic response. Edema in the mucous tissue of the upper windpipe (laryngeal edema) can block the airway altogether. Epinephrine is the drug of choice for anaphylactic shock. Epinephrine constricts blood vessels to raise the blood pressure and relieve laryngeal edema and dilates the bronchioles, actions that reverse those of histamine (see Chapter 16).

THERAPEUTIC AGENTS: ANTIHISTAMINES

Mechanism of Action

Antihistamines (Table 29-1) have been available for more than 50 years. Although these drugs block some actions of histamine, they do not block the histamine-mediated secretion of acid in the stomach. There are two types of histamine receptors: the H_1 receptors, acting principally on blood vessels and the bronchioles, and the H_2 receptors, acting mainly on the GI tract. The older antihistamines described in this chapter are specific antagonists for the H_1 receptors. Antagonists specific for the H_2 receptor are cimetidine (Tagamet), famotidine (Pepcid), nizatidine (Axid), and ranitidine (Zantac). These drugs, used primarily to decrease stomach acid, are discussed in Chapter 26. In this chapter, the term *antihistamine* refers to drugs that specifically block the H_1 receptors.

Pharmacokinetics

Antihistamines are given orally and are well absorbed. Their action is seen in 10 to 30 minutes and lasts for 4 to 6 hours. Timed-release forms are active for 8 to 12 hours. Antihistamines are metabolized to inactive compounds by the liver and kidneys.

Table 29-1 Antihistamines for Allergies

Generic Name	Trade Name	Administration/Dosage	Comments
astemizole	Hismanal*	ORAL: *Adults and children >12 yr*—10 mg once a day. *Children 6-12 yr*—5 mg once a day. *Children 2-6 yr*—2 mg/10 kg body weight. FDA pregnancy category C.	Nonsedating antihistamine. Take on an empty stomach. Available over the counter in Canada.
azatadine maleate	Optimine*	ORAL: *Adults and children >12 yr*—1-2 mg twice daily. FDA pregnancy category B.	Drowsiness is most common side effect.
azelastine hydrochloride	Astelin	INHALATION: *Adults and children >12 yr*—2 sprays per nostril 2 times/day.	For treating seasonal allergic rhinitis. May cause drowsiness and a bitter taste.
brompheniramine maleate	Dimetane* Various others	ORAL: *Adults*—4-8 mg 3-4 times/day or 8-12 mg of sustained-release form 2-3 times/day. FDA pregnancy category B. *Children >6 yr*—½ adult dose. *Children <6 yr*—0.5 mg/kg/day divided into 3-4 doses.	Drowsiness is most common side effect. Over-the-counter preparations available in the United States and Canada.
cetirizine hydrochloride	Reactine† Zyrtec*	ORAL: *Adults and children >6 yr*—5-10 mg once a day. *Children 2-6 yr*—5 mg once a day.	Nonsedating antihistamine but with modest incidence of drowsiness.
chlorpheniramine maleate	Aller-Chlor Chlor-Trimetron Various others	ORAL: *Adults*—4 mg 3-4 times/day or 8-12 mg of sustained-release form 2-3 times/day. FDA pregnancy category B. *Children 6-12 yr*—2 mg 3-4 times/day or 8 mg of sustained-release form once daily. *Children 2-6 yr*—1 mg 3-4 times/day.	Low incidence of drowsiness. A common ingredient in cold remedies. Many formulations available over the counter in the United States and Canada.
clemastine fumarate	Tavist*	ORAL: *Adults*—2.68 mg 3 times/day. Not intended for children. FDA pregnancy category B.	Low incidence of drowsiness. Very weak anticholinergic effects. Especially effective to relieve itching. Available over the counter in the United States and Canada.
cyproheptadine hydrochloride	Periactin*	ORAL: *Adults*—4-20 mg/day, not more than 0.5 mg/kg. Dose is started at 4 mg 3 times/day. FDA pregnancy category B. *Children 7-14 yr*—4 mg 2-3 times/day to maximum of 16 mg/day. *Children 2-6 yr*—2 mg 2-3 times/day to maximum of 12 mg/day.	Used to relieve itching. Drowsiness is most common side effect. Stimulates appetite. Available over the counter in Canada.
dexchlorpheniramine maleate	Polaramine*	ORAL: *Adults*—1-2 mg 3 or 4 times/day or 4-6 mg 2 times/day or 6 mg of time-released form 3 times/day. FDA pregnancy category B. *Children <12 yr*—0.15 mg/kg/day divided into 4 doses.	Drowsiness is most common side effect. Available over the counter in Canada.
diphenhydramine	Benadryl Various others	ORAL: *Adults*—25-50 mg 3-4 times/day. FDA pregnancy category B. *Children >20 lb*—2.5-25 mg 3-4 times/day. *Children <12 yr*—5 mg/kg in 4 divided doses each day.	High incidence of drowsiness with little paradoxical stimulation in children. Also used to treat motion sickness and mild parkinsonism. Also used as antitussive. May be used with epinephrine in treating anaphylactic reaction. Available over the counter in the United States and Canada.
doxylamine succinate	Unisom	ORAL: *Adults*—12.5-25 mg every 4-6 hr. *Children 6-12 yr*—75 mg divided into 4-6 doses daily. *Children <6 yr*—2 mg/kg body weight divided into 4-6 doses daily. Decapryn available without prescription.	High incidence of drowsiness. Often included in nonprescription sleeping aids.
fexofenadine	Allegra*	ORAL: *Adults and children >12 yr*—60 mg twice a day. FDA pregnancy category C.	Nonsedating antihistamine for seasonal allergic rhinitis.
loratadine	Claritin*	ORAL: *Adults*—10 mg once a day. FDA pregnancy category B.	Nonsedating antihistamine for seasonal allergic rhinitis.
methdilazine hydrochloride	Tacaryl	ORAL: *Adults*—8 mg 2-4 times/day. *Children >3 yr*—4 mg 2-4 times/day.	A phenothiazine derivative used primarily to relieve itching. Incidence of drowsiness is less than with other phenothiazines.
phenindamine tartrate	Nolahist	ORAL: *Adults*—25 mg every 4-6 hr as needed. *Children 6-12 yr*—12.5 mg every 4-6 hr.	Used for seasonal allergic rhinitis. Available over the counter.
pyrilamine maleate	Nisaval	ORAL: *Adults*—25-50 mg 4 times/day. *Children 6-12 yr*—½ adult dose.	Low incidence of drowsiness. Available over the counter.
trimeprazine tartrate	Panectyl† Temaril	ORAL: *Adults*—2.5 mg 4 times/day or 5 mg of sustained-release form every 12 hr. *Children >3 yr*—	A phenothiazine derivative. Drowsiness is most common reaction. Used primarily

*Available in Canada and the United States.
†Available in Canada only.

Continued

Table 29-1 Antihistamines for Allergies—cont'd			
Generic Name	Trade Name	Administration/Dosage	Comments
		2.5 mg at bedtime or up to 3 times/day (children >6 yr can take 5 mg of sustained-release form once a day). *Children 6 mo-3 yr*—1.25 mg at bedtime or up to 3 times/day.	to relieve itching of neurodermatitis, contact dermatitis, and chicken pox.
tripelennamine citrate or hydrochloride	PBZ-SR Pyribenzamine† Various others	ORAL: *Adults*—25-50 mg every 4-6 hr or 100 mg of sustained-release form every 12 hr. *Children >5 yr*—50 mg of sustained-release form every 12 hr. *Children and infants*—5 mg/kg daily divided into 4-6 doses.	Dizziness is common side effect. Available over the counter in Canada.
triprolidine hydrochloride	Myidil	ORAL: *Adults*—2.5 mg 3-4 times/day. FDA pregnancy category B. *Children >6 yr*—½ adult dose. *Children <6 yr*—0.3-0.6 mg 3-4 times/day.	Low incidence of side effects, with drowsiness being most common.

*Available in Canada and the United States.
†Available in Canada only.

Uses

Antihistamines and Allergic Reactions. Antihistamines such as **chlorpheniramine** are primarily effective in decreasing the discomfort of acute allergic reactions that involve the upper respiratory system (e.g., hay fever) or the skin (e.g., hives). Hay fever is most successfully treated when the antihistamine therapy is begun while the pollen count is still low. Sneezing, runny nose, and swollen eyes are reduced in more than 70% of patients. Antihistamines reduce the swelling and itching (pruritus) of urticaria and related conditions.

Antihistamines block only histamine receptors. Therefore some allergic responses are not effectively treated with antihistamines. Anaphylaxis represents a true emergency for which an antihistamine is inadequate because it neither acts fast enough nor reverses the histamine reactions. Epinephrine acts rapidly, and its pharmacologic actions reverse those of histamine.

Antihistamines do not prevent or treat colds, although they are combined with a decongestant in many over-the-counter (OTC) and prescription cold remedies. Because most antihistamines have anticholinergic actions, they can dry up a runny nose and relieve the symptoms of a cold.

Antihistamines do not treat asthma, probably because substances other than histamine are responsible for the prolonged bronchiole constriction characteristic of asthma. Antihistamines can relieve allergic rhinitis often associated with asthma.

Nonsedating Antihistamines. Recently antihistamines have been developed that blunt allergic reactions effectively without the sedation commonly associated with the older antihistamines. These new antihistamines include astemizole (Hismanal), cetirizine (Zyrtec), fexofenadine (Allegra), and **loratadine** (Claritin). These drugs are available only by prescription. They are widely prescribed for the relief of allergic symptoms.

Antihistamines as Sedatives. Sedation is a common side effect of antihistamines, some of which are used principally for this purpose. Many OTC sleeping aids use an antihistamine as the active agent. The antihistamines approved as sleep-aid ingredients are pyrilamine, doxylamine succinate, and **diphenhydramine**. Hydroxyzine (Atarax, Vistaril) is an antihistamine often used as an antianxiety agent (see Chapter 57).

Antihistamines as Antiemetics and Antiparkinsonism Agents. Selected antihistamines have other uses. Some antihistamines prevent nausea and vomiting, particularly from motion sickness and vertigo. These antihistamines are discussed in Chapter 25. Antihistamines that suppress the tremors of parkinsonism are discussed in Chapter 62.

Adverse Reactions and Contraindications

Although the antihistamines are so named because they specifically compete with histamine for the H_1 receptors, they have other pharmacologic properties. The main secondary action is an anticholinergic or atropine-like action. This is the origin of side effects such as inhibition of secretions, blurred vision, urinary retention, fast heart rate (tachycardia), and constipation. In the central nervous system (CNS) the anticholinergic effect can cause insomnia, tremors, nervousness, and irritability. These effects are particularly predominant in children. Sedation and drowsiness, the central antihistaminic effects, are more common in adults. The spectrum of antihistaminic and anticholinergic properties depends on the drug, the dosage, and the individual. Most antihistamines have a local anesthetic effect, which might relieve the itching of skin rashes. Antihistamines are rarely used for this purpose because they tend to be good antigens, thereby causing skin rashes themselves.

Antihistamines are contraindicated for nursing mothers because the drugs are secreted in milk. Antihistamines taken by young children can cause paradoxical excitement, whereas older adult patients are sensitive to the sedative actions.

Toxicity

Antihistamine overdose can cause CNS depression or stimulation, the latter being more common in children. The atropine-like symptoms (flushed skin and fixed, dilated pupils) are also prominent. Management maintains an airway and treats hypotension. In children a high tempera-ture is common, which can be reversed with ice packs and sponge baths. If the antihistamine is not a phenothiazine, vomiting is induced, gastric lavage is carried out, and cathartics are used to empty the GI tract of remaining drug. Vomiting should not be induced with phenothiazines because they can cause uncoordinated movements of the head and neck, which could cause aspiration of vomitus. Antihistamines that are phenothiazine derivatives are identified in the drug tables.

Interactions

The main drug interaction associated with antihistamines is the additive depression of the CNS when taken with alcohol, hypnotics, sedatives, antipsychotics, antianxiety drugs, or narcotic analgesics. Because of their atropine-like effects, antihistamines should be used with caution in patients with glaucoma, hyperthyroidism, cardiovascular disease, or hypertension.

Nursing Process Overview

Antihistamines for Allergic Reactions

Assessment

Assess vital signs, respiratory and cardiovascular status, relevant history of previous allergy, exposure to possible allergens, subjective symptoms, and objective data such as the extent and type of rash, or nasal exudate, difficulty breathing through nose, headache, and sore throat for respiratory allergy. Anaphylaxis is an emergency; the more delayed and chronic responses may represent a source of annoyance to the patient but may never progress to an acute phase.

Nursing Diagnoses

- Risk for injury related to drowsiness related to antihistamine therapy
- Possible altered bowel elimination: constipation related to antihistamine use

Patient Outcomes

The patient will state subjective improvement in symptoms of allergy and will not experience serious side effects.

Planning/Implementation

Anaphylaxis requires immediate diagnosis and treatment, usually with 1:1000 epinephrine injected subcutaneously or in-tramuscularly, followed by parenteral antihistamines. Supportive care is symptomatic and based on rapid assessment of the cardiovascular and respiratory response. Management of the less acute allergic response is not an emergency. Monitor the vital signs, respiratory status, cardiovascular status, platelet count, and white blood cell count. Observe for side effects of drug therapy, especially drowsiness; monitor fluid intake and output to check for urinary retention; and monitor the frequency of bowel movements to assess for constipation.

Evaluation

Before discharge, determine that patients can explain why and how to take the prescribed medication, what side effects may appear and which of these to report immediately, and what to do for specific side effects such as dry mouth, constipation, hypotension, and drowsiness. If specific allergens are identified, patients should be able to name them. Verify that patients understand the importance of wearing a medical identification tag or bracelet listing specific allergens.

Nursing Implications Summary

Antihistamines
Drug Administration

➤ Monitor blood pressure, pulse, and intake and output. Auscultate breath sounds. Inspect for development of rash. Monitor complete blood count, white blood cell count and differential, and platelet count. Supervise ambulation, especially of older adult patients. Keep siderails up and a nightlight on. Monitor smoking. Assess for urinary retention (difficulty initiating voiding and feeling of incomplete bladder emptying). Palpate the bladder.

Intramuscular Administration

➤ Use large muscle masses (see Chapter 5). Record and rotate injection sites. Aspirate before injecting medication to prevent accidental intravenous (IV) administration. Warn the patient that intramuscular (IM) injection of antihistamines may burn as the medication is injected.

➤ Read drug labels carefully. Some forms are for IM use only and should not be used for IV administration. Antihistamines may be prescribed with narcotic analgesics for pain relief. They may decrease nausea and may potentiate CNS depression, but they do not enhance the analgesic effect of the narcotic. It may be necessary to lower the dosage of one of the drugs because of the hypotension, sedation, and other side effects that may occur when both drugs are used.

Intravenous brompheniramine

➤ May be given undiluted, but further dilution is preferred. Do not use the concentrated solution (100 mg/ml) for IV administration. Check with the pharmacist about compatibility

Continued

Nursing Implications Summary—cont'd

with other drugs. Administer a single bolus injection over at least 1 minute.

Intravenous chlorpheniramine

➤ May be given undiluted. Do not use the concentrated solution (100 mg/ml) for IV administration. Administer at a rate of 10 mg over 1 minute or longer if possible.

Intravenous diphenhydramine

➤ May be given undiluted. Administer at 25 mg/min or longer if possible.

Nursing in the Community

➤ Warn the patient to avoid driving or operating hazardous equipment if drowsiness, blurred vision, or dizziness occurs. Instruct the patient to notify the physician if blurred vision develops.

➤ Review the Patient Problems boxes on constipation (Chapter 24), dry mouth (Chapter 23), orthostatic hypotension (Chapter 13), and photosensitivity (Chapter 58).

➤ Instruct the patient to report fever, sore throat, rash, unexplained bleeding, or bruising because these may be signs of rare but serious hematologic side effects.

➤ Instruct the patient to take oral doses with meals or a light snack to decrease gastric irritation, except for astemizole, which should be taken on an empty stomach.

➤ Instruct the patient to swallow sustained-release forms whole, without crushing or chewing. Scored tablets may be broken before swallowing. Capsules may be opened and contents poured into soft food for ease in taking. The patient should chew gum forms for 15 minutes or longer (see manufacturer's literature). Review administration technique for patients using suppository forms.

➤ Teach the patient correct IM administration technique if this route is prescribed for self-administration.

➤ For motion sickness, doses should be taken 30 to 60 minutes before beginning travel. Patients traveling by car should face forward in the center of the front seat if possible.

➤ Instruct the patient to avoid the use of alcohol and other CNS depressants.

➤ Remind the patients to keep all health care providers informed of all medications being used, even OTC preparations. Regular use of antihistamines may mask side effects developing from other drugs, such as ringing in the ears from salicylates.

➤ Instruct the patient to read labels of OTC preparations carefully. Patients using remedies for colds, hay fever, insomnia, and other problems may be taking unnecessary drugs or taking the same drug in two or more combination products and should consult the pharmacist for assistance.

➤ Remind the patient that antihistamines may also cause allergies. Encourage the patient to report any unexpected sign or symptom to the physician.

➤ Encourage patients with allergies to wear a medical identification tag or bracelet indicating the nature of the allergies. Pregnant women should not take any medication without the approval of the physician; some of the antihistamines are contraindicated during pregnancy because of potential harm to the fetus. Remind patients to keep these and all drugs out of the reach of children.

➤ A potentially fatal cardiotoxic effect may occur when astemizole or loratadine and itraconazole, metronidazole, miconazole, or ketoconazole are taken. Remind the patient to inform all health care providers of all medications being used.

 ## CHAPTER REVIEW

Application

1. Describe the origin, location, and role of histamine.
2. What factors mediate histamine release?
3. What are five pharmacologic actions of antihistamines?
4. What are the drug interactions and contraindications for the antihistamines?
5. Describe three clinical uses of the H_1 receptor antihistamines.
6. How does cimetidine differ from the H_1 receptor antihistamines?
7. Give examples of five situations in which patients may manifest allergic reactions or require antihistamines. One example is when a transfusion reaction occurs; name four others.

Critical Thinking

1. Ideally, all antihistamines would be effective, without side effects. Yet, many antihistamines are in common use with known side effects such as drowsiness and dry mouth. Why are antihistamines that cause these side effects still in common use?

2. Antihistamines can be found in OTC sleep remedies. Older adults are more sensitive than younger individuals to the side effects of antihistamines. As a home health nurse, you learn that your older adult patient is taking a sleeping aid containing an antihistamine. What suggestions can you give the patient to try that might help the patient get to sleep without relying on medication?

Drugs to Control Bronchial Secretions

OBJECTIVES

After studying this chapter, you should be able to do the following:

■ *Discuss the action of the alpha-adrenergic agonists, the imidazolines, and the antihistamines in relieving nasal congestion.*

■ *Differentiate between expectorants, antitussives, and mucolytic agents in treating a cough.*

■ *Develop a nursing care plan for a patient receiving a nasal decongestant or a drug to treat a cough.*

CHAPTER OVERVIEW

Many of the drugs covered in this chapter are available over the counter (OTC) for treatment of colds and coughs. Nasal decongestants are covered in the first section, and drugs to treat a cough are covered in the second section.

THERAPEUTIC RATIONALE: NASAL CONGESTION

Nasal congestion results when the blood vessels in the nasal passage become dilated as a result of infection, inflammation, allergy, or emotional upset. Dilation increases capillary permeability and allows fluid to escape into the nasal passage.

THERAPEUTIC AGENTS: NASAL DECONGESTANTS

Alpha-Adrenergic Agonists

Mechanism of Action

Nasal decongestants are alpha-adrenergic agonists and mimic the action of the neurotransmitter norepinephrine (see Chapter 12). These agents stimulate alpha-receptors and cause blood vessels to constrict, thereby relieving the congestion.

Pharmacokinetics and Uses

Several alpha-adrenergic agonists are applied topically as drops or sprays. Because these nasal decongestants have im-

mediate and direct contact with the nasal mucosa, they act rapidly and provide temporary symptomatic relief by opening the nasal passages.

When a nasal decongestant is applied as drops into the nostril, the patient should be lying on a bed with the head hanging over the edge and turned to one side. The drops are instilled into the upper nostril. After a few seconds the head is turned to allow administration to the other nostril. Use of this lateral, head-low position allows the drops to coat the nasal mucosa without being immediately swallowed.

Orally active alpha-adrenergic agonists commonly found in cold remedies include phenylpropanolamine, phenylephrine, and pseudoephedrine. Cold remedies are syrups, tablets, or capsules that may also include an antihistamine, an analgesic, or other miscellaneous ingredients. Cold remedies are discussed in Chapter 7.

Adverse Reactions, Contraindications, and Toxicity

Nasal decongestants may cause a stinging or burning sensation or induce sneezing when sprayed into the nose. **Rebound congestion** is a common side effect. This occurs when

Table 30-1   Nasal Decongestants

Generic Name	Trade Name	Administration/Dosage	Comments
oxymetazoline hydrochloride	Afrin Dristan* Various others	TOPICAL: *Adults*—2-3 drops or 2-3 sprays of 0.05% solution in each nostril at morning and at bedtime. *Children >6 yr*—as for adults. *Children 2-5 yr*—0.025% solution is used as above.	An imidazoline. Long acting. Side effects are mild and generally safe.
phenylephrine hydrochloride	Neo-Synephrine hydrochloride* Various others	TOPICAL: *Adults*—drops of 0.25%-1% solution in each nostril (head in lateral, head-low position) every 3-4 hr. Nasal spray or jelly may be used. *Children >6 yr*—as for adults. *Infants and young children*—0.125% solution is used as above.	Less potent and longer action than epinephrine. No central nervous system stimulation but can cause transient hypertension, headaches, and palpitations.
phenylpropanolamine hydrochloride	Various combination drugs	ORAL: *Adults*—25 mg every 3-4 hr or 50 mg every 6-8 hr. *Children 8-12 yr*—20-25 mg 3 times/day. Not recommended for children <8 yr.	Similar to ephedrine but with less central nervous system stimulation. Widely available over the counter.
pseudoephedrine hydrochloride	Sudafed* Various others	ORAL: *Adults*—60 mg every 4-6 hr. *Children*—4 mg/kg body weight in 4 divided doses.	Stereoisomer of ephedrine with lesser incidence of central nervous system stimulation and hypertension than ephedrine. Useful for relief of runny nose or congestion leading to earache.
xylometazoline hydrochloride	Otrivin* Neo-Synephrine II Various others	TOPICAL: *Adults and children >12 yr*—2-3 drops or inhalations of 0.1% solution/spray in each nostril every 8-10 hr. *Children 2-12 yr*—2-3 drops of 0.05% solution in each nostril every 8-10 hr.	An imidazoline. A relatively safe, long-acting decongestant but should not be used excessively or for more than a few days. Do not use in atomizers with aluminum parts.

*Available in Canada and the United States.

the effect of the drug wears off. If topical nasal decongestants are used with increasing frequency, they have less and less effect. The drug ultimately irritates the nasal passages and causes the congestion to become worse rather than better. Therefore topical decongestants are most effective when used only occasionally and for no longer than 3 to 5 days. Nasal decongestants are available without a prescription.

With repeated use of a topical nasal decongestant, more of the drug is absorbed, and systemic effects become possible. The symptoms of an overdose are those expected from a sympathomimetic drug (see Chapter 12), including nervousness, dizziness, palpitation, and transient high blood pressure readings. Children are especially vulnerable to overdoses of nasal decongestants and may have reactions that include sweating, drowsiness, shock, or coma.

Interactions

Patients with hyperthyroidism, diabetes mellitus, hypertension, or heart disease are vulnerable to the sympathomimetic side effects of nasal decongestants and should avoid these drugs. A hypertensive reaction to a nasal decongestant may occur in patients taking a monoamine oxidase inhibitor. Patients receiving tricyclic antidepressants are vulnerable to the cardiac effects of sympathomimetic agents.

Specific Sympathomimetic Drugs

Summary information on sympathomimetic drugs is presented in Table 30-1.

oxymetazoline

Oxymetazoline (Afrin, others) is a long-lasting nasal spray available OTC. It is safe for use in children older than 2 years.

▼ phenylephrine

Phenylephrine (Coricidin, Neo-Synephrine, others) is a potent alpha-adrenergic agonist that is administered orally or topically. It is available both alone and in many combination cold preparations.

phenylpropanolamine

Phenylpropanolamine (Prolamine) is used mainly in oral combination cold remedies. An alpha-adrenergic agonist, it acts indirectly, releasing norepinephrine from nerve terminals.

pseudoephedrine

Pseudoephedrine (Novafed, Sudafed, others) is included in many oral combination cold remedies. It is a beta- and an alpha-agonist.

xylometazoline

Xylometazoline (Otrivin, Neo-Synephrine II, others) is a long-lasting nasal spray available OTC. It is safe for use in children older than 2 years.

Other Drugs to Relieve Nasal Congestion

Nasal congestion is common in allergies such as hay fever. As discussed in Chapter 29, antihistamines treat hay fever because they block the receptors for histamine on the blood vessels and thereby prevent the dilation that causes nasal congestion. Antihistamines are also commonly included in cold remedy preparations. The anticholinergic action characteristic of antihistamines aids in reversing the vasodilation of the nasal blood vessels. Several corticosteroids are available as nasal sprays for treating congestion arising from allergies. These agents depress the inflammatory response causing nasal congestion and are discussed in Chapter 41.

THERAPEUTIC RATIONALE: RESPIRATORY SECRETIONS

Origin of Secretions

Respiratory secretions in the trachea, bronchi, and bronchioles originate from the goblet cells and bronchial glands (Figure 30-1). The goblet cells lie on the surface, making up part of the epithelial layer. The tracheal epithelium consists of about 20% goblet cells, and the bronchiolar epithelium consists of 2% goblet cells. These cells produce a gelatinous mucus that they periodically secrete. It is unknown what factors normally control the goblet cells, but chronic exposure to irritants increases their size, number, and activity. An example is the phlegm coughed up by smokers. The bronchial glands lie several layers beneath the epithelium. The grapelike (acinar) cells are controlled by the cholinergic nervous system; when stimulated, acinar cells secrete a plentiful watery fluid into a duct that empties onto the surface.

The secretions of the goblet cells and bronchial glands combine to form a mucus called the **respiratory tract fluid.** Much of the water in the respiratory secretions evaporates to humidify the air taken into the lungs. If too much water is lost to humidification, the mucus forms thick plugs that cannot be readily eliminated. Normally, the respiratory tract fluid forms a lining that is swept upward by the action of the ciliary hairs into the throat (pharynx), where it is swallowed. This activity, the **mucociliary escalator,** provides a cleansing mechanism for the lungs because foreign particles or bacteria are trapped in this viscous layer and eliminated. If the ciliary hairs are paralyzed by tobacco smoke or alcohol, secretions cannot be cleared naturally and give rise to the "smoker's cough."

Cough

A **cough** is a protective reflex initiated by irritation in the airway. As long as material is being brought up by the cough, it is beneficial. Several situations cause an unproductive cough. The air of heated rooms can dry the airway enough to cause irritation. A sore throat can produce an unproductive cough and can be self-perpetuating when the cough further irritates the throat. A cough can result from irritants responsible for asthma or pulmonary edema, which also stimulate the cough receptors. Congestion of the nasal mucosa results in postnasal drip, which irritates the throat and produces the cough associated with a cold or the flu.

When a cough is not productive and disrupts sleep and rest, relief is sought. Therapy for a cough depends on the cause. If the air is dry, a vaporizer or steamer may sufficiently liquefy the secretions so that they do not become irritating. A dehydrated state limits respiratory secretions, so having the patient drink plenty of fluids prevents or overcomes the dehydration that accompanies common illnesses. Patients

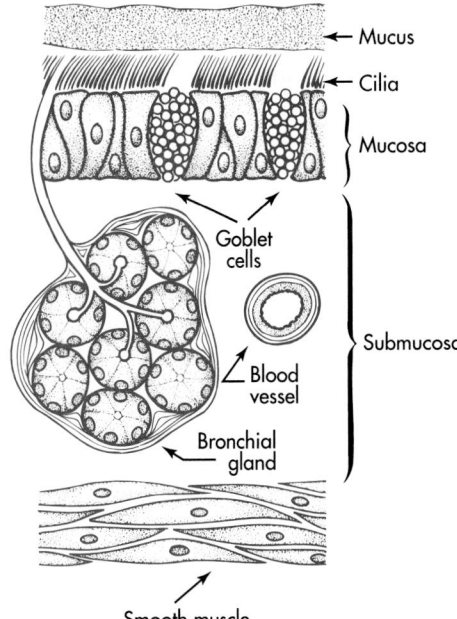

Figure 30-1 Mucous layer at top is lumen of airway. Relative position of goblet cells and bronchial glands, secretions of which make up mucus, are shown. Mucous layer is normally swept up toward throat by cilia to cleanse airway.

with sore throats can suck hard candies to increase saliva flow to coat the throat. If these simple measures do not eliminate the cough, expectorants may be used. An **expectorant** increases the output of respiratory tract fluid to coat the trachea and bronchi. In addition, a cough suppressant or antitussive drug may be taken. Expectorants and antitussive drugs are widely available as OTC drugs.

THERAPEUTIC AGENTS: EXPECTORANTS, ANTITUSSIVES, AND MUCOLYTIC AGENTS

Expectorants

Although many drugs have been used as expectorants, no expectorant has been proven effective. The only agent currently used as an expectorant is guaifenesin.

▼ guaifenesin

Guaifenesin (glyceryl guaiacolate) is a widely used expectorant. It stimulates the secretion of respiratory tract fluid through vagal reflex, thereby keeping respiratory secretions fluid and more readily removed through coughing. However, the true effectiveness of this activity is unclear. Guaifenesin is available as a single agent but is also commonly combined with other agents in cold and cough formulations.

Miscellaneous Expectorants

Other agents added as expectorants to cough suppressant mixtures include terpin hydrate, citric acid, sodium citrate, and calcium iodide.

Antitussives

Tussis is the Latin word meaning cough, and cough suppressants are called **antitussives.** These drugs are listed in Table 30-2. Opioids are effective antitussives, but only codeine and hydrocodone are used for this effect. Nonopiate antitussives include chlophedianol, dextromethorphan, and diphenhydramine.

codeine and hydrocodone

Codeine and hydrocodone are good antitussives, but they are opiates and therefore are capable of producing drug dependence. Hydrocodone has a greater potential than codeine for producing drug dependence. Most preparations containing codeine or hydrocodone are prescription drugs. Some preparations are available as schedule V drugs and may be obtained by signing for them with a registered pharmacist. The opiates suppress a cough by directly inhibiting the medullary center for the cough reflex. The doses required to suppress a cough are smaller than those to produce analgesia or respiratory depression. Side effects at antitussive doses are uncommon but include nausea, dizziness, and constipation.

chlophedianol

Chlophedianol (Ulone) is a centrally acting antitussive with some local anesthetic and anticholinergic action. Use of this drug may cause some patients to become excited and hyperirritable. Large doses cause sedation. Chlophedianol is available in Canada but not in the United States.

▼ dextromethorphan hydrobromide

Dextromethorphan hydrobromide is the most widely used antitussive in OTC cough mixtures. It is related to the opiates but has no analgesic effect and causes no drug dependence.

Table 30-2 Expectorants, Antitussives, and Mucolytic Agents

Generic Name	Trade Name	Administration/Dosage	Comments
Expectorant			
guaifenesin (glyceryl guaiacolate)	Anti-tuss Glycotuss Robitussin* Various others	ORAL: *Adults*—200-400 mg every 3-4 hr. *Children 6-12 yr*—100 mg every 3-4 hr. *Children 2-6 yr*—50 mg every 3-4 hr.	Use for symptomatic relief of dry, unproductive cough. Occasionally causes nausea or drowsiness. Available without prescription. Found in many cough/cold preparations.
Antitussives			
chlophedianol	Ulo† Ulone†	ORAL: *Adults*—25 mg 3-4 times/day. *Children 6-12 yr*—12.5-25 mg 3-4 times/day. *Children 2-6 yr*—12.5 mg 3 or 4 times/day.	Prescription drug. Side effects include drowsiness and nausea.
codeine, codeine phosphate, codeine sulfate		ORAL: *Adults*—10-20 mg every 4-6 hr; no more than 120 mg in 24 hr. *Children 6-12 yr*—½ adult dose. *Children 2-6 yr*—¼ adult dose.	Schedule II drug. Codeine is included in some schedule III and schedule V combination formulations, usually including a decongestant, an antihistamine, and an expectorant. For adverse effects, see Chapter 32.
dextromethorphan hydrobromide	Benylin* Robitussin DM Various others	ORAL: *Adults*—10-20 mg every 4 hr or 30 mg every 6-8 hr. *Children 6-12 yr*—½ adult dose. *Children 2-6 yr*—¼ adult dose.	Nonnarcotic, available without prescription. No tolerance develops. Has no analgesic or hypnotic effect and does not depress respiration. Does not cause constipation as readily as codeine.
diphenhydramine hydrochloride	Benylin Cough Syrup* Benadryl*	ORAL: *Adults*—25 mg every 4 hr, no more than 100 mg in 24 hr. *Children 6-12 yr*—½ adult dose. *Children 2-5 yr*—¼ adult dose.	An antihistamine. Side effects include drowsiness and a drying effect.
hydrocodone bitartrate	Hycodan Robidone Various others	ORAL: *Adults*—5-10 mg every 6-8 hr. *Children*—0.6 mg/kg body weight daily in divided doses.	Schedule II drug. Hydrocodone is included in some schedule III and schedule V combination formulations, usually including a decongestant, an antihistamine, and an expectorant. For adverse effects, see Chapter 32.
Mucolytic			
acetylcysteine	Mucomyst* Mucosil	NEBULIZATION: (using face mask, mouthpiece, or tracheostomy): 1-10 mg of 20% solution or 2-20 ml of 10% solution every 2-6 hr. DIRECT INSTILLATION: 1-2 ml of 10% or 20% solution as often as every hour.	Has odor of rotten eggs, which may cause gastrointestinal upset. Solutions can be diluted with sterile water for nebulization. Reacts with iron, copper, and rubber, so nebulization equipment should not contain these materials.

NOTE: Only those expectorants available alone are listed. Other drugs included in cough or cold mixtures as an expectorant include potassium guaiacolsulfonate, ammonium chloride, terpin hydrate, ipecac, calcium iodide, potassium iodide, and citric acid.
*Available in Canada and the United States.
†Available in Canada only.

Dextromethorphan is an effective cough suppressant that inhibits the medullary center for the cough reflex. It is well tolerated and only occasionally causes drowsiness or dizziness.

diphenhydramine

Diphenhydramine (Benylin) is an antihistamine with antitussive action. Adverse effects include drowsiness common to the antihistamines and the anticholinergic drying effect that hinders a productive cough.

Mucolytic

Water, taken as liquid or inhaled as vapor, keeps the mucus from becoming too viscous. An expectorant stimulates the watery secretion of the bronchial glands. A **mucolytic** breaks up viscous mucus so that it can be coughed up or otherwise drained. Viscous mucus is most likely to occur in the patient with a pulmonary infection or with chronic obstructive lung disease in which the normal mechanisms for clearing the lungs are compromised. Table 30-2 lists dosages and administration of the mucolytic drug currently available.

acetylcysteine

Acetylcysteine (Mucomyst, Mucosil) is a sulfhydryl compound that can break disulfide bonds. Viscous mucus has long molecules linked by disulfide bonds; when these disulfide bonds are broken, the molecules separate, reducing the viscosity.

Acetylcysteine is administered by nebulizer through a face mask, mouthpiece, or tracheostomy. Acetylcysteine has a rotten egg odor and may irritate the nasal passages.

Nursing Process Overview

Drugs Modifying Respiratory Secretions

Assessment

Perform a general assessment of the patient in addition to focusing on subjective complaints. An appropriate history asks about the onset of symptoms, possible irritants for symptoms, times of the day when symptoms are worse (e.g., a cough that is more troublesome at night), therapies used by the patient that have successfully relieved the symptoms, and the history of irritants or environmental conditions that may aggravate the symptoms. Objective data include the respiratory rate, vital signs, character and quantity of secretions, assessment of the lungs, and examination of the nose, throat, and ears.

Nursing Diagnoses

- Ineffective airway clearance related to suppressed ability to cough
- Altered health maintenance related to misuse or overuse of nasal decongestants

Patient Outcomes

The patient will successfully clear airway by learning to cough effectively; any infection present will be resolved. The patient will use nasal decongestants only 3 to 5 days and only as often as ordered.

Planning/Implementation

Monitor symptoms, vital signs, and in some patients, fluid intake and output. Identify nonmedical solutions for troublesome symptoms. For patients receiving the mucolytic agent, have a suction machine at the bedside if there is doubt that the patient can adequately handle secretions.

Evaluation

These drugs are successful if symptoms are relieved. Before discharge, patients should be able to explain how to take the drugs correctly, what side effects might occur that would require notification of the physician, why the drugs should be discontinued after symptoms have improved, and what actions to take if the symptoms return or do not improve.

Nursing Implications Summary

Nasal Decongestants
Drug Administration
➤ Monitor blood pressure and pulse. Monitor blood glucose levels in diabetic patients.
➤ Assess for gastrointestinal (GI) symptoms. Persistent or severe GI tract symptoms indicate a need to change drug or dosage.
Nursing in the Community
➤ Review side effects with the patient. Instruct the patient to choose OTC remedies appropriate for their symptoms and to read product labels. Hundreds of OTC products contain two or more of the following: antihistamines, antitussives, analgesics, expectorants, and decongestants. The patient should use products only as directed and should consult the pharmacist in choosing an appropriate remedy for a specific problem.
➤ Remind the patient to keep all health care providers informed of all drugs being used, even OTC preparations. In particular, patients with thyroid disease, diabetes mellitus, hypertension, or heart disease should use nasal decongestants only with physician approval.

Continued

Nursing Implications Summary—cont'd

➤ Remind the patient to keep all drugs out of the reach of children, even nasal sprays and drops. Only pediatric preparations and pediatric doses should be used for children. To prevent the spread of infection, do not share applicators. Each person should have a separate bottle or applicator.

➤ Review Chapter 5 for information about using nosedrops and nose sprays correctly. To prevent contamination of equipment, family members should not share droppers or spray applicators. Instruct the patient to rinse and dry applicators after each use.

➤ To prevent insomnia, instruct the patient to take the last dose of the day around the time of the evening meal. If photophobia occurs, instruct the patient to avoid brightly lit areas and to wear sunglasses.

➤ Instruct the patient how to use nasal jelly (phenylephrine and others): First, blow the nose. Wash hands. Place a pea-sized amount of jelly in each nostril. Sniff well to move jelly back into nose. Wipe off the tip of the tube with a tissue and replace the cap.

Expectorants and Antitussives
Nursing in the Community

➤ Instruct the patient about the difference between an antitussive and an expectorant.

➤ Remind the patient to read labels carefully on OTC preparations to avoid taking unnecessary medications and to consult the pharmacist for assistance as needed.

➤ Remind the patient to keep these and all drugs out of the reach of children. Only products for pediatric use and in pediatric doses should be administered to children.

➤ Remind the patient to avoid driving or operating hazardous equipment if drowsiness is a problem.

➤ Instruct patients with a cough to stay well hydrated (daily fluid intake of at least 2500 ml for an adult), avoid smoking, and keep the room air moist by using a vaporizer or humidifier.

➤ Instruct patients to drink a glass of water after each dose of medication to help loosen mucus.

➤ For preparations containing iodide, question the patient about history of allergy to iodine or shellfish before administering. Instruct the patient to swallow enteric-coated tablets whole, without chewing or crushing, and take them with a full glass (8 ounces) of liquid. Liquid preparations should be diluted with water, milk, or juice. Teach patients to take doses with meals or a snack to reduce gastric irritation. Discuss signs of chronic iodine poisoning such as headache, swelling of eyelids, metallic taste in the mouth, nausea, vomiting, diarrhea, skin changes, and mouth ulcers. Remind the patient to report any unexpected sign or symptom to the physician.

➤ Codeine and hydrocodone have the same potential for side effects as all narcotics; see Chapter 32.

Mucolytic
Drug Administration/Nursing in the Community

➤ Supervise the patient receiving acetylcysteine during and after treatment to see that the airway is still patent in the presence of increased pulmonary secretions. Have a suction machine at the bedside of patients who are older adults, immobilized, or intubated or anyone who may not be able to handle secretions.

➤ Before using a mucolytic agent with a patient for the first time, review the purpose and desired effects of the drug. Instruct the patient to cough up and expectorate loosened secretions.

➤ Because the drug may cause bronchospasm, supervise patients with asthma who are receiving acetylcysteine. If bronchospasm develops, discontinue nebulization; if severe, notify the physician. Assess for other common side effects including stomatitis, rhinorrhea, and nausea.

➤ Acetylcysteine is administered orally to treat acetaminophen overdose. The dose is based on the time since acetaminophen ingestion and the serum level of acetaminophen. The regimen involves a loading dose, followed by 17 doses at 4-hour intervals. Dilute doses in juice or cola beverages before administering. The drug has an unpleasant odor. Chill diluted dose by pouring over ice and administer it from a covered container through a straw. If the patient vomits within 1 hour after receiving a dose, the dose should be repeated; consult the physician. For additional information, see the manufacturer's insert.

CHAPTER REVIEW

Application

1. Explain how alpha-adrenergic agonists relieve nasal congestion.
2. Describe the technique for administering topical nasal decongestants.
3. What are the side effects, drug interactions, and contraindications for nasal decongestants?
4. What is rebound congestion?
5. Describe the origin and function of mucus.
6. List expectorants and their mechanisms of action.
7. Describe the mucolytic drug and its mechanism of action.
8. List antitussives and their mechanisms of action.
9. What are the nonmedicinal approaches for treating a cough?

Critical Thinking

1. As a home health nurse, you determine that your patient is using an OTC nasal spray 6 to 8 times per day. What more should you assess? If your patient states inability to stop using the nasal spray, what should you do next?

2. Many OTC cough and cold remedies contain both an expectorant and an antitussive. What are advantages or disadvantages to such a combination?

Reference

Self T, Alloway RR, Dempster JS: Treatment of rhinitis, *J Am Acad Nurse Pract* 8(3):135-147, 1996.

31

Aspirin, Acetaminophen, NSAIDs, and Drugs to Treat Gout

OBJECTIVES

After studying this chapter, you should be able to do the following:

■ *Differentiate between the actions, side effects, and uses of aspirin and acetaminophen.*

■ *Discuss drug therapy with nonsteroidal antiinflammatory drugs (NSAIDs) and differentiate between individual drugs.*

■ *Discuss drug therapy for gout.*

■ *Develop a nursing care plan for a patient receiving one of the drugs discussed in this chapter.*

CHAPTER OVERVIEW

This chapter covers analgesic-antipyretic drugs, including the NSAIDs. Aspirin is the prototype drug. It is used to reduce a fever (antipyresis), to provide analgesia for mild to moderate pain, and to reduce inflammation. Aspirin and acetaminophen are commonly found in over the counter (OTC) and prescription combination drugs that are marketed for relief of colds and allergies. Like acetaminophen and aspirin, the NSAIDs are also antipyretics and analgesics. Except for ibuprofen, ketoprofen, and naproxen, NSAIDs are prescription drugs used primarily to treat inflammation and resulting pain.

This chapter also covers drugs to treat gout. Gout is a metabolic disease in which crystals of uric acid may form in a joint, typically the base of the big toe. Agents are available to reduce the pain and inflammation associated with gout.

THERAPEUTIC RATIONALE: PAIN, FEVER, AND INFLAMMATION

Synthesis of Prostaglandins

The important role of prostaglandin E_2 as a mediator of pain, fever, and inflammation is well recognized. The prostaglandins belong to a chemical family called eicosanoids, which are derived from 20 carbon essential fatty acids found in cell membranes. The precursor of eicosanoids is arachi-

donic acid. This important fatty acid is released from cell membranes in response to a variety of cell signals—physical, chemical, and hormonal. The fate of arachidonic acid depends on the local enzymatic profile. Arachidonic acid is rapidly converted either by lipoxygenase to leukotrienes or by cyclooxygenase to prostaglandins and their products.

Cyclooxygenase is now recognized to come in at least two forms. Cyclooxygenase-1 (COX-1) is constantly in low levels. It is especially prevalent in blood vessels, stomach, and kidney. Cyclooxygenase-2 (COX-2) is not present normally but is induced by a number of agents such as cytokines and growth factors. It is the induction of COX-2 that is responsible for the production of prostaglandins associated with inflammation.

Research has now focused on how the inhibition of COX-1 and COX-2 explains the various actions of acetaminophen, aspirin, and the NSAIDs. Acetaminophen is a weak inhibitor of cyclooxygenase and therefore devoid of antiinflammatory activity. Aspirin is an effective inhibitor of both COX-1 and COX-2 and therefore is effective as an antiinflammatory as well as an analgesic and antipyretic. The inhibition of COX-1 is associated with stomach damage leading to ulcers and, to a lesser extent, kidney damage. The relative specificity of the various NSAIDs for inhibiting COX-1 and COX-2 has not yet been worked out.

The current goal is the development of agents that specifically inhibit COX-2 with little or no activity against COX-1. Several COX-2 inhibitors are being tested in human trials. The first two COX-2 inhibitors to become available were celecoxib (Celebrex) and rofecoxib (Vioxx). Such drugs are especially needed for the treatment of the painful joint inflammation associated with various kinds of arthritis. Serious gastric side effects are associated with the use of many current NSAIDs for arthritis, but COX-2 inhibitors would avoid stomach and kidney damage. Treatment of precancerous intestinal polyps with COX-2 inhibitors may be an important mechanism for preventing colon cancer. High levels of COX-2 in intestinal polyps are believed to promote mutation of polyps to cancerous tissue. Finally, the progression of Alzheimer's disease may be blunted by COX-2 inhibitors. This role is suggested by recent studies on patients with Alzheimer's disease in which those receiving NSAIDs seem to have decreased progression of the disease.

Role of Prostaglandins in Pain, Fever, and Inflammation

Analgesia refers to the relief of pain. The analgesics discussed in this chapter inhibit the enzyme cyclooxygenase. This enzyme is key to the synthesis of a family of compounds called eicosanoids. Eicosanoids act as local mediators and include prostaglandin E_2 and prostaglandin F_{2alpha}, which sensitize pain receptors to mechanical and chemical stimulation. By blocking cyclooxygenase, these mediators are not produced. Therefore, objective pain, pain arising from stimulation of peripheral nerve endings, is not felt. This mechanism contrasts that of the opioids, which interfere with subjective pain at the level of the central nervous system (CNS) (see Chapter 32).

Antipyresis refers to the reduction of fever. The balance between heat production and heat dissipation is regulated by the brain. An area of the preoptic anterior hypothalamus is the thermostat of the body. Fever results from an increase in the set point of this hypothalamic center. An endogenous fever-producing agent (pyrogen) is released by white cells engulfing foreign matter (phagocytic leukocytes). This pyrogen enters the CNS and stimulates the synthesis of prostaglandin E_2. This prostaglandin is the mediator elevating the temperature set point in the hypothalamus. The cyclooxygenase inhibitors prevent the synthesis of prostaglandin E_2.

Inflammation is the result of a complex series of events triggered by such stimuli as heat, physical injury, infectious agents, ischemia, and antigen-antibody interactions. The early reaction is a local vasodilation and increased capillary permeability. This is followed by an infiltration of leukocytes and phagocytes. The final stage is a chronic proliferative phase of tissue degeneration and fibrosis. Prostaglandin E_2 plays a major role in the early phase of inflammation.

Prostaglandin production is associated with a variety of conditions characterized by pain and inflammation. These conditions include inflammatory arthritic conditions and musculoskeletal injury. How prostaglandins affect pain receptors is unknown. The actions of prostaglandin E_2 include vasodilation and increased bone resorption. Large amounts of prostaglandin E_2 have been present in the synovial fluid of affected joints in patients with rheumatoid arthritis, synthesized by cells in the mesenchymal synovial lining. Presumably this production of prostaglandin E_2 contributes to the swelling and eventual bone erosion of rheumatoid arthritis.

Dysmenorrhea (menstrual cramps) appears to be caused by the overproduction of prostaglandins by the uterus at the time of menstruation. The prostaglandins can cause the uterus to contract to the point of cramping, producing dysmenorrhea.

Inflammatory bowel disease is associated with high production of prostaglandins. Sulfasalazine and olsalazine degrade to 5-aminosalicylic acid in the colon. This compound is effective in blocking the synthesis of prostaglandins in the colon.

THERAPEUTIC AGENTS: DRUGS TO TREAT PAIN, FEVER, AND INFLAMMATION

Many of the drugs presented in this chapter are commonly available OTC for relief of pain or fever. In particular, aspirin and acetaminophen are widely used by themselves or in combination with other agents to treat specific conditions such as headaches, colds, and allergies. Some aspirin-related compounds are absorbed through the skin and available as creams and ointments for relief of muscle and joint pain.

NSAIDs were developed to treat muscle and joint pain and inflammation, especially that associated with arthritis. These were all originally prescription drugs, but in recent years low-dose forms of ibuprofen, ketoprofen, and naproxen have become available as OTC medications. These relieve common problems such as headaches, musculoskeletal pain—especially associated with strains or sprains, and dysmenorrhea. In prescription form, the NSAIDs are the mainstay of treating pain and inflammation associated with rheumatic diseases and osteoarthritis.

▼ acetaminophen

Mechanism of Action

Acetaminophen (Datril, Tylenol, Panadol, others) is believed to act principally by inhibiting prostaglandin synthesis in the CNS. The extent of its activity in the periphery is unclear. Acetaminophen has very weak antiinflammatory action.

Pharmacokinetics

Elixirs, solutions, suspensions, chewable tablets, wafers, tablets, caplets, and capsules are available. Unlike aspirin, acetaminophen can be formulated as a liquid for infants and young children. Acetaminophen is rapidly and completely absorbed from the gastrointestinal (GI) tract. Analgesia is usually apparent within 20 minutes, and peak plasma concentrations are reached in 30 to 60 minutes. The duration of action is 3 to 4 hours. Acetaminophen is metabolized in the liver to glucuronide and sulfate conjugates, which are eliminated in the urine.

Uses

Acetaminophen is a drug of choice for mild pain and fever. It is also an effective analgesic for tension-type headache, muscle and joint pain, postpartum pain, postoperative pain, and the chronic pain of cancer. Acetaminophen is often combined with codeine to provide analgesia for moderate to severe pain (Table 31-1).

The advantages of acetaminophen are that it does not interfere with blood coagulation and platelet function or irritate the stomach. In addition, acetaminophen is not associated with Reye's syndrome when administered to children or adolescents with flu or chicken pox.

Acetaminophen has minimal antiinflammatory activity and therefore is not useful for dysmenorrhea, sunburn, rheumatic diseases, or juvenile arthritis.

Adverse Reactions and Contraindications

Persons with a known glucose-6-phosphate dehydrogenase deficiency can develop hemolytic anemia if they take acetaminophen. Chronic daily ingestion of acetaminophen is reportedly associated with an increased risk of renal disease.

Toxicity

In adults, overdose of acetaminophen causes liver damage. Alcoholics are especially prone to this problem. Children rarely experience permanent liver damage from the drug, but adults who take more than 2.6 g in 24 hours may show mild symptoms of liver damage such as loss of appetite, nausea, vomiting, and slight jaundice. In deliberate overdoses of 10 g or more, adults are highly susceptible to severe liver damage; death has been reported after ingestion of 15 g. This toxicity arises because the liver normally conjugates toxic metabolites of acetaminophen with a sulfhydryl compound, glutathione, to produce an inactive, readily excreted compound. The amount of glutathione available for conjugation is exceeded when large amounts of acetaminophen are ingested. The unconjugated metabolites then bind to and destroy liver cells. Acetylcysteine is most effective if administered within 8 hours of an acetaminophen overdose. Cimetidine, which inhibits hepatic metabolism of acetaminophen, is being tested as an additional antidote for overdose.

Acetylcysteine (Mucomyst) prevents liver damage caused by excessive acetaminophen. Acetylcysteine degrades bronchial mucus in respiratory therapy (see Chapter 30). When given to counteract acetaminophen, it provides the sulfhydryl groups needed to conjugate and inactivate the toxic metabolites of acetaminophen. Treatment should begin within 12 hours after overdose. The stomach is first emptied by lavage or induced vomiting. An initial dose of 140 mg/kg is given as a 5% solution; doses of 70 mg/kg are then administered every 4 hours for approximately 17 doses. Because acetylcysteine has the pervasive flavor of rotten eggs, it must be disguised in a flavored iced drink and preferably drunk through a straw to minimize contact with the mouth.

Damage to the kidneys in the form of renal tubular necrosis has also been associated with acetaminophen overdose, especially in conjunction with liver damage.

▼ aspirin

Mechanism of Action

Aspirin (acetylsalicylic acid) is the prototype of the NSAIDs. Aspirin inhibits both forms of the enzyme cyclooxygenase, the key enzyme regulating the formation of prostaglandins. Prostaglandins are involved in inflammatory pathways and can cause pain, fever, edema, and erythema.

Pharmacokinetics

Aspirin is rapidly absorbed from the stomach and upper small intestine. Once aspirin is absorbed, 50% to 90% binds loosely to plasma albumin. Aspirin is rapidly hydrolyzed in the blood. The acetyl group of aspirin is readily transferred to the enzyme cyclooxygenase of the blood platelets.

Salicylic acid is the other product of the hydrolysis of aspirin. Salicylate (the basic salt to which salicylic acid dissociates at the pH of blood) is an analgesic-antipyretic and a reversible inhibitor of prostaglandin synthesis. Salicylate does not affect platelet aggregation, and therefore a salicylate salt is sometimes used in place of aspirin.

In acidic urine, salicylic acid is uncharged and therefore diffuses back into the blood. Vitamin C (ascorbic acid) maintains an acidic urine when taken in large doses and can therefore delay the excretion of salicylic acid. This interaction can be dangerous if large doses of aspirin are being taken, such as for arthritis. In alkaline urine, salicylic acid dissociates to salicylate, which is charged, cannot diffuse back into the blood, and is therefore eliminated in the urine. Salicylate is metabolized to inactive salicyluric acid by the liver. However, a 325-mg aspirin tablet saturates this liver inactivation system, thus the liver cannot readily metabolize large doses of aspirin.

Buffering agents are present in several aspirin brands to hasten dissolution of the tablet and to reduce gastric irritation from the tablet. The advantages of buffering agents are

Table 31-1   Nonsteroidal Antiinflammatory Drugs

Generic Name	Trade Name	Administration/Dosage	Comments
Acetaminophen			
acetaminophen	Tylenol* Datril Panadol* Liquiprin Various others	ORAL: *Adults*—325-650 mg every 4 hr. No more than 2.6 g in 24 hr. *Children 7-12 yr*—½ adult dose. *Children 3-6 yr*—⅙ adult dose. Available without prescription.	Acts as analgesic and antipyretic only. Has little antiinflammatory action and no inhibition of platelets. Contraindicated in patients with glucose-6-phosphate dehydrogenase deficiency. Nonprescription.
Aspirin and Other Salicylates and Salicylate Derivatives			
aspirin (acetylsalicylic acid)	A.S.A. Aspergum Bayer Aspirin Children's Aspirin Ecotrin*	*For analgesia or antipyresis:* ORAL, RECTAL: *Adults*—650 mg every 4 hr, or 1.3 g of timed-release form every 8 hr. *Children*—65 mg/kg over 24 hr in divided doses, every 4-6 hr.	Oral doses should be taken with large glass of water or milk to decrease stomach irritation. Some patients may need to take aspirin after a meal to avoid gastrointestinal distress. Nonprescription.
aspirin (acetylsalicylic acid), buffered	Alka-Seltzer Bufferin Various others	Same as for aspirin. There are no smaller dose tablets for children.	Alka-Seltzer contains 1.9 g sodium bicarbonate and 1 g citric acid per tablet. To avoid acid-base disturbances, limit ingestion to occasional use only. Remaining products contain magnesium and aluminum antacid salts. These salts are not absorbed systemically to any great extent. Nonprescription.
aspirin (acetyl salicylic acid)	Bayer Timed-Release Bufferin, Arthritis Strength Various others	ORAL: *Adults*—For arthritis: 2.6-5.2 g/day in divided doses (every 8 hr for timed-release forms). *For acute rheumatic fever:* Up to 7.8 g/day in divided doses. *Children*—65 mg/kg over 24 hr in divided doses every 6 hr. Available without prescription.	Dosage needed to achieve blood levels for antiinflammatory activity of 20-30 mg/dl may vary from person to person. Doses given are average ones. Children who have viral illness and are given aspirin have increased risk of developing Reye's syndrome.
choline salicylate	Arthropan	ORAL: *Adults and children >12 yr*—870 mg (1 teaspoon) every 3-4 hr, up to 6 times/day. Available without prescription.	Mint-flavored liquid formulated for patients with arthritis.
diflunisal	Dolobid*	ORAL: *Adults*—500-1000 mg/day, taken as 2 doses. Maximum dose is 1.5 g/day. Prescription drug. FDA pregnancy category C.	Long-acting salicylic acid derivative. Has lower incidence of same side effects as aspirin.
magnesium salicylate	Doan's* Magan Sero-Gesic†	Same as aspirin. No pediatric forms. Prescription drug. FDA pregnancy category C.	Contains no sodium; low incidence of gastrointestinal upset. Contraindicated in renal failure.
olsalazine	Dipentum	ORAL: *Adults and adolescents*—1 g/day divided in 2 doses.	Prophylaxis for inflammatory bowel disease for patients intolerant to sulfasalazine.
salsalate	Amigesic Disalcid*	ORAL: *Adults only*—1 g 3 times/day. Prescription drug. FDA pregnancy category C.	Dimer of salicylate. Absorption is from intestine only after hydrolysis to salicylic acid. Delayed onset compared with free salicylic acid.
sodium salicylate	Dodd's Pills† Generic	Same as aspirin. Available without prescription. Injectable form is available by prescription.	Less effective than equal dose of aspirin. May be tolerated by patients with allergic reaction to aspirin. Does not affect platelet function but does retain vitamin K antagonist effect, which can increase prothrombin time.
sulfasalazine	Azulfidine PMS-Sulfasalazine†	ORAL: *Adults*—For rheumatoid arthritis: 500 mg-1 g daily for first week, then increase by 500 mg each week up to maintenance dose of 2-3 g/day. *For inflammatory bowel disease:* 1 g every 6-8 hr; maintenance, 500 mg every 6 hr.	Primary use is for treating inflammatory bowel disease; also used for treating rheumatoid arthritis.
Propionic Acid Derivatives			
fenoprofen	Nalfon*	ORAL: *Adults*—For rheumatoid arthritis: 300-600 mg 3 or 4 times/day. *For pain or dysmenorrhea:* 200 mg every 4-6 hr.	For mild to moderate pain, dysmenorrhea, and rheumatoid arthritis.

*Available in Canada and the United States.
†Available in Canada only.

Continued

Table 31-1   Nonsteroidal Antiinflammatory Drugs—cont'd

Generic Name	Trade Name	Administration/Dosage	Comments
Propionic Acid Derivatives—cont'd			
floctafenine	Idarac†	ORAL: *Adults*—200-400 mg every 6-8 hr.	For mild to moderate pain and inflammation.
flurbiprofen	Ansaid* Froben†	ORAL: *Adults*—*For arthritis:* 100-200 mg daily in 3 or 4 divided doses. *For dysmenorrhea:* 50 mg 4 times/day. FDA pregnancy category B.	For arthritis or dysmenorrhea.
ibuprofen	Advil Motrin* Nuprin Various others	ORAL: *Adults*—*For mild pain, fever, or dysmenorrhea:* 200-400 mg every 4-6 hr. *For antiinflammatory response:* 1.2-3.2 g/day in 3 or 4 divided doses.	Nonprescription for mild pain, fever, or dysmenorrhea. Higher dosages available in prescription form for arthritis.
ketoprofen	Orudis*	ORAL: *Adults*—150-300 mg/day divided into 3 or 4 doses. Available in capsules, delayed-release capsules, and suppositories. FDA pregnancy category B.	For rheumatoid arthritis and dysmenorrhea.
naproxen	Anaprox* Naprosyn* Various others	ORAL: *Adults*—*For rheumatoid arthritis:* 250-750 mg 2 times/day. *For mild to moderate pain, including dysmenorrhea:* 500 mg initially, then 250 mg every 6-8 hr. *For acute gout:* 750 mg initially, then 250 mg every 8 hr. FDA pregnancy category B.	For dysmenorrhea, mild to moderate pain, acute gout, and rheumatoid arthritis.
oxaprozin	Daypro	ORAL: *Adults*—1200 mg/day initially, then adjust according to patient tolerance and response. FDA pregnancy category C.	For rheumatoid arthritis and osteoarthritis. Patients with renal impairment should be started at half dose.
tiaprofenic acid	Surgam†	ORAL: *Adults*—600 mg/day divided into 2 or 3 doses.	For rheumatoid arthritis and osteoarthritis.
Other Nonsteroidal Antiinflammatory Drugs (NSAIDs)			
diclofenac	Novo-Difenac† Voltaren* Various others	ORAL: *Adults*—150-200 mg/day divided into 2-4 doses. Also available in extended-release form for once-daily administration. Available in Canada in suppository form. FDA pregnancy category B.	For rheumatoid arthritis, osteoarthritis, and ankylosing spondylitis.
etodolac	Lodine	ORAL: *Adults*—*For osteoarthritis:* 800-1200 mg/day. *For pain:* 400 mg, then 200-400 mg every 6-8 hr as needed. Daily dose should not exceed 20 mg/kg of body weight or 1200 mg, whichever is less. FDA pregnancy category C.	For pain and osteoarthritis.
indomethacin	Apo-Indomethacin† Indocid† Indocin Novomethacin†	ORAL: *Adults*—25 mg 2-3 times/day. If necessary, total daily dose can be increased by 25-50 mg/day at weekly intervals, but total daily dose should not exceed 200 mg. *Children*—1.5-2.5 mg/kg body weight/day, divided into 3 or 4 doses. Maximum dose is 4 mg/kg of body weight/day or 200 mg/day, whichever is less. *Premature infants*—0.3-0.6 mg/kg/24 hr to close ductus arteriosus. Available in capsules, extended-release capsules, oral suspension, and suppositories.	Administer with meals or with antacids to minimize gastric irritation. For acute inflammatory episodes. Also given to premature infants to close ductus arteriosus.
ketorolac tromethamine	Toradol	ORAL: *Adults*—10 mg every 4-6 hr, up to maximum of 40 mg/day. INTRAMUSCULAR: *Adults*—60 mg initially, followed by 30 mg every 6 hr. Maximum, 120 mg daily.	NSAID with analgesia equivalent to morphine. Useful for outpatient surgery.
meclofenamate	Meclomen	ORAL: *Adults*—200 mg/day divided into 3 or 4 doses. May be increased up to 400 mg/day if necessary.	For rheumatoid arthritis. Not available in Canada.
mefenamic acid	Ponstel Ponstan†	ORAL: *Adults*—500 mg initially, then 250 mg every 6 hr as needed. FDA pregnancy category C.	For mild to moderate pain. Administer after meals to avoid gastric irritation.
nabumetone	Relafen	ORAL: *Adults*—Initially 1000 mg/day, taken as single dose. May increase dose to 1500 or 2000 mg, taken as single dose or in 2 divided doses. FDA pregnancy category C.	For rheumatoid arthritis and osteoarthritis.

*Available in Canada and the United States.
†Available in Canada only.

Table 31-1   Nonsteroidal Antiinflammatory Drugs—cont'd

Generic Name	Trade Name	Administration/Dosage	Comments
Other Nonsteroidal Antiinflammatory Drugs (NSAIDs)—cont'd			
phenylbutazone	Butazolidin* Butazone Novobutazone Various others	ORAL: *Adults*—Initially, 300-600 mg/day divided into 3 or 4 doses. Maintenance dose is 100 mg 1-4 times/day. *For acute gout:* 400 mg initially, then 100 mg every 4 hr for 4 days or a maximum of 1 wk. Available in capsules, tablets, and delayed-release and buffered tablets. FDA pregnancy category C.	For rheumatoid arthritis and acute attacks of other arthritic conditions, including gout. Administer after meals to avoid gastric irritation.
piroxicam	Apo-Piroxicam† Feldene* Novopirocam†	ORAL: *Adults*—20 mg once a day or 10 mg twice a day.	For rheumatoid arthritis and osteoarthritis. Administer after meals to avoid gastric irritation.
sulindac	Apo-Sulin† Clinoril* Novo-Sundae†	ORAL: *Adults*—150-200 mg twice daily, not to exceed 400 mg/day.	For rheumatoid arthritis, acute gout, and bursitis.
tenoxicam	Mobiflex†	ORAL: *Adults*—20 mg once daily.	For rheumatoid arthritis, acute gout, and bursitis.
tolmetin	Tolectin*	ORAL: *Adults*—Initially, 400 mg every 8 hr, then 600-1800 mg/day, divided into 3 or 4 doses. FDA pregnancy category C.	For rheumatoid arthritis, osteoarthritis, ankylosing spondylitis, juvenile arthritis, and psoriatic arthritis.

*Available in Canada and the United States.
†Available in Canada only.

minimal, and if several doses are taken, the buffering agents may cause loose stools. Alka-Seltzer contains so much sodium and bicarbonate that it should be used only on a short-term basis.

Uses

Small doses of aspirin (325 to 650 mg or 1 to 2 adult tablets) reduce fever and relieve mild pain. Two aspirin tablets are the analgesic equivalent of 60 mg of codeine. Aspirin is an effective analgesic for most common mild to moderate headaches and generalized mild muscular aches. Aspirin or aspirin-codeine combinations also treat mild-to-moderate pain of tooth extractions, episiotomies, cancer, and bone fractures. A dosage of 1.2 g/day of aspirin produces the maximum analgesic effect. At much higher dosages (3 to 6 g/day), aspirin treats the inflammation of rheumatoid arthritis. At this concentration, aspirin is the prototype for the NSAIDs (see Table 31-1).

Because aspirin inhibits platelet aggregation, it is also widely taken as a prophylactic agent to prevent myocardial infarction (MI), stroke, and other thromboembolic conditions. A unique property of aspirin is that it irreversibly acetylates cyclooxygenase of blood platelets, an effect that persists for the 3- to 7-day lifetime of the platelet. Acetylated cyclooxygenase is inactive, and synthesis of the prostaglandin thromboxane A_2 is therefore blocked. Thromboxane A_2, a potent agent promoting platelet aggregation, is normally synthesized by platelets as they begin to aggregate. Even one aspirin tablet inhibits blood clotting by inhibiting platelet aggregation.

Aspirin administered at high dosages is often the initial treatment to control the symptoms of inflammatory arthri-

tis. Dosages of 2.6 to 7.8 g/day are required to produce the plasma concentrations of 20 to 30 mg/dl needed for an effective antiinflammatory response. These dosages are associated with considerable gastric irritation with or without bleeding, salicylism, decreased platelet aggregation, and interactions with other drugs. Aspirin must be taken continuously for at least 2 weeks before an improvement may be noted. Timed-release or enteric-coated formulations may improve patient compliance by decreasing the number of times aspirin must be taken each day and by bypassing the stomach, thereby reducing gastric irritation (see Table 31-1).

Adverse Reactions and Contraindications

Approximately 2% to 10% of those taking an occasional aspirin tablet experience GI upset. This effect may be felt as heartburn or nausea. Aluminum and calcium-urea salts of aspirin have been formulated to be less irritating to the stomach than aspirin. When aspirin is taken regularly in large doses for arthritis, this incidence becomes 30% to 50% and may be the factor limiting the use of aspirin. Sometimes antacids are prescribed to minimize stomach irritation, but antacids also raise the pH of the urine and increase the rate of excretion of salicylic acid. Alternatively, enteric-coated or timed-release preparations may be tried to decrease gastric irritation.

Aspirin is directly irritating and damaging to gastric mucosal cells. This is now believed to be a result of the inhibition of COX-1 with the result that protective prostaglandins are not synthesized. Because alcohol also has gastric effects, aspirin should not be taken when alcohol is in the stomach. The combination of alcohol and aspirin is greater than additive in producing gastric bleeding. Patients with active peptic ulcers should be advised not to use aspirin.

Long-term aspirin ingestion can cause the loss of 10 to 30 ml of blood daily from GI irritation. This loss may lead to iron deficiency anemia in women with heavy menses. Rarely, massive GI bleeding occurs in patients who take aspirin on a long-term basis.

Some people develop an allergy to aspirin. The most common form of aspirin intolerance is manifested as a rash. Patients with a skin rash caused by aspirin may tolerate other salicylates. A few people develop nasal polyps and sometimes later develop an asthma that is triggered by aspirin.

Patients sensitive to aspirin may be sensitive to a variety of other compounds. Most commonly, individuals sensitive to aspirin may show cross-sensitivity to salicylin-containing foods (e.g., apples, oranges, bananas), processed foods or drugs containing tartrazine dye or sodium benzoate, iodide-containing substances, various other NSAIDs, or tartrazine (see Patient Problems box on tartrazine allergy). As can be seen from these items, the origin of these cross-sensitivities is not always the classic cross-reactivity caused by structural similarities of the agents.

Aspirin is contraindicated to treat children and teenagers who have an acute febrile illness such as flu or chicken pox because aspirin puts them at increased risk for contracting **Reye's syndrome.** Reye's syndrome is rare but serious. It is characterized by vomiting and rapidly progressive encephalopathy. Acetaminophen and other NSAIDs have not been so implicated. Nonprescription aspirin products now contain a warning against administration to children and teenagers who manifest chicken pox or flu symptoms.

Toxicity

Mild intoxication with aspirin is called **salicylism** and is commonly experienced when the daily dosage is more than 4 g. Tinnitus (ringing in the ears) is the most common effect and may be accompanied by a degree of reversible hearing loss. Because salicylate stimulates the respiratory center, hyperventilation (rapid breathing) may occur. Fever may result because salicylate interferes with the metabolic pathways coupling oxygen consumption and heat production.

The plasma levels of salicylate reflect the level of toxicity (see Patient Problems box on aspirin toxicity). Acute overdose of aspirin causes serious disturbances in the body's acid-base balance. A child is more likely than an adult to die from a large overdose of aspirin. Fatalities among children have been dramatically reduced since 1970, when the Poison Prevention Packaging Act required that orange-flavored baby aspirin (81-mg tablets) be limited to 36 tablets per bottle and that safety caps be used. If a child has ingested more than 150 mg/kg (36 baby tablets [one bottle] or 9 adult tablets for a 45-lb child), vomiting may be induced, or gastric lavage may be used to eliminate undissolved tablets. Because charcoal absorbs about half its weight in aspirin, it is given orally to reduce absorption of aspirin.

PATIENT PROBLEMS

Tartrazine Allergy

THE PROBLEM
Tartrazine (FD&C yellow dye #5) is used by many drug companies in manufacturing their drugs. Ingestion of this dye may cause an allergic reaction in susceptible individuals. This rare reaction is seen more often in persons with aspirin hypersensitivity. Example drugs containing tartrazine include Pronestyl procainamide film-coated tablets, Choloxin 2-mg dextrothyroxine tablets, and Nicolar 500-mg niacin tablets.

SOLUTIONS
- Instruct patients with a known allergy to tartrazine to wear a medical identification tag or bracelet.
- Assess patients with an allergy to aspirin for associated allergy to tartrazine before giving medications that contain tartrazine.
- Instruct patients to warn the pharmacist of tartrazine allergy before prescriptions are filled so that tartrazine-containing products can be avoided. Instruct patients with this allergy not to switch brands of a drug without consulting the pharmacist to avoid accidental exposure to tartrazine.

Tartrazine is known to be associated with allergic reactions, but many other dyes, fillers, and preservatives are used in the manufacture of drugs. Patients who experience an unusual reaction to a drug may be manifesting an allergic response to an ingredient used in its manufacture. Read ingredient labels carefully. Take a thorough drug history. Consult the pharmacist.

PATIENT PROBLEMS

Aspirin Toxicity

TOXIC SALICYLATE PLASMA CONCENTRATIONS

Mild	45-65 mg/dl
Moderate	65-90 mg/dl
Severe	90 mg/dl
Usually fatal	>120 mg/dl

TREATMENT STEPS
1. Undissolved tablets are removed through induced vomiting or absorption with charcoal.
2. Plasma salicylate, acid-base, glucose, sodium, and potassium concentrations are determined every 4 to 5 hours.
3. Hyperthermia is treated with sponge baths, and dehydration is treated with fluid replacement.
4. Fluids are administered as required to treat electrolyte imbalances and acidosis.
5. If salicylate concentration is dangerously high or does not fall with supportive treatment, dialysis or exchange transfusions may be used.

Children, particularly those younger than 4 years of age, can rapidly develop metabolic acidosis. This condition may result because of the acidic nature of aspirin and its metabolites and because salicylate inhibits metabolism in a manner that favors the accumulation of organic acids, which would normally have been metabolized to carbon dioxide and water. The hyperthermia that is also produced with this metabolic block must be treated with sponge baths. Profuse sweating can produce dehydration. The supportive treatment of aspirin toxicity therefore consists of careful monitoring of the acid-base and electrolyte levels and appropriate fluid administration. Intravenous (IV) sodium bicarbonate can counter the tendency toward metabolic acidosis and produce an alkaline urine that hastens the excretion of salicylate. Osmotic diuretics or dialysis may be necessary in extreme cases to remove salicylate. Salicylate is a weak vitamin K antagonist and in large doses acts like an oral anticoagulant. A day or two after massive aspirin ingestion, increased bleeding tendency and signs of minor hemorrhaging may be noted.

Interactions

The drug interactions characteristic of aspirin are especially important because of its widespread and uncritical use. Drug interactions arise because aspirin enhances the potential for GI bleeding and ulcers with glucocorticoids, alcohol, and phenylbutazone. Aspirin can displace oral anticoagulants, oral hypoglycemic drugs, phenytoin, and methotrexate. Because the unbound drug is the effective concentration, free drug may reach toxic levels when displaced by aspirin. Aspirin also antagonizes the uricosuric effect of probenecid and sulfinpyrazone.

Other Salicylates and Salicylate Derivatives

diflunisal

Diflunisal (Dolobid) is a fluoridated derivative of salicylic acid with a long duration of action. It is not converted to salicylic acid. Because it does not penetrate the CNS, it does not lower a fever. A prescription drug, it relieves the symptoms of rheumatoid arthritis and osteoarthritis. Diflunisal does not cause tinnitus and has a lesser incidence of GI and antiplatelet side effects than aspirin.

olsalazine

Olsalazine (Dipentum) is an alternative to sulfasalazine in patients with ulcerative colitis. It is cleaved in the colon to two molecules of 5-aminosalicylate. Olsalazine does not have the sulfa component that causes intolerance in some patients. Currently, olsalazine is only indicated as prophylactic therapy for patients in remission from ulcerative colitis who do not tolerate sulfasalazine.

methyl salicylate

Methyl salicylate (oil of wintergreen) is used only topically. It causes vasodilation in the applied areas and thereby creates a warmth that relieves muscle or joint stiffness.

salsalate

Salsalate (Disalcid) is a dimer of salicylic acid. It is slowly hydrolyzed to two molecules of salicylic acid in the small intestine and absorbed into the bloodstream. It is less likely to cause gastric bleeding. Salicylic acid does not have a significant effect on platelet aggregation. Salsalate is used primarily to treat rheumatic diseases.

salicylamide

Salicylamide is a chemically modified form of salicylate and is not hydrolyzed to salicylic acid. It is used only in combination with other drugs.

salicylate salts

Sodium salicylate, magnesium salicylate, and choline salicylate are all salicylate salts that produce less GI upset than aspirin. They do not alter platelet function as does aspirin. Salicylates bind to plasma albumin and displace other drugs, particularly the oral anticoagulants.

Salicylate salts are available OTC. Sodium salicylate is marketed as an analgesic and antipyretic. Magnesium and choline salicylates are also marketed for the relief of muscle aches. Prescription strengths are used to treat rheumatic diseases.

sulfasalazine

Sulfasalazine (Azulfidine, PMS-Sulfasalazine, others) is degraded to its active component, 5-aminosalicylate, in the colon, where it blocks the conversion of arachidonic acid to eicosanoids by both cyclooxygenase and lipoxygenase pathways. The major use of sulfasalazine is in the treatment of inflammatory bowel disease. Sulfasalazine is also used occasionally for the treatment of rheumatic diseases. The active principal for rheumatic diseases may be the sulfapyridine component, which has suppressive effects on lymphocytes.

Nonsteroidal Antiinflammatory Drugs

Mechanism of Action

The primary mechanism of action of the NSAIDs is the inhibition of the enzyme cyclooxygenase so that prostaglandins are not formed.

Recent studies have clarified other mechanisms of the NSAIDs that contribute to their action. These include inhibition of various other enzymes, inhibition of transmembrane ion fluxes, and inhibition of the chemoattractant binding that affects the inflammatory process.

Pharmacokinetics

NSAIDs are generally well absorbed after oral administration and are effective for the relief of pain in 30 to 60 minutes. When used to treat arthritis, significant relief of other inflammatory symptoms may take several days. The duration of action depends on the NSAID, generally from 4 to 12 hours. Metabolism by the liver is the common route of degradation, with elimination of metabolites in the urine.

Uses

NSAIDs are widely used as first-line therapy for inflammatory types of arthritis, including rheumatoid arthritis, ankylosing spondylitis, and juvenile arthritis. Osteoarthritis is not characterized by a high level of inflammation, and lower analgesic dosages of NSAIDs can be used to treat pain associated with osteoarthritis. NSAIDs are also useful in treating pain and inflammation in athletic injuries, bursitis, synovitis, and other soft tissue injuries involving strains and sprains.

NSAIDs are effective analgesics for mild to moderate pain from a variety of conditions, including dental, obstetric, or orthopedic surgery.

NSAIDs are effective in averting menstrual cramps, particularly if therapy is begun a few days before the start of menses.

Ibuprofen and naproxen are used to reduce a fever.

Adverse Reactions and Contraindications

The major side effect of the NSAIDs is gastric irritation leading to an increase in peptic ulcers. Prostaglandins protect the gastric mucosa by inhibiting gastric acid secretion. GI irritation commonly caused by aspirin and other NSAIDs may arise because this protection is absent when these drugs, which inhibit prostaglandin synthesis, are present in the stomach. These effects can be minimized by taking the drugs with meals. All prescription NSAIDs now carry a warning to reflect concern about the GI side effects seen with their long-term use.

Misoprostol (Cytotec) controls gastric irritation associated with aspirin and other NSAIDs. Misoprostol, an analog of prostaglandin E$_1$, is protective by inhibiting excessive gastric acid secretion. Thus it replaces the prostaglandin that is suppressed by the NSAIDs (see Chapter 26 and Table 26-2).

Inhibition of platelet aggregation is another common side effect of the NSAIDs. Although this effect is irreversible with aspirin, it is reversible with the other NSAIDs. The inhibition of prostaglandin synthesis is responsible also for the platelet phenomenon.

Patients who develop a rash or other allergic reactions to one of the NSAIDs may be intolerant of the others. This is especially true of patients who have experienced bronchospasm that results from aspirin ingestion or who are sensitive to aspirin because they have asthma.

Older adult patients are more likely to develop GI distress, liver toxicity, or renal damage while taking NSAIDs and should be carefully monitored. In addition, patients with clinical conditions such as congestive heart failure, cirrhosis, and renal insufficiency are at risk for impaired renal function when taking NSAIDs. These patients require the local synthesis of vasodilating prostaglandins to maintain renal perfusion. NSAIDs, by inhibiting these prostaglandins, can allow unopposed vasoconstriction. This renal ischemia can lead to a deterioration of renal function.

Interactions

In general, the NSAIDs are bound to protein and displace other drugs, particularly hydantoins, sulfonamides, sulfonylureas, and calcium channel blockers, leading to exacerba-

tion of side effects because of these drugs. NSAIDs may increase the risk of renal damage if acetaminophen is used concurrently over long periods. The risk of GI complications, especially ulceration or hemorrhage, is increased if NSAIDs are taken concurrently with alcohol, anticoagulants, thrombolytics, or glucocorticoids. NSAIDs may diminish the effectiveness of diuretics and intensify the risk of renal failure. They potentiate drugs that inhibit platelet aggregation. NSAIDs should be discontinued when a gold compound or methotrexate is administered to treat rheumatoid arthritis because of their potential for renal damage.

Propionic Acid Derivatives

About half the NSAIDs are propionic acid derivatives. These include fenoprofen (Nalfon), floctafenine (Idarac), flurbiprofen (Ansaid), ibuprofen (Advil, Medipren, Motrin, Nuprin, others), ketoprofen (Orudis), naproxen (Anaprox, Naprosyn), oxaprozin (Daypro), and tiaprofenic acid (Surgam). They provide good analgesic and antiinflammatory action. They often treat dysmenorrhea, rheumatoid arthritis, osteoarthritis, and gout (see Table 31-1).

fenoprofen

Fenoprofen (Nalfon) is used for treating various forms of arthritis, including rheumatoid arthritis, osteoarthritis, ankylosing spondylitis, and psoriatic arthritis. It is also used to treat the pain of gout and to relieve vascular headaches and dysmenorrhea. It is taken orally every 6 to 8 hours.

floctafenine

Floctafenine (Idarac) is primarily used as an analgesic. It is taken orally every 6 to 8 hours. It is available in Canada but not in the United States.

flurbiprofen

Flurbiprofen (Ansaid) is used to treat rheumatoid arthritis, osteoarthritis, ankylosing spondylitis, musculoskeletal disorders, and dysmenorrhea. It is taken orally every 6 to 12 hours. An extended-release form is available for once-a-day dosage. Flurbiprofen has also been formulated as a solution for ophthalmic use.

▼ ibuprofen

Ibuprofen (Advil, Motrin, many others) is available OTC. It is rapidly absorbed and has a plasma half-life of 2 hours. It is generally well tolerated. GI irritation and bleeding occur less often than with aspirin and may be decreased by taking the drug with meals. In addition to its use as an analgesic and antipyretic, ibuprofen is effective in treating dysmenorrhea. In prescription strength, it is used to treat rheumatoid arthritis, osteoarthritis, juvenile arthritis, psoriatic arthritis, and gouty arthritis. It is also used to treat and prevent vascular headaches.

ketoprofen

Ketoprofen (Actron, Orudis KT) is available OTC in the United States as an analgesic, especially for headaches and dysmenorrhea. In prescription strength, it is used to treat rheumatoid arthritis, osteoarthritis, juvenile arthritis, psoriatic arthritis, and gouty arthritis. It is taken every 4 to 6 hours. Extended-release forms are available for once-a-day dosage. Patient with impaired renal function and the elderly have a longer half-life for the drug and may require a lower dosage.

naproxen

Naproxen (Aleve) is available OTC as an analgesic, especially for musculoskeletal pain, headaches, and dysmenorrhea. It is longer acting than aspirin or ibuprofen and can be taken twice a day. Naproxen is well tolerated. In prescription strength, it is used to treat rheumatoid arthritis, osteoarthritis, juvenile arthritis, psoriatic arthritis, and gouty arthritis. Elderly persons and those with impaired renal or hepatic function should receive lower dosages.

oxaprozin and tiaprofenic acid

Oxaprozin (Daypro) and tiaprofenic acid (Surgam) are long acting and require only once-a-day dosage. They are used for treating rheumatoid arthritis and osteoarthritis. Oxaprozin is a potent inhibitor of platelet aggregation and should be discontinued 1 to 2 weeks before elective surgery.

Oxaprozin is available in the United States but not in Canada. Tiaprofenic acid is available in Canada but not in the United States.

Other Nonsteroidal Antiinflammatory Drugs

diclofenac

Diclofenac (Voltaren) treats rheumatoid arthritis, osteoarthritis, and ankylosing spondylitis. An extended-release form is available for once-a-day dosage. The immediate release form must be taken in three or four daily doses. This formulation is used for analgesia and dysmenorrhea.

etodolac

Etodolac (Lodine) treats osteoarthritis and pain. It may also be used to treat acute gouty attacks, dysmenorrhea, vascular headaches, and musculoskeletal conditions. Etodolac is administered two to four times daily.

indomethacin

Indomethacin (Indocin, Indocid, others) is prescribed for its analgesic and antiinflammatory actions. It is administered two to four times daily. A suppository formulation is available. An extended-release form is also available for once-a-day dosage. GI disturbances such as nausea, vomiting, loss of appetite, indigestion, and diarrhea are common but can be reduced by taking the drug after meals. Occasionally, indomethacin can cause ulceration along the GI tract that may become serious if bleeding or perforation results.

Headaches and dizziness are the most common side effects. These can often be minimized if the dosage is lowered and then increased gradually. Other CNS disturbances that can limit the use of indomethacin include confusion, light-headedness, fainting, or drowsiness.

ketorolac tromethamine

Ketorolac tromethamine (Toradol) is a new NSAID, equivalent in potency to morphine. It is given by intramuscular (IM) injection for the short-term management of moderate to severe pain, particularly in postoperative patients. The lack of mental effects is especially beneficial in outpatient surgery.

meclofenamate and mefenamic acid

Meclofenamate (Meclomen) and mefenamic acid (Ponstel, Ponstan) are fenamate derivatives. Mefenamic acid is prescribed for mild to moderate pain. However, therapy with this drug is limited to 1 week because of the common occurrence of toxicity associated with the GI, kidney, and blood-forming systems. Side effects may include GI upset, diarrhea, and rash.

Meclofenamate is prescribed for rheumatoid arthritis and osteoarthritis. Side effects are similar to those of mefenamic acid.

nabumetone

Nabumetone (Relafen) treats rheumatoid arthritis and osteoarthritis. This is a prodrug that undergoes hepatic biotransformation to the active substance. It requires only once-a-day dosage, although larger doses may be divided.

phenylbutazone

Phenylbutazone (Azolid, Butazolidin, Butazone) is a potent antiinflammatory drug with a long plasma half-life of 2 to 3 days. It binds strongly to plasma albumin and can displace other bound drugs, particularly oral anticoagulant and oral hypoglycemic drugs. Phenylbutazone causes fluid retention and gastric irritation and prolongs platelet function, thereby inhibiting blood clotting. Occasionally, phenylbutazone causes liver damage or bone marrow suppression. Because of these problems, it is commonly prescribed for only 1 to 2 weeks to treat an acute inflammatory response.

piroxicam and tenoxicam

Piroxicam (Feldene) is well absorbed and has a long half-life of 45 hours, making once-a-day dosing adequate. Piroxicam is rapidly excreted in the urine as a glucuronide. Piroxicam is prescribed principally for rheumatoid arthritis and osteoarthritis.

Tenoxicam (Mobiflex) is derived from the same chemical family as piroxicam. Tenoxicam is available in Canada but not in the United States for treatment of rheumatoid arthritis, osteoarthritis, ankylosing spondylitis, bursitis, and tendinitis.

sulindac and tolmetin

Sulindac (Clinoril) and tolmetin (Tolectin) are chemically related to indomethacin. In general, their side effects are similar to those of aspirin, although the incidence is less than with aspirin. Sulindac has a plasma half-life of 8 hours and can be taken less often than indomethacin or tolmetin. It is a prodrug, activated after conversion by the liver. The active drug is excreted in the bile and reabsorbed from the intestine. Tolmetin induces fewer side effects in the CNS than does indomethacin. Tolmetin is absorbed rapidly and has a plasma half-life of only 1 hour.

Novel Therapies for Osteoarthritis

Hyaluronate Injections into the Knee

Synovial fluid surrounding a joint contains hyaluronate, a material that acts as a lubricant and shock absorber. In osteoarthritis of the knee, the synovial fluid may be deficient in hyaluronate. New agents have been developed to replace the synovial fluid of the osteoarthritic knee. This therapy is reserved for patients experiencing pain that is not relieved by analgesics.

Hylan G-F 20 (Synvisc) is an injectable elastic and viscous mixture of hylan polymers that is injected into the synovial fluid of the knee. The rationale is that the excess synovial fluid is first removed and then three doses are administered over 15 days. Side effects of mild local pain and swelling are rare. The therapeutic effect is pain relief that persists for several months.

Sodium hyaluronate (Hyalgan) is a solution of hyaluronate, which has elastic and viscous properties. Five injections into the knee are administered a week apart. Many patients experience pain relief for 6 months or longer.

ALTERNATIVE THERAPIES

Relief of Arthritis Pain

GLUCOSAMINE SULFATE AND CHONDROITIN SULFATE
Glucosamine is an amino sugar found in the body. Amino sugars are structural components in complex macromolecules that provide structure to tissues. Chondroitin sulfate is composed of repeating units of glucosamine with attached sugar molecules.

The use of glucosamine sulfate alone or in combination with chondroitin sulfate has become popular as a natural remedy providing symptomatic relief from the pain of arthritis, particularly osteoarthritis. The rationale is that these agents represent the components that the body uses to build new cartilage. Glucosamine is reported to retard the degradation of cartilage by inhibiting proteolytic enzymes and by stimulating the synthesis of new carridge.

There have been small clinical studies on the use of glucosamine in the treatment of osteoarthritis. Short-term benefits have been reported in symptomatic relief of pain and joint mobility. However, these have not been well-designed studies, nor have they evaluated long-term benefits or examined the course of the underlying cartilage degradation.

Glucosamine sulfate and chondroitin sulfate are available without prescription as nutritional supplements through health food stores and mail order distributors.

Nursing Process Overview

Analgesic-Antipyretic Drugs and Nonsteroidal Antiinflammatory Drugs

Assessment

Fever is not a disease; it is a symptom. Monitor temperature and other vital signs; note the presence of diaphoresis, chills, or seizures; and assess the level of consciousness and the fluid intake and output. Assess the patient for possible causes of fever, such as pulmonary infections, wound infection, and urinary tract infection. With NSAIDs, assess temperature, pulse, respiration, blood pressure, blood counts, and other laboratory data relevant to the possible or probable diagnosis. Perform a brief neurologic examination. Assess the patient's ability to perform activities of daily living to assist in planning for discharge.

Nursing Diagnoses

- Risk for impaired home maintenance management related to knowledge deficit of safe use of antipyretic agents
- Risk for GI distress or bleeding (with NSAIDs)
- Potential complication: hematologic disorders

Patient Outcomes

The patient will self-medicate appropriately with antipyretics and will not experience drug side effects. The patient will not experience GI distress or bleeding. The nurse will minimize and manage complications of hematologic disorders.

Planning/Implementation

The treatment of fever is twofold: to reduce the fever and to determine its cause. Administer antipyretics when the temperature exceeds the ordered upper limit or every 4 hours around the clock, as ordered. Monitor the patient's temperature every 4 hours, ensure adequate fluid intake, monitor fluid intake and output, and monitor blood counts and other vital signs. Maintain patient comfort. Use additional measures such as cool water baths and hypothermia mattresses if needed. If aspirin is used, monitor the patient for bruising or bleeding.

With NSAIDs, develop a plan with the patient to reach the goals of drug therapy. Reinforce the importance of other therapies, including other medications, heat or cold application, immobilization, special exercises, and restricted activity. Monitor vital signs and subjective and objective data related to the specific problem and the laboratory data appropriate to the problem and the drug therapy.

Evaluation

Ensure that the patient can explain why and how to take the prescribed drugs, what other therapies are being used to treat the problem, and which other drugs should be avoided while receiving therapy. Verify that patients know that alcohol should be avoided, what reasonable expectations of drug therapy are (e.g., will joint pain disappear or only diminish, will fever lessen), and what the possible side effects are and what to do if they occur. Finally, verify that the patient knows when to return for follow-up or assistance.

THERAPEUTIC RATIONALE: GOUT

Gout is a metabolic disease in which total body pools of uric acid (a product of DNA and RNA degradation) are elevated. The uric acid crystallizes in joints or, less commonly, in tendons or bursae. The joint at the base of the big toe is most commonly affected. During an attack of acute gouty arthritis there is a marked inflammation of the joint accompanied by significant pain. This acute attack is treated with the drug colchicine, which relieves the pain, with indomethacin or another of the NSAIDs already discussed, or with intraarticular injections of corticosteroids (see Chapter 41).

Some patients develop a tophus in a joint (crystals of uric acid with fibrous tissue surrounding them). Patients with tophi or recurrent attacks of gouty arthritis must receive long-term treatment, often for the rest of their lives, with drugs that will reduce uric acid levels in the body. With drug therapy, tophi, if present, often regress with long-term therapy, restoring the joint to a normal range of function. About 25% of such patients overproduce uric acid. These patients are treated with the drug allopurinol, which prevents the formation of uric acid from xanthine and hypoxanthine, the purine metabolites of DNA and RNA metabolism. Other patients are treated with a uricosuric drug, probenecid, or sulfinpyrazone. These drugs increase the renal excretion of uric acid by inhibiting its reabsorption from the proximal kidney tubule.

THERAPEUTIC AGENTS: DRUGS TO TREAT GOUT

Gout is a type of arthritis caused by a specific metabolic disorder leading to elevated concentrations of uric acid in the body. Patients with gout are advised to limit the intake of foods containing purine, a precursor of uric acid (see Dietary Considerations box). If gout is diagnosed early and therapy begun promptly, the disease can be arrested and complications of the disease prevented. Drugs used to treat gout are listed in Table 31-2.

allopurinol

Allopurinol (Zyloprim) inhibits the formation of uric acid from xanthine or hypoxanthine, so xanthine or hypoxanthine is excreted instead. A patient whose morning urine has a ratio of uric acid to creatinine greater than 0.75 or whose 24-hour urine contains more than 600 mg of uric acid is classified as an overproducer of uric acid. These overpro-

ducers and patients with renal uric acid crystals or impaired renal function are those for whom allopurinol will be most effective. It is also effective for patients with gout resulting from drug therapy that increases uric acid production, particularly cancer therapy. Side effects are rare; they appear to be allergic reactions. There are some drug interactions. Allopurinol inhibits the degradation of azathioprine, 6-mercaptopurine, antipyrine, coumarins, and cyclophosphamide, leading to higher plasma concentrations and potentially toxic concentrations of these drugs.

▼ colchicine

Mechanism of Action

Colchicine inhibits the phagocytosis of urate crystals by neutrophils and interferes with the inflammatory response.

Pharmacokinetics

Colchicine is administered orally, first with a dose of 1 mg and followed by a dose of 0.5 mg every 2 hours until a total dose of 8 mg has been administered or until abdominal distress and diarrhea have developed. It may also be given intravenously, but there is a much higher risk of toxic side effects. Because it causes severe tissue inflammation, it is diluted before IV administration to minimize the effect of any drug leakage. Elimination is primarily through the bile.

Uses

Colchicine provides relief from the pain of an acute attack of gouty arthritis, usually within 24 hours. The earlier in an episode colchicine is taken, the more effective it is. (Similarly, antiinflammatory drugs are more effective if taken early in an acute episode.)

Colchicine may be continued at reduced dosages once the acute episode is over. Continuance of colchicine is most common if a drug to reduce uric acid is begun. A sudden

DIETARY CONSIDERATIONS

Purine

Uric acid is produced when purine is catabolized. Gout is a problem of elevated uric acid. Formerly, a mainstay of gout therapy was purine restriction in the diet. With better drug therapy, purine restriction is a less significant component of therapy. Patients should probably modify their diets to limit excessive purine intake, unless more severe restriction is indicated on an individual basis. High purine foods to avoid or limit include the following:

- Organ meats
- Roe
- Sardines
- Scallops
- Anchovies
- Broth and consomme

- Mincemeat
- Herring
- Shrimp
- Mackerel
- Gravy
- Yeast

Table 31-2 Drugs to Treat Gout

Generic Name	Trade Name	Administration/Dosage	Comments
allopurinol	Lopurin Zyloprim*	ORAL: *Adults*—200-300 mg/day as single dose; maximum, 800 mg/day. Dose is reduced if there is renal insufficiency. FDA pregnancy category C.	Inhibits formation of uric acid from hypoxanthine or xanthine; these are excreted instead.
colchicine	Generic	ORAL: *Adults*—0.5-0.6 mg hourly or 1-1.2 mg initially and 0.5-0.6 mg every 2 hr. This regimen is for acute gouty attack and is continued until pain subsides or gastrointestinal symptoms appear. Maximum dose, 7-8 mg. *For prophylaxis:* 0.5-1 mg/day.	Terminates acute gouty attack. Appearance of gastrointestinal distress usually limits amount given.
		INTRAVENOUS: *For acute attack:* 1-2 mg initially, then 0.5 mg every 3-6 hr or 1 dose of 3 mg; maximum dose, 4 mg. FDA pregnancy category D.	Dilute drug 10-fold with sterile saline solution before injecting to minimize tissue damage.
probenecid	Benemid* Benuryl† Various others	ORAL: *Adults*—250 mg 2 or 3 times/day in first week, 500 mg twice daily thereafter. May increase to 2 g/day if necessary.	Inhibits reabsorption of uric acid by kidney. Prophylactic drug to reduce existing tophi and to prevent recurrence of gouty attack.
sulfinpyrazone	Anturan† Anturane	ORAL: *Adults*—100-200 mg twice daily with meals or with milk at bedtime. Dosage is raised as needed to control blood urate levels (400-800 mg/day). Dosage is then reduced to minimum effective level, usually 300-400 mg/day.	Acts like probenecid. May also prevent recurrence of myocardial infarction.

*Available in Canada and the United States.
†Available in Canada only.

change in body uric acid concentration often precipitates a new acute attack of gouty arthritis. This effect can often be avoided with prophylactic colchicine.

Adverse Reactions, Contraindications, and Toxicity

Colchicine commonly causes nausea, vomiting, and diarrhea, effects that limit the dosage tolerated. Elderly patients and those with hepatic or renal disease need a lower dosage to avoid toxic reactions. The onset of acute toxicity is seen in 24 to 72 hours, and the first sign is commonly a fever. A burning feeling may be noted in the throat or GI tract. Hair loss may be experienced 10 days after an overdose. When colchicine is given intravenously, there is a greater risk bone marrow suppression, kidney and renal damage, and injury to the CNS.

Interactions

Phenylbutazone, radiation therapy, and drugs causing bone marrow depression all increase the potential bone marrow depression of colchicine and should not be administered concurrently.

probenecid and sulfinpyrazone

Probenecid (Benemid) and sulfinpyrazone (Anturane) inhibit the reabsorption of uric acid by the kidney tubules and thereby promote the excretion of uric acid in the urine. The patient should drink at least eight glasses of water daily to keep the uric acid dilute so that it does not crystallize in kidney tubules or the bladder. Because these drugs flood the kidney tubules with uric acid, they are contraindicated in patients with renal failure or with a history of renal stones.

Probenecid is generally well tolerated but occasionally causes GI upset or an allergic reaction. It interferes with the renal excretion of many compounds.

Sulfinpyrazone is also well tolerated. The incidence of GI upset is higher with sulfinpyrazone than with probenecid. Recent studies show that sulfinpyrazone decreases the incidence of sudden death in the first 8 months after an MI. This effect is believed to be caused by decreased platelet aggregation. Because many patients with gout also have conditions such as diabetes, hypertension, or coronary artery disease (high-risk factors for MI), sulfinpyrazone may be more desirable than probenecid despite the higher incidence of GI upset.

A number of factors diminish the effectiveness of the uricosuric drugs probenecid and sulfinpyrazone. A diet high in purines produces too much uric acid (see Dietary Considerations box earlier in this chapter) and should be avoided.

The effectiveness of uricosuric drugs is diminished by several agents. Heavy alcohol consumption produces enough lactic acid to inhibit uric acid secretion. Aspirin and other salicylates at low dosages (300 to 650 mg) inhibit uric acid secretion. Acetaminophen should be substituted for simple pain relief. Diuretics, particularly the thiazides, furosemide, ethacrynic acid, triamterene, and spironolactone, inhibit uric acid secretion.

In addition, the uricosuric drugs inhibit the secretion or degradation of several medications. Probenecid inhibits the renal secretion of penicillin, indomethacin, methotrexate, sulfonylureas (oral hypoglycemics), sulfinpyrazone, salicylates, and rifampin, keeping their plasma levels high. Sulfinpyrazone inhibits the degradation of sulfonamides, particularly sulfadiazine and sulfisoxazole, sulfonylureas, and coumarins.

Nursing Process Overview

Drugs to Treat Gout

Assessment

Assess vital signs, weight, history of previous attacks, family history of gout, subjective complaints, and objective data. Monitor blood work, including the serum uric acid level. X-ray films and joint aspiration may be required.

Nursing Diagnoses

- Risk for impaired home maintenance management related to the need to increase daily fluid intake to 2500 ml
- Risk for GI distress

Patient Outcomes

The patient will successfully incorporate an increased fluid intake into daily life. The patient will not experience GI distress.

Planning/Implementation

Encourage a high urinary output (2000 to 3000 ml/day) to prevent the formation of kidney stones; this requires a high fluid intake. Monitor fluid intake and output until certain that the high fluid output is being maintained. Monitor vital signs, blood pressure, condition of affected joints, subjective complaints, objective signs, and appropriate laboratory work.

Evaluation

Before discharge, ensure that the patient can describe the disease, the medications that have been prescribed and their actions, the administration of the drugs to achieve maximum benefit, and the possible side effects and the ones that should be reported immediately. In addition, verify that the patient can demonstrate how to plan meals within any prescribed dietary restrictions and explain how to maintain a fluid intake that will ensure adequate urinary output.

Nursing Implications Summary

acetaminophen
Nursing in the Community

➤ When used in usual doses, few side effects are associated with this drug. Notify the physician if jaundice, diarrhea, nausea or vomiting, blood in the stools, unusual bleeding or bruising, or pinpoint red spots develop on the skin. Instruct the patient to report the development of any new sign or symptom to the physician.

➤ Remind the patient to keep these and all drugs out of the reach of children. Never encourage children to take medications by telling them that drugs are candy. Do not give children younger than 12 years of age more than five doses a day. Tell parents to seek medical help immediately if overdose is suspected, even if there are no apparent symptoms. Tell the patient to be alert to signs of acute toxicity such as nausea, vomiting, and abdominal pain. Severe poisoning may result in CNS stimulation, excitement, and delirium followed by CNS depression, stupor, hypothermia, rapid shallow breathing, tachycardia, hypotension, and circulatory failure.

➤ Teach the patient to read labels of all medications carefully. Many OTC products for pain and sinus problems or colds contain acetaminophen alone or in combination with other drugs, including caffeine or aspirin. Tell the patient to avoid taking several drugs simultaneously unless necessary.

➤ Fever that persists beyond 3 days, pain that persists longer than 10 days in an adult or 5 days in a child, or sore throat that persists longer than 2 days or worsens may signal a more serious health problem. Instruct the patient to seek medical help rather than to self-medicate indefinitely. Remind the

patient to take only the recommended dosage; too much may cause liver or kidney damage.

➤ Review with parents the dosages appropriate for children of various sizes and ages. Assist the parents in finding a drug form that is easy to administer. Note that absorption from a rectal suppository is variable and there may be rectal irritation; this route may be the least desirable.

➤ To take effervescent preparations, pour the granules into a glass. Fill the glass with 4 ounces of cool water. Drink all of the contents of the glass, whether still fizzing or not.

➤ To take oral powders, open the number of capsules needed for the prescribed dose, and pour the contents into 1 teaspoon water or other liquid. Drink all of the liquid and follow with more. The contents of the capsules may also be mixed with a small amount of applesauce, pudding, ice cream, or other soft food.

➤ To take oral granules, just before taking the dose, open the number of packets needed for the dose. Mix the granules with a small amount of applesauce, jam, pudding, or other soft food. Eat the granules along with the food.

➤ Teach the patient to avoid taking aspirin-containing products or NSAIDs while taking acetaminophen unless specifically directed to do so by the physician.

➤ Teach diabetic patients that acetaminophen may cause false results with blood glucose tests. Check with the physician before changing diet or insulin dosage if test results change, especially if diabetes is not well controlled.

➤ Emphasize the importance of avoiding alcoholic beverages while taking acetaminophen.

Continued

Nursing Implications Summary—cont'd

➤ Remind patients to inform all health care providers of all drugs they take.

➤ Acetylcysteine is discussed in Chapter 30.

aspirin and Related Drugs
Drug Administration

➤ Monitor platelet count and hematocrit level. Regularly check stools for presence of blood or guaiac. With long-term or high-dose therapy, monitor serum salicylate concentration. For patients taking choline and magnesium salicylates, monitor serum magnesium levels.

Nursing in the Community

➤ Instruct the patient to report the development of rash, tinnitus, unexplained bleeding or bruising, severe or persistent gastric irritation, or blood in the stool. Salicylates other than aspirin do not affect platelet aggregation.

➤ Warn parents to avoid the use of aspirin and other salicylates to treat fever and discomfort of the flu or chicken pox in children and teenagers because aspirin is associated with the development of Reye's syndrome. Acetaminophen is preferred over aspirin to treat childhood flu and chicken pox symptoms.

➤ Remind the patient to keep these and all drugs out of the reach of children. Never encourage children to take medications by telling them that drugs are candy. Instruct parents to seek medical help immediately if overdose is suspected, even if symptoms are not apparent.

➤ Teach the patient to read labels of all medications carefully. Many OTC products for pain and for sinus problems or colds contain salicylates alone or in combination with other drugs, including antihistamines or acetaminophen. Instruct the patient to avoid taking several drugs simultaneously unless necessary. Aspirin in combination with caffeine may provide better or faster pain relief in some patients.

➤ To reduce gastric irritation, teach the patient to take oral doses with a full glass (8 ounces) of fluid or with meals or a snack. Also, teach the patient to avoid lying down for 15 to 30 minutes after taking oral forms.

➤ Pain or fever that persists beyond 3 to 5 days may signal a more serious health problem. Instruct the patient to seek medical help rather than self-medicate indefinitely. Teach the patient to take only the recommended dosage; too much medication may result in salicylism or other complications.

➤ Remind the patient to keep all health care providers informed of all medications being taken, including aspirin; this includes dentists and oral surgeons. In addition, instruct the patient to avoid the use of aspirin for 7 days after tonsillectomy or oral surgery.

➤ Instruct the patient not to take aspirin products that smell strongly of vinegar because they may have broken down and may not be effective.

➤ To take effervescent preparations, pour the granules into a glass. Fill the glass with 4 ounces of cool water. Instruct the patient to drink all the contents of the glass, whether still fizzing or not.

➤ Instruct the patient to swallow enteric-coated preparations whole, without chewing or crushing. Chewable aspirin tablets may be crushed, chewed, or swallowed whole. Chew aspirin chewing gum for several minutes (or as directed on the package label) for the best effect. Break extended-release preparations along scored lines; some should not be chewed or crushed; consult the pharmacist about specific brands. Mix choline and magnesium salicylates oral solution with fruit juice just before taking, and follow dose with a full glass (8 ounces) of water.

➤ Instruct the patient to avoid alcoholic beverages while taking aspirin or salicylates. Buffered aspirin and choline and magnesium salicylates should not be taken at the same time as tetracyclines. Patients who take one of these drugs and tetracycline should allow 1 to 2 hours between doses. Do not take doses of ketoconazole within 3 hours of doses of buffered aspirin. Do not take laxatives containing cellulose within 2 hours of doses of salicylates.

➤ Patients receiving long-term therapy may find extended-release preparations helpful, particularly at night, because morning blood levels of aspirin may not be so low.

➤ Teach patients who take aspirin for arthritis and other musculoskeletal conditions that the best effect is achieved through regular use of the drug as prescribed. Several weeks of therapy may be needed to achieve full benefit.

➤ Warn diabetic patients that chronic or excessive use of aspirin-containing products may cause false urine sugar results. Monitor blood glucose levels. Consult the physician or pharmacist.

➤ Low-dose aspirin may be used for its antiplatelet effect. It may be prescribed to decrease the incidence of thromboembolism in immobilized patients and postoperative orthopedic patients. It is also used to prevent other vascular problems (see Chapter 20). Instruct patients to take the dose prescribed and not to increase the dose unless directed to do so by the physician.

➤ Teach women to avoid the use of aspirin during the last trimester of pregnancy unless first approved by the physician.

➤ Encourage patients who are allergic to aspirin to wear a medical identification tag or bracelet indicating this.

Nonsteroidal Antiinflammatory Drugs
Drug Administration

➤ Monitor vital signs, blood pressure, and weight. Monitor the complete blood count (CBC), differential, platelet count, serum potassium, blood urea nitrogen level (BUN), serum creatinine level, and liver function tests. Check stools for presence of blood. If diarrhea or vomiting is severe or persistent, monitor intake and output.

➤ Question the patient about a possible history of allergy to other drugs before administering the drug. If unsure that an

Nursing Implications Summary—cont'd

allergy to an NSAID exists, consult the physician before administering the first dose.

➤ In patients with cardiovascular, renal, or hypertensive disease, assess for possible fluid retention. Auscultate lung sounds. Assess for jugular venous distension. Monitor daily weight.

Nursing in the Community

➤ Review anticipated benefits and possible side effects of drug therapy. Instruct the patient to report the development of bruising, bleeding gums, nosebleeds, blood in stool, fever, rash, sore throat, mouth ulcers or irritation, jaundice, right upper quadrant abdominal pain, and malaise. Instruct the patient to notify the physician if unexpected symptoms develop.

➤ Tell patients with long-term musculoskeletal problems that several weeks of therapy may be necessary before full benefit is seen. Best effects are seen if the drugs are taken regularly, as ordered. Instruct patients not to discontinue or increase therapy without consulting the physician.

➤ Teach the patient to take doses with meals, a snack, or milk to reduce gastric irritation. Doses are taken with a full glass (8 ounces) of fluid. Tell the patient not to lie down for at least 15 to 30 minutes after an oral dose.

➤ The physician may want the patient to take doses with an antacid. This practice is especially important with indomethacin, mefenamic acid, phenylbutazone, or piroxicam. The best kind of antacid is one containing magnesium and aluminum hydroxides. Do not mix liquid forms of NSAIDs with the liquid antacid.

➤ Teach patients taking mefenamic acid to notify the physician if diarrhea develops.

➤ Review the other medications and drug interactions noted in the text; counsel patients as appropriate. Remind the patient to keep all health care providers, including dentists and oral surgeons, informed of all drugs they take. Tell the patient not to take OTC products without consulting the physician. This applies especially to products that contain aspirin or acetaminophen.

➤ Warn the patient to avoid driving or operating hazardous equipment if visual changes, dizziness, fatigue, confusion, drowsiness, or weakness occur and to notify the physician.

➤ Instruct the patient to avoid drinking alcoholic beverages while taking NSAIDs.

➤ NSAIDs may cause photosensitivity. Warn the patient to limit time in the sun or under sun lamps until the effects of the drug can be evaluated (see the Patient Problems box in Chapter 58 on photosensitivity).

➤ NSAIDs may be used to treat fever, even in children.

➤ Long-term use of these drugs is associated with visual changes. Encourage the patient to have recommended ophthalmic examinations.

➤ Instruct the patient to swallow enteric-coated forms whole, do not chew or crush them. Capsules may be opened and the contents mixed with food. Some tablets may be crushed and mixed with food. Work with the patient to find a form that he or she can take. Consult the pharmacist for information about crushing, breaking, or mixing an individual product.

➤ Instruct patients taking nonprescription NSAIDs to review the manufacturer's literature supplied with the package.

➤ Emphasize the importance of continuing with other prescribed therapies, which might include other medications, a prescribed exercise program, weight reduction, application of heat and cold, and physical therapy.

➤ Some of these drugs cause fluid retention. Assess the patient's ability, resources, and other health problems (e.g., hypertensive, cardiovascular, or renal disease). If appropriate, teach the patient to monitor and record weight daily. Report weight gain in excess of 2 lb/day or 5 lb/wk to the physician.

➤ Remind pregnant or lactating women to avoid all drugs unless prescribed by the health care provider.

➤ NSAIDs are also available for ophthalmic use (see Chapter 74). Instruct the patient to avoid wearing soft hydrogel contact lenses during treatment with diclofenac eye drops.

allopurinol

Drug Administration

➤ Inspect the patient to detect rash and skin changes. Assess vision. Monitor serum creatinine level, BUN level, uric acid levels, CBC, differential, platelet count, and liver function tests.

Nursing in the Community

➤ Review anticipated benefits and possible side effects of drug therapy. Instruct the patient to report bruising, bleeding, nosebleeds, blood in stool, fever, sore throat, malaise, jaundice, or abdominal pain. Encourage the patient to notify the physician of GI discomfort. Tell patients to notify the physician if rash, hives, or itching develop.

➤ Tell adult patients to maintain daily fluid intake sufficient to ensure a daily urinary output of at least 2 L; this may require an intake of 2500 ml/day (about ten 8-ounce glasses of water). Check with the physician for guidelines for children.

➤ Caution the patient to avoid analgesics containing salicylates unless approved by the physician.

➤ Remind patients to inform all health care providers of all drugs they take. Allopurinol may interfere with the effects of other drugs.

➤ Instruct the patient to take oral doses with meals or a snack to reduce gastric irritation.

➤ Review the Dietary Considerations box on purine earlier in this chapter.

➤ Teach the patient to limit the intake of alcoholic beverages. Tell the patient not to take vitamin C concurrently with allopurinol because it may increase urine acidity and promote the formation of kidney stones.

➤ Warn the patient to avoid driving or operating hazardous equipment if drowsiness or dizziness develops.

Continued

Nursing Implications Summary—cont'd

➤ For missed doses, instruct the patient to take the missed dose as soon as remembered, unless it is almost time for the next dose, then omit missed dose and resume regular dosing schedule.

colchicine

Drug Administration

➤ Inspect the patient to detect hair loss and skin changes. Assess for GI discomfort. Monitor serum creatinine level, BUN level, CBC, differential, platelet count, liver function tests, and uric acid levels.

Intravenous colchicine

➤ Dilute with 10 to 20 ml of 0.9% sodium chloride without a bacteriostatic agent. Administer over 2 to 5 minutes. Avoid extravasation or IM administration. Check that IV line is patent before administering. Do not administer via lines infusing with D5W, solutions containing a bacteriostatic agent, or fluids that might change the pH of the drug, because precipitation might occur. Contact pharmacist with questions.

Nursing in the Community

➤ Review anticipated benefits and possible side effects of drug therapy. Review dosage instructions, which are different for prophylactic treatment of gout and for treatment of an acute attack. Toxicity depends on the total dose given over time, so it is important to teach patients who take the higher dosages needed for an acute attack to take the drug only as prescribed and not to increase the dosage or change the dosage regimen without checking with physician.

➤ Instruct the patient to report a change in the color of urine (hematuria), bruising, bleeding, nosebleeds, blood in stool, fever, sore throat, malaise, jaundice, or abdominal pain. GI discomfort is common. Encourage the patient to notify the physician of any GI discomfort.

➤ Instruct the patient to take oral doses with meals or a snack to reduce gastric irritation.

➤ Caution the patient to avoid the use of analgesics that containing salicylates without approval of the physician.

➤ Remind patients to inform all health care providers of all drugs they take. Colchicine may interfere with the desired effect of other drugs.

➤ Review the Dietary Considerations box on purine earlier in this chapter.

➤ Remind the patients to limit intake of alcoholic beverages.

probenecid

Drug Administration

➤ Inspect for development of skin changes. Monitor blood pressure. Monitor liver function tests and serum creatinine, BUN, and uric acid levels.

➤ Probenecid is sometimes used concurrently with some antibiotics such as penicillins and cephalosporins; the probenecid helps increase the plasma and tissue antibiotic concentration.

Nursing in the Community

➤ Review the anticipated benefits and possible side effects of drug therapy. Instruct the patient to report malaise, jaundice, or abdominal pain. GI discomfort is common. Encourage the patient to notify physicians of GI discomfort.

➤ Tell the patient to maintain daily fluid intake sufficient to ensure a daily urinary output of at least 2 L; this may require an intake of 2500 ml/day (about ten 8-ounce glasses of fluid).

➤ Warn the patient to avoid driving or operating hazardous equipment and to notify the physician if dizziness occurs. Warn the patient that flushing may occur after drug ingestion. Caution the patient to avoid analgesics that contain salicylates without the physician's approval. In addition, tell the patient to avoid alcoholic beverages while taking probenecid.

➤ Remind patients to inform all health care providers of all drugs they take. Probenecid may interfere with the desired effect of other prescribed drugs.

➤ Alkalinization of urine helps prevent crystallization of uric acid. Sodium bicarbonate, potassium citrate, or other alkalinizing agent may be prescribed concurrently.

➤ Review the Dietary Considerations box on purine earlier in this chapter.

➤ Tell diabetic patients that probenecid may interfere with copper sulfate urine sugar tests.

➤ Some products contain colchicine and probenecid. Review side effects of both drugs with patients.

sulfinpyrazone

Drug Administration

➤ Assess for development of tinnitus and changes in hearing or GI distress. Inspect for skin changes or rash.

➤ Monitor serum uric acid, CBC, serum creatinine, and BUN.

Nursing in the Community

➤ Review the anticipated benefits and possible side effects of drug therapy. Instruct the patient to report bruising, bleeding, nosebleeds, or blood in stool; fever, sore throat, malaise, or tinnitus. GI discomfort is common. Encourage the patient to notify the physician of any GI discomfort.

➤ Teach the patient to take oral doses with milk, meals, or snacks to reduce gastric irritation.

➤ Tell the patient to maintain daily fluid intake sufficient to ensure daily urinary output of at least 2 L; this may require an intake of 2500 ml/day (about ten 8-ounce glasses of fluid).

➤ Caution the patient to avoid the use of analgesics that contain salicylates without obtaining the physician's approval.

➤ Remind patients to inform all health care providers of all drugs they take. Sulfinpyrazone may interfere with the desired effect of other drugs taken.

➤ Review the Dietary Considerations box on purine earlier in this chapter.

➤ Remind the patient to limit intake of alcoholic beverages.

CHAPTER REVIEW

Application

1. List the three pharmacologic actions characteristic of aspirin.
2. How do the nonnarcotic analgesics produce analgesia?
3. What is the mechanism of antipyresis?
4. What are the side effects of acetaminophen?
5. What is the mechanism of acetaminophen toxicity?
6. What is the dosage difference between aspirin taken for analgesia-antipyresis and for an antiinflammatory response?
7. What factors determine the metabolism and excretion of salicylate?
8. Describe salicylism. Describe aspirin toxicity.
9. What pharmacologic actions are characteristic of the NSAIDs?
10. Why is phenylbutazone used for 2 weeks or less?
11. What are the major side effects of indomethacin?
12. Describe the uses of NSAIDs.
13. Describe the role of colchicine in treating gout.
14. Describe the mechanisms of allopurinol, probenecid, and sulfinpyrazone for lowering the uric acid concentration of the body.

Critical Thinking

1. Why is acetaminophen considered safer than aspirin? Why should children not take aspirin?
2. How does aspirin affect the stomach? How does aspirin affect platelets? Describe nursing care considerations related to these effects.
3. Develop a nursing care plan for a patient receiving one or more of the drugs in this chapter.

References

Courts NF: Salicylism in the elderly: "a little aspirin never hurt anybody!" *Geriatr Nurs* 17(2):55-59, 1996.
Johnson W: Childhood fevers: advising parents on management. *Community Nurse* 2(2):20, 22-23, 1996.

32

Opioids (Narcotic Analgesics)

OBJECTIVES

After studying this chapter, you should be able to do the following:

- *Explain the action of morphine in the central nervous system (CNS) and the periphery.*
- *Describe the role of endogenous opioid peptides and the three types of opioid receptors in providing pain relief.*
- *Discuss tolerance and dependence with opioids.*
- *Describe the symptoms and treatment of acute opioid toxicity.*
- *Develop a nursing care plan for the patient receiving an opioid.*

CHAPTER OVERVIEW

Analgesics are drugs that relieve pain. The NSAID (nonsteroidal antiinflammatory drug) analgesics are covered in Chapter 31. This chapter presents the opioids, formerly referred to as narcotic analgesics. The nature of pain and its treatment with opioids are described. The pharmacology of morphine, the prototype for the opioids, is reviewed, followed by a discussion of the specific characteristics of clinically used opioids and the opioid antagonists. This chapter concludes with an examination of the nature and treatment of opioid tolerance and dependence.

THERAPEUTIC RATIONALE: PAIN AND THE USE OF OPIOIDS

History of Opioids

Analgesics are drugs that relieve pain. Opium has been used to produce analgesia and euphoria throughout history. The word *opium* comes from the Greek *opion,* meaning poppy juice, and the source of morphine today is still the sticky brown gum (opium) collected from the seed pod of *Papaver somniferum,* a variety of poppy. About 10% of the content of opium is morphine. Codeine can also be extracted from opium, although in such small amounts that most medicinal codeine is derived by chemically modifying morphine. Morphine was isolated in 1803 by a German pharmacist and named after Morpheus, the Greek god of sleep. Morphine was the first pure chemical substance that mimicked the pharmacologic effects of the natural product after extraction from the natural product.

Drug dependence as a property of morphine was not realized in the United States until the Civil War, when morphine was widely used to treat wounded soldiers, whose addiction subsequently became a significant social problem. Opium and morphine were readily available and were often ingredients of patent medicines. By the late 1800s, attempts were made to modify the structure of morphine to keep the analgesic property but eliminate the addictive potential. The first semisynthetic drug was heroin, but heroin produces drug dependence more readily than morphine. Today heroin is not a legal drug in the United States or Canada, although it is in other countries. Most opioids come under the Controlled Substances Act (United States) or are listed as controlled substances (schedule G) under the Canadian Food and Drugs Act (see Chapter 3).

Morphine is the prototype for the opioids. Opioids were formerly referred to as narcotic analgesics because they allowed patients in severe pain to sleep (*narcotic* means stupor). The term **opioid** includes all agents derived from morphine and those synthetic compounds with morphine-like activity. The first purely synthetic morphine-like compound was meperidine (Demerol), which came into clinical use in the 1940s. Because meperidine was not a chemical modification of morphine, widespread belief held that meperidine did not cause drug dependence. Today, meperidine is considered a drug with high abuse potential (schedule II) similar to morphine. The most recent examples of opioids with abuse potential that was not originally recognized are pentazocine (Talwin) and propoxyphene (Darvon), which are now classified as drugs of low abuse potential (schedule IV). The characteristics of opioid dependence and its treatment are discussed later in this chapter.

Overview of Pain

Pain is classified into two major components. Objective pain represents the stimulation of peripheral nerve endings when tissue is damaged. Nonopioids such as aspirin and acetaminophen act by inhibiting the synthesis of local mediators, the prostaglandins, that are released in damaged tissue to stimulate the nerve endings. In the presence of NSAID analgesics, pain is not felt because the nerves are not stimulated, and the pain message therefore is never delivered to the CNS. NSAID analgesics are discussed in Chapter 31. Subjective pain represents how a person reacts to pain, usually with fear, anxiety, and withdrawal. The subjective level of pain involves the spinal cord and brain, which collect and process the painful stimuli. The opioids blunt this subjective pain, allowing the individual to tolerate pain. With high dosages of these drugs, individuals become unaware of pain and become indifferent to all unpleasant stimuli.

Acute Pain

The major use of opioids is for the short-term treatment of severe acute pain such as that associated with trauma, surgery, or burns. Opioids are commonly classified by the level of pain they can relieve: severe, severe to moderate, and mild pain (Table 32-1). These are not specifically defined categories, however.

The pain of some specific conditions is effectively treated with opioids. These conditions include myocardial infarction, pulmonary edema, labor, preanesthesia and postanesthesia, and sickle cell crisis. Under some circumstances, pain associated with gastrointestinal (GI) and urinary tract disorders may be treated with an opioid.

In treating acute pain, opioids are administered in sufficient doses to relieve pain and at intervals frequent enough to prevent the recurrence of pain. Each patient must be evaluated frequently to determine the need for dosage adjustment. There is little danger of producing drug addiction in treating acute pain because psychologic dependence on opioids is unlikely under most medical circumstances. Most patients are able to discontinue medication with little difficulty.

A more common problem is the undermedication of patients in acute pain by health care providers unduly concerned about causing addiction. The usual 10-mg dose of morphine produces effective analgesia in only two thirds of

Table 32-1 Comparison of Opioids

Level of Pain	Drug	Equivalent Analgesic Dose (mg) Given Intramuscularly or Subcutaneously	Time for Peak Effect (min)	Duration (hr)	Schedule United States	Canada
Severe	morphine	10	30-90	3-7	II	N
	buprenorphine (Buprenex)	0.5	15	4-6	V	*
	dezocine (Dalgan)	10	60-120	3-6	†	*
	hydromorphone hydrochloride (Dilaudid)	1.5	3-90	4-5	II	N
	levorphanol tartrate (Levo-Dromoran)	2-3	60-90	5-8	II	N
	oxymorphone (Numorphan)	7.5-10	60-120	3-6	II	N
Moderate to severe	butorphanol (Stadol)	1.5-3.5	30	3-4	†	C
	meperidine (Demerol)	75-100	30-60	2-4	II	N
	nalbuphine (Nubain)	10	30	3-6	†	C
	oxycodone (Roxicodone)	15	60	3-4	II	N
	pentazocine (Talwin)	40-60	30-60	2-3	IV	N
Mild to moderate	codeine phosphate	120	60-90	4-6	II	N
	propoxyphene (Darvon)	180-240	60	4-6	IV	N

*Not available in Canada.
†Not scheduled as a controlled drug.

patients. Recent studies have found that effective pain relief has benefits with minuscule risk of addiction. Patients who received effective pain relief recover faster. Only 1 in 3000 patients receiving opioids for acute pain becomes addicted. Even chronic pain patients have a low rate of addiction to opioids, and those who become addicted mainly have a prior history of drug abuse.

Chronic Pain

Opioids are used to treat the chronic pain associated with cancer. Special care must be used to keep the dosage as low as possible to prolong the effectiveness of the drug and to keep the patient alert. Nonmedical aspects of patient comfort, including physical, social, mental, and spiritual measures, should be considered. Often, aspirin, acetaminophen, or other NSAIDs are effective analgesics. The treatment of chronic pain associated with cancer requires an individualized regimen that should be evaluated frequently. If opioids are used, increasing the dosage is usually preferable to increasing the frequency of administration. Because cross-tolerance of opioids is limited, a different opioid may be tried if the one being used must be discontinued because of adverse effects associated with increased dosage.

Anesthesia

Additional uses of opioids include preanesthetic medication and surgical anesthesia. As preanesthetic medication, opioids relieve anxiety and provide sedation so that the patient is not in a fearful state before surgery. More potent analgesic, including morphine, meperidine, fentanyl, and hydromorphone, are widely used as components of surgical anesthesia with nitrous oxide. Nitrous oxide by itself is not potent enough for surgical anesthesia but is potentiated by an opioid. A muscle relaxant such as tubocurarine is also used. This combination of opioid, nitrous oxide, and muscle relaxant is called balanced anesthesia (see Chapter 36). Duration of anesthesia is controlled by the duration of action of the opioid used.

THERAPEUTIC AGENTS: OPIOIDS

Pharmacology of Opioids

The pharmacology of morphine provides the standard for describing and comparing the actions of all opioids. The general activities of morphine are described in depth, including the biochemical basis of action and the central and peripheral physiologic effects. The clinical use of morphine and other opioids is detailed separately, and this chapter concludes with a discussion of opioid dependence and its treatment.

Mechanism of Action

Opioid Receptors. In the early 1970s, scientists demonstrated that specific receptors for opioids exist in the brain, spinal cord, and gut. These receptors did not recognize any of the known neurotransmitters. This finding suggested that a previously unknown, naturally occurring substance that is mimicked by morphine exists in the brain, spinal cord, and gut. Such compounds have now been found. So far, three classes of naturally occurring neuropeptides have been characterized: endorphins, enkephalins, and dynorphins.

Beta-endorphin is a large peptide derived from the prohormone for adrenocorticotropic hormone (ACTH) and is found in the pituitary gland. The **dynorphins** are also peptides derived from a larger peptide and found in the pituitary. The **enkephalins** are pentapeptides (five amino acids) and seem to be neurotransmitters associated with (1) mediation of pain and analgesia; (2) release of growth hormone, prolactin, and vasopressin from the pituitary; (3) modulation of locomotor activity; (4) regulation of mood; and (5) regulation of gut motility.

Three types of opioid receptors have been characterized. The mu-receptor mediates central analgesia, euphoria, respiratory depression, and physical dependence. The mu-receptor is associated with classic morphine effects and with beta-endorphin and the enkephalins. The kappa-receptors mediate spinal analgesia, miosis, sedation, and appetite regulation. Pharmacologic properties have been assigned to two subtypes of kappa-receptors. The kappa$_1$-receptor is associated with spinal analgesia, whereas the kappa$_3$-receptor is associated with analgesia in regions of the brain associated with pain modulation. The kappa-receptors are sensitive to opioids with mixed agonist-antagonist activity and to the naturally occurring dynorphins. Unlike the euphoria associated with the mu-receptor, the kappa-receptors are associated with disoriented and/or depersonalized feelings. The delta-receptor appears to mediate analgesia both spinally and in brain structures. It is thought to be the primary receptor for the enkephalins.

The properties and pharmacology of opioid receptor subtypes are actively being studied. Future research should clarify the nature of analgesia and the development of the opioid type of drug dependence and provide the basis for understanding the role of these opioid peptides in mental disorders, seizure activity, and behavior patterns involving the reward system, eating, and drinking.

Agonist/Antagonist Classification of Opioids. With the characterization of subtypes of opioid receptors, opioids are found to act as agonists or antagonists at the receptor subtypes. Full agonist opioids are those that like morphine fully activate the mu-receptor and produce analgesia. Other full agonist opioids are alfentanil, fentanyl, hydromorphone, levorphanol, meperidine, methadone, oxymorphone, and sufentanil. Partial agonist opioids cannot fully activate the mu-receptor and moreover can displace full agonists. Partial agonist opioids include codeine, diphenoxylate, hydrocodone, oxycodone, and propoxyphene. Mixed agonist-antagonist opioids produce agonist effects at one opioid receptor subtype while acting as an antagonist at another receptor subtype. Mixed agonist-antagonist opioids include buprenorphine, butorphanol, nalbuphine, and pentazocine. Antagonists block opioid activity at all receptor subtypes. The opioid antagonists are nalmefene, naloxone, and naltrexone.

Central Nervous System Actions

Analgesia. The analgesia produced by morphine has three characteristics. Morphine raises the threshold for pain perception, making patients less aware of pain. It also reduces anxiety and fear, the emotional reactions to pain. Finally, morphine induces sleep, even in the presence of severe pain.

The biochemical mechanism of pain relief by the opioids is their ability to mimic beta-endorphin, which acts through mu-opioid receptors at many sites in the brain to modify the perception of and reaction to pain. This direct action at the mu-opioid receptor also leads to the release of the various endogenous opioids that also act at delta- and kappa-receptors.

Opioids also exert a powerful analgesic action in the spinal cord. The spinal cord has all three opioid receptors. These receptors are found in both the spinal cord pain transmission neurons and on the afferent neurons that feed into them. The action of opioid agonists is to inhibit the release of excitatory neurotransmitters from the afferent neurons and to inhibit dorsal horn pain transmission directly.

The biochemical basis of the placebo response and the effectiveness of acupuncture appear to lie in the release of beta-endorphin. The antagonist naloxone, which blocks the activity of beta-endorphin, also blocks the placebo response and the effectiveness of acupuncture.

Medullary actions. Morphine affects several medullary centers. The most important is the **respiratory center,** which becomes less sensitive to carbon dioxide in the presence of morphine. Tolerance develops to this effect, so those individuals who abuse one of the opioids can tolerate doses of opioids that would cause fatal respiratory depression in nondependent individuals. Death from an opioid overdose is commonly caused by respiratory arrest; the victim stops breathing. Similarly, the most important drug interactions with morphine are those arising from a synergistic depression of the respiratory center such as with any of the sedative-hypnotic drugs, antianxiety agents, alcohol, general anesthetics, or phenothiazines. Tolerance does not develop to the respiratory depression produced by these latter drug classes. An individual who is abusing an opioid and a drug of another class such as alcohol or one of the other sedative-hypnotic drugs can readily succumb to drug-induced respiratory depression.

The **cough center** is the second medullary center depressed by morphine. Morphine seldom is prescribed as a cough suppressant, as is a related drug such as codeine. Cough suppressants (antitussive drugs) are described in Chapter 30. The **chemoreceptor trigger zone** is the third major medullary center affected by morphine. Morphine stimulates this center to produce nausea and vomiting. This effect is transient, so repeated doses do not usually cause nausea and vomiting. Individuals vary in their sensitivity to this emetic action.

Mental state. The effect of morphine on behavior depends on the mental state of the individual. Euphoria may be experienced if the individual has been in pain or has been fearful and anxious. Therapeutic doses produce minimum sedation, but larger doses cause drowsiness, sleep, or in large doses, coma. A few individuals become excited rather than depressed.

Peripheral Actions

Gastrointestinal System. Morphine has a profound depressant effect on the GI tract; constipation is a common side effect of morphine administration. Although morphine is not used to treat nonspecific diarrhea, related drugs such as codeine or diphenoxylate are used. The common medicinal use of opium historically was to stop diarrhea.

Gastric, biliary, and pancreatic secretions are inhibited by morphine. Morphine treats the pain associated with biliary colic but may exacerbate rather than relieve the pain in some patients because the biliary tract may go into painful spasms in the presence of morphine.

Urinary Retention. Urinary retention is another side effect of morphine. Morphine stimulates the release of vasopressin (an antidiuretic hormone); therefore more water is absorbed in the kidney tubules, decreasing urine volume. The drug also reduces perception of the need to void.

Cardiovascular Effects. Morphine commonly causes hypotension. This effect may be a result of depression of the vasomotor center in the medulla. In addition, morphine causes histamine release, and histamine is a potent vasodilator. The concurrent administration of a phenothiazine or atropine can intensify the hypotension. In large doses morphine slows the heart rate.

Ocular Effect. A classic effect of morphine is to reduce pupillary size. A pinpoint pupil is one characteristic of an opioid overdose. However, if the victim is near death, hypoxia causes the release of epinephrine, which dilates the pupil.

Adverse Reactions and Contraindications

The common adverse reactions of morphine and the other opioids are those predicted by the pharmacologic actions of morphine, including nausea and vomiting, constipation, urinary retention, itching, and hypotension resulting from histamine release.

Some actions characteristic of morphine, including the respiratory depression caused by opioids, are undesirable in certain patients. Patients with impaired respiratory function may be severely compromised by an opioid because their respiratory drive is already impaired. Although in general the opioids relax bronchial smooth muscle, a few patients with asthma experience severe bronchoconstriction and die. These drugs also pass into the milk of a nursing mother and affect the infant.

Patients with a head injury should not be given an opioid because the decreased respiration increases carbon dioxide retention and carbon dioxide dilates the intracranial blood vessels, worsening the situation. In addition, sedative and behavioral effects obscure evaluation of the CNS. Because opioids can cause hypotension, they must be used cautiously in patients with shock or blood loss, conditions worsened by a hypotensive action.

Acute Toxicity

Respiratory depression is the usual cause of death from an acute overdose of an opioid. An overdose is likely to occur in an individual who buys drugs on the street. Because street drugs have an unknown purity and concentration, occasionally the drug content is higher than anticipated.

The overdosed individual is stuporous or in a deep sleep and initially is warm and has flushed wet skin. The next stage is coma, in which respiration is depressed. As the individual becomes hypoxic (starved for oxygen), the skin becomes cold, clammy, and mottled, and the pupils dilate. Death is then imminent.

Clinical Use of Opioids: Severe Pain

The opioids currently in use are compared with respect to efficacy, dosage, onset, and duration of action in Table 32-1. In addition to these drugs, alfentanil (Alfenta), fentanyl (Sublimaze), remifentanil (Ultiva), and sufentanil (Sufenta) are short-acting opioids used primarily in anesthesia. These are discussed in Chapter 36.

The major use of the opioids is for the relief of moderate to severe pain. These drugs are most effective in relieving the constant dull pain associated with trauma, surgery, heart attack, biliary or ureteral colic, inflammation, and cancer. Isolated sharp pain is not as effectively relieved by opioids.

A summary of the most commonly used opioids is presented in Table 32-2.

▼ morphine

Morphine has already been described as the prototype for the opioids. Chemically, morphine is a base that is positively charged at the pH in the GI tract and therefore is not readily absorbed when taken orally. In the hospital, morphine is commonly given by intramuscular (IM) or subcutaneous (SC) routes. Because morphine is readily metabolized within the gut and by the liver, larger doses may be required when given orally. Older adult patients usually require a smaller dose because they do not metabolize morphine as readily as do younger patients.

Morphine or meperidine treats the pain of an acute myocardial infarction. At analgesic dosages, morphine not only relieves the pain but also reduces the anxiety without altering the cardiovascular system. If undue reduction in respiration, heart rate, or blood pressure occurs as a result of morphine administration, it can be reversed by administering naloxone, the opioid antagonist.

Morphine is the drug of choice in pulmonary edema. The beneficial actions of morphine include relief of anxiety and vasodilation, which reduces the workload of the heart so that it pumps more efficiently. This increased cardiac efficiency relieves the pulmonary edema that arises when the left side of the heart cannot adequately pump the blood being supplied by the pulmonary veins. This inefficiency gives rise to hypertension and edema in the pulmonary system.

dezocine

Dezocine (Dalgan) is a chemically different mixed agonist-antagonist opioid that acts as a partial agonist at the mu-opioid receptor. It is administered by IM or intravenous (IV) routes. Dezocine does not seem to have the dysphoria side effects characteristic of pentazocine. Dezocine does not adversely affect cardiac performance. When dezocine is given at higher dosages, respiratory depression is not as severe as with morphine.

hydromorphone

Hydromorphone (Dilaudid) is a semisynthetic derivative of morphine. A full opioid agonist, it is more potent but shorter acting than morphine. Oral doses require more time to become effective but are longer acting than parenteral doses. The actions of hydromorphone are identical to those of morphine.

levorphanol

Levorphanol (Levo-Dromoran) is a full agonist opioid that has actions identical to those of morphine. The effective dose is about one fourth that of morphine.

▼ methadone

Methadone (Dolophine) is a full agonist opioid with actions similar to those of morphine. Methadone can be taken orally. Although the onset of action for a single analgesic dose is similar to that for morphine, methadone is highly bound to protein and is not readily metabolized. Methadone has a half-life of 25 hours.

Methadone, 40 to 120 mg/day, substitutes for other opioids in drug-dependent individuals and prevents withdrawal symptoms. Methadone currently is used in the treatment of opioid dependence because it is effective orally and only one dose per day is necessary. In addition, the long plasma half-life more easily allows the gradual reduction in dosage without side effects.

Methadone is a second-line opioid for the management of cancer pain and can be very effective. It is best administered by an experienced professional because of its high potency, long half-life, and the unpredictable individual response.

oxymorphone

Oxymorphone (Numorphan) is a semisynthetic derivative of morphine with full agonist activity that has all the actions of morphine except the antitussive action. Oxymorphone is more potent than morphine but must also be given by injection or rectally.

Clinical Use of Opioids: Moderate to Severe Pain

Summary information about opioids is presented in Table 32-2.

Table 32-2 Opioids (Narcotic Analgesics)

Generic Name	Trade Name	Administration/Dosage	Comments
buprenorphine hydrochloride	Buprenex	INTRAMUSCULAR: *Adults*—0.3-0.6 mg, repeat every 6-8 hr as required.	Mixed agonist-antagonist opioid for moderate to severe pain. Schedule V drug.
butorphanol tartrate	Stadol* Stadol NS*	INTRAMUSCULAR: *Adults*—1-4 mg every 3-4 hr. INTRAVENOUS: *Adults*—0.5-2 mg every 3-4 hr. INHALATION: *Adults*—1 spray per nostril.	Mixed agonist-antagonist opioid for moderate to severe pain. Scheduled drug in the United States. Used in treating severe migraine.
codeine sulfate; codeine phosphate	Generic	ORAL, INTRAMUSCULAR, SUBCUTANEOUS: *Adults*—30-60 mg every 4-6 hr. FDA pregnancy category C. *Children*—0.5 mg/kg body weight every 4-6 hr.	Partial agonist opioid for mild pain. Schedule II drug.
dezocine	Dalgan	INTRAMUSCULAR: *Adults*—5-20 mg every 3-6 hr as needed. Maximum daily dose: 120 mg. INTRAVENOUS: *Adults*—2.5-10 mg every 2-4 hr. FDA pregnancy category C.	Mixed agonist-antagonist opioid for severe pain. Not a scheduled drug.
hydromorphone hydrochloride	Dilaudid* Hydrostat IR PMS-Hydromorphone	ORAL: *Adults*—2 mg every 3-6 hr. FDA pregnancy category C. INTRAMUSCULAR, SUBCUTANEOUS: *Adults*—1-2 mg every 3-6 hr. May be given by slow IV injection or as a suppository.	Full agonist opioid for severe pain. Schedule II drug.
levorphanol tartrate	Levo-Dromoran*	ORAL, SUBCUTANEOUS: *Adults*—2 mg.	Full agonist opioid for severe pain. Schedule II drug.
meperidine hydrochloride	Demerol*	ORAL, INTRAMUSCULAR, SUBCUTANEOUS, SLOW INTRAVENOUS: *Adults*—50-150 mg every 3-4 hr. *Children*—1-1.5 mg/kg body weight; maximum, 100 mg, every 3-4 hr.	Full agonist opioid for severe pain. Schedule II drug.
methadone hydrochloride	Dolophine Methadose	ORAL, INTRAMUSCULAR, SUBCUTANEOUS: *Adults*—2.5-10 mg. For pain relief, repeat every 4-8 hr.	Full agonist opioid for severe pain. Used as replacement drug for opiate dependence or to facilitate withdrawal. Schedule II drug.
morphine sulfate	MSIR Statex† Many others	ORAL: *Adults*—10-30 mg every 4 hr. FDA pregnancy category C. INTRAMUSCULAR, SUBCUTANEOUS: *Adults*—5-20 mg every 4 hr. *Children* (subcutaneous only)—0.1-0.2 mg/kg body weight; maximum, 15 mg. INTRAVENOUS: *Adults*—4-10 mg in 5 ml water, injected over 4-5 min. *Children*—0.1-0.2 mg/kg.	Full agonist opioid for severe pain. Not well absorbed orally. Schedule II drug.
nalbuphine hydrochloride	Nubain*	INTRAMUSCULAR, SUBCUTANEOUS, INTRAVENOUS: *Adults*—10 mg every 3-6 hr; maximum single dose, 20 mg; maximum daily dose, 160 mg.	Mixed agonist-antagonist opioid for severe to moderate pain. Not a scheduled drug.
oxycodone	Roxicodone Supeudol†	ORAL: *Adults*—5 mg every 3-6 hr or 10 mg 3 or 4 times/day as needed. May be increased for severe pain.	Partial agonist opioid for severe pain. Schedule II drug.
oxymorphone hydrochloride	Numorphan*	INTRAMUSCULAR, SUBCUTANEOUS: *Adults*—1-1.5 mg every 3-6 hr. INTRAVENOUS: *Adults*—0.5 mg. RECTAL: *Adults*—5 mg every 4-6 hr.	Full agonist opioid for severe pain. Schedule II drug.
pentazocine hydrochloride	Talwin*	ORAL: *Adults*—50 mg every 3-4 hr; maximum daily dose, 600 mg. (U.S. formulation contains naloxone.)	Mixed agonist-antagonist opioid for moderate to severe pain. Schedule IV drug.
pentazocine lactate	Talwin*	INTRAMUSCULAR, SUBCUTANEOUS, INTRAVENOUS: *Adults*—30 mg every 3-4 hr. Subcutaneous route is not recommended (tissue damage may occur).	Mixed agonist-antagonist opioid for moderate to severe pain. Schedule IV drug.
propoxyphene hydrochloride	Darvon 642†	ORAL: *Adults*—65 mg every 4 hr.	Partial agonist opioid for mild pain. Schedule IV drug.
propoxyphene napsylate	Darvon-N*	ORAL: *Adults*—100 mg every 4 hr.	Partial agonist opioid for mild pain. Schedule IV drug.
tramadol hydrochloride	Ultram	ORAL: *Adults*—50-100 mg every 6 hr as needed. Patients with impaired renal function should receive dose every 12 hr.	Not an opioid, but acts at opioid receptor. For moderate to severe pain. Not a scheduled drug.

*Available in Canada and the United States.
†Available in Canada only.

buprenorphine

Buprenorphine (Buprenex) is a mixed agonist-antagonist opioid. Its abuse potential appears low; it is a schedule V drug in the United States. Buprenorphine is administered intramuscularly. The onset of action is 15 minutes, and the duration of action is about 6 hours. Buprenorphine is effective for moderate to severe pain associated with surgery, cancer, neuralgias, labor, renal colic, and myocardial infarction. The respiratory depression produced by buprenorphine is not readily reversed by naloxone or nalmefene, suggesting that buprenorphine binds tightly to opioid receptors.

butorphanol

Butorphanol (Stadol) has a mixed agonist-antagonist opioid. Its abuse potential appears low, but it was recently put on the controlled substance list in the United States. Administered intramuscularly, butorphanol has an onset of action of 10 to 30 minutes with a duration of action of about 4 hours. It is also available in a nasal spray formulation that is especially useful for patients with migraine. In general, its actions resemble those of morphine, except that butorphanol increases pulmonary arterial pressure and the cardiac workload, which makes it undesirable for treating the pain of a myocardial infarction.

hydrocodone

Hydrocodone (Hycodan, Robidone) is a semisynthetic derivative of morphine and a partial agonist opioid. In Canada it is available as a syrup for cough suppression and in tablet form for analgesia or cough suppression. In the United States hydrocodone is commercially available only in combination with aspirin or acetaminophen.

meperidine

Meperidine (Demerol) was the first of the synthetic opioids. It is a full agonist opioid. It is shorter acting than morphine and does not have an antitussive effect. Meperidine is widely used for obstetric and surgical analgesia. It is more likely than most opioids to cause side effects associated with histamine release, convulsions, and constipation. Meperidine is metabolized to normeperidine, which is active and also neurotoxic. If meperidine is administered for several days, especially to patients with impaired renal or hepatic function, symptoms of normeperidine toxicity may be seen. These symptoms include significant mood changes (paranoia and hallucinations), increased irritability, quivering, fever or convulsions, and sinus tachycardia.

nalbuphine

Nalbuphine (Nubain) is a semisynthetic derivative of morphine and is a mixed agonist-antagonist opioid. The uses and limitations of nalbuphine are primarily those of meperidine or morphine. Nalbuphine may be preferable for treating the pain of a myocardial infarction because it appears to reduce the oxygen needs of the heart without reducing blood pressure. Nalbuphine is a stronger antagonist than pentazocine, which suggests that the degree of tolerance and drug dependence should be low. However, withdrawal symptoms are seen when nalbuphine is abruptly discontinued, and it causes withdrawal symptoms when administered to an individual already dependent on one of the more common opioids.

oxycodone

Oxycodone (Roxicodone) is a semisynthetic derivative of morphine and is a partial agonist opioid. It is taken orally. Oxycodone has an onset of action in 10 to 15 minutes and a duration of action of 3 to 6 hours. In the United States and Canada, oxycodone is also available as a combination product with aspirin or acetaminophen.

pentazocine

Pentazocine (Talwin) is a mixed agonist-antagonist opioid. For several years after pentazocine was introduced, it was believed not to produce drug dependence. Pentazocine is now a schedule IV drug, reflecting a low potential for producing drug dependence. Pentazocine causes respiratory depression in the fetus. Unlike morphine, pentazocine increases blood pressure and cardiac workload, making it less desirable than morphine for treating the pain of myocardial infarction or pulmonary hypertension. Pentazocine causes dysphoria rather than euphoria. Dysphoria can include nightmares, feelings of depersonalization, and visual hallucinations. Large doses induce seizures. Although there are reports of individuals with drug dependence for pentazocine, its administration to a person dependent on the other opioids results in withdrawal symptoms because of its antagonistic properties. In the United States pentazocine is also available as a combination product with aspirin or acetaminophen.

tramadol

Tramadol (Ultram) is a centrally acting analgesic that is not chemically an opioid. Tramadol has about one tenth the analgesic potency of morphine. The mechanism of action for tramadol is not well understood. The mechanism may include binding to the mu-opioid receptor and also inhibition of norepinephrine and serotonin uptake. Tramadol and its metabolite are effective in suppressing a cough. Tramadol is indicated for pain after orthopedic and gynecologic procedures. It is being evaluated in the long-term treatment of such chronic pain syndromes as cancer pain, low back pain, neuropathic pain, and orthopedic and joint conditions. Unlike NSAIDs, tramadol does not have antiinflammatory activity.

Clinical Use of Opioids: Mild Pain

A summary of information about opioids is presented in Table 32-2.

codeine

Codeine is a partial agonist opioid. An oral dose of 32 or 65 mg of codeine is equivalent to 2 aspirin tablets (650 mg).

At these low dosages codeine seldom produces side effects. At high dosages the side effects of codeine are similar to those of morphine. In the United States and Canada, codeine is available as a combination product with acetaminophen or aspirin.

Because codeine causes significant histamine release if given intravenously, it is given only intramuscularly or orally. A portion of codeine dose is metabolized to morphine in the liver. Codeine is a schedule II drug when given in analgesic doses. It is also formulated with the NSAID analgesics for pain relief, and these are usually schedule III drugs. Codeine is an effective cough suppressant at low dosages and is available for this purpose in dilute solutions as a schedule V drug.

propoxyphene

Propoxyphene (Darvon), an opioid related to methadone, is not a very potent analgesic. It is a partial agonist opioid. A 65-mg dose of propoxyphene is the analgesic equivalent of 2 tablets (650 mg) of aspirin or acetaminophen. Propoxyphene is commonly prescribed in combination with aspirin or acetaminophen. Alone or in combination, propoxyphene is a schedule IV drug. Side effects are uncommon at analgesic dosages. Propoxyphene has low abuse potential but has been implicated as a cause of death when abused in combination with alcohol and other CNS depressant drugs. In the United States propoxyphene is available as a combination product with acetaminophen or aspirin. In Canada a combination product with aspirin is available.

Therapeutic Agents for Opioid Overdose

Opioid antagonists produce few effects when used by themselves under usual circumstances. Their clinical use is to treat an opioid overdose. A summary of information about opioid antagonists is presented in Table 32-3.

nalmefene

Nalmefene (Revex) is an opioid antagonist that has a longer duration of action than naloxone. Nalmefene is intended for the management of known or suspected opioid overdose. It will bring a complete or partial reversal of the effects of various opioids, including respiratory depression, and will precipitate withdrawal symptoms in persons with opioid dependence. Nalmefene is usually administered intravenously with a reversal of respiratory depression apparent in 2 to 5 minutes. It may also be administered by IM or SC injection, but the effect requires 5 to 15 minutes. Nalmefene administered in partially reversing doses (1 μg/kg body weight) will have a duration of action of 30 to 60 minutes. If administered in fully reversing doses (14 μg/kg body weight or 1 mg/70 kg), the duration is many hours. A test dose of 0.1 mg/70 kg body weight is administered if opioid dependency is suspected.

▼ naloxone

Naloxone (Narcan) is a pure antagonist for the opioid receptors, which makes it especially useful in the emergency room. When a comatose patient is brought to the emergency department because of a drug overdose, the first goal is to support respiration and the second is to determine which drug was used. If an opioid is suspected, a specific test is used. Naloxone is administered intravenously, and if the overdose is a result of an opioid, the patient will respond in 2 to 3 minutes with improved respiration and will return to consciousness. Naloxone displaces the opioid from the

Table 32-3	**Opioid Antagonists**			
Generic Name	Trade Name	Administration/Dosage		Comments
nalmefene	Revex*	INTRAVENOUS, INTRAMUSCULAR, SUBCUTANEOUS: *Adults—For respiratory depression caused by narcotic overdose:* 0.5 mg/70 kg body weight; administer second dose of 1 mg/70 kg body weight if needed. Repeat in 2-5 minutes if necessary, up to 3 doses. *For narcotic depression of respiration after surgery:* 0.25 μg/kg body weight every 2-5 minutes as necessary. FDA pregnancy category B.		Pure narcotic antagonist used to reverse respiratory depression from narcotic overdose; produces no respiratory depression of its own.
naloxone hydrochloride	Narcan*	INTRAVENOUS, INTRAMUSCULAR, SUBCUTANEOUS: *Adults—For respiratory depression caused by narcotic overdose:* 0.4 mg. Repeat in 2-3 minutes if necessary, up to 3 doses. *For narcotic depression of respiration after surgery:* 0.1-0.2 mg every 2-3 minutes as necessary. FDA pregnancy category B. INTRAVENOUS: *Neonates*—0.01 mg/kg body weight.		Pure narcotic antagonist used to reverse respiratory depression from narcotic overdose; produces no respiratory depression of its own.
naltrexone	ReVia*	ORAL: *Adults*—Initial dose 25 mg. If there are no symptoms of withdrawal, rest of daily dose may be given. Usual daily dose is 50 mg, but it may also be administered as 100 mg every other day or 150 mg every third day. FDA pregnancy category C.		Adjunctive therapy for drug rehabilitation from opioids. Patients should have completed a withdrawal program and should be free of opioids for 7-10 days.

*Available in Canada and the United States.

receptor but produces no effect of its own. The result is a dramatic reversal of the drug overdose. The patient must still be monitored carefully, however, because naloxone has a short duration of action and its effect may wear off before the overdosed drug has been sufficiently eliminated. If the patient again becomes comatose, naloxone must be given again.

Multiple drug abuse is common, and naloxone reverses only the depression resulting from the opioid. Naloxone has no effect when the overdose is not caused by an opioid.

naltrexone

Naltrexone (ReVia) is an opioid antagonist. It has little pharmacologic activity but reverses opioid activity. Naltrexone is orally effective and long acting. It is prescribed for individuals detoxified of opioids. Because naltrexone blocks the effects of opioids, it is used in behavioral therapy to discourage resumption of opioid use. Naltrexone precipitates withdrawal symptoms when administered to an individual addicted to opioids.

Therapeutic Agents for Opioid Tolerance and Dependence

Drug Tolerance

Drug tolerance occurs when repeated use of a drug results in a lesser response unless the dosage is increased. Tolerance to the euphoric effect of the opioids develops rapidly. Individuals who abuse opioids keep increasing the dosage to maintain the good feeling associated with the drug. Patients who receive an opioid for severe pain over a limited period may also develop tolerance. Patients are unlikely to become drug dependent because as the pain subsides, so will the need and use of the drug. Tapering the dosage of the drug is usually sufficient for a patient to discontinue opioid therapy. However, individuals who abuse an opioid to achieve its euphoric effect increase the dosage and become drug dependent rapidly. Daily use of an opioid can produce drug dependence in 3 weeks. Little or no tolerance develops to the pupillary constriction or to the constipating effect of the opioids.

Drug Dependence

Drug dependence has complex psychologic and social components. In addition to the physical dependence produced by drug tolerance, there is a psychic dependence characterized by a continued desire or craving for the drug. Detoxification of addicted individuals is rarely sufficient to prevent relapse. Medications such as methadone may help in a drug rehabilitation program, but educational and psychosocial interventions are also needed (see Drug Abuse Alerts box).

Symptoms of Withdrawal Syndrome

Drug-dependent persons experience distinct physical reactions if the drug is suddenly discontinued. Opioid withdrawal syndrome after the sudden cessation of morphine or heroin use is predictable. The individual has a runny nose (rhinorrhea), gooseflesh (piloerection), tearing (lacrimation), sweating, and yawning 16 hours after the last dose. The pupils do not react readily to light. Over the next 20 hours the individual becomes restless, cannot sleep, and experiences muscle twitching. Hot and cold flashes and abdominal cramping occur. By 36 hours the individual feels nauseous, vomits, and has diarrhea. Withdrawal symptoms are generally the reverse of the drug effects described for the opioids. The body overcompensates when the drug is removed.

clonidine for Withdrawal Treatment

Clonidine is an antihypertensive drug that activates central alpha$_2$-adrenergic receptors (see Chapter 13). This activity reduces sympathetic overactivity. Because of this reduction in centrally mediated sympathetic activity, clonidine is useful in treating opioid withdrawal symptoms, reducing symptoms without producing a withdrawal syndrome.

methadone for Maintenance and Detoxification

In the United States the most widely used treatment for addiction to opioids is to substitute methadone, which can be given orally in a daily dose. Because tolerance already has developed to the "kick" from heroin in these individuals, the methadone maintains this tolerance while protecting against withdrawal symptoms. The goal of maintenance is to discourage the individual from continuing to seek drugs and to participate instead in rehabilitation programs. If detoxification (elimination of drug) is the goal, methadone is administered first when withdrawal symptoms appear, and then the dosage of methadone gradually is reduced to zero over 1 to 3 weeks. Because methadone has a long half-life in the body, the withdrawal symptoms are not as severe as with morphine or heroin.

DRUG ABUSE ALERTS

Heroin and Other Opioids

BACKGROUND
Heroin and other opioids are abused to achieve euphoria. Once self-administered only by intravenous injection, heroin is now also self-administered by sniffing/snorting or smoking.

PHARMACOLOGY
Heroin is an illegal opioid in the United States and Canada. Side effects include restlessness, vomiting, and drowsiness.

HEALTH HAZARDS
Heroin causes a high degree of physical and psychologic dependence. An overdose produces slow, shallow breathing, clammy skin, convulsions, and coma. Death can result. Withdrawal symptoms include nausea, cramps, chills and sweating, panic, tremors, irritability, and loss of appetite. Repeated injections may lead to infection of heart tissues, skin abscesses, and congested lungs.

Because of needle and syringe sharing, intravenous drug abuse is associated with a high incidence of transmission of human immunodeficiency virus (HIV) and has become a major risk factor for contracting acquired immunodeficiency syndrome (AIDS).

Nursing Process Overview

Opioids

Assessment

Assess the history, nature, and location of pain. Use an objective tool such as a visual analog scale or a numerical rating such as 1 to 10, with 1 representing mild pain and 10 representing the worst possible pain. Include objective data on the patients position, facial expression, medical history, vital signs, and age. Perform a brief neurologic examination. Pay close attention to the subjective complaints of pain.

Nursing Diagnoses

- Altered bowel elimination: constipation as drug side effect
- Altered comfort: nausea and vomiting as drug side effect
- Altered thought processes related to drug side effect

Patient Outcomes

The patient will have regular bowel elimination. The patient's nausea and vomiting will resolve. The patient's drug regimen will be manipulated until the patient's mentation is not clouded by the medications.

Planning/Implementation

Regular use of opioids at identified intervals usually provides better relief of pain than use on a prn (as-needed) basis. No patient who needs medication for pain should be denied it, but augment medication use with nursing care measures to promote comfort, including positioning, distracting, and touching the patient, and introducing relaxation techniques. Monitor vital signs, level of consciousness, and frequency of bowel movements; check for nausea, vomiting, and urinary retention. Some side effects necessitate discontinuing therapy, decreasing the dosage, or using additional kinds of treatments. Have opioid antagonists available. If antiemetics or other drugs are ordered, monitor side effects; also check compatibilities before administering two or more drugs in the same syringe. Use a microdrip administration set and an infusion monitoring device for constant IV infusion.

Evaluation

Before discharge, verify that the patient can explain the name and dose of drugs to be taken, the possible side effects and how to treat them, the signs indicating too large a dose, what to do if the pain worsens, and what drugs to avoid. Determine that the patient knows to avoid alcohol while taking these drugs.

Nursing Implications Summary

Opioids

Drug Administration

➤ Analgesics, especially opioids, constitute one of the most useful classes of medications because they permit individuals to tolerate short- and long-term pain and thus tolerate surgery and trauma and perhaps to face death more peacefully. Failure of the health care team members to be knowledgeable about adequate drug doses, frequency of drug administration, and choice of appropriate medication results in patients receiving inadequate treatment for pain.

➤ Assess the patient thoughtfully before administering pain medication. If the decision is made to use an opioid, use adequate doses and administer often enough to maintain a therapeutic blood level of medication. Administer medications 30 to 60 minutes before painful activities such as dressing changes, physical therapy, and whirlpool.

➤ Although opioids are useful, they should be used as adjuncts to other nursing measures such as massage, distraction, deep breathing and relaxation exercises, application of heat or cold, or just being there to provide care and comfort. Include effective nursing measures in the nursing care plan, and keep the care plan updated.

➤ Monitor respiratory rate as an indicator of CNS depression. If the rate is less than 12 breaths/min in an adult, with-

hold additional doses unless ventilatory support is being provided.

➤ Monitor pulse. If bradycardia develops (pulse less than 60 beats/min in an adult or 110 beats/min in an infant), withhold the dose and notify the physician.

➤ Monitor blood pressure. Hypotension is more common in older adults, the immobilized, and patients receiving other medications that have hypotension as a side effect. It may also be a sign of sepsis or shock.

➤ Auscultate breath sounds every 2 to 4 hours. Because opioids suppress the cough reflex, continue activities to prevent atelectasis and pneumonia, such as turning, deep breathing, and incentive spirometry.

➤ Have opioid antagonists, oxygen, and resuscitation equipment available in settings in which opioids are administered.

➤ Monitor level of consciousness and mental status. Evaluate findings carefully. For example, restlessness may be caused by pain, hypoxia, shock, or an unusual reaction to the analgesic.

➤ Keep siderails up, keep a night-light on, supervise ambulation, and discourage smoking.

➤ Monitor intake and output and weight. If nausea and vomiting occur, a switch to another analgesic may be appropriate; consult the physician. If nausea occurs, it may be

Continued

Nursing Implications Summary—cont'd

appropriate to administer an antiemetic concomitantly with the opioid. The peak and duration of many antiemetics may be at a different time from that of the opioid; if so, the drugs should be on a different dosing schedule. In addition, antiemetics may potentiate CNS depression, but they do not potentiate analgesic effects. Sedation and hypotension may be pronounced.

➤ Assess for urinary retention. It may be more pronounced in older adult patients, the immobilized, and men with preexisting prostatic hypertrophy. Question the patient about difficulty in voiding, pain in the bladder area, or sensations of inadequate bladder emptying. Palpate the bladder for distension. Suggest that the patient void before each dose of opioid.

➤ Although the theoretic possibility of opioid addiction exists for all patients who receive opioids, only a very small percentage of them become dependent. Patients who persist in requesting frequent or large doses of pain medication beyond the average time postoperatively should not be automatically characterized as becoming addicted. Pain is a warning signal, and its unexpected persistence should be investigated.

➤ Some postoperative patients fear requesting any medication for pain because they fear addiction. Reassure the patient that the use of opioids in decreasing amounts over a typical postoperative course will not cause addiction and that recovery will be easier if the pain is reduced.

➤ Use of aspirin, acetaminophen, or an NSAID along with opioids may increase pain relief. Consult the physician.

➤ Record carefully the patient's response to pain and the response to opioid administration.

➤ Check the physician's orders carefully. Note that some drugs are available in short-acting formulations and extended-release formulations. Do not interchange these without an adjustment of the dosage. Observe agency policy regarding expiration date of controlled substances.

➤ In addition to the standard oral, IM, IV, and SC routes, opioids may be administered via the intrathecal or intraspinal route, with patient-controlled analgesia (PCA) devices and with implanted pumps. Become familiar with the equipment in use. Consult the current literature for additional information. Review the manufacturer's directions and patient instruction information. Ascertain that the patient understands the advantages and uses of the various routes and equipment being used.

➤ For PCA use, the initial loading dose, continuous rate of infusion, patient self-administered dose, lock-out interval, and total doses per hour must be ordered by the physician.

➤ Transdermal dosage forms are now available for some drugs (see Fentanyl in Chapter 36). This route is not appropriate for relief of acute pain. See the manufacturer's insert.

➤ Use preservative-free morphine for intrathecal and intraspinal or epidural use.

➤ Dilute doses of meperidine syrup in at least a half a glass of water. When taken undiluted, it may cause temporary mucous membrane anesthesia.

➤ Dilute doses of methadone oral concentrate with water to a volume of at least 30 ml for treatment of chronic pain, and to a volume of 90 ml in treatment of opioid addiction. Dilute dispersible tablets in at least 120 ml of water, orange juice, citrus flavor (Tang brand) drink, or other acidic fruit beverage. Complete dispersion occurs in about 1 minute.

➤ For continuous infusion, use microdrip tubing and an infusion-controlling device to keep the rate of administration steady.

➤ PCA and epidural analgesia are discussed in Chapter 34.

Intravenous butorphanol
➤ May be given undiluted. Administer at a rate of 2 mg or less over 3 to 5 minutes.

Intravenous dezocine
➤ May be given undiluted. Administer at a rate of 5 mg over 2 to 3 minutes.

Intravenous hydromorphone
➤ Dilute dose with 5 ml of sterile water or normal saline solution for injection. Administer at a rate of 2 mg or less over 3 to 5 minutes. May be further diluted and administered as a constant infusion and may be titrated to degree of pain relief and respiratory rate.

Intravenous levorphanol
➤ Dilute dose with 5 ml of sterile water or normal saline for injection. Administer at a rate of 2 mg or less over 4 to 5 minutes.

Intravenous meperidine
➤ Must be diluted. Dilute in at least 5 ml of sterile water or normal saline for injection. Administer dose over 4 to 5 minutes. For infusion in an opioid syringe infuser system, dilute each 10 mg in at least 1 ml compatible IV fluid. May be further diluted in normal saline, D5W, D5NS, or other compatible solution for constant infusion. May also be diluted to 1 mg/ml and given as a constant infusion under the observation of an anesthesiologist.

Intravenous morphine sulfate
➤ Dose should be diluted in at least 5 ml of sterile water or normal saline, or other IV solutions, for injection. Administer at a rate of 15 mg or less over 4 to 5 minutes (direct injection). May also be diluted for infusion.

Intravenous nalbuphine
➤ May be given undiluted. Administer 10 mg or less over 3 to 5 minutes.

Intravenous oxymorphone
➤ Dilute dose with 5 ml of sterile water or normal saline for injection. Administer dose over 2 to 5 minutes.

Intravenous pentazocine
➤ May be given undiluted, but dilution is preferable. Dilute each 5 mg with at least 1 ml of sterile water for injection. Administer 5 mg or less over 1 minute.

Nursing in the Community
➤ Review the anticipated benefits and possible side effects of drug therapy. Encourage the patient to phone with any questions that arise.

Nursing Implications Summary—cont'd

➤ Review the Patient Problems boxes on constipation (Chapter 24), dry mouth (Chapter 23), and orthostatic hypotension (Chapter 13). With regular use of most opioids, constipation will develop, and the physician may prescribe stool softeners to help prevent it.

➤ Patients should take oral doses with milk or a snack to reduce gastric irritation.

➤ If the patient is to self-administer via injection, infusion, transdermal patch, or other route, teach the administration technique and have the patient give a return demonstration.

➤ Instruct the patient to avoid drinking alcoholic beverages while taking opioids.

➤ Teach the patient to avoid the use of other medications that may also cause CNS depression, such as barbiturates, antiemetics, antihistamines, or tranquilizers, unless first approved by the physician.

➤ Warn the patient to avoid driving or operating hazardous equipment if dizzy or drowsy.

➤ If a combination drug product has been prescribed, review the side effects associated with each of the drugs in the combined product.

➤ Remind the patient to keep these and all medications out of the reach of children. Accidental overdose with opioids in children may quickly lead to death.

➤ Remind patients to keep all health care providers informed of all medications being used.

Opioid Antagonist: nalmefene and naloxone

Drug Administration

➤ Monitor blood pressure, pulse, and respiratory rate every 5 minutes initially, tapering to every 15 minutes, then every 30 minutes until stable. Attach acutely ill or comatose patients to electrocardiogram (ECG) monitor. Have a suction machine available.

➤ Auscultate breath sounds. If respiratory symptoms are severe or persistent, notify the physician.

➤ Monitor intake and output; auscultate bowel sounds.

➤ Have drugs, equipment, and personnel available for resuscitation if needed. Do not leave the patient unattended until stable.

➤ Continue to monitor the patient closely for several hours after initial treatment because the effects of the opioid antagonist may wear off before the effects of the opioid wear off, causing the patient to again display signs of opioid overdose.

➤ These drugs are rarely used outside of the acute-care setting. Keep patient and family informed of the patient's condition, as appropriate.

Intravenous nalmefene

➤ Available in two dilutions. Blue label form contains 100 μg/ml and is used primarily for reversing postoperative narcotic depression. Green label form contains 1.0 mg/ml and is used primarily to reverse suspected narcotic overdose. May be given undiluted, but a 1:1 dilution with normal saline or sterile water is recommended, especially in patients with an increased risk of cardiovascular complications. Administer initial dose over 15 to 30 seconds. Extend time in patients with renal failure

Intravenous naloxone

➤ May be given undiluted, diluted with sterile water for injection, or diluted for infusion with NS or D5NS or D5W. Administer at a rate of 0.4 mg over 15 seconds. Infusion is usually titrated to patient response. In neonates the dose may be given via the umbilical vein.

Opioid Antagonist: naltrexone

Drug Administration

➤ Assess for CNS effects. It may be difficult to differentiate between effects caused by naltrexone and those caused by the emotional effect of opioid withdrawal. If insomnia is present, administer doses in the morning.

➤ Obtain baseline measurement of blood pressure, pulse, and ECG tracing, then monitor pulse and blood pressure daily, tapering to monthly if no abnormalities are noted.

➤ Monitor bowel sounds and keep a record of bowel movements. If abdominal discomfort is severe or persistent, notify the physician.

➤ Monitor respiratory rate and auscultate breath sounds. If respiratory symptoms are severe or persistent, notify the physician.

➤ Inspect for rash.

➤ Monitor liver function tests.

➤ Naltrexone therapy should not be initiated until the patient has completed detoxification and has been free of opioids for 7 to 10 days.

➤ Before administering oral naltrexone, the patient may be given a naloxone challenge test. In this test an SC or IV dose of naloxone is administered, and the patient then is observed for signs of opiate withdrawal, including nasal stuffiness, rhinorrhea, tearing, sweating, tremor, abdominal cramps, vomiting, goose flesh, and myalgia. If symptoms of withdrawal appear, the patient is not sufficiently drug free to begin naltrexone therapy. The challenge test may be repeated daily until the patient is opiate free.

➤ Monitor the patient carefully for at least 1 hour after the first dose of naltrexone for withdrawal symptoms.

➤ Naltrexone should be used only as a component of a medically supervised behavior modification program designed to help the patient maintain an opioid-free state.

Nursing in the Community

➤ Review with the patient the anticipated benefits and possible side effects of therapy. Instruct the patient to report unexpected side effects.

➤ Emphasize the importance of returning to the physician for follow-up visits and the importance of other aspects of treatment, including individual therapy and support groups.

➤ Tell the patient to take oral doses with meals or a snack to lessen gastric irritation.

Continued

Nursing Implications Summary—cont'd

➤ Review with the patient the need to avoid ingestion of opioids via any route of administration while taking naltrexone; this may include antidiarrheal medications and cough syrups. Also instruct patients not to try to overcome the effects of naltrexone by taking narcotics. Finally, instruct patients that naltrexone will not reverse the effects of alcohol, so it should not be used to try to improve ability to drive or perform other potentially dangerous activities while under the influence of alcohol.

➤ Remind patients to inform all health care providers of all medications they are taking, including naltrexone. Instruct patients not to share naltrexone with others.

➤ Instruct patients to wear a medical identification tag or bracelet indicating they are receiving naltrexone.

➤ There are a variety of treatment regimens for this drug. Have the patient discuss with the physician what to do about missed doses.

CHAPTER REVIEW

Application

1. What are the two components of pain? Which is affected by opioids?
2. Which diseases are associated with chronic pain that the nurse might administer opioids to treat?
3. What are endorphins, enkephalins, and dynorphins? Which actions do enkephalins mediate?
4. What are the three characteristics of the analgesia produced by morphine?
5. What are the three major actions of morphine in the medulla?
6. What actions does morphine have on tissues outside the CNS?
7. What five common adverse reactions to morphine should you monitor?
8. What opioids might you administer to relieve severe pain?
9. What opioids might you administer to relieve moderate to severe pain?
10. What opioids are used to relieve mild pain?
11. Which opioids have antagonist and agonist activity?
12. Which opioids are significant in treating pulmonary edema? pain of a heart attack?

Critical Thinking

1. Why is naloxone a good drug for treating acute opioid toxicity?
2. What properties of methadone make it useful for maintaining or withdrawing from opioid dependence?
3. What role do opioids have in anesthesia?

References

Barber D: The physiology and pharmacology of pain: a review of opioids, *J Perianesth Nurs* 12(2):95, 1997.

Lay TD, et al: Analgesics prescribed and administered to intensive care cardiac surgery patients: does patient age make a difference? *Prog Cardiovasc Nurs* 11(4):17-24, 1996.

Puntillo K, Casella V, Reid M: Opioid and benzodiazepine tolerance and dependence: application of theory to critical care practice, *Heart Lung J Acute Crit Care* 26(4):317, 1997.

Skobel SW: Epidural narcotic administration: what nurses should know, *Oncol Nurs Forum* 23(10):1555-1562, 1996.

Willliams C: Patient-controlled analgesia: a review of the literature, *J Clin Nurs* 5(3):139-147, 1996.

Chapter 33

Drugs to Treat Headaches

OBJECTIVES

After studying this chapter, you should be able to do the following:

- *Describe chronic tension, migraine, and cluster headaches.*
- *Identify lifestyle factors that may contribute to the development of headaches.*
- *Explain the rationale for using analgesic combinations, ergot-containing drugs, triptans, and methysergide in treating headaches.*
- *Develop a nursing care plan for a patient experiencing a headache.*

KEY TERMS

chronic tension headaches, p. 395
classic migraine, p. 396
cluster headache, p. 396
common migraine, p. 396

KEY DRUG ▼

sumatriptan, p. 399

CHAPTER OVERVIEW

A headache is a common type of pain. It is estimated that 40% of individuals experience a severe headache at least annually. Common headaches are often associated with stress and anxiety. Patients commonly self-treat these headaches and seek medical attention only if this tension-type headache becomes chronic.

Headaches that are severe or disabling require medical assessment. In about 10% of cases, a severe or chronic headache is a symptom of a serious illness such as a brain tumor, glaucoma, or giant cell arteritis. These headaches are secondary headaches, symptoms of a primary disorder. More commonly, headaches are the primary problem. The two principal varieties of primary headaches that are severe and recurring are migraine and cluster headaches.

This chapter presents drugs to treat severe migraine and cluster headaches. Common tension headaches are commonly relieved by relaxation and a mild analgesic such as acetaminophen, aspirin, ibuprofen, or naproxen, as discussed in Chapter 31.

THERAPEUTIC RATIONALE: HEADACHE

The International Headache Society has classified 129 different types of headache. Practically, most headaches for which patients seek medical help are one of three types: chronic tension headache, migraine, or cluster headache. Each of these three types are briefly described.

A tension headache can be occasional or chronic. The pain is commonly a throbbing, tight pain felt in the front part of the head, especially around the eyes, and lasts a half-hour or more. Most patients self-treat a tension headache with an over-the-counter analgesic such as acetaminophen, aspirin, ibuprofen, or naproxen. These drugs are discussed in

Chapter 31. People with tension headaches may seek medical help if the headaches last for many days and/or recur frequently (**chronic tension headaches**). These headaches are often associated with fatigue, stress, or excessive use of tobacco or alcohol. The treatment should emphasize lifestyle changes. Biofeedback training may be helpful for those needing help with stress management.

Migraine is a clinical classification for a periodic headache that lasts from 4 to 24 hours. The pain is on one side of the head and can be nondescript and throbbing or a severe stabbing pain. Nausea and vomiting are common, as is sensitivity to light, scalp tenderness, and light-headedness. Dark surroundings and sleep can bring some relief.

About 8 million Americans experience recurrent migraines. Attacks are commonly associated with specific stimuli, such as odors and foods. The **classic migraine** is associated with an aura that may precede the headache by several minutes to an hour. Usually the aura is visual, but the aura may be any sensory or motor symptom. Migraine without an aura is called **common migraine** and accounts for about 80% of migraine cases. Migraines occur at all ages, but commonly begin before the age of 40 years, with the highest incidence being in children and young adults. Seventy-five percent of migraine sufferers are women. The attacks may be related to the menstrual cycle and commonly stop during last trimester of pregnancy.

Each patient with migraine tends to have a characteristic pattern for the onset and duration of the migraine. A migraine is currently seen as the outcome of a complex series of events in the brain. The first phase involves the brainstem, which, after some unknown trigger, generates alterations in cerebral blood flow. This leads to a second phase in which arteries on the inside and outside of the brain contract or dilate. Blood flow studies indicate that the initial change is a modest decrease in blood flow. The third phase of a migraine is activation of the cells that process pain in the head and face (medullary trigeminal nucleus caudalis). Vasoactive peptides are released and produce swelling through dilation of blood vessels.

A **cluster headache** begins suddenly, reaching a peak in a few minutes and persisting for 30 to 120 minutes. The pain is described as sharp, boring, and excruciatingly severe. Pain is clustered on one side of the head around the eye, with lacrimation, eyelid drop, runny nose, congestion, and facial sweating. The common pattern is for one to three attacks per day to occur for a 4- to 8-week duration, followed by a year's remission. However, the pattern may be chronic. Attacks tend to come at the same time each day, and the time set may be during the day or at night while sleeping. Men between the ages of 20 and 50 years are the most commonly affected. Alcohol is commonly a precipitating factor in launching a bout of cluster headaches.

THERAPEUTIC AGENTS: DRUGS TO TREAT HEADACHES

Drug development for the treatment of severe migraine headaches focuses on the key role of the neurotransmitter serotonin. A current view of migraine is that it represents a hereditary perturbation of serotonergic neurotransmission. There are at least four main families of serotonin receptors and each receptor family has several subtypes. Serotonin receptor types 1A and 1D are found in the areas of the brain believed involved in migraine attacks. These are autoreceptors on the neurons releasing serotonin. When these autoreceptors are stimulated, serotonin is not released. Ergotamine and the triptans, drugs that can stop a migraine and are also effective for cluster headaches, act on these 1A and 1D receptors. The presumption is that the decrease in synaptic serotonin concentration resulting from this drug action is a key mechanism in aborting the migraine attack.

Treatment of migraines is divided into two phases: acute treatment and prophylactic treatment. Treatment of the acute attack seeks to stop or at least ameliorate the attack. Analgesics are used in the treatment of mild to moderate migraines as well as patients with tension headaches. Severe migraine may be treated with ergotamine or one of the new triptans. An antiemetic is often administered to counteract both the nausea of the headache as well as the nausea caused by ergotamine. Promethazine (Phenergan), prochlorperazine (Compazine), and metoclopramide (Reglan) are the antiemetics most commonly used (see Chapter 25). Patients with severe migraines often benefit from prophylactic treatment with one of a number of drugs.

Treatment of cluster headaches is also divided into acute treatment and prophylactic treatment. Because a cluster headache has a sudden and explosive onset, acute treatment is difficult. Sublingual ergotamine or parenteral dihydroergotamine may be useful. Subcutaneous sumatriptan may also be effective, but often the doses needed are above those recommended. Inhalation of 100% oxygen (7 to 9 L/min) for 15- to 20-minute periods with a 5-minute rest between periods may be helpful. The patient should be seated and leaning forward. Prophylactic treatment of cluster headaches begins with avoidance of alcohol and smoking. A number of medications, including lithium, prednisone, ergotamine, and divalproex sodium, can be tried as prophylactic agents.

Analgesics for Migraine

acetaminophen, aspirin, and Nonsteroidal Antiinflammatory Drugs

Patients with mild to moderate migraines usually respond to acetaminophen, aspirin, or one of the nonsteroidal antiinflammatory drugs (NSAIDs), especially an analgesic formulated with caffeine and the sedative butalbital. The mild nausea common to migraine is treated with an antiemetic. The analgesics used to treat migraine are listed in Table 33-1. These drugs are discussed more completely in Chapter 25 (Antiemetics), Chapter 31 (Aspirin, Acetaminophen, NSAIDs, and Drugs for Treating Gout), and Chapter 32 (Opioids).

butorphanol

Butorphanol (Stadol) is an opioid administered either by intramuscular (IM) injection or by nasal inhalation (see Chapter 32). It can provide rapid relief of migraine pain not controlled by other medications. Butorphanol is now a controlled substance. Reports of abuse have become more common since the nasal spray form became available in 1992.

lidocaine hydrochloride

Lidocaine (Xylocaine) is a local anesthetic (see Chapter 35). Administered as nosedrops, lidocaine can often bring quick relief to a cluster headache. Recent studies indicate that lidocaine may also be useful in treating acute migraines.

Table 33-1   Analgesic Combinations Used to Treat Headaches

Trade Name	Constituents/Dosage	Administration/Dosage	Comments
Aspirin Free Excedrin Bayer Select Maximum Strength Headache Pain Relief	acetaminophen 500 mg caffeine 65 mg	ORAL: *Adults*—1 tablet every 4-6 hr as needed; maximum daily dose acetaminophen: 4 g/day (short term) or 2.6 g/day (long term).	Chronic use can lead to caffeine dependence. Caution patients not to drink alcohol with acetaminophen (increased risk of liver damage).
Extra Strength Excedrin Others	acetaminophen 250 mg aspirin 250 mg caffeine 65 mg	ORAL: *Adults*—1 tablet every 4-6 hr as needed; maximum daily dose aspirin and acetaminophen: 4 g/day (short term) or 2.6 g/day (long term).	Chronic use can lead to caffeine dependence. Caution patients not to drink alcohol with acetaminophen (increased risk of liver damage) or aspirin (gastric damage)
Phrenilin Sedapap	acetaminophen 325 mg butalbital 50 mg	ORAL: *Adults*—1 or 2 tablets every 4 hr as needed, not to exceed 6 tablets/day.	Frequent use can lead to abuse and to rebound headaches when the medication is discontinued.
Esgic Fioricet Others	acetaminophen 325 mg butalbital 50 mg caffeine 40 mg	ORAL: *Adults*—1 or 2 tablets every 4 hr as needed, not to exceed 6 tablets/day.	Frequent use can lead to abuse and to rebound headaches when the medication is discontinued.
Fioricet with Codeine	acetamiophen 325 mg butalbital 50 mg caffeine 40 mg codeine phosphate 30 mg	ORAL: *Adults*—1-2 capsules every 4 hr as needed, not to exceed 6 capsules/day.	Frequent use can lead to abuse and to rebound headaches when the medication is discontinued.
Norgesic Others	orphenadrine citrate 25 mg aspirin 385 mg caffeine 30 mg	ORAL: *Adults*—1 or 2 tablets 3-4 times/day.	Orphenadrine is a skeletal muscle relaxant. Caution patients to avoid alcohol and other central nervous system depressants.
Midrin Migrex Others	acetaminophen 325 mg dichloralphenazone 100 mg isometheptene mucate 65 mg	ORAL: *Adults*—1 or 2 capsules every 4 hr as needed, up to 8 capsules/day.	Isometheptene is an indirect-acting sympathometic vasoconstrictor. Dichloralphenazone is a mild sedative and relaxant.
Darvocet N50 Darvocet N100	propoxyphene napsylate 50, 100 mg acetaminophen 325, 650 mg	ORAL: *Adults*—1 tablet every 4 hr as needed.	Propoxyphene is an opioid (schedule IV).
Darvon Compound 65	propoxyphene hydrochloride 65 mg aspirin 389 mg caffeine 32.4 mg	ORAL: *Adults*—1 capsule every 4 hr as needed, up to 8 capsules/day.	Propoxyphene is an opioid (schedule IV).
Vicodin	hydrocodone bitartrate 5 mg acetaminophen 325 mg	ORAL: *Adults*—1 or 2 tablets every 4-6 hr as needed, up to 8 tablets/day.	Hydrocodone is an opioid.
Endocet* Oxycocet† Percocet* Roxicet*	oxycodone hydrochloride 5 mg acetaminophen 325 mg	ORAL: *Adults*—1 tablet every 4-6 hr as needed.	Oxycodone is an opioid (schedule II).
Endodan* Oxycodan† Percodan* Roxiprin*	oxycodone hydrochloride 4.5 mg oxycodone terephthalate 0.38 mg aspirin 325 mg	ORAL: *Adults*—1 or 2 tablets every 4-6 hr as needed.	Oxycodone is an opioid (schedule II).

NOTE: Drugs are listed in increasing order of analgesia.
*Available in Canada and the United States.
†Available in Canada only.

Ergot Derivatives: dihydroergotamine (D.H.E. 45), ergotamine (Ergostat, Ergomar)

Mechanism of Action

Ergot derivatives have both agonistic and antagonistic activity for alpha-adrenergic, serotonergic, and dopaminergic receptors. The mechanism underlying the effectiveness of ergot derivatives in treating an acute migraine or cluster headaches is to decrease firing of serotonergic neurons. Two classes of serotonergic receptors are involved. Ergot derivatives activate the serotonin 1D receptors. Activation of these presynaptic autoreceptors on specific brain neurons prevents the release of serotonin. The prophylactic mechanism is believed to be antagonist activity at the serotonin 2 receptors. The serotonin 2 receptors are postsynaptic and their blockade prevents excitation of the postsynaptic cell by serotonin. These drugs are listed in Table 33-2.

Pharmacokinetics

Dihydroergotamine is administered parenterally and is well absorbed. A nasal spray is also available. Dihydroergotamine is extensively metabolized by the liver, and the primary metabolite is pharmacologically active. Metabolites are excreted primarily in the feces. Relief of the headache is achieved in 15 minutes to 2 hours.

Table 33-2   Drugs to Treat Severe Headaches

Generic Name	Trade Name	Administration/Dosage	Comments
Ergot-Containing Drugs			
dihydroergotamine mesylate	D.H.E. 45	INTRAMUSCULAR, SUBCUTANEOUS: *Adults*—1 mg at the start of an attack. May repeat in 1 hr if needed. Maximum daily dose: 3 mg. INTRAVENOUS: *Adults*—0.5 mg at the start of an attack. Given with an antiemetic. May repeat in 1 hr if needed. Maximum daily dose: 2 mg.	Has less arterial vasoconstrictive action than ergotamine.
	Migranal*	INHALATION: *Adults*—1 spray in each nostril; repeat in 15 min if needed.	New spray form must be prepared as needed and discarded after use.
ergotamine tartrate	Ergostat Ergomar† Gynergen† Medihaler Ergotamine†	ORAL,† SUBLINGUAL: *Adults*—1-2 mg at the start of an attack, repeated at 30-min intervals if needed. Maximum daily dose: 6 mg. INHALATION†: 1 metered spray at the start of an attack, repeated at intervals of at least 5 min, up to 6 metered sprays daily. FDA pregnancy category X.	Oral preparation without caffeine has a slower onset of action.
ergotamine tartrate with caffeine	Cafergot* Wigraine Others	ORAL: *Adults—For migraine:* 1-2 mg at the start of an attack, repeated at 30-min intervals if needed. Maximum daily dose: 6 mg ergotamine. *Children 6-12 yr*—1 mg initially, repeated up to 2 times. Maximum daily dose: 3 mg ergotamine. *For cluster headache:* 1-2 mg 1-3 times/day, 1-2 hr before the time attacks usually occur. *For nighttime attacks:* 1-2 mg 1-2 hr before bedtime. RECTAL: *Adults*—¼-1 suppository initially, repeated at 30-min intervals if needed. Maximum daily dose: 2 suppositories (4 mg ergotamine). *Children 6-12 yr*—¼-½ suppository at the start of an attack. Maximum daily dose: ½ suppository (1 mg ergotamine). FDA pregnancy category X.	To reduce the risk of dependence on ergotamine, use not more than 2 times/wk, preferably 5 days apart.
ergotamine tartrate with caffeine, belladonna†	Wigraine†	ORAL: *Adults—For migraine or cluster:* 1-2 mg at the start of an attack, repeated at 30-min intervals if needed. Maximum daily dose: 6 mg ergotamine. *Children 6-12 yr*—1 mg initially, repeated up to 2 times. Maximum daily dose: 3 mg ergotamine.	To reduce the risk of dependence on ergotamine, use not more than 2 times/wk, preferably 5 days apart.
Triptans			
naratriptan hydrochloride	Amerge	ORAL: *Adults*—1-2.5 mg as a single dose. May take a second dose after 4 hr if only partial response.	New antimigraine drug like sumatriptan.
rizatriptan benzoate	Maxalt Maxalt-MLT	ORAL: *Adults*—5 or 10 mg as a single dose. May take an additional dose 2 hr later. Maximum daily dose: 30 mg.	New antimigraine drug like sumatriptan. MLT formulation is mint-flavored and dissolves rapidly in the mouth.
sumatriptan	Imitrex	ORAL: *Adults*—100 mg. If there is a beneficial response in 4 hr, may repeat if the pain returns or increases in severity. Maximum daily dose: 300 mg. SUBCUTANEOUS: *Adults*—6 mg. If there is a beneficial response in 1-2 hr, may repeat if the pain returns or becomes more severe. Maximum daily dose: 12 mg.	Should not administer within 24 hr after ergotamine because of the risk of severe vasoconstriction. Should be administered only after headache pain begins. If the first dose is not effective, do not administer additional doses.
zolmitriptan	Zomig*	ORAL: *Adults*—2.5 mg or lower. May repeat in 2 hr if needed, up to 10 mg in 24 hr. FDA pregnancy category C.	New antimigraine drug like sumatriptan.
Serotonin Antagonist			
methysergide	Sansert*	ORAL: *Adults*—4-6 mg/day in divided doses.	Prophylactic treatment for migraine and cluster headaches.

*Available in Canada and the United States.
†Available in Canada only.

Ergotamine is administered orally but is poorly absorbed. There is considerable patient variation, in part because migraines are often accompanied by a sluggish gastric motility. Caffeine increases the rate and extent of absorption. Without caffeine, the onset of action is about 2 hours, but with caffeine the onset of headache relief is reduced to about 1 hour. Another additive can be metoclopramide, which stimulates gastrointestinal motility and thereby increases ergotamine absorption. Metoclopramide also has an antiemetic action.

Ergotamine and caffeine may also be administered rectally, a route that has more extensive absorption and produces less nausea. The onset of action is about 60 minutes. Sublingual ergotamine is slowly absorbed.

Like dihydroergotamine, ergotamine is extensively metabolized by the liver and excreted in the feces.

Uses

Dihydroergotamine is available for parenteral administration only. It is used to treat acute, severe migraine or chronic headache associated with dependence on ergotamine or analgesics.

Ergotamine is administered orally for the treatment of acute migraine or prophylactic treatment of cluster headaches. In addition to being formulated with caffeine to speed absorption, different Canadian formulations include the anticholinergic belladonna, the sedative pentobarbital, or an antihistamine such as cyclizine, dimenhydrinate, or diphenhydramine.

Adverse Reactions and Contraindications

The major side effects of ergot derivatives are nausea and vasoconstriction. The antiemetic metoclopramide is commonly given 20 to 30 minutes before administration of dihydroergotamine to minimize nausea. Some preparations of ergotamine are formulated with an antiemetic such as belladonna alkaloids, cyclizine, dimenhydrinate, or diphenhydramine.

The vasoconstrictive action of the ergot derivatives can lead to transiently cold fingers and toes, often accompanied by tingling or numbness. Dihydroergotamine produces less vasoconstriction than ergotamine.

Use of ergot derivatives is contraindicated during pregnancy because these agents stimulate the uterus. Ergotamine is a potent uterine stimulant. Also, the reduced uterine blood flow may be harmful to the fetus. Ergot derivatives are distributed into breast milk and can produce adverse effects in the infant, including vomiting, diarrhea, unstable blood pressure, and seizures.

Medical conditions that may be aggravated by ergot derivatives include coronary artery disease, hypertension, peripheral vascular disease, and impaired renal function. Patients with angina are at risk, and nitroglycerin is less effective as a vasodilator. Patients with impaired liver function may not metabolize the drug readily leading to toxicity.

Toxicity

The classic toxicity associated with ergot alkaloids is ergotism, called St. Anthony's fire in the middle ages. Ergot alkaloids are produced by a fungus, *Claviceps purpurea,* that flourishes in damp grains, especially rye. Epidemics of ergotism from contaminated grain are part of recorded history. Symptoms included hallucinations, fiery pain, prolonged vasoconstriction leading to gangrene, miscarriages, and seizures. Ergotamine poisoning from medicinal use can occur. Severe vasoconstriction can be treated with nitroprusside infusion until the ergotamine is eliminated by the body.

Interactions

Drugs that have a vasoconstrictor action are contraindicated. These drugs include cocaine, epinephrine, metaraminol, methoxamine, norepinephrine, and phenylephrine. Smoking increases the risk of vasoconstrictive side effects.

Triptans

Sumatriptan (Imitrex) is the first commercially available drug of a new class of serotonergic drugs called the triptans. Naratriptan (Amerge), rizatriptan (Maxalt), and zolmitriptan (Zomig) are now in the U.S. market and other new drugs in this class are anticipated.

Mechanism of Action

Triptans stimulate the serotonin 1D receptor. Stimulation of this presynaptic receptor causes vasoconstriction of cerebral blood vessels and inhibits the release of pain-producing inflammatory neuropeptides.

Pharmacokinetics

Sumatriptan is rapidly absorbed after oral or subcutaneous administration. However, the bioavailability is low after oral administration because of first-pass metabolism by the liver as well as by incomplete absorption. Although sumatriptan is widely distributed in the body, passage through the blood-brain barrier is low. Naratriptan and zomitriptan are administered orally to abort a migraine.

The onset of action for migraine relief is 10 minutes after subcutaneous administration and 30 minutes after oral administration. The duration of action is 24 to 48 hours. Sumatriptan is extensively metabolized by the liver and excreted in the urine.

Uses

Sumatriptan has become the drug of choice for relief of acute migraine headaches. It is not for prophylactic or chronic treatment. However, because many patients know when a migraine is starting, an injection of sumatriptan or oral dose of any triptan can abort the acute attack. The use of sumatriptan in aborting attacks of cluster headache has not been established.

Adverse Reactions and Contraindications

Triptans commonly produce only mild and transient side effects, namely nausea, malaise, dizziness, and weakness. However, these are also symptoms of the migraine itself. A tingling sensation may be noted.

The major concern is the vasoconstriction caused by triptans. Patients are screened for active or potential underlying cardiovascular disease, including angina, hypertension, diabetes, obesity, and smoking. The first dose of sumatriptan is given subcutaneously under medical supervision to monitor for unexpected cardiovascular response. All patients on triptans are monitored for cardiovascular changes during therapy.

The risk of triptans to pregnancy is unknown. Overdoses of triptans have not been described.

Interactions

Triptans should not be administered within 24 hours of dihydroergotamine or ergotamine because of the risk of severe vasoconstriction.

Serotonic Antagonist: methysergide

Mechanism of Action

Methysergide (Sansert) is a serotonin antagonist. The inhibition of serotonin at postsynaptic receptors is believed to account for the mechanism of action.

Pharmacokinetics

Methysergide is administered orally in divided doses. The duration of action is 1 to 2 days. Some of the drug is metabolized in the liver, and unchanged drug and its metabolites are excreted in the urine.

Uses

Methysergide is indicated for the prophylactic treatment of migraine and cluster headaches. If a response has not occurred after 3 weeks, treatment is discontinued.

Adverse Reactions and Contraindications

The major side effect of methysergide is peripheral ischemia, which can produce abdominal pain; chest pain; itching of the skin; numbness and tingling of the toes, fingers and face; or pale and cold hands and feet. Occasionally there are changes in vision, peripheral edema, and rashes. Orthostatic hypotension may be noted as dizziness or light-headedness.

A rare side effect after a longer duration of therapy is fibrosis, which may occur in cardiac, penile, pleuropulmonary, and/or retroperitoneal tissues. Because of this risk, methysergide should be administered for no longer than 6 months, with a drug-free interval of 3 to 4 weeks.

Patients with any comorbid cardiovascular, pulmonary hepatic, or renal conditions are at greater risk for side effects. Methysergide is not recommended for mothers who breastfeed, for children, or for the elderly.

Toxicity

Methysergide is chemically related to the hallucinogen LSD. Signs of an overdose include changes in vision and symptoms of central nervous system (CNS) stimulation such as excitement, difficulty in thinking, a feeling of being outside the body, or hallucinations and nightmares. The patient may show clumsiness or unsteadiness. The drug should be discontinued and the patient carefully monitored, especially for impaired respiration and convulsions. If the patient has ingested an overdose, gastric lavage may be needed. Severe peripheral vasospasm may require treatment with nitroprusside.

Interactions

Methysergide should not be administered with ergot alkaloids or other vasoconstrictive agents. Smoking increases the likelihood of peripheral vascular ischemia.

Prophylactic Agents for Migraine and/or Cluster Headaches

Selected drugs are used as prophylactic agents in the treatment of migraine or cluster headache. Prophylactic treatment is reserved for patients with two or three disabling or one or more prolonged migraines a month. A prophylactic agent is tried for a month for efficacy. Once the patient has been stabilized, the drug is continued for about 6 months, and the dose is then tapered down. Remission is achieved in some patients. Although a number of agents are used as prophylactic agents for migraine, most patients are managed successfully with propranolol or amitriptyline. These prophylactic agents have other primary uses, so their use for the treatment of headaches only is described here.

Antidepressants

Amitriptyline is the most widely used antidepressant for prophylactic treatment of migraine. Side effects include sedation, dry mouth, orthostatic hypotension, and arrhythmias. Amitriptyline and propranolol work together synergistically in the prophylactic treatment of migraine. Amitriptyline and other antidepressants inhibit the neuronal reuptake of serotonin, leading to a decrease in serotonin receptors over time. Other antidepressants used as prophylactic treatment for migraine include nortriptyline, imipramine, desipramine, doxepin, trazodone, and fluoxetine. Antidepressants are discussed in detail in Chapter 59.

Beta-Adrenergic Blockers

Beta-adrenergic blockers prevent arterial dilation and taken prophylactically can decrease the frequency, duration, and intensity of migraines. Propranolol is the most widely used beta-adrenergic agent for migraine prophylaxis, but nadolol, atenolol, and timolol have also been used successfully. The major side effects are hypotension, weight gain, depression, insomnia, nightmares, impotence, and bradycardia. Beta-adrenergic blockers are discussed in detail in Chapter 13.

Calcium Channel Blockers

Verapamil is used in the United States as a prophylactic agent for migraine. In Canada flunarizine is available as a cerebral selective calcium channel blocker for the prophylactic treatment of migraine. Calcium channel blockers are discussed in Chapter 13.

divalproex sodium

Divalproex (Depakote) is an anticonvulsant drug for the treatment of seizures (see Chapter 61). It is occasionally used for prophylactic treatment of severe migraine, although this use is not an approved indication for the drug.

lithium

Lithium (Eskalith, others) has proven effective in the prophylactic treatment of cluster headaches. The major use of lithium is in the treatment of manic-depressive disorder (see Chapter 59).

Nursing Process Overview

Drugs to Treat Headaches

Assessment

Perform a complete assessment. Rarely, a headache is a symptom of a more serious problem. Question the patient about previous headaches, recognized triggers, or aura, if any, and previous treatments that have been successful. Note the location of the headache, and ask the patient to describe the pain. Use a pain rating scale to quantify the degree of pain (see Chapter 34). Assess for ptosis (drooping of the upper eyelid), tearing or redness of the eyes, photophobia, nasal congestion, or runny nose. Question patients about alcohol, tobacco, and caffeine intake, and recent changes in schedule or diet. Assess menstruating women about their monthly schedule. Obtain a drug history of all medications currently in use, and ask about any allergies.

Nursing Diagnoses

- Acute pain related to headache as evident by patient description of pain, patient holding head, and crying
- Sleep pattern disturbance related to frequent awakenings secondary to headaches as evident by statements of "I'm afraid to fall asleep because I'm having two or three headaches each night."
- Potential complication: migraine headaches or cluster headaches

Patient Outcomes

The patient will state relief of pain. The patient will identify techniques to induce sleep. The patient will describe less frequent and/or less intense headaches.

Planning/Implementation

Because the severity, frequency, and cause of headaches vary widely, the implementation phase will vary from patient to patient. Continue to monitor the patient's pain, using a pain rating scale or other objective tool. Instruct the patient about the use and side effects of prescribed medications. Teach the patient about nondrug strategies that may be helpful: relaxation techniques, biofeedback, massage, and application of heat or cold. Refer patients to smoking cessation groups or other community resources as requested. Provide emotional support as needed.

Teach patient about drug administration techniques for IM, subcutaneous, rectal, or intranasal dosage forms if needed, including proper disposal of contaminated syringes and needles. Teach the patient how to keep a journal or record of headaches and possible contributing factors, if appropriate. Encourage patient to return for regular follow-up.

Evaluation

Continue to monitor for expected effects and drug side effects. Most patients will not be hospitalized for their headaches, so they will need routine assessment in the office setting. Routinely reevaluate drug administration techniques if needed. Verify that the patient can state when to call the physician.

Nursing Implications Summary

GENERAL GUIDELINES: DRUGS FOR HEADACHES

➤ Teach patients about the prescribed medications. Recognize that many products contain multiple drugs (see Table 33-1) and that the patient needs to know about all of the component drugs. All of the component drugs in Table 33-1 are discussed elsewhere in this text, except for isometheptene, dichloralphenazone, and butalbital.

➤ Review the dosing schedule with the patient. Emphasize the importance of taking doses as ordered for best effect, but not increasing the dose or frequency of dosing unless approved by the physician. Many of these drugs are habit-forming.

➤ Many of these drugs cause drowsiness or dizziness. Caution the patient to avoid driving or engaging in potentially dangerous activities until the effects of the medication are known. Remind patients to avoid alcohol or other drugs that depress the CNS (sleeping pills, sedatives, and antihistamines) unless approved by the physician. Remind patients to

avoid self-medicating with over-the-counter preparations unless first approved by the physician. Tell patients to keep all health care providers informed of all medications being used.

➤ These drugs should be avoided during pregnancy and breast-feeding unless approved by the physician.

➤ Many of these medications will be more effective if the patient can lie down in a darkened room immediately after taking the prescribed dose. Also try limiting noise in the environment and applying a cold washcloth to the forehead.

➤ Remind patients to keep these and all medications out of the reach of children.

➤ Instruct patients to seek medical help immediately if overdose with any of these medications is suspected.

butalbital

➤ This drug is a barbiturate, so it resembles other drugs in the class (see Chapter 57).

Continued

Nursing Implications Summary—cont'd

➤ This drug usually causes drowsiness, but in some children and elderly, it may cause excitation.

dichloralphenazone
➤ This drug is related to chloral hydrate (see Chapter 57).

isometheptene
➤ The mechanism of action is unclear for this drug, but it is an indirect-acting sympathomimetic drug that causes vasoconstriction (see Chapter 16).

Ergot-Containing Drugs
Drug Administration/Nursing in the Community
➤ See general guidelines. Monitor blood pressure. Examine extremities and monitor peripheral pulses. Instruct the patient to report the development of chest pain.
➤ Teach patient appropriate drug administration techniques: IM, subcutaneous, sublingual, inhalation, or rectal, depending on the drug. Review patient instruction leaflets provided by manufacturer. Use of metered-dose inhalers is described in the nursing care section of Chapter 28. If rectal suppositories must be divided to obtain correct dose, instruct patient to cut lengthwise. Refrigerate suppositories to make cutting and insertion easier.
➤ Instruct patients to avoid alcohol, which may aggravate headaches, and avoid smoking and cold temperatures, which may intensify vasoconstriction.
➤ These drugs may cause nausea and vomiting. In some patients, this may subside with use, but antiemetics may be prescribed concurrently.
➤ Remind patients not to share medications with anyone else.

Intravenous dihydroergotamine mesylate
➤ Administer 500 μg (0.5 mg) over 1 minute.

sumatriptan
Drug Administration/Nursing in the Community
➤ See general guidelines. Swallow oral doses whole without breaking or chewing. Take doses with a full glass (8 ounces) of water.
➤ Review the patient instruction leaflet supplied with injectable form. After dose administration, discard used cartridge, but not the autoinjector unit, which can be refilled and reused.
➤ Monitor blood pressure. Examine extremities and monitor peripheral pulses. Instruct the patient to report the development of chest pain.
➤ Instruct patients to avoid alcohol, which may aggravate headaches.

methysergide
Drug Administration/Nursing in the Community
➤ See the general guidelines. Monitor blood pressure. Examine extremities and monitor peripheral pulses. Instruct the patient to report the development of chest pain.
➤ Instruct patients to avoid alcohol, which may aggravate headaches, and to avoid smoking and cold temperatures, which may intensify vasoconstriction.
➤ Instruct patients to take oral doses with milk or snack to reduce gastric irritation.
➤ If orthostatic hypotension develops, instruct patients to move slowly from lying or sitting to standing positions.

 CHAPTER REVIEW

Application

1. Differentiate among the four kinds of headache described in this chapter.
2. What kinds of medications are included in the combination products listed in Table 33-1? Why are these ingredients included?
3. Why are ergot derivatives contraindicated during pregnancy?
4. Why are the elderly at greater risk for side effects from vasoconstricting drugs?
5. What kinds of nondrug therapies might be helpful to a patient experiencing a headache?

Critical Thinking

1. This chapter discusses four kinds of headaches but makes reference to the International Headaches Society listing of 129 types of headaches. What types of headaches have you or your family members experienced that do not seem to fit the four described here?
2. If you have an acquaintance who experiences migraine headaches, ask him or her to describe their headaches to you. Does it include an aura? Are there triggers? What does it feel like? How does it disrupt his or her life?

References

Barrett E: Primary care for women: assessment and management of headache, *J Nurse Midwife* 41(2):75-79, 117-124, 1996.

Green CA: Nursing rounds: is this headache serious? *Am J Nurs* 97(2):Contin Care Extra Ed:45-6, 55, 1997.

Headache Classification Committee of the International Headache Society: Classification and diagnostic criteria for headache disorders, cranial neuralgias and facial pain, *Cephalgia* 8(suppl 7):1, 1988.

Management of the Patient in Pain

KEY TERMS

epidural analgesia, p. 412

patient-controlled analgesia (PCA), p. 411

transdermal fentanyl patch, p. 411

OBJECTIVES

After studying this chapter, you should be able to do the following:

- *Describe methods for assessing a patient's pain.*
- *Discuss selected nonpharmacologic therapies for pain relief.*
- *Discuss the use of medications in pain relief.*
- *Describe challenges to assessment and management of pain in children and older adults.*
- *Develop a plan of care for the patient in pain.*

CHAPTER OVERVIEW

Nursing management of the patient in pain can be challenging and complicated. Drugs are an important part of the treatment plan for many kinds of pain. Nonnarcotic drugs for pain are discussed in Chapter 31, and opioids (narcotic analgesics) are discussed in Chapter 32. The major focus of this chapter is the use of medications with the patient in pain.

IS PAIN A PROBLEM?

Most people experience pain at times during their lifetime. Many kinds of pain disappear without treatment. Other kinds of pain resolve after treatment of the associated infection, obstruction, or other cause. Nevertheless, many patients seek assistance from the health care team for help in pain relief. Many strategies are available to help patients in pain, including medications, surgery, exercises, traction, nerve blocks, surgery to alleviate pain, massage, and application of heat or cold. Despite this list of treatments, many times, patients do not receive adequate pain relief.

Unrelieved pain may contribute to a variety of problems. The patient in pain is less likely to remain active and therefore may develop decreased mobility. The patient may be reluctant to cough and may retain secretions, which can lead to pneumonia. Immobility may contribute to slowed gastric function and constipation. Because the patient in pain may not wish to be around others, the pain may contribute to the patient developing social isolation.

The Meaning of Pain to the Patient

Pain may mean many things to patients. For an athlete, muscle or joint pain may signal that the athlete will be removed from the game or competition. A soldier wounded in action may not even notice pain until the battle is over, then may recognize the pain as a legitimate reason for leaving the high-stress battlefield. For a weekend sportsman, pain may be the signal that it is time to stop playing basketball, soccer, or football. For some patients the occurrence of pain may remind them they are aging or signal a recurrence of cancer or other chronic problem.

Patients may also have different expectations of pain and its expression. Some patients may feel it is "unmanly" to complain of pain, whereas others may come from a background where free expression of pain is the norm. Some may fear pain and therefore ignore it, whereas others fear that if they do not express pain they will be ignored. Patients are also influenced by personal experiences with pain in themselves or in those around them.

Factors That May Interfere with Pain Relief

Even when the health care team is working with the patient to help produce pain relief, certain factors may interfere. Patients may not have the same goal as the health care team has. For example, the patient may assume that complete pain relief is possible in a given situation, whereas the health care team may assume that the patient is willing to tolerate a degree of short-term discomfort in an effort to achieve a long-term goal.

Sometimes patients do not understand how a specific therapy is expected to work and therefore do not use it correctly. A few patients sometimes feel that they "deserve" pain or that there is a religious meaning to pain. These patients may feel that they are not "permitted" to experience pain relief, so they refuse to carry out prescribed therapies. Other patients may not understand how a prescribed activity could help, so they do not use it.

Pain and the Nurse

Research continues to demonstrate that some nurses, physicians, and other members of the health care team are inadequately prepared to help patients with pain relief. Studies have shown that some nurses hold misconceptions about patients and their pain. These misconceptions include the belief that many patients exaggerate their pain, that all patients with the same medical diagnosis have the "same amount" of pain and should all require the same treatment, that men should be stoic and women may freely show pain, or that all individuals from a specific ethnic or racial group respond to pain the same way.

The nurse's personal life experiences influence the view of pain. A nurse who had a difficult, painful labor and childbirth may feel everyone has an equally painful one, or conversely, that no one's could be as bad as her own. A nurse who had a pain-free arthroscopic examination of a knee may be intolerant of patients who complain of pain after a similar examination. Health care workers may also have misconceptions about a patient's behavior. For example, it is incorrect to assume that if a patient is sleeping, the patient is not experiencing pain, or that if a child can enjoy playing, the child is not in pain.

ASSESSMENT OF PAIN

Objective Assessment

Objective data are important in defining changes in the patient's situation and in providing additional information about problems that the patient may have. Obtain baseline vital signs and blood pressure, and monitor these periodically. Pain may cause an increase in respiratory rate, blood pressure,

and pulse. The patient may perspire or have dilated pupils. In time, as the patient adapts to pain, these signs will return to normal. Assess the patient's mood: crying, grimacing, calm, agitated, pacing, or restless. Does the patient have full range of movement, or is the patient guarding or protecting a joint, limb, or other area of the body? Assess the patient's gait.

Observe the area of pain, if localized, for redness or discoloration, swelling, and temperature differences. Is there any exudate or drainage? If there is a recent incision, is it healing as anticipated? Assess for other objective indicators of pain that the patient might have. For example, some patients with migraine headaches will develop reddened, swollen eyes as the headache continues. Do the results of diagnostic tests provide information?

Assessment of Subjective Data

McCaffery, one of the leading nurse researchers in the field of pain, taught that "Pain is whatever the experiencing person says it is and exists whenever he says it does."* This guideline continues to be appropriate. Ask the patient about the pain: Where is it? How long has it been there? Are there any aggravating factors? Ask the patient to describe the pain. Typical descriptors of pain include sharp, dull, throbbing, stabbing, and crushing. Ask the patient if there is a pattern to the pain: time of day or month, duration, and frequency. Are there other accompanying symptoms, such as nausea and vomiting, itching, or numbness?

What does the patient think the cause of the pain may be? Has the patient experienced this pain before, and what has the patient done about it? Question the patient about interventions used to relieve the pain and determine whether they were successful.

Several tools for assessing a patient's pain have been developed. One is described in Box 34-1, and another is shown in Figure 34-1. There are several advantages to using a pain assessment tool: the patient's ratings over time can be compared, the nurse can record the level of the patient's pain, and finally, using a tool or scale gives both the nurse and the patient a way to communicate about current pain and goals for pain alleviation.

The Pediatric Patient

Assessing the pediatric patient can be difficult. Objective data include crying, changes in vital signs, fretfulness, or general changes in behavior. On physical examination, the infant may indicate apparent pain or discomfort on movement of extremities or systematic palpation. As the infant grows older, the ability of the child to provide more specific indicators improves. Observe the child for clues about pain; for example, the child may avoid certain movements, pull at one or both ears, or refuse to do certain activities that were previously done. Question parents and caregivers about changes in the child's behavior.

---

*McCaffery M: *Nursing management of the patient with pain*, Philadelphia, 1972, JB Lippincott, p. 219.

INITIAL PAIN ASSESSMENT TOOL

Date _____

Patient's Name_____ Age _____ Room _____

Diagnosis_____ Physician _____

Nurse _____

I. LOCATION: Patient or nurse mark drawing.

II. INTENSITY: Patient rates the pain. Scale used _____

    Present: _____

    Worst pain gets: _____

    Best pain gets: _____

    Acceptable level of pain: _____

III. QUALITY: (Use patient's own words, e.g., prick, ache, burn, throb, pull, sharp) _____

_____

IV. ONSET, DURATION, VARIATIONS, RHYTHMS: _____

_____

V. MANNER OF EXPRESSING PAIN: _____

_____

VI. WHAT RELIEVES THE PAIN? _____

_____

VII. WHAT CAUSES OR INCREASES THE PAIN? _____

_____

VIII. EFFECTS OF PAIN: (Note decreased function, decreased quality of life.) _____

    Accompanying symptoms (e.g., nausea) _____

    Sleep _____

    Appetite_____

    Physical activity_____

    Relationship with others (e.g., irritability) _____

    Emotions (e.g., anger, suicidal, crying) _____

    Concentration _____

    Other _____

IX. OTHER COMMENTS: _____

_____

X. PLAN: _____

_____

Figure 34-1   Initial pain assessment tool. *(From McCaffery M, Pasero C: Pain: clinical manual, St Louis, 1999, Mosby, p. 60. Used with permission.)*

Box 34-1   Examples of Pain Rating Scales

There are several tools that are variations of the visual analog scale (VAS). The VAS is a straight line marked or calibrated to represent increasing pain. For example, a 10-cm line on a piece of paper could be drawn, as shown below.

**No   Worst possible
pain   pain**

The patient is asked to mark on the line at the point that represents the current level of pain. That point is measured, and a "level" can be attached to it. For example, a mark at 4.2 cm from the left is a pain level of 4.2 out of a possible 10.

   Sometimes, the VAS is marked at 1- or 2-cm intervals, with or without accompanying descriptors.

No pain   Mild pain   Moderate pain   Severe pain   Very severe pain   Worst possible pain

Another variation is to ask patients to rate their pain from 1 to 10, with 0 representing "No pain" and 10 representing the "Worst possible pain," but no visual scale is shown to the patient. Variations of VAS are available to measure distress and pain intensity.

Box 34-2   Examples of Tools to Assess Pain in Children

WONG-BAKER FACES PAIN RATING SCALE*

0	1	2	3	4	5
No Hurt	Hurts Little Bit	Hurts Little More	Hurts Even More	Hurts Whole Lot	Hurts Worst

Explain to the person that each face is for a person who feels happy because he has no pain (hurt) or sad because he has some or a lot of pain. **Face 0** is very happy because he doesn't hurt at all. **Face 1** hurts just a little bit. **Face 2** hurts a little more. **Face 3** hurts even more. **Face 4** hurts a whole lot. **Face 5** hurts as much as you can imagine, although you don't have to be crying to feel this bad. Ask the person to choose the face that best describes how he is feeling.

   Rating scale is recommended for persons age 3 years and older.

Another way to assess pain in children as young as 4 years old is to use the Hester Poker Chip Scale.†
1. Use four red poker chips.
2. Align the chips horizontally in front of the child on the bedside table, a clipboard, or other firm surface.
3. Tell the child, "These are pieces of hurt." Beginning at the chip nearest the child's left side and ending at the one nearest the right side, point to the chips and say, "This (the first chip) is a little bit of hurt and this (the fourth chip) is the most hurt you could ever have."
For a young child or for any child who does not comprehend the instructions, clarify by saying, "That means this (the first chip) is just a little hurt; this (the second chip) is a little more hurt; this (the third chip) is more hurt; and this (the fourth chip) is the most hurt you could ever have."
4. Ask the child, "How many pieces of hurt do you have right now?" Children without pain will say they don't have any.
5. Clarify the child's answer by words such as "Oh, you have a little hurt? Tell me about the hurt."
6. Record the number of chips selected on the bedside flow sheet.
Regardless of the tool used in an agency, better results will be obtained if everyone uses the same tool and the results of the assessment are recorded and used for planning purposes.

*From Wong D: *Whaley and Wong's Essentials of Pediatric Nursing*, ed 5, 1997, p. 1215. Copyrighted by Mosby, Inc. Reprinted by permission.
†Poker Chip Tool instructions developed in 1975 by Nancy O. Hester, University of Colorado Health Sciences Center, Denver, CO. Spanish instructions by Jordan-Marsh M, Hall D, Yoder L, Watson R, McFarlane-Sosa G, Garcia M: *The Harbor-UCLA Medical Center Humor Project for Children*, Los Angeles, 1990, Harbor-UCLA Medical Center.

As a child grows older, assessment becomes gradually easier. The child can begin to answer simple questions or respond to directions. The nurse may ask "Does it hurt?" followed by asking the child to point to where it hurts. Certain assessment tools can be used with children (Box 34-2). Some of these tools may be used with children as young as 4 years of age.

In working with children, remain calm and unhurried. Children may need more time to develop some trust with the nurse and to feel comfortable in talking with the nurse, who is often a stranger to the child. Some children respond better with a parent present, whereas other children should be assessed without parents present. Offering a young child a toy to hold or play with during assessment may cause the child to relax so that examination of the child is easier. Some children may respond if dolls or puppets are used.

The Older Adult

Avoid making assumptions about older adults. Reported assumptions about this age group include assuming that older adults do not experience pain to the degree that younger adults do or assuming that older adults do not mind pain. Other misconceptions include assuming that pain is a natural part of the aging process or assuming that approaches used with younger patients (e.g., exercises, relaxation, narcotics) cannot be used with older individuals.

Assessing older adults may pose special challenges. Some older adults have communication problems because of hearing or vision loss. Older adults who have had strokes or have some aphasia may not be able to communicate clearly. Patients with Alzheimer's disease or other dementias may not be able to provide accurate subjective data. Careful objective assessment may provide important data. Ask family members or caregivers about changes in the patient's behavior, activity level, and ability to perform activities of daily living. Do not assume that patients immediately think to complain of pain, depending on their own expectations about discomfort.

Many of the strategies suggested for children are helpful in working with some older adults. Remain calm and unhurried. If possible, sit down with the patient. Some older adults respond better if questions are kept simple and sufficient time is allowed to formulate an answer. Try to eliminate background noise by turning off the television or radio or shutting the door. Remain within the patient's vision. Of course, these strategies are appropriate with all patients but may be especially helpful with older adult patients.

NURSING DIAGNOSES AND PATIENT OUTCOMES

Once the initial assessment is completed, develop the nursing diagnoses appropriate for the patient. Analysis of the data may indicate several appropriate diagnoses for the patient. "Pain related to . . ." may be the primary diagnosis, but other diagnoses are commonly seen when a patient has pain, such as (1) anxiety (potential or actual), (2) altered health maintenance, (3) impaired physical mobility, (4) sleep pattern disturbance, (5) fatigue, and (6) fear.

Work with the patient and/or family to develop appropriate outcomes. It would seem obvious that the goal is for the patient to be pain free, but that may not be immediately possible. One advantage of a pain rating scale is that the nurse and patient can share a common language about pain. If the patient currently describes a pain level of 5 out of a possible 10, the nurse can determine the level that is satisfactory to the patient. Together the patient and nurse can develop specific strategies to achieve this.

In the course of developing outcomes, the nurse may also be able to provide some guidance, based on the nurse's expertise and experience. For example, the nurse may conclude that a patient's nausea may be caused by an analgesic currently being used by the patient, so the nurse could explain to the patient that changing the current medication may be helpful in relieving pain and relieving nausea. For another patient the nurse may conclude that nausea is actually a manifestation of the patient's pain, and relieving the pain will help in relieving the nausea.

PATIENT EDUCATION

Patient education must be included throughout the development and implementation of the plan of care. First, acknowledge the patient's pain. Then let the patient know that the health care team will work with him or her to relieve the pain. As more data are obtained about the patient's specific situation, the nurse may be able to explain the cause(s) of some or all of the pain. Knowing the cause of the pain does not relieve the pain, but it may help decrease a patient's anxiety. Keep the patient informed as the physical examination continues, diagnostic tests are performed, and medications are administered.

Present each therapy used for pain relief in a positive way. A nurse who suggests "I don't really think this will help much, but . . ." will not elicit the same outcome as a statement like "Some of my patients have found this helpful, and I would like to try it with you." Most patients are not interested in the physiologic explanation of pain relief strategies but would like to know what will happen; how long the therapy, treatment, or intervention will take; if it works, how soon relief will begin; and if it does not work, what next? Reassure patients that the health care team will continue to work together with the patient as long as needed to help solve the problem.

Anxiety often accompanies pain, but the patient may not identify anxiety as a problem. Strategies to relieve pain may help lessen anxiety, and efforts to lessen anxiety may also result in more effective pain relief. Keeping the patient informed about what is going on and what will happen to the patient will help lessen his or her anxiety.

THE PLAN OF CARE: SELECTED NONPHARMACOLOGIC MEASURES FOR PAIN RELIEF

As the data are analyzed, the diagnoses determined, and the hoped-for patient outcomes decided, the plan begins to emerge. As with all care plans, this one should be specific and be developed by the health care team working together. The more the team shares common goals and common understanding about pain and its management, the more likely the plan will succeed. If one member of the team believes primarily in cognitive-behavioral approaches and another prefers medicinal approaches, implementation of the plan may be uneven.

Once the plan is developed, it is important to monitor its effectiveness. One way to do this is to use a flow sheet to record the patient's response, as shown in Figure 34-2. The column headings can be modified to meet the patient's individual situation.

Many patients profit from an approach that combines several approaches such as combining a cognitive-behavioral approach with medication or combining two kinds of physical agents. Cognitive-behavioral measures for pain relief are especially helpful in giving patients a sense of involvement and control over their pain. Patients can become active in personal pain assessment and can become knowledgeable about how to control their own pain. These strategies may help patients alter their pain behavior. Some of these strategies are well suited for patients who have long-term pain or who do not want or should not have strong or sedating drugs. Some patients, however, will be resistant to these measures, even after efforts to present them in a positive, therapeutic manner. Cognitive-behavioral measures include relaxation (Box 34-3), distraction (see Research Highlights

---

Box 34-3   Example Instructions for a Relaxation Exercise

Help the patient assume a comfortable position. Tell the patient the following:
1. Clench your fists; breathe in deeply and hold it a moment.
2. Breathe out slowly and go limp as a rag doll.
3. Start yawning.

Yawning becomes spontaneous and is contagious, so others may begin yawning and relaxing too.

From McCaffery M, Pasero C: *Pain: clinical manual,* St Louis, 1999, Mosby. Used with permission.

RESEARCH HIGHLIGHTS

Ameliorating Adults' Acute Pain during Phlebotomy with a Distraction Intervention

—Cason CC, Grissom NL: *Appl Nurs Res* 10(4):168-173, 1997.

PURPOSE

Patients who have a venipuncture and blood withdrawn (phlebotomy) experience transitory but acute pain with the procedure. Pharmacologic intervention to decrease pain is rarely used for such a brief episode of pain. Nondrug therapies for pain that can be inexpensively and quickly administered would be ideal for this type of pain. One nondrug approach to pain relief is distraction, which can be a highly effective coping strategy with adults. This study was designed to evaluate the distraction intervention of viewing a kaleidoscope on adults' perception of pain associated with phlebotomy. A second purpose was to correlate measures of pain on one of three pain assessment tools with the measures on the two other tools.

METHODS

A two-group quasiexperimental design was used. Before phlebotomy, subjects were randomly assigned to one of two groups. Subjects in the experimental group used a kaleidoscope during phlebotomy, while subjects in the control group did not. The kaleidoscope used was lightweight and could be handled easily with the free arm; it is pictured in the article. Before phlebotomy, subjects rated anticipated pain on each of three instruments, the Wong-Baker FACES Pain Scale, the visual analog scale (VAS), and the Present Pain Intensity (PPI) Scale. After phlebotomy, subjects rated how painful phlebotomy was, using the same three scales. Subjects were patients at a family practice clinic. There were 45 subjects in the experimental group, and 51 subjects in the control group. The two groups had the same average age, and

same mix of subjects by gender, with women outnumbering men 3 to 1. Both groups had the same average education and similar phlebotomy histories.

RESULTS

The average time for phlebotomy was 86 seconds, with a range of 22 to 442 seconds. Multivariate analysis of covariance (MANCOVA) revealed a significant difference in scores between the two groups ($F(3, 89) = 55$, $p = 0.00$; power = 0.93), with the experimental group reporting less discomfort. The correlations among the three assessment tools indicated validity for the FACES instrument when used to study adults' responses to painful stimuli.

IMPLICATIONS

The kaleidoscope used in this study demanded sufficient attention from subjects to serve as a useful distraction strategy. Its use may be helpful during other short-term procedures such as intramuscular injection, urinary catheter insertion, and colposcopy. This study also indicated that the FACES pain scale is an appropriate measure of pain perception among adults. This scale does not require literacy and may also be used with non-English speaking patients.

CRITICAL THINKING: What are some short-term procedures associated with patient discomfort that are performed in your clinical setting? Could the kaleidoscope strategy be used there? Can you think of other simple, inexpensive methods of distraction?

FLOW SHEET—PAIN

Patient _____ Date _____

*Pain rating scale used _____

Purpose: To evaluate the safety and effectiveness of the analgesic(s)

Analgesic(s) prescribed: _____

Time	Pain rating	Analgesic	R	P	BP	Level of arousal	Other†	Plan & comments

*Pain rating: A number of different scales may be used. Indicate which scale is used and use the same one each time. For example, 0-10 (0 = no pain, 10 = worst pain).
†Possibilities for other columns: bowel function, activities, nausea and vomiting, other pain relief measures. Identify the side effects of greatest concern to patient, family, physician, and nurses.

Figure 34-2   A flow sheet to track the effectiveness of pain management. *(From McCaffery M, Pasero C:* Pain: clinical manual, *St Louis, 1999, Mosby. Used with permission.)*

box on distraction intervention), music therapy, imagery, and prayer.

In addition to cognitive-behavioral approaches to pain control and management, many physical agents or approaches can be used. One physical agent is heat, including applying hot compresses, soaking in warm water, and using a hot water bottle, heating pad, or heat lamp. Another physical agent is cold, which can be applied in moist forms (e.g., soaking foot or hand in ice water; applying towels dipped in ice water and then wrung out) or dry forms (applying a waterproof bag filled with ice, frozen gel packs, or a bag of frozen green peas or corn). Other forms of physical agents include massage, exercise, and transcutaneous electrical nerve stimulation (TENS).

USE OF MEDICATIONS FOR PAIN RELIEF

Medications remain a mainstay of pain relief. Usually, begin with less potent drugs before moving to more potent. The initial drug should be aspirin, acetaminophen, or a nonsteroidal antiinflammatory drug (NSAID) (see Chapters 31 and 32). There are other situations in which it is not appropriate to begin with any of these drugs. In many postoperative situations, oral nonnarcotics are not a satisfactory choice for the immediate postoperative period because the patient is not yet ready to resume oral intake.

Next, use an adequate dose and decide on the frequency of doses. Recommended dosages are based on studies done on large numbers of patients and reflect the dosage that is effective for the average patient. Any individual patient may require more or less. Use an appropriate pain assessment tool and monitor the effectiveness of the dosage. Work with the physician to determine whether prn (as-needed) or around-the-clock doses are better for the specific patient and situation.

Anticipate pain rather than waiting until the patient is obviously uncomfortable. Assess the patient frequently. If it appears that the patient's pain level is increasing, med-

Table 34-1 Equianalgesic Chart of Opioid Analgesics Commonly Used for Severe Pain

Drug Name	Equianalgesic IM Dose (mg)	Equianalgesic Oral Dose (mg)	Comments
Morphine-Like Agonists			
morphine	10	20-30 (every 3-4 hr, around the clock) 60 (single dose or intermittent)	Available in sustained-release preparation (MS Contin) and a rectal suppository.
codeine	120 (rarely used at this dose)	200 (not recommended)	Doses needed to relieve severe pain may cause nausea, vomiting, and severe constipation.
hydromorphone (Dilaudid)	1.5	7.5	Slightly shorter duration than morphine; available as rectal suppositories.
levorphanol (Levo-Dromoran)	2	4	Accumulates on days 2-3.
meperidine (Demerol)	75 (irritating with repeated IM injections)	300 (not recommended)	Normeperidine (toxic metabolite) accumulates with repetitive dosing, causing central nervous system excitation; avoid in patients with impaired renal function or those who are receiving monoamine oxidase inhibitors.
oxycodone (Roxicodone; also in many combination drugs, e.g., Tylox, Percocet)	Not available	30	
oxymorphone (Numorphan)	1-1.5	Not available	Available as a rectal suppository; 5 mg of rectal suppository = 5 mg of morphine IM.
Mixed Agonist-Antagonists			
butorphanol (Stadol)	2	Not available	Like IM pentazocine.
nalbuphine (Nubain)	10	Not available	Like IM pentazocine but incidence of psychotomimetic effects is lower than with pentazocine.
pentazocine (Talwin)	60 (irritating to tissues with repeated IM injection)	150-180	Used orally for less severe pain; mixed agonist-antagonists may cause psychotomimetic effects; may precipitate withdrawal in narcotic-dependent patients; contraindicated in myocardial infarction.
Partial Agonist			
buprenorphine (Buprenex)	0.3-0.4	Not available	Sublingual form not yet available in the United States; less likely to produce psychotomimetic effects; may precipitate withdrawal in narcotic-dependent patients.

IM, Intramuscular.

icate the patient. Anticipate that the patient will experience pain during certain activities, and medicate the patient before activities such as physical therapy or postoperative ambulation.

The usual approach is to begin with a nonnarcotic and then to change to oral narcotics when nonnarcotics are no longer effective. Even if a patient requires a narcotic, a combination of a narcotic and nonnarcotic such as aspirin or acetaminophen is more effective than a low dosage of a narcotic alone. This is the logic behind combination products such as Percocet (oxycodone plus acetaminophen), Tylenol #3 (acetaminophen and codeine), and Percodan (oxycodone and aspirin).

Narcotics for Pain Relief

Narcotic analgesics are the most potent drugs for pain, short of general or local anesthesia (see Chapter 32). Even when used in appropriate situations, however, patients are sometimes forced to endure excessive waiting periods between doses, inadequate doses, or insensitivity on the part of members of the health care team. Drug addiction or psychologic dependence that develops into drug abuse is rare in patients receiving medication for pain. Remember that opioid tolerance and physical dependence are predictable consequences of long-term opioid use and are not signs of drug abuse or drug addiction (see Chapter 8). Opioid tolerance may develop in a relatively short period and is simply a problem to deal with, not a reason to withhold medication or label a patient inappropriately. When narcotics are used beyond a few days, anticipate the development of some side effects, including constipation, and develop a plan to deal with the side effect.

Many patients who require narcotics for pain relief are initially titrated on intravenous (IV) forms. Once the patient is more comfortable, the health care team can work with the patient to develop a plan for pain relief that relies on routes of administration that are easier to self-administer. An important concept in switching a patient from one drug to another is understanding equianalgesic dosages (Tables 34-1 and 34-2). As the tables illustrate, a patient who requires 10 mg of morphine will require 75 to 100 mg of meperidine to achieve the same degree of pain relief.

Generally, patients prefer oral drug forms to injectable forms because of the ease of administration. Once a patient achieves pain relief from IV narcotics, the physician usually tries to switch the patient to oral forms. Another approach is to prescribe a **transdermal fentanyl patch** (see Nursing Implications Summary, Chapter 36) augmented with oral doses of a second drug for breakthrough pain. The transdermal form is effective in providing a constant blood level of drug but is slow to achieve this blood level because it is transdermal. Narcotics are available in oral, rectal, transdermal, nasal spray, IV, intramuscular (IM), and epidural routes; patients in severe pain may require concurrent administration via several routes of administration.

Patient-Controlled Analgesia

Patient-controlled analgesia (PCA) is a special use of IV narcotics. With PCA, a mechanical pump containing a reservoir of an IV narcotic, usually morphine, is attached to a continuous IV infusion. The patient is given a small control device activated by pressing a button. When the patient is uncomfortable or needs something for pain, the patient pushes the button and a preset dose of the narcotic is infused into the IV line. The pump has controls to set for the minimum time between doses, the maximum number of doses per time period (e.g., 1-hour period), and amount of each dose. The pump may also keep a running record of number of doses used by the patient.

Table 34-2 **Comparison Doses of Selected Oral Drugs for Pain**	
Analgesic	Oral Dose (mg)
Nonopioid Analgesics	
acetaminophen (Datril, Tylenol)	650-975 (2-3 325-mg tablets)
aspirin (ASA)	650-975 (2-3 325-mg tablets)
Opioid Analgesics	
codeine	30-60
meperidine (Demerol)	50
hydrocodone (Vicodin, which also contains acetaminophen)	5
pentazocine (Talwin) (opioid agonist-antagonist)	60
propoxyphene hydrochloride (Darvon)	65
propoxyphene napsylate (Darvon-N)	100
Selected Nonsteroidal Antiinflammatory Drugs	
ibuprofen (Advil, Motrin, others)	200 (superior to ASA in analgesic efficacy at this dose)
naproxen sodium (Anaprox)	275 (comparable to ASA; 550 is superior)
indomethacin (Indocin)	25-50 (comparable to ASA)
ketoprofen (Orudis)	25 (comparable to ASA; 50 superior)
piroxicam (Feldene)	20 (comparable in efficacy, slower onset, longer duration than ASA)

Using PCA has many advantages: The patient controls the frequency of medication administration and does not have to wait for the nurse to prepare and administer a requested dose of medication. Each dose of medication may be small, but the patient can repeat doses within the time limits programmed into the pump. Patients are also given a sense of control over their own pain relief. Currently PCA is widely used for postoperative patients, but it can be used any time IV narcotics are appropriate (see Research Highlights box on PCA). The patient in severe pain may be receiving a constant infusion of narcotics, with PCA for breakthrough pain.

Epidural Analgesia

Morphine or other opioids may be administered via epidural catheters. With this approach smaller doses of medication can be used to provide widespread analgesia without motor blockade or excessive central nervous system (CNS) depression. For **epidural analgesia** a catheter is inserted into the thoracic or lumbar epidural space and secured. Intermittent or continuous medication may be administered. Drugs used include morphine, meperidine, fentanyl, and sufentanil (see Chapters 32 and 36). A PCA pump may also be attached to allow the patient to control drug delivery. Because of the location of the catheter, it must be inserted by an anesthesiologist or nurse anesthetist.

Assess the patient regularly for side effects and degree of pain relief. Monitor the rate and depth of respirations, pulse oximeter, and degree of sedation. Monitor bladder distension and lower extremity muscle strength.

lidocaine and prilocaine cream for Topical Analgesia

A medication formed from mixing the solid pure bases of lidocaine and prilocaine (eutectic mixture of local anesthetics, or EMLA) is available to provide local anesthesia to the skin before diagnostic tests, venipunctures, and other painful activities. This local anesthetic cream is applied thickly over the prescribed area. The area is then covered with an occlu-

---

RESEARCH HIGHLIGHTS

A Comparison of Two Regimens of Patient-Controlled Analgesia for Children with Sickle Cell Disease

—Trentadue NO, Kachoyeanos MK, Lea G: J Pediatr Nurs *13*(1):15-19, 1998.

PURPOSE

The vasoocclusive crisis of sickle cell disease is associated with excruciating pain. Morphine is the drug of choice in treating this pain. Patient-controlled analgesia (PCA) is widely used as a strategy to help patients maintain better control over their pain, and thus gradually decrease the amount of medication needed as the degree of pain lessens. One of many dosage regimens includes a continuous, basal infusion of morphine with patient-controlled additional doses of morphine as needed (within the parameters prescribed by the physician). The purpose of this study was to compare two regimens of PCA for treatment of sickle cell crisis in terms of safety, efficacy, and cost.

METHODS

A retrospective chart review of pediatric patients with a diagnosis of "Sickle Cell Pain Crisis" was done. A total of 84 records were reviewed, with PCA used for 26 children over 60 separate admissions. There were 11 males and 15 females between the ages of 11 and 18 years. There were 30 patients (episodes) in each group, comparing high dosages of PCA with low basal infusion dosages (HPCA/LBI) and low dosages of PCA with high basal infusion dosages (LPCA/HBI). HPCA/LBI was defined as a PCA dosage of at least 0.25 mg/kg/dose with a low basal infusion at nighttime of 0.01 to 0.03 mg/kg/hr; patients in this group with unrelieved pain received increases in the PCA dosages. LPCA/HBI received PCA dosages of 0.01 to 0.02 mg/kg/dose with a basal infusion of 0.05 to 0.2 mg/kg/hr; patients in this group with unrelieved pain received increases in the continuous infusion dosage. A linear analog pain rating scale was used to compare the degree of pain relief.

RESULTS

Children in group 1 (HPCA/LBI) used significantly less morphine compared with group 2 (LPCA/HBI), $p = 0.0130$. Children in group 1 averaged significantly fewer days of PCA (4.9 days) than group 2 (6.16 days), $p = 0.0112$. Children in group 1 averaged fewer days of hospitalization (5.0333 days) than group 2 (7.1833 days), $p = 0.0012$. Total costs for group I were significantly less than for group 2 because group 1 needed fewer days of PCA pump rental, fewer syringes for the PCA pump, fewer days of hospitalization, and fewer days of nursing care. There was no significant difference in pain scores on day 1 between the two groups, but on day 2 there was a statistically significant difference between the highest pain score reported for group 1 compared with group 2 (group 1 significantly lower), and for the lowest reported pain score (group 1 significantly lower).

IMPLICATIONS

Data support the use of generous morphine dosages administered via PCA for control of pain associated with sickle cell crisis in pediatric patients over the age of 10 years. Further research is needed using prospective methodologies, larger sample size, and different dosing regimens.

CRITICAL THINKING: What pain control problems have you encountered in practice? Are there populations who are not using PCA who could use PCA if taught? What are potential hazards to continuous narcotic infusion?

sive dressing and left for an hour or longer. Before the procedure the dressing and cream are removed, and the area is cleaned with an antiseptic solution. Although the agent is applied topically, the same precautions used with injected local anesthetics apply to EMLA. This ointment is not recommended for use in infants younger than 3 months of age. Other forms of topical analgesics are also being developed and tested. Nurses who use these forms with their patients should review the manufacturer's literature for specific directions about their use.

Special Considerations for the Pediatric Patient

A child may not understand explanations about pain and therapies that are going to be tried. Sometimes the frequent discomfort of repeated tests causes a child great distress, and his or her crying and uncooperative behavior upset the family and the health care team. Other times diagnostic tests or other activities require that the child remain as still as possible for accuracy purposes; however, if the procedure is painful, the child is unlikely to remain still.

There are ongoing controversies about some pediatric problems. For example, one area of controversy is the use of analgesics for circumcision of newborns. Questions continue about the extent of pain the infant perceives and the best way to relieve the pain. Some argue that the procedure takes so little time that analgesics are unnecessary. Others argue that some pain relief measures (e.g., injection of local anesthetics) are as painful as the procedure itself so should not be used. The nurse working with pediatric patients should keep up-to-date with research related to specific pediatric problems.

With children, topical or local anesthetics may be used before painful tests. Oral or IV anxiety-reducing drugs such as benzodiazepines may be given to calm down a child in preparation for procedures. Nitrous oxide or ketamine may be administered (by trained personnel) before procedures. IV drugs for pain may be chosen over IM or subcutaneous forms to avoid repeated injections. Different routes of administration for drugs may be needed for a child, depending on a child's age. There has been recent work on the development of a lollipop-form of narcotic analgesic to use in infants and small children.

Special Considerations for the Older Adult Patient

Older adults in pain present special challenges. Because these patients often take many medications for their health problems, the nurse should monitor for drug interactions. Older adults have increased sensitivity to the sedating effects and hypotensive effects of many drugs. In addition, older patients may have diminished liver and/or kidney function, putting them at greater risk for drug toxicity. Finally, although the aging process alone does not reduce the serum proteins, poor nutrition and chronic disease may contribute to reduced serum albumin, and therefore circulating free-drug levels of protein-bound drugs may be higher, contributing to potential drug toxicity. These factors suggest that frequent assessment, use of smaller drug doses, and less frequent drug administration are appropriate approaches to older adult patients.

CASE STUDY
Chronic Pain

Warren H. is a 68-year-old patient who has recently been readmitted to the oncology unit with shortness of breath and progressive pain in his back and right hip. He was diagnosed with small cell lung cancer 6 months ago. He underwent chemotherapy as well as radiation therapy at that time. He also has a history of cigarette smoking and emphysema. Warren tells his nurse that his pain was initially managed with acetaminophen and ibuprofen. After a month, however, his pain increased and Warren's physician prescribed hydrocodone, acetaminophen, and buspirone (an antianxiety agent). Two months before this admission, however, Warren began to experience increasing pain. His physician discontinued the hydrocodone and added to Warren's pain management regimen MS Contin, a controlled-release oral morphine, 90 mg every 12 hours. This worked well until recently, when Warren began to experience recurrent breakthrough pain.

1. Considering that it was expected that Warren's pain would progress, why did his physician initially prescribe the oxycodone and acetaminophen, as opposed to starting him on the morphine?

2. Why was the antianxiety agent buspirone added to Warren's medication regimen?

3. Warren tells his nurse "I don't understand why these pain medications aren't working anymore. I'm afraid I'm becoming addicted to them." How should the nurse respond?

4. Warren's treatment plan includes additional radiation therapy and switching his morphine from the oral to the intravenous route. The physician orders a patient-controlled analgesia (PCA) pump with the following settings: morphine 2 mg/hr continuous with a 2-mg bolus every 10 minutes prn. The nurse sets up the PCA pump for Warren. What assessment data is important to obtain before initiating this drug therapy?

5. What is the advantage of the PCA over nurse-administered analgesics? Why has the physician ordered the PCA to administer continuous morphine doses instead of "on-demand" dosing only?

6. What are the common adverse effects of morphine? Because Warren has been taking opioids for some time, what is his risk for developing these adverse effects?

7. What nonpharmacologic pain management strategies might be effective for Warren?

8. A week later Warren is being discharged home. Discharge medications include a fentanyl patch and prn hydromorphone orally for his pain management. Why has this regimen been chosen?

Use of Placebos

Occasionally, a physician orders a normal saline injection for a patient in pain. If the patient responds positively to this placebo, the patient may be incorrectly labeled as malingering, as not having real pain, or as addicted to medications. A positive response to a placebo is generally meaningless in the patient with pain because it provides no information about the pain. In addition, it is deceitful to administer a placebo when the patient believes that a different drug is being administered. Placebos are used appropriately in double-blind drug research studies, but in those studies the patient has given informed consent that placebos may be used. For more information about placebos, consult texts about pain and review the American Nurses' Association Code for Nurses. See the end of the chapter for additional sources of information about pain.

Other Drugs Used in Management of the Patient with Pain

Carbamazepine (see Chapter 61) is recognized as the drug of choice to treat the pain of trigeminal neuralgia (tic douloureux). Sumatriptan is used in the treatment of migraine headaches (see Chapter 33). Local anesthetics (see Chapter 35) are used to treat many kinds of surface pain. Ergot-derivative–containing combination products are used to treat or prevent vascular headaches, including cluster headaches (see Chapter 33).

Many patients in pain also experience nausea, and antiemetics are often used to control this annoying symptom in patients (see Chapter 25). Some patients in pain have their anxiety treated with an antianxiety agent (see Chapter 57). Muscle relaxants may be prescribed to treat muscle spasms (see Chapter 63). The antidepressants amitriptyline, doxepin, imipramine, and desipramine may have analgesic properties distinct from their effects on depression. In addition, these drugs may help patients sleep better at night and may reduce anxiety (see Chapter 59).

PAIN MANAGEMENT PROGRAMS

Sometimes patients do not achieve an acceptable degree of pain relief with usual approaches and should be referred to a pain management program. Pain management programs may be inpatient, outpatient, or comprehensive. There is often a team approach, with physicians, nurses, psychologists, social workers, physical and occupational therapists, rehabilitation counselors, clergy, and others available. The treatment plan may be complex and may include strategies already mentioned as well as behavioral modification, hypnosis, biofeedback, and acupuncture. Anesthesiologists are available to pain centers to perform nerve blocks, insert spinal catheters, administer intrathecal medications, and so on.

Nursing Process Overview

The Patient in Pain

Assessment
Perform a complete physical assessment. Monitor vital signs. Observe the behavior and gait of the patient. Use an assessment tool appropriate for the patient, and have the patient rate the degree of pain. Obtain the patient's subjective description of pain.

Nursing Diagnoses
- Pain related to (specify)
- Anxiety related to (specify)
- Sleep pattern disturbance related to unrelieved pain

Patient Outcomes
The patient will state that pain is relieved or that the persisting pain is at an acceptable level. The patient will discuss feelings of anxiety and will relate that anxiety is decreased. The patient will state that uninterrupted periods of sleep have increased in length.

Planning/Implementation
Acknowledge that the patient is in pain. Work with the patient to define the goal of pain relief. Combine nursing care measures with drugs or other therapies for pain relief. Present pain relief measures in a positive manner. Administer medications, if prescribed, in doses and frequencies appropriate for the patient's age and condition and for achieving pain relief. Provide medication to patients in anticipation of painful activities. Anticipate side effects when medications are used, and develop interventions to prevent or control them, such as preventing constipation when narcotics are used. Remember that the patient is the greatest authority in the degree of pain he or she has and when pain relief has occurred.

Evaluation
Nursing care of the patient in pain is effective if the patient's pain is relieved to a degree that is satisfactory to the patient. Before discharge, the patient should know how to administer prescribed medications and/or perform other therapies. The patient should know how to treat side effects and when to call the health care team for additional help in pain relief.

CHAPTER REVIEW

Application

1. What are some possible outcomes of unrelieved pain in patients?
2. What are some examples of what pain might mean to a patient?
3. What are some misconceptions the nurse might have about pain? What are misconceptions about pain in children? the older adult?
4. How might a nurse's personal experiences interfere with providing effective pain relief to a patient?
5. What are some objective signs that may indicate that a patient is in pain?
6. What are some subjective signs of pain in a patient?
7. Give examples of tools used for assessing a patient's pain.
8. Give examples of possible nursing diagnoses that might be seen in patients with pain.
9. How does patient education play a role in helping a patient in pain?
10. What groups of drugs are used for pain relief (see also Chapters 31 and 32)?
11. What is EMLA, and when is it used?
12. What is PCA, and when is it used? What are the advantages and disadvantages of PCA?
13. Describe special considerations for pediatric patients and older adult patients.
14. Discuss reasons against using placebos outside of formal drug testing.
15. Why would antidepressants be used for patients in pain?

Critical Thinking

1. Compare and contrast oral, transdermal, IM or subcutaneous, IV, and epidural administration of drugs. Consider the following: ease of administration, ease of preparing the correct dose, speed of achieving therapeutic serum drug levels, degree of sedation, kinds of side effects, and ease of self management at home.
2. What is epidural analgesia? What are the advantages and disadvantages of this approach? Is it used in your local agencies? Are there agency protocols in place?
3. Compare and contrast the cost of PCA and epidural analgesia. (Call your local pharmacist and/or hospital for cost information.)
4. Compare and contrast the cost of the following: aspirin, acetaminophen, and an NSAID (pick any one); oral and IV morphine; and transdermal and epidermal fentanyl.

References

Berkowitz CM: Epidural pain control—your job, too, *RN* 60(8):22-28, 1997.

Bral EE: Caring for adults with chronic cancer pain, *Am J Nurs* 98(4):26-33, 1998.

Dellasega C, Keiser CL: Pharmacologic approaches to chronic pain in the older adult, *Nurse Pract* 22(5):20, 22-24, 26 passim, 1997.

Dossey BM: Holistic modalities & healing moments, *Am J Nurs* 98(6):44-47, 1998.

Ferrell BR, McCaffery M: Nurses' knowledge about equianalgesia and opioid dosing, *Cancer Nurs* 20(3):201-212, 1997.

McCaffery M: Analgesics: mapping out pain relief, *Nursing* 26(1):41-46, 1996.

McCaffery M: Pain management handbook, *Nursing* 27(4):42-45, 1997.

Pasero CL: Managing pain in addicted patients, *Am J Nurs* 97(4):17-18, 1997.

Pasero CL: Nondrug measures for painful procedures, *Am J Nurs* 97(8):18-20, 1997.

Pasero CL: Pain during circumcision, *Am J Nurs* 97(10):21-22, 1997.

Pasero CL: Transdermal fentanyl for chronic pain, *Am J Nurs* 97(11):17-18, 1997.

Pasero CL: Using breathing to supplement pain control, *Am J Nurs* 97(2):16, 1997.

Pasero CL: When does 'drug seeking' behavior signal addiction? *Am J Nurs* 97(5):17-18, 1997.

Pasero CL: Pain control: when the physician prescribes a placebo, *Am J Nurs* 98(1):52-53, 1998.

Vessey JA, Carlson KL: Nonpharmacological interventions to use with children in pain, *Iss Compr Pediatr Nurs* 19(3):169-182, 1996.

Resources

American Society of Pain Management Nursing (ASPMN), telephone 888-342-7766, e-mail: ASPMN@aol.com.

Oncology Nursing Society, telephone 412-921-7373, e-mail: customer.service@ons.org.

Mayday Pain Resource Center, telephone 626-359-8111, ext. 3829, e-mail: mayday_pain@smtplink.coh.org.

Local Anesthetics

OBJECTIVES

After studying this chapter, you should be able to do the following:

■ *Describe the mechanism of action of local anesthetics.*

■ *Describe the side effects and adverse reactions of local anesthetics.*

■ *Explain the differences between agents for surface anesthesia and those injected to produce local anesthesia.*

■ *Differentiate among infiltration, nerve block, epidural, caudal, and spinal anesthesia.*

■ *Develop a nursing care plan for a patient who has received local anesthesia.*

CHAPTER OVERVIEW

Local anesthetics reversibly block nerve conduction, leading to loss of sensation and preventing muscle activity. In addition to topical anesthesia, local anesthetics can be infiltrated to various nerve sites, producing anesthesia over a wide area.

Cocaine was the first local anesthetic used clinically, after the observation in the late 1880s that when cocaine was administered orally to patients, their tongues and throats became numb. Its main use as a local anesthetic was to desensitize the cornea to allow local surgery without a general anesthetic. It was quickly recognized that cocaine had a high potential for abuse, and it was replaced by procaine (Novocain) in 1905. Today lidocaine (Xylocaine), introduced in the 1940s, is the most versatile and widely used local anesthetic. More than 15 local anesthetics are available, but they vary in their suitability for different applications.

THERAPEUTIC RATIONALE: LOCAL ANESTHESIA

Many medical and dental procedures require anesthesia of only a portion of the body. Local anesthesia is achieved by drugs that reversibly inhibit nerve conduction to produce both a loss of sensation and a loss of muscle activity. The local anesthetic is administered at the desired site of action. The inhibition of nerve conduction persists until the drug diffuses and enters the circulation for subsequent degradation and excretion. All neurons in the area of administration, whether pain, motor, or autonomic, are affected, so in addition to the loss of pain, loss of sensory, motor, and autonomic activities occurs. The size of the nerve fiber determines its sensitivity to local anesthetics; smaller fibers are the most sensitive. Because sensory fibers are smaller than motor fibers, loss of sensation precedes loss of motor activity, and conversely, motor activity is regained before sensory function.

The choice of local anesthetic depends on the route of administration and the desired duration of action.

THERAPEUTIC AGENTS: LOCAL ANESTHETICS

Local Anesthetics: General Characteristics

Mechanism of Action

Chemically, most local anesthetics are weak bases, being secondary or tertiary amines. This means that under physiologic conditions, most molecules carry a positive charge and are not lipid soluble. However, it is the uncharged form that diffuses across the nerve membrane and then reequilibrates to charged and uncharged forms. The positively charged form binds to a receptor near the intracellular end of the sodium channel. The result is that nerve conduction is blocked because the voltage-gated sodium channels are blocked. Because the action potential is generated by the influx of sodium ions, the local anesthetic depresses the action potential so that it is not propagated. The resting potential of neurons is not affected by local anesthetics.

Pharmacokinetics

Local anesthetics eventually enter the systemic circulation and can affect other organs, limiting their safety. The relative safety of procaine and chloroprocaine results from their rapid hydrolysis in the plasma by pseudocholinesterases. Other local anesthetics are slowly degraded by the liver and have a longer plasma half-life.

The rate at which local anesthetic is removed from the infiltrated area depends largely on the degree of vascularization. The duration can be increased by 50% to 100% with the inclusion of epinephrine, 1:200,000, or phenylephrine to cause vasoconstriction and thereby restrict systemic absorption. However, epinephrine is contraindicated for infiltration of areas with end arteries (fingers, toes, ears, nose, and penis) because the resultant ischemia may lead to tissue death. Similarly, the addition of a vasoconstrictor is contraindicated in epidural anesthesia in labor because of the potential vasoconstriction of the uterine blood vessels with a resultant decrease in placental circulation. Epinephrine is also contraindicated for patients with severe cardiovascular disease or thyrotoxicosis, in whom cardiac function would be compromised by added vasoconstrictors.

Uses

In general, local anesthetics can be divided into those applied topically to provide surface anesthesia and those injected into an area to produce local anesthesia. Only **lidocaine** (Xylocaine), dibucaine (Nupercaine), and tetracaine (Pontocaine) are used both topically and by injection.

Surface Anesthesia. Those local anesthetics applied as drops, sprays, lotions, creams, or ointments, also called **surface anesthetics,** are listed in Table 35-1. Distinction is made between those drugs safely applied to the eyes, skin, and mucosal areas. Only tetracaine (Pontocaine) is suitable for application to all three sites.

Most drugs for surface anesthesia are effective when applied to the skin. These drugs are poorly soluble, so little systemic absorption occurs when they are applied to the skin to relieve itching or the pain of mild burns. The main potential toxicity of local anesthetics applied to the skin is allergy, usually contact dermatitis. Because several chemical classes are represented by local anesthetics, a drug from a different chemical group can be substituted if an allergy develops.

Mucosal membranes of the nose, mouth, and throat (bronchotracheal mucosa) and of the urethra, rectum, and vagina are highly vascular and allow ready absorption of the local anesthetic into systemic circulation. Application of excessive amounts of local anesthetics to mucosal surfaces is the most common cause of systemic toxicity with local anesthetics. A local anesthetic is often used to eliminate the gag reflex when inserting an endotracheal tube or to limit the discomfort of endoscopic procedures. The lowest concentration possible of the local anesthetic should be used on mucosal surfaces to avoid systemic toxicity, and the total amount of drug should be recorded and matched against recommended total doses.

Local Anesthetics Administered by Injection. Local anesthetics used by injection are listed in Table 35-2. The potency and the duration of action increase together with the lipid solubility of the drug. The onset of anesthesia is determined by the concentration of drug and the size of the nerve. Before infiltrating an area with a local anesthetic, the syringe should first be aspirated to ensure that a blood vessel has not been entered. This step is necessary because the concentration of drug is high and could prove fatal if injected systemically.

The area affected by a local anesthetic depends on how and where it is injected. The anesthesia produced is described by the technique of injection: infiltration, nerve block, epidural, and spinal. These techniques are described with their potential for producing toxic side effects.

Infiltration anesthesia refers to the superficial application of a local anesthetic. To suture a cut or to perform dental procedures, local anesthetic is injected superficially in small amounts to block the small nerves and to numb the area. To work on the scalp or to make an incision in the skin, the anesthetic is infused around the area. Small incisions require a small volume and a low concentration of drug, so little toxicity is associated with these uses. However, systemic toxicity from local anesthetics is commonly seen in the emergency room when large cuts are infiltrated with local anesthetic.

Nerve block anesthesia refers to the injection of a local anesthetic along a nerve before it reaches the surgical site. The volume and concentration of a local anesthetic for a nerve block must be larger than in infiltration anesthesia to penetrate the larger nerve.

Intravenous regional anesthesia (Bier's block) is an anesthetic technique used for surgery to the forearm and hand or foot and distal leg. The limb is cannulated and then exsanguinated with an elastic bandage. A tourniquet is applied and inflated to 100 to 150 mm Hg above the systolic blood pressure. The local anesthetic, usually lidocaine, is then applied through the cannula. Anesthesia takes about 5 to 10 minutes. The duration must be limited to 2 hours to avoid ischemic nerve injury. The advantage of the technique is that it can be terminated by deflation of the tourniquet with rapid return of sensation. However, toxic levels of local anesthetic may be released if the tourniquet is not left in place for a minimum of 15 to 30 minutes.

The most extensive field of local anesthesia is achieved by applying the local anesthetic around the nerve roots near the spinal cord to produce epidural or spinal anesthesia. As

Table 35-1 **Local Anesthetics for Surface Anesthesia**

Generic Name	Trade Name	Eyes	Mucous Membranes‡	Skin	Comments
benzocaine	Americaine Dermoplast*	0	+	+	Widely used. Included in many nonprescription preparations to relieve sunburn, itching, and mild burns. Long acting and poorly absorbed.
butamben		0	+	+	Mucosal formulation includes benzocaine and tetracaine. Also a nonprescription ointment to relieve itching and burning.
cocaine hydrochloride		+	+	0	Schedule II drug. Medically used in ear, nose, and throat procedures when vasoconstriction and shrinking of mucous membranes are desired. Ophthalmic preparations anesthetize cornea and conjunctiva.
dibucaine hydrochloride	Nupercaine*	0	+	+	Nonprescription skin ointment or cream; also cream for relieving hemorrhoids.
dyclonine hydrochloride	Duclone Sucrets	0	+	+	Lozenges relieve a sore throat. Topical suppresses gag reflex and lessens discomfort of genitourinary endoscopy. Precipitated by iodine of contrast media used in pyelography and should not be used.
lidocaine	Xylocaine*	0	+	+	Widely used for topical anesthesia in ear, nose, and throat procedures; upper digestive tract procedures; and genitourinary procedures. Rapid onset and intermediate duration. Not irritating and low incidence of hypersensitivity.
lidocaine hydrochloride	Xylocaine hydrochloride*	0	+	+	
pramoxine hydrochloride	Fleet Relief Tronothane*	0	+§	+	Nonprescription cream or ointment primarily used to relieve pain of itching, burns, and hemorrhoids.
proparacaine hydrochloride	Ophthaine*	+	0	0	Applied topically to eye to anesthetize cornea and conjunctiva.
tetracaine hydrochloride	Pontocaine*	+	+	+	Topically, onset is 5 min, and duration is 45 min. Usual topical dose is 20 mg; maximum is 50 mg because of toxicity and slow degradation. Ophthalmic preparations are dilute solutions for instillation.

+, Suitable site for application; 0, site not suitable for application.
*Available in Canada and the United States.
‡Mucous membranes include the oral esophageal mucosa, bronchotracheal mucosa, and the mucosa of the urethra, rectum, and vagina.
§Not for application to the bronchotracheal mucosa.

shown in Figure 35-1, the spinal cord proper ends at the lumbar region. The spinal cord is surrounded by three membranes: first the pia mater, then the arachnoid, and finally the outer membrane, the dura mater. These membranes extend below the spinal cord proper to form a sac in the lumbar and sacral region. The dura mater and arachnoid membranes are close together, and the subarachnoid space is between the arachnoid and pia mater. Cerebrospinal fluid fills the subarachnoid space throughout the spinal cord.

For **epidural anesthesia,** the local anesthetic is administered outside the dura mater (see Figure 35-1) so that the nerve roots are blocked at the point after they emerge from the dura mater. The extent of anesthesia depends on the volume and concentration of local anesthetic used. **Caudal**

anesthesia is another form of epidural anesthesia and is achieved by administering the local anesthetic epidurally at the base of the spine (see Figure 35-1). The extent of anesthesia affects only the pelvic region and legs. Caudal anesthesia is used for obstetrics and for surgery on the rectum, anus, and prostate gland.

Spinal anesthesia is achieved by injecting local anesthetic into the subarachnoid space between the arachnoid and pia mater membranes in the lumbar area, usually between the second lumbar and first sacral vertebrae and well below the spinal cord proper. This method blocks the nerve roots for the entire lower body. If the solution containing local anesthetic has the same density (isobaric) as cerebrospinal fluid and is administered slowly, it will stay where it is injected

Table 35-2 Local Anesthetics for Injection

Generic Name	Trade Name	Local Infiltration or Nerve Block or Epidural Block	Spinal Block (Subarachnoid)	Duration‡	Comments
bupivacaine hydrochloride	Marcaine‡ Sensorcaine-MPF	+	+	Long§	Provides long-acting epidural anesthesia in labor with no reported effects on fetus. Maximum dose is 200 mg.
chloroprocaine hydrochloride	Nesacaine	+	0	Short	Little systemic toxicity because of rapid hydrolysis in plasma. No effects reported on fetus after epidural anesthesia in mother. Maximum dose is 800 mg.
etidocaine hydrochloride	Duranest	+	0	Long	Highly lipid soluble. Onset for epidural block is 5 min. Profound muscle relaxation is desirable for abdominal surgery but not for labor.
lidocaine	Xylocaine*	+	+	Intermediate	Widely used local anesthetic. Maximum dose is 300 mg (4.5 mg/kg body weight). Can cause drowsiness, fatigue, and amnesia.
mepivacaine	Carbocaine*	+	0	Intermediate	Chemically related to lidocaine. Maximum dose is 400 mg (7 mg/kg body weight).
prilocaine	Citanest*	+	0	Intermediate	Used for dental procedures. Maximum dose is 400 mg.
procaine hydrochloride	Novocaine*	+	0	Short	Noted for its safety because of its rapid hydrolysis in plasma. Maximum dose is 600 mg (10 mg/kg body weight). Duration of epidural block is unreliable.
propoxycaine and procaine	Ravocaine and Novocain with Neo-Cobefrin	+	0	Short to intermediate	Used for dental procedures. Dose is 4 mg propoxycaine and 20 mg procaine.
ropivacaine	Naropin*	+	0	Long	Used for epidural, field block, and major nerve block anesthesia. Dose is 20-40 mg.
tetracaine	Pontocaine*	0	+	Long	Most widely used drug for spinal anesthesia. Onset is 5 min. Dose for spinal anesthesia is 2-15 mg. Available in hyperbaric, isobaric, and hypobaric solutions.

+, Suitable use; *0,* use not suitable.
*Available in Canada and the United States.
‡Duration without epinephrine: short, 1 hr; intermediate, 2 hr; long, 3 hr (approximations).
§Duration of bupivacaine in nerve block is 6-13 hr.

and will only slowly diffuse into the rest of the cerebrospinal fluid. The solution of local anesthetic can be made more dense (hyperbaric) by diluting the local anesthetic into 5% dextrose. The solution will then move downward (toward the ground). If the patient is on a tilt bed with feet high and head low, the hyperbaric solution will travel up the spinal cord toward the head and anesthetize more of the body. The solution of local anesthetic also can be diluted with distilled water to be less dense (hypobaric). In patients positioned on the tilt bed, this solution would move to the end of the dura mater and anesthetize only the lower part of the body. Pro-

cedures using hypobaric and hyperbaric solutions of local anesthetic require skill in positioning patients. If the level of anesthesia is adjusted to block more of the spinal cord than just the lumbar and sacral regions, there is danger of paralyzing the intercostal and phrenic nerves, thereby paralyzing spontaneous respiration.

If the patient is seated when the local anesthetic is administered as a low spinal anesthetic, only those nerves affecting the parts of the body that would be in contact with a saddle are affected; hence the name **saddle block.** This procedure is used principally in obstetrics for vaginal delivery.

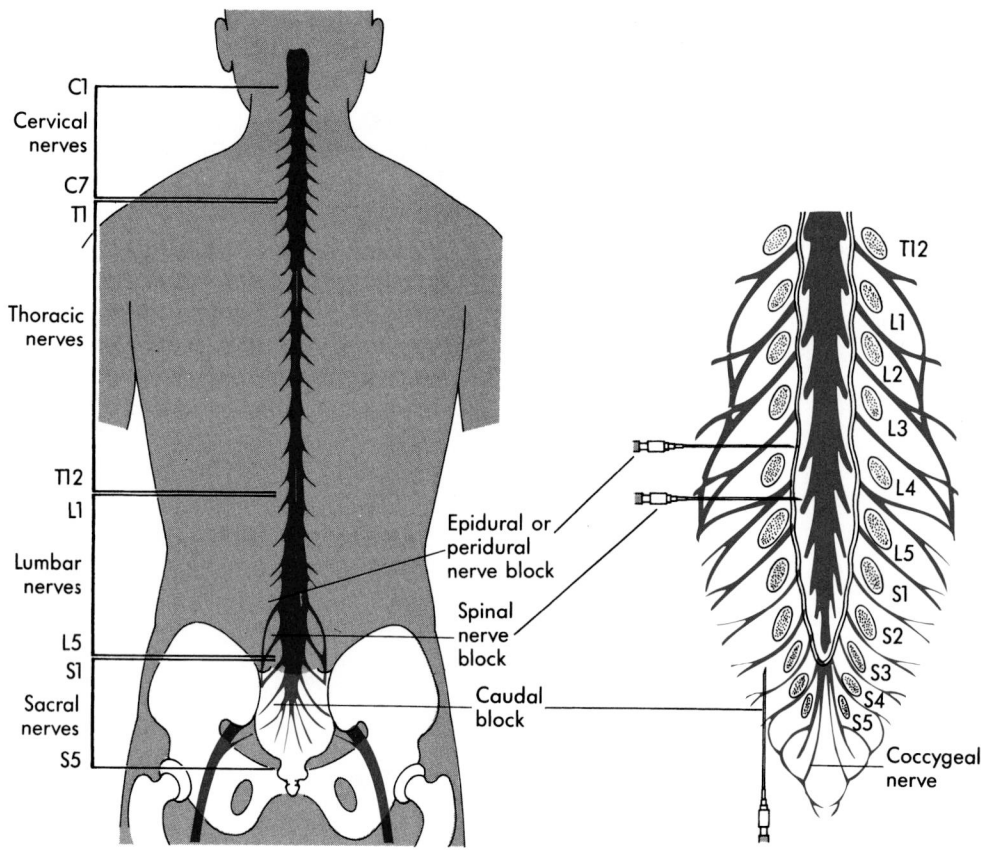

Figure 35-1   Sites for injection of local anesthetic to achieve spinal, epidural, and caudal anesthesia.

With spinal anesthesia the patient is awake, breathing and cardiovascular function are not immediately affected, and good muscle relaxation is present. These are advantages for patients with heart and lung disease or for older adults. However, the sympathetic fibers to the blood vessels are blocked, so vasodilation with hypotension is a common side effect of spinal anesthesia. Spinal anesthesia is therefore considered hazardous for abdominal surgery in poor-risk patients because of the potential for sudden vasodilation and hypotension. Spinal anesthesia is widely used in obstetrics, particularly for cesarean sections.

Adverse Reactions, Toxicity, and Contraindications

Although cocaine is unique in causing euphoria, all local anesthetics act as central nervous system (CNS) stimulants if absorbed systemically, producing symptoms such as anxiety, tingling (paresthesia), tremors, and ringing in the ears (tinnitus). This CNS stimulation may ultimately result in convulsions. Intravenous (IV) diazepam (Valium) in 2.5-mg increments or small doses of an ultrashort-acting barbiturate such as thiopental (Pentothal), thiamylal (Surital), or methohexital (Brevital) are given to stop these convulsions.

A high plasma concentration of a local anesthetic causes CNS depression, with or without prior symptoms of CNS stimulation. Depression of CNS function is serious because vasomotor control is lost, resulting in profound hypotension, respiratory depression, and coma.

In addition to the CNS effects, direct cardiovascular effects of local anesthetics are important. The electrical properties of the heart reflect in part the activity of sodium channels. The local anesthetics lidocaine and procainamide are also used as antiarrhythmic drugs. High systemic levels of local anesthetics decrease electrical excitability. If local anesthetics are inadvertently administered intravenously, plasma levels toxic to the heart may result. Bupivacaine and etidocaine are especially cardiotoxic. Ropivacaine has low cardiotoxicity.

Local anesthetics cause direct vasodilation, increasing blood flow and favoring removal of the drug. Thus epinephrine is sometimes added to the local anesthetic because it causes vasoconstriction and prolongs the time the local anesthetic remains at the injection site. Cocaine is unique among the local anesthetics in being a potent vasoconstrictor. Prolonged abuse of cocaine by insufflation (sniffing) can cause loss of nasal septa caused by tissue death after ischemia (insufficient blood flow). Local anesthetics are cardiac depressants. Lidocaine is used to depress cardiac arrhythmias (see Chapter 19).

Local anesthetics that are esters (chloroprocaine, procaine, and tetracaine) can cause an allergic response. Anaphylaxis is rare, and more commonly, the topical use of a local anesthetic with an ester bond leads to skin rash (contact dermatitis).

Spinal anesthesia can cause variable hypotension because the neurons controlling vasomotor tone are in the spinal tract. A severe headache may be experienced after spinal anesthesia and may last for hours or days after the anesthetic has worn off. This postspinal headache is believed to reflect a drop in the pressure of the cerebrospinal fluid caused by a leak where the dura mater was penetrated. Incidence of a spinal headache is reduced when patients are kept flat on their backs and instructed not to raise their heads for 12 hours after spinal anesthesia. This minimizes the hydrostatic pressure of the cerebrospinal fluid on the head.

Nursing Process Overview

Local Anesthesia

Assessment

Assess vital signs and temperature, history of allergies, response to previous surgery, and overall condition.

Nursing Diagnoses

- Risk for urinary retention and inability to void related to spinal anesthesia
- Impaired swallowing and loss of gag reflex related to local anesthesia

Patient Outcomes

The patient will void completely, without difficulty. The patient will not aspirate because of the effects of local anesthetics.

Planning/Implementation

For minor or brief procedures such as suturing or dental work, careful observation of the patient may be sufficient. For longer procedures or when spinal anesthesia is used, monitor vital signs and other parameters of patient function. With spinal anesthesia, position the lower extremities carefully. Insert a Foley catheter to allow urinary output. Monitor the level of consciousness. Allergic responses are possible when local anesthetics are used by any route; have epinephrine and equipment for resuscitation available to treat possible anaphylaxis. When used for labor and delivery, monitor the mother and the baby; assess fetal heart tones.

Evaluation

All anesthetics require time to wear off, and specific nursing care depends on the area that has been anesthetized. For example, if the throat has been anesthetized for bronchoscopy, evaluate ability to swallow, position the patient on the side to reduce the possibility of aspiration, restrict oral intake until the patient can swallow, and have a suction machine available at the bedside. After spinal anesthesia, keep the patient flat for 12 to 24 hours. Check the position of the lower extremities to prevent pressure areas, and keep the patient in bed until sensation returns to the lower extremities. Monitor vital signs and intake and output.

If the patient is still under the effects of the local anesthetic at discharge, verify that the patient can explain any restrictions in activity or diet to be followed until the anesthesia wears off. If analgesic medications are prescribed for use after the anesthesia wears off, the patient should be able to explain their use (see Chapters 31 and 32). If a local anesthetic is prescribed for outpatient use, determine that the patient can explain how and with what frequency to use the medication and what to do if it is ineffective.

Nursing Implications Summary

General Guidelines: Local Anesthesia
Drug Administration
- Obtain a careful history of previous response to local anesthetics. Remember that the term *Novocain* is often used by patients to refer to any local anesthetic, regardless of the specific drug. Monitor the blood pressure and pulse. If epidural, nerve block, or spinal anesthesia is used, monitor respirations. If anesthesia is used during labor and delivery, assess fetal heart tones.
- Keep the patient flat up to 12 hours after spinal anesthesia. Transfer the patient flat from the stretcher to the bed. Use a thin pillow.
- Assess the patient who has had epidural, nerve block, or spinal anesthesia for ability to void or for a distended bladder. Monitor intake and output. If the patient has not voided in 8 hours after surgery or delivery, notify the physician.
- Assist the patient who has received epidural, nerve block, or spinal anesthesia when ambulating for the first time.
- Position the patient carefully in bed after epidural, nerve block, or spinal anesthesia because the patient has no sensation to warn of wrinkles, tight sheets, or other skin irritants.
- Apply heat or cold to anesthetized area with extreme caution because the patient will be unable to indicate if irritation or burning occurs. If applying heat or cold is necessary, shield

Continued

Nursing Implications Summary—cont'd

the skin well from the heat or cold source and check the patient and the skin surfaces every 5 to 15 minutes. This applies after oral or dental anesthesia also.

➤ Although serious systemic reactions are rare with local anesthetics, have drugs, equipment, and personnel available to treat acute allergic reactions in settings where these drugs are used.

➤ A patient in the operating or delivery rooms who is receiving local anesthesia may be drowsy from preoperative medications but will usually be alert and able to understand conversation in the room. Keep conversation and noise to a minimum. Avoid discussing other patients, complications, pathology reports, or other topics that might alarm the patient.

➤ After bronchoscopy or other procedures in which surface anesthesia may have been applied to the back of the throat, assess the gag reflex and ability to swallow. Do not leave the patient unattended until the patient can safely handle secretions.

➤ Consult the state board of nursing or other regulatory agency for clarification of questions related to the scope of practice for nurses and the administration of injected local anesthetics.

Nursing in the Community

➤ After injection of anesthetics into tongue, lips, and gums, or after topical application of liquid, lozenges, or other agents causing numbness to the throat or mouth, caution the patient to avoid eating or chewing until sensation returns to avoid biting the tongue or cheek and to avoid choking.

➤ Tell the patient to report any rash or skin irritation occurring as a result of application of a local anesthetic.

➤ If the patient develops an allergic or untoward response to a local anesthetic, instruct the patient to wear a medical identification tag or bracelet indicating the causative agent.

➤ Instruct the patient to use surface anesthetics as instructed and not to increase the frequency of application or to use the preparation on skin surfaces for which it was not designed. Before discharge, review any limitations the patient may have until the effects of the anesthetic wear off. For example, a patient who has had local anesthesia to a joint may be instructed to avoid use of the joint for a certain number of hours or until the anesthesia has worn off.

➤ Dental anesthetics: Children and the elderly may be especially sensitive to the effects of dental anesthetics. Read labels carefully, and use as directed. Tell parents to be alert to this possibility.

➤ Dental paste: See manufacturer's instructions. Instruct the patient to use an applicator to apply small amounts to the sore areas and not to rub with fingers while applying because the medication will crumble.

➤ Anesthetic lozenges: Instruct the patient to allow the lozenge to dissolve in the mouth and not to bite them, swallow them whole, or chew them. Warn family to make certain the child understands how to use a lozenge correctly before giving it to a child.

➤ Benzocaine film-forming gel: Review manufacturer's instructions. Instruct the patient to dry the area with a swab where the medication is to be applied, apply gel to a second swab, then roll gel over the specified area. Instruct the patient to try to keep mouth open and dry for 30 to 60 seconds after applying gel. The gel will form a film that should not be removed; it will slowly disappear over several hours.

➤ Viscous lidocaine or other thick liquid form: Follow physician's instructions. The drug may be applied to specific areas in the mouth with an applicator, or a specified amount may be poured into a medicine cup and swished around in the mouth and throat. Remind the patient to use only the amount prescribed and to measure the dose carefully. The patient should not swallow the liquid unless instructed to do so by physician.

➤ Aerosol forms sprayed in the mouth: Instruct the patient to avoid inhaling the spray and to avoid spraying the back of the throat unless specifically instructed to do so.

➤ Gel or liquid forms of dental anesthetics: Unless otherwise instructed, the patient should apply medication with fingertip, applicator, or piece of gauze to sore area. Instruct the patient to wait until tenderness or pain disappears before putting dentures or appliances in mouth and not to apply directly to dentures or oral appliances.

➤ Ophthalmic forms: Instruct the patient to apply ointment or solution as directed and not to rub the eye until the anesthetic has worn off because inadvertent eye injury may occur.

➤ Rectal forms: Read the manufacturer's instructions carefully. For creams or ointments that are to be inserted into rectum, instruct the patient to use applicators provided by the manufacturer and to be careful not to insert the cap into the rectum. For rectal aerosol form, instruct the patient not to insert the container itself into the rectum and to use the applicator provided by the manufacturer. For topical forms applied to the area around the rectum: clean the area with soap and water or a cleansing wipe, then dry the area. Use a tissue, gauze, glove, or finger cot to apply a small amount of medication to the area.

➤ Topical application to the skin: Instruct the patient to use only as directed and to read the product label carefully: some products contain alcohol. Caution the patient to not use products containing alcohol while smoking or near an open flame to avoid possible fire hazard. Caution the patient to avoid using any product near eyes, nose, or mouth.

➤ Butamben ointment: This ointment may stain clothing permanently and discolor hair. Instruct the patient to avoid touching clothing or hair while applying medication and to cover the area when medication has been applied with a loose bandage.

➤ Lidocaine film-forming gel: Dry area with a clean cloth. Apply medication as directed. A clear film should form within about 1 minute.

CHAPTER REVIEW

Application

1. What is the mechanism of action of local anesthetics?
2. What property of procaine and chloroprocaine makes them relatively safe?
3. What are toxic effects of systemic absorption of local anesthetics?
4. To what three types of surfaces are local anesthetics applied?
5. Describe the areas of anesthesia achieved by infiltration, nerve block, epidural, and spinal anesthesia.

Critical Thinking

1. What hazards are associated with spinal anesthesia?
2. How is the duration of local anesthetics prolonged?

General Anesthetics

OBJECTIVES

After studying this chapter, you should be able to do the following:

- *Describe the characteristics of inhalation anesthetics, intravenous anesthetics, balanced anesthesia, and neuroleptanesthesia.*
- *Explain minimum alveolar concentration.*
- *Outline the characteristics of the different agents described in this chapter.*
- *Develop a nursing care plan for the patient receiving a specific general anesthetic agent or a combination of agents.*

CHAPTER OVERVIEW

Modern surgery did not begin until the introduction of nitrous oxide, ether, and chloroform as general anesthetics in the late 1800s. The agents used today as general anesthetics include gases (nitrous oxide), volatile liquids (diethyl ether, halothane, methoxyflurane, enflurane, and isoflurane), and intravenous (IV) agents (ketamine and opioids). The ultrashort-acting barbiturates, benzodiazepines, and etomidate are used intravenously for induction of anesthesia.

THERAPEUTIC RATIONALE: GENERAL ANESTHESIA

General anesthetics act on the central nervous system (CNS) to abolish the perception of pain and the reaction to painful stimuli. The use of general anesthetics requires specifically trained personnel to monitor the level of anesthesia and the patient's vital signs while under anesthesia.

THERAPEUTIC AGENTS: GENERAL ANESTHETICS

Inhalation Anesthetics: General Characteristics

Mechanism of Action

Inhalation anesthetics are gases or volatile liquids administered as gases. They are unusual in their mechanism of action because they do not appear to act by a receptor mechanism. The historic mechanism attributed to inhalation anesthetics is that they alter the lipid structure of cell membranes, so physiologic functions are impaired. Current research suggests a receptor-associated mechanism involving the inhibitory transmitters gamma-aminobutyric acid (GABA) and glycine. These neurotransmitters activate receptors that conduct chloride ions into neurons, making them less likely to fire action potentials. There is evidence that anesthetics potentiate this inhibitory action.

The network of neurons making up the CNS is especially vulnerable to anesthetics because alteration of membrane structure interrupts the complex intercommunication necessary for function. The most sensitive system to such alterations is the ascending reticular activating system, the neuronal formation monitoring incoming stimuli and determining what information is to be sent to the brain for processing and response. Consciousness is lost when the ascending reticular activating system ceases to transmit information effectively.

Pharmacokinetics

The effective concentration of an inhalation anesthetic in the brain does not depend on the solubility of the anesthetic in blood or tissue. Rather, effective concentration depends on the partial pressure of the anesthetic or effective pressure of the gas in the atmosphere. If a constant partial pressure of anesthetic is inhaled, partial pressure in the alveoli rises toward the inhaled level. If the gas is not soluble in blood, little gas is removed by the blood circulating around the alveoli, and the partial pressure of the gas in the blood quickly reaches the inhaled partial pressure. This anesthetic has a rapid onset of action. If the gas is soluble in blood, however, partial pressure of the gas in the alveoli quickly drops because the gas is being removed more rapidly by the blood than can be replenished by breathing. A long time is required to equilibrate the blood with the gas to where the partial pressure matches that coming into the alveoli. To shorten the time to reach this steady state, anesthesia is induced using a high partial pressure of the gas and then lowering the partial pressure to maintain anesthesia.

The potency of an inhalation anesthetic is determined by the **minimum alveolar concentration (MAC)** that produces insensitivity to a skin incision (anesthesia) in 50% of patients. For instance, MAC of 10% is equivalent to a partial pressure of 0.1 atmosphere or 76 mm Hg at standard conditions (sea level). MAC of 10% means that when air in the alveoli has equilibrated with the body and incoming air, all of which are 10% anesthetic gas, the patient has a 50-50 chance of being unreactive to a skin incision. Surgery is conducted at about 1.4 times the MAC value of the anesthetic chosen.

The depth of anesthesia was traditionally defined by four stages of anesthesia based on the action of diethyl ether as follows: I, analgesia; II, excitement; III, surgical; and IV, medullary depression. Today so many ancillary drugs are administered that these stages are not useful for observation purposes. The most reliable indication of stage III surgical anesthesia is the loss of the eyelash reflex in which the eye blinks when the eyelash is stroked and the establishment of a respiratory pattern that is regular in depth and in rate.

The distribution of the anesthetic is determined by the blood flow; thus the brain, liver, and kidneys reach equilibrium first. Excretion of the inhalation anesthetics is largely through the lungs. The anesthetic that is in solution is metabolized by the liver to a variable degree. Certain halogenated hydrocarbons (e.g., enflurane, halothane, methoxyflurane) are metabolized to products that may damage the liver and kidney.

Emergence is the time during which the patient regains consciousness after the anesthetic has been discontinued. The duration of emergence from the inhaled anesthetics depends on the same factors as induction. The patient's vital signs are carefully monitored in a recovery room, and symptoms of pain or nausea and vomiting must be watched for and treated appropriately.

Uses

Nitrous oxide, desflurane, and isoflurane are the most widely used inhalation anesthetics in the United States. Halothane is often used for pediatric anesthesia but is not often used for adults. Enflurane is occasionally used for adult patients but is not often used for pediatric patients. Methoxyflurane is sometimes used for obstetric anesthesia. Diethyl ether is not used in the United States.

Adverse Reactions and Contraindications

In general, pediatric patients require higher concentrations of inhalation anesthetics and geriatric patients require lower concentrations. Geriatric patients are also more likely to react with hypotension and circulatory depression.

Inhalation anesthetics vary in the degree to which they affect the cardiovascular system. Halothane and enflurane have the more pronounced effects, which include reduced blood pressure and myocardial depression.

All inhalation anesthetics except nitrous oxide are respiratory depressants. They decrease the ventilatory response to hypoxia. Both during surgery and recovery, ventilatory assistance and increased oxygen are needed.

Kidney function is affected by inhalation anesthetics. Glomerular filtration rate and renal plasma flow are decreased. Blood flow to the liver is also decreased by inhalation anesthetics.

The inhalation anesthetics aside from nitrous oxide are uterine muscle relaxants. This effect can assist fetal manipulation during delivery, but increases bleeding during a dilation and curettage (D&C) procedure.

Shivering is a common reaction during recovery. It represents a response to heat loss and to the recovery of neurologic functions.

Toxicity

Hepatotoxicity has been associated with enflurane, halothane, and methoxyflurane; however, this association is weak and may reflect a susceptible subpopulation of individuals who have a defect in their hepatic cell membranes.

Nephrotoxicity is associated with methoxyflurane because of the level of inorganic fluoride resulting from its metabolism. This is a major reason that methoxyflurane is not widely used. Enflurane and halothane carry a low risk of nephrotoxicity.

Malignant hyperthermia is a rare toxic reaction to inhaled anesthetics and occurs in genetically susceptible patients. Symptoms include tachycardia, hypertension, acidosis, hyperkalemia, muscle rigidity, and hyperthermia. Treatment includes administering IV dantrolene, lowering the body temperature, and restoring electrolyte and acid-base balance.

Chronic toxicity caused by anesthetic exposure in operating room personnel has been suggested. In particular an increased incidence of miscarriages has been reported. The evidence is not considered strong, however. Most operating rooms have vents to remove anesthetics.

Specific Inhalation Anesthetics

Table 36-1 lists specific inhalation anesthetics and their properties.

diethyl ether

Diethyl ether is a volatile liquid that is flammable and explosive. Although it was the first widely used anesthetic, it is no longer used. The MAC is 1.92%. A long time is required for induction and emergence when ether alone is used because it is highly soluble in blood. In addition, ether is unpleasant to inhale because it has a noxious and pungent odor, irritates the respiratory tract, and stimulates secretions. An anticholinergic drug may be administered to minimize these secretions. The explosive hazard and the noxious, pungent odor account for the rare use of ether in modern surgery. Nevertheless, ether is used in areas of the world where sophisticated equipment is unavailable for monitoring the patient. Ether has a wide margin of safety and has few effects on the cardiovascular system, allowing it to be administered without sophisticated control of concentration. Ether produces good analgesia and muscle relaxation, making extra medication unnecessary.

desflurane

Desflurane (Suprane) is the newest inhalation anesthetic. It is a halogenated hydrocarbon and chemically related to isoflurane. Desflurane is a nonflammable liquid that is administered with a special heated vaporizer. The MAC is 7.3%, but this decreases when combined with benzodiazepines or opioids. The sensitivity to desflurane also increases with age. One drawback of desflurane is that it irritates the respiratory tract to produce coughing, apnea, laryngospasm, and increased secretions. Induction is therefore usually accomplished with an IV drug. However, induction and emergence are rapid (5 to 7 minutes), making desflurane useful for ambulatory surgery. Cardiac output tends to remain stable, although the heart rate may increase and blood pressure may decrease.

enflurane

Enflurane (Ethrane) is a halogenated hydrocarbon and a nonflammable liquid. MAC is 1.68%, and induction is fairly rapid. Enflurane is one of the stimulant anesthetics that produce muscle contractions and seizurelike brain wave patterns at high concentrations. Enflurane is usually administered with nitrous oxide to avoid high concentrations, which can cause CNS stimulation and cardiovascular depression. Enflurane causes a decrease in blood pressure resulting from depressed cardiac output and decreased peripheral resistance. Emergence is usually uneventful except for shivering. About 2.5% of enflurane is metabolized to release a low concentration of fluoride ion. The amount of fluoride ion is not harmful, except in patients with preexisting kidney damage.

halothane

Halothane (Fluothane) is a nonflammable liquid halogenated hydrocarbon and was widely used for many years. MAC is 0.77%, and induction is fairly rapid. Postoperative nausea and vomiting are not problems. Halothane is a direct myocardial depressant and causes a dose-dependent reduction in cardiac output with no change in heart rate, a combination of effects that lowers blood pressure. Halothane also sensitizes the myocardium to exogenously administered catecholamines. This sensitization means that a sympathomimetic drug must be used cautiously during surgery to maintain blood pressure because sympathomimetic drugs may precipitate arrhythmias. Catecholamines may be used topically, such as on the brain or in irrigation of the bladder to stop bleeding. Halothane does not give adequate muscle relaxation; a separate muscle relaxant must be used.

Rarely (1:800,000 patients) halothane is responsible for fatal hepatitis. Current theory is that free radical metabolites,

Table 36-1 Properties of Inhalation Anesthetics

Generic Name	Trade Name	Properties	Comments
desflurane	Suprane	Nonflammable liquid. Rapid onset. MAC: 7.3%. Eliminated through lungs with little metabolism by liver.	Minimum cardiovascular effects. Good muscle relaxation. Irritating to airways.
enflurane	Ethrane	Nonflammable liquid. Rapid onset. MAC: 1.68%. Eliminated through lungs with 2%-5% metabolized by liver. FDA pregnancy category B.	Decreases blood pressure and sensitizes heart to catecholamines. Good muscle relaxation. Causes low body temperature, hypothermia, and shivering.
halothane	Fluothane	Nonflammable liquid. Rapid onset. MAC: 0.77%. Eliminated through lungs with 20% metabolized by liver. FDA pregnancy category C.	Decreases blood pressure. Fair muscle relaxation. Sensitizes heart to catecholamines. Poor analgesia.
isoflurane	Forane	Nonflammable liquid. Rapid onset. MAC: 1.30%. Eliminated through lungs with little metabolism by liver. FDA pregnancy category C.	Minimum cardiovascular effects. Good muscle relaxation. Excellent analgesia. Widely used.
methoxyflurane	Penthrane	Nonflammable liquid. Slow onset. MAC: 0.16%. Some elimination through lungs but 70% metabolized by liver. FDA pregnancy category C.	Decreases blood pressure. Good muscle relaxation. Excellent analgesia. High incidence of nephrotoxicity at anesthetic levels.
nitrous oxide	Generic	Nonflammable gas. Very rapid onset. MAC: 101%. Eliminated through lungs.	Widely used with other drugs for anesthesia. Good analgesia. Minimum cardiovascular effects.

which are very reactive compounds, may be produced by the liver and may damage liver cells.

▼ isoflurane

Isoflurane (Forane) was introduced in 1981 and is currently the most widely used inhalation anesthetic. It is a chemical isomer of enflurane, but unlike enflurane, isoflurane is a depressant anesthetic similar to halothane. MAC is 1.3%. Induction is smooth and rapid, and muscle relaxation is adequate. The heart is not sensitized to catecholamines, but the blood pressure falls because of a decrease in the peripheral resistance of blood vessels. Only 0.25% of isoflurane is metabolized.

methoxyflurane

Methoxyflurane (Penthrane) is a nonflammable liquid halogenated hydrocarbon. It produces analgesia adequate for obstetrics. MAC is 0.16%. Methoxyflurane depresses the cardiovascular system but does not sensitize the heart to catecholamines. Methoxyflurane that is not exhaled is metabolized extensively (70%) by the liver to fluoride ion. Prolonged anesthesia with methoxyflurane may result in high-output renal failure because in the presence of the fluoride ion, the kidney loses its concentrating ability so that urine volume is high. This renal failure is usually reversible. However, the potential for nephrotoxicity limits the use of methoxyflurane.

▼ nitrous oxide

Nitrous oxide is a nonexplosive gas that is widely used. The major limitation of nitrous oxide is that the maximum concentration allowable, 65% to 70% N_2O and 30% to 35% O_2, does not produce surgical anesthesia because MAC is 101%. Nevertheless, nitrous oxide produces good analgesia and is used for this purpose in dental and obstetric procedures. In addition, nitrous oxide is widely used with other anesthetics to produce surgical anesthesia. Its effect is additive with other anesthetics, so a 50% MAC concentration of nitrous oxide and a 50% MAC concentration of another inhalation anesthetic produces surgical anesthesia. In addition, nitrous oxide is widely used as one component of **balanced anesthesia,** in which an opioid, a skeletal muscle relaxant, and nitrous oxide are used together to produce surgical anesthesia.

Nitrous oxide has been shown to increase the incidence of spontaneous abortions in women and to decrease spermatogenesis in men who work in operating rooms. Scavenging equipment must now be used in the operating room to remove nitrous oxide. The gas is 34 times more soluble than nitrogen in the blood, so pockets of trapped gas in the patient expand as nitrogen leaves and is replaced by larger amounts of nitrous oxide. Trapped gas is common in a blocked middle ear, pneumothorax, loops of intestine, lungs, renal cysts, and the skull after a pneumoencephalogram. These conditions represent contraindications for nitrous oxide because the large increases in pressure or volumes that may result after its administration may cause serious damage.

Intravenous Anesthetics: General Characteristics

Table 36-2 provides a summary of information on IV anesthetics.

Mechanism of Action

Diverse agents are used as **IV anesthetics,** including the ultrashort-acting barbiturates: thiopental (Pentothal) and methohexital (Brevital); two benzodiazepines: diazepam (Valium) and midazolam (Versed); and the agents ketamine (Ketaject), etomidate (Amidate), and propofol (Diprivan). In addition, the development of short-acting opioids, alfentanil (Alfenta), fentanyl citrate (Sublimaze), remifentanil (Ultiva), and sufentanil citrate (Sufenta), for use as IV agents has extended the use of multiple drugs for anesthesia.

Pharmacokinetics

It may seem paradoxical that an IV anesthetic would be so short acting when it must be metabolized to be excreted. The explanation is that the IV anesthetics are lipid soluble. Initially, they are distributed to the brain, liver, and kidneys, the organs with the largest blood flow, but later the drug is redistributed to body fat and skeletal muscle, which are less well perfused. This redistribution lowers the circulating concentration to that which no longer maintains anesthesia. This redistribution is responsible for the short duration of action. Metabolism of the drug proceeds as the drug passes through the liver.

Uses

The advantage of the IV agents is that they are effective seconds after administration. Only ketamine is a true anesthetic, abolishing the perception of and the reaction to pain. The barbiturates and benzodiazepines do not abolish reflex reaction to pain even when they are administered in doses large enough to render the patient unconscious. These drugs are used primarily as induction agents.

Conscious sedation is the use of IV benzodiazepines and opioid analgesics to confer amnestic, sedative and analgesic effects without complete loss of consciousness. This is useful for many diagnostic, therapeutic, and minor surgical procedures.

Deep sedation is achieved with thiopental, ketamine, propofol, and IV opioids. The patient is in a controlled state of anesthesia with decreased consciousness and is not easily aroused. There is a loss of protective reflexes, an inability to maintain a open airway, and lack of response to surgical stimuli.

Neuroleptanalgesia refers to the combination of fentanyl and droperidol to produce a quiet state with reduced motor activity, reduced anxiety, and indifference to the surroundings. Procedures such as endoscopy, radiologic studies, and changing burn dressings can be carried out. Concurrent

Table 36-2   **Injectable Drugs for Anesthesia**

Generic Name	Trade Name	Administration/Dosage	Comments
Barbiturates			
methohexital sodium	Brevital Sodium Brietal Sodium†	INTRAVENOUS: *Adults—For induction:* 5-12 ml of 1% solution no faster than 1 ml every 5 sec. Maintenance: 2-4 ml of 1% solution as required. FDA pregnancy category C.	Shortest duration of action (5-7 min) of barbiturates. Some patients develop hiccups after rapid injection. Schedule IV substance in the United States; G in Canada.
thiopental sodium	Pentothal*	INTRAVENOUS: *Adults—For induction:* 50-100 mg (2-4 ml) in 2.5% solution every 30-40 sec or 3-5 mg/kg body weight. Maintenance: 2-4 ml of 2.5% solution as required. *Children*—3-5 mg/kg as described for adults. FDA pregnancy category C.	Duration of action is about 15 min. May cause yawning, coughing, or laryngospasm. Schedule III substance in the United States; G in Canada.
Benzodiazepines			
diazepam	Valium*	INTRAVENOUS: *Adults*—0.1-0.2 mg/kg body weight to induce sleep; maximum dose: 10-20 mg. Basal sedation requires only 5-30 mg, so 2.5-5 mg is injected every 30 sec until light sleep or slurred speech is produced.	Do not mix with other liquids. Local anesthetic may be required for intravenous injection. Schedule IV substance.
midazolam	Versed*	INTRAMUSCULAR: *Adults—For preoperative sedation:* 70-80 μg/kg, 30-60 min before surgery. FDA pregnancy category D. *Children*—80-200 μg/kg. INTRAVENOUS: *Adults—For conscious sedation:* 2.5 mg administered over 2 min just before procedure. *For general anesthesia:* 200-350 μg/kg administered over 5-30 sec. *Children*—50-200 μg/kg.	Schedule IV substance. Older or debilitated patients should be administered smaller dose. Postoperative effects include somnolence, disorientation, and amnesia. Will further depress respiration if used with opioids.
Opioids			
alfentanil hydrochloride	Alfenta*	INTRAVENOUS: *Adults—For induction of anesthesia:* 130 μg/kg body weight. FDA pregnancy category C.	Schedule II substance in the United States, N in Canada. Potent, short-acting narcotic analgesic. Very short-acting (30-45 min) drug.
fentanyl	Duragesic	TRANSDERMAL: *Adults—For analgesia:* Apply to skin of upper torso every 72 hr. Initially, one 2.5 mg transdermal system. For maintenance, dosage may be adjusted every 3 days, according to patient response. Some patients require application every 48 hr.	Schedule II substance in the United States, N in Canada. Patients tolerant to opioids may require higher dosages. First opioid analgesic available in a transdermal system. Not for short-term relief of acute pain.
fentanyl citrate	Sublimaze*	INTRAVENOUS: *Adults and children >2 yr*—0.002-0.003 mg/kg body weight in divided doses over 6-8 min. Maintenance: 0.05-0.1 mg every 30-60 min. Onset: 1-2 min. FDA pregnancy category C.	Schedule II substance in the United States, N in Canada. Potent, short-acting narcotic analgesic. Used with droperidol and nitrous oxide for neuroleptic anesthesia and with nitrous oxide for balanced anesthesia.
remifentanil hydrochloride	Ultiva	INTRAVENOUS: *Adults—For induction of anesthesia:* 0.5-1 μg/kg/min; reduce by half or more for maintenance of anesthesia with nitrous oxide, isoflurane, or propofol.	Schedule II substance in the United States, N in Canada. Produces intense analgesia very rapidly. Metabolized by nonspecific esterases, so recovery is rapid and independent of dose or duration of infusion.
sufentanil citrate	Sufenta*	INTRAVENOUS: *Adults*—Initial dose is 1-8 mg/kg with nitrous oxide and oxygen. Additional doses are 10-25 mg/kg. Doses depend on severity of pain associated with surgery. *Children >2 yr—For cardiovascular surgery:* 10-25 mg/kg with oxygen and muscular relaxant. Additional doses are 25-50 mg (1-2 mg/kg). FDA pregnancy category C.	Schedule II substance in the United States, N in Canada. Potent, short-acting narcotic analgesic used with nitrous oxide for balanced anesthesia or alone with oxygen and muscle relaxant.
Miscellaneous Agents			
droperidol	Inapsine*	INTRAVENOUS: *Adults and children >2 yr*—0.15 mg/kg body weight. Onset: 10-15 min. Duration: 3-6 hr.	Antipsychotic drug. Used with fentanyl citrate and nitrous oxide to produce neuroleptanesthesia. May cause extrapyramidal symptoms.
etomidate	Amidate	INTRAVENOUS: *Adults and children >10 yr—For induction:* 0.3 mg/kg body weight injected over 30-60 sec; may vary between 0.2 and 0.6 mg/kg. FDA pregnancy category C.	Nonbarbiturate agent used for induction and sometimes maintenance of anesthesia. No cardiovascular effects. May cause involuntary muscle movements.
ketamine	Ketalar*	INTRAVENOUS: *Adults and children*—1-4.5 mg/kg body weight over 60 sec, ½ of initial dose used for maintenance as needed.	Produces dissociative anesthesia with good analgesia. Not a scheduled drug. Causes cardiovascular stimulation and increased

*Available in Canada and the United States.
†Available in Canada only.

Table 36-2	Injectable Drugs for Anesthesia—cont'd		
Generic Name	Trade Name	Administration/Dosage	Comments
Miscellaneous Agents—cont'd			
ketamine—cont'd		INTRAMUSCULAR: *Adults and children*—6.5-13 mg/kg body weight, ½ of initial dose for maintenance as needed.	cerebral blood flow. Patients may hallucinate during emergence.
propofol	Diprivan*	INTRAVENOUS: *Adults (up to 55 yr)—For induction of anesthesia:* Increments of approximately 40 mg every 10 sec until adequate anesthesia is achieved. Usual total dose is 2-2.5 mg/kg. Maintenance: 25-50 mg as required is given by intermittent bolus, or 0.1-0.2 mg/kg/min is infused. *Older adults and debilitated or hypovolemic patients:* Dose is reduced by ½. FDA pregnancy category B.	For induction of anesthesia. Rapid onset and recovery. Causes hypotension and respiratory depression. Not a scheduled drug.

*Available in Canada and the United States.
†Available in Canada only.

administration of 65% nitrous oxide in oxygen produces neuroleptanesthesia.

Balanced anesthesia refers to the combination of an opioid, nitrous oxide, and a skeletal muscle relaxant for surgical anesthesia. This is described under the entry for opioids.

Specific Intravenous Anesthetics

Barbiturates

Thiopental (Pentothal) and methohexital (Brevital) are ultrashort-acting barbiturates used primarily to induce anesthesia. Loss of consciousness occurs within 60 seconds. Thiopental is effective as the sole anesthetic for about 15 minutes. Methohexital is even shorter acting. Barbiturates provide no analgesia and can cause excitement or delirium in the presence of pain in an awake patient. Changes in blood pressure or cardiac output are uncommon unless the injection is made rapidly. Respiration is markedly depressed, and yawning, coughing, or laryngospasm may occur. Methohexital can cause hiccups.

Solutions of barbiturates should be injected only into veins. Arterial injections can cause inflammation and clotting. The barbiturate solution damages tissue if it leaks around the injection site, and this situation can lead to gangrene.

Benzodiazepines

Diazepam (Valium) is used occasionally as an induction agent but more commonly to sedate patients undergoing cardioversion or endoscopic or dental procedures. IV diazepam takes 60 seconds to become effective. Sedation, sleep, and amnesia are achieved with little depression of cardiovascular or respiratory functions. Unlike barbiturates, diazepam is metabolized to active products and has a long duration of action (see Chapter 57).

Midazolam (Versed) is a relatively short-acting benzodiazepine used as an IV anesthetic. It should be used only in hospital or ambulatory care settings where respiratory and cardiac functions can be monitored. Midazolam may be administered intravenously or intramuscularly to induce sedation or amnesia.

Midazolam is used alone or with an opioid to produce conscious sedation before such short diagnostic procedures as bronchoscopy, gastroscopy, cystoscopy, coronary angiography, and cardiac catheterization.

droperidol

Neuroleptanesthesia refers to the combination of droperidol (Inapsine), an antipsychotic drug of the butyrophenone class, an opioid (usually fentanyl), and nitrous oxide. A skeletal muscle relaxant may be used if needed. A fixed combination of the opioid fentanyl and droperidol is available as Innovar. Nitrous oxide produces loss of consciousness, and if it is discontinued, the patient becomes conscious but in an altered state of awareness. The patient may be confused or depressed. Neuroleptanesthesia is useful for older adult and poor-risk patients and for bronchoscopy and carotid arteriography. Innovar alone greatly facilitates intubation in awake patients.

Side effects of neuroleptanalgesia or neuroleptanesthesia are hypotension, a slow heart rate (bradycardia), and respiratory depression. The action of droperidol persists for 3 to 6 hours, whereas the analgesic effect of fentanyl persists for only 30 minutes. Droperidol has adrenergic-receptor blocking, antifibrillatory, antiemetic, and anticonvulsant actions. About 1% of patients who receive droperidol may have extrapyramidal muscle movements (see Chapter 58) for as long as 12 hours after administration of the drug. These movements may be controlled by administration of atropine or benztropine.

etomidate

Etomidate (Amidate) is an IV anesthetic for the induction of surgical anesthesia. An injection will induce sleep that lasts for about 5 minutes. Etomidate produces minimum cardiovascular or respiratory changes. Because etomidate does not produce analgesia, the short-acting narcotic-analgesic fentanyl citrate also may be infused for total IV anesthesia. The most common side effects of etomidate are pain at the injection site and transient, myoclonic skeletal muscle movements.

ketamine

Ketamine (Ketalar) is neither a barbiturate nor a benzodiazepine. Unlike those drug classes, ketamine produces a cataleptic anesthesia in which the patient appears to be awake but neither responds to pain nor remembers the procedure. This is sometimes called **dissociative anesthesia.** Ketamine is not a controlled substance and is readily available in emergency rooms. It is also used for repeated changes of dressing, radiologic procedures in children, and some cardiac surgical procedures. Ketamine is rapidly effective when administered intramuscularly and intravenously. Ketamine alone provides anesthesia for 5 to 10 minutes when given intravenously and for 10 to 20 minutes when given intramuscularly.

Ketamine enhances muscle tone and increases blood pressure, heart rate, and respiratory secretions. The major side effect is seen in the recovery period, when patients may experience vivid, unpleasant dreams or hallucinations. Adults are more prone than children to these experiences. It may also cause vomiting and shivering. It is chemically related to phencyclidine (PCP), an illicit hallucinogen.

Ketamine should be used cautiously in patients with convulsive disorders, psychosis, or mild hypertension or those who are undergoing eye surgery; it is contraindicated for patients with coronary artery disease, severe hypertension, cerebrovascular accident (stroke), or treated hypothyroidism.

Opioids

The ideal anesthetic would produce analgesia, unconsciousness, muscle relaxation, and reduction of reflex activity. This anesthetic would act promptly and would be rapidly eliminated, remaining unmetabolized and producing no unwanted effects in body tissues. Because no anesthetic has all these desirable properties, several drugs are used in combination to achieve these goals. For surgical anesthesia, one widely used combination of agents is referred to as **balanced anesthesia.** This combines an opioid, nitrous oxide, and a skeletal muscle relaxant. Anesthesia is induced, generally with a short-acting barbiturate or occasionally with diazepam or other agents, and then the opioid, nitrous oxide, and skeletal muscle relaxant are administered. Respiration must be controlled because the opioids are potent respiratory depressants, and patients are usually paralyzed by a skeletal muscle relaxant. Nitrous oxide is effective at a 65% concentration because of its synergism with the opioid. The skeletal muscle relaxant is necessary because neither the opioid nor the nitrous oxide provides the muscular relaxation necessary for surgery.

The choice of the opioid is determined by the anticipated length of surgery. Alfentanil (Alfenta), **fentanyl** citrate (Sublimaze), remifentanil (Ultiva), and sufentanil citrate (Sufenta) are short-acting opioids primarily used for surgery. Morphine has been used for cardiac and poor-risk patients.

The advantage of balanced anesthesia is that the cardiovascular system is neither depressed nor sensitized to catecholamines. Respiration is depressed, but controlled ventilation is readily available and opioid antagonists can be administered to reverse depressed respiration postoperatively. The incidence of postoperative nausea, vomiting, and pain is low. However, awareness during anesthesia and unpleasant postoperative recall are occasional side effects of balanced anesthesia.

▼ propofol

Propofol (Diprivan) is an IV anesthetic for rapid induction and maintenance of general anesthesia. It is also used with opioids and nitrous oxide in balanced anesthesia. Propofol can cause hypotension, and this is potentiated by opioid analgesics. Propofol is also a respiratory depressant. Recovery from anesthesia is rapid, with minimal psychomotor impairment. Propofol is also used for sedation during regional anesthesia or intensive care. The drug is inactivated in the liver.

Nursing Process Overview

General Anesthesia

Assessment

Perform a complete physical assessment, with focus on vital signs and respiratory system, laboratory data, and studies specific to known medical problems (e.g., coagulation studies in patients with liver disease or pulmonary function studies in patients with severe chronic obstructive pulmonary disease [COPD]).

Nursing Diagnoses

- Altered comfort: nausea and vomiting related to general anesthesia

- Ineffective airway clearance: inability to remove airway secretions related to general anesthesia

Patient Outcomes

The patient will experience no vomiting after general anesthesia, and any nausea will be treated. The patient will recover from surgery without aspiration or pneumonia.

Planning/Implementation

Delivery of general anesthesia requires knowledge and facility with management of the respiratory and cardiovascular systems, multiple drugs, and the immobilized unconscious patient. For further information, consult appropriate textbooks of nursing, medicine, and anesthesiology.

Evaluation

Perform frequent evaluations of vital signs, respiratory and cardiovascular status, level of consciousness, and ability to handle secretions. Assess degree of postoperative pain and medicate if appropriate. Assess wound, drainage, intake and output, and other parameters as indicated by the type of surgery performed.

Nursing Implications Summary

General Anesthesia
Drug Administration/Nursing in the Community

➤ Techniques of administration of general anesthesia are beyond the scope of this book; for further information consult appropriate textbooks of anesthesia.

➤ Obtain a careful drug history before surgery. Assess for allergic or unusual responses to previous anesthetic agents and for any current medications the patient is taking.

➤ Preoperative medications are an integral part of planned anesthesia. Administer them as ordered and on time.

➤ To prepare the patient for surgery, inform the patient and family about the surgical procedure and what to expect postoperatively. Have the patient give a return demonstration of any exercises or activities required, such as coughing and deep breathing. Provide the patient with an opportunity to ask questions of the anesthesiologist or nurse anesthetist. Schedule a visit to the intensive care unit, if appropriate. Provide emotional support.

➤ Malignant hyperthermia is a rare but potentially fatal syndrome that can develop in genetically susceptible patients, even if patients have had previous uneventful surgeries. It can develop when any volatile anesthetic is used, but the onset is usually more abrupt when succinylcholine is used. Symptoms include tachycardia or tachyarrhythmias, tachypnea, labile blood pressure, and flushing followed by cyanotic mottling. Blood pH may fall and serum potassium levels rise. Some patients develop muscle rigidity. Elevated temperature is a late sign, but the temperature rises to high levels (110° F [42° C]). Treatment includes discontinuing anesthesia, administering 100% oxygen and IV dantrolene, correcting acid-base imbalances, and cooling the patient. A similar syndrome in appearance is neuroleptic malignant syndrome (see Chapter 58). Teach patients who develop this syndrome to wear a medical identification tag or bracelet and to inform all health care providers that this syndrome has occurred.

Postoperative Care

➤ Monitor temperature, pulse, respirations, blood pressure, and pulse oximetry frequently. With the exception of temperature, this may be every 5 minutes initially, progressing to every 15 minutes, then every 30 minutes and longer. Auscultate lung sounds and check neurologic status. Do not leave the patient unattended unless the patient can call for assistance and can handle secretions safely.

➤ Position the patient on the side initially, if possible, to prevent aspiration if vomiting should occur. Keep a suction machine at the bedside and keep siderails up.

➤ Evaluate the patient for pain medication in the immediate postoperative period (first 2 to 4 hours after surgery). Factors to consider include the nature and location of surgery, vital signs, age, weight, level of consciousness, anesthetic agent(s) used, and whether analgesics were administered during surgery. The initial dose of analgesics may be one half to one fourth the ordered dose of analgesic, but make reductions in dose only after consultation with the physician.

➤ Begin nursing measures to prevent atelectasis and pneumonia as soon as the patient is able. This may include turning and deep breathing, coughing, and early ambulation.

➤ Effects of anesthesia persist even after the patient appears to be alert and awake. If it is necessary to give instructions about activity, diet, or medications, as in the outpatient or day-surgery setting, do so verbally and in writing to the patient and have at least one family member present.

➤ Do not permit patients in the outpatient setting to drive themselves home if they have received general anesthesia, IV barbiturates or benzodiazepines, or any drug that may alter response time or level of consciousness.

➤ Warn a patient who has a severe reaction or response to any anesthetic to carry the name of the agent at all times. If surgery is ever again needed, instruct the patient to tell the anesthetist of the previous severe response. Suggest that the patient wear a medical identification tag or bracelet indicating the severe reaction.

➤ See the nursing implications summary for narcotic analgesics in Chapter 32. Patients perform needed postoperative activities better if they are adequately medicated for pain.

ketamine

➤ Ketamine is associated with unpleasant dreams, emergence delirium, irrational behavior, disorientation, and hallucinations. These side effects may be lessened by providing the patient with a quiet wake-up period, perhaps in the quietest corner of the postanesthesia recovery room. Avoid excessive stimulation, although vital signs must be monitored. If psychic effects occur, provide calm reassurance and reorientation. Do not leave the patient unattended.

➤ Vivid dreams and hallucinations usually disappear upon awakening, but some patients may experience flashbacks for up to several weeks after surgery.

Continued

Nursing Implications Summary—cont'd

➤ Once the patient is returned to the room, keep it dimly lit and keep noise and stimulation to a minimum. Inform family members of the probable cause of the behavior and enlist their aid in patient reorientation and reassurance.

midazolam

➤ Conscious sedation with midazolam (Versed) is discussed at the end of Chapter 57.

fentanyl

➤ As noted, fentanyl is available in a transdermal form for treatment of pain. See Chapters 32 and 34 for a general discussion of analgesics and assessing and managing pain.

➤ Epidural analgesia is discussed in Chapter 34.

➤ The individual transdermal system ("patch") is designed to release fentanyl over a 72-hour period. Analgesic effect may persist for several hours after the system is removed. The onset of action is 12 to 24 hours, and the time to peak action for a single application is between 24 and 72 hours. Shorter-acting analgesics are used to control the patient's pain initially, then the patient is converted to an appropriate dose of fentanyl. The physician may prescribe a short-acting agent for breakthrough pain when the patient is using the fentanyl transdermal system.

➤ See the manufacturer's literature for information about determining the correct dose of fentanyl based on the patient's current use of morphine or other analgesic.

➤ Review application technique with the patient and family: Keep medication system in original sealed pouch until ready to apply. Apply to clean, dry skin. Site may be washed before application, but use clear water only, no soaps, lotions, alcohol, or other agents. Let area dry completely. Avoid hairy areas, or clip hair before applying; do not shave the area. Remove covering from adhesive surface and press on to skin surface; hold in place firmly for about 30 seconds to ensure good adhesion. If two or more patches are to be applied, they may be applied near each other but should not touch. Wash hands to remove any drug that may have come in contact with skin surface. Remove old patches and discard by folding each one in half, adhesive sides toward each other, and flush down toilet. Do not place in trash or any place where children or pets could come in contact with drug. Wash hands.

➤ Instruct the patient to notify physician if transdermal form appears to be causing skin irritation or if rash or itching develop.

➤ Teach the patient that the full effect of transdermal form cannot be evaluated for at least 24 hours after first dose is applied. Monitor blood pressure and respirations. Caution patients to avoid driving or operating hazardous equipment while using this drug, until effects in an individual patient are understood. Instruct the patient to avoid the use of alcohol or other CNS depressants unless their use is approved by the physician.

➤ Forewarn the patient that nausea, vomiting, constipation, and sedation may occur. Depending on the situation, it may be appropriate for the patient to use antiemetics; consult the physician. See the Patient Problems box in Chapter 24 on constipation.

➤ Review with the patient the importance of using the transdermal system as prescribed. Tell the patient not to increase or double doses without consulting physician and not to share supply with others.

➤ Instruct patients that they may swim, bathe, or shower with the patch on but that they should dry off the area around the patch carefully. Instruct the patient to remove and replace the patch if is torn or comes loose. The newly applied patch should be removed after 72 hours.

➤ Caution the patient to avoid using a heating pad or sunlamp or taking long, hot baths or showers because heat may increase the chance of side effects or overdose.

➤ Instruct the patient not to discontinue use of transdermal fentanyl without consulting physician. Remind the patient to keep all health care providers informed of all drugs being used, including transdermal drugs.

➤ Review with the patient and family the signs of overdose: cold, clammy skin; deep sedation in which it is difficult to arouse the patient; fewer than 8 respirations per minute, hallucinations, difficulty speaking, or a change in vision. Instruct the patient to seek medical help immediately if overdose is suspected and to contact the physician if any unexpected sign or symptom develops.

CHAPTER REVIEW

Application

1. What is MAC?
2. What factors determine induction and emergence? Outline your responsibilities during the emergence period.
3. Why is diethyl ether seldom used in the United States?
4. Which inhalation anesthetics sensitize the heart to catecholamines?
5. Which inhalation anesthetics are metabolized to some degree?
6. Which inhalation anesthetics lower blood pressure during surgery?
7. What factor limits the use of nitrous oxide alone as an anesthetic? How is this limitation overcome?
8. What are the hazards of nitrous oxide to patients and to operating room personnel?

9. Which barbiturates are used as IV induction agents for anesthesia? How is their action effectively terminated?
10. Which benzodiazepines are used as IV induction agents for anesthesia?
11. Describe balanced anesthesia.
12. Describe neuroleptanesthesia.

Critical Thinking

1. How are general anesthetics believed to work?
2. What measurement determines the effective concentration of an inhalation anesthetic? How does this differ from the concentration based on total solubility?

3. Which inhalation anesthetics are halogenated hydrocarbons? What needs to be monitored in a patient who has received a halogenated hydrocarbon?
4. What is the nature of anesthesia with ketamine? What nursing care activities might be needed with a patient who has received ketamine?
5. What are the properties of an ideal anesthetic?

References

Burns LS: Advances in pediatric anesthesia, *Nurs Clin North Am* 32(1):45-71, 1997.

Vermette E: Malignant hyperthermia, *Am J Nurs* 98(4):45, 1998.

Walker JR: What is new with inhaled anesthetics: part I, *J Perianesth Nurs* 11(5):330, 1996.

Chapter

37

Neuromuscular-Blocking Drugs

KEY TERMS

depolarizing neuromuscular-
blocking drug, p. 438
neuromuscular-blocking
drugs, p. 434
nondepolarizing or competitive blocking drugs, p. 434

KEY DRUGS ▼

succinylcholine, p. 438
tubocurarine, p. 434

OBJECTIVES

After studying this chapter, you should be able to do the following:

- *Discuss the action of neuromuscular-blocking drugs.*
- *Differentiate between nondepolarizing and depolarizing neuromuscular-blocking drugs.*
- *Develop a nursing care plan for patients receiving neuromuscular-blocking drugs.*

CHAPTER OVERVIEW

Motor neurons are single neurons originating in the spinal cord and terminating on the muscle. The neuromuscular-blocking drugs occupy the receptors for acetylcholine on muscles, thus preventing muscle contraction. These drugs produce muscular relaxation for intubation and surgical procedures.

THERAPEUTIC RATIONALE: NEUROMUSCULAR BLOCKADE

As shown in Figure 37-1, **neuromuscular-blocking drugs** produce complete muscle relaxation by preventing muscular contraction. Assisted ventilation should be available for short-acting succinylcholine and is mandatory when administering long-acting neuromuscular blockers. Skeletal muscle relaxants do not inhibit pain or provide amnesia.

Neuromuscular-blocking drugs provide muscle relaxation during surgery, particularly relaxation of the abdominal muscles, without using deep general anesthesia, which would relax abdominal muscles by depressing the spinal cord. Neuromuscular blockers are also used with light anesthesia to allow a tube to be passed down easily to the trachea (endotracheal intubation), to relieve spasm of the larynx, to prevent convulsive muscle spasms during electroconvulsive therapy for depression, and to allow breathing to be controlled totally by a respirator (controlled ventilation) during surgery.

THERAPEUTIC AGENTS: NEUROMUSCULAR-BLOCKING DRUGS

Most neuromuscular-blocking drugs are nondepolarizing, which means they competitively bind to the receptor without depolarizing the muscle membrane. Tubocurarine is the prototype for these agents. Only succinylcholine is a depolarizing agent, and is presented separately.

Table 37-1 summarizes neuromuscular-blocking drugs and their administration.

▼ tubocurarine

Mechanism of Action

Neuromuscular-blocking drugs produce complete muscle relaxation by binding to the receptor for acetylcholine at the neuromuscular junction. **Tubocurarine** (curare) is the prototype for the **nondepolarizing or competitive blocking drugs,** which bind to the receptor without initiating depolarization of the muscle membrane. Tubocurarine was originally isolated as the active principle of the South American

434

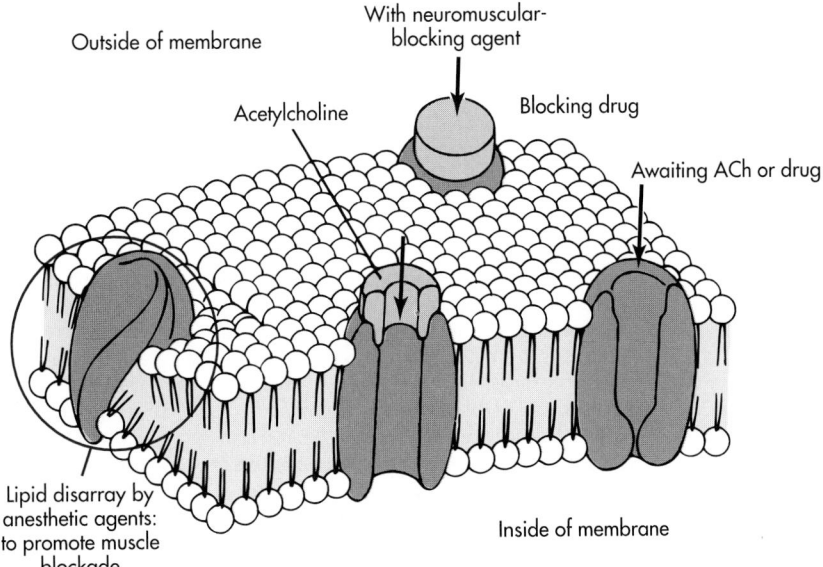

Outside of membrane

With neuromuscular-blocking agent

Acetylcholine

Blocking drug

Awaiting ACh or drug

Lipid disarray by anesthetic agents: to promote muscle blockade

Inside of membrane

Figure 37-1 Neuromuscular-blocking drugs block receptor, preventing acetylcholine *(ACh)* from binding to receptor and opening channel. Anesthesia caused by neuromuscular-blocking drugs differs from lipid disarray caused by general anesthetic drugs.

arrow poison. An animal hit with an arrow containing curare falls paralyzed a short time later. Curare is the classic acetylcholine blocker for the neuromuscular junction (see Chapter 11).

Pharmacokinetics

Curare is administered by slow (60 to 90 seconds) intravenous (IV) injection. Maximal paralysis occurs within 5 minutes and persists for 60 minutes (range: 25 to 90 minutes). The progression of paralysis begins with the eyelids, then the face, the extremities, and finally the diaphragm, resulting in the cessation of spontaneous breathing. Recovery from neuromuscular blockade can be assisted by injecting edrophonium, neostigmine, or pyridostigmine to increase the amount of acetylcholine at the neuromuscular junction.

About 40% of tubocurarine is excreted unchanged in the urine. Patients with renal failure or acidosis excrete tubocurarine less rapidly and require a smaller dose.

Uses

Tubocurarine produces muscle relaxation during surgery or electroconvulsive shock therapy, reduces muscle spasm in tetanus, and allows controlled ventilation.

Adverse Reactions, Contraindications, and Toxicity

Tubocurarine can cause release of histamine, which causes hypotension or bronchospasm (see Chapter 29). Hypotension can arise from ganglionic blockade by tubocurarine. Tubocurarine does not cross the placenta or blood-brain barrier.

Interactions

Many anesthetics, including halothane, ether, methoxyflurane, and enflurane, potentiate the action of tubocurarine. Antibiotics potentiating the action of tubocurarine include the aminoglycosides and the polymyxins (see Chapter 48), bacitracin, lincomycin, and clindamycin. Other drugs that potentiate the action of tubocurarine are the antiarrhythmic drugs, quinidine, ganglionic blockers, trimethaphan, and magnesium sulfate. Because patients with myasthenia gravis have an exaggerated response to tubocurarine, very small doses of tubocurarine can be used to diagnose myasthenia gravis if tests with edrophonium or neostigmine are inconclusive.

Other Nondepolarizing Neuromuscular Blockers

The following nondepolarizing neuromuscular-blocking agents belong to two general chemical classes. The benzylisoquinolines include atracurium, cisatracurium, doxacurium, and mivacurium.

The ammonio steroids include pancuronium, pipecuronium, rocuronium, and vecuronium. Gallamine is a distinct synthetic agent.

atracurium

Atracurium (Tracrium) is a nondepolarizing muscle relaxant. It is shorter in duration than tubocurarine, producing adequate relaxation for 15 to 20 minutes. Atracurium is inactivated by hydrolysis. At usual doses, atracurium does not produce cardiovascular side effects.

Table 37-1   Neuromuscular-Blocking Agents

Generic Name	Trade Name	Administration/Dosage	Comments
atracurium besylate	Tracrium*	INTRAVENOUS: *Adults*—0.4-0.5 mg/kg body weight; subsequent doses 0.08-0.1 mg/kg. FDA pregnancy category C.	Drug is not affected by renal or hepatic impairment and is relatively free of cardiovascular side effects. Doses given are for use with nitrous oxide. Other inhalation anesthetics may require smaller doses.
cisatracurium besylate	Nimbex*	INTRAVENOUS: *Adults—For skeletal muscle relaxation during surgery:* 0.15 mg/kg body weight initially. Maintenance infusion: 3 μg/kg body weight/min initially, decreasing to 1 or 2 μg/kg body weight/min. FDA pregnancy category B.	New neuromuscular blocker for skeletal muscle relaxation during surgery. Onset is 2 min; duration is about 60 min, but depends on surgical conditions. Duration is shorter for children.
doxacurium chloride	Nuromax	INTRAVENOUS: *Adults—For endotracheal intubation:* 0.05 mg/kg body weight will provide 100 min relaxation. *After succinylcholine-assisted endotracheal intubation:* 0.025 mg/kg body weight will provide 60 min relaxation; maintenance requires 0.005 mg/kg body weight for relaxation. FDA pregnancy category C. *Children*—0.03 mg/kg body weight initially for halothane anesthesia will provide 30 min relaxation.	Drug does not increase heart rate. Adult dosages must be decreased by one-third if used with enflurane, halothane, or isoflurane anesthesia. Dosages for older adult patients or patients with hepatic or renal disease may need to be reduced. Ideal body weight should be used for obese patients.
gallamine triethiodide	Flaxedil*	INTRAVENOUS: *Adults*—1-1.15 mg/kg body weight. Supplemental doses: 0.3-1.2 mg/kg. FDA pregnancy category C. *Children*—2.5 mg/kg initially. Supplemental doses: 0.3-1.2 mg/kg. *Newborns up to age 1 mo:* 0.25-0.75 mg/kg initially. Supplemental doses: 0.1-0.5 mg/kg.	Drug may cause increased heart rate. Drug is not used for patients in renal failure. Doses given are for use with nitrous oxide. Other inhalation anesthetics may require smaller doses.
metocurine iodide	Metubine*	INTRAVENOUS: *Adults*—0.1-0.3 mg/kg body weight. Supplemental doses: 0.02-0.03 mg/kg. FDA pregnancy category C.	See tubocurarine chloride. Doses given are for use with nitrous oxide. Other inhalation anesthetics may require smaller doses. Drug is not for use in patients with renal failure.
mivacurium chloride	Mivacron	INTRAVENOUS: *Adults—For endotracheal intubation and surgical relaxation:* 0.15-0.2 mg/kg body weight administered over 5-15 sec initially. Maintenance: 0.1 mg/kg body weight. FDA pregnancy category C. *Children 2-12 yr*—0.2-0.25 mg/kg body weight administered over 5-15 sec.	Drug has negligible direct effect on cardiovascular system. Metabolized by plasma cholinesterases. Renal and biliary elimination of inactive metabolites. Effective dose not affected by impaired hepatic or renal function.
pancuronium bromide	Pavulon*	INTRAVENOUS: *Adults and children*—0.04-0.1 mg/kg body weight initially. Supplemental doses: 0.01-0.02 mg/kg. Newborns may be very sensitive; use test dose of 0.02 mg. FDA pregnancy category C.	Drug does not cause hypotension. Drug may stimulate heart rate and cardiac output. Doses given are for use with nitrous oxide. Other inhalation anesthetics may require smaller doses.
pipecuronium bromide	Arduan	INTRAVENOUS: *Adults—For endotracheal intubation:* 0.07-0.085 mg/kg ideal body weight. *After succinylcholine-facilitated endotracheal intubation:* 0.05 mg/kg ideal body weight for 45 min of muscle relaxation or 0.07-0.085 mg/kg ideal body weight for 1-2 hr of muscle relaxation. *Maintenance during surgery:* 0.01-0.015 mg/kg ideal body weight. FDA pregnancy category C. *Children 1-14 yr*—0.057 mg/kg body weight.	Onset in 2.5-3 minutes. Long-acting, about 60 min, with wide variability depending on anesthetic used. Children recover more quickly. Drug has negligible direct effect on cardiovascular system. Metabolite has some activity; most of drug is excreted unchanged in urine; doses must be reduced for patients with renal function impairment.
rocuronium	Zemuron*	INTRAVENOUS: *Adults and children >3 mo—For endotracheal intubation:* 0.6 mg/kg ideal body weight. *Maintenance during surgery:* 0.01-0.012 mg/kg ideal body weight/min. FDA pregnancy category B.	Drug related to pancuronium. Onset in 1-1.5 min. Do not combine with alkaline intravenous barbiturate solutions.
tubocurarine chloride (curare)	Tubarine† Tubocurarine chloride*	INTRAVENOUS: *Adults and children*—0.2-0.4 mg/kg body weight initially. Supplemental doses: 0.04-0.2 mg/kg. *Diagnosis of myasthenia gravis:* ¹⁄₁₅-¹⁄₃ of above dose. FDA pregnancy category C.	Intravenous injection should be slow (1-1.5 min). Do not combine with alkaline intravenous barbiturate solutions. Doses given are for use with nitrous oxide. Other inhalation anesthetics may require smaller doses.

*Available in Canada and the United States.
†Available in Canada only.

Table 37-1	Neuromuscular-Blocking Agents—cont'd			
Generic Name	Trade Name	Administration/Dosage		Comments
vecuronium	Norcuron	INTRAVENOUS: *Adults—For intubation:* 0.07-0.14 mg/kg body weight. *For surgery:* 0.04-0.1 mg/kg initially, followed by 0.015-0.02 mg/kg as needed. FDA pregnancy category C.		Drug related to pancuronium but shorter (by ⅓ to ½) in duration. Drug is relatively free of cardiovascular side effects. Doses given are for use with nitrous oxide. Other inhalation anesthetics may require smaller doses.
Depolarizing Drug				
succinylcholine chloride	Anectine* Quelicin* Sucostrin	INTRAVENOUS: *Adults*—0.6-1.1 mg/kg body weight initially. *Continuous infusion:* 0.1% or 0.2% solution at rate of 0.5-10 mg/min. FDA pregnancy category C. *Children*—1.1 mg/kg body weight initially. Supplemental doses: 0.3-0.6 mg/kg. *Newborns*—2 mg/kg. Continuous infusion is not recommended for children and newborns.		Duration is only 5 min because of hydrolysis by plasma cholinesterase. This enzyme is missing genetically in some patients, and prolonged action is seen. Drug may cause cardiac arrhythmias. Doses given are for use with nitrous oxide. Other inhalation anesthetics require smaller doses.

*Available in Canada and the United States.
†Available in Canada only.

cisatracurium

Cisatracurium (Nimbex) is a stereoisomer of atracurium with many of the properties of atracurium. Cisatracurium releases less histamine from tissues.

doxacurium

Doxacurium (Nuromax) is a long-acting drug with minimal cardiovascular effects, desirable features for use in patients with coronary disease. It is used to facilitate endotracheal intubation in procedures lasting 90 minutes or longer and to induce skeletal muscle relaxation during surgical procedures. Doxacurium is excreted unchanged in the urine and should be used with caution in patients with renal failure.

gallamine triethiodide

Gallamine triethiodide (Flaxedil) is a synthetic drug similar in action to tubocurarine but with a shorter duration of action. Gallamine does not cause histamine release or ganglionic blockade. The major side effect of gallamine is an increase in heart rate (tachycardia), which is seen a few minutes after injection and then declines. Gallamine is excreted unchanged in the urine and should not be used in patients with renal failure.

metocurine (dimethyl tubocurarine) iodide

Metocurine iodide (Metubine), a semisynthetic derivative of tubocurarine, is two to three times as potent as tubocurarine but otherwise similar. Metocurine is excreted unchanged in the urine and should not be used in patients with renal failure.

mivacurium

Mivacurium (Mivacron) has a fast onset of action and is short acting. It does not accumulate because it is rapidly broken down by cholinesterases in the plasma.

pancuronium bromide

Pancuronium bromide (Pavulon) has a faster onset of action than tubocurarine, although the duration of action is similar. Pancuronium does not cause the histamine release or ganglionic blockade characteristic of tubocurarine. Heart rate, cardiac output, and atrial pressure are increased by pancuronium, effects that may be desired in cardiac surgery. Pancuronium is excreted in the urine, and doses must be decreased for patients with renal failure.

pipecuronium bromide

Pipecuronium bromide (Arduan) has a long duration of action and is used for procedures lasting 90 minutes or longer. Pipecuronium has no vagal blocking action to cause tachycardia, so it can be used in the presence of coronary artery disease in which tachycardia can be dangerous. Pipecuronium is also used to facilitate the management of patients undergoing mechanical ventilation.

rocuronium

Rocuronium (Zemuron) is a new nondepolarizing neuromuscular blocker with a rapid to intermediate onset of action. In some patients it causes tachycardia. Its elimination time is shorter in children than in adults. Patients with impaired hepatic function have an increased elimination time. Rocuronium is indicated as an adjunct to general anesthesia to facilitate tracheal intubation and to induce skeletal muscle relaxation during surgery or mechanical ventilation.

vecuronium

Vecuronium (Norcuron) is a nondepolarizing muscle relaxant chemically related to pancuronium. Vecuronium is shorter acting than pancuronium, and its effects are not cumulative with repeated administration. Unlike tubocurarine, the cardiovascular side effects arising from ganglionic or vagal blockade, interference with norepinephrine reuptake, or release of histamine are minimal with vecuronium. Vecuronium's intensity and duration of action are affected significantly by liver damage and modestly by renal failure.

▼ succinylcholine chloride

Mechanism of Action

Succinylcholine (Anectine and others) is the only **depolarizing neuromuscular-blocking drug** in use. It binds to the receptor for acetylcholine and causes depolarization of the muscle membrane.

Pharmacokinetics

Succinylcholine chloride has the briefest duration of action (5 minutes) of the neuromuscular-blocking drugs because plasma cholinesterases readily degrade succinylcholine. Longer action requires continuous infusion of succinylcholine, but then care must be taken to avoid desensitizing the muscle. The duration of action is increased by drugs that inhibit cholinesterases. Some patients have abnormal plasma cholinesterases that do not readily degrade succinylcholine. In these patients the action of succinylcholine is prolonged. Conditions that elevate plasma potassium concentration, such as burns, tetanus, massive trauma, or brain or spinal cord injury, prolong the action of succinylcholine.

Uses

Succinylcholine's short duration of action makes it a drug of choice for endoscopy, terminating laryngospasm, endotracheal intubation, orthopedic procedures, and electroconvulsive shock therapy.

Adverse Reactions, Contraindications, and Toxicity

Children are not as sensitive to succinylcholine on a weight basis as adults and require higher dosages. Children are more apt to show side effects of succinylcholine resulting from parasympathetic stimulation such as slow heart rate (bradycardia) and cardiac arrhythmias. Succinylcholine does not cross the blood-brain barrier or the placenta.

Succinylcholine initially causes fasciculations before the muscles are paralyzed. This effect is believed to cause the stiffness and soreness many patients experience 12 to 24 hours after they have received succinylcholine. Succinylcholine also transiently raises intraocular pressure and must be administered before eye surgery.

Nursing Process Overview

Neuromuscular-Blocking Drugs

Patients receive neuromuscular-blocking drugs when undergoing anesthesia, undergoing diagnostic studies that necessitate brief muscle relaxation, "bucking" ventilators, and undergoing electroconvulsive therapy.

Assessment

Monitor the patient's pulse, respiratory rate, and blood pressure. Assess the patient, focusing on the major problems being treated and the diagnostic or therapeutic procedure to be carried out.

Nursing Diagnoses

- Ineffective airway clearance related to drug effect
- Anxiety related to inability to swallow, ineffective airway clearance, and weakness

Patient Outcomes

The patient will recover from paralysis without aspiration or development of pneumonia. The patient will state reduced anxiety as the procedures are explained or as the drug wears off.

Planning/Implementation

Observe the rate, quality, and depth of respirations and provide ventilatory support as needed. Have equipment for intubation and suctioning at the bedside. Use an infusion monitoring device for IV administration. Neuromuscular blockers alone do not produce anesthesia; medicate the patient for pain if necessary. Position the patient carefully and check to see that instruments and bed linens are not causing unnecessary pressure on the patient's body. After the drug has been administered, it may take minutes to hours for the effect of the neuromuscular-blocking agents to wear off. Continue to assess the patient's ability to breathe unassisted, to cough, and to handle secretions. Use a peripheral nerve stimulator to monitor for drug effectiveness and to avoid overdose. Position patients on their sides and keep the siderails up. Do not leave patients unattended until they can adequately cough, handle secretions, and call for help.

Evaluation

These agents are successful if they produce sufficient muscle relaxation to allow the procedure or activity to proceed. These are all short-acting drugs and are not prescribed for use outside a hospital setting.

Nursing Implications Summary

General Guidelines: Neuromuscular Blockers

Drug Administration

➤ Neuromuscular blockers produce apnea. Have available a suction machine, oxygen, mechanical ventilator or resuscitation bag, and resuscitation equipment and drugs. Use these drugs only in a setting where personnel and equipment are available to provide immediate intubation.

➤ Monitor blood pressure, pulse, and respirations and auscultate lungs. Monitor arterial blood gases and electrocardiogram.

➤ When administering these drugs via constant infusion, use a microdrip tubing set and an infusion controlling device. Use a peripheral nerve stimulator to monitor effectiveness of the drug.

➤ Remember that neuromuscular blockers cause paralysis but not anesthesia. Unless a patient is also anesthetized, the patient can still hear, feel, and see if the eyelids are opened. Remember to remain professional in discussions within the patient's hearing, to explain sounds in the environment, to describe anticipated nursing care activities, and to use television or radio judiciously. Arrange for uninterrupted periods so that the patient can sleep.

➤ Avoid rough handling, position the patient in a comfortable position, offer backrubs if possible, and medicate for pain if appropriate. Keep the reversing agent or antagonist readily available.

➤ Consult the manufacturer's literature for specific guidelines regarding calculation of dosages. In many institutions, induction with a neuromuscular-blocking agent must be done by the anesthesiologist or nurse anesthetist; follow agency guidelines. Check with state board of nursing for any regulations that may apply.

➤ When discontinuing therapy, do not leave the patient unattended until sufficient muscle tone has returned so that the patient can breathe, handle secretions, and call for assistance if needed. In infants assess for the ability to hold up the legs. Keep the siderails up and the call bell within reach.

➤ Usually these drugs are not used for home management. Keep the patient and family informed of the patient's condition.

➤ IV atracurium: Initial dose may be given undiluted over 30 to 60 seconds. May be further diluted in normal saline, D5W, D5NS, and titrated to symptoms. For example dilute 20 mg (2 ml) with 98 ml diluted to make a concentration of 200 μg/ml (0.2 mg/ml). See manufacturer's literature for additional dilution guidelines. Antidote is pyridostigmine or neostigmine with atropine.

➤ IV cisatracurium: IV bolus may be given undiluted over 5 to 10 seconds. May be further diluted for infusion. See manufacturer's literature for guidelines on dilution. Antidote is neostigmine or edrophonium with atropine.

➤ IV doxacurium: See manufacturer's guidelines. Dosage must be adjusted based on specific inhalation agents, in the presence of obesity, electrolyte imbalances, or impaired renal function, and in the elderly or cachectic. Preferred antidote is neostigmine. Administer atropine or glycopyrrolate a few minutes before neostigmine.

➤ IV pancuronium: May be given undiluted over 60 to 90 seconds. Incompatible with diazepam. Antidote is pyridostigmine or neostigmine with atropine.

➤ IV pipecuronium: Must be reconstituted before administration. See manufacturer's literature. Antidote is atropine followed by neostigmine.

➤ IV rocuronium: Initial IV dose may be given undiluted or diluted in sterile water for injection, administered over 5 to 15 seconds. May also be further diluted for infusion; see manufacturer's instructions. Antidote is atropine followed by neostigmine or edrophonium.

➤ IV tubocurarine: The 3-mg/ml concentration may be given undiluted over 60 to 90 seconds. Dilute smaller doses with normal saline to facilitate administration. See manufacturer's literature; dosage adjustment is needed in many situations, including prematurity, acidosis, and hypothermia. Antidote is edrophonium or neostigmine with atropine.

➤ Tubocurarine for myasthenia gravis testing: Dilute dose to 4 ml with sterile normal saline and administer over 3 minutes. Anticipate apnea, and have antidote available at bedside.

➤ IV vecuronium: See manufacturer's literature. Each dose must be diluted.

➤ IV succinylcholine: May be given undiluted over 30 seconds; too rapid administration may cause bradycardia and, rarely, asystole. May be diluted for intermittent or constant infusion; see manufacturer's literature. Antidote is atropine and neostigmine.

 # CHAPTER REVIEW

Application

1. Make two lists of the neuromuscular-blocking drugs. Write the nondepolarizing agents on one list and the depolarizing agents on the other.

Critical Thinking

1. Describe the uses of tubocurarine.
2. What genetic alteration do some patients have that prolongs the action of succinylcholine? What supportive actions would you take?
3. How would you assess the patient's ability to handle secretions?

References

Hooper VD: Reversal agents to counteract muscle relaxation: nursing considerations, *DCCN* 15(6):284-295, 1996.

Hooper VD: Reversal of muscle relaxants: clinical implications for critical care nurses, *DCCN* 15(6):287, 296-297, 1996.

Chapter

38

Introduction to the Immune System

OBJECTIVES

After studying this chapter, you should be able to do the following:

- *Discuss the organs and cells of the immune system.*
- *Discuss the general function of cytokines.*
- *Describe the classes of immunoglobulins.*
- *Describe the uses of colony-stimulating factors.*

CHAPTER OVERVIEW

The immune system allows us to live safely in a world full of dangerous organisms that can invade the body and cause disease. This chapter describes the components of the immune system. Understanding the function and regulation of the various cells and organs in the immune system creates a foundation for understanding how pharmacologic manipulations can influence this vital body system.

IMMUNE SYSTEM

The immune system is a complex and diffuse system that is present throughout the body. It protects the body from damage caused by foreign environmental agents. Foreign agents include invading microorganisms such as bacteria, fungi, parasites, and viruses, as well as foreign tissue such as transplanted kidneys, hearts, and livers. Any foreign agent capable of inducing an immune response is termed an **antigen.** The immune system also protects the body, ridding it of malignant cells as they arise and preventing it from acting against its own tissues. Like all other body systems, the immune system can exhibit pathology and abnormal responses.

Innate and Acquired Immunity

Immunity is innate or acquired. Innate immunity is derived from all elements with which a person is born and that are always available on short notice to protect the body from challenges by foreign materials. Innate immunity is conferred by physical, cellular, and chemical barriers. Physical barriers include skin, mucous membranes, and the cough reflex. Phagocytic cells make up the cellular barrier. **Phagocytosis** is ingestion and destruction of foreign particles such as bacteria by individual cells of the immune system. Biologically active substances that include degradative enzymes, toxic free radicals, lipids, and low pH are chemical barriers to invasion by foreign agents.

Acquired immunity is not present at birth but develops as the individual grows and matures. Although a person has the capacity at birth for developing acquired immunity, this immunity is not exhibited until the person has had two sequential exposures to the same foreign agent. The first exposure initiates programming of a subset of lymphocytes to recognize and respond to the foreign substance. These "memory" cells are able to mount a rapid response when exposed to the foreign substance at a later time. Acquired immunity has two main arms, the humoral and the cellular immune response. Humoral immunity involves production of **antibodies,** which are soluble proteins present in normal serum that bind a foreign substance. Cellular immunity consists of responses such as the delayed type of hypersensitivity, which are mediated by cells rather than by soluble substances. Lymphocytes are the main providers of acquired immunity.

Cells of the Immune System

The immune system is comprised of six white blood cell types: lymphocytes, monocytes and macrophages, polymorphonuclear neutrophil leukocytes (PMNs), basophils, mast cells, and eosinophils. All these, as well as red blood cells and platelets, are derived from a common precursor cell type found in the bone marrow. This precursor cell type is the stem cell.

Monocytes and macrophages represent different states of cell maturation. Monocytes circulate freely within the body; with differentiation, they become macrophages. Macrophages may be fixed within the tissues, where they may persist for years; some, however, recirculate through secondary lymphoid organs. Fixed or recirculating macrophages can assist lymphocytes in generating immune responses and can phagocytize foreign particles. Macrophages can become activated to kill tumor cells.

Lymphocytes are subdivided into the thymus-derived cells or T cells and the bone marrow–derived cells or B cells. The B lymphocytes produce antibodies. T lymphocytes are further subdivided into helper T cells and cytotoxic T cells. Helper T cells assist B cells in responding to an antigen and mediate the delayed type of hypersensitivity. Cytotoxic T cells reject grafts and destroy virus-infected cells. The ratio of helper cells to cytotoxic cells normally ranges from 1.2:1 to 2:1. In the acquired immunodeficiency syndrome (AIDS), this ratio is usually reversed and can be as low as 0.2 (1:5).

PMNs are the predominant phagocytes within the circulation. They are usually the first cells to arrive at the site of an infection. Beside phagocytosis, the PMNs have two other means of killing foreign invaders. The oxidative burst of the PMNs leads to release of superoxide dismutase and hydrogen peroxide. Antimicrobial substances, including lysozyme, lactoferrin, cathepsin G, and defensins, are contained within azurophil granules and are released on activation of the PMNs.

Basophils participate in allergic and inflammatory responses. These cells contain densely staining granules in their cytoplasm. Within these granules are mediators of allergic and inflammatory responses such as histamine, complement components, and leukotrienes C and D. Degranulation occurs when antigen interacts with immunoglobulin E (IgE) molecules bound to the cell surface of the basophil.

Eosinophils participate in allergic reactions but also kill parasites. Contained within the cytoplasmic granules of the eosinophil are some of the same mediators found in basophil granules, such as leukotrienes C and D, and a number of proteins toxic to parasites. Eosinophils can also cause histamine to be released from mast cells and basophils. Eosinophils are also phagocytic, but their role as phagocytes is not as important as is that of the PMNs.

Mast cells are not circulating white blood cells, but they are important in immunity and especially in certain pathologic disorders. Like basophils, mast cells can participate in allergic reactions and inflammation and are thought to affect asthma. Mast cell granules contain histamine and a number of protease enzymes. Like basophils, mast cells can also synthesize leukotrienes C and D, as well as prostaglandin D_2. Also like basophils, mast cells degranulate when antigen interacts with IgE molecules bound to the cell surface. High numbers of mast cells can be found in the skin, lung, and intestinal mucosa. Subtypes of mast cells have been classified based on the types of proteases found within their granules. The tryptase-containing, or mucosal, mast cells are mainly located in mucosal areas as the name implies. Tryptase-chymase–containing, or connective tissue, mast cells are found in the skin. The connective tissue subtype contains more histamine than the mucosal variety. Depending on the microenvironment, mast cells can interconvert.

ALTERNATIVE THERAPIES

Immunity Enhancer

ECHINACEA

Echinacea appears to have some immunostimulating properties and is widely promoted today for prophylaxis of colds and flu at the onset of symptoms. The name *echinacea* refers to a prolific member of the daisy family (Asteracea) that grows wild throughout the Midwestern regions of the United States. North American Indians had long recognized the medicinal property of echinacea, and at least one American entrepreneur marketed it as a "patent medicine" cure-all and tonic toward the end of the nineteenth century. Echinacea was also widely marketed as an antiinfective medicine during the first half of the twentieth century. Its popularity and use faded with the discovery of sulfonamide antiinfective drugs, and all but disappeared completely, except as a folk remedy, in the age of antibiotics. The recently rekindled interest in old herbal remedies has renewed public interest in echinacea.

Although several species of echinacea exist, echinacea purpura, which is widely cultivated, seems to provide the largest source of the remedy in today's market. The medicinal properties of echinacea reside in the above-ground parts of the plant, where cichoric acid, alkylamides, polysaccharides, and an essential oil are found. It is not yet clear which, if any, of these constituents of the plant can be credited with the antiseptic and immunostimulant properties associated with echinacea.

Tablets, capsules, and liquid formulations are marketed for oral consumption. Ointments for topical application are promoted as an aid to wound healing.

Echinacea is contraindicated in tuberculosis, human immunodeficiency virus infections, multiple sclerosis, and other autoimmune diseases. Because the current food and drug laws cannot ensure strict quality control of herbal remedies sold as nutritional supplements, potential users of echinacea should choose their remedy only after carefully evaluating the manufacturer and supplier's reputation.

Organs of the Immune System

Organs of the immune system are classified as primary or secondary. The primary lymphoid organs are the thymus and the bone marrow. Maturation of lymphocytes occurs in these structures. The spleen, lymph nodes, and Peyer's patches are the secondary lymphoid organs. Peyer's patches are clusters of lymphocytes spread throughout the lining of the intestinal wall, tonsils, and appendix. Secondary lymphoid tissues trap and concentrate foreign substances and are the main sites of antibody production and generation of antigen-specific T lymphocytes.

IMMUNE RESPONSES

The previous section presented the cells and organs that make up the immune system. Each cell type plays one or more roles. The success of the immune system depends on an efficient and reliable system for cells to communicate and to act collectively and in harmony. The elements of the immune response consist of specialized cell functions to mount the immune response, the release of cytokines for communication and coordination among the cell types, and the production of antibodies and activation of the complement system to neutralize and eliminate foreign products.

Antigen-Presenting Cells

Generation of humoral or cellular immunity requires (1) activation, (2) proliferation, and (3) differentiation. Activation of T lymphocytes requires that antigen be processed and presented by specialized cells called **antigen-presenting cells.** The antigen-presenting cells also secrete soluble factors necessary for the proliferation of T cells. The major antigen-presenting cells are monocytes and macrophages. Other cells that can also present antigen include dermal Langerhans' cells, dendritic cells in various locations, and hepatic Kupffer's cells. The antigen-presenting cells take up antigen, process it, and then express it on the cell surface with histocompatibility antigens. T lymphocytes are activated by interaction with this complex of processed and histocompatibility antigen on the surface of the antigen-presenting cells. B lymphocytes are activated by interacting directly with unprocessed antigen via antibody molecules on their surface.

Major Histocompatibility Complex

The major histocompatibility complex (MHC) refers to the genes encoding the molecules that allow the immune system to differentiate self from nonself. Knowledge of the MHC arose from studies of why transplanted tissues are rejected. In humans, MHC is also called HLA for human leukocyte antigen genes. Two classes of MHC gene products play a major role in activation of T cells. Although antigens interact directly with antibody bound to B cells to activate B cells, a T-cell receptor must have antigen bound to a MHC class I or class II molecule on another cell, an antigen-presenting cell. The antigen-presenting cell must internalize the antigen, digest it, and process it to peptides that become associated with

an MHC molecule and transported in this complex to the cell surface. All nucleated cells have class I MHC. Class II MHC molecules are found primarily on B cells, Langerhans' cells, and dendritic cells. However, endothelial, synovial, and glial cells can present antigen.

T-Cell Subsets

T cells differentiate into two major subsets. The subset of T cells referred to as cytoxic T (T_C) cells are primarily characterized by a surface molecule, CD8. A T_C cell recognizes a cell presenting a foreign antigen by class I MHC molecule on the cell's surface. The T_C cell kills that cell. This is particularly effective in destroying cells infected by viruses or foreign tissue grafts. The subset called helper T (T_H) cells are distinguished by a surface molecule, CD4. One type of T_H cells, T_{H1} cells, stimulates a macrophage that has ingested a microbe to kill the microbe. Another type of T_H cells, T_{H2} cells, is able to select out B cells with MHC class II molecules presenting an antigen. The T_{H2} cells direct those B cells to make antibodies to the presented antigen.

Activated T and B Cells

Once activated, T and B lymphocytes express receptors for growth factors synthesized and released primarily by activated helper T cells. In response to these growth factors, the T and B cells proliferate. Having undergone proliferation, B and T cells can then respond to other soluble mediators secreted by activated helper T cells and will differentiate into functional effector cells. B lymphocytes differentiate into antibody-secreting plasma cells. T lymphocytes differentiate into cells capable of mediating a delayed type of hypersensitivity or killing virus-infected cells. Generation of humoral and cellular immune responses is summarized in Figure 38-1.

Cytokines

Communication within the immune system occurs mainly through release of soluble factors called **cytokines.** Cytokines are primarily released as a means of one immune cell influencing another immune cell. Cytokines are very important in controlling the development of the immune response. Many cytokines have more than one action, and more than one cytokine may be produced depending on the cell type. The result is a complex repertoire for the modulation of the immune response.

The names and major actions of the better characterized cytokines are summarized in Table 38-1. The genes for most of these cytokines have been cloned so that they can be produced outside the body in large amounts. These recombinant DNA techniques have made using those factors in clinical trials in humans possible. **Interleukins** are a diverse series of cytokines allowing one type of leukocyte to influence the function of other leukocytes. Some of these mediators can act on or be produced by cells outside of the immune system.

The interferons are a group of cytokines originally identified by their antiviral activity. Interferon-gamma (IFN-

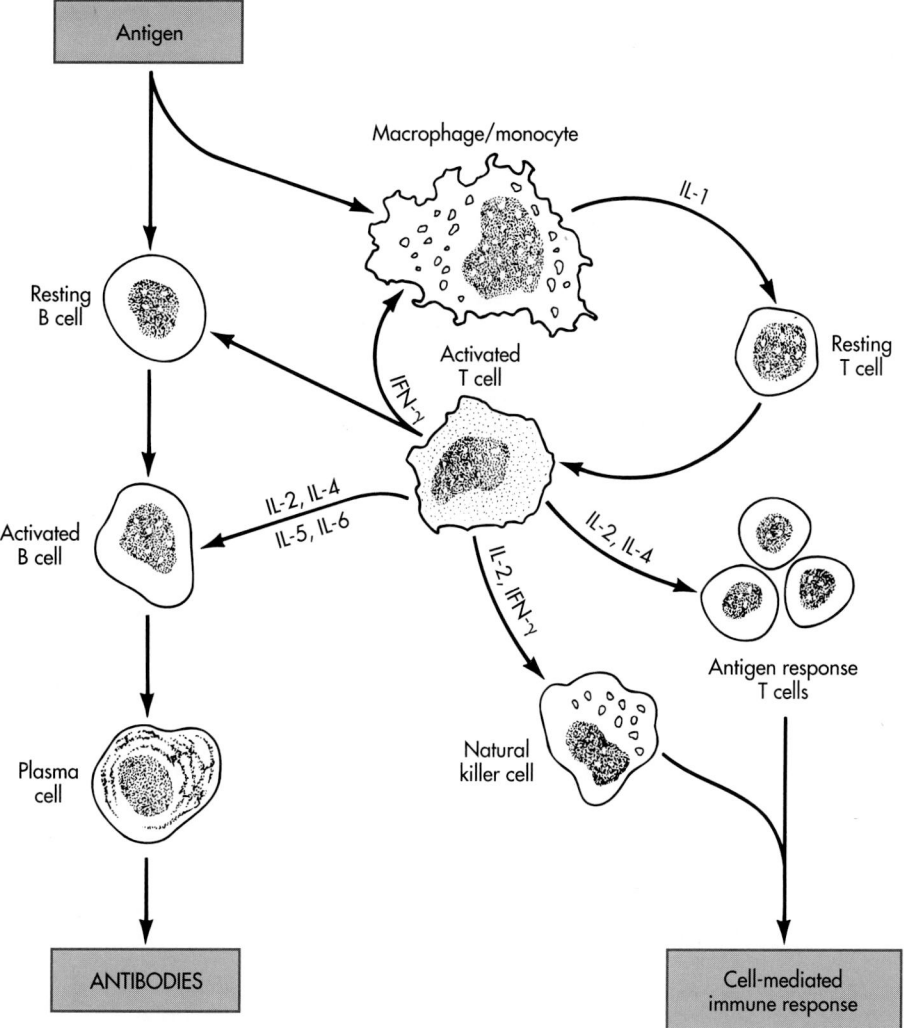

Figure 38-1 Generation of immune response. Key features of immune reaction include factors responsible for humoral immunity (shown on left) and factors responsible for delayed, cell-mediated immunity (shown on right). *IFN*, Interferon; *IL*, interleukin.

gamma) is produced mainly by the T_{H1} subset of activated T cells and natural killer cells to promote a cellular inflammatory response. IFN-gamma activates other immune cells and promotes inflammation by induction of MHC class I and MHC class II expression on macrophages and increasing natural killer cell activity. IFN-gamma is implicated in the pathogenesis of several autoimmune and chronic inflammatory conditions, including lupus and type I diabetes.

Tumor necrosis factor-alpha (TNF-alpha) is the principal cytokine produced in response to gram-negative bacteria. TNF-alpha is a mediator of both natural and acquired immunity and is also an important link between specific immune responses and acute inflammation. Overproduction of TNF-alpha leads to shock. Activated monocytes and macrophages are the major source of TNF-alpha whose activities include enhanced proliferation of activated T cells and B cells; induction of MHC class I and MHC class II ex-

pression; and expression of adhesion molecules on endothelial cells. TNF-alpha mediates several diseases, including septic shock syndrome, cachexia, AIDS, and certain autoimmune diseases. The role of TNF-beta is less clear. TNF-beta appears to play a critical role in the development of peripheral lymphoid organs.

Colony-stimulating factors control the differentiation of hematopoietic stem cells to produce new leukocytes. Table 38-2 summarizes the major colony-stimulating factors and the cells that develop from their action. The development of some immune cells can be directed by more than one of these factors.

Immunoglobulins (Antibodies)

Antibodies, the soluble mediators of humoral immunity, are specialized proteins called **immunoglobulins.** There are five classes of immunoglobulins: IgM, IgG, IgA, IgE, and IgD

Table 38-1   **Properties of Human Cytokines**

Cytokine	Biologic Properties
Interleukin-1 (IL-1)	Monocytes and macrophages are the main source for IL-1. Multifunctional pro-inflammatory activities through ability to affect expression of genes and surface receptors. Activates T cells; stimulates synthesis of other cytokines; increases natural killer cell activity; chemotaxin for neutrophils, lymphocytes, and macrophages.
Interleukin-2 (IL-2)	T-cell growth factor produced by activated T helper 1 cells. Augments cytokine production by T cells; activates cytotoxic T cells; increases natural killer cell activity.
Interleukin-3 (IL-3)	Multicolony colony-stimulating factor produced primarily by activated T cells. Supports growth of pluripotent bone marrow stem cells; promotes proliferation and maturation of committed granulocyte and macrophage progenitors.
Interleukin-4 (IL-4)	Produced by T cells, mast cells, and activated basophils to regulate B-cell responses: expression of class II histocompatibility antigens; expression of IgG and IgE; low-affinity Fc receptors for IgE. Also, induces proliferation of T cells and mast cells; regulated macrophage functions and hematopoietic progenitor cells.
Interleukin-5 (IL-5)	Produced by activated T cells. Induces differentiation of eosinophils; increases IgM and IgG secretion by activated B cells. Affects activity of IL-2 and IL-4.
Interleukin-6 (IL-6)	Produced by many cells. Induces proliferation of activated B cells, T cells, mesangial cells, keratinocytes, synovial fibroblasts, and Kaposi sarcoma cells. Induces differentiation of B cells and cytotoxic T cells.
Interleukin-7 (IL-7)	Produced by bone marrow stromal cells. Induces proliferation of immature lymphoid cells; cofactor for T-cell growth with IL-2; induces lymphokine-activated killer cells.
Interleukin-8 (IL-8)	Produced by many cell types. Major activities involve chemotaxis and activation of neutrophils.
Interleukin-9 (IL-9)	Produced by helper T cells. Promotes T-cell proliferation.
Interleukin-10 (IL-10)	Produced by T cells and B cells. Inhibits cytokine synthesis by Th1 cells, cytotoxic T cells, and natural killer cells; inhibits macrophage function. Stimulates B-cell proliferation and mast cell production.
Interleukin-11 (IL-11)	Growth factor for certain B cells and T cells.
Interleukin-12 (IL-12)	Major source is B cells and macrophages. Many activities, especially Th1 and cytotoxic T-cell proliferation and activation required for cell-mediated immune response.
Interleukin-13 (IL-13)	Produced by activated T cells. Stimulates B-cell proliferation and immunoglobulin production.
Interleukin-14 (IL-14)	Produced by T cells and some malignant cells. Stimulates differentiation and proliferation of mature B cells or memory B cells.
Interleukin-15 (IL-15)	Produced by several cell types. Stimulatory activities similar to those of IL-2.
Interleukin-16 (IL-16)	Chemoattractant factor for T cells, monocytes, and eosinophils. Also, induces IL-2 receptor in T cells.
Interleukin-17 (IL-17)	Induces IL-6 and IL-8 production.
Interleukin-18 (IL-18)	Also known as IGIF (interferon-gamma-inducing factor). Produced by Kupffer cells and activated macrophages. Like IL-12, regulates proliferation and activation of Th1 and cytotoxic T cells required for cell-mediated immune response.
Interferon-gamma (IFN-gamma)	Produced by T cells and natural killer cells in response to antigen stimulation. Exerts antiviral activity; induction of MHC class I and MHC class II expression on macrophages; decreases IgE synthesis by B cells; increases natural killer cell activity. Implicated in the pathogenesis of several autoimmune and chronic inflammatory conditions, including lupus and type 1 diabetes.
Tumor necrosis factor (TNF)	Activated monocytes and macrophages are the major source of TNF-alpha, whose activities include enhanced proliferation of activated T cells and B cells; induction of MHC class I and MHC class II expression and expression of adhesion molecules on endothelial cells. TNF-alpha mediates several diseases, including septic shock syndrome, cachexia, AIDS, and certain autoimmune diseases. Role of TNF-beta is less clear.

MHC, Major histocompatibility complex; *AIDS,* acquired immunodeficiency syndrome.

(Table 38-3). The immunoglobulin molecule is comprised of two light chains and two heavy chains. Figure 38-2 is a schematic diagram of an antibody molecule. The light chain is made up of a variable region (V) and a constant region (C). Heavy chains contain three or four constant regions and the variable region. Each variable portion of the immunoglobulin molecule includes three hypervariable regions, which vary widely in amino acid composition. The combination of these hypervariable regions makes up the antibody-combining site of the immunoglobulin molecule. This portion of the molecule binds the antigen against which the antibody was generated. Each antibody molecule has two combining sites. Five different constant regions define the major immunoglobulin classes. IgG is the major immunoglobulin in serum and has four subclasses. Two subclasses of IgA molecules exist. IgG, IgE, and IgD are

monomeric, each composed of one antibody molecule. IgM is composed of five antibody molecules, and IgA is composed of two. A protein, the J chain, joins the five basic molecules that make up the IgM molecule. A secretory component, synthesized by epithelial cells, connects the two IgA molecules that compose the dimer. Table 38-3 summarizes the immunoglobulin classes and their functions.

Complement System

The complement system is a group of enzymes found in serum that work together to "complement" the action of antibodies in destroying microorganisms. The major functions of the complement system include mediating inflammatory responses and opsonization, or coating, of antigenic particles (including microorganisms), which causes damage to the membrane of the microorganism and often results in ly-

Table 38-2 Colony-Stimulating Factors

Factor	Produced By	Colony-Stimulating Activity
Granulocyte-macrophage colony-stimulating factor (GM-CSF)	Activated T cells, B cells, mast cells, macrophages, fibroblasts, and endothelial cells	Stimulates production of granulocytes (basophils, eosinophil, neutrophils) and macrophages from bone marrow bipotential stem cells.
Granulocyte colony-stimulating factor (G-CSF)	Monocytes, fibroblasts, activated endothelial cells, and bone marrow cells	Stimulates production of granulocytes (basophils, eosinophil, neutrophils) in bone marrow culture.
Macrophage colony-stimulating factor (M-CSF)	Monocytes, fibroblasts, epithelial cells, and endothelial cells	Stimulates colonies of monocyte and macrophage precursors.
Multi-colony-stimulation factor, also called interleukin-3 (IL-3)	T cells and mast cells	Stimulates colonies of pluripotent stem cells. Promotes proliferation and maturation of committed granulocyte and macrophage progenitors.

Table 38-3 Major Classes of Immunoglobulins

Class	Distribution	Biologic Properties
IgG	Intravascular and extravascular	Responsible for most responses to antigens, including activation of complement, sensitization of target cells for destruction by killer cells, neutralization of toxins and viruses, and immobilization of bacteria. Can pass placenta.
IgM	Mostly intravascular	First type of antibody produced during primary immune response; activates complement well; efficient agglutinating antibodies; natural isohemagglutinins.
IgA	Intravascular and secretions	Most common antibody in secretions, where it protects mucous membranes; bactericidal in presence of lysozyme; efficient antiviral antibody.
IgE	On basophils and mast cells; in saliva and nasal secretions	Mediates hypersensitivity and allergic reactions; protects against parasite infections.
IgD	On surface of B lymphocytes; trace in serum	Serves as antigen-specific receptor on B cells; may be involved in differentiation of B lymphocytes.

sis of the microorganism. Nineteen distinct proteins make up the complement system. Proteins of the complement system interact such that the products of one reaction form the enzyme needed for the next step in the enzyme cascade. A small stimulus can be amplified to activate large amounts of complement.

Complement can be activated by the classic and the alternate pathway. The pathways share many components but differ in the ways they become activated. The classic pathway is activated by antigen-antibody complexes. The alternate pathway is activated by suitable surfaces or molecules, including cell walls of some bacteria, cell walls of yeast, endotoxin derived from cell walls of gram-negative bacteria, and aggregated IgA. Several steps in the complement cascade result in the release of a fragment of some of the proteins of the complement system. These small molecules are very potent mediators of a number of reactions. C3a and C5a are chemotaxins and anaphylatoxins. Chemotaxins cause phagocytic cells to migrate from an area where there is less chemotaxin to an area of higher concentration. Anaphylatoxins cause mast cell degranulation, smooth muscle contraction, and increased capillary permeability. C3b opsonizes anything to which it binds. C3b and C5b activate the lytic pathway, leading to the formation of the membrane attack complex, a series of proteins with detergent properties

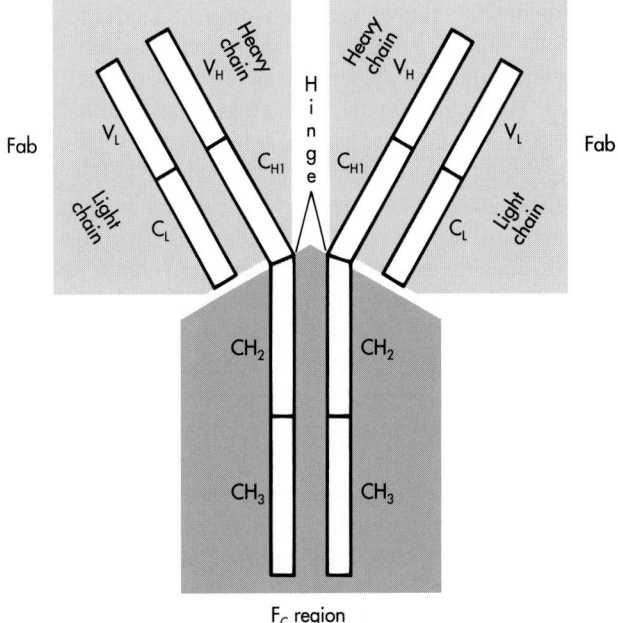

Figure 38-2 Schematic diagram of antibody molecule. Heavy and light chains composed of variable (V_H, V_L) regions and constant (C_H, C_L) regions. The Fab portions of molecule are responsible for antigen binding, and F_c portion mediates biologic activity.

that produce "holes" in the target cell membrane, resulting in lysis of the target cell.

ABNORMAL IMMUNE RESPONSES

Hypersensitivity (Allergy)

The role of the immune system is to recognize and inactivate foreign substances. However, after the individual develops an immune response to a substance, the reactivity may be altered so that there is a pathologic reaction on reexposure to the substance. Hypersensitivity, or allergy, refers to this pathologic, exaggerated reaction to a foreign substance.

Immediate Hypersensitivity

Immediate hypersensitivity refers to allergic responses that occur within minutes to hours. Three types of immediate hypersensitivity responses are recognized. These responses are initiated with an antibody and antigen combine but trigger tissue injury.

Type I hypersensitivity refers to the release of histamine from basophils or tissue mast cells. The antibody is IgE bound to the surface of the basophil or tissue mast cell and the antigen induces cross-linking of the IgE molecules, a process that leads to the release of histamine and other proinflammatory chemical mediators. Type I hypersensitivity is characteristic of asthma, hay fever, and hives (see Chapters 28 and 29). The most extreme reaction is classic systemic anaphylaxis, a generalized release of histamine leading to a profound fall in blood pressure and shock, as well as a constriction of the airways, which can be fatal if not treated immediately. Drug allergies that can give type I reactions include penicillins, cephalosporins, aspirin, and iodides. Other common causes of type I hypersensitivity include insect stings and antitoxins prepared from animal serum.

Type II hypersensitivity arises from an antigen on a cell surface that is complexed by IgM or IgG antibody. This complex may lead to tissue destruction through cell lysis by complement or phagocytosis. Examples are hemolytic responses during blood transfusions and the hemolytic response of an Rh-positive fetus to an Rh-negative mother. In these cases an antibody against a foreign red blood cell membrane antigen binds to the red blood cell and initiates complement-mediated destruction of the red blood cell. Some complexes lead to altered cell function without cell destruction as in Graves' disease. Substances can also bind to a red blood cell or other tissue membrane and act as an antigen, leading to type II hypersensitivity. Such drug reactions include hemolytic anemia induced by methyldopa and thrombocytopenic purpura induced by quinidine. Examples of autoimmune diseases involving type II hypersensitivity include autoimmune hemolytic anemia, autoimmune thrombocytopenia, Goodpasture's syndrome, pemphigus, phemigoid, pernicious anemia, myasthenia gravis, and Graves' disease.

Type III hypersensitivity, or immune complex disease, is characterized antigen-antibody complexes that become deposited in tissues such as kidney, skin, and serous membranes

and activate complement, leading to cell destruction. The reaction leads to increased vascular permeability and the recruitment of neutrophils. Depending on the location, the result can be skin rashes, glomerulonephritis, or arthritis. Normally, immune complexes are cleared by macrophages in the spleen and elsewhere. Serum sickness is a generalized immune complex reaction. Examples of immune complex diseases include systemic lupus erythematosus, polyarteritis nodosa, and poststreptococcal glomerulonephritis.

Delayed Hypersensitivity

Type IV hypersensitivity, or delayed hypersensitivity, is mediated by T cells, not antibodies. The reaction is seen 2 or 3 days after reexposure to the antigen, not minutes to hours. The classic delayed hypersensitivity reaction is the tuberculin test in which the test antigen is applied to the skin and the reaction read after 2 to 3 days. In delayed hypersensitivity the sensitized T cells release cytokines that recruit macrophages and neutrophils, which ultimately produce widespread tissue damage. Delayed hypersensitivity is a reaction to infections caused by intracellular pathogens such as *Mycobacterium tuberculosis* and *Leishmania*. Contact dermatitis is a common delayed hypersensitivity response to a variety of compounds, including such agents as poison ivy.

Autoimmune Diseases

Sometimes the immune system manufactures T cells and antibodies directed against the body's own cells. These T cells and autoantibodies contribute to such diseases as diabetes, rheumatoid arthritis, systemic lupus erythematosus, myasthenia gravis, multiple sclerosis, and Graves' disease (hyperthyroidism). The therapy of selected autoimmune diseases is presented in Chapter 42.

Immune Deficiencies

The immune system is tightly regulated to ensure optimal function. Disorders in the development of immune cells during the generation of immune responses or in the synthesis of the products of the immune system may cause immunologic disorders ranging in severity from mild to fatal. The disorders can be classified into deficiencies of immune cells or their soluble products and overproduction of immune cells or their products. Immune deficiencies are primary or secondary. **Primary immune deficiencies** are diseases in which the immune deficiency is the cause of the disease; they may be hereditary or acquired. **Secondary immune deficiencies** result from diseases. Patients with secondary immune deficiencies invariably experience recurrent infections; this development often leads to the diagnosis of an immune deficiency.

Primary Immune Deficiencies

B-cell deficiencies can result in the absence of one or all immunoglobulin classes. Persons with B-cell deficiencies experience mainly recurrent bacterial infections. Although immunoglobulin replacement therapy may maintain these patients for as long as 20 to 30 years, the prognosis is poor and many succumb to chronic lung disease.

T-cell deficiencies affect not only cell-mediated immune responses but also synthesis of antibody because T cells are necessary for most antibody responses. Patients with T-cell disorders are extremely susceptible to fungal, viral, and protozoal infections.

Severe combined immunodeficiencies result from defects in both T and B cells. These disorders are very serious. Untreated infants rarely survive beyond 1 year of age. Patients with combined immunodeficiencies are susceptible to every type of infection. Treatment with drugs alone is ineffective. Infants can be cured by bone marrow transplantation, provided the transplantation is done before irreversible complications of the disease arise.

Phagocytic cell dysfunctions also cause severe disorders because these cells affect both innate and acquired immunity. Defects may result from deficiencies of antibody, lymphokines, or complement deficiencies and can also result from cell defects.

Abnormalities in the complement system can lead to immunodeficiencies. Genetic defects affecting nearly all the individual components of the complement system have been documented.

Secondary Immune Deficiencies

Secondary immune deficiencies occur as complications of other diseases. The most common cause of these disorders is the deliberate immune suppression associated with the use of chemotherapeutic agents in cancer treatment or the immunosuppressive drugs used to prevent rejection of transplanted organs. The best known secondary immune deficiency is AIDS. This disease is caused by infection with human lymphotropic virus III, now called human immunodeficiency virus (HIV). The immune deficiency associated with AIDS is largely caused by the loss of helper T cells. These cells are not the only immune cells affected by the virus because the profound immune suppression associated with AIDS cannot be explained only on the basis of loss of helper T cells. Patients with secondary immune deficiencies experience severe recurrent infections by opportunistic organisms normally not pathogenic.

Gammopathies

Several neoplastic diseases arise from abnormal proliferation of B cells and plasma cells. These diseases are called gammopathies. The principal gammopathies are multiple myeloma, macroglobulinemia, and heavy chain disease.

Multiple myeloma is the most common of the gammopathies, resulting from the malignant proliferation of plasma cells. It is characterized by synthesis of large amounts of a given isotype of immunoglobulin and may be accompanied by the production of free light chains (called Bence Jones proteins). Multiple myeloma involves multiple organ systems, resulting from infiltration of them by malignant plasma cells. Patients are susceptible to recurrent bacterial and viral infections because of suppression of the synthesis of normal antibodies.

Macroglobulinemia occurs because of synthesis of large amounts of IgM. The excess immunoglobulin leads to increased viscosity of serum, which leads to decreased blood flow, thrombosis, disorders of the central nervous system (CNS), and bleeding. Decreased synthesis of the other immunoglobulin classes is observed, leading ultimately to hypogammaglobulinemia.

Heavy chain disease is characterized by the appearance of large amounts of protein in the serum and urine resembling the Fc portion of the immunoglobulin molecule. This disorder is uncommon. Patients have recurrent bacterial infections, anemias, and enlarged lymphoid organs.

 # CHAPTER REVIEW

Application

1. What is innate immunity?
2. What is acquired immunity?
3. What are the forms of acquired immunity?
4. What white blood cell types are responsible for phagocytosis?
5. What are T cells? Where are they formed?
6. What are B cells? Where are they formed?
7. What cell type forms antibodies?
8. What cell type produces the delayed type of hypersensitivity?
9. What are interleukins?
10. What are the five classes of antibodies?
11. What are the primary functions of each class of antibody?
12. What is the complement system?
13. What are the two major functions of the complement system?
14. Define primary and secondary immune deficiency.
15. Define gammopathy.

Critical Thinking

1. How does measurement of T cells and B cells provide information about the immune system?
2. How does analysis of a patient's white blood cell differential provide information about the bone marrow, possible infections, and immune status? What does "a shift to the left" mean?
3. Why is AIDS described as a "secondary immune deficiency?"
4. How does information about immunoglobulins relate to allergic reactions to drugs?

Chapter

39

Immunizations

OBJECTIVES

After studying this chapter, you should be able to do the following:

- *Discuss the difference between passive and active immunity.*
- *Develop a nursing care plan for the patient receiving an immunostimulant.*

CHAPTER OVERVIEW

Immunization, a way of modulating the action of the immune system to provide protection from specific infections, has been known for a long time. This chapter describes the immunizations currently available. Some of the common diseases that are now preventable through vaccination include chicken pox, hepatitis A and B, *Haemophilus influenzae* type b, influenza, measles, mumps, whooping cough, *Pneumococcal pneumonia,* polio, and rubella (German measles). Antivenin and immunoglobulins are available for temporary passive immunity following exposure to certain diseases or toxins.

THERAPEUTIC RATIONALE: IMMUNOSTIMULATION

Immunostimulation refers to the activation of T cells and B cells by an antigen. Once an antigen activates the immune system, some of the T cells and B cells become memory cells. The next time that antigen is encountered, the immune system can mount an active and vigorous response.

Immunity varies in its duration and effectiveness depending on how it was acquired. The fetus is protected from bacterial and viral infections and from microbial toxins by maternal immunoglobulin G (IgG) antibodies, which pass to the fetus through the placenta to confer passive immunity. IgG is the only antibody that can cross the placenta. Newborn infants do not have a fully functional immune system; human milk, however, contains factors that aid the newborn response against infectious agents. Some of these factors enhance the growth of beneficial intestinal flora, and others nonspecifically inhibit the growth of harmful microorganisms. The inhibitory factors include lysozyme, lactoferrin, interferon, and leukocytes. Antibodies are also found in

breast milk and are especially abundant in colostrum (first milk).

Active immunization to a disease organism is achieved through the administration of a vaccine. Worldwide vaccination programs have been successful in virtually eradicating smallpox and polio. Many diseases devastating to children are now rare because of the recommended immunization schedule for standard pediatric care and the requirement most school systems have for proof of immunization (Table 39-1). The most successful immunization programs are for those viral diseases in which few pathogenic strains exist and with which antigenic properties do not change. The vaccine for poliovirus fits these criteria. However, immunization against rhinoviruses has not been feasible because there are approximately 100 strains. Each strain induces a separate antibody in humans and the antibodies are not cross-reactive. Influenza vaccines are of value for a limited time because the viruses shift antigenic properties every few years, leaving the old vaccines ineffective.

Growing attention is being given to developing additional new adult vaccines. A new vaccine has been released for Lyme disease. The scope of vaccine research is expanding to develop therapeutic vaccines, especially against skin and other cancers.

Most current vaccines are administered by injection. Current research is aimed at new methods of vaccine delivery. A flu vaccine administered by nasal spray is being tested. Vaccine contained in slowly soluble microspheres may be injected to release small doses over a long period, eliminating the need for booster injections. It may be possible to administer DNA encoding antigenic material for incorporation into the body's own cells. The antigenic protein would be made over a long period and induce a strong, long-lasting immunity. Antigen material may be genetically engineered into plants, such as bananas or potatoes, to induce protective immunity when eaten.

Passive immunity consists of administering antibodies or serum taken from immunized humans or animals. This approach can offer immediate intervention in life-threatening exposures.

THERAPEUTIC AGENTS: VACCINES, IMMUNE SERUM, AND ANTIBODIES

Agents for Active Immunity

Mechanism of Action

Active acquired immunity involves **immunization**—administration of substances such as vaccines that stimulate the immune system to respond against a foreign material. **Vaccines** usually contain killed or attenuated bacteria or viruses, but protection can also be conferred with immunogenic proteins (toxoids) from the pathogen in question. Once the immune response has occurred, specific cells in the immune system "remember" the response, and a secondary immune response occurs rapidly on a subsequent encounter with the antigen. This principle is illustrated in Figure 39-1. Active immunity usually persists for years.

Table 39-1 Active Immunization Schedule Recommended in the United States

Age	Vaccine
2 months	DTaP (or DTP)-1, HB-1*, PV-1, Hib-1
4 months	DTaP (or DTP)-2, HB-2, PV-2, Hib-2
6 months	DTaP (or DTP)-3, PV-3, Hib-3
6-18 months	(PV-3), HB-3
12-15 months	MMR-1, Hib-4, Var
15 months	DTaP (or DTP)-4
4-6 years	DTaP (or DTP)-5, MMR-2
14-16 years	Td (MMR-2)
18-24 years	MMR if not previously administered
25-64 years	MMR if not previously administered and no childhood history of the disease; Td every 10 years
65 years and older	Annual influenza vaccination; single pneumococcal polysaccharide vaccination; Td every 10 years

DTaP, Diphtheria and tetanus toxoids and acellular pertussis vaccine (preferred over DTP); *DTP*, diphtheria, tetanus, and pertussis vaccine; *HB*, hepatitis B; *PV*, polio vaccine (two doses of killed poliovirus vaccine followed by two doses of live oral trivalent, *or* 4 doses live oral trivalent, *or* 4 doses of killed poliovirus vaccine); *Hib*, *Haemophilus influenzae* type b conjugate vaccine; *MMR*, measles, mumps, rubella virus live vaccine; *Td*, tetanus and diphtheria toxoids adsorbed for human use; *Var*, varicella (chicken pox).
*Begin within 12 hours of birth if mother is positive for hepatitis B.

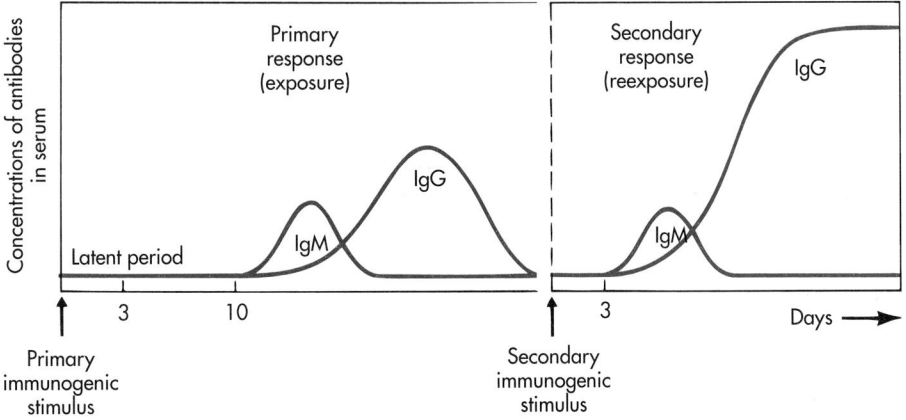

Figure 39-1 Time course of antibody release on first exposure versus subsequent exposure. *IgG*, Immunoglobulin G; *IgM*, immunoglobulin M.

Pharmacokinetics

Vaccines are administered by either intramuscular (IM) or subcutaneous (SC) injection. Oral polio vaccine and an oral typhoid vaccine are exceptions. Duration of protection is usually from 1 to 10 years. Because vaccines stimulate the immune system to respond actively rather than passively, protection persists after the injected agent has disappeared. Because vaccines are antigens and not antibodies, they are taken up and processed by antigen-presenting cells (see Chapter 38) for the generation of immune responses. Some of the injected agent is metabolized in this manner. Once antibodies have been produced, any remaining injected material can be complexed with the antibodies and cleared by phagocytes.

Uses

Childhood Immunization Schedule. A number of infectious diseases are almost completely preventable through routine childhood immunizations. The recommended childhood immunization schedule in the United States begins when the infant is 2 months of age and can mount an effective immune response on its own. Table 39-1 indicates the recommended schedule for active immunization throughout life. Recommended childhood immunizations include hepatitis B (HB-1); diphtheria, tetanus, and pertussis (DTP); *H. influenzae* type b (Hib); poliovirus (PV); measles, mumps, and rubella (MMR); and chicken pox (varicella-zoster virus [VZV]).

CASE STUDY
Childhood Immunizations

A young Hispanic woman comes into the emergency department with her toddler who seems to be very ill. The woman speaks very little English and indicates that her child is "so sick." When you ask her how old the child is and about the illness, she shrugs, frustrated, and begins to cry. The child is listless, with a temperature of 103° F, breathes with difficulty, and has a congested cough. When you ask her about the child's doctor, she says "No doctor!" The nurse practitioner who examines the child determines that he has bronchiolitis and asks about the child's immunization status. When you ask her about the child's "shots," she frowns and says "No hablo ingleses, no comprendo." She shows you a card that indicates that her husband has temporary employment in a local factory.

1. What can you do to improve your communication with this client?
2. If the child has had no immunizations, what resources may be available for referral for this client?
3. If the toddler is 13 months old, what immunizations have been missed so far?
4. What cultural implications are important to consider for this family?

Because some vaccines were introduced only in the 1990s, catch-up vaccination is indicated for children 11 to 12 years of age who were not previously vaccinated to hepatitis B and chicken pox (VZV).

Adult Immunizations. Adults who have no history of disease or active immunization against measles, mumps, rubella, and chicken pox should be immunized for these diseases because they are more severe diseases in adults than in children. Most adults in the United States have been immunized against polio. A booster for tetanus and diphtheria should be administered every 10 years throughout life. Adults older than 65 years are advised to have an annual influenza vaccination and at least one pneumococcal vaccination.

Special Situations. Women of childbearing age who do not have rubella immunity should be immunized when they are not pregnant, preferably during the immediate postpartum period. Travelers (especially to underdeveloped regions), military personnel, and health care workers should be immunized against hepatitis A and hepatitis B. Immunization against hepatitis B is also recommended for individuals living in the same household as an infected person, for individuals with multiple sex partners, and for intravenous (IV) drug users. Immunization against pneumococcal pneumonia is recommended not only for those older than 65 years but also for those with chronic disease or lowered immunity, alcoholics, organ transplant recipients, and those older than 50 years in group-living facilities. Vaccination against influenza is recommended not only for those older than 65 years but also for those who have chronic disease or lowered immunity, are nursing home residents, or have contact with high-risk people. Influenza vaccination must be repeated yearly.

Special immunizations are recommended for those at specific risk, as for cholera, meningococcal meningitis, plague, rabies, typhoid, or yellow fever.

Currently available agents are included in Table 39-2. Postexposure prophylaxis should be provided with exposures to *H. influenzae* type b, meningococcal infection, hepatitis A, hepatitis B, tuberculosis, and rabies.

Adverse Reactions and Contraindications

Live virus vaccines should not be used in patients receiving immunosuppressive therapy because these vaccines can cause progressive disease in immunocompromised patients. Live virus vaccines are also contraindicated in pregnant women because live virus vaccines can damage the fetus. These live virus vaccines include the Bacillus Calmette-Guérin (BCG) vaccine for tuberculosis, MMR vaccines, typhoid vaccine, chicken pox (varicella) vaccine, and yellow fever vaccine.

Individuals with an allergy to eggs may experience adverse reactions to viruses grown in eggs, such as influenza virus vaccines, MMR vaccine, and yellow fever vaccine.

In general, vaccines should not be administered when the individuals has a fever or febrile illness.

Table 39-2 **Agents for Active Immunization**

Generic Name (Trade Name)	Route	Duration of Effect	Indications
Bacillus Calmette-Guérin (BCG) vaccine Tice strain: TICE-BCG	PERCUTANEOUS: *Adults and children*—0.02-0.03 ml. Reduce dose by 50% for infants less than 1 month of age.	Protection rate variable; duration variable	For active immunization against tuberculosis (TB) of adults and children with negative tuberculin skin tests in high-risk households; also for health care workers exposed to resistant TB; travelers to endemic areas.
Cholera vaccine	INTRAMUSCULAR, SUBCUTANEOUS: *Adults and children >10 yr*—0.5 ml. *Children 5-10 yr*—0.3 ml. *Children 6 mo-4 yr*—0.2 ml; give second dose 1 wk-1 mo apart. INTRADERMAL: *Adults and children ≥5 yr*—0.2 ml.	6 mo	Only for individuals traveling to countries where cholera is endemic or vaccination is required. Previous allergic reaction to the vaccine is a contraindication.
Diphtheria and tetanus toxoids adsorbed, pediatric (DT)	INTRAMUSCULAR: *Children <12 mo*—3 0.5-ml injections administered at different sites at 4- to 8-wk intervals, followed by a fourth dose 6-12 mo later. *Children >12 mo*—2 doses 4-8 wk apart, third dose 6-12 mo later. Booster when child is 4-6 yr old.	10 yr	Not for primary immunization of a child unless there is a contraindication to pertussis vaccine. Do not administer to child with a fever or to a child who has a history of neurologic or severe hypersensitivity reaction to a previous dose.
Diphtheria and tetanus toxoids adsorbed for adult use (Td)	INTRAMUSCULAR: *Adults and children >7 yr*—2 injections of 0.5 ml 4-8 wk apart; reinforcing dose 6-12 mo later.	10 yr; booster required	Susceptible children >7 yr old and adults.
Diphtheria and tetanus toxoids and acellular pertussis vaccine adsorbed (DTaP) or Diphtheria and tetanus toxoids and pertussis whole cell adsorbed (DTwP) (Acel-Immune, Tri-Immunol, Tripedia)	INTRAMUSCULAR: *Children 2 mo-6 yr*—0.5 ml, followed by 2 more doses at 4- to 8-wk intervals; fourth dose at 15-18 mo and booster at 4-6 yr old.	10 yr; boosters required for tetanus toxoid	For children <7 yr of age only. Do not administer to child with a fever; do not administer if reaction to an earlier DTP administration was severe (fever of 105°F or higher, anaphylaxis, encephalopathy).
Diphtheria and tetanus toxoids and pertussis vaccine adsorbed and *Haemophilus influenzae* type b conjugate vaccine (DPT-Hib, Tetramune)	INTRAMUSCULAR: *Children 2-6 mo of age at first dose*—3 doses 2 mo apart, fourth dose at 12-18 mo or at least 6 mo after third dose.	See individual vaccines	For children <7 yr of age only. Coordinates administration of four recommended childhood immunizations.
H. influenzae type b polysaccharide vaccine (Act-Hib; Hibtiter; Pedvaxhib; Prohibit)	INTRAMUSCULAR: *Children 2 mo-5 yr*—Initial vaccination for infants at 1-2 mo, 2 additional doses at 2-mo intervals.	Unknown, probably 1½-3 yr	For all children and persons whose spleens have been removed. Do not administer if child has fever or active infection.
Hepatitis A vaccine, inactivated (Havrix, Vaqta)	INTRAMUSCULAR: *Adults*—1 dose in the deltoid region. *Children 2-18 yr*—2 doses 1 mo apart.	Booster dose after 6-12 mo	For persons at increased risk of infection by hepatitis A virus, including military and travelers to endemic areas. Bleeding disorder and febrile illness are contraindications.
Hepatitis B vaccine recombinant (HBV vaccine: Engerix B; Heptavax-B; Recombivax HB)	INTRAMUSCULAR: Dose depends on manufacturer and exposure to hepatitis. See package insert.	At least 5 yr	For all infants, preadolescents, and young adults; for persons with environmental or lifestyle risk, including hemophiliacs and patients receiving hemodialysis.
Influenza virus vaccine (FluShield; Fluviral; Fluvirin; Fluzone)	INTRAMUSCULAR: *Infant 6-35 mo*—0.25 ml. *Children >3 yr to adult*—0.5 ml. Type of vaccine depends on age, see package insert; children <8 yr need a second dose 4 wk or more later.	1 yr	For adults ≥65 yr, persons with asthma and other respiratory conditions, medical care personnel.
Japanese encephalitis virus vaccine (Je-Vax)	SUBCUTANEOUS: *Adults and children >3 yr*—1 ml on days 0, 7, and 30; booster after 2 yr. *Children 1-3 yr*—½ adult dose.	At least 2 yr after 3 doses	For adults and children who plan to travel or reside in areas endemic for Japanese encephalitis.
Measles virus vaccine live (Attenuvax)	SUBCUTANEOUS: *Children ≥15 mo*—Single dose (0.5 ml) into the outer aspect of the upper arm; second dose at least 1 mo later.	≥8 yr	For adults born after 1956 without a history of measles or live virus vaccination on or after their first birthday.

Continued

Table 39-2 **Agents for Active Immunization—cont'd**

Generic Name (Trade Name)	Route	Duration of Effect	Indications
Measles, mumps, and rubella virus vaccine live (M-M-R II)	SUBCUTANEOUS: *Children ≥15 mo*—Single dose (0.5 ml) into the outer aspect of the upper arm.	Years; second dose recommended at entry to grade school, middle school, or high school	For all children.
Measles and rubella virus vaccine live (M-R-VAX II)	SUBCUTANEOUS: *Adults and children ≥15 mo*—Single dose (0.5 ml) into the outer aspect of the upper arm.	≥8 yr	For immunization of susceptible persons >12 mo of age who have immunity to mumps.
Meningococcal polysaccharide vaccines (Menomune A/C/Y/W-135)	SUBCUTANEOUS: *Adults and children >2 yr*—0.5 ml as single injection; children <4 yr may require a booster.	Years; young children in endemic areas may require additional injections	For military recruits, persons without spleens or immunosuppressed, and those with household, institutional, or travel contact with meningococcal disease.
Mumps virus vaccine live (Mumpsvax)	SUBCUTANEOUS: *Adults and children ≥12 mo*—0.5 ml.	Permanent immunity (in 75%-90% of patients receiving vaccine)	For adults born after 1956 without a history of mumps or live virus vaccination on or after their first birthday.
Pertussis vaccine adsorbed	INTRAMUSCULAR: *Children 2 mo-6 yr*—3 doses (0.5 ml) 4-8 wk apart with fourth dose at 15-18 mo of age. Booster given at 4-6 yr of age. *Adults*—0.25 ml booster during pertussis epidemics.	4-6 yr	For unimmunized children or adults during pertussis epidemics.
Plague vaccine	INTRAMUSCULAR: *Adults and children >10 yr*—1-ml dose, followed in 4 wk by second dose of 0.2 ml; another 0.2-ml dose at 3-6 mo after first dose. *Children <10 yr*—Receive reduced doses, see manufacturer's instructions.	3 booster doses of 0.2 ml at 6-mo intervals; then at 1-2 yr	For laboratory personnel working with *Yersinia pestis,* persons in contact with rodents or fleas, and persons in endemic areas.
Pneumococcal polysaccharide vaccine (Pneumovax 23; Pnu-Imune 23)	SUBCUTANEOUS, INTRAMUSCULAR: 0.5 ml as a single dose.	Years	For adults >65 years and persons at increased risk, including people with weakened immune systems, cancers, organ transplants, or chronic diseases.
Poliovirus vaccine live oral trivalent (OPV, Sabine vaccine, TOPV)	ORAL: *Infants*—Administer at 2, 4, and 15-18 mo. *Children and adolescents*—2 doses 6-8 wk apart, third dose 1 yr later.	Years	For infants 6-12 wk, all children and adolescents up to 18 yr old, and adults at high risk. IPV preferred for adults.
Poliovirus vaccine inactivated (IPV)	SUBCUTANEOUS: *Infants*—Initial dose at 6-12 wk, second dose at 4-8 wk; third dose 6-12 mo after second dose.	Years; booster before entering grade school	For infants 6-12 wk, all children and adolescents up to 18 yr old, and adults at high risk. IPV preferred for adults.
Rabies vaccine, adsorbed (RVA)	INTRAMUSCULAR: *Adults*—1 ml in deltoid area on days 0, 3, 7, 14, and 28 for preexposure prophylaxis. *Children*—Same dose into anterolateral thigh. See package insert for postexposure doses.	Check antibody levels after 2 yr, give booster if necessary	Postexposure immunization against rabies infection; preexposure for persons at risk through animal handling.
Rabies vaccine, human diploid cell (HDCV: Imovax Rabies, Imovax Rabies ID)	INTRAMUSCULAR: *Adults*—1 ml in deltoid area on days 0, 3, 7, 14, and 28 for preexposure prophylaxis. *Children*—Same dose into anterolateral thigh. See package insert for postexposure doses.	Check antibody levels after 2 yr, give booster if necessary	Postexposure immunization against rabies infection; preexposure for persons at risk through animal handling.
Rabies vaccine, purified chick embryo cell culture (RabAvert)	INTRAMUSCULAR: *Adults*—1 ml in deltoid area on days 0, 3, 7, 14, and 28 for preexposure prophylaxis. *Children*—Same dose into anterolateral thigh. See package insert for postexposure doses.	Check antibody levels after 2 yr, give booster if necessary	Postexposure immunization against rabies infection; preexposure for persons at risk through animal handling.
Rubella virus vaccine live (Meruvax II)	SUBCUTANEOUS: *Adults and children ≥12 mo*—0.5 ml into the outer aspect of the upper arm.	Years; booster not recommended	Persons ≥12 mo, nonpregnant women, women postpartum with no history of immunization, and persons traveling to endemic areas.
Rubella and mumps virus vaccine live (Biavax II)	SUBCUTANEOUS: *Children 12 mo to puberty*—Single dose (0.5 ml) into the outer aspect of the upper arm.	Permanent	All susceptible persons ≥12 yr except pregnant women.

Table 39-2   **Agents for Active Immunization—cont'd**

Generic Name (Trade Name)	Route	Duration of Effect	Indications
Tetanus toxoid; tetanus toxoid adsorbed	INTRAMUSCULAR: *Adults and children*—4 injections (0.5 ml) with 4-8 wk between first, second, and third doses, and 6-12 mo between third and fourth doses.	10 yr; booster required	All children and adults.
Typhoid vaccine, inactivated Ty2 *S. typhi*	SUBCUTANEOUS: *Adults and children >10 yr*— 2 doses of 0.5 ml 4 wk or more apart or 3 doses of 0.5 ml at weekly intervals. *Children 6 mo-10 yr*—2 doses of 0.25 ml 4 wk or more apart or 3 doses at weekly intervals.	3 yr; boosters can be given when needed	For military personnel and other persons in or traveling to endemic areas.
Typhoid vaccine live oral TY21a (Virotif Berna)	ORAL: *Adults and children >6 yr*—1 capsule ingested with a cold or lukewarm drink 1 hr before a meal on days 1, 3, 5, and 7.	5 yr; repeat immunization schedule	For persons in or traveling to endemic areas.
Varicella virus vaccine live (Varivax)	SUBCUTANEOUS (deltoid region of the arm): *Adults and adolescents*—0.5 ml, followed by a booster dose of 0.5 ml 4-8 wk later. *Children 1-12 yr*—Single dose of 0.5 ml.	Unknown, new vaccine	For persons >12 mo, including adolescents and adults with no history of chicken pox.
Yellow fever vaccine (YF-Vax)	SUBCUTANEOUS: *Adults and children >9 mo*— 0.5 ml.	10 yr	For persons >9 mo who are living in or traveling to areas of South America or Africa where yellow fever is endemic.

Interactions

All immunosuppressive agents can interfere with the generation of active immunity induced by vaccines and toxoids. Corticosteroids, azathioprine, cyclosporine, and some agents used in cancer chemotherapy fall in this category.

Agents for Passive Immunity

Mechanism of Action

Passive acquired immunity involves administration of preformed substances such as immune serum or antibodies that can immediately combine with the foreign agent to which they are directed. Antivenins and antitoxins are prepared from the serum of horses inoculated with the toxin. The passive immunity conferred by immune sera, antibodies, or globulins lasts only weeks.

Pharmacokinetics

IM injection is the usual route of administration of the immune serums and globulins. Oral administration is usually impossible with these agents because the degradative processes in the digestive tract render them inactive before they can be absorbed. Distribution is fairly rapid after IM injection, but if very rapid therapy is required, these agents can be given intravenously, resulting in immediate distribution. The immunity provided by immune globulins and serums lasts from 1 to 6 weeks. Once injected, the antibodies interact with the entire organism against which they were generated, thus facilitating phagocytosis of the organism by monocytes or macrophages and polymorphonuclear neutrophil leukocytes (PMNs). Antibodies made against toxins of pathogenic microorganisms form complexes with the toxin, and these immune complexes are also cleared by phagocytes. Immunity is lost when the injected antibodies have been cleared from the system.

Uses

Antiserums and immune globulins are used prophylactically and therapeutically to provide temporary immunity against infectious agents, microbial exotoxins, and snake and insect venoms. Examples are antivenins for poisonous bites of snakes and spiders; antitoxins for botulism, diphtheria, and tetanus; and special immune globulin preparations for treatment of tetanus and rabies. These agents are listed in Table 39-3.

Adverse Reactions and Contraindications

Many side effects of immune serum or globulin injections are dose related. Patients may have pain at the injection site, mild chest pain, and chills. Less common side effects include malaise, headache, nausea and vomiting, dyspnea, syncope, and back pain. Hepatitis B immune globulin can also cause urticaria and angioedema. Varicella-zoster immune globulin injections can cause a mild rash, usually observed 10 to 14 days after immunization.

Toxicity

Immune sera, especially those using nonhuman proteins, can cause anaphylaxis in patients with a history of hypersensitivity reactions to immune globulin injections. This serum sickness results from an immune response directed against proteins in the injected serum. Massive immune complex formation occurs, followed by deposition of these complexes in the kidney and circulatory system, leading to nephritis and arteritis. The deposited immune complexes also initiate

Table 39-3   Antivenins, Antitoxins, and Other Immunoglobulins for Passive Immunity

Generic Name (Trade Name)	Route	Indications	Contraindications
Antivenin (Micrurus fulvius) North American coral snake	INTRAVENOUS: *Adults and children*—IV drip of 250-500 ml with 3-5 vials of antivenin (30-50 ml) added to tubing or to reservoir.	Neutralizes venom from Eastern and Texas coral snakes. Protection lasts for several days.	After first 1 or 2 ml, administered over 3-5 min, observe for anaphylactic reaction before proceeding. Severe hypersensitivity to equine serum.
Antivenin (Crotalidae) polyvalent Rattlesnake	INTRAVENOUS: *Adults and children*—Dose is based on extent of envenomation; see manufacturer's literature; most effective when given within 4 hr of bite.	Neutralizes venom from crotalid snakes, including rattlesnakes, copperheads, and moccasins. Protection lasts for several days.	
Antivenin (Latrodectus mactans) Black widow spider	INTRAMUSCULAR: *Adults and children*—1 container injected into anterolateral thigh. INTRAVENOUS: *Children <12 yr or in shock*—Dilute 1 container into 10-50 ml and administer over 15 min.	Neutralizes venom from black widow spider and related species. Protection lasts for several days.	Hypersensitivity to horse serum.
Botulism antitoxin trivalent	INTRAVENOUS: *Adults with symptomatic botulism and after sensitivity testing*—2 vials. INTRAMUSCULAR: *Adults after ingestion of contaminated food*—$\frac{1}{5}$-1 vial.	Neutralizes toxin of *Clostridium botulinum* from ingesting contaminated food. Protection lasts 5-7 days.	Sensitivity to equine serum.
Diphtheria antitoxin	IINTRAMUSCULAR: *Adults and children*—For prophylaxis of those not immunized who are in contact with patients: 2,000-10,000 units. INTRAMUSCULAR or INTRAVENOUS, slow infusion: *Adults and children with diphtheria*—20,000-120,000 units.	Prevention and treatment of respiratory diphtheria. Protection lasts about 3 wk.	Allergy to serum; pregnancy.
Hepatitis B immune globulin (HBIG: H-BIG, Hep-B-Gammagee, HyperHep)	INTRAMUSCULAR: *Adults and children*—0.06 ml/kg or 5 ml to adults, administered as soon as possible (within 7 days) after exposure. *Newborn infants*—0.5 ml as soon as possible after birth.	Protection of exposed newborns; prophylaxis postexposure for adults. Protection lasts weeks; immunization should begin as soon as possible after exposure.	Not for treatment of fulminant acute or chronic active hepatitis B.
Immune globulin intravenous (IGIV: Gamimune N; Gammagard; Gammar IV; Sandoglobulin I.V.)	INTRAVENOUS: See individual preparation for dosage.	Replacement therapy for antibody deficiency disorders, immune thrombocytopenic purpura, hypogammaglobulinemia in chronic lymphocytic leukemia, and Kawasaki disease. Protection lasts 3 wk.	History of anaphylactic reaction or severe systemic response to immune globulin.
Immune globulin (IG: Gammar IM)	INTRAMUSCULAR: *For hepatitis A postexposure prophylaxis*—0.02 ml/kg; for travel in areas where hepatitis A is common, 0.02 ml/kg for visits less than 2 mo; 0.06 ml/kg repeated every 5 mo for longer visits; also 0.25 ml/kg for prophylaxis against measles.	Pooled antibodies to protect those exposed to hepatitis A, measles, or rubella and for patients with immunoglobulin deficiency. Protects for months.	Not for postexposure prophylaxis of hepatitis B.
Palivizumab (Synagis)	INTRAMUSCULAR: 15 mg/kg body weight.	Prevention of serious lower respiratory tract infection caused by respiratory syncytial virus in infants and children with bronchopulmonary dysplasia and in infants with a history of premature birth.	Not for adolescents or adults.
Rabies immune globulin (Imogam Rabies-HT, BayRab)	INTRAMUSCULAR: 20 IU/kg; with half being infiltrated around wound.	Postexposure protection for those not immunized to rabies. Protects for 3 wk.	Thrombocytopenia.
Rh$_o$(D) Immune Globulin	INTRAMUSCULAR: 1 vial within 72 hr of term delivery or after spontaneous or induced abortion, miscarriage, or ectopic pregnancy.	For women who are Rh$_o$ negative and carrying a fetus. Suppresses active antibody response to Rh$_o$-positive infant after delivery.	History of systemic allergic reactions to preparations containing human immunoglobulins.
Tetanus immune globulin (TIG)	INTRAMUSCULAR: *Adults and children*—For prophylaxis: 250-500 units by deep IM injection. *For treatment: Adults*—3000-6000 units. *Children*—500-3000 units.	Prophylaxis and treatment of persons with wounds with no history of recent immunization. Protects for 14 wk.	Adverse reactions uncommon.

---

mediator release from platelets, basophils, and PMNs. This massive mediator release can be life-threatening. A local deposition of insoluble immune complexes at the site of injection produces the Arthus reaction, in which redness and edema occur near blood vessels. Use caution when repeating injections of foreign serum. Other signs of serum sickness include arthralgias, lymphadenopathy, and pruritus. In serious cases, abdominal pain, fever, headache, and malaise may occur. Use of immune sera may be contraindicated in patients with thrombocytopenia because excessive bleeding may occur at the injection site.

Interactions

There are no known drug interactions that are associated with the use of passive immunostimulants, immune serum, and globulins.

Table 39-3 Antivenins, Antitoxins, and Other Immunoglobulins for Passive Immunity—cont'd

Generic Name (Trade Name)	Route	Indications	Contraindications
Vaccinia immune globulin	INTRAMUSCULAR: *Adults and children*—0.3 ml/kg as soon as possible after exposure; doses larger than 10 mg should be injected at 2 or more sites.	For prevention or modification of vaccinia infection. Protects for weeks.	No benefit in patients with postvaccinal encephalitis.
Varicella-zoster immune globulin (human) (VZIG)	INTRAMUSCULAR: *Adults*—125 units/10 kg, maximum, 626 units, with each vial injected into a different site.	For prophylaxis of chicken pox. Protects for 10-28 days.	Only for individuals with four significant risk factors.

Nursing Process Overview

Immunization

Assessment
Perform a baseline assessment based on the patient's age, severity of presenting problems, acuity level, and planned drug intervention. Assess for history of any problems with previous immunizations.

Nursing Diagnoses
- Potential complication: serum sickness

Patient Outcomes
The patient will experience no side effects related to immunizations.

Planning/Implementation
Most patients receive immunizations as outpatients and have no subjective or objective problems related to the immunization other than a mildly sore arm. Some patients experience low-grade fever and malaise for a few days, depending on the specific immunization. If problems develop, monitor vital signs and assess the patient. For some childhood immunizations, routine use of acetaminophen every 4 hours for 24 hours after the immunization may lessen subjective symptoms; consult the physician.

Evaluation
Before discharge, teach patients about anticipated benefits and possible side effects of immunizations. Encourage patients to call if questions arise or new signs or symptoms develop.

Nursing Implications Summary

Immunizations
Drug Administration
➤ Any serum product containing proteins can cause acute allergic reactions and serum sickness. Review the signs and symptoms of serum sickness with the patient, and instruct the patient to notify the physician if it develops. Note that serum sickness may not develop for up to 6 to 12 days after immunization.

➤ Have available epinephrine 1:1000 solution when protein-containing products are administered. Have drugs, equipment, and personnel available to treat acute allergic reactions.

➤ Question patient (or parent) about response to previous immunizations. Assess for fever or acute infection before administering immunizations, and if present, check with physician before administering dose.

Nursing Implications Summary—cont'd

➤ Question the female patient about the possibility of pregnancy before administering vaccines. Live virus vaccines are contraindicated in pregnant women.

➤ Assess the patient for human immunodeficiency virus (HIV) or other compromised immune state. Patients with a compromised immune state may require postponement of immunizations or may require an adjusted dose; consult the physician.

➤ Review the manufacturer's insert for current information about contraindications, cross-sensitivities with other drugs or allergens, and sensitivity testing.

➤ For IM administration, use anatomic landmarks in selecting injection sites. Use the vastus lateralis muscle in infants and small children. Use the deltoid muscle for administration of most vaccines and similar medications in older children and adults. Usually, avoid injection sites in the gluteal area unless large-volume doses must be divided into two or more injections or the patient is receiving two or more drugs that cannot be administered in the same site. Aspirate before injecting the drug to avoid inadvertent IV administration; if blood is aspirated, withdraw the needle, discard the syringe and needle, and prepare a fresh dose. Record the injection site and rotate sites with subsequent doses.

➤ DTP immunizations: Administer each of the four primary immunizing doses in a different site (e.g., each deltoid muscle and each vastus lateralis).

➤ Polio vaccine: Administer the parenteral forms of polio vaccine via SC injection. Administer the oral form directly or mix with distilled water, chlorine-free tap water, approved syrups, or milk. It may also be applied to food such as bread, cake or cube sugar.

➤ *H. influenzae* type b vaccine: Read orders and labels carefully. There are both conjugate forms and polysaccharide forms.

➤ Hepatitis B vaccine: Administer via the IM route into the deltoid muscle of adults and older children. Use the vastus lateralis muscle in infants and small children.

➤ Influenza vaccine: Assess for history of allergy to eggs, aminoglycosides, sodium bisulfite, or thimerosal before administering.

➤ For agents used to confer passive immunity (immune globulins): Read manufacturer's literature for information about dilution, precautions, and administration.

➤ Review Tables 39-2 and 39-3 as needed.

Nursing in the Community

➤ Review the anticipated benefits and possible side effects of drug therapy with the patient. With small children, if regular immunizations usually cause a fever, suggest that the mother use acetaminophen to treat this side effect. Instruct the mother to consult the physician.

➤ Warn the patient to avoid scratching injection sites. Brief application of an ice pack may lessen irritation.

➤ When appropriate, review with the patient the schedule for additional immunizations.

➤ Refer the patient to the local health department if appropriate.

➤ Instruct patients who manifest an allergic response to wear a medication identification tag or bracelet listing the allergic response and to be cautious in taking vaccines or immunomodulators without consulting the physician.

Measles Virus (Live Vaccine), Mumps Virus (Live Vaccine), or Rubella Virus (Live Vaccine)

Drug Administration/Nursing in the Community

➤ See the general guidelines for immunizations.

➤ Caution the female patient to avoid pregnancy for 3 months after immunization to prevent possible birth defects.

➤ Instruct the patient to keep all health care providers informed about immunizations for the next 3 months. The patient should not receive blood transfusions or blood products within 2 weeks of this immunization, gamma-globulin or other globulins within 2 weeks, other live virus vaccines within 1 month, or tuberculin skin test within 6 to 8 weeks of this vaccine.

CHAPTER REVIEW

Application

1. Explain active acquired immunity and how it is achieved. How long does it last?
2. Explain passive acquired immunity and how it is achieved. How long does it last?
3. What immune protection does the fetus have?

4. What is a common side effect of immune serums? How should you assess this and teach patients about it?

Critical Thinking

1. Find out what immunizations are required by your local school system for children to enter public school.
2. What immunizations are required by your hospital for personnel who work with patients?

References

Borton D: Keeping measles at bay, *Nursing* 27(12):26, 1997.

Gardner J: Action stat: Rattlesnake bite, *Nursing* 27(6):33, 1997.

Lerner-Durjava L: Protecting against tetanus, *Nursing* 26(2):26-27, 1996.

Lerner-Durjava L: How to stop the pox [chicken pox], *Nursing* 27(4):20, 1997.

Immunomodulators and Care of Patients with Altered Immune Function

OBJECTIVES

After studying this chapter, you should be able to do the following:

- *Describe the clinical uses of immunosuppressants.*
- *Discuss the pharmacology of cyclosporine.*
- *Describe the types of patients who might receive immunostimulants.*
- *Develop a nursing care plan for a patient receiving an immunosuppressant or an immunostimulant.*

CHAPTER OVERVIEW

In Chapter 39 we considered the use of vaccines and antibodies to stimulate an immune response. These substances are mostly used in healthy individuals to prevent disease caused by exposure to a pathogen. In this chapter another class of immunostimulants is considered, drugs that are most often used to stimulate a faltering or failing immune system. In addition, this chapter discusses specific immunosuppressants that are used primarily in organ transplantation.

THERAPEUTIC RATIONALE: IMMUNOSTIMULATION

Modern medicine must deal with large numbers of patients whose immune systems are compromised directly by disease or indirectly as a side effect of drugs used to treat neoplastic disease, host-versus-graft disease, or other conditions. In the past these patients were managed by attempting to protect them from exposure to disease, but little else could be done. Today, recombinant engineering technology coupled with a growing understanding of the immune system has made available a number of agents that can partially restore immune function.

THERAPEUTIC AGENTS: COLONY-STIMULATING FACTORS AND CELL-STIMULATING AGENTS

Colony-Stimulating Factors

Colony-stimulating factors are proteins that regulate development of cells that are precursors to specific blood cells. The natural proteins are present in the body in very small amounts, but recombinant technology allows unlimited quantities of these human proteins to be made in *Escherichia coli* bacteria or in the yeast *Saccharomyces cerevisiae*. Two colony-stimulating factors are currently accepted for medical use. One stimulates the production of the granulocyte cell line and the other stimulates the production of both granulocyte and monocyte-macrophage lines. Table 40-1 lists specific dosages and other information for immunostimulant drugs.

▼ filgrastim and sargramostim

Mechanism of Action

Filgrastim (recombinant **granulocyte colony-stimulating factor**) binds to receptors on specific progenitor cells in bone marrow, causing them to increase production of neutrophil granulocytes. Neutrophils are polymorphonuclear leukocytes that play a key role in phagocytosis (see Chapter 38). Therefore the treatment with filgrastim promotes the return of cell-mediated immunity.

Sargramostim (recombinant **granulocyte-macrophage colony-stimulating factor**) binds to receptors on a less differentiated progenitor cell than filgrastim; therefore production of more than one type of cell is promoted. The most important cell types that increase in response to sargramostim are neutrophils and monocyte-macrophages.

Pharmacokinetics

Both filgrastim and sargramostim are rapidly absorbed from subcutaneous sites and achieve peak concentrations within hours. The effect of filgrastim on neutrophil production can be seen usually within a day, whereas the effects of sargramostim on leukocyte production occur over several days.

Uses

The primary use for filgrastim is to treat neutropenia that is induced by cancer chemotherapy, but it may also be used for congenital neutropenia or idiopathic neutropenia. Sargramostim is used primarily for promoting myeloid engraftment after bone marrow transplantation or to improve the yield of progenitor cells, but it may also be used to reverse chemotherapy-induced neutropenia.

Adverse Reactions and Contraindications

The most common adverse reaction to either filgrastim or sargramostim is pain in bone, joints, and muscles. Bone pain seems correlated with recovery of the bone marrow and increased production of neutrophils. Headache, skin rash, and redness at the site of injection are less common.

Patients who have a significant number of leukemic myeloid blasts are at risk for further leukemic progression when treated with colony-stimulating factors because these agents may promote proliferation of the precursor cells.

Serious allergic reactions are rare, but patients who are sensitive to proteins derived from *E. coli* are more likely to show signs of allergy to filgrastim, which is made by *E. coli* cells.

Sargramostim may cause capillary leak syndrome. Symptoms include peripheral edema, pleural effusion, and shortness of breath. Patients may also react to the first dose of sargramostim with an episode of flushing, hypotension, and syncope. This reaction usually does not recur with subsequent doses.

Patients with acquired immunodeficiency syndrome (AIDS) should not receive sargramostim unless they are also receiving a drug to control human immunodeficiency virus (HIV) proliferation. Some reports have indicated that sargramostim can promote proliferation of the virus.

Toxicity

Capillary leak syndrome and fever are dose-related responses to sargramostim. Overdosages can therefore lead to serious or life-threatening reactions.

Table 40-1 Immunostimulant Drugs

Generic Name	Trade Name	Administration/Dosage	Comments
aldesleukin	Proleukin	INTRAVENOUS: *Adults—For metastatic renal carcinoma:* 600,000 U/kg infused over 15 min every 8 hr for 14 doses. FDA pregnancy category C.	Recombinant interleukin-2 stimulates immune system at several points.
filgrastim	Neupogen*	INTRAVENOUS, SUBCUTANEOUS: *Adults—*5 μg/kg starting 24 hr or more after last dose of cytotoxic chemotherapy. FDA pregnancy category C.	Recombinant colony-stimulating factor increases numbers of neutrophils.
interferon-gamma	Actimmune	SUBCUTANEOUS: *Children—For chronic granulomatous disease:* 50 μg/m² 3 times weekly for children >0.5 m² surface area; smaller children receive 1.5 μg/kg 3 times weekly. FDA pregnancy category C.	Recombinant protein stimulates phagocyte functions.
levamisole	Ergamisol*	ORAL: *Adults—*50 mg every 8 hr for 3 days; repeat every 2 wk for a year. FDA pregnancy category C.	Immunostimulant used with fluorouracil for colorectal carcinoma.
pegademase	Adagen	INTRAMUSCULAR: *Children—*10 U/kg on day 1, 15 U/kg on day 8, 20 U/kg on day 15; then 20 U/kg weekly. FDA pregnancy category C.	Bovine adenosine deaminase corrects enzymatic defect and restores immune function.
sargramostim	Leukine	INTRAVENOUS, SUBCUTANEOUS: *Adults—To promote myeloid engraftment in bone marrow transplantation:* 250 μg/m² surface area daily for 14-21 days. First dose should begin 2-4 hr after bone marrow transplantation. FDA pregnancy category C.	Recombinant colony-stimulating factor increases numbers of granulocytes and monocyte-macrophages.

*Available in Canada and the United States.

Interactions

No specific toxicity or interactions have been documented for these drugs, perhaps because they are used in complex regimens involving many drugs, each with significant direct and secondary actions.

Cell-Stimulating Agents

Colony-stimulating factors stimulate progenitor cells in bone marrow to increase the numbers of leukocytes being formed, thus improving immune function. Another class of agents improves immune function by stimulating the activity of cells already formed.

aldesleukin

Mechanism of Action

Aldesleukin is a recombinant form of **interleukin-2 (IL-2)**, one of the major cytokines regulating function of the immune system (see Chapter 38). Multiple effects of aldesleukin contribute to stimulation of cell-mediated immunity.

Pharmacokinetics

Aldesleukin is used only by intravenous (IV) routes. The drug distributes well to many sites. Elimination involves hydrolysis of this protein into amino acids in the kidneys. The biologic effect of aldesleukin on immune function may persist for months.

Uses

Aldesleukin is indicated only for renal cell carcinoma. The very high risk of side effects limits use for other indications.

Adverse Reactions and Contraindications

Aldesleukin causes a wide array of potentially serious side effects. Central nervous system (CNS) effects include agitation, confusion, depression, dizziness, and fatigue. Pulmonary symptoms may include lung congestion, edema, and shortness of breath. Anemia may require blood transfusions. Arrhythmias are usually transient but may occasionally be life-threatening.

A skin rash with redness, itchiness, and peeling commonly appears within 2 or 3 days of the start of treatment and begins to resolve only after the drug is discontinued. Blisters on the skin may signal a more dangerous condition, exfoliative dermatitis, which can be fatal. Dizziness, nausea, and vomiting almost always occur.

Aldesleukin is contraindicated for patients with preexisting impairment of cardiac or pulmonary function. The drug is also avoided in patients with metastatic cancer in the CNS. Aldesleukin is not used in patients with transplanted organs because the immune stimulation produced by the drug may prompt organ rejection.

Toxicity

Capillary leak syndrome is more likely at higher dosages. Symptoms of capillary leak syndrome include peripheral edema, pleural effusion, and shortness of breath. This condition may be fatal.

Interactions

Drugs like daunorubicin or doxorubicin may cause dangerous additive cardiotoxicity with aldesleukin. Likewise the toxicity of bone marrow depressants, hepatotoxic drugs, and nephrotoxic medications may be worsened by aldesleukin. Corticosteroids may antagonize the actions of aldesleukin.

interferon-gamma

Mechanism of Action

Interferon-gamma (IFN-gamma) promotes the formation of reactive forms of oxygen in phagocytes. This and other actions improve phagocytosis.

Pharmacokinetics

The absorption of IFN-gamma from injection sites is slow but relatively efficient. Peak concentrations in blood occur in 4 to 7 hours. Mechanisms for biotransformation or elimination may involve both the liver and kidneys.

Uses

IFN-gamma is used in chronic granulomatous disease, a condition in which oxidative functions of phagocytic cells are impaired. Thus the direct actions of the drug tend to reverse the genetically induced defect, with the result that immune function is improved.

Adverse Reactions and Contraindications

IFN-gamma typically causes a flulike syndrome. Symptoms include achiness, chills, fever, headache, and joint pain. Diarrhea, nausea, and vomiting are also common and may contribute to weight loss. Rashes and dizziness may occur. IFN-gamma commonly causes leukopenia, but symptoms are rare.

The fever and chills caused by IFN-gamma cause stress on the cardiovascular system. Patients with preexisting cardiovascular disease may be unable to tolerate this added load. Patients with CNS disease may be at greater risk for serious reactions with use of IFN-gamma. A history of allergic reactions to *E. coli*–derived products may indicate an increased risk with recombinant IFN-gamma, which is produced in *E. coli*.

Toxicity

Leukopenia, CNS effects, and gastrointestinal (GI) tract side effects are dose-related reactions to IFN-gamma. These reactions are therefore worse with very high dosages.

Interactions

Any drugs that interfere with bone marrow function can influence the activity of IFN-gamma.

levamisole

Mechanism of Action

Levamisole returns leukocyte function to normal levels after chemotherapy or surgery. T cells, monocytes, macrophages, and neutrophils are influenced.

Pharmacokinetics

Levamisole is easily absorbed orally and undergoes extensive biotransformation in the liver. The drug persists in blood for several hours. Elimination of metabolites is primarily in urine.

Uses

Levamisole is used as an adjunct for surgery and chemotherapy of primary colorectal carcinoma. Metastatic disease does not respond.

Adverse Reactions and Contraindications

GI tract effects such as nausea and diarrhea are common with levamisole. Blood dyscrasias can also occur but usually cause no symptoms. A flulike syndrome may be related to onset of serious blood dyscrasias.

CNS impairment is rare but can include ataxia, blurred vision, confusion, mental changes, paresthesias, seizures, tardive dyskinesia, or tremors.

Bone marrow depression or infections may be worsened by levamisole; patients with these conditions should be carefully watched for serious reactions.

Toxicity

Many of the potentially serious effects of levamisole are allergic or idiosyncratic reactions and are therefore not dose related.

Interactions

Levamisole is often used in combination with fluorouracil; the drugs may have additive effects on blood cell counts. Leukopenia is usually transient with levamisole alone but when combined with fluorouracil, leukopenia may persist or develop into agranulocytopenia.

pegademase

Mechanism of Action

Pegademase is bovine adenosine deaminase, an enzyme that is required for removal of toxic metabolites of adenosine. Without this enzyme, lymphocytes die. The absence of this enzyme is the cause of severe combined immunodeficiency disease (SCID).

Pharmacokinetics

Pegademase is designed so that the adenosine deaminase is covalently linked to a larger molecule that allows the material to remain in the blood longer. The material may remain in circulation for several days. The onset of action on immune function is gradual and significant clinical improvement may not occur for as long as a year.

Uses

Pegademase is used only for adenosine deaminase deficiency, or SCID.

Adverse Reactions and Contraindications

Side effects are rare with pegademase but may include headache or pain at the site of injection. Pegademase is avoided in patients with thrombocytopenia because of the risk of bleeding.

Toxicity

Toxicity has not been documented with doses below 30 mg/kg.

THERAPEUTIC RATIONALE: IMMUNOSUPPRESSION

Organ transplantation has been made possible by the existence of drugs that can successfully control rejection of the transplanted tissue without compromising all immune function in the host. The arm of the immune system that must be controlled is cell-mediated immunity (see Chapter 38).

THERAPEUTIC AGENTS: IMMUNOSUPPRESSANT AGENTS

Several types of agents may be useful to control host-versus-graft disease. The following section covers cyclosporine, basiliximab, daclizumab, muromonab-CD3, mycophenolate, and tacrolimus, drugs not covered extensively elsewhere in this text. Azathioprine is covered in Chapter 42, and the corticosteroids are covered in Chapter 41. Table 40-2 lists specific dosages and other information for immunosuppressant drugs.

▼ cyclosporine

Mechanism of Action

Cyclosporine blocks the release of IL-2 from activated helper T cells. This action inhibits induction of cytotoxic T lymphocytes (see Figure 38-1). As a result, cell-mediated immunity is suppressed.

Pharmacokinetics

Oral absorption of cyclosporine is variable, and bioavailability is only about 30%. The drug is extensively metabolized by the liver. The half-life of the drug is long in adults, ranging from 10 to 27 hours but tends to be shorter in children. Elimination of the drug is through bile into the feces.

Uses

Cyclosporine is the most widely used drug for prevention of organ rejection after transplantation. It is often combined with corticosteroids.

Adverse Reactions and Contraindications

Cyclosporine commonly causes hypertension and nephrotoxicity, but symptoms are usually absent. These reactions may be monitored by checking blood pressure regularly and by following the blood urea nitrogen (BUN) and creatinine.

Gingival hyperplasia is also common with cyclosporine. This reaction and increased hair growth (hirsutism) are often troublesome to patients because self-image may be affected.

Table 40-2	**Immunosuppressant Drugs**		
Generic Name	Trade Name	Administration/Dosage	Comments
basiliximab	Simulect	INTRAVENOUS: *Adults*—20 mg infused over 20-30 min hr before transplant and 4 days later. FDA pregnancy category B. *Children*— 12 mg/m² up to maximum of 20 mg, on same schedule as adult.	Used in renal transplantation. Give initial dose within 2 hrs prior to transplant.
cyclosporine	Sandimmune* Neoral*	ORAL: *Adults and children*—12-15 mg/kg initially, then reduced by 5% weekly to maintenance of 5-10 mg/kg/day. FDA pregnancy category C.	Intravenous preparation is given 4-12 hr before transplant, but oral doses should be substituted as soon as possible after surgery.
	Sandimmune*	INTRAVENOUS: *Adults and children*—2-6 mg/kg daily until oral doses are possible.	
daclizumab	Zenapax	INTRAVENOUS: *Adults*—1 mg/kg infused over 15 min every 14 days for 5 doses. FDA pregnancy category C.	Used in renal transplantation. Give initial dose within 24 hr before transplant.
muromonab-CD3	Orthoclone OKT3*	INTRAVENOUS: *Adults*—5 mg by rapid injection daily for 10-14 days. FDA pregnancy category C. *Children*—0.1 mg/kg by rapid injection daily for 10-14 days.	Monoclonal antibody blocks immune cell activation.
mycophenolate	CellCept	ORAL: *Adults*—1 g 2 times/day, starting within 72 hr of renal transplant. FDA pregnancy category C.	Enzyme inhibitor blocks lymphocyte proliferation.
tacrolimus	Prograf*	ORAL: *Adults*—75 μg/kg every 12 hr. *Children*—150 μg/kg every 12 hr. INTRAVENOUS: *Adults*—50 μg/kg/day by continuous infusion. *Children*—100 μg/kg/day by continuous infusion.	Oral dose preferred.

*Available in Canada and the United States.
†Available in Canada only.

A variety of potentially serious reactions, including hepatotoxicity, pancreatitis, and electrolyte imbalances, are possible with cyclosporine. Alterations in elimination of potassium may lead to confusion, paresthesias, shortness of breath, and muscle weakness. Convulsions may also occur. Anaphylaxis is possible, especially with parenteral dosing. Because cyclosporine suppresses part of the immune system, the risk of serious infection is also increased.

Cyclosporine is used cautiously in patients with hepatic or renal damage, adjusting dosages carefully to avoid drug accumulation. Active infections may be worsened by the drug.

Toxicity

Several of the reactions to cyclosporine are dose related. Irreversible nephrotoxicity may occur with persistently high dosages. Tremors are another dose-related symptom that may signal overdose.

Interactions

Many drugs that are metabolized in the liver may interfere with the metabolism of cyclosporine and therefore cause accumulation of cyclosporine, leading to serious side effects. Drugs that may act in this way include androgens, cimetidine, danazol, diltiazem, erythromycin, estrogens, and imidazole antifungal agents.

The risk of hyperkalemia may be increased when medications containing potassium are used. Other drugs such as potassium-sparing diuretics and succinylcholine may also increase the risk.

Live virus vaccines should not be used with cyclosporine because the immune suppression caused by cyclosporine may allow an uncontrolled proliferation of the virus. Serious generalized disease may result.

Lovastatin may cause cell damage and renal failure in patients with cardiac transplants who receive cyclosporine.

daclizumab and basiliximab

Mechanism of Action

Daclizumab and basiliximab are monoclonal antibodies that bind to IL-2 receptors on lymphocytes. As a result of this binding, the response of lymphocytes to IL-2 is impaired. Without IL-2 activation of lymphocytes, cell-mediated immune reactions are diminished.

Pharmacokinetics

Because daclizumab and basiliximab are proteins, they must be administered intravenously. These recombinant antibodies persists in the body for up to a month, which is about the same as for natural antibodies.

Uses

Daclizumab and basiliximab are currently used only to prevent acute rejection of transplanted kidneys. The monoclonal antibodies are used in combination with other immunosuppressants such as cyclosporine and corticosteroids.

Adverse Reactions and Contraindications

Side effects with daclizumab include chest pain, edema, GI distress, shortness of breath, pain in the joints, and slow wound healing. In addition to these effects, basiliximab may cause headache, insomnia, dizziness, and tremor. The only absolute contraindication to these agents is a documented allergy to the proteins.

Toxicity/Interactions

No dose-related toxicity or drug interactions have been demonstrated.

muromonab-CD3

Mechanism of Action

Muromonab-CD3 is a monoclonal antibody that binds to the CD3 receptor on human T helper cells. The binding of the drug prevents the cell from responding to signals from activated macrophages or monocytes. As a result, T-cell function is inhibited and cell-mediated immune responses are blunted.

Pharmacokinetics

Muromonab-CD3 is a protein and must be given intravenously. The protein binds directly to helper T cells; therefore its action is almost immediate. Return to normal numbers of fully functional CD3 cells usually occurs within a week after muromonab-CD3 is discontinued.

Uses

Muromonab-CD3 is used to treat episodes of transplant rejection. The drug is usually combined with other immunosuppressants such as azathioprine, cyclosporine, or glucocorticoids.

Adverse Reactions and Contraindications

Muromonab-CD3 provokes release of cytokines in most patients. Symptoms include chills, diarrhea, dizziness, fainting, spiking fever, headache, malaise, muscle or joint pain, nausea, and vomiting. These symptoms may progress to more serious signs such as arrhythmias, chest pain, shortness of breath caused by pulmonary edema, trembling, and weakness. The cytokine release reaction usually appears 30 minutes to 48 hours after injection. Anaphylaxis may also produce similar symptoms but usually appears within 10 minutes of injection.

Many CNS signs may occur with muromonab-CD3. These include confusion, headache, hallucinations, sensitivity to light, and tiredness. More serious reactions include coma or seizures.

Muromonab-CD3 is avoided in patients with fluid overloads or heart failure because of the excessive risk of potentially fatal pulmonary edema. The drug is also avoided in patients with fever or infections.

Muromonab-CD3 is a mouse protein. Patients with strong allergies to mice should not receive the drug because the risk of a serious allergic reaction is increased.

Toxicity

Most of the reactions to muromonab-CD3 are caused by release of cytokines in the body. These effects may worsen with increases in dosage.

Interactions

When muromonab-CD3 is combined with other immunosuppressants, the risk of severe immune suppression is increased. Immune function should be monitored and dosages of both drugs adjusted as necessary. The patients should also be monitored for signs of infections.

Immunosuppressants should not be used with live virus vaccines because the immune suppression caused by the drug may allow an uncontrolled proliferation of the virus. Serious generalized disease may result.

mycophenolate

Mechanism of Action

Mycophenolate inhibits inosine monophosphate dehydrogenase, an enzyme required for synthesis of guanine nucleotides needed for DNA synthesis. Both T and B lymphocytes must maintain synthesis of DNA to proliferate normally. Therefore the result of treatment with mycophenolate is to block proliferation of T and B lymphocytes, thereby impairing cell-mediated immune responses that might promote rejection of transplanted organs.

Pharmacokinetics

Mycophenolate mofetil, the prodrug form that is actually administered, is adequately absorbed orally, and the prodrug is rapidly converted in the body to mycophenolic acid, the active metabolite. If the drug is taken with food or cholestyramine, blood levels may be decreased; therefore the drug is taken on an empty stomach. The drug is highly bound to plasma proteins and has a half-life of 17 to 18 hours. The drug appears to undergo extensive enterohepatic circulation (see Chapter 1). The liver forms inactive metabolites, including a glucuronide that is eliminated renally.

Uses

The only current indication for mycophenolate is to prevent rejection of allogeneic cardiac or renal transplants. The drug is combined with cyclosporine and glucocorticoids.

Adverse Reactions and Contraindications

GI tract symptoms are common and include abdominal pain, constipation or diarrhea, heartburn, nausea, and vomiting. Headache and general weakness are also common. Common reactions that are more serious include anemia, blood in urine, chest pain, edema, hypertension, and neutropenia. Neutropenia, which exposes the patient to increased risk of infection, peaks 1 to 6 months after transplantation and the start of immunosuppression.

Mycophenolate should be used with caution in patients with serious GI tract disease because the drug may increase the risk of hemorrhage or perforation. Patients with renal impairment may require lower dosages.

Toxicity

Overdoses have not been reported. Cholestyramine might be expected to assist in such cases by sequestering mycophenolate and promoting fecal excretion.

Interactions

Mycophenolate is used cautiously in combination with other immunosuppressants; the risk of excessive immunosuppression or development of lymphomas may be increased.

tacrolimus

Mechanism of Action

Tacrolimus is a macrolide that suppresses activation of the immune system, blocking production of IL-2. This action is similar to that of cyclosporine, but tacrolimus is much more potent than cyclosporine. In addition, tacrolimus may in a different way inhibit formation of several other cytokines, including granulocyte-macrophage colony-stimulating factor, tumor necrosis factor-alpha, and interleukins (IL-1, IL-3 through IL-6, and IL-8). All these actions contribute to inhibition of cell-mediated immunity.

Pharmacokinetics

Tacrolimus may be absorbed orally or may be used by IV infusion. Oral absorption is highly variable and may be diminished by food. Tacrolimus is metabolized by the CYP3A enzyme systems in liver (see Chapter 1). Very little drug is eliminated renally.

Uses

Tacrolimus is currently indicated only for treating tissue rejection in patients with transplanted livers. The drug is being tested for other applications, including use in inflammatory skin lesions.

Adverse Reactions and Contraindications

Adverse reactions may include serious nephrotoxicity and electrolyte imbalances such as hyperkalemia. Neurotoxicity may involve peripheral nerves, with tingling in hands and feet, or may involve CNS effects such as anxiety, confusion, depression, dizziness, hallucinations, headache, nervousness, seizures, sleep disorders, or tremors. GI disturbances and generalized weakness also occur.

Toxicity

Most of the reactions to tacrolimus are dose related and thus are worse with overdoses. Nephrotoxicity, neurotoxicity, and diabetes were the effects most often observed.

Interactions

Live virus vaccines may cause dangerous generalized disease in immunosuppressed patients and should be avoided in patients receiving tacrolimus.

Because tacrolimus is metabolized by CYP3A (see Chapter 1), tacrolimus may interact with other drugs such as rifampin, which induces CYP3A and thus increases metabolism of tacrolimus. Drugs such as danazol, erythromycin, and azole antifungals may compete with tacrolimus for the CYP3A enzyme and thus diminish the metabolism of tacrolimus.

Nursing Process Overview

Immunomodulators

Assessment

Assess vital signs. Perform a complete physical assessment. Obtain a history of previous infections. Monitor weight and assess for recent changes in weight. Auscultate lung sounds. If the patient has received a transplanted organ, take a history appropriate to the transplant.

Nursing Diagnoses

- Potential complication: infection

Patient Outcomes

The patient will not experience an infection, or if one occurs, the nurse will minimize and manage complications associated with the infection.

Planning/Implementation

Monitor vital signs. Assess for signs of infection. If an immunostimulant is prescribed, monitor for improvement in cell counts and subjective improvement. If an immunosuppressant is ordered, review with the patient the potential danger of infection. Teach the patient how to administer prescribed drugs at home.

Evaluation

Immunostimulants are effective if the patient develops more resistance to infections. Immunosuppressants are administered to prevent organ rejection after transplant. Evaluate signs of organ rejection and indicators of continuing function of the transplanted organ(s). The patient should be able to state how to administer ordered medications, the importance of returning for follow-up, and side effects that should be reported to the physician.

Nursing Implications Summary

COLONY-STIMULATING FACTORS

filgrastim
Drug Administration/Nursing in the Community
➤ Review side effects. Monitor vital signs. Assess for pain in joints, muscles, and bones. Analgesics may be needed for bone pain, and for some patients, narcotics may be required. Consult physician.
➤ If the patient is to self-administer at home, teach injection technique and proper handling of syringes and needles.
➤ For IV administration, see manufacturer's insert. Administer dose over at least 30 minutes, or a 4- to 24-hour infusion may be prepared.
➤ For subcutaneous injection, may be prepared for rapid injection or as a 24-hour continuous infusion.
➤ Depending on the concentration of the final dose, it may be necessary to add human albumin to the dextrose injection; consult manufacturer's literature.
➤ Monitor the complete blood count (CBC) and white blood cell (WBC) differential, platelet count, BUN and serum creatinine, and liver function tests.

sargramostim
Drug Administration/Nursing in the Community
➤ Review side effects. Monitor vital signs. Assess for fluid retention and monitor weight. Auscultate lung sounds. Assess for pain in joints, muscles, and bones. Monitor weight and assess hydration.
➤ Rarely, a first-dose reaction characterized by flushing, hypotension, and fainting may occur.
➤ If the patient is to self-administer at home, teach injection technique and proper handling of syringes and needles.
➤ Instruct the patient receiving granulocyte-macrophage colony-stimulating factor that fever, chills, headache, nausea and vomiting, weakness, and fatigue may occur. If persistent or severe, instruct the patient to notify the physician.
➤ For IV administration review the insert supplied by the manufacturer. Administer as a 2-hour infusion via a central venous line. Do not use an in-line filter.
➤ Monitor the CBC and WBC differential, platelet count, BUN and serum creatinine, and liver function tests.

CELL-STIMULATING AGENTS

aldesleukin
Drug Administration/Nursing in the Community
➤ Monitor vital signs. See the Patient Problems boxes in Chapter 54 on bleeding tendencies and leukopenia. Instruct the patient that side effects are common. The patient should stay in close contact with the physician and report the development of any new sign or symptom.
➤ Monitor weight and assess for edema. Auscultate lung sounds and assess for shortness of breath. Assess for skin changes.
➤ Consult the manufacturer's literature for current guidelines about drug administration.

➤ Monitor CBC, WBC differential, platelet count, thyroid function tests, liver function tests, BUN and serum creatinine, and pulmonary function tests including arterial blood gases.

IFN-gamma
Drug Administration/Nursing in the Community
➤ See the Patient Problems boxes in Chapter 54 on bleeding tendencies and leukopenia.
➤ Assess vital signs. Monitor weight.
➤ Fever and flulike symptoms may occur. Some physicians prescribe acetaminophen before doses.
➤ For self-administration, teach the patient injection technique and proper handling of syringes and needles. Use the deltoid muscle or anterior thigh for injections; see patient instruction leaflet.
➤ Monitor the WBC differential and platelet count, liver function tests, and lactate dehydrogenase.

levamisole
Drug Administration/Nursing in the Community
➤ See the Patient Problems boxes in Chapter 54 on leukopenia, bleeding tendencies, and stomatitis.
➤ Assess vital signs. Assess for CNS effects, including ataxia, tremors, blurred vision, confusion, and numbness or tingling in face, hands, or feet. Assess for tardive dyskinesia: lip smacking, wormlike movements of the tongue, or uncontrolled movements of the arms and legs.
➤ Caution the patient to avoid driving or operating hazardous equipment if blurred vision occurs.
➤ Monitor CBC, WBC differential, platelet count, serum electrolytes, carcinoembryonic antigen, and liver function tests.

pegademase
Drug Administration/Nursing in the Community
➤ Consult manufacturer's leaflet for current information, or contact pharmacist.
➤ Monitor trough plasma adenosine deaminase activity and red blood cell (RBC) deoxyadenosine triphosphate concentrations.
➤ Review with the patient the importance of continuing this medication for life.

IMMUNOSUPPRESSANT DRUGS

basiliximab
Drug Administration/Nursing in the Community
➤ Monitor blood pressure and vital signs. Monitor weight.
➤ Assess for abdominal pain, excessive fatigue or loss of energy, back pain, white patches in the mouth or throat, cough, dyspnea, edema, tremor, signs of infection, changes in vision, itching, blood in stool, stomatitis, and urinary retention.
➤ Advise women of childbearing age to use contraceptive measures during treatment with basiliximab and for at least 2 months after the drug is stopped.

Nursing Implications Summary—cont'd

➤ See manufacturer's insert for current information about preparing dose and administration requirements.

➤ Encourage the patient to obtain regular dental care and to maintain good oral hygiene (brushing, flossing).

➤ Instruct the patient to avoid driving or operating hazardous equipment if changes in vision or dizziness develop; the patient should notify the physician.

➤ Instruct the patient to notify the physician of any unexpected sign or symptom that develops.

cyclosporine
Drug Administration

➤ See information on side effects.

➤ Monitor blood pressure and pulse. Monitor intake, output, and weight. Inspect teeth and gums regularly. Assess for skin changes and hair growth.

➤ Monitor CBC and WBC differential, liver function tests, BUN, serum creatinine levels, serum cyclosporine concentrations, serum uric acid levels, and serum electrolytes.

➤ Review the manufacturer's instructions when preparing oral doses because doses must be measured with a dropper, then diluted in a glass container with milk, chocolate milk, or orange juice. Review instructions with the patient.

➤ IV cyclosporine: Review the manufacturer's instructions regarding preparation. Infuse properly diluted doses over 2 to 6 hours. Monitor vital signs.

Nursing in the Community

➤ Review the anticipated benefits and possible side effects of drug therapy. Encourage the patient to have teeth cleaned and dental caries repaired before starting therapy. Emphasize the importance of thorough teeth brushing and flossing and regular professional teeth cleaning treatment and prevention of gingival hyperplasia.

➤ Warn the patient that tremor may develop.

➤ Warn the patient to avoid driving or operating hazardous equipment if confusion develops; the patient should notify the physician.

➤ See the Patient Problems box in Chapter 54 on leukopenia. Instruct the patient to avoid having any immunizations while taking cyclosporine. In addition, instruct others living in the patient's household to avoid oral polio vaccine while the patient is taking cyclosporine. If the patient must be near someone who has recently had the oral polio vaccine, have the patient wear a mask that covers the nose and mouth.

➤ Instruct the patient not to stop therapy without consulting the physician.

daclizumab
Drug Administration/Nursing in the Community

➤ Monitor blood pressure and vital signs. Monitor weight.

➤ Assess for chest pain, cough, dyspnea, edema, tremor, and signs of infection.

➤ Advise women of childbearing age to use contraceptive measures during treatment with daclizumab and for at least 2 months after the drug is stopped.

➤ See manufacturer's insert for current information about preparing dose and administration requirements.

➤ Encourage the patient to obtain regular dental care and to maintain good oral hygiene (brushing, flossing).

➤ Instruct the patient to notify the physician of any unexpected sign or symptom that develops.

muromonab-CD3
Drug Administration/Nursing in the Community

➤ Monitor blood pressure and pulse. Remain with the patient for 15 to 30 minutes after the first dose to monitor for anaphylaxis. Chest pain may follow the first dose but is rare thereafter. Monitor patient for up to 48 hours for cytokine release syndrome: chest pain, rapid or irregular heartbeat, shortness of breath, trembling, and weakness.

➤ Assess for side effects that commonly occur such as fever, chills, dyspnea, wheezing, nausea, vomiting, tremor, headache, and tachycardia.

➤ Forewarn the patient that trembling and shaking of the hands after the first dose is common.

➤ Monitor intake, output, and weight. Auscultate breath sounds.

➤ See the manufacturer's literature for current guidelines about dose preparation. Administer the prepared dose as a bolus over 1 minute.

➤ See the Patient Problems box in Chapter 54 on leukopenia. Instruct the patient to avoid having any immunizations while taking muromonab-CD3. In addition, instruct others living in the patient's household to avoid oral polio vaccine while the patient is taking muromonab-CD3. If the patient must be near someone who has recently had the oral polio vaccine, have the patient wear a mask that covers the nose and mouth.

➤ Monitor the CBC, WBC differential, platelet count, liver function tests, BUN and serum creatinine, and muromonab-CD3 concentrations.

mycophenolate
Drug Administration/Nursing in the Community

➤ See the Patient Problems boxes in Chapter 54 on leukopenia and bleeding tendencies (thrombocytopenia).

➤ Assess for peripheral edema, oral moniliasis (white patches in mouth, throat), and tremor. Monitor weight.

➤ Advise the patient to take doses on an empty stomach and to swallow capsules whole, without chewing, crushing, or opening. Instruct the patient to take doses with a full glass (8 ounces) of water. Tell the patient not to take doses at the same time as taking antacids.

➤ Monitor the CBC and WBC differential.

➤ Emphasize the importance of returning to the physician for regular follow-up. Instruct the patient to notify the physician

Continued

Nursing Implications Summary—cont'd

of severe or persistent constipation or diarrhea, headache, nausea and vomiting, skin rash, or weakness.

➤ Caution the patient to avoid driving or operating hazardous equipment if dizziness develops.

➤ Advise women of childbearing age to use contraceptive measures during treatment with mycophenolate and for at least 2 months after the drug is stopped.

tacrolimus
Drug Administration/Nursing in the Community

➤ Review anticipated benefits of drug. Emphasize importance of taking the drug as ordered and not discontinuing the drug without consulting the physician.

➤ See the Patient Problems box in Chapter 54 on leukopenia. Instruct the patient to avoid having any immunizations while taking tacrolimus. In addition, instruct others living in

the patient's household to avoid oral polio vaccine while the patient is taking tacrolimus. If the patient must be near someone who has recently had the oral polio vaccine, have the patient wear a mask that covers the nose and mouth.

➤ Instruct the patient to avoid raw oysters or shellfish while taking tacrolimus.

➤ Instruct the patient to avoid grapefruit and grapefruit juice while taking tacrolimus.

➤ Monitor the CBC, WBC differential, platelet count, serum electrolytes, liver function tests, BUN, and serum creatinine.

➤ IV tacrolimus: See the manufacturer's insert for latest information. Remain with the patient for 30 minutes after the first dose to monitor for allergic reaction. Have epinephrine, oxygen, and personnel available to treat acute allergic reactions when this drug is administered.

CHAPTER REVIEW

Application

1. What is the function of colony-stimulating factors? How may they be used clinically?

2. What is the most common adverse reaction patients experience with filgrastim?

3. Why is filgrastim avoided in patients with leukemic myeloid blasts?

4. Why does sargramostim increase more types of cells than filgrastim?

5. If a patient with AIDS is to receive sargramostim, what should you confirm before administering the drug?

6. How do the actions of aldesleukin and IFN-gamma differ from those of the colony-stimulating factors?

7. What is the most common reaction with IFN-gamma?

8. What is the clinical use of levamisole?

9. Why is cyclosporine effective at preventing organ rejection?

10. What organ systems may be affected by cyclosporine?

11. What might tremors signify in a patient receiving cyclosporine? What should you do?

12. Why should a patient taking cyclosporine not receive a live virus vaccine? What vaccines might be included?

13. Why are estrogens and other drugs that are metabolized by the liver usually avoided in patients receiving cyclosporine?

14. What is the mechanism of action of muromonab-CD3?

15. Why are allergies to mice associated with greater risk of allergy to muromonab-CD3?

16. What symptoms associated with cytokine release are caused by muromonab-CD3?

17. Why does mycophenolate interfere with lymphocyte proliferation?

18. What is the mechanism of action of tacrolimus?

Critical Thinking

1. How would you evaluate for capillary leak syndrome in a patient receiving sargramostim?

2. Aldesleukin can be expected to cause skin rashes. What sign would lead you to consider that a patient was experiencing a more serious skin reaction? What should you do?

3. A patient receiving levamisole develops a flulike syndrome. What other potentially more serious reaction would this prompt you to look for in this patient? How would you do this evaluation?

4. A patient receiving tacrolimus is given itraconazole to treat a fungal infection. You are monitoring blood concentrations of tacrolimus. What do you expect to see happen to the blood concentration of tacrolimus when this azole antifungal agent is added? Explain your answer.

References

Baquiran DC, Dantis L, McKerrow J: Monoclonal antibodies: innovations in diagnoses and therapy, *Semin Oncol Nurs* 12(2):130-141, 1996.

Macey WH: Interferon: an overview for dermatology nurses. *Dermatol Nurs* 8(3):155-159, 1966.

Shultz SL, Meriney DK: Cyclosporine and tacrolimus: a comparison of immunosuppressants used for liver transplantation, *DCCN* 15(4):187-197, 1996.

Chapter

41

Glucocorticoids to Treat Inflammatory Conditions

KEY TERMS

cushingoid appearance,
 p. 471
glucocorticoid activity, p. 467

KEY DRUG ▼

hydrocortisone, p. 472

OBJECTIVES

After studying this chapter, you should be able to do the following:

- *Describe the use of glucocorticoids for inflammatory and immune disorders.*
- *Compare and contrast the antiinflammatory and sodium-retaining activity of the systemic glucocorticoids.*
- *Describe the side effects associated with long-term glucocorticoid use.*
- *Develop a nursing care plan for patients receiving glucocorticoids.*

CHAPTER OVERVIEW

Glucocorticoids are used clinically for a wide variety of clinical inflammatory and immune conditions. The systemic and local uses of glucocorticoids are summarized. The serious toxic effects that limit usage are reviewed.

THERAPEUTIC RATIONALE: INFLAMMATORY AND IMMUNE DISORDERS

Inflammation is a nonspecific response of tissues to a stimulus or insult. In this chapter inflammatory conditions for which glucocorticoids are used clinically will be considered.

The inflammatory response includes the migration of various leukocytes to the area and their release of various humoral agents. These humoral agents include complement 5a, leukotrienes, interleukin-8, and transforming growth factor-beta. These agents not only have effects of their own but also serve to attract additional leukocytes to the inflammatory site, augmenting the inflammatory response.

Inflammation and an immune response are closely linked. The inflammatory response focuses on the release of hu-

moral agents to affect a given site. The immune response refers to the mobilization and interactions of the various immune cells, such as lymphocytes, macrophages, neutrophils, eosinophils, basophils, and mast cells.

Glucocorticoids inhibit the access of leukocytes to inflammatory sites, interfere with their function, and suppress the production and effects of humoral agents. At high physiologic concentrations, **glucocorticoid activity** suppresses the inflammatory response, whether the initiating event is an infection, physical or chemical injury, or an immune reaction. A number of conditions have an inflammatory or immune response that can be suppressed by glucocorticoids. However, glucocorticoids themselves are rarely curative and their prolonged systemic use leads to serious adverse effects.

467

THERAPEUTIC AGENTS: GLUCOCORTICOIDS FOR INFLAMMATORY SUPPRESSION

Glucocorticoids: General Characteristics

Mechanism of Action

Glucocorticoids enter a target cell and bind to a steroid receptor in the cell cytoplasm. The binding of the glucocorticoid activates the receptor, which allows the complex to enter the nucleus. In the nucleus the complex binds to selected DNA sites known as glucocorticoid response elements (GREs). This promotes or inhibits the transcription of specific mRNAs. In turn the synthesis of the respective proteins is promoted or inhibited.

There is also a mineralocorticoid receptor with a high affinity for aldosterone. However, cortisol and cortisone, the naturally occurring glucocorticoids, also have low affinity for the mineralocorticoid receptor. A weak or absent affinity for the mineralocorticoid receptor is a characteristic of the intermediate-acting and long-acting glucocorticoids as indicated in Table 41-1.

Glucocorticoids suppress lymphocyte functions, suppressing inflammation and immune reactions. Glucocorticoids are also an important regulator of metabolism in other tissues. In muscle, glucocorticoids decrease the use of glucose and mobilize amino acids from the breakdown of protein. In the liver, glucocorticoids promote the synthesis of glucose and its storage as glycogen. At low or baseline physiologic concentrations, glucocorticoids are important in regulating metabolism of skeletal and connective tissue. At high pharmacologic concentrations, glucocorticoids impair extracellular collagen and matrix formation. This leads to delayed wound healing and tissue maintenance. High pharmacologic concentrations of glucocorticoids also decrease bone formation and increase the urinary excretion of calcium and phosphorus, actions leading to bone loss.

Pharmacokinetics

Oral preparations are commonly used for systemic glucocorticoid therapy because they are well absorbed from the gastrointestinal (GI) tract. Peak plasma concentrations are reached in 1 to 2 hours. Glucocorticoids are lipophilic and readily cross plasma membranes. Cortisone and prednisone are converted to the active forms, hydrocortisone and prednisolone, by the liver. Hydrocortisone and prednisolone bind to a plasma protein, corticosteroid-binding globulin (CBG), and albumin, which keeps them from being readily cleared from the plasma.

A major factor in the overall potency of the various glucocorticoids is their relative rate of metabolism by the liver. The intermediate- and long-acting glucocorticoids have structural changes that not only decrease their mineralocorticoid activity but also slow their rate of metabolism. Severe liver disease has multiple effects on bioavailability of glucocorticoids. Hydrocortisone and prednisolone are preferred because they do not require hepatic metabolism to an active form. The hypoalbuminemia of severe liver disease increases the free concentration of hydrocortisone and prednisolone. The metabolism of all glucocorticoids may be impaired. In general severe liver disease increases the biologic and toxic effects of glucocorticoids.

Glucocorticoids are also metabolized by the placenta in pregnant women, limiting exposure of the fetus. However, very high dosages of glucocorticoids can suppress fetal adrenal function.

Because the action of glucocorticoids depends on the promotion or inhibition of new protein synthesis, the onset of action is in hours to days and the duration of action is in days to weeks. The eight glucocorticoids used systemically vary in their duration of action depending both on the chemical characteristics of the glucocorticoid and also on the formulation and route of administration. These points are summarized in Table 41-2.

Table 41-1 Comparison of Systemic Glucocorticoids

Drug	Activity Relative to Hydrocortisone		Equivalent Dose (mg)
	Antiinflammatory	Sodium-Retaining	
Short-Acting			
hydrocortisone	1.0	1.0	20.0
cortisone	0.8	0.9	25.0
Intermediate-Acting			
methylprednisolone	5.0	0	4.0
prednisolone	4.0	0.8	5.0
prednisone	3.5	0.8	5.0
triamcinolone	5.0	0	4.0
Long-Acting			
betamethasone	25.0	0	0.6
dexamethasone	30.0	0	0.75
paramethasone	10.0	0	2.0

Oral glucocorticoid therapy usually begins with one or more daily doses to control symptoms. When symptoms are under control, treatment can often be continued with alternate-day administration of prednisone, prednisolone, or methylprednisolone. The advantage of alternate-day therapy is that the suppression of the hypophysial-pituitary-adrenal axis is less. Growth rate in children is maintained and bone loss in all individuals is less.

A number of glucocorticoids have been developed specifically for local administration. Glucocorticoids formulated for local administration are listed in Table 41-3. Local uses of glucocorticoids include bronchial inhalation for asthma; dental pastes; various creams, ointments, and other preparations for use on the skin; nasal sprays; drops for the eyes and ears; and ointments and suppositories for rectal administration.

Uses

Glucocorticoids are used to treat a number of diseases and conditions, many of which are detailed below. For systemic use in treating inflammatory conditions, the intermediate-acting glucocorticoids (methylprednisolone, prednisone, prednisolone, and triamcinolone) are generally used because they have low mineralocorticoid activity and can be administered in a way to lessen adverse reactions. Prednisone is the most commonly used glucocorticoid of this group because of its long history of reliable use and low cost.

Allergic States. Glucocorticoids may be used as adjunct therapy in treating acute, severe episodes of asthma, angioedema, transfusion reactions, and serum sickness. Inhaled glucocorticoids have become a preferred prophylactic treatment of

---

Table 41-2 Glucocorticoids Used Systemically

Generic Name	Trade Names (Representative)*	Route	Onset	Duration
bethamethasone	Betnesol,* Celestone	PO	1 hr	3 days
betamethasone sodium phosphate	Selestoject	IV, IM	Rapid	Short
betamethasone acetate/sodium phosphate	Celestone Soluspan	IM, IA, IL, IS, ST	1-3 hr	1-2 wk
cortisone acetate	Cortone acetate	PO	Rapid	1-1½ days
		IM	Slow	>2 days
dexamethasone	Decadron, Deronil*	PO	1 hr	3 days
dexamethasone acetate	Dalalone LA	IM	<8 hr	6 days
		IA, ST, IL	Slow	1-3 wk
dexamethasone sodium phosphate	Decadrol, Hexadrol†	IV, IM	Rapid	Short
		IA, IS, IL, ST	Slow	3-21 days
hydrocortisone	Cortef	PO	<1 hr	1½ days
	Cortenema	PR	3-5 days	
hydrocortisone acetate	Hydrocortone acetate	IA, IS, IB, IL, ST	<24 hr	3-28 days
	Cortef	PO	1 hr	
hydrocortisone cypionate	Cortef	IM	<4 hr	Days
hydrocortisone sodium phosphate	Hydrocortone phosphate	IV, IM	Rapid	Short
hydrocortisone sodium succinate	Solu-Cortef	IV, IM	Rapid	Variable
methylprednisolone	Medrol	PO	<1 hr	1½ days
methylprednisolone acetate	Depo-Medrol	IM	6-48 hr	1-4 wk
methylprednisolone sodium succinate	Solu-Medrol	IV, IM	Rapid	Intermediate
prednisolone	Prelone	PO	<1 hr	1½ days
prednisolone acetate	Key-Pred, Predaject, Predcor, Predicort	IM	Slow	1-3 days
prednisolone acetate/sodium phosphate	Generic	IM, IB, IS, IA, ST	Slow	3-28 days
prednisolone sodium phosphate	Hydeltrasol, Key-Pred SP, Predicort-RP	IV, IM	<1 hr	Short
prednisolone tebutate	Hydeltra T.B.A., Nor-Pred T.B.A., Predcor T.B.A.	IA, IL, ST	1-2 days	1-3 wk
prednisone	Apo-Prednisone,* Deltasone,† Meticorten, Orasone, others	PO	<2 hr	1½ days
triamcinolone	Aristocort	PO	<2 hr	2 days
triamcinolone acetonide	Kenalog	IM	1-2 days	1-6 wk
		IB, IA, IS, IL, ST	Slow	Weeks
triamcinolone diacetate	Kenacort	PO	<2 hr	Intermediate
	Aristocort forte	IM	Slow	4-28 days
		IL	Slow	1-2 wk
		IA, IS, ST	Slow	1-8 wk
triamcinolone hexacetonide	Aristospan	IA, IL	Slow	3-4 wk

IA, Intraarticular; *IB,* intrabursal; *IL,* intralesional; *IM,* intramuscular; *IS,* intrasynovial; *IV,* intravenous; *PO,* oral; *PR,* rectal; *ST,* soft tissue.
*Available in Canada and the United States.
†Available in Canada only.

Table 41-3 **Glucocorticoid Preparations for Nonsystemic Use**

Preparations	Trade Names
Inhalation: Inflammation, Asthma	
beclomethasone dipropionate, metered spray	Beclodisk,† Beclovent,* Vanceril*
budesonide†	Pulmicort,† Nubuamp, Turbohaler
flunisolide, metered spray	AeroBid, Bronalide†
fluticasone propionate, metered spray	Flovent
triamcinolone acetonide, metered spray	Azmacort*
Nasal: Polyps, Rhinitis	
beclomethasone dipropionate, metered spray	Beconase,* Vacenase†
budesonide,† metered spray	Rhinocort,† Turbohaler, Aqua
flunisolide, metered spray	Nasalide, Rhinalar†
fluticasone propionate, nasal spray	Flonase
mometasone	Nasonex
triamcinolone acetonide, metered spray	Nasacort*
Ophthalmic: Allergic, Inflammation	
betamethasone sodium phosphate† solution	Betnesol†
dexamethasone solution, ointment	Maxidex*
dexamethasone sodium phosphate solution, ointment	AK-Dex, Baldex, Decadron,* others
fluorometholone suspension, ointment	FML,* Fluor-Op
fluorometholone acetate suspension	Eflone, Flarex*
hydrocortisone acetate ointment†	Cortamed†
loteprednol etabonate suspension	Altrex, Lotemax
medrysone suspension	HMS Liquifilm*
olopatadine hydrochloride suspension	Patanol
prednisolone acetate suspension	Pred Mild,* Pred Forte,* others
prednisolone sodium phosphate solution	AK-Pred, Inflamase,† I-Pred, Ocu-Pred, Pedair†
rimexolone	Vexol
Otic: Inflammation of External Auditory Meatus	
betamethasone sodium phosphate†	Betnesol*
dexamethasone	AK-Dex,* Decadron*
hydrocortisone acetate ointment†	Cortamed†
Topical: Skin Disorders, Rectal Disorders, Oral Lesions	
alclometasone dipropionate cream, ointment	Aclovate
amcinonide cream, lotion, ointment	Cyclocort*
beclomethasone dipropionate† cream, lotion, ointment	Propraderm†
betamethasone benzoate cream, gel, lotion	Uticort
betamethasone dipropionate cream, gel, lotion, ointment	Alphatrex, Diprolene,* Diprosone,* Maxivate, Teladar, Topilene,† Topisone†
betamethasone valerate cream, lotion, ointment	Betacort,† Betaderm,† Betatrex, Beta-Val, Valisone
clobetasol propionate cream, solution, ointment	Dermovate,† Temovate
clobetasone butyrate† cream, ointment	Eumovate†
clocortolone pivalate cream	Cloderm
desonide cream, lotion, ointment	DesOwen, Tridesilon*
desoximetasone cream, gel, ointment	Topicort*
dexamethasone gel, aerosol	Aaeroseb-Dex, Decaderm, Decaspray
dexamethasone sodium phosphate cream	Decadron
diflorasone diacetate cream, ointment	Florone,* Maxiflor, Psorcon
diflucortolone valerate† cream, ointment	Nerisone†
flumethasone pivalate cream, ointment†	Locacorten†
fluocinolone acetonide cream, ointment, topical solution	Bio-Syn, Fluocet, Fluoderm,† Flurosyn, Synalar,* Synemol
fluocinonide cream, gel, ointment, topical solution	Fluocin, Licon, Lidex,* Lidemol,† Lyderm†
flurandrenolide cream, lotion, ointment, tape	Cordran, Drenison†
fluticasone propionate cream, ointment	Cutivate
halcinonide cream, ointment, topical solution	Halog*
halobetasol propionate cream, ointment	Ultravate
hydrocortisone acetate dental paste	Orabase-HCA
hydrocortisone rectal cream, rectal ointment, suppositories	Proctocort, Rectocort†

*Available in Canada and the United States.
†Available in Canada only.

Table 41-3 **Glucocorticoid Preparations for Nonsystemic Use—cont'd**	
Preparations	Trade Names
Topical: Skin Disorders, Rectal Disorders, Oral Lesions—cont'd	
hydrocortisone acetate rectal cream, suppositories	Anucort-HC, Anusol-HC, Corticaine, Cortiment,† Hemril
hydrocortisone cream, lotion, ointment, topical solution for skin	Allercort, Bactine, Cort-Dome, Cortrate,† many others
hydrocortisone acetate cream, topical aerosol, lotion, ointment for skin	Cortacet,† Corticaine, Lanacort, many others
hydrocortisone butyrate cream, ointment for skin	Locoid
hydrocortisone valerate cream, ointment for skin	Westcort
mometasone furoate cream, lotion	Elocon*
triamcinolone acetonide dental paste	Kenalog in Orabase, Oracort, Oralone
triamcinolone acetonide cream, lotion, ointment topical aerosol for skin	Aristocort,* Kenalog, others

chronic asthma to suppress inflammation of the bronchioles. Dermatologic reactions such as severe reactions to poison ivy can be blunted with oral glucocorticoids.

Dermatologic Disorders. Various types of dermatitis and pemphigus are treated with glucocorticoids. Topical glucocorticoids are used for keloids, lichen planus, lichen simplex chronicus, discoid lupus, and severe psoriasis.

Gastrointestinal Disorders. Inflammatory bowel diseases, including ulcerative colitis, regional enteritis (Crohn's disease), and ulcerative proctitis, are treated with glucocorticoids.

Hematologic Disorders. Large doses of glucocorticoids suppress the immune processes, destroying blood cells in acute phases of autoimmune hemolytic anemia and thrombocytopenia. Lower dosages maintain remission.

Joint Inflammation. Injection of glucocorticoids into inflamed joints gives symptomatic relief in bursitis.

Neoplastic Diseases. Glucocorticoids are administered with antineoplastic agents to produce remissions for leukemias and lymphomas. The antilymphocytic action of glucocorticoids aids in destroying lymphoid cancers.

Ophthalmic Diseases. Steroids may be applied directly to the eye to treat allergic conjunctivitis, chorioretinitis, iritis, iridocyclitis, and keratitis. The antiinflammatory action reduces permanent eye damage and controls acute symptoms.

Rheumatic Diseases. Acute inflammatory episodes of various types of arthritis (ankylosing spondylitis, psoriatic arthritis, rheumatoid arthritis) respond to glucocorticoids. Modest dosages are sometimes used to maintain inhibition of the inflammatory and autoimmune processes. Glucocorticoids are used to control flares of systemic lupus erythematosus.

Adverse Reactions and Contraindications

The adverse actions of glucocorticoids limit their long-term use. High dosages of glucocorticoids administered for a few days have relatively few undesirable side effects. However, prolonged therapy with even low dosages of glucocorticoids suppresses the hypothalamic-pituitary-adrenal axis regulating the natural production of cortisol (see Chapter 66). This means that glucocorticoids cannot be abruptly discontinued. Rather, the dosage must be gradually tapered to allow the adrenal gland to resume functioning, thereby avoiding an adrenal crisis.

Higher than physiologic dosages of glucocorticoids leads to altered metabolism of a number of tissues and organs. These changes include muscle wasting from the negative nitrogen balance induced by glucocorticoids and increased fat tissue, especially in the central portion of the body and around the face. The result is a **cushingoid appearance:** moon face, thin limbs, and fat on the trunk of the body. Other effects of glucocorticoids include changes in behavior and personality, usually marked by euphoria, but occasionally psychotic episodes are seen. Growth is suppressed in children. Long-term use of glucocorticoids leads to osteoporosis. Osteonecrosis is also more common. The metabolic effects of glucocorticoids can lead to impaired glucose tolerance and frank diabetes mellitus.

Glucocorticoids are classified in the Food and Drug Administration (FDA) pregnancy category C. Glucocorticoids are found in breast milk; however, as long as the mother is taking small doses of glucocorticoids, the small amount in the breast milk poses no risk for her infant.

Toxicity

Toxic reactions to long-term glucocorticoid therapy are listed in Box 41-1. The frequency of side effects is related to the duration of therapy. Common effects appearing after a relatively short duration of days to weeks include weight gain, mood changes, glucose intolerance, and transient adrenal suppression. Occasionally, hypertriglyceridemia, peptic ulcers, or acute pancreatitis occur. After months of glucocorticoid therapy, weight is redistributed, producing central obesity; the skin becomes fragile; muscle atrophies; the adrenal gland is suppressed; and bone loss occurs. Occasionally, long-term therapy produces cataracts, glaucoma, hypertension, or avascular necrosis. Opportunistic infections are more common.

Box 41-1 Undesirable Glucocorticoid Effects

Common	Sporadic
Early Effects (Days to Weeks)	
Weight gain: from changes in lipid metabolism	*Anaphylactoid reactions:* hypersensitivity reaction
Mood changes: euphoria most common, also increased appetite, insomnia; uncommonly, psychoses	*Hypertriglyceridemia:* from changes in lipid metabolism
Glucose intolerance: from gluconeogenic effects; resulting diabetes is usually mild and reversible	*Peptic ulcers:* may be induced or masked by glucocorticoids
Transient adrenal suppression: physiologic feedback on hypothalamic-pituitary-adrenal axis	*Acute pancreatitis:* may result from changes in lipid metabolism
Potassium/sodium changes: glucocorticoids with mineralocorticoid activity may cause decreased serum potassium and increased sodium concentrations.	
Later Effects (Months to Years)	
Central obesity: classic cushingoid appearance from altered lipid metabolism	*Aseptic necrosis of bone:* most commonly affects femoral head
Skin fragility: from inhibitory effects on synthesis of collagen and extracellular matrix; also, changes in hair	*Cataracts:* cause unknown; seen with systemic or local therapy
Myopathy: from protein breakdown; more pronounced with fluoride derivatives such as triamcinolone	*Glaucoma:* from interference with normal aqueous outflow; greater risk in diabetic patients
Osteoporosis: from increased bone resorption; patients with arthritis and postmenopausal women at greatest risk.	*Hypertension:* more of a problem with cortisone and hydrocortisone, which have significant mineralocorticoid activity
Growth failure: from inhibition of growth hormone action; limits use in children	*Opportunistic infections:* from suppression of immune functions

---

Interactions

A number of clinically important adverse drug interactions occur with glucocorticoids. Drugs that slow the metabolism or clearance of glucocorticoids include antibiotics, cyclosporine, estrogen, isoniazid, and ketoconazole. The dosage of glucocorticoids should be decreased.

Drugs that increase the metabolism or clearance of glucocorticoids include aminoglutethimide, carbamazepine, cholestyramine, phenobarbital, phenytoin, and rifampin. The dosage of glucocorticoids should be increased.

Glucocorticoids affect the metabolism or clearance of some other drugs, requiring adjustment of their dosages. These drugs include antianxiety agents, antipsychotics, anticholinesterases, anticoagulants, antihypertensive agents, cyclosporine, hypoglycemic drugs, liver or killed virus vaccine, pancuronium, salicylates, and sympathomimetic agents.

Glucocorticoids: Specific Drugs

betamethasone

Betamethasone (Betnelan, Celestone) is a long-acting glucocorticoid with no mineralocorticoid effect. It is available in preparations for oral and rectal administration. In addition, injectable preparations are available. Long-term use in children inhibits growth.

cortisone

Cortisone (Cortone) is a short-acting glucocorticoid that is converted by the liver to its more active form, hydrocortisone (cortisol). Cortisone has significant mineralocorticoid activity. It is available in preparations for oral administration and for intramuscular injection.

dexamethasone

Dexamethasone (Decadron, Deronil, Dexasone, Dexone, others) is a long-acting glucocorticoid with no mineralocorticoid effect. It is used as a diagnostic aid for Cushing's syndrome and for endogenous depression. Dexamethasone can also be effective as an antiemetic for cancer chemotherapy. Long-term use in children inhibits growth.

▼ hydrocortisone

Hydrocortisone (cortisol) (Cortef, Hydrocortone, Solu-Cortef) is the naturally occurring glucocorticoid. It is short acting and has significant mineralocorticoid activity. Hydrocortisone is available in preparations for oral and rectal administration, as well as in various injectable formulations.

methylprednisolone

Methylprednisolone (Depo-Medrol, Medrol) has more potent antiinflammatory activity than prednisolone with almost no mineralocorticoid activity. It is available in oral and injectable formulations. Methylprednisolone is used in treating multiple sclerosis.

prednisolone

Prednisolone (Delta-Cortef, Predcor, Prelone, others) has equivalent potency to prednisone with both antiinflammatory and some mineralocorticoid activity. It is available in a variety of salt forms that provide different onset of action and allow various routes of administration.

prednisone

Prednisone (Apo-Prednisone, Deltasone, Meticorten, Orasone, others) is metabolized to prednisolone and has the same antiinflammatory and mineralocorticoid activity. Prednisone is inexpensive and is widely used for replacement therapy and to treat flares of various rheumatic disorders. Prednisone is available only for oral administration.

triamcinolone

Triamcinolone (Aristocort) is similar to methylprednisolone in being an intermediate-acting glucocorticoid with essentially no mineralocorticoid activity. Salt forms are available for long-acting injections.

Nursing Process Overview

Glucocorticoids

Assessment

Perform a complete patient assessment. Monitor temperature, pulse, respirations, blood pressure, and weight, and check blood and urine glucose. Assess skin carefully, notice color and characteristics of skin, distribution of body mass, the presence of bruises or petechiae, and the condition of hair and nails. Assess signs and symptoms of other health problems.

Nursing Diagnoses

- Body image disturbance related to weight gain and change in weight distribution related to chronic glucocorticoid administration
- Potential complication: electrolyte abnormalities
- Potential complication: fragile bones resulting in increased susceptibility to fractures

Patient Outcomes

The patient will share feelings related to body image. The nurse will minimize and manage complications associated with electrolyte abnormalities. The patient will not experience fractures related to the effects of glucocorticoids on the bones.

Planning/Implementation

Glucocorticoids are one of the most commonly used groups of drugs. Monitor the blood pressure, weight, serum electrolytes, and blood glucose. Remember that wound healing will be slowed and infection may be masked. Improvement in appetite and sense of well-being may be a result of drug therapy. Drug-induced diabetes mellitus may require treatment with insulin. In planning for discharge, determine with the physician the discharge dose and schedule of drugs, and begin teaching the patient.

Evaluation

Before discharge, ascertain that the patient can explain why the drug has been prescribed, the desired goals of therapy, how to take the drug correctly, and side effects that may occur. Verify that the patient can explain additional therapies needed such as antacid therapy, dietary restrictions, and exercise or physical therapy. Ensure that the patient can explain when to notify the physician; for example, if the patient is too sick to take ordered doses. Patients must know not to discontinue or decrease the dosage of long-term glucocorticoids without physician approval. Verify that the patient can explain if any parameters should be monitored at home, such as weight, blood pressure, or blood glucose.

Nursing Implications Summary

Glucocorticoids

Drug Administration

- ➤ See Box 41-1 for a list of side effects associated with long-term glucocorticoid therapy.
- ➤ Assess vital signs and blood pressure, lung sounds, weight, history of any weight gain or loss, and dependent areas for edema. Assess for nausea and vomiting and perform a mental status examination. Assess skin for striae (reddish-purple lines), thin skin, unusual or excessive bruising, change in skin color, change in amount of hair growth, and acne.
- ➤ Monitor height and growth pattern in children receiving long-term therapy.
- ➤ With long-term therapy, suggest ophthalmologic examinations at periodic intervals to monitor for cataracts, increased intraocular pressure, and glaucoma.
- ➤ Assess for signs of depression including lack of interest in personal appearance, withdrawal, insomnia, and anorexia.
- ➤ Check stools for presence of occult blood.
- ➤ Monitor complete blood count (CBC) and differential and serum electrolytes and blood glucose. After long-term therapy monitor hypothalamic-pituitary-adrenal axis function to determine whether there will be normal adrenal function.

- ➤ Use care in moving and positioning immobilized patients receiving long-term therapy to prevent fractures and bruising. Pad siderails as appropriate. Avoid using adhesive tape on fragile skin.
- ➤ Glucocorticoids are given via many routes (see Tables 41-2 and 41-3). Read labels carefully. Ascertain that the preparation can be given via the ordered route.

Intravenous betamethasone sodium phosphate
- ➤ May be given undiluted or diluted. Administer undiluted dose over at least 1 minute.

Intravenous dexamethasone sodium phosphate
- ➤ May be given undiluted. Administer dose over 1 minute.

Intravenous hydrocortisone sodium phosphate
- ➤ May be given undiluted. Always use a separate syringe. Administer 25 mg or less over 1 minute.

Intravenous hydrocortisone sodium succinate
- ➤ Reconstitute as directed on label of vial. Administer direct IV at a rate of 500 mg or less over 1 minute.

Intravenous methylprednisolone sodium succinate
- ➤ Reconstitute as directed on label of vial. Administer direct IV at a rate of 500 mg or less over 2 to 3 minutes or longer.

Intravenous prednisolone sodium phosphate
- ➤ May be given undiluted at a rate of 10 mg or less over 1 minute. Always use a separate syringe for Hydeltrasol brand.

Continued

Nursing Implications Summary—cont'd

Nursing in the Community

➤ Review anticipated benefits and possible side effects of drug therapy. With short-term use (over 7 to 10 days), side effects may be minimal, if noticeable. With long-term use, some side effects will usually develop. Instruct the patient to report any new side effects.

➤ Instruct the patient to take oral doses with meals or a snack to lessen gastric irritation. Some physicians prescribe antacids or other drugs prophylactically to lessen the risk of ulceration. Instruct the patient to avoid alcoholic beverages while taking this medication because the combination may contribute to increased stomach irritation.

➤ For missed doses, when the dosage regimen is once every other day, the patient should take the missed dose as soon as remembered if remembered on the day it was to be taken. If not remembered until the next day, the patient should take the dose, then readjust the dosage schedule to be every other day from the day the most recent dose was taken. Instruct the patient to not double up for missed doses.

➤ For missed doses, when dose is taken once a day, the patient should take the missed dose as soon as remembered unless not remembered until the next day. In that case the patient should omit the missed dose and resume the regular dosing schedule. Instruct the patient not to double up for missed doses.

➤ For missed doses, when doses are taken more than once a day, the patient should take the missed dose as soon as remembered. If not remembered until the next dose is due, the patient should take both doses at that time and resume regular dosing schedule.

➤ See the Patient Problems box in Chapter 24 on constipation.

➤ If weight gain is excessive, counsel the patient about weight reduction diets; consult the physician about a change in glucocorticoid or dose. Other dietary modifications may include decreasing sodium intake and increasing potassium intake. See the Dietary Considerations boxes on potassium sources (Chapter 14) and sodium and hypertension (Chapter 13). Encourage the patient to increase protein intake.

➤ Warn diabetic patients to monitor blood glucose levels carefully because glucocorticoids increase blood glucose levels. A change in diet or insulin may be necessary.

➤ Instruct the patient to notify the physician if any of the following develop: blood in stool; black, tarry stools; mood changes, depression, or insomnia; changes in vision, headache, or weight gain in excess of 2 pounds per day or 5 pounds per week; menstrual irregularities; irregular heartbeat; excessive fatigue; severe or persistent stomach or abdominal pain; or any serious injury or infection.

➤ Instruct the patient to avoid rough activities if skin becomes fragile and easily bruised.

➤ Warn patients receiving long-term therapy to take doses every day as ordered, even if they are sick. Failure to take ordered doses, even for a few days, may result in adrenocortical insufficiency in susceptible patients. Remind the patient

not to discontinue long-term steroid therapy without consulting the physician; tapering the dosage may be necessary.

➤ Remind the patient to inform all health care providers of all medications being used and to not take any medications unless approved by the physician.

➤ Warn the patient not to increase or decrease the dosage without consulting the physician.

➤ Update immunizations before the start of therapy if possible. Instruct the patient to avoid immunizations during therapy and for at least 3 months after therapy and to check with the physician for questions. Instruct the patient to avoid contact with anyone who has received oral polio vaccine recently or to wear a mask covering the nose and mouth if contact is unavoidable.

➤ Instruct the patient to avoid skin testing unless approved by the physician.

➤ Instruct the patient to avoid contact with anyone who has measles or chicken pox while taking glucocorticoids.

➤ Encourage the patient receiving long-term therapy to wear a medical identification tag or bracelet indicating that glucocorticoids are being used.

➤ Menstrual difficulties may develop with long-term therapy. Instruct women to keep a record of menstrual periods. Counsel about contraceptive methods as appropriate. Warn the patient to notify the physician if pregnancy is suspected.

➤ Large doses of glucocorticoids increase susceptibility to infection and mask the symptoms of infection. Warn the patient about this side effect. Instruct the patient to notify the physician of fever, cough, sore throat, malaise, and injuries that do not heal. Instruct the patient to avoid contact with individuals with active infections.

➤ Review the drug and route of administration prescribed for the patient. Review the manufacturer's instruction for administration. Ascertain that the patient can administer the ordered drug correctly (see Chapter 5).

➤ Remind the patient not to share medications with others. Remind the patient to keep all medications out of the reach of children.

➤ If this drug is injected into a joint, remind the patient to use the joint only as directed by physician. Too much use, too soon may stress the joint.

Nasal Solution

➤ Review the manufacturer's instruction sheet. The patient should blow the nose. With nosepiece in the nostril, the patient should aim the spray toward the inner corner of the eye, then spray and sniff. Encourage the patient to save the inhaler, which may be reusable.

Aerosol Metered Dose

➤ Review the manufacturer's instruction sheet. If an adrenergic bronchodilator such as albuterol, metaproterenol, or terbutaline is also prescribed via the inhalation route, instruct the patient to use the bronchodilator first, wait 5 minutes, then use the adrenocorticoid. The patient should not increase the number of sprays unless directed to do so by the

Nursing Implications Summary—cont'd

physician. Remind the patient to avoid spraying medication in the eyes.

➤ The aerosol metered dose form of glucocorticoids may cause hoarseness, throat irritation, and infection in the mouth. Gargling or rinsing the mouth after each drug use may help prevent these problems. Warn the patient not to swallow the water after gargling or rinsing. The physician may also want the patient to use a spacer, which is a tube that fits on the inhaler.

➤ Instruct the patient to rinse the mouth with water after each dose to help prevent dry mouth and clean the mouthpiece of the inhaler every day. See the manufacturer's instructions.

➤ If the canister is cold, instruct the patient to warm it between the hands before administering the dose.

➤ Encourage the patient not to discard the inhaler because it may be possible to use it with refill canisters; check with the pharmacist. Remind the patient to use the inhaler for this drug only with this drug, not with any others, even if other canisters fit the inhaler.

➤ Instruct the patient to use this drug only as prescribed and to not increase the frequency or dose of medication without consulting with the physician.

➤ Encourage the patient to limit or stop smoking if possible.

➤ Several weeks of therapy may be needed to see full benefit.

Eyedrops and Eye Ointment

➤ Emphasize the importance of using the eyedrops or ointment as directed, even if no symptoms are present.

➤ Using this drug while wearing contact lenses may increase the chance of infection. The physician may want the patient to avoid wearing contact lenses while taking this drug and for several days after completing the course of eyedrop therapy. Check with the physician.

➤ See Chapter 5 for information about administering eyedrops or ointment. Instruct the patient to wash hands after administration to keep medication from being absorbed through skin.

➤ For missed doses, instruct the patient to apply the missed dose as soon as remembered unless it is almost time for the next dose, then omit the missed dose and resume regular dosing schedule. The patient should not double up for missed doses.

➤ Administration of eyedrops or ointment may make vision blurry or cloudy for a few minutes; warn the patient not to drive or operate hazardous equipment until vision is clear.

➤ Instruct the patient to notify the physician if eye pain or irritation develops.

➤ Instruct the patient to use eyedrops or ointment as prescribed but not longer than the time ordered because side effects may begin to develop. Also, instruct the patient not to use steroid eyedrops for eye problems that may develop in the future unless directed to do so by the physician.

Otic (Ear) Solutions

➤ See Chapter 5 to review administration technique. Instruct the patient to put a cotton ball in as a plug if desired. The physician may want eardrops put onto the cotton plug be-

fore it is put into the ear. Try to avoid touching the ear with the dropper. The dropper may be wiped off but should not be rinsed with water.

➤ Instruct the patient to use the drops as prescribed but not to use leftover medication to treat ear problems that may develop in the future unless directed to do so by the physician.

➤ Instruct the patient to notify the physician if stinging, itching, or burning of the ear develops.

Otic (Ear) Ointment

➤ Review administration technique. Instruct the patient to use a finger or piece of gauze to apply a small amount of ointment just inside the ear canal. Instruct the patient not to use a cotton-tipped swab unless directed to do so by the physician. Instruct the patient to use the ointment as prescribed but not to use leftover medication to treat ear problems that may develop in the future unless directed to do so by the physician. Instruct the patient to notify the physician if stinging, itching, or burning of the ear develops.

Enema

➤ Review with the patient the manufacturer's instruction leaflet. Each bottle contains one dose; the entire contents of the bottle should be used unless otherwise directed by the physician. Inform the patient to use the enema after having a bowel movement. Instruct the patient to lie down on the left side when administering the enema and to insert tip of applicator slowly to prevent injury. After administering the medication, the patient should remain on the left side for 30 minutes to allow the medication to work. If possible, the patient should retain the enema all night.

Rectal Aerosol Form

➤ Review with the patient the manufacturer's instruction leaflet. Instruct the patient to insert the applicator tip only into the rectum and not to insert the aerosol container.

Topical Corticosteroids

➤ Assess the area being treated for irritation, lesions, redness, and swelling. After beginning use of topical medication, assess for improvement or signs of possible skin irritation caused by the medication.

➤ Instruct the patient and family to wear gloves to apply the dose or to wash fingers off with soap and water after application to avoid absorbing medication through the skin or accidentally getting medication in the eyes.

➤ Instruct the patient to use topical corticosteroids only as prescribed. Several kinds of skin problems should not be treated with topical corticosteroids. Instruct the patient to read the package labels carefully and check with the physician before treating skin problems.

➤ Instruct the patient not to wrap the skin being treated unless directed to do so by the physician. Also, if used in the diaper area, tight-fitting diapers or plastic pants should not be used unless directed to do so by the physician.

➤ There may be temporary stinging after gel, solution, lotion, or aerosol forms are applied.

Continued

Nursing Implications Summary–cont'd

➤ For aerosol topical forms, see the manufacturer's insert supplied with the medication. Instruct the patient to apply the medication carefully and to avoid getting medication in the eyes or breathing in fumes. Instruct the patient to rinse the eyes with copious amounts of water if medication gets in the eyes.

➤ For missed doses, instruct the patient to apply a missed dose as soon as remembered unless almost time for next dose; then omit the missed dose and resume the regular dosing schedule. The patient should not double up for missed doses.

➤ Children or teenagers should not use topical corticosteroids over large areas of skin or for longer than 2 weeks without checking with the physician.

➤ Instruct the patient to notify the physician if any of the following develop: worsening of skin condition, redness, itching, or blisters.

➤ Occasionally, systemic side effects may develop if gel, ointment, cream, lotion, solution, or tape is applied to large areas or at high dosages. These possible side effects include depression, weight gain, acne, oily skin, blurred vision, stretch marks on skin, increased hair growth, excessive fatigue, and increased blood pressure. Instruct the patient to keep all health care providers informed of all medications being used and to notify the physician if any unusual signs or symptoms develop.

➤ Flurandrenolide tape: Review the manufacturer's instructions supplied with the product.

Dental Paste

➤ Instruct the patient to use a cotton-tipped swab to apply a small amount of the paste to the prescribed area. Instruct the patient not to rub the paste but to press the paste in place until a smooth, slippery film forms. Recommend that the patient apply paste at bedtime so that it can work during the night. Instruct the patient to use the paste as prescribed but not to use leftover medication to treat oral problems that may develop in the future unless directed to do so by the physician. Instruct the patient to notify the physician if stinging, irritation, itching, or burning of the mouth develops.

CHAPTER REVIEW

Application

1. What is the difference between an inflammatory response and an immune response?
2. How do glucocorticoids suppress the inflammatory response?
3. How does liver disease influence the effects of the glucocorticoids?
4. What is the advantage of alternate-day therapy with systemic glucocorticoids?
5. What are some diseases or conditions that may be treated with glucocorticoids?
6. What are the early and late effects of long-term glucocorticoid administration?
7. What are the signs and symptoms of adrenal crisis?

Critical Thinking

1. Why should a patient receiving long-term glucocorticoid therapy consult the physician before discontinuing glucocorticoid therapy?
2. Study Table 41-1. Why is dexamethasone a better choice for treating increased intracranial pressure than cortisone?
3. The patient receiving long-term glucocorticoid therapy should not have allergy skin testing. Why?

Reference

Brenner ZR, Cannito M: Administering steroids, *Nursing* 28(3):34-44, 1998.

Chapter 42

Drug Treatment of Selected Autoimmune Diseases

OBJECTIVES

After studying this chapter, you should be able to do the following:

For myasthenia gravis:
■ *Describe the action of acetylcholinesterase inhibitors.*

■ *Develop a nursing care plan for patients receiving drug treatment for myasthenia gravis.*

For rheumatoid arthritis:
■ *Describe the use and limitations of the various disease-modifying antirheumatic drugs (DMARDs).*

■ *Develop a nursing care plan for patients receiving drug treatment for rheumatoid arthritis.*

For systemic lupus erythematosus:
■ *Describe the drugs used to control symptoms of systemic lupus erythematosus.*

■ *Develop a nursing care plan for patients receiving drug treatment for systemic lupus erythematosus.*

For multiple sclerosis:
■ *Describe the drugs used to control symptoms of multiple sclerosis.*

■ *Develop a nursing care plan for patients receiving drug treatment for multiple sclerosis.*

CHAPTER OVERVIEW

The immune system is normally able to distinguish the body's own components from invading bacteria, viruses, and other foreign organisms. However, **autoimmune diseases** represent the immune system turned against some component of the hosts body. Some of the factors explaining why this happens are beginning to emerge. One component involves the way antigens are handled, with human lymphocyte antigen (HLA) (or major histocompatibility complex [MHC]) molecules presenting antigens to T cells. The antigens picked for presentation may be the same as the body's own naturally occurring antigens (molecular mimicry). Such self-reactive T cells are normally eliminated by the thymus during development, but this elimination may be bypassed by viral or bacterial infection. Certain HLA genes appear to increase the likelihood of certain autoimmune diseases. For instance, HLA-DR4 is associated with an increased prevalence of rheumatoid arthritis, HLA-DR2 with multiple sclerosis, and HLA-DR3 and HLA-DR4 with type one diabetes mellitus.

Current research is revealing new knowledge about the complex origins of autoimmune diseases, but therapeutic options remain relatively limited. However, better characterization of these diseases with more aggressive intervention has lead to improved outcomes for people with these chronic conditions.

Figure 42-1 Myasthenia gravis is often first indicated by a drooping eyelid (paresis of levator palpebrae superioris muscle). Only one upper eyelid may be affected. Disease may stay limited to this muscle group. *(From Newell FW: Ophthalmology: principles and concepts, ed 7, St Louis, 1992, Mosby.)*

THERAPEUTIC RATIONALE: MYASTHENIA GRAVIS

Myasthenia gravis is a disease in which the skeletal muscles quickly show weakness and become fatigued. Muscles controlling facial movements are most commonly involved. One early sign of myasthenia gravis is a drooping eyelid (ptosis) (Figure 42-1). As the disease progresses, chewing and swallowing become increasingly difficult, and the voice becomes less distinct. Death can result if the intercostal muscles and the diaphragm, muscles essential for breathing, become affected.

Myasthenia gravis affects about 25,000 people in the United States. The incidence among women is greatest between 20 and 30 years of age; in men from ages 50 through 70 years of age.

Myasthenia gravis is the best understood of the autoimmune diseases. The basic defect in myasthenia gravis is a reduction by 70% to 90% in the available receptors for acetylcholine at the neuromuscular junction (Figure 42-2). This reduction is caused by autoantibodies against the neuromuscular receptors for acetylcholine. These autoantibodies block the active site for acetylcholine of the neuromuscular (nicotinic) receptor and also increase the rate at which the receptors are degraded by the cell.

Although at one time fatal or disabling, myasthenia gravis is now effectively treated in most patients. The first line of medical management is anticholinesterase drugs. Most patients achieve significant improvement with these drugs. Thymectomy, removal of the thymus, is a common procedure performed on patients with myasthenia gravis. About 75% of patients with myasthenia gravis have an abnormal thymus, commonly hyperplasia or thymomas. Also, muscle-like cells in the thymus are thought to be a major source of the autoantigen-stimulating antibody production. Removal of the thymus brings overall improvement for about 85% of patients with essentially no complications.

When anticholinesterase drugs are not adequate to treat myasthenia gravis, immunosuppressive therapy is indicated. Prednisone, azathioprine, and cyclosporine are the agents used for long-term immunosuppressive therapy. Plasmapheresis to remove antibodies from circulation is another therapy. It produces only short-term improvement and is used for patients in myasthenic crisis or those undergoing thymectomy.

A number of drugs have weak anticholinergic effects of their own and are contraindicated for the patient with myasthenia gravis. These drugs, listed in Box 42-1, can dangerously weaken the patient with myasthenia gravis but do not noticeably block the neuromuscular receptor of a healthy person.

> **Box 42-1   Drugs That May Weaken a Patient with Myasthenia Gravis**
>
> Adrenocorticotropic hormone and glucocorticoids
> Anesthetics
>   diethyl ether
>   halothane (Fluothane)
>   lidocaine IV (Xylocaine)
> Antiarrhythmics
>   procainamide (Pronestyl)
>   propranolol (Inderal)
>   quinidine
> Antibiotics
>   bacitracin (Bacitracin)
>   colistimethate (Coly-Mycin M)
>   colistin (Coly-Mycin S)
>   gentamicin (Garamycin)
>   kanamycin (Kantrex)
>   lincomycin (Lincocin)
>   neomycin (Mycifradin, Neobiotic)
>   netilmicin (Netromycin)
>   paromomycin (Humatin)
>   polymyxin B (Aerosporin, Polymyxin B)
>   streptomycin (Streptomycin)
>   viomycin (Viocin)
> Anticonvulsants
>   magnesium sulfate
> Antimalarials
>   quinine
> Diuretics and other drugs or circumstances promoting hypokalemia (low blood potassium concentration)
> Muscle relaxants
>   gallamine (Flaxedil)
>   metocurine (Metubine)
>   pancuronium (Pavulon)
>   succinylcholine (Anectine)
>   tubocurarine
> Sedatives, especially those with respiratory depressant effects, such as barbiturates, narcotics, and tranquilizers
> Thyroid compounds

THERAPEUTIC AGENTS: DRUGS TO TREAT MYASTHENIA GRAVIS

Acetylcholinesterase Inhibitors: General Characteristics

Mechanism of Action

Drugs that inhibit the degradation of acetylcholine, **acetylcholinesterase inhibitors** (anticholinesterases), are the first line of treatment for myasthenia gravis. These drugs are listed in Table 42-1. As seen in Figure 42-2, the enzyme acetylcholinesterase is present throughout the neuromuscular junction, where it rapidly degrades acetylcholine after release. Acetylcholinesterase inhibitors allow acetylcholine to accumulate at the neuromuscular junction, ensuring that available receptors are activated.

Pharmacokinetics

Anticholinesterase drugs are positively charged compounds that are not lipid soluble. These drugs are therefore not readily absorbed orally; the oral dose is 30 times the parenteral dose. The most widely used anticholinesterases are pyridostigmine and neostigmine. The anticholinesterases are metabolized by plasma esterases and by hepatic enzymes to inactive compounds. The drugs and their metabolites are excreted in the urine.

The effective dose must be individualized for each patient. Stress and infection can increase the requirement. Women in the premenstrual part of their cycle may require higher dosages. Very ill patients may become unresponsive to their medication, but temporary reduction or withdrawal of the dose over a 3-day period may restore their responsiveness. Parenteral administration may be required.

Uses

Acetylcholinesterase inhibitors used to treat myasthenia gravis are also used to reverse the effects of competitive neuromuscular-blocking drugs used in surgery.

Adverse Reactions and Contraindications

Side effects arising from overstimulation of neuromuscular (nicotinic) receptors include muscle cramps, rapid small contractions (fasciculation), and weakness. Acetylcholinesterase inhibitors can also act at sites other than neuromuscular sites. At muscarinic sites they produce side effects classic for parasympathetic stimulation such as excessive salivation, perspiration, abdominal distress, and nausea and vomiting. Patients often develop a tolerance to the muscarinic effects of the anticholinesterases.

Anticholinesterase drugs are contraindicated for patients with intestinal or urinary tract obstruction. These drugs should be used cautiously in patients with bronchial asthma. Persons sensitive to bromide should be given neostigmine methylsulfate or ambenonium chloride instead of more commonly used bromide-containing anticholinesterases.

Acetylcholinesterase Inhibitors: Specific Drugs

ambenonium

Ambenonium (Mytelase) is slightly longer acting than pyridostigmine or neostigmine. Patients may experience side effects not seen with pyridostigmine or neostigmine, such as jitteriness, headaches, confusion, and dizziness. Ambenonium is not a bromide salt, unlike pyridostigmine and

Figure 42-2 Acetylcholine *(ACh)* is neurotransmitter released by nerve to occupy nicotinic receptors on muscle; it thereby initiates biochemical events causing muscle to contract. ACh is rapidly degraded by acetylcholinesterase *(AChE)*, present throughout synapse. In myasthenia gravis, the number of receptors is greatly decreased. AChE inhibitors prevent rapid breakdown of ACh. With more ACh present, fewer receptors are needed and loss of receptors is partially compensated.

neostigmine. It is therefore the preferred drug for patients allergic to bromides.

edrophonium

Edrophonium (Tensilon) is a short-acting acetylcholinesterase inhibitor used as a diagnostic agent. When a new patient with suspected myasthenia gravis is given 2 mg of edrophonium intravenously, an increase in muscle strength should be seen in 1 to 3 minutes. If no response occurs, another 4 to 10 mg of edrophonium is given over the next 2 minutes, and muscle strength is again tested. If no increase in muscle strength occurs with this higher dosage, the muscle weakness is not caused by myasthenia gravis. Patients receiving injections of edrophonium commonly show a drop in blood pressure and feel faint, dizzy, and flushed.

A second diagnostic use for edrophonium is to help physicians determine treatment when a patient being treated for myasthenia gravis becomes weaker. The problem is to identify whether the patient is reacting to an overdose of medication (cholinergic crisis) or an increasing severity of the disease (myasthenic crisis). An edrophonium injection makes the patient in cholinergic crisis temporarily worse (negative Tensilon test) but temporarily improves the condi-

tion when the patient is in myasthenic crisis (positive Tensilon test).

neostigmine

Neostigmine (Prostigmin) can be used to diagnose and treat myasthenia gravis. As a diagnostic tool, an intramuscular (IM) injection of neostigmine should improve the patient's muscular strength in 10 minutes, and this improvement should last 3 to 4 hours. Neostigmine is also prescribed to relieve the symptoms of myasthenia gravis. Because neostigmine is irregularly absorbed from the gastrointestinal (GI) tract, it can be difficult to establish effective drug levels with oral administration. Muscarinic side effects, particularly salivation, cramps, and diarrhea, are common enough to limit the long-term use of neostigmine. If neostigmine is used, atropine may also be prescribed to block the muscarinic effects.

▼ pyridostigmine

Pyridostigmine (Mestinon) is the preferred drug for the treatment of myasthenia gravis. Compared with neostigmine, pyridostigmine is better absorbed from the GI tract and is longer acting. Adverse effects such as miosis, sweating,

---

Table 42-1   Cholinomimetic Drugs for Myasthenia Gravis

Generic Name	Trade Name*	Administration/Dosage	Comments
ambenonium chloride	Mytelase	ORAL: *Adults*—5 mg 3 or 4 times/day increased every 1-2 days as required. *Children*—0.3 mg/kg body weight/day in divided doses, increased gradually if necessary to maximum of 1.5 mg/kg/day.	Mytelase is an acetylcholinesterase inhibitor that is rapidly absorbed.
edrophonium chloride	Tensilon* Enlon*	*For diagnosis of myasthenia gravis:* INTRAVENOUS: *Adults*—2 mg injected over 15-30 sec. If no response, 8 mg is given. May repeat test after 30 min. *Children*—2 mg initially as above followed by 5 mg (if <75 lb) or up to 10 mg (if >75 lb).	Tensilon is a very short-acting acetylcholinesterase inhibitor. Diagnosis is positive if muscle strength increases within 3 min (duration 5-10 min).
		To differentiate myasthenic from cholinergic crisis: 1-2 mg.	Cholinergic crisis if muscle strength decreases (lower medication dosage). Patient in cholinergic crisis may require ventilatory assistance after injection.
neostigmine bromide	Prostigmin bromide*	ORAL: *Adults*—15 mg every 3-4 hr initially, then adjust upward as required. *Children*—begin with 2 mg/kg body weight/day in divided doses.	Prostigmin bromide is an acetylcholinesterase inhibitor with a high incidence of side effects.
neostigmine methylsulfate	Prostigmin methylsulfate*	INTRAMUSCULAR, SUBCUTANEOUS: *Adults*—0.5 mg, with subsequent doses based on patient's response. *Children*—0.01-0.04 mg/kg body weight (with 0.01 mg/kg atropine, intramuscularly).	Prostigmin methylsulfate is an injectable form for diagnosis of myasthenia gravis.
pyridostigmine bromide	Mestinon* Regonol†	ORAL: *Adults*—30-60 mg every 3 or 4 hr initially, increased as necessary. *Children*—7 mg/kg in divided doses as required. INTRAMUSCULAR, INTRAVENOUS: *Adults*—1/30 of oral dose. *Newborn infants of myasthenic mothers*—0.05-0.15 mg/kg body weight.	Mestinon is an acetylcholinesterase inhibitor; it is the drug of choice for controlling muscular weakness of myasthenia gravis.

*These drugs are available in Canada and the United States.
†Available in Canada only.

Nursing Process Overview

Myasthenia Gravis

Assessment

Patients who have or who are suspected of having myasthenia gravis require acetylcholinesterase inhibitors (anticholinesterases). Symptoms range from mild ptosis and easy fatigue to acute muscular weakness. Assess the temperature, pulse, respiration, blood pressure, vital capacity, ability to swallow, muscle strength, and degree of ptosis. Assess the results of peripheral nerve stimulation. Assess the patient's ability to perform activities of daily living. Finally, assess the patient for additional medical problems that may influence treatment.

Nursing Diagnoses

- Risk for ineffective airway clearance related to medication dosage adjustments
- Risk for impaired swallowing related to inadequate doses of acetylcholinesterase inhibitors
- Anxiety related to frequent swings between myasthenic and cholinergic crises and apparent inability to obtain adequate drug control of myasthenia gravis

Patient Outcomes

The patient will state a decrease in anxiety as the medication treatment plan is developed. The nurse will manage and minimize ineffective airway clearance and impaired swallowing until control by medications is achieved. The patient will learn to self-manage at home.

Planning/Implementation

Monitor signs of myasthenia gravis such as ptosis, ability to swallow, vital capacity, muscle strength, and vital signs. Use a peripheral nerve stimulator to monitor effectiveness of drug therapy until stabilized. Administer medications on time. Keep a suction machine at the bedside if the patient displays any inability to swallow secretions adequately. Keep edrophonium, pyridostigmine, atropine, neostigmine, and syringes at the bedside. Have equipment for intubation readily available. Teach the patient and family about myasthenia gravis management in the home. Refer the patient to other members of the health care team for physical therapy, home nursing care, or social services. Refer the patient and family to local and national myasthenia support and research groups.

Evaluation

Successful drug therapy helps the patient maintain as normal a lifestyle as possible but does not cure the disease. Patient compliance and understanding are essential to good control of the symptoms. Before discharge the patient should be able to explain how and why the medication should be taken, signs and symptoms of medication overdose and underdose, symptoms that require physician notification, other measures to assist in managing the disease (e.g., using an alarm clock with battery back-up to awaken the patient for nighttime doses of medication), and medications to avoid.

---

salivation, GI distress, and slow heart rate are less common with pyridostigmine than with neostigmine.

THERAPEUTIC RATIONALE: RHEUMATOID ARTHRITIS

Rheumatoid arthritis is an autoimmune disease that primarily involves the synovial membrane. The synovial membrane is the inner layer of the articular capsule surrounding a freely movable joint, such as the knee and joints of the finger. This tissue, which normally is smooth and shiny and secretes a thick fluid that lubricates the joint, becomes inflamed, painful, and the joint is swollen with fluid. The inflammatory process leads to the production of cytokines such as interleukin-1 and tumor necrosis factor-alpha that trigger the production of proteinases that eventually destroy cartilage and bone.

Rheumatoid arthritis occurs in about 1% of the population (more than 2 million people in the United States); it affects women about three times more often than men. Although the disease can occur at any age, the peak onset is in women between the ages of 20 and 45 years, and the incidence of clinical illness is greatest among those 40 to 60 years.

What triggers the autoimmune process is unknown. Several bacteria have been implicated, including *Streptococcus*, *Mycoplasma*, and more recently, *Borrelia*, the agent of Lyme disease. No definitive causes have been documented. Because only a 5 amino acid sequence in a protein is required to trigger an autoimmune response, it is difficult to identify a key antigen for rheumatoid arthritis.

The onset of rheumatoid arthritis is typically slow and insidious, with swelling of the small joints in the hands and feet being common, although large joints, especially the knees, may also be involved. Fever and fatigue may be present. Rheumatoid arthritis is a chronic progressive disease characterized by remissions, during which symptoms subside, and flares, during which symptoms become worse. Therapy is directed at reducing inflammation and slowing progression.

THERAPEUTIC AGENTS: DRUGS TO TREAT RHEUMATOID ARTHRITIS

Rheumatoid arthritis is a highly variable disease process. It often goes into remission for months or years. In early rheumatoid arthritis only the synovial membranes are inflamed, causing painful swelling. Aspirin and the other nonsteroid antiinflammatory drugs (NSAIDs) (see Chapter 31) may be sufficient to control symptoms. The antiinflammatory effect added to the analgesic effect eases the pain and increases the mobility of the affected joint. However, it has become widely appreciated that at the high dosages of NSAIDs required to control inflamed joints, a common serious adverse effect is the appearance of bleeding stomach ulcers caused by the inhibition of prostaglandin production in the stomach lining. NSAIDs can be combined with misoprostol, a prostaglandin, to protect the stomach lining when high dosages of NSAIDs are taken.

Disease-modifying antirheumatic drugs (DMARDs) (Table 42-2) were originally reserved for patients with severe, difficult-to-manage rheumatoid arthritis. These drugs include azathioprine, gold therapy, hydroxychloroquine, methotrexate, penicillamine, and sulfasalazine. However, some rheumatologists believe that more aggressive therapy should be initiated earlier in the course of treatment, especially for progressive cases.

Hydroxychloroquine has relatively low toxicity and suppresses symptoms in about 50% of patients treated. Methotrexate at low dosages has emerged in recent years as a relatively safe and effective drug for treating progressive rheumatoid arthritis. It is currently widely used to treat rheumatoid arthritis not controlled by NSAIDs. Glucocorticoids have a restricted role in treating severe exacerbations of rheumatoid arthritis. All antirheumatic drugs have potentially serious side effects that must be monitored carefully.

Although an NSAID may be continued, DMARDs are not generally combined with each other. Many have potentially severe side effects that must be monitored. However, some clinicians are reporting that a combination of methotrexate, sulfasalazine, and hydroxychloroquine led to improvement in patients with rheumatoid arthritis unresponsive to methotrexate alone.

A number of novel new drugs are being widely tested for treating rheumatoid arthritis. One such agent is etanercept (Enbrel), which blocks the action of tumor necrosis factor-alpha (TNF-alpha), a key cytokine of inflammation. Avakine, or cA2, is a monoclonal antibody to neutralize TNF-alpha. "Super" aspirins, the cyclooxygenase-2 (COX-2) inhibitors, act selectively on COX-2, the form inducible in inflammation, and leave the stomach cyclooxygenase alone. Such drugs may be safer and more effective than NSAIDs. Two COX-2 inhibitors include celecoxib (Celebrex) and rofecoxib (Vioxx). Also under testing are antiinflammatory agents that block the recruitment of neutrophils into inflammatory lesions and agents that block the activity of interleukins. A different approach is the feeding of collagen to induce oral tolerance. Leflunomide (Arava) inhibits pyrimidine synthesis and may be an alternative to methotrexate. Hopefully some of these new agents will provide superior therapeutic results for patients with rheumatoid arthritis.

azathioprine

Mechanism of Action

Azathioprine (Imuran) is an antimetabolite for purines and interferes with the metabolism of DNA and RNA. The exact mechanism of its immunosuppressive activity is unknown, but T cell–mediated immunity is affected more than B cell–mediated immunity.

Pharmacokinetics

Azathioprine may be given orally or by injection. It is well absorbed and rapidly converted by the liver to the active metabolites, 6-mercaptopurine and 6-thioinosinic acid, which account for the actual effects of azathioprine. The actual plasma half-life of the drug and its active metabolites is 5 hours. Metabolites are excreted in the bile. The onset of immunosuppressive action is much longer, 4 to 8 weeks. The clinical effects can persist for some time after the drug is discontinued.

Uses

A major use of azathioprine is to prevent organ transplant rejection. The dosages administered to prevent rejection begin with 3 to 5 mg/kg body weight per day initially with maintenance dosages of 1 to 2 mg/kg body weight per day.

For autoimmune diseases, including rheumatoid arthritis, systemic lupus erythematosus, and myasthenia gravis, the initial dosage is about 1 mg/kg body weight per day, generally 50 or 100 mg, as one or two doses. This dosage is increased by 0.5 mg/kg body weight daily after 4 weeks. A usual dose for azathioprine is 50 to 200 mg taken as a single dose. A clinical response should be seen in 12 weeks or therapy is discontinued. If a satisfactory clinical response is achieved and no adverse reactions occur, therapy may be continued with careful monitoring of the patient.

Adverse Reactions and Contraindications

The most common adverse reactions to azathioprine are nausea, vomiting, diarrhea, and abdominal pain. These are usually just annoying and do not require that therapy be discontinued.

More serious side effects include liver injury and low blood cell counts. In particular, low platelet counts may lead to bruising and bleeding. If the white blood cell (WBC) count is significantly depressed, the number of infections experienced may increase. In particular, viral infections such as herpes zoster and chicken pox are more common. Jaundice can indicate liver damage. Severe vomiting may indicate mucosal ulcers.

Less common side effects include skin rash, drug fever, loss of hair, and pancreatitis.

Azathioprine should not be used by pregnant or nursing women because of potential effects on the fetus or infant. Azathioprine is contraindicated for patients with chicken pox, herpes zoster, gout, renal function impairment, or hepatic function impairment.

Table 42-2   **Disease-Modifying Antirheumatic Drugs (DMARDs)**

Generic Name	Trade Name	Administration/Dosage	Comments
auranofin	Ridura*	ORAL: *Adults*—6 mg once daily or 3 mg twice daily. FDA pregnancy category C.	Dosage may be increased to 9 mg/day after 6 mo if inadequate response for another 3 mo. If response is still inadequate, discontinue. Complete blood count and urinalysis should be performed every 2-4 wk. Less toxic than injectable gold.
aurothioglucose	Solganal	INTRAMUSCULAR: *Adults*—10 mg first wk; 25 mg second and third wk; then 25-50 mg once a wk until a total dose of 800-1000 mg has been given. Maintenance: 25 or 50 mg every 2 wk for 2-20 wk, then 25 or 50 mg every 3 or 4 wk. INTRAMUSCULAR: *Child 6-12 yr*—2.5 mg first wk, 6.25 mg second and third wk; then 12.5 mg weekly until a total dose of 200-250 mg has been given; then 6.25 or 12.5 mg every 3 or 4 wk. FDA pregnancy category C.	Onset of action is usually 6-8 wk; may cause nitroid reactions and temporary joint pain after an injection. Gluteal injection is preferred.
azathioprine	Imuran*	ORAL: *Adults*—1 mg/kg body weight/day, increasing by 0.5 mg/kg body weight/day after 6-8 wk, then every 4 wk as necessary for a maximum dose of 2.5 mg/kg body weight/day. Maintenance: Reduce to the minimum effective dose in steps of 0.5 mg/kg body weight/day at 1- to 2-mo intervals. FDA pregnancy category D.	Complete blood count should be performed weekly for the first mo; twice monthly second and third mo; monthly thereafter. Liver function tests should be performed every 1-3 mo.
gold sodium thiomalate	Myochrysine*	INTRAMUSCULAR: *Adults*—10 mg first wk; 25 mg second and third wk; then 25-50 mg once a wk until a total dose of 1000 mg has been given. Maintenance: 25 or 50 mg every 2 wk for 2-20 wk, then 25 or 50 mg every 3 or 4 wk. INTRAMUSCULAR: *Child 6-12 yr*—10 mg first wk, then 1 mg/kg body weight, up to 50 mg/dose, until desired therapeutic response or until toxicity occurs. FDA pregnancy category C.	Gluteal injection preferred. If therapy has been halted because of mild adverse reactions, an initial dose of 5 mg is given and if tolerated, increased in 5- to 10-mg increments at weekly to monthly intervals until a dose of 25-50 mg is reached.
hydroxychloroquine sulfate	Plaquenil*	ORAL: *Adults*—Up to 6.5 mg/kg lean body weight/day, with meals or a glass of milk.	If the usual initial dosage produces side effects, reduce dosage for 5-10 days, then gradually increase. Eye examination should be performed initially and after 6 mo.
methotrexate	Rheumatrex*	ORAL: *Adults*—2.5-5 mg every 12 hr for 3 doses each wk, increasing if necessary by 2.5 mg weekly up to 20 mg weekly. INTRAMUSCULAR, INTRAVENOUS: *Adults*—10 mg once a wk, increasing dosage if necessary up to 25 mg weekly. FDA pregnancy category X.	Oral route is associated with less toxicity. Complete blood count and liver function tests should be performed every 2 wk initially, then every 1-3 mo. Onset of action is 1-2 mo.
penicillamine	Cuprimine*	ORAL: *Adults*—125-250 mg once a day, increasing if necessary by 125-250 mg daily every 2-3 mo if necessary, up to 1.5 g/day.	Side effects are common; complete blood count and urinalysis should be performed every 2 wk initially, then every 1-3 mo.
sulfasalazine	Azulfidine PMS Sulfasalazine† Salazopyrin†	ORAL: *Adults*—500 mg-1 mg/day for first wk, may increase by 500 mg each wk, up to maintenance dose of 2 mg/day. May be divided into 2 doses. FDA pregnancy category B.	Complete blood count should be performed periodically. Not for persons allergic to sulfa drugs.

*Available in Canada and the United States.
†Available in Canada only.

Toxicity

About 28% of patients who take azathioprine have hematologic reactions, including anemia and a decrease in WBC and thrombocyte counts. Long-term administration of azathioprine may increase the risk of developing cancer or leukemia.

Interactions

Allopurinol, an inhibitor of purine metabolism used to treat gout, greatly increases the activity and toxicity of azathioprine. Live virus vaccines should not be given to patients who take azathioprine because the lowered immune activity will not allow an adequate immune response and the virus may cause illness. Azathioprine should not be administered with other immunosuppressive agents because of the risk of infections and neoplasms.

Azathioprine also has a steroid-sparing effect, which allows a reduction in steroid dosage when the two are combined for treating chronic inflammatory diseases.

Glucocorticoids

Glucocorticoids dramatically relieve inflammation and the accompanying pain of arthritis and flares of systemic lupus erythematosus. Because of the profound side effects, the use of glucocorticoids is reserved to control severe cases of rheumatoid arthritis. The use of glucocorticoids for immune and inflammatory conditions is described in detail in Chapter 41.

When used in rheumatoid arthritis, a low oral dosage of prednisone daily or on alternate days is sometimes used in conjunction with another slower-acting drug such as gold, methotrexate, hydroxychloroquine, sulfasalazine, or azathioprine. Prednisone either is gradually decreased as the slower-acting drug starts to have an effect or may be continued longer at the smallest possible dose.

Gold Compounds

Mechanism of Action

Although gold compounds have both antiinflammatory and immunosuppressive activity, the exact mechanism of action is unknown. They appear to decrease the release of enzymes that degrade the joint. Gold compounds are capable of retarding progression of rheumatoid arthritis and even inducing a remission.

Pharmacokinetics

Aurothioglucose and gold sodium thiomalate are administered by weekly IM injection. The onset of action is very slow. Gold is stored in the body, particularly the reticuloendothelial system, and only slowly excreted, over about 6 months, through the kidney and feces.

Auranofin is a gold compound that can be taken orally. Clinical trials indicate that auranofin is as effective as the injectable gold drugs in inducing remission in rheumatoid arthritis, although less effective for severe cases. Auranofin is taken twice daily.

Uses

Gold is administered to reduce joint pain and to induce a remission in patients with rheumatoid arthritis.

When given intramuscularly to adults, 10 mg is given the first week, 25 mg the second week, and 50 mg the third week and thereafter until 800 to 1000 mg total has been administered. If no response is seen, the drug is discontinued. If joint pain decreases, the injections are continued. When the clinical status stabilizes, the dosage can be reduced to 25 to 50 mg every 2 weeks and then to monthly injections. After a year of remission, some doctors will discontinue the drug; others will continue at a reduced dosage. Only 30% to 60% of patients treated with gold respond over a 2- to 3-year course of treatment.

Gold may also be administered to patients with juvenile rheumatoid arthritis, although there are not good data that gold is effective for these patients. The initial dosage is 0.2 mg/kg, 0.5 mg/kg the second week, and 1 mg/kg weekly thereafter. No single dose is more than 50 mg.

When administered orally, the adult dose is 6 mg/day as a single or divided dose. If an adequate response is not achieved in 6 months, the dosage may be raised to 9 mg/day, but therapy is discontinued if there is still no response after an additional 3 months.

Adverse Reactions and Contraindications

Gold compounds either are well tolerated or produce toxic effects that lead to their discontinuance.

The most common reason for discontinuing successful gold therapy is the appearance of serious side effects such as skin reactions, mouth ulcers, fever, kidney damage, or abnormalities in the blood count. About 40% of patients develop an adverse reaction. These effects can occur at any time during therapy but are more common after a cumulative dose of 400 to 800 mg. Skin reactions and mouth ulcers are the most common side effects. If these are mild, gold therapy may be halted temporarily and then tried again. A complete blood count (CBC) and a urinalysis to measure protein should be done before each dose early in gold therapy and continued periodically throughout therapy.

Contraindications for gold therapy include uncontrolled diabetes mellitus, renal disease, hepatic dysfunction, congestive heart failure, hypertension, and blood dyscrasia. Patients who take other immunosuppressive drugs should not receive gold therapy. Because gold crosses the placenta and also appears in breast milk, pregnant and nursing women should not receive gold therapy.

Toxicity

Early symptoms of toxic reactions include a rash, purple blotches, pruritus, mouth lesions, and a metallic taste. Patients should be questioned about these before each injection. Because toxicity can appear even after therapy has been discontinued, the patient should be followed for at least the next 6 months for gold toxicity.

About 20% of patients experience dermatitis or lesions of the mucous membranes, usually in the first 6 months of therapy. The first sign of a skin reaction is often pruritus, and therapy may be temporarily discontinued to avoid severe dermatitis. Sunlight can aggravate skin reactions.

Severe hematologic reactions are rare, but therapy should be discontinued if the WBC count falls below 3500/mm^3. Renal damage is manifested by proteinuria. Urinary protein estimates should be done before any gold injection and the injection withheld if protein is found. About 70% of patients with proteinuria have that condition resolve when gold therapy is discontinued. Glucocorticoids should not be used to treat this kidney damage.

Interactions

Penicillamine is a chelating agent and should not be given with gold salts. Drug interactions are uncommon with gold therapy.

Gold Compounds: Specific Drugs

auranofin

Auranofin (Ridaura) is the one gold preparation that is given orally rather than by injection. It is considered less effective than injectable gold for severe cases of rheumatoid arthritis. GI reactions, including diarrhea, abdominal pain, nausea, and loss of appetite, are common early in therapy but usually subside in the first 3 months. Skin reactions occur in about 30% of patients but are generally mild.

aurothioglucose

Aurothioglucose (Solganal) is a suspension in sesame oil, administered intramuscularly once a week. It is used for active adult rheumatoid arthritis. NSAIDs are usually continued until improvement with gold therapy is seen. Dermatitis is the most common side effect and is worsened by sunlight. Mouth ulcers are also common and may be preceded by a metallic taste in the mouth.

gold sodium thiomalate

The vehicle for gold sodium thiomalate (Myochrysine) may give an anaphylactoid type of reaction with flushing, fainting, dizziness, sweating as well as nausea, vomiting, and weakness.

▼ hydroxychloroquine

Mechanism of Action

Hydroxychloroquine (Plaquenil) is an antimalarial drug. The mechanism of action in treating rheumatic diseases is unclear. It appears to have immunosuppressive effects and may also indirectly inhibit collagen and cartilage breakdown.

Pharmacokinetics

Hydroxychloroquine is readily absorbed after oral administration. The plasma half-life is up to 30 days because the drug is deposited in tissues, especially the eye, liver, lungs, and kidney, and only slowly released. Metabolites are excreted in the urine and may be found months or years after the drug is discontinued.

Uses

Hydroxychloroquine, an antimalarial drug, is also effective in treating rheumatic diseases, especially systemic lupus erythematosus and rheumatoid arthritis. A response may not be seen for 3 to 6 months after the start of therapy, and therapy is discontinued after 1 year if no response is seen. About 70% of patients with rheumatoid arthritis experience at least moderate relief of symptoms. Hydroxychloroquine is used for patients with systemic lupus erythematosus to control arthritis, skin rashes, and mouth ulcers.

Chloroquine is also occasionally used, but it has a higher incidence of pigment changes to the eye.

Adverse Reactions, Toxicity, and Contraindications

Hydroxychloroquine can produce GI upset, dry skin, and pruritus. These effects are usually mild. Opthalmic examination is recommended and therapy should be discontinued if pigment changes are noted. Rarely, emotional changes or muscle weakness are noted.

Hydroxychloroquine is fairly toxic to children; doses of 750 mg to 1 g are fatal. However, hydroxychloroquine has been successfully used to treat juvenile rheumatoid arthritis. The drug crosses the placenta and is not recommended for use during pregnancy. Use by nursing mothers is not recommended because of the greater toxicity in children, although no adverse actions have been reported.

Contraindications for hydroxychloroquine include blood dyscrasia, severe neurologic disorders, hepatic function impairment, and a history of retinal or visual field changes.

Interactions

Hydroxychloroquine should not be combined with penicillamine because the penicillamine plasma concentrations are increased with a higher incidence of adverse reactions.

▼ methotrexate

Mechanism of Action

Methotrexate (Rheumatrex) is a folic acid antagonist. It inhibits DNA, RNA, and protein synthesis and thereby slows rapidly growing cells. It has many antiinflammatory actions, including reduction of leukotrienes, suppression of cell-mediated immunity, inhibition of gene expression for collagenase, and reduced proliferation of synovial fibroblasts and endothelial cells.

Pharmacokinetics

Methotrexate is variably absorbed and has a half-life of 3 to 10 hours. Most of the drug is excreted unchanged in the urine in the first 24 hours.

Uses

At high dosages (75 to 150 mg/wk), methotrexate is used to treat various carcinomas and leukemia. At low dosages (5 to 20 mg/wk), methotrexate can be effective in treating psoriasis and rheumatoid arthritis. Improvement is noted in 2 to 6 weeks and plateaus at about 6 months. Although many DMARDs become ineffective after a couple of years, methotrexate remains effective over time. Although methotrexate originally was used only for severe cases of rheumatoid arthritis, this drug is becoming more widely used in preference to other DMARDs because at low dosages it has proven to be effective and well tolerated.

Adverse Reactions, Toxicity, and Contraindications

Side effects include nausea, mucositis, GI discomfort, rash, diarrhea, and headaches. Toxic reactions are possible but most are reversible if detected early; possible reactions include liver damage, lung disease, bone marrow depression, severe diarrhea, and ulcerative stomatitis. Baseline studies include blood chemistry, renal function, liver function, and chest x-ray films; these are repeated periodically throughout treatment. However, serious side effects with low dosages of methotrexate are uncommon. There have been rare reports of non-Hodgkin's lymphoma and other lymphomas. Contraindications to the use of methotrexate include pregnancy and nursing, alcoholism, blood dyscrasia, immunodeficiency syndromes, and hypersensitivity to the drug.

Interactions

Methotrexate given concurrently with phenylbutazone increases the risk of developing agranulocytosis. Probenecid can inhibit renal excretion of methotrexate and increase its toxicity. Because of immunosuppression, live viral vaccines may have increased adverse effects and may not be effective in producing immunity. Alcohol and drugs with potential hepatotoxicity can increase the risk of damage to the liver.

penicillamine

Mechanism of Action

Penicillamine (Cuprimine, Depen) is a chelating agent. It has an immunosuppressive action through suppression of T-cell activity, but the mechanism for this effect is unknown.

Pharmacokinetics

Penicillamine is administered orally and has a peak plasma concentration in 2 hours. The drug should be taken on an empty stomach about 1 hour before a meal. It is metabolized extensively with most metabolites excreted in the feces.

The onset of action for relieving symptoms of rheumatoid arthritis may take 2 to 3 months. To minimize side effects, the dosage is kept low, 125 to 250 mg once a day, for at least a month, and then increased stepwise monthly in 125- to 250-g increments. If remission does not occur after 4 months of therapy at 1000 to 1500 mg/day, therapy is discontinued. Otherwise therapy is continued. The maximum therapeutic effect is usually seen after 6 to 9 months.

Uses

Penicillamine is used to treat rheumatoid arthritis that has not responded to other drugs. It is also used to treat Wilson's disease, a disease of excessive copper deposition in tissues. As a chelating agent, penicillamine is also used to treat heavy metal toxicity, especially from mercury, lead, copper, and iron, by forming soluble complexes that are readily excreted in the urine. Penicillamine also combines chemically with cystine to prevent the formation of renal cystine calculi and to dissolve existing stones.

Adverse Reactions and Contraindications

Penicillamine has a high incidence of adverse actions. The most common side effects include pruritus, rash, loss of appetite, nausea, vomiting, alteration in taste, and diarrhea. More serious side effects include mouth ulcers, bone marrow depression, leukopenia, and thrombocytopenia. Blood tests should be performed initially, every 2 weeks during the first 6 months of therapy, and monthly thereafter. Possible damage to the kidney should also be monitored with urinary protein excretion, blood urea nitrogen (BUN), and creatinine levels.

Penicillamine can occasionally trigger another autoimmune disease, including lupus, pemphigus, Goodpasture's syndrome, myasthenia gravis, and dermatomyositis. These are usually reversible if penicillamine is discontinued. Penicillamine is contraindicated for individuals with any of these autoimmune diseases.

Contraindications for penicillamine include impaired renal function and pregnancy. Persons allergic to penicillin should not receive penicillamine.

Interactions

Penicillamine should not be given with gold therapy or other immunosuppressants except glucocorticoids. Phenylbutazone can cause serious hematologic and renal toxicity when combined with penicillamine. Iron supplements should be avoided.

sulfasalazine

Mechanism of Action

Sulfasalazine (Azulfidine, Salazopyrin, others) is metabolized to a salicylate and acts as an NSAID.

Pharmacokinetics

Sulfasalazine is composed of a sulfa compound and a 5-aminosalicylic acid. In the colon the drug is metabolized by bacteria to the component drugs.

Uses

Sulfasalazine is particularly effective in the treatment of inflammatory bowel disease. The effectiveness of sulfasalazine in treating rheumatoid arthritis is about equal to that of hydroxychloroquine or penicillamine. Sulfasalazine is also effective in treating ankylosing spondylitis.

Adverse Reactions, Toxicity, and Contraindications

Side effects include dizziness and GI disturbances. The more serious side effects include hypersensitivity and photosensitivity. Patients with elevated hepatic enzymes should not take sulfasalazine. CBCs should be done periodically to monitor for agranulocytosis and neutropenia.

Interactions

Sulfasalazine can potentiate the activity of anticoagulants and oral antidiabetic agents by displacing them from protein binding. Methotrexate, phenylbutazone, and sulfinpyrazone can also be potentiated.

Nursing Process Overview

Rheumatoid Arthritis

Assessment

Obtain a careful history of the presenting problem in addition to vital signs, weight, and subjective and objective data related to the complaint and the patient's overall condition. Monitor laboratory work, including hematocrit and hemoglobin level, blood counts, tests to confirm the diagnosis or to monitor diseases such as the rheumatoid factor, antinuclear antibody (ANA), complement, erythrocyte sedimentation rate (ESR), and tests to monitor the activity or side effects of drugs the patient is taking. Assess joint function, mobility, and ability to perform activities of daily living.

Nursing Diagnoses

- Risk for stomatitis (with gold compounds)
- Potential complication: hematologic disorders
- Potential anxiety related to chronic disease, changing medical therapies, and use of drugs with high potential for causing side effects

Patient Outcomes

The patient will state improved function and less discomfort. The nurse will minimize and manage blood dyscrasias. The patient will take drugs as ordered but will seek medical assistance if side effects develop.

Planning/Implementation

No drug can cure rheumatoid arthritis. Goals of drug therapy are to provide analgesia, to reduce inflammation and decrease pain, and to maintain or increase joint function. Monitor the patient's response to the therapeutic regimen, including pain, joint function, subjective and objective data related to the patient's complaints, new signs and symptoms possibly because of the therapy, and laboratory work specific for the drugs in use or the patient's problems. Plan goals so that patient management is directed to a mutually satisfactory outcome. Teach the patient that maintaining ideal weight is less stressful to joints in cases of arthritis; dietary restriction and instruction may be necessary. Refer to occupational therapy, physical therapy, and visiting nurses.

Evaluation

Ascertain that the patient understands the disease process and the specific drugs being used, is aware of possible side effects of the drugs and what action to take if they should appear, knows how to take ordered drugs correctly, understands the need for frequent follow-up and data that will be obtained at these visits to monitor for effectiveness and side effects, and recognizes the need to avoid self-medication with over-the-counter (OTC) drugs unless approved by the physician.

THERAPEUTIC RATIONALE: SYSTEMIC LUPUS ERYTHEMATOSUS

Systemic lupus erythematosus (SLE, or simply lupus) is a chronic, inflammatory multisystem disorder of the immune system that affects about 1 in 2000 persons in the United States. It usually develops in young women; it is nine times more common in women than in men. Persons of African or Hispanic background and those with relatives having SLE are more likely to develop SLE. Lupus varies greatly in severity, from mild cases that require minimal intervention to those with significant damage to the lungs, heart, kidney, and brain. No two cases are exactly alike. SLE is also characterized by exacerbation of activity (flares) with periods of remission that may last weeks to years.

The autoimmune disorder underlying lupus is not well understood. It is characterized by an overproduction of autoantibodies. Tissue damage results from inflammatory response to deposition of immunoglobulins and complement. Early symptoms of lupus are vague, nonspecific, and easily confused with other disorders. Profound fatigue is an almost universal symptom. Other symptoms that are commonly seen can include arthralgia, arthritis, fever higher than 100° F, skin rashes, anemia, kidney involvement, pleurisy, malar rash, photosensitivity, hair loss, Raynaud's phenomenon, seizures, and mouth or nose ulcers. Lupus flares are eruptions of symptoms and often have erratic patterns. Potential life-threatening complications include damage to the kidney, central nervous system, and vascular system.

Use of certain drugs may induce a lupuslike syndrome with a positive ANA test, pleuropericardial inflammation, fever, rash, and arthritis. The symptoms subside when the drug is discontinued. Drugs that have definitely been associated with drug-induced lupus include chlorpromazine, hydralazine, isoniazid, methyldopa, and procainamide. Drugs with possible association include beta-blockers, captopril, carbamazepine, cimetidine, diphenylhydantoin, ethosuximide, methimazole, penicillamine, perphenazine, and quinidine.

THERAPEUTIC AGENTS: DRUGS TO TREAT SYSTEMIC LUPUS ERYTHEMATOSUS

Drug therapy for lupus is directed at controlling symptoms to prevent or control serious complications as a result of organ damage by the inflammatory processes. The drugs most commonly used include NSAIDs, glucocorticoids, hydroxychloroquine, and azathioprine (Table 42-3). Cyclophosphamide is primarily used to treat lupus nephritis.

azathioprine

The major use of azathioprine (Imuran) for lupus is for the glucocorticoid-sparing effect. Azathioprine potentiates the immunosuppressive action of glucocorticoids and thereby allows a lower dosage of glucocorticoid to have a greater immunosuppressive action. See Table 42-1 and the earlier section on rheumatoid arthritis.

cyclophosphamide

Cyclophosphamide (Cytoxan, Endoxan) is a cytotoxic drug used to treat a number of cancers. The role of cyclophosphamide in lupus is the immunosuppressive treatment of diffuse proliferative nephritis and other organ inflammation unresponsive to glucocorticoids. Its use is reserved for severe cases because of the many adverse side effects. Cyclophosphamide is administered intravenously once a month (pulse therapy) for 6 months, and the results are evaluated. Cytotoxic drugs to treat cancer are covered in Chapter 55.

Glucocorticoids

Glucocorticoids are used at high dosages to treat exacerbations of the lupus and at low dosages to control lupus symptoms when other drugs do not work. Glucocorticoids are discussed in detail in Chapter 41. It is important for patients on glucocorticoids to take supplemental calcium and vitamin D to minimize bone loss.

▼ hydroxychloroquine

The antimalarials, particularly **hydroxychloroquine** (Plaquenil), are prescribed for the control of lupus arthritis, skin rashes, and mouth ulcers (see previous section on rheumatoid arthritis). Continuous treatment with antimalarials may prevent the recurrence of flares.

Nonsteroidal Antiinflammatory Drugs

Salicylates and NSAIDs are commonly prescribed for patients with lupus, especially to control fever and arthralgia (see Chapter 31).

THERAPEUTIC RATIONALE: MULTIPLE SCLEROSIS

Multiple sclerosis (MS) is a crippling autoimmune disease in which the myelin sheath of nerve fibers of the brain and spinal cord become inflamed, damaged, and sometimes scarred or destroyed. Without an intact myelin sheath, nerve conduction is inefficient or disabled.

MS affects about 300,000 people in the United States, two thirds of them women. MS is common in European and North American Caucasian populations but is practically nonexistent in Asian and African populations. Most commonly, MS begins slowly, usually in young adulthood, with a series of attacks followed by complete or partial remissions. This common clinical course is classified as relapsing-remitting MS. However, about one third of MS patients have a progressive form of the disease.

Table 42-3	**Agents for Systemic Lupus Erythematosus**		
Generic Name	**Trade Name***	**Administration/Dosage**	**Comments**
azathioprine	Imuran*	ORAL: *Adults*—1 mg/kg body weight/day, increasing by 0.5 mg/kg body weight/day after 6-8 wk, then every 4 wk as necessary for a maximum dose of 2.5 mg/kg body weight/day. Maintenance: Reduce to the minimum effective dosage in steps of 0.5 mg/kg body weight/day at 1- to 2-mo intervals. FDA pregnancy category D.	Complete blood count should be performed weekly for the first mo; twice monthly second and third mo; monthly thereafter. Liver function tests should be performed every 1-3 mo. Can be used with prednisone or another glucocorticoid to reduce dosage as needed to control symptoms.
cyclophosphamide	Cytoxan*	INTRAVENOUS: *Adults*—For lupus nephritis: 0.5-1 g/M² once monthly for 6 mo. FDA pregnancy category D.	Pulse therapy decreases mortality when lupus nephritis develops. Ovulation is inhibited and may be permanently impaired.
hydroxychloroquine sulfate	Plaquenil*	ORAL: *Adults*—Up to 6.5 mg/kg lean body weight/day, with meals or a glass of milk.	If the usual initial dosage produces side effects, reduce dosage for 5-10 days, then gradually increase. Eye examination should be performed initially and after 6 mo.
prednisone	Apo-Prednisone† Deltasone* Orasone Others	ORAL: *Adults*—1-10 mg once a day for maintenance or higher dosages to control active disease. FDA pregnancy category C.	Side effects are related to dosage and length of therapy.

*Available in Canada and the United States.
†Available in Canada only.

Nursing Process Overview

Systemic Lupus Erythematosus

Assessment

Complete a total assessment. Pay special attention to history of fever, weight loss, fatigue, joint pain, dyspnea, cough, pleuritic pain, lung sounds, and presence of edema. Assess for rash, purpura, and alopecia. Assess vital signs and weight. Monitor CBC, renal function tests, and urinalysis. Assess electrocardiogram (ECG), if available. Question the patient about ability to perform activities of daily living and activity tolerance.

Nursing Diagnoses

- Activity intolerance and/or fatigue related to disease progression
- Fluid volume excess related to renal failure and/or drug side effects
- Anxiety related to variable course of disease

Patient Outcomes

The patient will achieve optimal activity level (describe level appropriate for patient). The patient will describe methods to decrease edema. The patient will state a lessened degree of anxiety.

Planning/Implementation

The course of SLE is highly variable and characterized by remissions and exacerbations. Management will depend on the patient's situation. Provide emotional support. Instruct the patient about prescribed drug regimen. Depending on drugs being used and presence of renal dysfunction, instruct the patient about concomitant dietary modifications that may be helpful, such as limiting calories and sodium intake and increasing intake of protein and potassium if the patient is taking glucocorticoids. Work with the patient to modify the daily routine to permit periods of rest, if needed. Emphasize the importance of regular medical follow-up visits to monitor the progress of disease and effectiveness of therapy.

Evaluation

At present, no cure exists for SLE. Ascertain that the patient understands the disease process and the specific drugs being used and is aware of possible side effects of the drugs and what action to take if they should appear. Determine whether the patient understands the need for regular follow-up. If fatigue or activity intolerance are present, evaluate the efforts of the patient to increase strength and incorporate regular periods of rest into daily activities.

Common early symptoms of MS are vision changes, including blurred or double vision, red-green distortion, or even blindness in one eye. The visual problems arise from inflammation of the optic nerve. A common symptom is muscle weakness in the extremities. The first signs are tingling (paresthesia) in the extremities or on one side of the face. Later symptoms include emotional lability, abnormal reflexes, ataxia, and difficulty in bladder and bowel control. Because of the periods of remission and the vagueness of the symptoms, diagnosis of MS is difficult and involves ruling out other diseases.

A mouse model for MS has been developed by injecting myelin basic protein to produce an autoimmune disease in susceptible mice, experimental allergic encephalomyelitis (EAE). This model has helped researchers understand some of the autoimmune events underlying MS. MS appears to be a T cell–mediated autoimmune disease. The trigger for autoimmunity may be a virus. Recent evidence suggests that the human herpesvirus 6, found in about 90% of Americans, may be a trigger. This virus causes childhood roseola.

Another advance in understanding MS has been the application of magnetic resonance imaging (MRI) to visualize lesions in the brain produced by MS. These studies have indicated that brain inflammation and damage continue even when MS patients are feeling well, dispelling notions that remission means periods of no disease activity. As the disease progresses, MRI scans show atrophy of the brain. Autopsy of brains from those who had MS show that axons appear to have been cut.

THERAPEUTIC AGENTS: DRUGS TO TREAT MULTIPLE SCLEROSIS

Treatment options are increasing for MS (Table 42-4). Recent trials with interferon-beta (IFN-beta) have shown that this agent can increase the time between relapses and can slow progression of MS. A new drug, glatiramer, has also decreased the relapse rate of MS in clinical trials.

The standard therapy for managing acute attacks of MS is adrenocorticotropic hormone (ACTH) or methylprednisolone. However, these agents do not have a long-term therapeutic effect except for the treatment of optic neuritis.

Trials with other immunosuppressive drugs have been conducted. Cyclophosphamide and cyclosporine have shown no therapeutic benefit for MS. Azathioprine shows modest benefit. Methotrexate is the most promising of the immunosuppressive drugs in slowing the neurologic impairment of MS. None of these immunosuppressive agents is currently standard therapy for MS.

corticotropin

Corticotropin (ACTH) is the hormone released by the pituitary to act on the adrenal cortex and increase the natural production of corticosteroids (see Chapter 66). A regimen of high-dose intravenous (IV) or IM corticotropin may improve the recovery from an acute relapse of MS. This therapy is conducted in the hospital. In one regimen, 80 units is given intravenously in 500 ml of 5% dextrose over 6 to 8 hours and repeated the next 2 days. In another regimen, 40 units of ACTH gel is administered intramuscularly every

12 hours for 7 days and the dosage is then tapered over the following month. Patients commonly are treated with lithium carbonate for the manic reaction to the high level of corticosteroids in the body.

glatiramer acetate

Mechanism of Action

Glatiramer acetate (Copaxone), also called copolymer-1, is a mixture of synthetic polypeptides containing four naturally occurring amino acids. This agent is able to interfere with the binding of myelin proteins to MHC molecules, thereby suppressing T-cell activation and the subsequent inflammatory response.

Pharmacokinetics

Glatiramer acetate is administered subcutaneously twice a day. Much of the drug is believed to be hydrolyzed locally by proteases. Presumably some of the material reaches the lymphatic circulation and regional lymph nodes to exert its response.

Uses

Glatiramer acetate is approved for the treatment of relapsing-remitting MS. Clinical trials indicate that the relapse rate for patients was decreased by 29%. No direct comparison has been made of glatiramer with IFN-beta therapy.

Adverse Reactions, Contraindications, and Interactions

The main side effects of glatiramer acetate are pain, erythema, and itching at the injection site. About 10% of patients have a general reaction that includes flushing, chest pain, palpitation, anxiety, difficulty in breathing, constriction of the throat, and urticaria. These reactions have not led to serious consequences. However, hypersensitivity to glatiramer acetate remains a potential contraindication.

The long-term effects of glatiramer acetate are unknown. Because of its immune-modulating response, effects on the immune system will need to be followed. An increase in immunoglobulin G (IgG) levels has been documented, but with no associated adverse effects.

▼ interferon-beta

Interferon-beta is available in two forms: IFN-beta-1a (Avonex) and IFN-beta-1b (Betaseron). These drugs are manufactured through recombinant DNA technology. IFN-beta-1a is identical to natural human interferon. IFN-beta-1b differs by a single amino acid from the natural human form and is not glycosylated.

Mechanism of Action

Interferons are cytokines that inhibit the proliferation of certain cell types. IFN-beta is a type 1 interferon that is produced by fibroblasts and epithelial cells in response to a viral infection. IFN-beta inhibits cell proliferation and increases the expression of MHC molecules on the cell surface, promoting antiviral activity. IFN-beta antagonizes the expression of MHC class II molecules in glial cells, an activity that would suppress an inflammatory response to autoantigens in MS.

Pharmacokinetics

IFN-beta-1a is administered intramuscularly once a week. IFN-beta-1b is administered by subcutaneous injection every other day. The serum levels are undetectable.

Uses

IFN-beta-1 is indicated for patients who have the relapsing-remitting form of MS. In clinical trials this drug significantly reduced the frequency and intensity of relapses. In addition, the onset of disability is delayed.

Table 42-4 **Agents for Multiple Sclerosis**			
Generic Name	Trade Name*	Administration/Dosage	Comments
corticotropin (ACTH)	Acthar*	INTRAVENOUS: *Adults*—See text. INTRAMUSCULAR: *Adults*—80-120 USP units/day for 2 or 3 wk. See text. FDA pregnancy category C.	For acute exacerbations of multiple sclerosis.
glatiramer acetate (copolymer-1)	Copaxone	SUBCUTANEOUS: *Adults*—20 mg/day.	For prophylactic treatment of multiple sclerosis when there are recurrent attacks followed by partial or complete remission.
interferon-beta-1a	Avonex Rebif†	INTRAMUSCULAR: *Adults*—30 μg once a wk. FDA pregnancy category C.	For prophylactic treatment of multiple sclerosis when there are recurrent attacks followed by partial or complete remission.
interferon-beta-1b	Betaseron	SUBCUTANEOUS: *Adults*—0.25 mg every other day. FDA pregnancy category C.	For prophylactic treatment of multiple sclerosis when there are recurrent attacks followed by partial or complete remission.
methylprednisolone sodium succinate	Solu-Medrol*	INTRAMUSCULAR, INTRAVENOUS: *Adults*—160 mg/day for 1 wk, followed by 64 mg every other day for 1 mo. FDA pregnancy category C.	For acute exacerbations of multiple sclerosis.

*Available in Canada and the United States.
†Available in Canada only.

Adverse Reactions and Contraindications

Reactions at the injection site are fairly common with IFN-beta-1b but not with IFN-beta-1a. Other common reactions include flulike symptoms of fever, chills, myalgia, malaise, and sweating. Women may experience menstrual disorders. Less common reactions include palpitations, hypertension, tachycardia, and peripheral vascular disorders.

Blood studies should be performed, especially to monitor the neutrophil count and serum levels of bilirubin and alanine amino transferase (ALT). The drug should be discontinued if the absolute neutrophil count is less than 750/mm³ or if AST (aspartate amino transferase)/ALT levels exceed 10 times the upper limit of normal. Some patients may experience confusion and anxiety. Signs and symptoms of depression should be monitored because a few patients have become suicidal while taking the drug.

IFN-beta-1 is contraindicated for pregnant women because spontaneous abortions have been reported.

Interactions

No drug interactions have been reported with the use of IFN-beta-1.

methylprednisolone

Methylprednisolone is one of the intermediate-acting glucocorticoids presented in Chapter 41. An alternative to ACTH, high-dose IV administration of methylprednisolone improves the recovery from acute exacerbations of MS, although there is no long-term improvement in the disease. The usual regimen is to administer 1 g of methylprednisolone in 500 ml of 5% dextrose intravenously over 4 to 6 hours in the morning every day for 3 days, followed by 500 mg/day for 3 days and finally 250 mg/day for 3 days.

Nursing Process Overview

Multiple Sclerosis

Assessment

Perform a complete assessment. MS is highly individualized: what is a problem for one patient may not affect another. Monitor vital signs and weight. Auscultate lung sounds. Obtain a history of ability to perform activities of daily living, presence of fatigue, or activity intolerance. Question the patient about changes since the last visit.

Nursing Diagnoses

- Anxiety related to presence of chronic disease, specific symptoms, or inability to maintain usual level of daily activities
- Risk for self-concept disturbance related to loss of usual role responsibilities

Patient Outcomes

The patient will learn strategies to optimize physical abilities (specify). The patient will discuss anxiety. The patient will discuss recent changes in role and feelings about those changes.

Planning/Implementation

At present, no cure exists for MS. The course is highly variable from person to person. Provide emotional support as needed. Seek assistance as needed from other members of the health care team, including the physical or occupational therapist, home care nurses, and social worker. Teach the patient about the disease itself and about any prescribed medications. Emphasize the importance of regular follow-up to monitor disease process and effectiveness of any medications or treatments.

Evaluation

Ascertain that the patient understands the disease process and what drugs are being used, is aware of possible drug side effects, and knows what action to take if they should appear. Verify that the patient can state the importance of regular follow-up visits to monitor progress.

Nursing Implications Summary

Drugs for Diagnosis and Treatment of Myasthenia Gravis

Drug Administration

➤ Assess the patient for signs of myasthenic crisis (inadequately treated myasthenia gravis) such as positive Tensilon test; increased blood pressure and pulse; difficulty chewing, swallowing, and coughing; bladder and bowel incontinence; increasing ptosis; difficulty breathing; and cyanosis. Differentiate symptoms of myasthenic crisis from those of cholinergic crisis (overtreated myasthenia gravis) such as negative Tensilon test; abdominal cramps; diarrhea; fasciculations; and nausea, vomiting, and blurred vision. The following may be seen in myasthenic or cholinergic crisis: generalized weakness; increased salivation, tearing, and bronchial secretions; general feeling of apprehension; restlessness; and difficulty breathing. Have a suction machine at the bedside.

Continued

Nursing Implications Summary—cont'd

➤ Keep edrophonium, pyridostigmine, atropine, neostigmine, syringes, and a tourniquet at the patient's bedside or in a convenient place on the patient care unit for rapid treatment of a myasthenic or cholinergic crisis.

➤ Assess the patient's ability to swallow before preparing an ordered oral dose of anticholinesterase. If the ability to swallow is deteriorating, it may be necessary to administer a parenteral dose of medication. Obtain written orders for oral and parenteral doses at the time of admission so that time is not lost if the patient can no longer swallow.

➤ Schedule off-unit diagnostic studies and therapies for the patient with myasthenia gravis so that medication administration is not delayed while the nurse waits for the patient to return. If the patient is not present when a medication is due, take the dose of the medication to the patient.

➤ Assess blood pressure, pulse, vital capacity, presence and degree of ptosis, muscle strength, and ability to swallow as indicators of adequate drug control.

➤ When one of these drugs is used as an antidote for tubocurarine or other neuromuscular-blocking agents, administer via slow IV push. Continue appropriate ventilatory support until the patient is breathing well unassisted. Have atropine at the bedside. If the pulse is less than 80 beats/min, administer atropine before the neostigmine.

➤ For constant infusion of anticholinesterases, use a volume control device and microdrip tubing. Monitor respiratory and cardiovascular status. The dosage may be titrated to peripheral nerve stimulator response.

Intravenous edrophonium

➤ May be given undiluted at a rate of 2 mg (0.2 ml) over 15 to 30 seconds. A physician or nurse anesthetist should be present. Read drug labels carefully: Enlon contains edrophonium, whereas Enlon-Plus contains edrophonium and atropine. The dosage may be titrated to peripheral nerve stimulator response.

Intravenous neostigmine

➤ Read the drug label: must be for IV use. May be given undiluted at a rate of 0.5 mg or less over 1 minute. A physician or nurse anesthetist should be present. The dosage may be titrated to peripheral nerve stimulator response.

Intravenous pyridostigmine

➤ May be given undiluted at a rate of 0.5 mg or less over 1 minute. A physician or nurse anesthetist should be present. The dosage may be titrated to peripheral nerve stimulator response.

➤ When used as an antagonist for muscle relaxants, the dosage is significantly higher; administer atropine first.

Nursing in the Community

➤ Teach the patient and family about the signs and symptoms of myasthenia gravis, myasthenic crisis, and overdose with anticholinesterases.

➤ Teach the patient and family to take medications exactly as ordered. Forgetting, omitting, or doubling a dose of medication may cause the patient's condition to deteriorate.

➤ Encourage the patient to keep a daily log of medication use and response to the medication.

➤ No medication, whether prescription or OTC, should ever be taken without the approval of the physician. In addition, give the patient a list of drugs known to be contraindicated for patients with myasthenia gravis (see Box 42-1). Suggest that the patient plan a medication schedule that includes taking doses of anticholinesterases 30 to 60 minutes before meals to increase strength for chewing and swallowing. Instruct the patient to take anticholinesterases with milk or a snack to reduce gastric irritation. Use a reliable alarm clock with battery back-up to wake the patient for early morning or nighttime doses of medication.

➤ Keep careful watch on supplies of drugs on hand, and refill prescriptions before they run out. Reinforce to the patient and family the need to seek medical assistance immediately if the patient's condition seems to be deteriorating. Encourage the patient to wear a medical identification tag or bracelet and to carry a list of the names and dosages of medication being taken. Refer the patient and family to local, state, or national myasthenia gravis support groups.

➤ If IM forms are prescribed for self-administration, teach injection technique to the patient and family members.

THERAPEUTIC AGENTS FOR RHEUMATOID ARTHRITIS
azathioprine
Drug Administration

➤ Assess vital signs. Monitor CBC, WBC differential, and platelet count.

➤ There may be some risk to personnel who prepare and administer immunosuppressant drugs. Check agency procedures and handle parenteral form as a cytotoxic agent. When preparing doses, use a biologic containment cabinet, and wear disposable gloves and masks. Use careful technique in the handling and administration of these medications. Dispose of vials, syringes, needles, IV equipment, and unused medication in biohazard containers.

➤ Monitor CBC and differential, platelet count, and liver function tests.

➤ Assess for signs of hepatitis, including right upper quadrant abdominal pain, jaundice, fever, malaise, nausea, vomiting, and anorexia. Tell the patient to report these signs and symptoms if they develop.

Intravenous azathioprine

➤ Reconstitute by adding 10 ml of sterile water for injection to the vial and swirling to dissolve drug. May be further diluted in at least 50 ml of 0.9% sodium chloride injection, D5W, or 5% dextrose in normal saline. Incompatible with preservatives such as parabens and phenol. Administer a diluted dose over at least 30 to 60 minutes, but rate may vary from 5 minutes to 8 hours depending on use, volume of fluid, and the patient's size and age.

Nursing Implications Summary—cont'd

Nursing in the Community

➤ Review the reasons for using this drug with the patient. See the Patient Problems boxes in Chapter 54 on bleeding tendencies and leukopenia.

➤ Emphasize the importance of returning for regular follow-up and not discontinuing the medication without consulting the physician.

➤ Remind the patient to take doses after meals or at bedtime if the drug causes nausea. If the patient vomits shortly after taking a dose, have the patient contact physician to see whether the dose should be repeated.

➤ Instruct the patient to avoid immunizations unless first discussed with the physician. Others in the patient's house should avoid immunization with oral poliovirus vaccine. If the patient must be in contact with someone who has received the polio vaccine, tell the patient to limit close contact and wear a protective mask that covers the nose and mouth.

➤ For missed doses, if the ordered dose is once a day, omit the missed dose, and resume the regular dosing schedule the next day. Do not double up for missed dose. If doses are ordered more than once a day, take the missed dose as soon as remembered. Contact the physician with questions.

➤ Teach injection technique if required. Refer the patient to a home nursing care agency for follow-up.

➤ Use of azathioprine during pregnancy is not recommended. Instruct patient as needed about birth control measures. Instruct patient to notify physician immediately if pregnancy is suspected.

Gold Compounds

Drug Administration

➤ Assess respiratory rate and auscultate lung sounds. Monitor intake and output, and weight. Monitor CBC and differential, platelet count, BUN level, serum creatinine level, and liver function tests. Monitor urinalysis to detect proteinuria and hematuria. Inspect the skin and mouth for presence of rashes, ulcers, stomatitis, and irritation.

➤ For IM injection, use large muscle masses. Record and rotate injection sites. Aspirate before administering dose to prevent inadvertent IV administration. Keep the patient supine for at least 15 minutes after dose. Monitor vital signs and blood pressure. Have available drugs, equipment, and personnel to treat an acute allergic reaction when parenteral gold compounds are administered.

Intramuscular aurothioglucose

➤ This drug form is an oil-based suspension (see Box 5-3).

Nursing in the Community

➤ Review the anticipated benefits and possible side effects of drug therapy with the patient. Instruct the patient to notify the physician if severe or persistent vomiting or diarrhea, rashes, skin irritation, itching, mouth ulcers, oral irritation, stomatitis, metallic taste, unexplained bruising, bleeding of gums, bleeding in stool, nosebleeds, jaundice,

right upper quadrant abdominal pain, malaise, fever, sore throat, eye irritation, or visual changes develop. Reinforce the importance of reporting new signs or symptoms to the physician.

➤ Instruct the patient to take oral compounds with meals or a snack to lessen gastric irritation.

➤ Review oral hygiene with the patient if stomatitis develops. See the Patient Problems box in Chapter 54 on stomatitis, and review the Patient Problems box in Chapter 58 on photosensitivity.

➤ Explain that weeks to months of therapy may be necessary before full benefit of gold therapy can be seen. Emphasize the importance of continuing other prescribed therapies, including prescribed exercise program, weight reduction, application of heat and cold, and physical therapy.

➤ For patients receiving the injectable forms: Immediately after the injection, dizziness, feeling faint, nausea and vomiting, increased sweating, or weakness may develop, but these symptoms should resolve in a short time. The patient should lie down after injection in anticipation of these effects. If these symptoms worsen or other symptoms develop within 10 minutes of the injection, notify the physician. Joint pain may occur for 1 or 2 days after each injection but should diminish after several doses.

➤ Teach the patient injection technique if gold preparations are to be self-administered.

➤ For missed doses (oral form) ordered once a day, instruct the patient to take the missed dose when remembered, unless not remembered until the next day, then omit the missed dose. For missed doses when doses are ordered more than once a day, instruct the patient to take the missed dose as soon as remembered, unless almost time for the next dose, then omit. Do not double up for missed doses.

➤ Gold preparations are not recommended during pregnancy. Instruct the patient about birth control measures before initiating gold therapy.

GLUCOCORTICOIDS: PREDNISONE AND METHYLPREDNISOLONE

➤ See Chapter 41 for a detailed discussion of these drugs.

hydroxychloroquine

➤ See Chapter 53 for a detailed discussion of this drug, also used to treat malaria.

methotrexate

➤ See Chapter 55 for a detailed discussion of this drug, used at higher dosages to treat cancer.

penicillamine

Drug Administration

➤ Monitor weight and blood pressure. Auscultate lung sounds. Inspect for presence of skin rashes and lesions. Monitor

Continued

Nursing Implications Summary—cont'd

CBC and differential, platelet count, serum creatinine level, BUN level, and liver function tests. Monitor urinalysis to detect proteinuria.

➤ Assess penicillin allergy before administering. Cross-sensitivity between the two drugs is possible although rare.

➤ Penicillamine is a copper-chelating agent and is also used in the treatment of Wilson's disease, a disorder of copper metabolism. Teach patients with Wilson's disease to avoid foods higher in copper, including chocolate, nuts, shellfish, mushrooms, liver, molasses, broccoli, and copper-enriched cereals.

Nursing in the Community

➤ Review the anticipated benefits and possible side effects of drug therapy. Instruct the patient to notify the physician if severe or persistent vomiting or diarrhea, skin rashes, lesions, scaling, dermatitis, hair loss, fever, inflamed mouth, mouth lesions, stomatitis, swelling or edema, bruising, bleeding, nosebleeds, blood in stool, malaise, sore throat, jaundice, or abdominal pain develops. Explain that side effects may develop any time during therapy. Tell the patient to report new signs and symptoms to the physician.

➤ Review the Patient Problems box in Chapter 54 on stomatitis.

➤ Emphasize the importance of taking drugs as ordered. Sporadic or intermittent use (unless prescribed by the physician) may contribute to further allergic reactions.

➤ Capsules may be opened and contents mixed with 15 to 30 ml of chilled applesauce, other puréed foods, or fruit juice for ease in administering.

➤ When used for prevention of kidney stones, tell the patient to take the bedtime dose with at least two 8-ounce glasses of water, and to drink two more 8-ounce glasses of water during the night. Take daytime doses with a full glass (8 ounces) of water.

➤ Teach patients taking oral iron preparations to allow at least 2 hours to elapse between the two drugs.

➤ Penicillamine increases the body's requirement for pyridoxine. If pyridoxine is also prescribed, emphasize the importance of taking this supplement. See the Dietary Considerations box in Chapter 17 on vitamins for dietary sources of pyridoxine.

➤ Penicillamine may lead to impaired taste. For all patients except those with Wilson's disease, normal taste may be returned with administration of copper each day (e.g., several drops of cupric sulfate solution diluted in fruit juice); check with the physician.

➤ Women of childbearing age may wish to use some form of birth control while taking penicillamine; discuss this issue before initiating therapy.

➤ Emphasize that weeks to months of therapy may be necessary before full benefit of penicillamine can be seen. Reinforce the importance of continuing other prescribed therapies, which might include a prescribed exercise program, weight reduction, application of heat and cold, and physical therapy.

➤ For treatment of arthritis, teach the patient to take doses 1 hour before or 2 hours after meals, and 1 hour before or after other medications, food, or milk.

➤ For treatment of Wilson's disease, instruct the patient to take doses on an empty stomach, 30 to 60 minutes before or 2 hours after meals.

➤ For treatment of lead poisoning, teach the patient to take doses on an empty stomach, 2 hours before or 3 hours after meals.

➤ Teach patients with Wilson's disease to avoid multivitamin preparations that contain copper. Teach the patient to use distilled or demineralized water for drinking if the patient's water supply contains more than 0.1 mg of copper per liter.

sulfasalazine

Nursing in the Community

➤ Assess the patient for allergy to other sulfonamides, furosemide, thiazide diuretics, salicylates, carbonic anhydrase inhibitors, or sulfonylureas (see Chapter 49).

➤ Do not give this drug to children younger than 2 years of age unless specifically directed to do so by the physician.

➤ Teach the patient to take doses with meals or a snack to lessen gastric irritation.

➤ Instruct the patient to take enteric-coated tablets whole, without chewing or crushing.

➤ Instruct the patient to take doses with a full glass (8 ounces) of water and to maintain a daily fluid intake of at least 2000 to 2500 ml.

➤ Caution the patient to avoid driving or operating hazardous equipment if dizziness occurs.

➤ See the Patient Problems boxes on photosensitivity (Chapter 58), leukopenia (Chapter 54), and bleeding tendencies (Chapter 54).

➤ Encourage regular dental care and good dental hygiene (flossing and brushing). Leukopenia and thrombocytopenia may contribute to gum infections and bleeding gums.

➤ Teach the patient to return to the physician if symptoms, including diarrhea, do not improve in 4 to 6 weeks. Encourage the patient to return for regularly scheduled follow-up visits.

➤ This drug may cause the skin or urine of some patients to turn yellow-orange. This discoloration does not need medical attention.

THERAPEUTIC AGENTS FOR SYSTEMIC LUPUS ERYTHEMATOSUS

cyclophosphamide

➤ See Chapter 55 for a discussion of this drug, which is also used to treat cancer.

THERAPEUTIC AGENTS FOR MULTIPLE SCLEROSIS

corticotropin (ACTH)

➤ See Chapter 65 for a discussion of this drug.

glatiramer

Drug Administration/Nursing in the Community

➤ See manufacturer's insert for current information.

Nursing Implications Summary—cont'd

➤ Assess the patient for anxiety, joint pain, chest pain, difficulty breathing, lymphadenopathy, chills, flu-like symptoms, fever, chills, and peripheral edema. Inspect skin for injection-site reactions, including hard lumps, and hives, redness, rash, and skin nodules. Instruct the patient to report the development of new signs and symptoms to the physician.

➤ Reconstitute as directed in manufacturer's instructions. Administer subcutaneously immediately after preparing dose.

➤ For home management, teach the patient self-administration, including injection technique and proper handling and disposal of syringes and needles. Refer to a community-based nursing care agency for follow-up.

interferon-beta-1
Drug Administration
➤ See the manufacturer's insert for detailed information about this drug.

➤ Monitor blood chemistry, liver function tests, CBC and differential, and platelet count.

➤ Assess for excessive or unusual fatigue or weakness, diarrhea, fever, chills, flulike symptoms, headache, muscle aches, and signs of depression. Inspect the skin for hives, skin lesions, and redness and swelling at the injection site. Assess blood pressure and heart rate.

➤ To prepare dose, allow vial of drug and diluent to come to room temperature. Reconstitute with the diluent provided by the manufacturer. Use within 3 hours of reconstituting drug. Use immediately or refrigerate dose and use within 6 hours. Administer intramuscularly.

Nursing in the Community
➤ For home management, teach the patient self-administration, including injection technique and proper handling and disposal of syringes and needles.

➤ Refer to a community-based nursing care agency for follow-up.

➤ Emphasize the importance of returning for follow-up visits to monitor drug effectiveness and side effects. Remind the patient not to discontinue medications without consulting the physician.

CHAPTER REVIEW

Application

1. Describe the mechanism by which acetylcholinesterase inhibitors increase activation of the neuromuscular junction.
2. What muscarinic side effects of neostigmine and pyridostigmine would you observe? Which drug would you administer as an antidote for neostigmine?
3. Describe two diagnostic uses of edrophonium.
4. Develop a teaching plan for the patient taking anticholinesterases.
5. What is meant by disease-modifying agents for rheumatic diseases (DMARDs)? Which drugs are classified as DMARDs?

6. Which drugs are commonly used to treat lupus? Which drug is used to treat lupus nephritis?
7. Which drugs are used as therapeutic agents for MS?

Critical Thinking

1. Autoimmune diseases are chronic disease for which no cures exist. They are marked by periods of remission, but over time they may become progressively more debilitating. Research one of these diseases and describe some of the challenges in working with a patient not only related to adjusting medications but also to other aspects of care.

References

Boyden KM: Copolymer-1 in the treatment of multiple sclerosis, *J Neurosci Nurs* 30(2):135-141, 1998.

Frizzell J: Antinuclear antibody testing, *Am J Nurs* 97(12):14-15, 1997.

Mahat G: Perceived stressors and coping strategies among individuals with rheumatoid arthritis, *J Adv Nurs* 25(6):1144-1150, 1997.

Chapter 43

Introduction to the Use of Antiinfective Agents

KEY TERMS

acquired resistance, p. 498

antimicrobial spectrum, p. 498

bactericidal, p. 497

bacteriostatic, p. 497

eucaryotic cells, p. 497

minimum bactericidal concentration (MBC), p. 498

minimum inhibitory concentration (MIC), p. 498

plasmids, p. 498

procaryotic cells, p. 497

selective toxicity, p. 497

superinfections, p. 500

OBJECTIVES

After studying this chapter, you should be able to do the following:

- *Discuss the principle of selective toxicity.*
- *Describe the difference between bactericidal and bacteriostatic agents.*
- *Explain why antibiotic resistance can be passed between bacteria.*
- *Describe the factors that influence the outcome of antibiotic therapy.*
- *Explain why antibiotics should not be discontinued until the prescribed therapy is complete.*
- *Outline important patient teaching points related to general use of antiinfective agents.*

CHAPTER OVERVIEW

The preceding chapters presented the use of drugs intended to alter processes that occur naturally in the body. For example, diuretics alter existing patterns of water and ion movement in the kidneys; the therapeutic goal of increasing water excretion is achieved by this direct action of the drug. In contrast, antiinfective agents ideally do not directly affect any physiologic process in the patient. These drugs may be considered selective poisons because the goal of their use is to poison invading pathogenic microorganisms without poisoning the patient.

This chapter presents concepts that apply to all antiinfective agents. Microbiologic principles are reviewed, general mechanisms by which these drugs act are discussed, and major problems associated with antimicrobial therapy are presented.

THERAPEUTIC RATIONALE: INFECTIOUS DISEASES

Although the world of microbes was discovered by Anton Van Leeuwenhoek in 1676, the impact of these tiny organisms on human lives was not appreciated until the last third of the nineteenth century. During this period Louis Pasteur and Robert Koch, working in separate laboratories and on different microorganisms, showed that bacteria could cause human disease. After these discoveries microbiologists and physicians began to classify human diseases in terms of the organism that produced the disease. By the early twentieth century, microorganisms that cause cholera, typhoid, bubonic plague, gonorrhea, leprosy, malaria, syphilis, and other diseases were identified.

This new knowledge put therapy of microbially induced diseases on a more rational basis. The first attempts at controlling diseases caused by microorganisms involved immunization. This approach allowed certain diseases to be prevented, but immunization was not effective for all diseases nor was it effective once the disease was established. Thus chemists sought agents that could eradicate invading

496

pathogens in a living patient. A leader in this area was Paul Ehrlich, who in 1912 introduced salvarsan, a drug for syphilis. Salvarsan and a related drug, neosalvarsan, established the validity of drug therapy for infectious diseases. In 1935 a synthetic agent that could cure streptococcal infections was discovered, and in 1939 development was begun on an extract of culture fluid from the mold *Penicillium*. These discoveries marked the beginnings of sulfonamides and penicillins. The search for more effective antimicrobial agents has not ceased. As subsequent chapters illustrate, that search has been extraordinarily fruitful.

Antimicrobial agents are possible because bacterial pathogens differ significantly from their human hosts. Bacteria are **procaryotic cells,** which have genetic material that exists in contact with the cell protoplasm. Human cells are **eucaryotic cells** and have membrane-bounded nuclei that contain the genetic material. Other distinguishing characteristics include the procaryotic cell wall composed in part of peptidoglycan, a complex molecule that contains amino acids and sugars. Human cells have no cell wall but only a cell membrane. Single-celled eucaryotic organisms such as algae and fungi may possess complex rigid cell walls, but these walls do not contain peptidoglycan.

Procaryotes and eucaryotes also differ in certain internal functions. For example, ribosomes in eucaryotes are larger than those in procaryotes, and the two forms differ in their response to certain chemicals (see Chapters 46 through 48). Likewise, folic acid metabolism may differ. Many procaryotes cannot use folic acid from the environment but must synthesize the vitamin from simpler starting materials (see Chapter 49). In contrast, eucaryotes cannot synthesize folic acid but must absorb it from the diet.

The structural and metabolic differences between procaryotes and eucaryotes form the basis for **selective toxicity.** Selective toxicity is the selective poisoning of an invading disease-causing organism by means of an agent that has no effect on the person in whom the disease exists.

No drug that is a perfectly selective agent is yet available; at some dosage every antiinfective agent currently available may cause a direct effect on the host. One way to evaluate the degree of selective toxicity that may be achieved with a drug is by means of the therapeutic index (see Chapter 1). The therapeutic index (TI) is the ratio of the dose of a certain drug that kills 50% of the test animals to the dose of that drug that is effective in 50% of the animals ($TI = LD_{50}/ED_{50}$). A drug that is relatively nontoxic may be given in very large doses before it kills animals. If the drug is also potent, it may require small doses to achieve the desired clinical effect, which in this case is to cure the infection. Such a drug would have a large TI and would be considered to display good selective toxicity: it attacks the pathogen at doses much smaller than those that are dangerous to the host. In contrast a drug with low TI would not have good selective toxicity. A drug with a TI of 1 would be equally toxic to the bacteria and to the patient.

The TI is derived from studies on laboratory animals. Because correlating animal studies with the clinical effectiveness of a drug is sometimes difficult, other indices of selective toxicity have been used to indicate clinical experience with a drug. For example, the safety margin of a drug is the percentage increase above the standard therapeutic dose that is required to produce serious toxic reactions in a certain percentage of patients. This evaluation is based entirely on clinical experience.

A drug with a large TI and a wide safety margin may be given to patients in larger-than-normal doses without causing significant toxicity in most patients. The antibiotics gentamicin and penicillin G can be used to illustrate this principle. Gentamicin must be given in carefully controlled doses because it can damage the kidneys if the concentration in blood becomes too high. Gentamicin has such a low TI and narrow safety margin that increasing the dose by 50% may cause significant toxicity (see Chapter 48). In contrast penicillin G has a very wide safety margin and a high TI. Direct toxicity with this drug is low, and doses three or four times the standard dose may be administered with little risk of toxic reactions in most patients (see Chapter 44).

THERAPEUTIC AGENTS: ANTIMICROBIAL DRUGS

Most antibiotics achieve selective toxicity by acting on microorganisms in one of the following five ways: inhibiting cell wall formation, blocking protein synthesis, disrupting cell membranes, interfering with nucleic acid synthesis, or preventing synthesis of folic acid. Each mechanism of action exploits a biochemical difference between eucaryotic and procaryotic cells.

Antibiotics not only may be classified by specific mechanisms, but also may be broadly classified as **bacteriostatic** or **bactericidal.** Bactericidal drugs directly kill bacteria. For example, antibiotics that interfere with cell wall synthesis may cause the bacterium to explode because the osmotic forces generated by the cytoplasm can no longer be contained by the defective cell wall. Likewise, antibiotics that disrupt the bacterial cell membrane allow the cytoplasmic contents of the bacterium to leak out, and it dies. Bacteriostatic drugs halt bacterial reproduction without directly killing the bacteria. With bacteriostatic drugs, bacteria removed from exposure to the drug can resume growth. The host's immune system must immobilize and kill the pathogens for therapy with bacteriostatic drugs to achieve a long-term cure. In theory, cures can be effected with bactericidal drugs independent of immune function, but such cures are not easily achieved. In immunosuppressed patients cures of bacterial infections are much more difficult to achieve than in patients with normal immune function, even with appropriately prescribed bactericidal drugs. These observations suggest that cures of bacterial disease in ordinary persons depend strongly on immunologic factors.

To classify a drug as exclusively bactericidal or bacteriostatic may be misleading. Many antibiotics are bacteriostatic or bactericidal depending on dose, site of infection, and the causative organism. For example, sulfonamides, which prevent folic acid synthesis in sensitive bacteria, might be considered bacteriostatic for a systemic infection, but because of the high drug concentration in urine, they may be bactericidal in urine. Other examples are cases in which two types of microorganisms differ greatly in sensitivity to a certain antibiotic. For the more sensitive organism, the serum and tissue levels achievable with normal dosage may be sufficient for bactericidal action, whereas the more resistant organism may simply suffer growth inhibition, a bacteriostatic effect, at that same antibiotic concentration.

The **antimicrobial spectrum** is the range of microbes against which the drug is effective. Table 43-1 lists common pathogenic microorganisms according to criteria set by microbiologists. A drug effective against only a few of these organisms has a narrow spectrum, such as penicillin G, which is primarily effective against gram-positive bacteria. In contrast a drug that can be used against several groups of organisms has a broad spectrum, such as tetracycline, which is effective against gram-positive and gram-negative bacteria, as well as against *Rickettsia* and *Chlamydia*.

Minimum inhibitory concentration (MIC) and **minimum bactericidal concentration (MBC)** relate to the antimicrobial spectrum. For each antibiotic and microorganism, it is possible to determine in the laboratory the amount of that drug required to halt the growth of the organism and the amount required to kill the organism. The concentrations are the lowest ones at which growth inhibition or cell death can be observed. A consideration of these figures and determination of safe blood levels for an antibiotic help determine an effective therapeutic regimen. For example, a blood concentration above the MBC is desirable, but whether that concentration can be obtained depends on the pharmacologic properties governing drug absorption and elimination and the threshold for toxicity produced by the drug in the host.

Table 43-1 Microbial Pathogens of Humans

Organisms	Common Diseases Produced
Viruses	
Influenza	Flu and upper respiratory tract infection
Herpes simplex	Skin, eye, and brain infections
HIV	Immunodeficiency, AIDS
Chlamydia	Psittacosis; eye and genital infections
Rickettsia	Typhus, Q fever, and Rocky Mountain spotted fever
Spirochetes	Syphilis and yaws
Eubacteria, Gram-Negative	
Haemophilus	Meningitis
Escherichia	Urinary tract infections
Proteus	Urinary tract infections
Klebsiella	Urinary tract infections and pneumonia
Pseudomonas	Urinary tract infections and meningitis
Neisseria	Meningitis and gonorrhea
Salmonella	Typhoid and gastroenteritis
Shigella	Dysentery
Eubacteria, Gram-Positive	
Staphylococcus	Soft tissue infections
Streptococcus	Upper respiratory tract infections
Mycobacteria	Tuberculosis, leprosy
Actinomycetes	Organ lesions and abscesses
Fungi	
Candida	Minor skin, mild respiratory, and severe systemic infections
Cryptococcus	
Histoplasma	
Blastomyces	

HIV, Human immunodeficiency virus; *AIDS,* acquired immunodeficiency syndrome.

FACTORS AFFECTING OUTCOME OF ANTIBIOTIC THERAPY

Microbial Resistance to Antibiotics

Not all microorganisms are sensitive to all antibiotics. Resistance to antibiotics may be inherent or acquired. Inherent resistance to an antibiotic is a stable genetic trait. For example, *Pseudomonas aeruginosa* is resistant to penicillin G in part because the drug cannot penetrate the cell wall complex of this organism. This property of the bacteria does not change significantly over time or on exposure to penicillin G.

In contrast **acquired resistance** represents a genetic change that converts a previously drug-sensitive bacteria to a drug-resistant one. *Staphylococcus aureus* is a good example of the clinical importance of acquired resistance. Strains of this bacteria isolated from clinical infections during the 1940s, before penicillin use became widespread, were almost always penicillin sensitive, whereas today clinically isolated *S. aureus* strains are mainly penicillin resistant. Resistance can also be acquired on a much shorter time scale. An example is the drug ciprofloxacin. When originally introduced, this drug was active against many gram-negative bacteria, including *P. aeruginosa*, and against gram-positive bacteria, including methicillin-resistant *S. aureus*. Within a year some institutions reported widespread resistance to the drug.

One particularly important mechanism for acquiring antibiotic resistance involves plasmids. **Plasmids** are small circular pieces of DNA separate from the bacterial chromosome. Many different kinds of plasmids exist and not all bacteria contain them. The most important plasmids of concern to medicine are those that contain genes for antibiotic resistance. Because plasmids may be rapidly passed between bacterial cells, antibiotic resistance can spread rapidly through an entire bacterial population. This mechanism for acquired resistance usually results in serious therapeutic difficulty because resistance to several antibiotics may occur simultaneously.

Microbiologists have recently discovered that plasmids can be shared between distantly related bacteria normally found in the human gastrointestinal (GI) tract. This fact leads us to the unsettling realization that if any bacteria is resistant to a drug, the gene for that resistance may be acquired by many bacteria, given time and exposure to the drug.

The mechanisms by which microorganisms achieve resistance to an antibiotic may be divided into three categories. Destruction of the antibiotic by the microorganism usually involves enzymes that chemically alter and thereby inactivate the drug. Examples of this process include penicillinase, which destroys penicillin and the acetylase, phosphorylase, and adenylating enzymes that inactivate the aminoglycoside antibiotics.

Bacteria may also achieve antibiotic resistance by reducing the uptake of the drug into the bacterial cell. Many antibiotics freely enter and in some cases are concentrated within bacterial cells. Resistance is achieved by blocking this uptake. An example of this type of resistance is with tetracyclines, which can freely enter sensitive bacteria but not resistant strains.

The third mechanism for resistance involves a mutation or an alteration in the target of the antibiotic in the microorganism. For example, erythromycin inhibits protein synthesis by binding to certain sites on the bacterial ribosome. Certain resistant microorganisms form altered ribosomes that do not bind erythromycin and are therefore resistant to its inhibitory action. A more clinically important example of this type of resistance is methicillin-resistant *S. aureus* (Box 43-1).

Identifying Bacteria Causing the Infection

The first step in antibiotic therapy is proper identification of the microorganism causing the disease. In some infections the symptoms are clear enough to allow accurate diagnosis with a physical examination only. In other cases culturing must be done to identify the organism. At some institutions nursing personnel are trained to take specimens for culture, whereas in others laboratory personnel or physicians perform this function. The second step in treatment is the selection of the proper antibiotic, a process that depends on knowledge of the pathogen involved. This decision may be based entirely on clinical experience or may be aided by antibiotic susceptibility testing carried out in

---

> **Box 43-1   Are We Losing the Battle against Infectious Disease?**
>
> The question of whether we are losing the battle against infectious disease has been posed often in newspapers and magazines in the last few years. The answer is not simple. It is true that for most patients receiving antibiotics for acute conditions, therapy is effective. For a small but increasing number of patients, however, therapy fails and often fails spectacularly. The most worrisome failures are when the infection is caused by a well-known organism with a new pattern of resistance. For example, *Staphylococcus aureus*, a gram-positive bacterium that causes serious soft tissue infections, first developed resistance to penicillin. Then strains resistant to methicillin, a drug specifically designed for *S. aureus*, began to appear and spread. Now in many places, the only antibiotic still effective against *S. aureus* is vancomycin, but vancomycin resistance has appeared in enterococci and other bacteria. Genes for vancomycin resistance are carried on plasmids and are passed between strains of enterococci. It is expected that the genes for vancomycin resistance will in time pass to *S. aureus*, and in the not too distant future, an outbreak of totally drug-resistant *S. aureus* could occur. The race is on to see whether new drugs can be developed and tested in time to meet this challenge.

---

the microbiology laboratory on the pathogen isolated from the patient.

Site of Infection

Even when the proper drug has been selected, several factors influence effectiveness of therapy. One is the site of infection. For example, meningitis is difficult to treat partly because many antibiotics do not penetrate the blood-brain barrier very well, making an effective drug concentration difficult to obtain at the infection site. Similarly, many abscesses or soft tissue infections are not easily treated because the areas of infections are poorly perfused, and many drugs do not penetrate well into these areas. Healing is often hastened by surgical drainage.

Other Drugs

Other drugs the patient is receiving may influence the outcome of antibiotic therapy. Immunosuppressant drugs, for example, limit antibiotic effectiveness by depressing immune mechanisms that ordinarily assist in clearing the infection. Large doses of glucocorticoids cause significant immunosuppression. The use patterns of antibiotics can also influence resistance. For example, resistance to ciprofloxacin was more likely in settings where ciprofloxacin or its chemical relatives were widely used.

Clinical Status of the Patient

The patient's clinical status can alter the outcome of antibiotic therapy. For example, renal function is important because many antibiotics are excreted by the kidney. If renal function is impaired, drugs eliminated through the kidney may accumulate. Likewise, hepatic disease may cause accumulation of drugs that are eliminated primarily by liver mechanisms. Patients with insufficiencies in these organ systems must be watched closely for signs of drug toxicity, which may occur at lower dosages than would be expected in normal persons. Resistance to antibiotics is also more common in patients with certain chronic diseases such as cystic fibrosis. These patients are likely to have received multiple courses of antibiotic therapy, which also increases the risk of developing antibiotic resistance.

PROBLEMS IN ANTIBIOTIC THERAPY

Side Effects of Antibiotics

Direct Toxicity

Each antibiotic should be considered for its potential toxicity to the patient when it is administered. The signs of direct toxicity are often highly characteristic for a given class of drugs. For example, any aminoglycoside antibiotic can cause kidney damage and loss of hearing or equilibrium. When these drugs are given, patients should be observed closely for these toxic signs. Even drugs with a high TI occasionally cause direct toxic reactions. For example, at high enough dosages penicillin can have direct effects on the central nervous system. Nurses should be alert to these signs. Direct toxic reactions to antibiotics are often dose dependent and would be expected to be more common and serious when high dosages of drugs are given or when drug accumulation occurs in patients with renal or hepatic impairment.

Allergic Reactions

Allergies commonly occur with several antibiotics. The penicillins can produce allergic reactions that range from simple rashes to anaphylactic shock. Allergies occur in patients who have previously been exposed in the medical setting or in the environment to the antibiotic or compounds chemically related to it. Environmental exposure may be direct, as in workers in the antibiotic industry, or more subtle. For example, animals intended for immediate slaughter may not be treated with antibiotics also used in humans, but meat occasionally has contained sufficient residues of antibiotics to sensitize some people who consumed it.

Superinfections

Superinfections are infections that arise during antibiotic therapy. By definition, they involve microorganisms resistant to the antibiotic originally used; thus superinfections are often serious and difficult to treat. Such infections are more common with broad-spectrum than narrow-spectrum antibiotics. The reason is that broad-spectrum antibiotics eliminate much more of the natural bacterial flora and upset the ecologic controls that normally keep resistant pathogens in check. With tetracyclines, for example, yeasts such as *Candida* are often involved in superinfections.

Misuse of Antibiotics

Viral Infections

One common misconception is that antibiotics can cure any type of infectious disease, including those caused by viruses. In fact, no effective drugs exist to treat minor viral infections such as colds or sore throats (see Chapter 52). It is not always easy to distinguish these viral infections from bacterial infections that might respond to antibiotics, and patients often request antibiotics for every cold or sore throat they experience.

Early Discontinuation of Antibiotics

Many infections resolve quickly once appropriate antibiotics are administered. Thus it is tempting for patients to discontinue medication as soon as they feel better. This practice is dangerous for several reasons. Antibiotics with bacteriostatic action inhibit growth of bacteria, but the bacteria remain alive, at least until the immune system can eliminate them. Therefore if therapy is stopped too early, these organisms may again proliferate and relapse may occur. Not only does this prolong recovery, but it may also make the disease more difficult to treat. If we consider that the organisms most resistant to the drugs being used are the ones that probably survive longest, we can appreciate that these resistant organisms may cause the relapse. Therapy may therefore be difficult because some degree of drug resistance has occurred.

One excuse often given when patients stop antibiotic therapy early is that they wish to have the drug on hand in case they ever need it again. This practice is dangerous not only for the reasons just discussed but also because it assumes that patients can diagnose future illnesses accurately. Self-medication with old, unused antibiotic prescriptions may delay proper medical attention and prolong or worsen the patient's disease. Once medication has been started, culture results become unreliable and proper diagnosis may be impossible. Thus patients should be discouraged from saving previously prescribed antibiotics to take them "just until I can get to the doctor."

Instability of Stored Antibiotics

Many drugs require special storage conditions and do not remain active for long when exposed to the warm, humid environment of most bathroom medicine cabinets. Drugs stored for weeks or months under such conditions may be inactive or may convert to forms that are more toxic. For example, tetracyclines tend to be light-sensitive and break down to toxic compounds.

Potential Dangers to Children

Any drug that remains in the household may be a hazard to children. Proper use and disposal of drugs is important to protect children from accidental poisoning. In addition, young children may be much more sensitive than adults to certain antibiotics. Antibiotics should never be given to children without first consulting a physician.

Nursing Process Overview

Antiinfective Therapy

Assessment

Perform a complete physical assessment. Assess for fever, drainage, elevation of the white blood cell count, and signs of inflammation such as redness, swelling, or tenderness. Monitor vital signs. Assess for symptoms appropriate to the problem being treated: cough, production of phlegm, or nasal drainage; difficulty or pain while urinating; and frequent urination. Obtain a history of any exposure to infecting organisms and preexisting medical condition. Obtain the ordered cultures.

Nursing Diagnoses

- Altered bowel elimination: diarrhea and cramping related to antiinfective use
- Risk for vaginal superinfection with *Candida*

Patient Outcomes

The patient will complete the course of antiinfective therapy with minimal GI discomfort. The patient will have oral or vaginal superinfection diagnosed early if it occurs and will complete a course of appropriate drug therapy to treat it.

Planning/Implementation

Obtain additional data relevant to the antibiotic prescribed, such as renal function or liver function studies, and assessment of possible ototoxicity. Monitor vital signs, blood count, culture reports, and the patient's subjective and objective signs of infection. Maintain adequate nutritional and fluid intake, and use other therapies appropriate to the problem being treated: warm soaks, debridement of infected areas, and special wound-cleaning procedures. Use agents for patient comfort such as antipyretics for fever or bladder analgesics for bladder discomfort. Assess for side effects and for superinfection.

Evaluation

Before discharge, ascertain that the patient can explain why and how to take the prescribed drug, why it is necessary to continue the course of therapy as prescribed, what side effects may occur and which ones warrant contacting the physician, and what symptoms indicate that the medication is not effective.

Nursing Implications Summary

Antiinfective Agents

Drug Administration

➤ Assess for history of allergy to antibiotics or antiinfectives before administering dose. Phrase questions appropriately. For example, "Are there any medicines you should not take and why?" may elicit more information than "Are you allergic to any antibiotics?" Have the patient describe previous problems. A gastric upset is probably a side effect; the development of hives is probably an allergic reaction. If there is a question about whether the patient is allergic to a medication, consult the physician before administering the dose.

➤ Label the patient's health record, chart, medication record, and armband (per agency procedure) if the patient is allergic to any medications. In some hospitals patients with allergies wear a second specially marked or colored identification bracelet indicating allergies.

➤ Observe all patients receiving antiinfective agents for possible allergic reactions. Monitor vital signs. Have equipment and personnel available to treat acute allergic reactions. Have drugs such as epinephrine, antihistamines, and steroids available to treat allergic reactions.

➤ Nurses who are allergic to any antiinfective agent should wear gloves and should consider wearing protective eye covering and a mask when preparing or administering doses of that drug.

➤ Read the physician's orders and drug labels carefully. Within a class of antiinfectives, several drugs may have similar names.

➤ Reconstitute parenteral forms as directed by the label or in the manufacturer's literature. Date and initial the vial if some of the drug will be saved for later use. Do not use undated reconstituted medications. Observe expiration dates.

➤ For intramuscular (IM) administration, use large muscle masses (see Chapter 5). Aspirate before administering to prevent inadvertent intravenous (IV) administration. Record and rotate injection sites. If the ordered dose is a large volume of medication, divide the dose and administer in two injections.

Nursing in the Community

➤ Review the anticipated benefits and possible side effects of drug therapy with the patient. Instruct the patient to report the development of any unexpected sign or symptom.

➤ Encourage patients with a known allergy to any drug to wear a medical identification tag or bracelet indicating allergies.

➤ Instruct the patients to take antiinfective agents for as long as prescribed (usually 7 to 10 days), even if they begin to feel better. Emphasize the following points: Do not share drugs with other family members. Do not save remaining doses to treat later infections. Do not administer drugs prescribed for adults to children.

Continued

Nursing Implications Summary—cont'd

➤ Antiinfectives work best when taken at evenly spaced intervals throughout the day. Discuss with the patient an appropriate dosing schedule based on the prescribed drug frequency.

➤ Tell pregnant or lactating women not to take any antiinfective agents without consulting the physician.

➤ Remind the patient to shake suspensions thoroughly before pouring dose and to use the same spoon or same size medicine cup to ensure the same dosage each time.

➤ Some oral liquids are dispensed in bottles with droppers, although the medicine is to be taken orally; review this with patients.

➤ Remind the patient that chewable tablets should be chewed and swallowed for best effect.

➤ Tell the patient to swallow enteric-coated preparations whole, without crushing or chewing. Consult the pharmacist if in doubt.

➤ Review with the patient any restrictions about taking the drug with meals, milk, or a snack and special storage considerations such as refrigeration. Pharmacists usually label drugs that must be refrigerated.

➤ If a dose is missed, tell the patient to take it as soon as remembered, unless it is almost time for the next dose, in which case the missed dose should be omitted. Exact guidelines vary depending on the frequency of doses. Instruct the patient not to double up for missed doses.

➤ Remind parents to keep drugs out of the reach of children. Pediatric dosage forms are often disguised in pleasant-tasting syrups and diluents, and children may want to take more than ordered doses. Tell parents to give children only drugs and dosages prescribed for children.

➤ Instruct the patient to keep all health care providers informed of all drugs being taken. Review all drugs a patient is taking. If questions about drug incompatibilities arise, consult the physician or pharmacist.

➤ In the home, check drug containers for expiration dates and encourage the patient to discard expired medications. Assess the area where the patient stores medications, and make recommendations if needed.

CHAPTER REVIEW

Application

1. What is the principle of selective toxicity?
2. Why is selective toxicity possible to achieve?
3. How is selective toxicity achieved? How is it measured?
4. What is the difference between a bacteriostatic and a bactericidal drug?
5. What is the antimicrobial spectrum of a drug?
6. Define minimum inhibitory concentration (MIC) and minimum bactericidal concentration (MBC).
7. What is the difference between inherent and acquired resistance?
8. What are the three ways microorganisms resist the action of antibiotics?
9. Name five factors that influence the outcome of antibiotic therapy.
10. What problems may arise during antibiotic therapy?
11. What two dangers are associated with saving leftover antibiotics in the home?

Critical Thinking

1. How would you assess for superinfections?
2. What are some of the common misuses of antibiotics? What should you teach patients to help avoid these problems?
3. What are the dangers associated with premature cessation of antibiotic therapy? What would you teach patients about this problem?

References

Cohen FL, Tartasky D: Microbial resistance to drug therapy: a review, *Am J Infect Cont* 25(1):51-64, 1997.

DeGroot-Kosolcharoen J: Culture and sensitivity testing, *Nursing* 26(9):33-38, 1996.

Kayley J: Use of IV antibiotics at home, *Community Nurse* 2(7):15-16, 1996.

Pilling M, Walley T: Parenteral antibiotics at home in cystic fibrosis: experiences and attitudes of recipients, *Health Social Care Comm* 5(3):209-212, 1997.

Penicillins, Cephalosporins, and Related Drugs

OBJECTIVES

After studying this chapter, you should be able to do the following:

- *Explain the specific antibacterial effects of penicillins and cephalosporins.*
- *Describe the classes of penicillins.*
- *Explain mechanisms of resistance that bacteria develop to penicillins and cephalosporins.*
- *Describe the most common reactions to penicillins and cephalosporins.*
- *Develop a nursing care plan for a patient receiving one of the drugs discussed in this chapter.*

CHAPTER OVERVIEW

This chapter introduces the most widely used family of antibiotics in medical practice, the beta-lactam antibiotics, of which penicillins and cephalosporins are the most important representatives. These agents share many properties, but individual drugs also have some important distinguishing characteristics.

THERAPEUTIC RATIONALE: BACTERIAL INFECTIONS

Infections caused by bacteria take many forms, ranging from mild local infections to life-threatening systemic disease. The large family of **beta-lactam antibiotics** includes agents that are effective against most commonly encountered pathogens. The name *beta-lactam* comes from the highly reactive beta-lactam ring system that is shared by all members of this class and is required for antibacterial activity. **Penicillins** are named for the mold *Penicillium* that was the first discovered source of a beta-lactam antibiotic. **Cephalosporins** were discovered later, originally in extracts of the mold *Cephalosporium*.

THERAPEUTIC AGENTS: DRUGS TO TREAT BACTERIAL INFECTIONS

Beta-Lactam Antibiotics

Mechanism of Action and Bacterial Resistance

Penicillins, cephalosporins, and other beta-lactam antibiotics are irreversible inhibitors of a bacterial enzyme called transpeptidase. This enzyme cross-links strands of cell wall material called peptidoglycan. When cross-linking occurs, peptidoglycan becomes rigid and is an effective cell wall. When cross-linking is blocked by beta-lactam antibiotics, cell wall synthesis continues, but the unreinforced strands formed cannot resist the osmotic forces within the bacterial cell. The bacterium may explode. Because exposed bacteria may be directly killed, beta-lactam antibiotics are classified as bactericidal drugs. However, even at dosages below those required to kill bacteria, penicillins and cephalosporins may disrupt the bacterial cell wall enough to make the bacteria more liable to elimination by the immune system of the host.

Beta-lactam antibiotics prevent formation of new, intact cell wall and thus are most effective against actively multiplying bacteria. These drugs are highly selective because they attack a process that does not exist in mammalian cells.

Resistance to penicillins and cephalosporins develops in microorganisms. The most common mechanism for resistance involves enzymes called **beta-lactamases.** These enzymes are usually referred to as penicillinases or cephalosporinases, depending on which type of drug the enzyme is most effective against. These enzymes destroy the penicillin or cephalosporin molecule, rendering the drug inactive. Some organisms possess these enzymes as part of their normal metabolic makeup and therefore are intrinsically resistant to beta-lactam antibiotics. Other organisms may acquire the enzyme and thus be converted from antibiotic sensitivity to resistance. Clinically important examples of acquired penicillin resistance are *Staphylococcus aureus* and *Neisseria gonorrhoeae.* Although 25 years ago both organisms could routinely be considered sensitive to penicillin G, today significant resistance to penicillin G exists for both organisms. In some hospitals, more than 90% of *S. aureus* strains are resistant.

Although resistance to penicillins is most commonly acquired by developing beta-lactamase, other important forms of resistance are known. The most clinically relevant example may be **methicillin-resistant *Staphylococcus aureus*** (MRSA). In this organism, resistance is conferred by altered penicillin targets. Altered targets are also the basis for resistance of *Streptococcus pneumoniae* to penicillin, which is an increasingly common clinical problem today.

Pharmacokinetics

Most penicillins and cephalosporins are excreted renally, by a combination of glomerular filtration and active tubular secretion. Exceptions are cefotaxime, cephalothin, and cephapirin, which are metabolized in liver to a significant degree. Both metabolites and unchanged drug are eliminated in urine. Nafcillin, ceftriaxone, cefpodoxime, and cefoperazone are also exceptions in that they are eliminated mostly in bile.

Penicillins, cephalosporins, and other beta-lactam antibiotics may accumulate in patients with impaired renal function. Therefore the dosage of many of these drugs may be reduced when renal function is lower than normal. Dosage is adjusted based on creatinine clearance, according to guidelines in the package insert for each individual drug.

Uses

The primary clinical uses of the beta-lactam antibiotics are summarized in Table 44-1 and in the following sections on individual drugs.

Adverse Reactions and Contraindications

Allergies are the most common adverse reaction to penicillins. Many patients experience skin rashes or urticaria, but anaphylaxis is a much more dangerous allergic response. Injections of penicillin are responsible for most anaphylactic episodes, but any form of exposure to penicillin may produce anaphylaxis in sensitive individuals. Cephalosporins are good allergens much like penicillins, and many patients experience similar allergic reactions. Many patients who are allergic to penicillins are also allergic to cephalosporins and vice versa.

Allergic rashes and drug fevers usually appear after several days of therapy, but the onset of anaphylaxis is nearly always within 10 minutes. A patient beginning therapy with a beta-lactam antibiotic should remain under medical supervision for 30 minutes after the injection so that if anaphylaxis develops, help is immediately available. If anaphylaxis occurs, medical personnel first should administer subcutaneous epinephrine. Anaphylaxis involves profound vasomotor collapse, and laryngeal edema may further complicate resuscitation efforts. Steroids may be required, as well as a tracheostomy and oxygen under positive pressure. All of these emergency supplies should be on hand in any clinical setting where antibiotics are administered.

An estimated 3% to 5% of the general population is allergic to penicillin, but 10% of those who have previously received penicillin in a medical setting may be allergic. Patients about to receive penicillin must be asked if they have ever been given penicillin before and if they have ever had a rash or other allergic symptom during drug therapy. This information, although necessary, is somewhat unreliable. Many patients cannot recall what drugs they have received. Other patients may report past allergy to penicillin, yet they do not experience allergic reactions when reexposed. In these cases the original reaction may not have been a true penicillin allergy. Ampicillin, for example, may cause a benign macular eruption rather than a urticarial reaction. This toxic rash is not a sign of allergy but may be reported as an allergy by the patient.

Despite the uncertainties in assessing past allergic responses, a medically documented prior allergic response to a penicillin, a cephalosporin, or penicillamine is the only contraindication to the use of most beta-lactam antibiotics.

The second most common reaction to beta-lactam antibiotics is gastrointestinal (GI) tract distress. Oral penicillin or cephalosporin preparations are the most likely to cause this side effect. Reactions include irritation and inflammation of the upper GI tract, nausea, vomiting, and diarrhea. Severe reactions may include antibiotic-associated pseudomembranous colitis. This condition arises when normal bacterial flora of the bowel are destroyed by an antibiotic, allowing *Clostridium difficile* to flourish. This anaerobic organism releases a toxin that causes the symptoms of pseudomembranous colitis, which include violent watery diarrhea and sloughing of tissue lining the GI tract.

Table 44-1   Primary Uses of Beta-Lactam Antibiotics

Organism	Typical Infections	Beta-Lactam Antibiotics Used*
Gram-Positive Bacteria		
Streptococcus pneumoniae	Otitis media, sinusitis, pneumonia, meningitis	PENICILLIN G, PENICILLIN V, amoxicillin, ampicillin, piperacillin
Group A streptococci (e.g., *S. pyogenes*)	Pharyngitis, scarlet fever, impetigo, rheumatic fever	PENICILLIN G, PENICILLIN V, amoxicillin, ampicillin, cephalosporins, piperacillin
Group B streptococci (e.g., *S. agalactiae*)	Neonatal sepsis, postpartum infections, meningitis	AMOXICILLIN, AMPICILLIN, MEZLOCILLIN, PENICILLIN G, PENICILLIN V, PIPERACILLIN, cephalosporins
Enterococci	Endocarditis, urinary tract infections, nosocomial infections	AMPICILLIN, PENICILLIN G, imipenem, penicillin V
Staphylococcus aureus nonpenicillinase	Boils, wound infections, skin infections, bone infections, endocarditis, meningitis	FIRST-GENERATION CEPHALOSPORINS, penicillin G, penicillin V, amoxicillin, ampicillin, imipenem
Staphylococcus aureus penicillinase strains	Boils, wound infections, skin infections, bone infections, endocarditis, meningitis	FIRST-GENERATION CEPHALOSPORINS, CLOXACILLIN, DICLOXACILLIN, METHICILLIN, NAFCILLIN, OXACILLIN, imipenem
Gram-Negative Bacteria		
Haemophilus influenzae	Pneumonia, bacteremia, tissue infections, meningitis, otitis media	AMOXICILLIN, AMPICILLIN, CEFUROXIME, THIRD-GENERATION CEPHALOSPORINS (parenteral), aztreonam
Neisseria gonorrhoeae	Gonorrhea, pelvic inflammatory disease	CEFTRIAXONE, CEFIXIME, amoxicillin
Neisseria meningitidis	Meningitis	PENICILLIN G, amoxicillin, ampicillin, cefotaxime, ceftriaxone, cefuroxime
Escherichia coli	Diarrhea, wound infections, urinary tract infections	CEPHALOSPORINS, LORACARBEF, amoxicillin, ampicillin, aztreonam, imipenem, mezlocillin, piperacillin
Klebsiella pneumoniae	Pneumonia, urinary tract infections	CEPHALOSPORINS (except cefadroxil, cefprozil, cephalexin), aztreonam, imipenem
Serratia, Providencia	Bacteremia, nosocomial infections	CEFOPERAZONE, CEFOTETAN, CEFTAZIDIME, CEFTIZOXIME, ceftriaxone
Pseudomonas aeruginosa	Urinary tract infections, burn infections, wound infections, pneumonia	MEZLOCILLIN, PIPERACILLIN, TICARCILLIN, aztreonam, ceftazidime, imipenem
Bacteroides fragilis	Abscesses, infections at anaerobic sites	AMPICILLIN + SULBACTAM, IMIPENEM, TICARCILLIN + CLAVULANATE, mezlocillin, piperacillin, ticarcillin
Spirochetes		
Treponema pallidum	Syphilis	PENICILLIN G, BENZATHINE PENICILLIN G
Borrelia burgdorferi	Lyme disease	CEFOTAXIME, CEFTRIAXONE, AMOXICILLIN

*Primary drugs are set in UPPER CASE; alternative drugs are set in lower case.

Toxicity

Direct drug toxicity with penicillins is low; massive doses have been given with no ill effects. The tissue most sensitive to direct effects is the central nervous system (CNS). Intrathecal injection (into the subarachnoid space or cerebrospinal fluid [CSF]) may produce convulsions. Convulsions also occur occasionally in patients given high dosages intramuscularly or intravenously, especially if renal impairment exists and the drug accumulates. A relatively high concentration must be achieved in the CSF before convulsions occur. This complication could occur in older adult patients being treated for serious infections such as streptococcal endocarditis. These patients may receive 25 to 40 million units of penicillin daily to maintain continuous bactericidal drug concentrations. Healthy persons can readily eliminate these large amounts through their kidneys, but older adults may have diminished renal function (see Geriatric Considerations box). Therefore drug accumulation may oc-

 GERIATRIC CONSIDERATIONS

Penicillins and Cephalosporins

THE PROBLEM
Most beta-lactam antibiotics are excreted primarily through the kidneys, with biliary excretion as an alternative route. If renal function is impaired, excretion may be slowed, and the drug can accumulate. Healthy geriatric patients may have significantly lower renal function than younger adults and perhaps should be considered as renally impaired.

SOLUTIONS
When administering these drugs to older adult patients, it is important to monitor renal function. Dosages should be adjusted for renal function as prescribed or as described in the package insert.

cur, and penicillin may enter the CNS. The first sign may be loss of consciousness or myoclonic movements. Generalized seizures may follow.

Another group of patients with reduced ability to excrete penicillin are newborn infants. Because of this limitation, neonates receive carefully adjusted penicillin dosages based on their body weight and reduced clearance of penicillin.

Interactions

Penicillins and cephalosporins require care in handling and diluting for intramuscular (IM) or intravenous (IV) therapy. Many penicillins require properly buffered solutions for stability; thus not all are compatible with common IV fluids. The nurse should check the package insert or ask the pharmacist before adding penicillins or cephalosporins to any IV fluid.

Beta-lactam antibiotics are also incompatible in solution with aminoglycoside antibiotics. Both drugs are inactivated. When patients must receive both drugs, they are given at least 1 hour apart at separate sites.

Probenecid is sometimes used with penicillins to increase their effective duration of action by slowing active tubular secretion in the kidney. Probenecid may cause toxic reactions that are difficult to distinguish from a penicillin reaction. For example, probenecid may cause chills, fever, rash, GI tract irritation, and anemia. Probenecid also blocks renal excretion of some, but not all, cephalosporins.

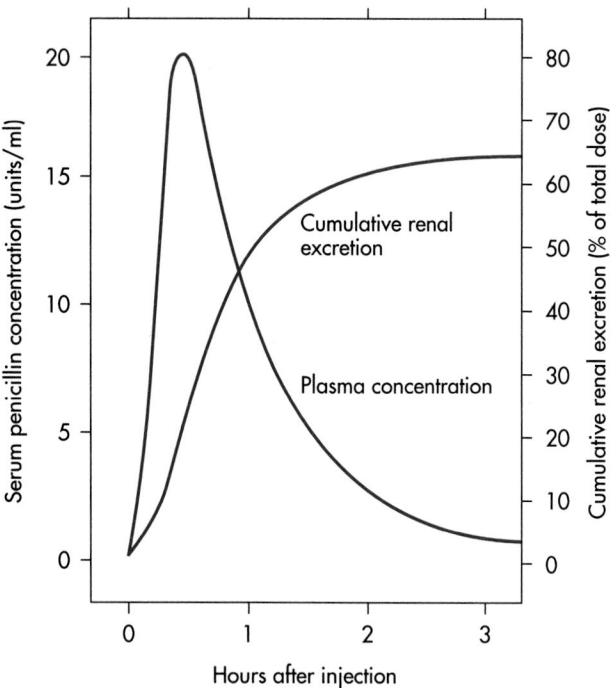

Figure 44-1 Serum concentration and urinary excretion of intramuscular (IM) dose of penicillin G. Penicillin G is efficiently and rapidly absorbed after IM injections. Peak plasma concentrations of drug appear 20 to 30 minutes after injection. Penicillin G is actively secreted by renal tubules, accounting for rapid elimination half-time of about 20 to 30 minutes. Most of drug dose ends up in urine as unaltered penicillin.

Many penicillins and cephalosporins may block excretion of methotrexate because these drugs may compete for elimination by active tubular secretion. If methotrexate accumulates, significant toxicity may result.

Individual penicillins and cephalosporins occasionally have specific interactions with other drugs. These are listed under the individual antibiotics in the following sections.

Narrow-Spectrum Penicillins

▼ penicillin G and penicillin V

Mechanism of Action and Bacterial Resistance

All beta-lactam antibiotics share the same bactericidal mechanism of action: they inhibit bacterial cell wall biosynthesis. Resistance to **penicillin G** and penicillin V (Table 44-2) is often caused by penicillinases, enzymes that destroy the antibiotic. Examples include *S. aureus* and *N. gonorrhoeae*. Resistance in *S. pneumoniae* is mediated by changes in the penicillin target protein that render them impervious to inhibition by the antibiotic.

Pharmacokinetics

The penicillin molecule must remain intact to retain antibacterial activity. At least one bond in the molecule is sensitive to acid, which explains the lability of penicillin G in the stomach. Approximately 30% of an oral dose is absorbed, the rest being destroyed in the stomach or retained in the intestine and destroyed by bacteria in the large bowel. Because of the incomplete and somewhat variable absorption of penicillin G by this route, oral doses of penicillin G are not recommended.

Attempts to improve the oral absorption of penicillin G led to the development of penicillin V. Penicillin V is more acid stable and thus more efficiently absorbed from the GI tract than penicillin G; however, penicillin V is less potent as an antibacterial agent. Penicillin V should be given 1 hour before or 2 hours after meals because food can interfere with absorption.

Penicillin G is rapidly and completely absorbed after IM injection, so serum concentrations reach a peak 20 to 30 minutes after injection (Figure 44-1). This peak concentration persists for only a short time, primarily because the kidney so efficiently removes penicillin from the blood. Within 2 to 3 hours after IM injection, about 60% of the penicillin dose appears in urine. The drug in urine is unchanged and still possesses antibacterial activity. Penicillin enters urine by active secretion in the renal tubule.

Penicillin G is distributed to many tissues, with high concentrations found in blood, liver, kidney, and bile. Very little drug is found in brain or CSF in healthy persons. If the meninges are inflamed, as in meningitis, penicillin can enter the CNS in significant amounts.

Uses

Penicillin G is a narrow-spectrum antibiotic; the organisms against which it is effective are summarized in Table 44-1. Most of the sensitive organisms are gram-positive bacteria.

Table 44-2 Common Dosages of Representative Penicillins

Generic Name	Trade Name	Administration/Dosage
amoxicillin	Amoxil* Polymox	ORAL: *Adults*—250-500 mg every 8 hr. *Infants and children 8-20 kg*—6.7-13.3 mg/kg body weight every 8 hr.
amoxicillin + K clavulanate	Augmentin Clavulin†	ORAL: *Adults*—250 or 500 mg amoxicillin + 125 mg clavulanate every 8 hr. FDA pregnancy category B. *Infants up to 40 kg*—Amoxicillin 6.7-13.3 mg/kg body weight + 1.7-3.3 mg clavulanate every 8 hr.
ampicillin	Ampicin† Omnipen Polycillin Principen	ORAL: *Adults*—250-500 mg every 6 hr. FDA pregnancy category B. *Infants*—12.5-25 mg/kg body weight every 6-12 hr. INTRAMUSCULAR, INTRAVENOUS: *Adults*—Same as for oral. *Infants*—25-50 mg/kg body weight every 6-12 hr.
ampicillin + sulbactam	Unasyn	INTRAMUSCULAR, INTRAVENOUS: *Adults*—1-2 g ampicillin and 0.5-1 g sulbactam every 6 hr. FDA pregnancy category B.
bacampicillin	Penglobe† Spectrobid	ORAL: *Adults*—400-800 mg every 12 hr. FDA pregnancy category B. *Children*—12.5-25 mg/kg every 12 hr.
benzathine penicillin G	Megacillin† Bicillin-LA*	ORAL: *Adults*—200,000-500,000 units every 4-6 hr. FDA pregnancy category B. *Children*—25,000-90,000 units/kg/day, divided into 3, 4, or 6 doses. INTRAMUSCULAR: *Adults*—1.2 million units every 2-4 wk. *Children*—50,000 units/kg body weight up to 1.2 million units every 1-4 wk.
carbenicillin	Geopen* Pyopen†	INTRAMUSCULAR, INTRAVENOUS: *Adults*—1-2 g every 6 hr. Doses increased for life-threatening infections but should not exceed 40 g/day. FDA pregnancy category B. *Children*—25-75 mg/kg body weight every 6-12 hr.
carbenicillin indanyl sodium	Geocillin	ORAL: *Adults*—0.5-1 g (1 or 2 tablets) every 6 hr.
cloxacillin	Orbenin† Tegopen	ORAL: *Adults*—0.25-0.5 g every 6 hr. FDA pregnancy category B. *Infants*—6.25-12.5 mg/kg body weight every 6 hr. Administer 1 hr before or 2 hr after meals.
dicloxacillin	Dycill Dynapen	ORAL: *Adults*—0.125-0.25 g every 6 hr. FDA pregnancy category B. *Children*—3.125-6.25 mg/kg body weight every 6 hr. Administer 1 hr before or 2 hr after meals.
methicillin	Staphcillin	INTRAMUSCULAR: *Adults*—1 g every 4-6 hr. FDA pregnancy category B. *Children*—25 mg/kg body weight every 6 hr. Higher dosages used for meningitis. INTRAVENOUS: *Adults*—1 g every 6 hr. *Children*—Same as for intramuscular.
mezlocillin	Mezlin	INTRAMUSCULAR, INTRAVENOUS: *Adults*—3-4 g every 4-6 hr; do not exceed 24 g/day. FDA pregnancy category B. *Children*—50 mg/kg body weight every 4 hr.
nafcillin	Nafcil Nallpen Unipen*	ORAL: *Adults*—0.25-1 g every 4-6 hr. FDA pregnancy category B. *Children*—6.25-12.5 mg/kg body weight every 6 hr. *Neonates*—10 mg/kg body weight every 6-8 hr. INTRAMUSCULAR: *Adults*—500 mg every 4-6 hr. *Children*—25-50 mg/kg body weight every 8-12 hr. INTRAVENOUS: *Adults*—0.5-1 g every 4 hr. *Children*—20-40 mg/kg body weight every 8 hr.
oxacillin	Bactocill Prostaphlin	ORAL: *Adults*—0.5-1 g every 4-6 hr. FDA pregnancy category B. *Children*—12.5-25 mg/kg body weight every 6 hr. Administer 1 hr before or 2 hr after meals. INTRAMUSCULAR, INTRAVENOUS: *Adults*—0.25-2 g every 4-6 hr. *Children*—12.5-25 mg/kg body weight every 6 hr.
penicillin G		ORAL: *Adults*—200,000-500,000 units every 4-6 hr taken ½ hr before or 2 hr after meals. FDA pregnancy category B. *Children*—25,000-90,000 units/kg body weight daily in 3-6 doses. INTRAMUSCULAR, INTRAVENOUS: *Adults*—1-5 million units every 4-6 hr. *Children*—12,500-25,000 units/kg body weight every 6 hr. Higher dosages used for meningitis.
penicillin V	Pen-Vee K V-Cillin-K*	ORAL: *Adults*—125-500 mg every 6-8 hr. FDA pregnancy category B. *Children*—3.75-12.5 mg/kg body weight every 4-8 hr.
piperacillin	Pipracil*	INTRAMUSCULAR, INTRAVENOUS: *Adults*—3-4 g every 4-6 hr; do not exceed 24 g/day. FDA pregnancy category B. *Neonates*—For bacterial meningitis only: 50 mg/kg every 6-12 hr depending on age and body weight.
piperacillin + tazobactam	Zosyn Tazocin†	INTRAVENOUS: *Adults*—3-4 g piperacillin and 0.375-0.5 g tazobactam every 6-8 hr. FDA pregnancy category B.
procaine penicillin G	Crysticillin Wycillin*	INTRAMUSCULAR: *Adults and children*—600,000-1.2 million units every 12-24 hr. FDA pregnancy category B. *Infants*—50,000 units/kg body weight once daily.
ticarcillin	Ticar*	INTRAMUSCULAR: *Adults*—1 g every 6 hr. FDA pregnancy category B. *Children*—50-75 mg/kg body weight every 6 hr. INTRAVENOUS: *Adults and children*—For bacterial meningitis: 75 mg/kg body weight every 6 hr. *Neonates*—75 mg/kg body weight every 6-12 hr depending on age and body weight.
ticarcillin + clavulanate	Timentin*	INTRAVENOUS: *Adults and adolescents* >60 kg—3 g ticarcillin and 100 mg of clavulanic acid every 4-6 hr. FDA pregnancy category B. *Children 1 mo-12 yr old*—50 mg ticarcillin and 1.7 mg clavulanic acid per kg body weight every 4-6 hr.

*Available in Canada and the United States.
†Available in Canada only.

These bacteria are characterized by thick, peptidoglycan-rich cell walls, which react with the Gram stain. Some of these gram-positive organisms, such as *S. aureus, Streptococcus* species, and *S. pneumoniae,* cause common infections of the upper respiratory tract and soft tissues, as well as more serious infections. Other rare gram-positive organisms, such as the ones that cause anthrax, gas gangrene, tetanus, and diphtheria, are also sensitive to penicillin G.

Among gram-negative organisms, clinically significant sensitivity to penicillin G is seen only with *N. meningitidis* (meningococcus) and *N. gonorrhoeae* (gonococcus). Other common gram-negative organisms normally found in the bowel and those commonly responsible for urinary tract infections are clinically resistant to penicillin G. In the laboratory some of these gram-negative bacteria can be affected by high dosages of penicillin G, but these high drug levels cannot routinely be achieved in patients.

Although penicillin G is not effective against pathogens that commonly cause urinary tract infections, it is effective against syphilis and gonorrhea. Syphilis is often treated effectively with single-dose penicillin G therapy. Gonorrhea was at one time also treated with a single dose of penicillin G but the organism that causes gonorrhea (*N. gonorrhoeae*) has gradually developed resistance to penicillins. Therefore cephalosporins or other drugs are now preferred.

The uses of penicillin V are restricted to conditions in which oral antibiotic therapy is appropriate. Mild to moderately serious infections caused by penicillin-sensitive organisms may be treated with penicillin V. Penicillin V also may be used in prophylaxis, especially in patients who have had rheumatic fever. In these patients, penicillin V prophylaxis may prevent recurrent streptococcal infections, which could lead to heart or kidney damage.

Adverse Reactions and Contraindications

Rashes and other allergic reactions are the primary side effects with narrow-spectrum penicillins. Because anaphylaxis, although rare, is potentially lethal, a medically documented allergy is a contraindication to the use of these drugs.

Toxicity

Massive doses of penicillins may cause CNS toxicity, including seizures, in susceptible individuals, the elderly, and those with renal failure. In addition, potassium or sodium included in drug formulations may cause difficulties for some patients. For example, 1 million units of penicillin G and penicillin V may contain 1.5 mEq of potassium. Given at high enough dosages for long enough periods, potassium intoxication and cardiac arrhythmias may occur. Some preparations of penicillin G contain high concentrations of sodium, which may cause difficulties in patients with preexisting cardiac or renal dysfunction.

Interactions

Active secretion of penicillins involves a specific renal transport system for which several drugs may compete. Physi-

cians may take advantage of this trait by using another actively secreted drug such as probenecid to block penicillin excretion, thereby increasing peak penicillin concentration in the serum and increasing its effective duration.

Potassium supplements should be discontinued when potassium penicillin G or potassium penicillin V is being used to avoid potassium toxicity.

Repository Penicillins

procaine penicillin G and benzathine penicillin G

Mechanism of Action and Bacterial Resistance

The repository penicillins (see Table 44-2) contain penicillin G as the active ingredient and therefore have the same mechanism of action.

Pharmacokinetics

Repository penicillins were designed for slow absorption from IM injection sites, creating a long duration of action. Once drug is absorbed from depot sites, it is hydrolyzed to release penicillin G, which is the active agent.

Slower absorption of drug means that peak concentrations are lower and take longer to achieve. For example, procaine penicillin G yields peak drug concentrations in serum 3 to 4 hours after injection, and significant serum concentrations may persist for 48 hours. A single dose of 300,000 units of aqueous penicillin G gives peak serum levels of 6 to 8 units/ml within 30 minutes of injection, but procaine penicillin G at that same dose produces peak concentrations of only 1 to 2 units/ml. Benzathine penicillin G is absorbed even more slowly; thus peak serum levels occur 8 hours after injection, and useful serum levels persist for at least 2 weeks. An adult dose of 1.2 million units of benzathine penicillin G produces peak serum levels of only 0.1 to 0.3 units/ml.

Uses

Repository penicillins are not appropriate for serious infections when high serum concentrations of drug are required. Rather, these drugs are best used to maintain modest serum levels for relatively long periods. These conditions occur when very sensitive organisms are involved in mild to moderately serious infections or when prophylaxis is required.

Adverse Reactions and Contraindications

Procaine penicillin G is associated with CNS side effects because of the procaine content of the formulation. After injection, procaine may be released in significant amounts into the blood and may produce anxiety, lowered blood pressure, respiratory depression, and convulsions. These CNS reactions to procaine are usually transient, lasting less than 1 hour.

As with any penicillin, allergies can also occur, and documented prior allergies to beta-lactam antibiotics or penicillamine are a contraindication.

Toxicity

Repository penicillins are intended for deep muscular injections. Both preparations are stabilized suspensions of relatively insoluble forms of penicillin and contain up to about 2% weight/volume of emulsifying agents in addition to buffers. Such preparations should never be given by IV routes. Care must be taken on IM injection to prevent the accidental entry of these preparations into blood vessels because occlusion of blood vessels may result.

Penicillinase-Resistant Penicillins

cloxacillin, dicloxacillin, methicillin, nafcillin, and oxacillin

Mechanism of Action and Bacterial Resistance

Penicillinase-resistant penicillins retain the same mechanism of action as other penicillins, interfering with cell wall biosynthesis. These drugs were developed to resist the penicillinase produced by *S. aureus,* and thus are useful in many situations in which infections are caused by penicillinase-producing strains of that organism. Cloxacillin, dicloxacillin, and oxacillin are more potent than methicillin but are less potent than penicillin G.

Although these drugs resist penicillinase, other mechanisms of resistance may develop. A good example is methicillin, in which case resistance to the drug involves developing altered targets that render *S. aureus* tolerant to the drug. When methicillin resistance occurs, the organism also becomes resistant to all beta-lactam antibiotics and other antibiotics as well. Treatment of MRSA is a difficult clinical problem because of the limited number of effective drugs.

Pharmacokinetics

Methicillin is destroyed by stomach acid and therefore must be given parenterally. The other penicillinase-resistant penicillins are more stable in acid and thus may be used orally. Although nafcillin is sometimes used orally, it is not as well absorbed as oxacillin, cloxacillin, and dicloxacillin. With these latter drugs, oral absorption can be approximately doubled by fasting.

Nafcillin is unique among the penicillins in being excreted primarily in bile. All other penicillins are excreted primarily by the kidneys.

Uses

Penicillinase-resistant penicillins are primarily used in initial therapy when a penicillinase-producing gram-positive bacteria is suspected. In all other penicillin-sensitive infections penicillin G is preferred because it is more potent than penicillinase-resistant drugs. One of the dangers in too frequent use of penicillinase-resistant penicillins is that the unusual drug-tolerance type of resistance may increase in bacterial populations. This type of resistance then affects all beta-lactam antibiotics and makes the resistant organism difficult to eradicate.

Adverse Reactions and Contraindications

As with any oral antibiotics, GI tract disturbances may occur. Methicillin and oxacillin can cause significant blood dyscrasias and interstitial nephritis. These reactions are uncommon with other penicillins.

Toxicity

Allergies may occur, and documented prior allergic reactions to beta-lactam antibiotics or penicillamine are a contraindication.

Hepatotoxicity is associated with cloxacillin, dicloxacillin, and oxacillin more than with other penicillins. Hepatotoxicity may be more prevalent in patients with human immunodeficiency virus (HIV).

Interactions

Drug interactions seldom influence the use of these drugs.

Extended-Spectrum Penicillins

▼ ampicillin, amoxicillin, and bacampicillin

Mechanism of Action and Bacterial Resistance

Amoxicillin, ampicillin, and bacampicillin have the same mechanism of action as other beta-lactam antibiotics, in that they interfere with bacterial cell wall biosynthesis. Resistance to these drugs is commonly mediated by penicillinases.

Pharmacokinetics

Ampicillin is used orally, but only 35% to 50% of an oral dose is absorbed. Bacampicillin, a prodrug, is more rapidly and completely absorbed than ampicillin and releases ampicillin on breakdown in the body. Amoxicillin is more acid stable than ampicillin and therefore better absorbed orally.

Uses

The penicillins discussed previously have narrow antimicrobial spectra, being primarily useful against gram-positive bacteria (see Table 44-1). The development of ampicillin and related drugs broadened the penicillin spectrum to include several common gram-negative pathogens. These drugs penetrate gram-negative cell walls better and are therefore more effective than penicillin G against these organisms. The extended-spectrum penicillins are not resistant to penicillinase, so they may not be effective against *S. aureus* strains resistant to penicillin G.

Fixed combinations of ampicillin with sulbactam and amoxicillin with clavulanic acid are available. Sulbactam and clavulanic acid are inhibitors of beta-lactamases. Inclusion of these inhibitors in fixed combinations protects the active drugs from destruction, allowing their use against some organisms that would otherwise be resistant.

Adverse Reactions and Contraindications

All beta-lactam antibiotics have the potential to cause allergic reactions and are avoided in patients with reported penicillin allergies.

CASE STUDY
Child with Otitis Media

Name: Jay Doyle **Age**: 3 years **Weight**: 33 pounds
Height: 34 inches
Vital Signs: HR: 95 Respiratory Rate: 26
Blood Pressure: 78/40 Temperature: 100.8° F

REASON FOR VISIT
Fever of 102.6° F last night, congestion with runny eyes and nose, noisy breathing at night, and irritable behavior

HEALTH HISTORY
Born 5 weeks prematurely. Weighed 6 pounds, 14 ounces. APGAR scores of 8 and 9. Was transferred to special care nursery 12 hours after birth and placed on a ventilator for 2 days for episodes of apnea and bradycardia; was also given a course of antibiotics (mother does not remember name of drug). Discharged home with an apnea monitor, which he had for 5 months. Had several colds the first 6 months of life but began to have multiple episodes of otitis media when placed in a day-care situation. Treated seven times during the period between 6 months and 18 months for ear infections with six different antibiotics (see medication history below). At 2½ years, had bilateral myringotomy tubes placed and has had two documented cases of otitis media since that time. Continues to have high incidence of colds and congestion, and the question of allergies has been raised. Family practice doctor has referred child to an ear, nose, and throat (ENT) doctor for possible tonsillectomy and adenoidectomy.

SOCIAL HISTORY
Lives with parents, two cats, and one dog. Both parents smoke, as do several of their close friends. Also goes to maternal aunt's and uncle's house frequently, and they both smoke. Goes to a day-care center because both parents work. Dad is a house painter, and mom manages a liquor store. They own their own home, and Jay has his own room.

FAMILY HEALTH HISTORY
Father and mother in good health. Father has history of "sensitive skin" and has recurrent boils and dry skin conditions. He is allergic to bromide in swimming pools. Fraternal grandfather with cerebrovascular accident, hypertension, and colon-rectal cancer. Maternal grandmother with history of diabetes, emphysema, and depression.

PREVIOUS ANTIBIOTICS (IN ORDER)
For otitis: Amoxil X 2; Ceclor, Suprax, Augmentin, Cefzil, (Tubes) Bactrim
   For swollen tonsils: Amoxil

PHYSICAL EXAMINATION
Cervical lymph nodes enlarged; tonsils 3+, no exudate; clear nasal discharge, mouth breathing; tympanic membranes erythematous, tubes in place bilaterally draining pus; Tympanogram flat; no other significant findings, no lab values to consider

ASSESSMENT
Bilateral otitis media, upper respiratory infection

PLAN
Antibiotic, decongestant, fluids, and education of parent

1. What additional information should you gather in planning care for this child?
2. What is the likely bacteria or virus that is causing his otitis media?
3. What elements in Jay's history and physical examination might help you explain his apparent propensity for ear infections?
4. What problems can you identify that need nursing interventions?
5. What antibiotic would be indicated to treat his otitis media? Why? What would be an appropriate dosage?
6. What other pharmacologic or nonpharmacologic interventions might be ordered?
7. What points need to be covered in the educational plan for the parents? What criteria will you use to follow up on Jay's treatment?

Ampicillin commonly causes GI tract complaints and is one of the leading causes of antibiotic-associated colitis. In its worst form, this condition progresses to pseudomembranous colitis, which is associated with destruction of the GI tract lining by a toxin formed by *C. difficile*.

Toxicity

Ampicillin commonly causes a rash that is not allergic in origin, called a toxic rash. This rash appears 8 to 10 days after the start of therapy. Incidence of rash is greatly increased in patients with mononucleosis.

Interactions

Ampicillin and amoxicillin may reduce effectiveness of oral contraceptives by effects on steroid metabolism. Alternate birth control may be sought during the cycle when the antibiotics are used.

Ampicillin and bacampicillin may increase the incidence of rashes in patients receiving allopurinol.

The interaction of ampicillin and amoxicillin with sulbactam and clavulanic acid produces synergistic antibacterial action, as described previously (see discussion of uses).

Anti-*Pseudomonas* Penicillins

carbenicillin, mezlocillin, piperacillin, and ticarcillin

Mechanism of Action and Bacterial Resistance

Like all other penicillins the anti-*Pseudomonas* penicillins interfere with bacterial cell wall synthesis in susceptible bacteria. These drugs are sensitive to penicillinases, including the one produced by *S. aureus*.

Pharmacokinetics

These drugs must be administered parenterally. For carbenicillin, an indanyl ester is available, which allows the drug to be used orally. However, indanyl carbenicillin does not produce high enough serum levels of carbenicillin to make the drug effective for most infections. Therefore it is reserved for use in urinary tract infections because the drug does accumulate to high concentrations in urine after oral dosage.

Uses

One pathogenic organism that is not sensitive to extended-spectrum penicillins is *Pseudomonas aeruginosa*. This gram-negative bacterium is responsible for certain urinary tract infections, bacteremias, and infections in burn patients and is unusually resistant to many antibiotics. Thus the anti-*Pseudomonas* drugs were developed specifically for use against this organism. Anti-*Pseudomonas* penicillins may be used with gentamicin or another anti-*Pseudomonas* aminoglycoside (see Chapter 43) to treat severe *Pseudomonas* infections.

Adverse Reactions and Contraindications

Carbenicillin, piperacillin, and ticarcillin often interfere with platelet function. This problem is worse in uremic patients because they have preexisting platelet dysfunction as a result of their renal disease.

Toxicity

Anti-*Pseudomonas* penicillins and especially preparations of ticarcillin contain high concentrations of sodium, which may cause difficulties in patients with preexisting cardiac or renal dysfunction.

Interactions

Gentamicin or other aminoglycosides must never be directly mixed in the syringe or IV bottle with any beta-lactam antibiotic because the two classes of drugs inactivate each other.

Cephalosporins

Mechanism of Action and Bacterial Resistance

Cephalosporins (Table 44-3) share the same mechanism as penicillins; both types of drugs inhibit the action of transpeptidase enzymes that cross-link bacterial cell wall peptidogly-can. The drugs are considered bactericidal because the weakened cell wall can rupture, leading to death of the bacteria.

Resistance to cephalosporins occurs most often because bacteria produce beta-lactamases that destroy the antibiotic. The enzymes that attack cephalosporins are often different from those that destroy penicillins. For example, the beta-lactamase of *S. aureus* that confers resistance to many penicillins does not attack cephalosporins.

Pharmacokinetics

Several cephalosporins are currently available for oral use (see Table 44-3). These preparations are well absorbed and produce effective serum concentrations of antibiotic. Absorption of cephalosporins from the GI tract is slowed by food in the stomach, but about the same amount of drug is ultimately absorbed as in a fasting patient.

Most cephalosporins are given parenterally because they are well absorbed from IM sites. The elimination half-times of all these drugs are about twice as long as that of penicillin G and are roughly equivalent to those of ampicillin or the penicillinase-resistant penicillins.

Cephalosporins are distributed in the body in a manner similar to that of penicillins, except that first-generation and most second-generation cephalosporins do not penetrate the CNS well enough to be used in meningitis. Cephalosporins, with the exception of cefoperazone, cefpodoxime, and ceftriaxone, are excreted primarily by the kidneys and are highly concentrated in urine, making them useful in treating common types of urinary tract infections.

Uses

The cephalosporins are divided into subgroups called generations. Among the first-generation cephalosporins, cephalothin and cefazolin are the most widely used parenteral agents, and cephalexin is the most widely used oral agent, although other members of this class differ little from these three. Second-generation cephalosporins differ from the first-generation drugs by having slightly extended activity against gram-negative bacteria. For example, some second-generation cephalosporins are especially active against *Haemophilus*. Third-generation cephalosporins generally have lower activity against gram-positive organisms than first-generation drugs, but some third-generation cephalosporins have significant activity against the gram-negative pathogen *P. aeruginosa*. They are the only cephalosporins to possess such activity. In addition, several third-generation cephalosporins are distributed reliably into the CNS.

The primary usefulness of cephalosporins is based on the differences in the antimicrobial spectra of penicillins and cephalosporins. First-generation cephalosporins resemble ampicillin in their effectiveness against gram-negative bacteria. Unlike ampicillin, however, cephalosporins resist the action of staphylococcal penicillinase and can be used when the organism is resistant to penicillin G. Cephalosporins are not effective against MRSA. Second- and third-generation cephalosporins are used for specific, serious infections

Table 44-3   Common Dosages of Representative Cephalosporins

Generic Name	Trade Name	Administration/Dosage‡
First Generation		
cefadroxil	Duricef*	ORAL: *Adults*—0.5-1 g every 12 hr. Maximum daily dose: 4 g. *Children*—15 mg/kg body weight every 12 hr.
cefazolin	Ancef* Kefzol*	INTRAMUSCULAR, INTRAVENOUS: *Adults*—250 mg every 8 hr, up to 1.5 g every 6 hr. Maximum daily dose: 6 g. *Children*—6.25-25 mg/kg body weight total every 6 hr.
cephalexin	Keflex*	ORAL: *Adults*—250-500 mg every 6 hr. *Children* >1 yr—6.25-25 mg/kg body weight every 6 hr.
cephalothin	Keflin*	INTRAVENOUS, INTRAMUSCULAR: *Adults*—0.5-2 g every 4-6 hr. *Children*—20-40 mg/kg body weight every 6 hr.
cephapirin	Cefadyl	INTRAMUSCULAR, INTRAVENOUS: *Adults*—0.5-1 g every 4-6 hr. *Children* >3 mo—10-20 mg/kg body weight every 6 hr.
cephradine	Velosef	ORAL, INTRAMUSCULAR, INTRAVENOUS: *Adults*—1-4 g total daily dose. *Children* >9 mo—6.25-12.5 mg/kg body weight every 6 hr. Maximum daily dose: 4 g.
Second Generation		
cefaclor	Ceclor*	ORAL: *Adults*—250-500 mg every 8 hr. *Children*—10-20 mg/kg body weight, not to exceed 1 g/day.
cefamandole	Mandol*	INTRAMUSCULAR, INTRAVENOUS: *Adults*—500 mg-2 g every 4-8 hr. Maximum daily dose: 12 g. *Children*—8.3-33.3 mg/kg body weight every 4-8 hr.
cefonicid	Monocid	INTRAMUSCULAR, INTRAVENOUS: *Adults*—1-2 g once daily. No more than 1 g should be given at single intramuscular site.
cefotetan	Cefotan*	INTRAMUSCULAR, INTRAVENOUS: *Adults*—1-3 g every 12 hr. Maximum daily dose: 6 g.
cefoxitin	Mefoxin*	INTRAVENOUS: *Adults*—1-2 g every 4-8 hr. *Children*—20-40 mg/kg body weight every 6-8 hr. Maximum daily dose: 12 g.
cefprozil	Cefzil*	ORAL: *Adults*—250-500 mg every 12 hr. *Children* >6 mo—7.5-15 mg/kg every 12 hr. Maximum daily dose: 1 g.
cefuroxime	Kefurox* Zinacef*	INTRAMUSCULAR, INTRAVENOUS: *Adults*—0.75-1.5 g every 8 hr. *Children* >1 mo—12.5-33.3 mg/kg body weight every 6-8 hr.
cefuroxime axetil	Ceftin*	ORAL: *Adults*—250-500 mg every 12 hr. *Children*—125-250 mg every 12 hr.
Third Generation		
cefepime	Maxipime*	INTRAVENOUS, INTRAMUSCULAR: *Adults*—0.5-1 g every 12 hr. Doses of 2 g every 8-12 hr by IV only.
cefixime	Suprax*	ORAL: *Adults*—200 mg every 12 hr or 400 mg once daily. *Children*—4 mg/kg body weight every 12 hr or 8 mg/kg body weight once daily.
cefoperazone	Cefobid	INTRAVENOUS: *Adults*—2-4 g every 8 hr. Daily dose not to exceed 12 g.
cefotaxime	Claforan*	INTRAVENOUS: *Adults*—1-2 g every 4-12 hr; maximum daily dose 12 g. *Neonates*—50 mg/kg body weight every 8 hr. *Infants* >1 mo to 50 kg—12.5-45 mg/kg every 6 hr. INTRAMUSCULAR: *Adults*—250 mg as single dose for uncomplicated gonorrhea.
cefpodoxime	Vantin	ORAL: *Adults*—100-400 mg every 12 hr. *Children* >5 mo—5 mg/kg every 12 hr.
ceftazidime	Fortaz* Tazicef	INTRAMUSCULAR, INTRAVENOUS: *Adults*—0.5-1 g every 8-12 hr. Doses of 2 g every 8 hr by IV only. *Children*—30-50 mg/kg body weight every 8-12 hr. Maximum daily dose: 6 g.
ceftibuten	Cedax	ORAL: *Adults*—400 mg once daily; do not exceed this dose. *Children* 6 mo-12 yr—9 mg/kg body weight once daily.
ceftizoxime	Cefizox*	INTRAVENOUS: *Adults*—1-4 g every 8-12 hr. *Adults* >65 yr— Dose should not exceed 1.5 g. *Children* >6 mo—50 mg/kg body weight every 6-8 hr. INTRAMUSCULAR: *Adults*—0.5-1 g once; frequency and dosage on follow-up depend on disease and renal function.
ceftriaxone	Rocephin*	INTRAMUSCULAR, INTRAVENOUS: *Adults*—1-2 g every 24 hr. *Children*—25-37.5 mg/kg body weight every 12 hr. Higher dosages for meningitis.

*Available in Canada and the United States.
‡ All drugs in this table are FDA pregnancy category B.

caused by gram-negative bacteria. For example, the third-generation drugs cefotaxime and ceftriaxone are now considered first-line drugs for typhoid fever.

Adverse Reactions and Contraindications

Many cephalosporins cause pain at the injection site. When given intravenously, these drugs cause phlebitis or thrombophlebitis and pain along the affected vein. Orally administered cephalosporins may cause gastric irritation, nausea, and vomiting. Superinfections may arise when these relatively broad-spectrum drugs are used, the most common being oral or vaginal candidiasis (yeast infections). Allergies to cephalosporins may take the form of rashes, serum sickness, hemolytic anemia, Stevens-Johnson syndrome, or anaphylaxis.

Cefamandole, cefoperazone, and cefotetan have been associated with platelet dysfunction. Patients should be observed for signs of unusual bleeding or bruising. The bleeding time or prothrombin time may require monitoring. Patients with bleeding disorders should not receive these drugs.

The only contraindication to the use of cephalosporins is a history of serious allergic reaction to penicillamine, a penicillin, or a cephalosporin. Caution should be used if these drugs must be given to patients with hepatic disease or renal impairment, and dosages may require reduction. Patients with GI tract disease may be more likely to develop antibiotic-associated pseudomembranous colitis.

Toxicity

Overdoses of cephalosporins may cause seizures. The drugs should be discontinued if seizures occur; specific treatment for controlling seizure activity may be required.

Interactions

Interstitial nephritis is sometimes seen with these drugs. Synergistic nephrotoxicity may occur when a cephalosporin is given with other nephrotoxic agents such as an aminoglycoside antibiotic or the diuretics furosemide or ethacrynic acid. Despite this risk, third-generation cephalosporins such as ceftazidime or cefoperazone may be given with an aminoglycoside such as amikacin, netilmicin, tobramycin, or gentamicin when synergistic activity is required to treat serious infections caused by *P. aeruginosa.*

Probenecid may prolong the persistence of cephalosporins in the body by blocking renal tubular secretion. Probenecid has no effect on the duration of action of cefoperazone, ceftriaxone, or ceftazidime because these three drugs depend less on active tubular secretion for elimination than do the other cephalosporins.

Cefamandole, cefoperazone, and cefotetan are a chemically related subset of cephalosporins that may cause excessive bleeding if used with anticoagulants or platelet-aggregation inhibitors such as aspirin. These drugs are also more likely than other cephalosporins to cause a disulfiram reaction if alcohol is ingested while the drugs are being taken.

Other Beta-Lactam Antibiotics

aztreonam

Mechanism of Action and Bacterial Resistance

Aztreonam (Table 44-4) acts in a way similar to other beta-lactam antibiotics, interfering with bacterial cell wall synthesis. Unlike most penicillins and cephalosporins, aztreonam inhibits or destroys primarily gram-negative aerobic bacteria. Aztreonam is ineffective for gram-positive or anaerobic bacteria because the drug fails to bind to critical targets in those organisms.

Pharmacokinetics

Aztreonam must be administered parenterally to obtain useful concentrations in plasma. The drug is distributed well to many body tissues and fluids but is relatively low in CSF. Excretion is primarily via the kidneys, and only minor amounts of drug are eliminated by hepatic mechanisms.

Uses

Aztreonam is given to treat urinary tract infections, septicemia, infections of the lower respiratory tract, intraabdominal or gynecologic infections, and soft tissue infections. These infections are typically caused by gram-negative bacteria, including *Pseudomonas.*

Adverse Reactions and Contraindications

The principal adverse reactions to aztreonam include pain or phlebitis at the injection site in up to 2.4% of patients. GI tract symptoms (including nausea, diarrhea, or vomiting) occur in up to 1.3% of patients. Rash and other symptoms of allergic reactions occur, as with all beta-lactam antibiotics.

The only contraindication to the use of aztreonam is prior allergic reaction to a beta-lactam antibiotic, but caution should be used when the drug must be given to patients with cirrhosis or renal impairment. Dosages may require reduction in these conditions.

imipenem and meropenem

Mechanism of Action and Bacterial Resistance

Imipenem and meropenem (see Table 44-4) inhibit bacterial cell wall synthesis in a manner similar to other beta-lactam antibiotics. Both drugs have broad antimicrobial spectra that include gram-positive, gram-negative, and anaerobic bacteria. Imipenem and meropenem are remarkably resistant to penicillinases and many cephalosporinases.

Resistance to imipenem has begun to appear in MRSA and *P. aeruginosa. Enterococcus faecium* is also resistant to imipenem. In some cases, unusual beta-lactamases are involved in resistance, but other mechanisms of resistance also occur.

Table 44-4	**Clinical Summary of Other Beta-Lactam Antibiotics**		
Generic Name	**Trade Name**	**Administration/Dosage**	
aztreonam	Azactam	INTRAMUSCULAR, INTRAVENOUS: *Adults*—0.5-2 g every 6-8 hr. Maximum daily dose: 8 g. FDA pregnancy category B.	
imipenem-cilastatin	Primaxin*	INTRAVENOUS: *Adults*—1-4 g/day, divided into 3 or 4 equal doses. FDA pregnancy category C.	
loracarbef	Lorabid	ORAL: *Adults*—200-400 mg every 12 hr. FDA pregnancy category B. *Children*—7.5 mg/kg body weight every 12 hr.	
meropenem	Merrem	INTRAVENOUS: *Adults*—1 g every 8 hr. FDA pregnancy category B. *Children*—>3 mo—20 mg/kg every 8 hr, not to exceed 2 g in 8 hr.	

*Available in Canada and the United States.

Pharmacokinetics

Imipenem is well distributed to many tissues but is low in cerebrospinal fluid. Excretion is through the kidneys. When given alone, imipenem is hydrolyzed in the kidneys and excreted as inactive products. The clinical preparation includes cilastatin, an agent chemically related to imipenem but with little antibacterial activity. Cilastatin inhibits destruction of imipenem in the kidneys and allows active imipenem to accumulate in renal tissue and urine.

In contrast to imipenem, meropenem metabolism is insignificant: 70% of a dose appears unchanged in urine. Meropenem distributes to key tissues, including the CNS.

Uses

Because imipenem has such a broad antimicrobial spectrum, it is used to treat a variety of infections at many sites. *P. aeruginosa* is usually sensitive, but resistant strains may occur. Meropenem is used to treat intraabdominal infections and meningitis.

Adverse Reactions and Contraindications

Imipenem or meropenem may cause allergic reactions. CNS reactions, including seizures, may also occur. GI disturbances are common, and pseudomembranous colitis may occur.

Toxicity

Dosages of imipenem greater than 2 g/day increase the risk of seizures. Imipenem is more likely than other beta-lactam antibiotics to cause seizures.

Interactions

Imipenem is used in fixed combination with cilastatin to avoid destruction of imipenem in the kidneys (see discussion of pharmacokinetics). Probenecid is avoided with meropenem because meropenem may accumulate to toxic levels.

Table 44-5 Direct Infusion Rate for Penicillins, Cephalosporins, and Related Drugs

Drug	Recommended Dilution*	Rate of Administration†
Penicillins		
ampicillin	500 mg/at least 5 ml diluent	1 dose/10-15 min
ampicillin + sulbactam	1.5 g/3.2 ml diluent, then further diluted in at least 50 ml compatible diluent	1 dose/15-30 min
carbenicillin	Dilute as directed on vial, then further dilute each gram in at least 5 ml diluent	1 g/5 min
methicillin	500 mg reconstituted drug in at least 25 ml diluent	10 ml/min
mezlocillin	1 g in at least 10 ml diluent	1 dose/3-5 min
nafcillin	Desired amount of drug in 15-30 ml diluent	500 mg/5-10 min
oxacillin	1 g/10 ml diluent	1 ml/min
piperacillin	1 g/5 ml diluent	1 dose/3-5 min
piperacillin + tazobactam	Dose/5 ml diluent, then further dilute in desired volume	1 dose/30 min
ticarcillin	1 g in at least 4 ml diluent, then further diluted to 1 g/10 ml	1 g/5 min
ticarcillin + clavulanate	3.1 g/13 ml diluent; further diluent; further dilute in 50-100 ml of fluid	1 dose/30 min
Cephalosporins		
cefamandole	1 g/10 ml diluent	1 g/3-5 min
cefazolin	1 g/10 ml diluent	1 g/5 min
cefepime	500 mg/5 ml, then further dilute in 50-100 ml	1 dose/30 min
cefonicid	0.5 g/2 ml diluent	1 dose/3-5 min
cefoperazone	1 g/5 ml diluent, then dilute further	1 dose/15-30 min
cefotaxime	1 dose/10 ml diluent	1 dose/3-5 min
cefotetan	1 g/10 ml diluent	1 dose/3-5 min
cefoxitin	1 g/10 ml diluent	1 g/3-5 min
ceftazidime	0.5 g/5 ml	1 dose/3-5 min
ceftizoxime	1 g/10 ml diluent	1 dose/3-5 min
ceftriaxone	250 mg/2.4 ml; further dilute in 500-100 ml of fluid	1 dose/15-30 min
cefuroxime	750 mg/8 ml diluent	1 dose/3-5 min
cephalothin	1 g/10 ml diluent	1 g/3-5 min
cephapirin	1 g/10 ml diluent	1 g/5 min
cephradine	500 mg/5 ml diluent	1 g/3-5 min
Others		
aztreonam	1 dose/6-10 ml diluent	1 dose/3-5 min
imipenem and cilastatin	1 dose/10 ml diluent; further dilute in 100 ml fluid	500 mg/20-30 min
meropenem	Dilute to a concentration of 50 mg/ml	1 g/3-5 min

*For information about appropriate diluents, preparations for constant infusion, compatibilities with infusion fluids, storage conditions, and other questions, consult the pharmacist and the manufacturer's information. Because the cephalosporins are so irritating to the vein, diluting these drugs more than is indicated in the table is preferable, when possible.
†These rates are for direct intravenous push unless otherwise noted. When diluted in 50 to 100 ml or more, the rate is determined in part by the total volume.

Nursing Process Overview

Penicillins, Cephalosporins, and Related Drugs

Assessment

Assess the patient and monitor for clinical signs of infection. Assess history of allergy to antiinfectives. Monitor renal function.

Nursing Diagnoses

- Possible complication: allergic reaction
- Risk for diarrhea related to drug side effects

Patient Outcomes

Ideally, the patient will not experience an allergic reaction; but if one occurs, the nurse will manage and minimize complications associated with the allergic response. The patient will not experience diarrhea related to drug side effects.

Planning/Implementation

Observe the patient closely for possible allergic response for 20 to 30 minutes after the first dose is administered. Have available drugs and equipment for resuscitation. In preparation for discharge, review with the patient the need to take the prescribed drug for the full course of therapy and to try to space doses evenly throughout the 24-hour day.

Evaluation

Penicillins, cephalosporins, and related drugs seldom cause long-term side effects. Before discharge, ascertain that the patient can judge improvement in the infection and describe possible side effects and situations that warrant consulting the physician.

Nursing Implications Summary

Penicillins, Cephalosporins, and Related Drugs

Drug Administration

- ➤ Review the Nursing Implications Summary in Chapter 43.
- ➤ Assess for history of allergy before administering these drugs.
- ➤ Monitor vital signs and temperature. Inspect for rash.
- ➤ Monitor serum creatinine and blood urea nitrogen (BUN) levels, liver function tests, complete blood count (CBC), and differential count. Monitor serum electrolyte level of patients with hypertensive, renal, or cardiovascular disease and in patients receiving drugs high in potassium or sodium. With cephalosporins, it may be necessary to monitor bleeding time and/or prothrombin time.
- ➤ For IV administration, consult the manufacturer's literature or Table 44-5 for the approximate rate of IV push administration. Too rapid administration of penicillins has resulted in the occurrence of seizures. Too rapid administration of the cephalosporins contributes to venous irritation and patient discomfort.
- ➤ Warn patients that IM injection may be painful. Use large muscle masses. Record and rotate injection sites. See Chapter 5 for a description of IM injection sites.
- ➤ Penicillins and cephalosporins are incompatible with aminoglycosides (see text).
- ➤ Read drug labels and orders carefully. Products containing procaine, benzathine, or a combination of these are never given by IV routes. Occasionally, patients are sensitive to procaine; symptoms include anxiety, confusion, agitation, fear of impending doom, and convulsions.

Nursing in the Community

- ➤ Review the Nursing Implications Summary in Chapter 43.
- ➤ The following drugs should be taken on an empty stomach, 1 hour before or 2 hours after meals, with a full glass (8 ounces) of water: ampicillin, liquid bacampicillin, car-

benicillin, cloxacillin, dicloxacillin, flucloxacillin, nafcillin, oxacillin, and penicillin G.

- ➤ The following drugs may be taken with food or on an empty stomach: amoxicillin, amoxicillin and clavulanate, the tablet form of bacampicillin, penicillin V, pivampicillin, pivmecillinam, and oral cephalosporins.
- ➤ Instruct the patient to take amoxicillin suspension straight or mix with formula, milk, fruit juice, ginger ale, or other cold drink. Instruct the patient to take the dose immediately after mixing it.
- ➤ Instruct the patient to avoid acidic fruit juices or beverages within 1 hour of taking a dose of penicillin G.
- ➤ Cefuroxime axetil should be taken with food or snack and may be crushed and mixed with food to ease taking and to help disguise the taste.
- ➤ Liquid forms may be dispensed with a calibrated measuring device or may be in the form of pediatric drops. Review measurement and administration of the dose with the patient and family.
- ➤ The penicillins, cephalosporins, and related drugs may cause false-positive reactions with copper sulfate urine glucose tests. Advise the diabetic patient to check with the physician before changing insulin or diet. Instruct the patient to monitor blood glucose levels.
- ➤ If chewable tablets are prescribed, encourage the patient to chew or crush the tablets before swallowing them.
- ➤ Penicillins, cephalosporins, and related drugs may cause diarrhea. Instruct the patient to notify the physician if diarrhea is severe or persistent. For mild diarrhea, only medicines containing kaolin or attapulgite should be used.
- ➤ Warn the patient taking cefamandole, cefoperazone, or cefotetan to avoid the use of alcohol while taking these drugs and for several days after completing the course of therapy.

Continued

Nursing Implications Summary—cont'd

Ingestion of alcohol may cause a disulfiram-type of reaction (see the Patient Problems box in Chapter 57 on alcohol use and disulfiram).

➤ For patients with phenylketonuria (PKU): Cefprozil contains phenylalanine; patients with PKU should not use this drug.

➤ Warn the female patient taking ampicillin, amoxicillin, or penicillin V that oral contraceptives containing estrogen may not work during the course of antiinfective drug therapy. Female patients should use an alternate or additional form of birth control while taking these antiinfectives; advise the patient to consult the physician or a pharmacist.

CHAPTER REVIEW

Application

1. What is the mechanism of action of penicillins and cephalosporins?
2. What is the most common mechanism by which bacteria gain resistance to beta-lactam antibiotics?
3. What is the mechanism of excretion for most penicillins and cephalosporins?
4. Name the most common toxic reaction to penicillins or cephalosporins. What should you watch for?
5. What is the purpose of skin tests for penicillin allergies?
6. What is the effect of penicillin on the CNS?
7. Name two groups of patients most at risk for accumulating penicillins given at normal doses.
8. What type of patient would be most at risk from the potassium and sodium contained in many penicillin and cephalosporin preparations? What tests should you monitor?
9. Why is probenecid sometimes administered with penicillin G?
10. Why is penicillin G absorbed erratically from the GI tract?
11. When does the peak concentration of penicillin G appear in the blood after an IM dose of the drug?
12. What is the elimination half-time for penicillin G in normal patients?
13. How does the penetration of penicillin G into the CSF differ in healthy patients and in those with meningitis?
14. Why do procaine penicillin G and benzathine penicillin G have longer durations of action than penicillin G?
15. What is the risk to patients from accidentally administering repository penicillins by IV routes?
16. What advantage does penicillin V have over penicillin G?

17. Why is methicillin useful in treating infections caused by penicillinase-producing *S. aureus*?
18. How do bacteria become resistant to methicillin?
19. What advantages do oxacillin, cloxacillin, and dicloxacillin have over methicillin?
20. How does the antimicrobial spectrum of ampicillin and amoxicillin differ from that of penicillin G?
21. What advantage does amoxicillin possess over ampicillin?
22. Why is clavulanic acid or sulbactam included in fixed combination with ampicillin, amoxicillin, or ticarcillin?
23. Infections caused by what pathogen are appropriately treated with carbenicillin or ticarcillin?
24. How does carbenicillin indanyl sodium differ from carbenicillin?
25. Why are first-generation cephalosporins not useful in treating meningitis?
26. What is the most common reaction expected from most cephalosporins when administered by IV routes?
27. How does the antimicrobial spectrum of cephalosporins differ from that of penicillin G?
28. What is the antimicrobial spectrum of aztreonam?
29. What is the antimicrobial spectrum of imipenem?
30. Why is imipenem given with cilastatin?

Critical Thinking

1. Which would produce a higher serum concentration of antibiotic: 1 million units of penicillin G or 1 million units of procaine penicillin G?
2. Compare and contrast one drug from each generation of cephalosporins. Consider spectrum of activity, route of administration, frequency of dose, and cost.
3. What are the main points of a nursing care plan for patients receiving drugs covered in this chapter?
4. What teaching points are important for patients receiving one of the antiinfective agents discussed in this chapter?

References

Degnan R: Pharmacology in practice: antibiotics, *RN* 60(10):49-55, 1997.

Porterfield LM: Problem Rx: the risk of cross-sensitive drug reactions, *RN* 58(10):72, 1995.

Sharts-Hopko NC: STDs in women: what you need to know, *Am J Nurs* 97(4):46-53, 1997.

45

Quinolones

OBJECTIVES

After studying this chapter, you should be able to do the following:

- *Explain the unique mechanism of action of fluoroquinolone antibiotics.*
- *Discuss the side effects that are most common with fluoroquinolones.*
- *Explain why fluoroquinolones are generally not used in children.*
- *Explain why fluoroquinolones may be avoided in patients with a history of seizures.*
- *Develop a nursing care plan for a patient receiving ciprofloxacin.*

CHAPTER OVERVIEW

This chapter introduces a new group of potent antibiotics that were developed from older agents such as nalidixic acid, which was too weak for use in systemic infections. The newer agents are sometimes referred to as **fluoroquinolones** because the greater antibacterial potency of the new agents comes from a fluorine substitution on the quinolone ring. This chapter focuses on these newer drugs.

THERAPEUTIC RATIONALE: BACTERIAL INFECTIONS

Infections caused by bacteria range from mild local infections to life-threatening systemic disease. Infections caused by gram-positive bacteria are associated with many infections of the throat and ears, as well as soft tissue infections and pneumonia. Gram-negative bacteria are likely to be the cause of urinary tract infections (UTIs). These organisms may also cause pneumonia, especially in hospitalized or chronically ill patients. The newer quinolone antibiotics are especially useful against gram-negative pathogenic bacteria.

THERAPEUTIC AGENTS: DRUGS TO TREAT BACTERIAL INFECTIONS

Fluoroquinolone Antibiotics

Mechanism of Action and Bacterial Resistance

Fluoroquinolones interfere with DNA replication in bacteria by inhibiting the proper functioning of **topoisomerases,** enzymes involved in DNA replication, transcription, repair, and recombination. In gram-negative bacteria the primary target is a topoisomerase II known as DNA gyrase. DNA gyrase is the enzyme that allows bacterial DNA to unwind (relax) so that replication may proceed. In gram-positive bacteria, the primary target may be topoisomerase IV, an enzyme with actions related to those of topoisomerase II. By interfering with the activity of these enzymes, fluoroquinolones block bacterial reproduction and may cause breaks in double-stranded DNA. These agents are bactericidal at concentrations achieved in blood.

Resistance to fluoroquinolones can occur, but plasmid-mediated resistance is not yet significant. One mechanism of resistance seems to involve antibiotic transport out of bacterial cells. Mutations of the topoisomerases may also confer resistance.

Pharmacokinetics

Fluoroquinolones (Table 45-1) are generally well absorbed when given orally, with oral bioavailabilities ranging from 70% to essentially 100%. Tissue penetration and persistence in plasma is greatest with the new drugs grepafloxacin and sparfloxacin, with half-lives ranging from 16 to 30 hours. For other fluoroquinolones, the half-lives range from 3 to 12 hours.

Portal circulation carries absorbed fluoroquinolones directly to the liver, where metabolism may occur. Grepafloxacin and sparfloxacin are extensively metabolized, primarily to glucuronides which may be excreted renally. For ciprofloxacin, norfloxacin, and trovafloxacin, hepatic metabolism accounts for 20% to 25% of a dose. Levofloxacin, lomefloxacin, and ofloxacin undergo little hepatic metabolism.

Trovafloxacin is used orally, but when intravenous (IV) doses are required, the prodrug alatrofloxacin is used. Upon entry into the body, the prodrug is rapidly cleaved to release trovafloxacin.

Levofloxacin, lomefloxacin, and ofloxacin rely almost solely on renal mechanisms for elimination, with little contribution by hepatic metabolism or biliary excretion. The half-lives of these drugs range up to 8 hours. From 60% to 87% of an oral dose of these drugs appears unchanged in urine.

Dosages of many fluoroquinolones may require adjustment in patients with renal impairment because the kidneys are the primary organ of excretion of active drug or metabolites. Typically, doses are cut in half and/or the dosing interval is doubled when creatinine clearance falls below about 50% of normal values. In addition, the dosage of grepafloxacin or trovafloxacin requires lowering when hepatic function is significantly impaired.

Uses

The fluoroquinolone antibiotics are potent agents with activity against a variety of bacteria. They are especially useful for infections caused by gram-negative organisms. Thus fluoroquinolones like **ciprofloxacin** that penetrate adequately into the urogenital tract may be useful for UTIs, gonorrhea, urethritis, cervicitis, prostatitis, or pelvic inflammatory disease (see Table 45-1). Fluoroquinolones are also highly effective for typhoid fever.

Many fluoroquinolones distribute well to the lung and other soft tissues. Therefore they may be effective against bronchitis, pneumonia, and skin infections (see Table 45-1), which are often caused by gram-positive bacteria. Strains of gram-positive bacteria that produce penicillinase or methicillin-resistant *Staphylococcus aureus* (MRSA) can be susceptible to fluoroquinolones, but resistance in gram-positive bacteria may develop rapidly. Occasionally, streptococcal pneumonia has developed or progressed during therapy with ciprofloxacin or other fluoroquinolones. This risk of resistance has limited the application of fluoroquinolones to serious infections caused by gram-positive bacteria when other antibiotics are contraindicated.

Adverse Reactions and Contraindications

Fluoroquinolones have two major side effects. The first involves the central nervous system (CNS). Symptoms include headache, dizziness, tinnitus, insomnia, shakiness, changes in vision, and seizures. These drugs are used cautiously in patients with preexisting CNS disease, such as prior seizure activity, because they can worsen the problem. The second side effect shared by the fluoroquinolones is a tendency to damage cartilage, especially in the young (see Pediatric Considerations box). This reaction has been observed in the young of several animal species and has led to permanent damage and lameness. Therefore fluoroquinolones are not given to children. Tendonitis, especially of the Achilles tendon, has also been noted occasionally in adults receiving these drugs.

In addition to the serious side effects already noted, fluoroquinolones, like many other oral antibiotics, can cause

Table 45-1	**Fluoroquinolones**		
Generic Name	**Trade Name**	**Administration/Dosage‡**	**Comments**
ciprofloxacin	Cipro*	ORAL: *Adults*—500-750 mg every 12 hr. INTRAVENOUS: *Adults*—400 mg infused over 1 hr every 8-12 hr.	For bacterial diarrhea, bone and soft tissue infections, bronchitis, gonorrhea, pneumonia, and urinary tract infections.
grepafloxacin	Raxar	ORAL: *Adults*—400-600 mg once daily.	For bronchitis, cervicitis, gonorrhea, pneumonia, and urethritis.
levofloxacin	Levaquin	ORAL, INTRAVENOUS: *Adults*—250-500 mg once daily.	For bronchitis, pneumonia, sinusitis, soft tissue infections, and urinary tract infections.
lomefloxacin	Maxaquin	ORAL: *Adults*—400 mg once daily.	For bronchitis and urinary tract infections.
norfloxacin	Noroxin*	ORAL: *Adults—For urinary tract infections:* 400 mg every 12 hr. *For gonorrhea:* 800 mg as single dose.	For gonorrhea, prostatitis, and urinary tract infections.
ofloxacin	Floxin*	ORAL, INTRAVENOUS: *Adults*—200-400 mg every 12 hr.	For bronchitis, chlamydial infection, gonorrhea, pneumonia, prostatitis, soft tissue infections, and urinary tract infections.
sparfloxacin	Zagam	ORAL: *Adults*—400 mg once, then 200 mg once daily.	For bronchitis and pneumonia.
trovafloxacin	Trovan	ORAL: *Adults*—100-200 mg once daily. INTRAVENOUS: *Adults*—200-300 mg as the prodrug alatrofloxacin once daily.	For bronchitis, cervicitis, gonorrhea, pelvic infections, perioperative prophylaxis, prostatitis, sinusitis, soft tissue infections, and urinary tract infections.

*Available in Canada and the United States.
‡ All drugs in this table are FDA pregnancy category C.

mild to moderate gastrointestinal (GI) tract symptoms, including nausea, vomiting, and diarrhea.

Allergies to fluoroquinolones are uncommon but can be severe. Symptoms include rashes, itching, shortness of breath, serum sickness, and Stevens-Johnson syndrome. Allergy to nalidixic acid or any other fluoroquinolone may be a contraindication for receiving any fluoroquinolone because cross-allergenicity does exist.

Two of the newer fluoroquinolones, grepafloxacin and sparfloxacin, cause a prolongation of the QTc interval on the electrocardiogram. This action may slow the heart rate and produce symptoms, including fainting. These two drugs are avoided in patients with preexisting conditions that prolong the QTc interval.

Toxicity

Overdoses may require gastric lavage or induction of emesis. High dosages of any fluoroquinolone may cause signs of CNS toxicity, including tremors or seizures. High dosages of ciprofloxacin or norfloxacin may cause renal difficulties because both drugs are relatively insoluble, especially in alkaline urine. Most people have slightly acidic urine, but strict vegetarians and persons taking certain drugs (see the following discussion) may have alkaline urine. Under these conditions the drug may crystallize in the urinary tract, causing pain and obstruction. The risk for this complication, called **crystalluria,** can be lessened by acidifying the urine and maintaining an adequate fluid intake.

Overdoses of grepafloxacin or sparfloxacin may cause cardiac arrhythmias; patients should be carefully observed for any changes in heart rate or rhythm.

Interactions

Antacids containing aluminum or magnesium compounds can block absorption of fluoroquinolones. Lower plasma and urinary concentrations of antibiotic and loss of antibacterial effectiveness result. To avoid this interaction the antibiotics should be taken 2 hours before the antacids. Didanosine, a drug used against human immunodeficiency virus (HIV), reduces absorption of ciprofloxacin and possibly other fluoroquinolones because the didanosine preparation contains aluminum. These combinations should be avoided.

Sodium bicarbonate, citrates, carbonic anhydrase inhibitors, and antacids containing calcium may alkalinize urine, which renders ciprofloxacin and norfloxacin less soluble. Avoiding these agents and maintaining an adequate fluid intake lessen the risk of crystalluria developing.

Ciprofloxacin, grepafloxacin, and norfloxacin lower hepatic clearance of the asthma medication theophylline, which can cause theophylline to accumulate. As serum theophylline levels increase, so does the risk of CNS toxicity; nausea, vomiting, tremors, restlessness, agitation, and palpitations may occur. Most case reports of seizure activity in patients receiving fluoroquinolones have involved patients who were also receiving theophylline. Caffeine clearance can also be slowed by some fluoroquinolones. Levofloxacin, lomefloxacin, ofloxacin, sparfloxacin, and trovafloxacin have little or no effect on caffeine or theophylline clearance and thus are not subject to this interaction.

Warfarin anticoagulation may be increased by ciprofloxacin or norfloxacin and possibly other fluoroquinolones. Prothrombin times should be monitored in patients receiving warfarin and a fluoroquinolone to avoid bleeding episodes.

Grepafloxacin and sparfloxacin must be avoided in patients receiving medications that can increase the QTc interval, such as disopyramide, erythromycin, phenothiazines, and tricyclic antidepressants. These combinations put patients at risk of the potentially fatal condition called torsade de pointes.

PEDIATRIC CONSIDERATIONS

Fluoroquinolones

THE PROBLEM
Fluoroquinolones, as well as nalidixic acid and cinoxacin, have damaged cartilage in tests in young animals, leading to permanent joint impairment.

SOLUTIONS
- Avoid these drugs in children or younger teenagers.
- Remind adults not to share drugs with children, even if symptoms appear to be the same; some drugs should not be given to children.

Table 45-2 Antibiotics Related to Quinolones

Generic Name	Trade Name	Administration/Dosage	Comments
cinoxacin	Cinobac	ORAL: *Adults*—250 mg every 6 hr or 500 mg every 12 hr. FDA pregnancy category C.	For urinary tract infections only.
enoxacin	Penetrex	ORAL: *Adults*—200-400 mg every 12 hr. FDA pregnancy category C.	For gonorrhea and urinary tract infections.
nalidixic acid	NegGram*	ORAL: *Adults*—1 g 4 times/day for 7-14 days. FDA pregnancy category C.	For urinary tract infections only; emergence of resistant bacterial strains often causes treatment failure.

*Available in Canada and the United States.

THERAPEUTIC RATIONALE: URINARY TRACT INFECTIONS

Infections of the urinary tract are common and often involve gram-negative bacteria. Most infections are uncomplicated and will resolve easily with appropriate therapy. Others are more difficult, especially when there is a mechanical obstruction to urine flow. Successful treatment involves assessing and correcting any underlying conditions leading to UTIs, as well as selection of an antibiotic that has the correct antimicrobial spectrum and achieves high concentrations in tissues and fluids of the urinary tract.

THERAPEUTIC AGENTS: CINOXACIN, ENOXACIN, AND NALIDIXIC ACID

Mechanism of Action and Bacterial Resistance

Nalidixic acid, cinoxacin, and enoxacin (Table 45-2) are older agents related in structure to fluoroquinolones. Like fluoroquinolones, these drugs inhibit topoisomerase activity but are much less potent than fluoroquinolones.

Pharmacokinetics

Nalidixic acid is the most extensively metabolized drug of this group, with glucuronide and hydroxylated derivatives being formed. The hydroxylated form of nalidixic acid is biologically active and comprises a significant proportion of the active drug in blood or urine. More than 90% of nalidixic acid in blood is bound to serum proteins. Little enters most body tissues. The only organs in which drug concentration exceeds the plasma concentration are the kidneys. Nalidixic acid has the lowest plasma concentration of any drug in this group.

Cinoxacin and enoxacin are primarily excreted renally. In addition, 40% of cinoxacin administered and 20% of enoxacin is metabolized by liver.

Uses

Cinoxacin, enoxacin, and nalidixic acid are active against many gram-negative pathogens causing common UTIs, but they are not active against *Pseudomonas aeruginosa*. Nalidixic acid and cinoxacin are used exclusively for UTIs, but enoxacin may be used for gonorrhea as well as UTIs. These three agents are not appropriate for systemic infections.

Adverse Reactions and Contraindications

Like the fluoroquinolones, cinoxacin, enoxacin, and nalidixic acid may cause CNS toxicity, with dizziness, headache, drowsiness, or insomnia. GI distress is relatively common.

Interactions

Nalidixic acid interacts with anticoagulants such as warfarin (Coumadin), causing an increase in the anticoagulant effect because the anticoagulants are displaced from protein-binding sites by nalidixic acid.

Enoxacin is especially effective at decreasing metabolism of caffeine and theophylline, leading to increases in toxicity with these compounds.

Nursing Process Overview

Quinolones

Assessment
Assess vital signs and signs and symptoms of presenting problem. Assess for history of allergy to antiinfective drugs, and in women assess for pregnancy. Check complete blood count (CBC), liver function tests, and renal function tests. Obtain baseline weight.

Nursing Diagnoses
- Knowledge deficit related to need to increase fluid intake while taking quinolones

Patient Outcomes
The patient's infection will resolve, and the patient will increase fluid intake to 2500 ml/day while taking a quinolone.

Planning/Implementation
Continue to monitor presenting symptoms. Assess for GI tract disturbance, skin changes, and CNS side effects. Encourage fluid intake. Monitor renal function and weight.

Evaluation
Ascertain that the patient understands the need to maintain an adequate fluid intake, the major side effects, and how to take the prescribed medication correctly.

Nursing Implications Summary

Drug Administration
- See Nursing Implications Summary in Chapter 43.
- Assess for pregnancy or history of allergy before administering drug.

- Assess for CNS side effects such as headache, dizziness, tinnitus, insomnia, shakiness, and changes in vision. Assess for GI discomfort, diarrhea, nausea, or vomiting. Assess for heel pain or Achilles tendinitis.

Nursing Implications Summary—cont'd

➤ Monitor CBC and differential, platelet count, blood urea nitrogen (BUN) level, serum creatinine level, and liver function tests.

➤ IV ciprofloxacin: Available pre-mixed and ready to hang for infusion, or may be diluted with normal saline or D5W to a final concentration of 0.5 to 2 mg/ml. Administer dose evenly over 60 minutes.

➤ IV ofloxacin: Available premixed and ready to hang for infusion, or may be diluted to a final concentration of 4 mg/ml. See manufacturer's literature for acceptable diluents. Administer dose evenly over 60 minutes. Monitor blood pressure.

➤ IV trovafloxacin: Withdraw dose and dilute as directed in manufacturer's package insert. Administer dose over 60 minutes.

Nursing in the Community

➤ See Nursing Implications Summary in Chapter 43.

➤ Review the anticipated benefits and possible side effects of drug therapy with the patient. Instruct the patient to report any new sign or symptom.

➤ Reinforce the importance of not giving fluoroquinolones or cinoxacin to children or adolescents (see Pediatric Considerations box earlier in this chapter).

➤ Instruct the patient to take oral doses with a full glass (8 ounces) of water or fluid and to increase daily intake of water by several 8-ounce glasses a day. Instruct the patient to take doses of ciprofloxacin, levofloxacin, lomefloxacin, sparfloxacin, trovafloxacin, or nalidixic acid on a full or empty stomach. Instruct the patient to take doses of enoxacin, norfloxacin, or ofloxacin on an empty stomach 1 hour before or 2 hours after meals.

➤ See the Patient Problems boxes on UTIs (Chapter 49), photosensitivity (Chapter 58), and dry mouth (Chapter 23).

➤ Note the drug interactions. Instruct the patient to take ofloxacin, norfloxacin, or trovafloxacin 2 hours before or 2 hours after taking antacids containing aluminum or magnesium or taking sucralfate. Instruct the patient to take ciprofloxacin or lomefloxacin 2 hours before or 4 hours after taking theses antacids or sucralfate. Instruct the patient to take enoxacin 8 hours after or 2 hours before taking these antacids or sucralfate. Review the patient's other medications, and counsel as necessary. Remind the patient to inform all health care providers of all drugs being used.

➤ IV morphine administered concurrently with oral trovafloxacin significantly reduces the absorption of the trovafloxacin. Administer IV morphine 2 hours after oral trovafloxacin taken on an empty stomach (fasting), or at least 4 hours after oral trovafloxacin taken with food.

➤ Caution the patient to avoid driving or operating hazardous equipment if CNS symptoms develop. Advise the patient to report dizziness, tinnitus, and visual changes to the physician.

➤ If photophobia develops (eyes have increased sensitivity to light), instruct the patient to wear sunglasses and to avoid bright lights and sunlight.

➤ Inform diabetic patients taking nalidixic acid that the drug may interfere with urine glucose results. Inform diabetic patients not to change diet or insulin dosage without consulting the physician. Instruct diabetic patients to monitor blood glucose level.

CHAPTER REVIEW

Application

1. What is the mechanism of the antibacterial effect of fluoroquinolones?

2. By what routes are fluoroquinolones given?

3. What is the major route of excretion of levofloxacin, lomefloxacin, and ofloxacin?

4. How does the elimination of grepafloxacin and sparfloxacin differ from that of other fluoroquinolones?

5. What side effects are associated with fluoroquinolones?

6. What side effects of grepafloxacin and sparfloxacin differ from other members of the class?

7. What types of patients are most likely to develop seizures when they receive fluoroquinolones?

8. Why are fluoroquinolones not used in children?

9. Why is it important to know the renal status of a patient receiving a fluoroquinolone antibiotic?

10. What special precaution may be required in an asthmatic patient using theophylline who is given ciprofloxacin?

11. What process should be monitored when warfarin is given with ciprofloxacin?

12. Why are nalidixic acid and cinoxacin restricted to use in UTIs?

Critical Thinking

1. Patients taking one of the fluoroquinolones should increase their fluid intake to at least 2400 ml/day. Think of specific suggestions to give to patients to help them remember to do this.

2. A patient who is receiving a fluoroquinolone reports pain and tenderness in his right heel and lower calf, along with swelling. What nursing diagnoses should you consider and what should you do?

Reference

Degnan R: Pharmacology in practice: antibiotics, *RN* 60(10):49-55, 1997.

Macrolides, Clindamycin, and Miscellaneous Penicillin Substitutes

OBJECTIVES

After studying this chapter, you should be able to do the following:

- *Explain the common indications for a macrolide antibiotic (e.g., erythromycin).*
- *Describe common side effects of macrolides.*
- *Develop a nursing care plan for a patient receiving a macrolide.*
- *Explain the common indications for clindamycin, vancomycin, and spectinomycin.*
- *Describe common side effects of clindamycin and vancomycin.*
- *Develop a nursing care plan for a patient receiving clindamycin or vancomycin.*

CHAPTER OVERVIEW

This chapter introduces several antibiotics that are effective against the same gram-positive bacteria covered by narrow-spectrum penicillins. Because of this property, these drugs are sometimes grouped together as **penicillin substitutes**. Despite this similarity in antibacterial spectrum, these drugs have different mechanisms of action and pharmacokinetics.

THERAPEUTIC RATIONALE: BACTERIAL INFECTIONS

Infections caused by bacteria range from mild local infections to life-threatening systemic disease. Infections caused by gram-positive bacteria are associated with many infections of the throat and ears, as well as soft tissue infections and pneumonia. Certain gram-negative bacteria are also associated with specific pneumonias or other respiratory tract infections. The macrolides may be especially useful for these conditions, but the other drugs covered in this chapter are primarily used as substitutes for narrow-spectrum penicillins.

THERAPEUTIC AGENTS: DRUGS TO TREAT BACTERIAL INFECTIONS

▼ Macrolides: azithromycin, clarithromycin, dirithromycin, and erythromycin

Mechanism of Action and Bacterial Resistance

Macrolides are large molecules that contain lactone rings substituted with various sugars and amino sugars. These antibiotics bind to bacterial ribosomes and thus prevent bacterial protein synthesis. At low concentrations this effect is bacteriostatic, but at high concentrations the drugs may be bactericidal. For example, azithromycin is bactericidal against

Streptococcus pyogenes, S. pneumoniae, and *Haemophilus influenzae,* organisms that commonly cause respiratory infections or pharyngitis.

Bacteria are resistant to **erythromycin** by two mechanisms. Gram-negative bacteria from the bowel, such as *Escherichia coli,* seem to be relatively impermeable to erythromycin and are therefore intrinsically resistant. Cell wall–deficient forms of these bacteria (L-forms) are permeable to erythromycin and are highly sensitive to the drug. In contrast, gram-positive bacteria acquire resistance by chemically altering their ribosomes so that the ribosomes no longer bind erythromycin; thus protein synthesis is not inhibited. This ribosomal alteration is catalyzed by an enzyme that is synthesized from genes carried on a bacterial plasmid. Plasmids are discrete circular molecules of DNA that are separate from the bacterial chromosome (see Chapter 43). These plasmids can be transferred directly from one bacterial cell to another. Therefore resistance to erythromycin may spread rapidly throughout a bacterial population.

The mechanism of resistance to the other macrolides is similar to that of erythromycin, but the spread of resistance has not been fully assessed for these newer drugs.

Pharmacokinetics

Erythromycin is sensitive to acid and therefore may be extensively degraded in the stomach. Thus erythromycin base is formulated with acid-resistant coatings so that the drug will pass intact through the stomach and be dissolved and absorbed in the small intestine. This tactic is based on the knowledge that the pH of the duodenum is near neutrality (see Chapter 1).

Certain chemical forms of erythromycin are used clinically primarily because of their increased resistance to acid and their better oral absorption. These compounds are the stearate, ethylsuccinate, and estolate esters of erythromycin (Table 46-1). Erythromycin stearate and erythromycin ethylsuccinate are absorbed more rapidly and completely from the gastrointestinal (GI) tract than erythromycin base. Free erythromycin apparently is absorbed from the duodenum with these agents after hydrolysis of the esters. With erythromycin estolate, much better absorption of drug is achieved, and serum levels may be four times higher than with other forms of erythromycin. However, with erythromycin estolate, most of the drug in the serum is actually the ester, and controversy exists regarding whether this form of the drug has biologic activity. Many physicians prefer erythromycin

Table 46-1 Summary of Macrolides

Generic Name	Trade Name	Drug Form	Administration/Dosage
azithromycin	Zithromax*	Capsules, tablets, oral suspension	ORAL: *Adults and children >16 yr*—500 mg on first day, then 250 mg once daily. *For chlamydial infections:* 1000 mg as single dose. FDA pregnancy category B. *Children 6 mo-12 yr (oral suspension)*—10-12 mg/kg up to 500 mg on day 1; 5-12 mg/kg on days 2-5.
		Solution for injection	INTRAVENOUS: *Adults and children >16 yr*—500 mg/day for 1 or 2 days; switch to oral.
clarithromycin	Biaxin*	Tablets, oral suspension	ORAL: *Adults*—250-500 mg every 12 hr. FDA pregnancy category C. *Children >6 mo*—7.5 mg/kg body weight every 12 hr; do not exceed 500 mg/dose.
dirithromycin	Dynabac	Tablets	ORAL: *Adults*—500 mg once daily. FDA pregnancy category C.
erythromycin base	ERYC E-Mycin* Erythromid†	Enteric or film-coated tablets or capsules	ORAL: *Adults*—250 mg 4 times/day; do not exceed 4 g/day. FDA pregnancy category B. *Children*—7.5-12.5 mg/kg every 6 hr or 15-25 mg/kg every 12 hr.
erythromycin base	Staticin*	Gel, solution, or swabs	TOPICAL: *Adults and children*—Apply to skin twice daily.
erythromycin base	Ilotycin*	Ophthalmic ointment	TOPICAL: *Adults and children*—Apply to conjunctiva 1-6 times/day.
erythromycin estolate	Ilosone*	Tablets, capsules, and suspension	ORAL: *Adults and children*—Same as for erythromycin base.
erythromycin ethylsuccinate	E.E.S.*	Oral suspension, chewable or film-coated tablets	ORAL: *Adults*—400 mg every 6 hr. FDA pregnancy category B. *Children*—Same as for erythromycin base.
erythromycin ethylsuccinate + sulfisoxazole	Pediazole*	Oral suspension	ORAL: *Children >2 mo*—12.5 mg erythromycin/kg body weight every 6 hr.
erythromycin gluceptate	Ilotycin*	Powder for reconstitution with sterile preservative-free water	INTRAVENOUS: *Adults*—250-500 mg base every 6 hr. Maximum daily dose: 4 g. FDA pregnancy category B. *Children*—3.75-5 mg/kg every 6 hr.
erythromycin lactobionate	Erythrocin*	Powder for reconstitution with sterile preservative-free water	INTRAVENOUS: *Adults and children*—Same as for erythromycin gluceptate.
erythromycin stearate	Erythrocin*	Film-coated tablets, oral suspension	ORAL: *Adults and children*—Same as for erythromycin base.

*Available in Canada and the United States.
†Available in Canada only.

estolate because of the high tissue and blood levels and note that many tissues and bacteria can hydrolyze the ester form of the drug to release free erythromycin at the infection site.

Oral bioavailability for the macrolides varies from 30% to 65%, depending on which preparation is used. Food may interfere with the oral absorption of most macrolides. Erythromycin estolate, erythromycin ethylsuccinate, and dirithromycin are exceptions, being well absorbed even when food is present.

Erythromycin is available as the lactobionate or the gluceptate for intravenous (IV) injection (see Table 46-1). These water-soluble products may be diluted with sterile water for injection but should not be diluted in sterile water containing preservatives. Erythromycin lactobionate and erythromycin gluceptate should be infused slowly into the vein to avoid pain. Intramuscular (IM) administration of erythromycin is avoided because injections are extremely painful.

Erythromycin readily distributes to tissues, where concentrations of drug may persist well beyond when it can be detected in serum. Erythromycin is especially concentrated in the liver and spleen. It enters fluids of the middle ear and pleural fluids but not cerebrospinal fluid (CSF) unless the meninges are inflamed. The drug does cross the placenta, but fetal blood levels are less than 20% of maternal blood levels. Erythromycin also enters breast milk, in which the concentrations may equal that of maternal serum.

Azithromycin, clarithromycin, and dirithromycin are more strongly concentrated in tissues than is erythromycin and therefore persist longer in the body. Azithromycin and dirithromycin in particular concentrate in the lungs and other organs. Macrolides do not accumulate in normal brain tissue, although this remains to be tested for dirithromycin.

The liver is the major excretory organ for macrolides. A large percentage of orally administered drug is concentrated in bile and excreted in feces. Some reabsorption from the intestine occurs in a process called enterohepatic circulation (see Chapter 1). For erythromycin, a significant proportion of the drug is inactivated in the liver. Less than 10% of orally administered erythromycin appears as active drug in urine; with IV dosages, about 15% of the dose appears in urine.

Dirithromycin is rapidly converted to its active form erythromycylamine. This conversion is not dependent on the liver or enzymes. There is little other metabolism of either the prodrug or the active form. Elimination is almost exclusively biliary.

Uses

Erythromycin is active against the same gram-positive bacteria that are usually susceptible to penicillin G, but erythromycin is chemically unrelated to penicillins and is not cross-allergenic with them. Therefore it is a useful substitute in patients allergic to penicillins. In addition, because penicillins and erythromycin act by entirely different mechanisms, bacteria that become resistant to one of these drugs may still be sensitive to the other. The newer macrolides—azithromycin,

clarithromycin, and dirithromycin—have equal or improved activity over erythromycin toward gram-positive organisms.

Erythromycin is the drug of choice for some atypical pneumonias such as those caused by *Mycoplasma pneumoniae* and *Legionella pneumophila* (Legionnaire's disease), but the other macrolides may be substituted in some cases. Erythromycin may be preferred over penicillin G for diphtheria because it eradicates the diphtheria carrier state. Erythromycin also may be useful in relapsing urinary tract infections; the relapse is commonly caused by L-forms of gram-negative organisms such as *E. coli* and *Proteus mirabilis*. These L-forms lack cell walls and are therefore resistant to penicillins. The L-form bacteria remain latent during penicillin therapy, revert to normal, and again produce disease when penicillin therapy is stopped. Because erythromycin penetrates these L-forms and blocks protein synthesis, the infection may be eradicated.

Adverse Reactions and Contraindications

The most common patient complaint with oral macrolides is some form of GI tract difficulty. Abdominal discomfort and cramping are dose-related reactions to these drugs. Severe pain and nausea may rarely indicate pancreatitis. At normal dosages, nausea, vomiting, and diarrhea often occur, as with other oral antibiotics. Headache or dizziness may also occur. In addition to these side effects, clarithromycin may occasionally cause thrombocytopenia, with bruising or bleeding. Azithromycin may cause interstitial nephritis, with fever, rash, and joint pain.

Clinical studies suggest that pregnant women have variable absorption of oral erythromycin, and many do not achieve effective serum concentrations of the drug. Erythromycin estolate also causes hepatotoxicity in about 10% of pregnant women. Therefore erythromycin, and especially erythromycin estolate, may not be recommended during pregnancy.

Toxicity

Rarely, patients who receive more than 4 g of erythromycin a day experience hearing loss. Loss of hearing is usually reversible and may appear at any time during therapy.

The most significant toxicity occurs with erythromycin estolate, which damages the liver by direct drug toxicity or an immune reaction. This reaction, called **cholestatic hepatitis**, usually appears 10 to 12 days after therapy is begun but may appear earlier in patients previously exposed to the drug. These patients may experience severe abdominal pain, liver enlargement, fever, and jaundice. In most patients these symptoms rapidly disappear when the drug is discontinued.

Interactions

Erythromycin is metabolized in the liver and therefore may compete with other drugs for the limited hepatic metabolic capacity. For example, alfentanil, carbamazepine, cyclosporine, warfarin, valproic acid, and theophylline must be eliminated by hepatic mechanisms; when erythromycin is given concurrently, these drugs are eliminated more slowly, serum levels rise, and the drugs may accumulate. Because these drugs have dose-related toxicity, erythromycin not only increases serum levels but also increases the risk of serious toxicity. Clarithromycin has also been shown to increase serum concentrations of carbamazepine, theophylline, and terfenadine. Dirithromycin does not act on hepatic enzymes and therefore shares none of these interactions.

Rarely, erythromycin may cause hepatotoxicity, especially when used at high dosages or for long periods. The risk of liver damage is increased if erythromycin is given concurrently with other hepatotoxic agents such as acetaminophen (at high dosages), anabolic steroids, androgens, estrogens, isoniazid, ketoconazole, phenothiazines, rifampin, sulfonamides, or valproic acid.

Macrolides can interact in several ways with other antimicrobial agents. Erythromycin and other macrolides can antagonize the antibacterial effects of clindamycin and chloramphenicol because they share the same target in bacteria and may displace each other from the target. Erythromycin should not be used concurrently with these antibiotics. Rifabutin, a drug used to treat *Mycobacterium avium-intracellulare* infections, significantly lowers serum concentrations of clarithromycin. Serum concentrations of zidovudine are significantly lowered by clarithromycin; the drugs must be taken at least 4 hours apart to avoid this interaction.

Erythromycin lactobionate or erythromycin gluceptate may be rapidly inactivated if added to fluids below pH 5.5. This sensitivity to extremes of pH makes erythromycin incompatible in solution with a number of other drugs. Before adding erythromycin to any other drug solution, compatibility of the agents should be verified with the pharmacist.

Few interactions have been noted with azithromycin. The major documented interaction involves aluminum and magnesium contained in antacids. These materials lower absorption of azithromycin and should be taken at least 2 hours before the antibiotic.

clindamycin

Mechanism of Action and Bacterial Resistance

Clindamycin inhibits the action of bacterial ribosomes in a manner similar to erythromycin. This drug halts bacterial protein synthesis and may be bacteriostatic or bactericidal, depending on drug concentrations. Bacterial resistance to clindamycin develops in several ways. Some organisms may become impermeable to the drugs, but others alter their ribosomes to prevent binding of clindamycin. With this latter mechanism, organisms may also become resistant to erythromycin or chloramphenicol. In practice, most clinically observed resistance to clindamycin develops in a gradual, stepwise manner.

Pharmacokinetics

Clindamycin is well absorbed orally, and oral absorption is not significantly impaired by food. Clindamycin palmitate is available as flavored granules to be used in suspension for oral administration. The palmitate is rapidly removed to release active clindamycin.

Clindamycin-2-phosphate may be injected intramuscularly, but clinical reports suggest that local pain after injection may occur. Absorption of drug by this route is good, with serum peaks being achieved 30 to 60 minutes after injection. These drugs are also suitable for IV use. By this route, clindamycin-2-phosphate causes pain and phlebitis. Clindamycin-2-phosphate is inactive as an antibiotic but is rapidly converted to clindamycin in the body.

Clindamycin is well distributed to most body tissues, with the exception of the central nervous system (CNS). Clindamycin does not appear in the CSF even when meningitis is present. Clindamycin appears in the milk of lactating women treated with this drug.

Clindamycin is extensively biodegraded in the body; the liver is the primary site of biotransformation. Because less than 20% of the total drug administered orally shows up as active antibiotic in urine or feces, these drugs are used at normal dosages in patients with renal insufficiency or failure. Clindamycin is not removed by hemodialysis.

Uses

Clindamycin has an antimicrobial spectrum similar to those of penicillin G and erythromycin, being primarily effective against gram-positive organisms. Clindamycin is not as effective as penicillin against *Neisseria gonorrhoeae* or other gram-negative cocci. Clindamycin is effective against several anaerobic organisms, particularly *Bacteroides fragilis*. Infections caused by these organisms are a major indication for clindamycin.

The dangers of severe colitis have largely restricted the use of clindamycin to cases in which patients are allergic to safer drugs or the pathogenic organism is demonstrated by the microbiology laboratory to be sensitive to these agents.

Adverse Reactions and Contraindications

The most serious reaction to clindamycin is colitis. Symptoms range from mild diarrhea to a severe, life-threatening condition called **pseudomembranous colitis.** Any increase in frequency of bowel movements or softness of the stools may be reason to discontinue the drug, especially in older adult patients. Significant diarrhea should prompt discontinuation of the drug and may be relieved by that measure alone. The appearance of blood or mucus in the stool may signal severe colitis.

Pseudomembranous colitis is caused by a toxin produced by *Clostridium difficile.* Overgrowth of this organism in the bowel can result from antibiotic disturbance of the bacterial flora in the bowel. This superinfection and its associated colitis may be treated with vancomycin. Fluid and electrolyte replacement and other supportive therapy also may be required. Agents that slow peristaltic action may worsen the condition or prolong it; thus opiates and diphenoxylate with atropine are not appropriate for use in these patients.

In addition to colitis, clindamycin may produce GI tract irritation ranging from nausea and vomiting to glossitis and stomatitis. This drug is usually avoided in patients with significant preexisting GI tract disease.

Allergies to clindamycin range from mild rashes to fever and anaphylactic shock. These reactions may occur in anyone but are more common in those with other allergies. The appearance of any allergic response is cause for discontinuing the drug.

Some reports suggest that blood dyscrasias and liver dysfunction occur during clindamycin therapy. Clindamycin dosages are often lowered when patients have significant preexisting hepatic disease to avoid clindamycin accumulation.

Toxicity

Direct toxicity of oral doses of clindamycin is low, except for the increased risk of GI tract symptoms arising from alteration of bacterial populations in the bowel. Direct infusion of clindamycin may also affect the cardiovascular system. Clindamycin should be administered in an IV solution no more concentrated than 0.6 g/dl at a rate no more rapid than 100 ml/20 min.

Interactions

Clindamycin is incompatible in solution with aminophylline, ampicillin, barbiturates, calcium gluconate, magnesium sulfate, and phenytoin. Chloramphenicol and erythromycin antagonize the antibacterial effect of clindamycin and lincomycin.

Because clindamycin has neuromuscular-blocking properties, it may enhance the action of various neuromuscular-blocking agents and inhalation anesthetics.

The use of kaolin-pectin antidiarrheal agents given at the time oral clindamycin is ingested significantly lowers the serum concentrations of the antibiotic.

vancomycin

Mechanism of Action and Bacterial Resistance

Vancomycin is a glycopeptide antibiotic that prevents synthesis of bacterial cell walls by blocking peptidoglycan strand formation. This site of action is different from the sites sensitive to penicillin and other antibiotics interfering with cell wall synthesis.

Resistance to vancomycin developed slowly, with the first strains of vancomycin-resistant enterococci (VRE) appearing in the United States in 1988, some 30 years after discovery of the drug. As the drug is used clinically, it is a rapidly bactericidal agent, which may partly explain why the low incidence of bacterial resistance to vancomycin persisted for so many years. Unfortunately, the resistance to vancomycin that has appeared is carried on plasmids that spread readily among strains of enterococci. By 1992 some hospitals reported VRE accounted for 10% of isolates of enterococci. Infections caused by VRE are difficult to treat. **Bacteremia** (bacteria shed into the blood) caused by VRE has a very high mortality rate.

Pharmacokinetics

Vancomycin is a complex glycopeptide that may be positively or negatively charged, depending on pH. Therefore vancomycin does not easily cross biologic membranes and is not significantly absorbed after oral administration (Table 46-2). Vancomycin is most often given by intermittent IV infusion but may rarely be given by mouth for intestinal infections. Bactericidal concentrations of drug are not obtained in systemic circulation with oral doses.

Vancomycin is well distributed throughout the body and reaches clinically effective concentrations in various body fluid compartments such as pericardial, synovial, and

Table 46-2 Summary of Clindamycin and Miscellaneous Penicillin Substitutes			
Generic Name	**Trade Name**	**Drug Form**	**Administration/Dosage**
clindamycin	Cleocin Dalacin C†	Capsules	ORAL: *Adults*—150-300 mg every 6 hr. *Children* >*1 mo*—2-5 mg/kg body weight every 6 hr.
clindamycin palmitate	Cleocin Pediatric Dalacin C†	Oral suspension	ORAL: *Children*—2-5 mg/kg body weight every 6 hr for children >10 kg. Smaller children should receive 37.5 mg every 8 hr.
clindamycin phosphate	Cleocin Dalacin C†	Solution with benzyl alcohol, di-sodium edetate, and hydrochloric acid or sodium hydroxide	INTRAMUSCULAR, INTRAVENOUS: *Adults*—300-600 mg every 6-8 hr to upper limit of 2.4 g/day (no more than 0.6 g/injection site intramuscularly). *Children* >*1 mo*—3.75-5 mg/kg body weight every 6 hr.
clindamycin phosphate	Cleocin T	1% topical gel, lotion, or solution	TOPICAL: *Adults and children*—For acne vulgaris: Apply thin film to affected area twice daily. FDA pregnancy category B.
spectinomycin	Trobicin*	Powder to be reconstituted with diluent (0.945% benzyl alcohol)	INTRAMUSCULAR: *Adults*—2 g in single dose.
vancomycin	Vancocin*	Powder to be reconstituted with sterile water	INTRAVENOUS: *Adults*—500 mg every 6 hr. *Children 1 mo-12 yr*—10 mg/kg body weight every 6 hr. FDA pregnancy category C.
vancomycin	Vancocin*	Oral solution, capsules	ORAL: Same as for intravenous. *Note:* This route is for intestinal infections only. FDA pregnancy category B.

*Available in Canada and the United States.
†Available in Canada only.

pleural fluids. It does not penetrate normal CSF but does enter the CNS when the meninges are inflamed.

Active vancomycin appears in very high concentrations in urine. The kidney is the major excretory organ for vancomycin, and nonrenal elimination is limited. In patients with renal insufficiency, vancomycin may accumulate unless drug dosages are reduced to compensate for loss of excretory efficiency. In patients who lack kidney function, vancomycin is usually given only once between dialysis treatments. Vancomycin is not cleared from the body by hemodialysis.

Uses

Vancomycin is most often used in serious or life-threatening staphylococcal or streptococcal infections. Because the drug is chemically unrelated to penicillins and has a different mechanism of action, it acts against organisms that resist penicillins, including methicillin-resistant *Staphylococcus aureus*. Because vancomycin and penicillin are not cross-allergenic, vancomycin is useful in patients allergic to penicillins. Vancomycin also has special utility in treating antibiotic-induced colitis, which arises from a superinfection with *C. difficile* in the bowel.

Adverse Reactions and Contraindications

IV infusion of vancomycin has produced nausea, flushing, and itching. These reactions are more likely when undiluted vancomycin is dripped directly into a running IV line rather than being properly diluted beforehand. The reaction, which is caused by generalized histamine release, is sometimes called red man syndrome because of the intense flushing reactions observed. If vancomycin inadvertently enters tissues around an IV site, local necrosis may develop.

Toxicity

Vancomycin causes deafness in some patients, especially when serum concentrations exceed 80 mg/ml serum. Patients with impaired renal function and older adult patients are more likely than healthy or younger persons to show drug accumulation (see Geriatric Considerations box) and should be watched closely for ringing in the ears (tinnitus) or hearing loss. Some patients have regained some hearing acuity when vancomycin was stopped. For others, hearing loss may persist.

Nephrotoxicity may occur, with symptoms of increased thirst, altered urination, anorexia, or weakness. Blood and protein in urine occasionally have been noted.

Interactions

Vancomycin is compatible with many common IV fluids. The major consideration in combining vancomycin with another drug should be to avoid administering another ototoxic or nephrotoxic drug, such as an aminoglycoside antibiotic, bumetanide, cisplatin, ethacrynic acid, or furosemide. Combining one of these drugs with vancomycin

may result in additive toxic effects. Complete loss of hearing or renal failure is possible.

spectinomycin

Mechanism of Action and Bacterial Resistance

Spectinomycin is an aminocyclitol antibiotic that inhibits protein synthesis in many bacteria, but the ability of spectinomycin to inhibit *Neisseria gonorrhoeae* is the basis for its clinical usefulness. On this basis, it is classified as a penicillin substitute. Resistance to spectinomycin may occur.

Pharmacokinetics

Spectinomycin is injected intramuscularly to treat gonorrhea (see Table 46-2). Absorption produces high serum concentrations of drug that are maintained long enough after a single injection to eradicate *N. gonorrhoeae* from the infection site. Within 2 days, nearly all the injected drug appears in an active form in urine.

Uses

Spectinomycin is used only for gonorrhea. It is not effective for chlamydial infections, which often occur along with gonorrhea.

Adverse Reactions and Contraindications

Single doses of spectinomycin have caused nausea, chills, and dizziness. Patients may report pain at the injection site, urticaria, or fever. Spectinomycin is contraindicated when known allergy to the drug exists.

Toxicity

No significant toxicity is noted with single doses in adults. The preparation is not used in children because benzyl alcohol included as a preservative is toxic in infants.

Interactions

No significant interactions occur with single doses used in adults.

 GERIATRIC CONSIDERATIONS

Vancomycin

THE PROBLEM
Patients older than 60 years of age have reduced renal function and therefore excrete vancomycin more slowly than do younger adults. The drug may accumulate because alternative paths of elimination are limited. Older adults also have some hearing loss because of their age.

SOLUTIONS
- Lower dosages to avoid accumulation.
- Monitor serum vancomycin concentration.
- Monitor renal function tests.
- Perform baseline auditory function tests; repeat during therapy.

Nursing Process Overview

Macrolides, Clindamycin, and Miscellaneous Penicillin Substitutes

Assessment

Perform a thorough patient assessment, focusing on the presenting problem. Depending on the antiinfective agent prescribed, obtain baseline hearing acuity. Monitor vital signs, complete blood count (CBC), and white blood cell (WBC) differential.

Nursing Diagnoses

- Potential complication: pseudomembranous colitis
- Potential complication: ototoxicity
- Knowledge deficit related to prevention of sexually transmitted diseases

Patient Outcomes

The patient's infection will resolve without side effects. If pseudomembranous colitis or ototoxicity develops, the nurse will manage and minimize side effects of these problems.

Planning/Implementation

Monitor renal function tests or liver function tests, depending on drug prescribed. Monitor serum drug levels, if available. Teach patients to report the development of side effects. Monitor vital signs and clinical signs of the initial infection.

Evaluation

Before discharge, verify that the patient can explain what drug reactions might be expected and when to notify the physician.

Nursing Implications Summary

Macrolides

Drug Administration
- See Nursing Implications Summary in Chapter 43.
- Assess for history of allergy before administering the drug.
- Assess baseline hearing acuity. Assess for GI tract symptoms and signs of liver dysfunction. Monitor intake and output and weight.
- Monitor liver function tests. Monitor the electrocardiogram, especially with high-dose parenteral forms.

Intravenous azithromycin
- See manufacturer's insert for current guidelines.

Intravenous erythromycin lactobionate or gluceptate
- Dilute each 500 mg with 10 ml of sterile water for injection without preservatives and further dilute as instructed in drug insert. Administer at a rate of 1 g diluted in 100 ml over 20 to 60 minutes. Monitor vital signs.

Nursing in the Community
- See Nursing Implications Summary in Chapter 43.
- Instruct the patient to report tinnitus or hearing loss, malaise, fever, jaundice, right upper quadrant abdominal pain, and change in the color or consistency of stools.
- Patients should take oral doses of erythromycin with meals or a snack to reduce gastric irritation. Instruct the patient to take doses of azithromycin on an empty stomach 1 hour before or 2 hours after meals. Instruct the patient to take doses of clarithromycin with meals or snack or on an empty stomach.
- Instruct the patient to take doses of dirithromycin with meals or food, or within 1 hour of eating. Tell the patient not to crush, cut, or chew dirithromycin tablets.
- Instruct the patient to swallow delayed-release capsules or tablets whole, without chewing or breaking.

clindamycin

Drug Administration
- See Nursing Implications Summary in Chapter 43.
- Assess for history of allergy before administering the drug.
- Assess for diarrhea or GI tract distress. Monitor intake and output and weight.
- Monitor CBC and WBC differential, platelet count, liver function tests, and serum electrolyte level.

Intravenous clindamycin
- IV clindamycin is available premixed, or each 18 mg must be diluted with at least 1 ml of suitable diluent; see drug insert. Administer at a rate of 300 mg or less over at least 10 minutes. Do not administer too rapidly. Monitor vital signs. Supervise ambulation.

Nursing in the Community
- Instruct the patient to report diarrhea to the physician. Warn the patient to not self-medicate for severe diarrhea; for mild diarrhea, the patient may self-medicate with antidiarrheal drugs containing kaolin or attapulgite. These medications should be taken 2 hours before or 3 to 4 hours after taking lincomycin or clindamycin.
- Instruct the patient to take oral capsules of clindamycin with a full glass (8 ounces) of fluid, with or without meals. Instruct the patient to measure doses of the oral liquid form with the dropper provided by the pharmacist.
- For topical administration of clindamycin, instruct the patient to apply carefully, avoiding the eyes, nose, mouth, and mucous membranes, and to apply over the entire affected area, not just to pimples. Instruct the patient to use the drug regularly for best effect and to use only water-based cosmetics. Instruct the patient to notify the physician if acne does not improve in 6 weeks, if skin irritation develops, or if any GI tract symptoms develop. The topical solution form contains alcohol, so teach the patient to wait 30 minutes after washing or shaving before applying medication to decrease stinging. The topical solution is dispensed in a bottle with an applicator tip. See manufacturer's instructions for correct technique of application.

Nursing Implications Summary–cont'd

➤ For vaginal cream, review administration technique with the patient. See the Patient Problems box in Chapter 51 on vaginal infections. Instruct the patient to wear a minipad or sanitary napkin to absorb leaking medication; the patient should not use tampons. Instruct the patient to avoid intercourse during the course of therapy and to avoid latex (rubber) contraceptives, diaphragms, or cervical caps during therapy and for 72 hours after completing the course of therapy because clindamycin may weaken the latex, causing it to be ineffective.

vancomycin

Drug Administration

➤ See Nursing Implications Summary in Chapter 43.

➤ Assess for history of allergy before administering the drug.

➤ Assess baseline hearing acuity.

➤ Monitor serum creatinine level, blood urea nitrogen (BUN) level, CBC, and WBC differential count. Monitor urinalysis. Monitor serum drug levels, if available.

Intravenous vancomycin

➤ Dilute each 500 mg with 10 ml of sterile water for injection. Further dilute with 100 ml of normal saline or D5W. Administer each diluted dose over 60 minutes. Monitor vital signs. Too rapid IV administration may be associated with hypotension, cardiac arrest, or red man syndrome (red neck syndrome): maculopapular or erythematous rash of the face, head, chest, and arms; fever; chills; fainting; nausea; vomiting; tachycardia; or itching.

Nursing in the Community

➤ See Nursing Implications Summary in Chapter 43.

➤ Instruct the patient to report tinnitus or hearing loss.

➤ Instruct the patient not to take oral doses within 4 hours of taking cholestyramine or colestipol.

➤ If vancomycin is prescribed to treat diarrhea caused by other antibiotics, caution the patient to avoid antidiarrheal medicine unless first approved by the physician.

spectinomycin

Drug Administration/Nursing in the Community

➤ See Nursing Implications Summary in Chapter 43.

➤ Caution the patient to avoid driving or operating hazardous equipment if dizziness develops; the patient should notify the physician.

➤ Warn the patient that IM injections may cause burning at the injection site. Use diluent supplied by the manufacturer. Dilute as directed on the vial label.

➤ If given to treat gonorrhea, warn the patient that the sexual partner may also need treatment to avoid passing the organism back and forth. Also instruct the patient about sexually transmitted diseases as appropriate. Caution the patient that the male sexual partner should wear a condom to prevent transmission of infection.

CHAPTER REVIEW

Application

1. Why are erythromycin, clindamycin, vancomycin, and spectinomycin called penicillin substitutes?
2. What advantages do the esters of erythromycin have over erythromycin base?
3. Which of the erythromycin esters is best absorbed orally and may be taken with meals?
4. Which forms of erythromycin can be used parenterally?
5. What property limits parenteral use of erythromycin?
6. What is the major route of excretion of macrolides?
7. What is the most common adverse reaction to macrolides?
8. What toxic reaction is unique to erythromycin estolate?
9. How does azithromycin differ from erythromycin in distribution in the body?
10. Bacterial resistance to clindamycin is associated with resistance to which other antibiotic?
11. What form of clindamycin is appropriate for parenteral use?
12. How is clindamycin eliminated from the body?
13. What is the limiting toxicity to clindamycin? What implications does this have for nursing care?
14. How is antibiotic-associated colitis best treated?
15. By what route is vancomycin usually administered?
16. What is the major route of excretion of vancomycin?
17. What toxic reactions are most common with vancomycin?
18. What are clinical uses for vancomycin?
19. What is the primary clinical indication for spectinomycin?
20. What pharmacologic property of spectinomycin makes it a useful replacement of penicillin in treating gonorrhea?

Critical Thinking

1. Develop a nursing care plan for a patient receiving erythromycin, clindamycin, or vancomycin.

References

Degnan R: Pharmacology in practice: antibiotics, *RN* 60(10):49-55, 1997.

Fitzgerald M: Macrolide antibiotics, *Clin Excellence Nurse Pract* 1(1):71-77, 1997.

Chapter 47

Tetracyclines and Chloramphenicol

OBJECTIVES

After studying this chapter, you should be able to do the following:

- *Describe how the antimicrobial spectra of tetracyclines and chloramphenicol differ from those of erythromycin (see Chapter 46) and penicillin G (see Chapter 44).*
- *Name the most common route of administration for tetracyclines and chloramphenicol.*
- *Explain how doxycycline and minocycline differ from other tetracyclines.*
- *Describe common side effects of tetracyclines.*
- *Describe the serious side effects of chloramphenicol.*
- *Develop a nursing care plan for a patient receiving doxycycline or chloramphenicol.*

CHAPTER OVERVIEW

This chapter introduces antibiotics with very broad antimicrobial spectra. The tetracyclines are a large family of chemically related compounds, many of which are clinically useful both in human and in animal medicine. Chloramphenicol is the only member of its chemical class approved for use in the United States.

THERAPEUTIC RATIONALE: MICROBIAL INFECTIONS

Infections caused by bacteria range from mild local infections to life-threatening systemic disease. Other organisms cause similar diseases. For example, *Chlamydia trachomatis* causes genitourinary tract infections, and various *Rickettsia* cause diseases such as typhus and Rocky Mountain spotted fever. A spirochete, *Treponema pallidum*, causes syphilis, and protozoans of the genus *Plasmodium* cause malaria. These nonbacterial diseases comprise the primary indications for tetracyclines today. Without treatment, these nonbacterial diseases are serious and potentially fatal.

THERAPEUTIC AGENTS: TETRACYCLINES AND CHLORAMPHENICOL

▼ Tetracyclines: demeclocycline, doxycycline, minocycline, oxytetracycline, and tetracycline

Mechanism of Action and Bacterial Resistance

Tetracyclines are a group of chemically related drugs that block bacterial growth by preventing ribosomes from binding messenger RNA, thereby preventing the start of protein synthesis. Members of this drug family are therefore bacteriostatic rather than bactericidal.

For tetracyclines to be effective, they must first be transported into bacteria via an energy-dependent transport system. Resistant bacteria lose the ability to take in tetracyclines, and the antibiotic does not come in contact with its intracellular target. Most tetracycline resistance involves a plasmid (see Chapter 43) that is transmitted from bacterium to bacterium and may therefore spread rapidly throughout bacterial populations. For example, families of patients treated on a long-term basis with low dosages of tetracyclines may lose the normal tetracycline-sensitive bacterial flora and gain tetracycline-resistant forms. Cross-resistance between the older tetracyclines is complete. Minocycline and **doxycycline** are more lipid soluble than the other drugs and are transported into bacteria by different mechanisms than the older drugs. These drugs may therefore penetrate bacterial cells that do not concentrate the older tetracyclines.

Pharmacokinetics

Tetracyclines are most often administered orally (Table 47-1), usually as a hydrochloride or as a phosphate salt to increase solubility and thereby increase absorption. Tetracyclines are variably absorbed from the gastrointestinal (GI) tract. Absorption is influenced by acid lability, water solubility, and lipid solubility. All tetracyclines except doxycycline and minocycline are acid labile and are partly destroyed by stomach acid. Tetracyclines are not highly water soluble, and this solubility may be further reduced by complex formation with metal ions or with solid material in the intestine. In these insoluble forms, drugs are not absorbed but remain in the intestine and are excreted in feces. Doxycycline and minocycline are exceptions; being highly lipid soluble, both drugs pass freely through GI tract membranes and are much more completely and rapidly absorbed than most other tetracyclines.

Absorption of tetracyclines from intramuscular (IM) sites is poor and often causes local tissue irritation and pain at the injection site. IM use of tetracyclines is therefore limited.

Tetracyclines may be used intravenously in serious infections. Oxytetracycline, doxycycline, and minocycline can be obtained in a form suitable for intravenous (IV) use. These drugs have low water solubility and must be diluted extensively before use by this route. When used intravenously, tetracyclines may cause thrombophlebitis. Improper dilution of the drug or repeated infusion into the same vein increases the likelihood of thrombophlebitis.

Tetracyclines are well distributed in most body tissues and fluids, appearing in liver, spleen, bone marrow, bile, and cerebrospinal fluid (CSF), even in the absence of inflammation. The drugs pass the placental barrier and enter fetal circulation in appreciable amounts. Tetracyclines also appear in the milk of nursing mothers.

Differences in lipid solubility among the tetracyclines affect their elimination. The more polar or water-soluble drugs are eliminated through the kidneys in greater amounts than are the lipid-soluble tetracyclines doxycycline and minocycline. All tetracyclines enter urine by passive glomerular filtration, but lipid-soluble drugs are more completely reabsorbed from kidney tubules than drugs that are charged at the acid pH of tubular fluid. This high degree of reabsorption is reflected in the longer elimination half-life for doxycycline and minocycline (12 to 15 hours) than those of less lipid-soluble tetracyclines such as oxytetracycline, tetracycline, and chlortetracycline (6 to 9 hours).

Table 47-1	Clinical Summary of Chloramphicol and Tetracyclines	
Generic Name	**Trade Name**	**Administration/Dosage**
chloramphenicol	Chloromycetin Chloroptic	ORAL: *Adults and children*: 12.5 mg/kg every 6 hr. *Infants up to 2 wk*—6.25 mg/kg every 6 hr. OPHTHALMIC: *Adults and children*—Apply solution or ointment to conjunctiva every 3 hr or more frequently.
chloramphenicol	Chloromycetin*	OTIC: *Adults and children*—Apply 2 or 3 drops to ear canal every 6-8 hr.
chloramphenicol palmitate	Chloromycetin	ORAL (suspension): *Children*—As for other oral forms.
chloramphenicol succinate	Chloromycetin*	INTRAVENOUS: As for oral.
demeclocycline	Declomycin*	ORAL: *Adults*—150 mg every 6 hr. FDA pregnancy category D. *Children >8 yr*—1.65-3.3 mg/kg every 6 hr.
doxycycline	Doryx* Vibramycin*	ORAL, INTRAVENOUS: *Adults*—100-200 mg/day. FDA pregnancy category D. *Children >8 yr*—1.1-2.2 mg/kg every 12 hr.
minocycline	Minocin*	ORAL, INTRAVENOUS: 200 mg initially, then 100 mg every 12 hr. FDA pregnancy category D. *Children >8 yr*—4 mg/kg initially, then 2 mg/kg every 12 hr.
oxytetracycline	Terramycin	ORAL: *Adults*—250-500 mg every 6 hr. *Children >8 yr*—6.25-12.5 mg/kg every 6 hr. INTRAMUSCULAR: *Adults*—100 mg every 8 hr. *Children >8 yr*—5-8.3 mg/kg every 8 hr. INTRAVENOUS: *Adults*—250-500 mg every 12 hr. *Children >8 yr*—5-10 mg/kg every 12 hr.
tetracycline	Achromycin* Sumycin Tetracyn*	ORAL: *Adults*—250-500 mg every 6 hr. *Children >8 yr*—6.25-12.5 mg/kg every 6 hr. INTRAMUSCULAR: *Adults*—100 mg every 8 hr. *Children >8 yr*—5-8.3 mg/kg every 8 hr, not to exceed 250 mg/day.

*Available in Canada and the United States.
†Available in Canada only.

The second major route of elimination is by biliary excretion. Tetracyclines are concentrated in liver and bile and carried into the intestine, where they may be reabsorbed by enterohepatic circulation. The liver is also the site for biotransformation of several tetracyclines. In general, the more lipid-soluble drugs penetrate liver cells and are more extensively biotransformed. In particular, minocycline is extensively biotransformed. The high lipid solubility of doxycycline and its tendency to form insoluble complexes with intestinal solids account for an unusual mode of elimination for this drug. Doxycycline diffuses directly into the intestine, where it is sequestered by complex formation with fecal material. Because of this unusual mechanism for excretion, doxycycline does not accumulate in renal failure.

Uses

Tetracyclines are clinically important because of their wide antibacterial spectrum. Most gram-positive organisms are sensitive to tetracyclines; however, most infections caused by these organisms are best treated by other agents because penicillins, cephalosporins, erythromycin, and clindamycin are equally or more effective against these organisms and are less toxic.

Gram-negative bacterial pathogens cause diseases including urinary tract infections (*Klebsiella* species) and pneumonia (*Haemophilus influenzae*) that may respond to tetracyclines. Gram-negative bacteria found in the bowel (e.g., *Escherichia coli*) may be susceptible to tetracyclines, but resistance does develop. *Serratia, Proteus,* and *Pseudomonas* strains are usually resistant. *Neisseria gonorrhoeae* is sensitive to tetracyclines. Clinically, tetracyclines are used to treat gonorrhea only when penicillin is contraindicated. Tetracyclines are clinically effective for a number of bacterial infections that are relatively rare in the United States, including chancroid (*Haemophilus ducreyi*), rabbit fever or tularemia (*Francisella tularensis*), black plague (*Yersinia pestis*), brucellosis (*Brucella* species), and cholera (*Vibrio cholerae*).

Tetracyclines are highly effective for diseases caused by **Rickettsia** (tick fever, Rocky Mountain spotted fever, typhus, and Q fever), **Chlamydia** (parrot fever or psittacosis, trachoma, lymphogranuloma venereum), and *Mycoplasma pneumoniae* (atypical, or "walking," pneumonia).

Tetracyclines are useful in treating Lyme disease, relapsing fever, syphilis, and yaws, which are all caused by **spirochetes.** Tetracyclines may have a useful role in treating amebic dysentery. Minocycline in particular may be useful in nocardial infections.

Tetracyclines are widely used to treat acne. Relatively low dosages may be prescribed over long periods. Although this treatment is effective for many patients, questions arise as to long-term adverse effects of the drugs and to the contribution this practice makes to the development of tetracycline-resistant bacterial populations.

Pharmaceutical formulations of tetracyclines are quite varied. These antibiotics are available in 50- to 500-mg tablets or capsules, syrups for pediatric use, ophthalmic ointments or drops, and various forms for topical use.

Adverse Reactions and Contraindications

Tetracyclines cause a wide variety of adverse reactions. The most common complaint is GI tract irritation. Many patients experience nausea, vomiting, or pain with oral tetracyclines. Diarrhea may occur as a result of irritation by unabsorbed tetracycline remaining in the bowel. Diarrhea may also result from changes in the intestinal flora. Occasionally, the effects of these broad-spectrum drugs on intestinal flora are so extensive that overgrowth of drug-resistant bacteria occurs. Life-threatening staphylococcal enterocolitis may result, producing bloody diarrhea and extensive damage to the intestinal epithelium. *Candida* infections of the throat, vagina, and bowel also occur occasionally.

Tetracyclines are also commonly associated with central nervous system (CNS) effects, causing dizziness or unsteadiness.

Allergies to tetracyclines are uncommon. Urticaria, morbilliform rashes, and dermatitis can occur, as well as more serious reactions such as asthma, angioedema, and anaphylaxis.

Tetracyclines are not entirely specific for bacterial ribosomes and may inhibit mammalian protein synthesis to a small degree. This may explain their toxic effect on various tissues. For example, kidney function may be impaired by tetracyclines, and the effects may be worse in a kidney already damaged by disease or by trauma. Renal function should therefore be watched carefully in patients receiving these drugs.

Tetracyclines may delay blood coagulation. The exact mechanism for this reaction is unknown, but it may involve binding the calcium that is required in coagulation.

The ability of tetracyclines to bind calcium also leads to their deposition in bones and teeth. In adults this binding produces little visible effect, but in children less than 8 years of age, the newly formed permanent teeth may be stained by the drug. This staining is irreversible. Binding of tetracyclines to bones may detectably slow bone growth in fetuses or young children. Infants may also display increased intracranial pressure with bulging fontanelles when given tetracyclines (see Pediatric Considerations box).

All tetracyclines can be degraded to toxic products by exposure to light, but demeclocycline most commonly causes these reactions. The drug is broken down by the action of ultraviolet light on the skin, and the toxic products released cause an intense sunburn reaction. Because tetracyclines other than demeclocycline can cause this reaction, patients receiving these drugs should be cautioned to limit their exposure to direct sunlight, especially in subtropical or tropical climates.

Outdated tetracycline preparations have sometimes led to severe adverse reactions, apparently caused by toxic breakdown products of the drugs. One such reaction is the Fanconi syndrome, which involves loss of amino acids, proteins, and glucose in urine, along with polyuria, poly-

PEDIATRIC CONSIDERATIONS

Tetracyclines

THE PROBLEM

Young children rapidly form bones and teeth, which are composed primarily of calcium phosphates. As this material is deposited, tetracyclines may be so tightly bound to the calcium in bones and teeth that it cannot be released. Fetal bone growth may be slowed. Over time, tetracyclines are degraded by light and exposure to chemicals. This process occurs even though the drug is incorporated into the solid matrix of teeth. The degraded tetracyclines appear as brown to gray-colored permanent stains on the teeth.

SOLUTIONS
- Avoid tetracyclines in the last half of pregnancy.
- Avoid tetracyclines in children younger than 8 years.

dipsia, acidosis, nausea, and vomiting. These reactions slowly disappear after the drug is discontinued. In other cases, patients show symptoms reminiscent of systemic lupus erythematosus.

Specific tetracyclines may cause unique adverse reactions. For example, minocycline can damage vestibular function, thereby impairing balance. Minocycline may also discolor skin and mucous membranes. Demeclocycline is the tetracycline most likely to induce nephrogenic diabetes insipidus, with weakness, thirst, and increased urination.

Toxicity

The liver may be sensitive to tetracyclines. Hepatotoxicity may progress to jaundice, fatty liver, and death unless the drug is discontinued at the first sign of difficulty. Pregnant women are most sensitive to this complication and should rarely, if ever, be given tetracyclines.

Older adult patients who are extremely debilitated or patients recovering from extensive surgery or traumatic injuries may experience metabolic derangement when given tetracyclines. These patients often show negative nitrogen balance. This reaction may result from tetracycline inhibition of mammalian protein synthesis.

Interactions

Several tetracycline interactions with other drugs result from the ability of tetracyclines to form insoluble complexes with metal ions. For example, oral tetracyclines often cause gastric irritation; therefore patients may wish to take antacids along with the antibiotic. This practice should be discouraged because common antacids include magnesium and aluminum salts, which complex with tetracyclines and prevent their absorption from the GI tract, reducing the antibacterial effect of the antibiotic. Likewise, iron-containing preparations such as vitamin or mineral supplements may prevent tetracycline absorption. Milk and other dairy products are high in calcium

and also impair absorption. Sodium bicarbonate taken with a tetracycline tablet may impede tablet dissolution in the stomach and thereby reduce absorption of the drug.

Food in the stomach impairs absorption of oral tetracyclines, with the exception of doxycycline and minocycline. These lipid-soluble tetracyclines are absorbed well even in the presence of food or milk products in the stomach.

Cholestyramine and colestipol bind tetracyclines and impair oral absorption of the antibiotics. As a result, effective blood concentrations may not be achieved with concurrent use of these drugs.

Several tetracyclines, especially doxycycline and minocycline, are metabolized to some degree in the liver. Drugs such as barbiturates, which increase hepatic drug-metabolizing enzymes, shorten the duration of action of doxycycline and minocycline. This action may decrease the antibacterial effectiveness of these agents.

Estrogen-containing contraceptives may be less effective when tetracyclines are used over prolonged periods. Metabolism of the estrogen may be influenced by tetracyclines.

The bacteriostatic mechanism of action of tetracyclines leads to specific interactions. For example, penicillins given with tetracyclines may be less effective than penicillin given alone. Penicillins are bactericidal and act against actively multiplying bacteria. By inhibiting bacterial growth, tetracyclines make the bacteria resistant to the action of penicillins.

Tetracycline nephrotoxicity may become significant and dangerous when these antibiotics are given with other nephrotoxic agents.

chloramphenicol

Mechanism of Action and Bacterial Resistance

Chloramphenicol is a very simple synthetic molecule that inhibits bacterial protein synthesis. The mechanism of action differs from that of tetracyclines in that chloramphenicol inhibits late rather than early steps in ribosomal function. Like tetracyclines, chloramphenicol is usually bacteriostatic rather than bactericidal.

Bacterial resistance to chloramphenicol nearly always involves destruction of the antibiotic by bacterial enzymes. These enzymes are not always present but may be induced by exposure of potentially resistant bacteria to sublethal doses of chloramphenicol. The genes required for synthesizing this enzyme are usually carried on plasmids, which exist separately from bacterial chromosomes. Plasmids may be transmitted from bacterium to bacterium, and resistance to chloramphenicol may thereby be transmitted widely throughout bacterial populations.

Pharmacokinetics

Chloramphenicol is nearly completely absorbed from the GI tract after oral administration. The peak serum concentration achieved by an oral dose is about the same as that produced by an equivalent dose given intravenously, although attainment of peak serum concentration is somewhat delayed with oral administration. IM injection produces lower blood levels than oral administration and therefore is not recommended. Seriously ill patients should receive chloramphenicol intravenously because oral absorption may be impaired in these patients. The succinate form of chloramphenicol is used for IV administration only, but chloramphenicol itself is used orally.

Chloramphenicol is well distributed throughout body tissues and fluids. Significant and effective concentrations of the drug enter the eye, joint (synovial), and pleural fluids. Unlike many other antibiotics, chloramphenicol enters CSF relatively easily, even when the meninges are not inflamed. Chloramphenicol also easily crosses the placenta and appears in human milk.

Most of a dose of chloramphenicol is inactivated in the liver. The drug is conjugated with glucuronic acid to form chloramphenicol glucuronide. This inactive drug form may be excreted in the kidneys by tubular secretion, whereas unaltered chloramphenicol is excreted solely by glomerular filtration. The actual concentration of active chloramphenicol in urine is high enough to be antibacterial, but active chloramphenicol in urine is only a small fraction of the total drug excreted via this route.

Uses

Because of dangerous toxic reactions, chloramphenicol is used only in serious infections. In addition, life-threatening infections such as bacteremias and meningitis may be treated with chloramphenicol when the pathogen has been tested and has proved sensitive to the drug. The antibacterial spectrum of chloramphenicol is similar to that of tetracyclines and includes gram-negative bacteria (except *Pseudomonas aeruginosa*), *Rickettsiae,* and *Chlamydia.* Chloramphenicol is especially effective against the important anaerobic pathogen *Bacteroides fragilis.* Although once the drug of choice for typhoid fever, chloramphenicol has been replaced by safer, more effective drugs.

Adverse Reactions and Contraindications

Chloramphenicol is an effective antibiotic, but its clinical use is limited by its potential for bone marrow toxicity. A reversible form of bone marrow depression causes leukopenia and a reduction of reticulocytes. These symptoms usually resolve quickly when chloramphenicol is discontinued. Patients receiving chloramphenicol should have routine blood tests performed during therapy to detect early signs of this toxic reaction.

Chloramphenicol may also induce irreversible bone marrow depression, which leads to **aplastic anemia,** a condition with high mortality. This condition is usually characterized by pancytopenia (loss of all forms of blood cells), but in some cases, one or more types of blood cells continue to be formed. Aplastic anemia, although rare, may appear weeks or months after chloramphenicol therapy. This time lag between drug administration and appearance of aplastic anemia complicates accurate calculation of drug-associated risk, especially considering that most patients have received more

than one other drug during the interim between chloramphenicol therapy and development of aplastic anemia. Best estimates of incidence suggest that roughly 1 in 30,000 chloramphenicol-treated patients will develop aplastic anemia. Although this incidence is low, the often fatal outcome is sufficient cause to restrict the use of chloramphenicol to the treatment of very serious infections.

Less severe problems also occur with chloramphenicol therapy. Allergies of various types and GI tract irritation may occur. Long-term therapy has been associated with neuritis, which may involve the optic nerve. Blindness has occurred in a few patients. CNS symptoms, including headache, mental confusion, depression, and delirium, are also seen in some patients.

Chloramphenicol crosses the placenta and may concentrate in fetal liver. Therefore the drug is not given to pregnant women near term.

Toxicity

Patients with reduced liver function are at risk of severe toxic reactions because of drug accumulation. The liver normally converts more than 90% of administered chloramphenicol, which is toxic, to a glucuronide, which is nontoxic. Therefore any reduction in the liver's ability to detoxify the drug may cause accumulation of the toxic drug, unless dosages are appropriately reduced. Neonates have an immature liver that lacks the enzyme to form glucuronides, increasing their risk for this complication. When these infants are given a weight-adjusted dosage based on adult doses, many develop gray syndrome. Drug accumulation proceeds without symptoms for 3 to 4 days, after which time the infant may develop abdominal distension, emesis, progressive pallid cyanosis, and irregular respiration. In a high percentage of cases, vasomotor collapse and death result. Infants receiving smaller doses are less likely to develop these symptoms. If early signs of the condition are noted by alert health care personnel and the drug is discontinued, most infants recover.

Interactions

Chloramphenicol can inhibit drug-metabolizing enzymes in the liver. This property may lead to dangerous interactions with drugs that have a low therapeutic index and are eliminated by microsomal hepatic enzymes. Drugs in this category include alfentanil, chlorpropamide, phenytoin, tolbutamide, and coumarin anticoagulants. When a patient receiving one of these drugs on a long-term basis is given chloramphenicol, these liver-metabolized drugs tend to accumulate. As a result, the patient's previously well-controlled conditions may escape control. For example, well-controlled diabetic patients may become hypoglycemic, successfully anticoagulated patients may develop spontaneous bleeding, or controlled epileptic patients may develop phenytoin toxicity.

Chloramphenicol competes with erythromycin and clindamycin for binding sites on bacterial ribosomes. As a result, the drugs may be antagonistic with one another and should not be combined.

Nursing Process Overview

Tetracyclines and Chloramphenicol

Refer to Chapter 43 for general guidelines on the nursing process with antibiotic therapy. The additional material in this chapter relates specifically to the tetracyclines and chloramphenicol.

Assessment

Carry out a thorough patient assessment. Monitor liver and kidney function. Monitor signs of clinical infection.

Nursing Diagnoses

- Potential complication: GI distress
- Potential complication: bone marrow depression

Patient Outcomes

The patient's infection will resolve without incident. The nurse will manage and minimize complications.

Planning/Implementation

Monitor renal and liver function. Assess for GI tract distress. Adjust timing of ordered doses to allow for interactions with food or other drugs (especially with tetracycline).

Evaluation

Before discharge, ascertain that the patient can take drugs as ordered and can explain signs and symptoms warranting consultation with the physician.

Nursing Implications Summary

Tetracyclines

Drug Administration

➤ See Nursing Implications Summary in Chapter 43.

➤ Assess for allergy to tetracyclines or "caine" drugs (e.g., lidocaine, procaine) before administering drug.

➤ Assess for dizziness and vertigo in patients receiving minocycline. Inspect for bruising, bleeding, or blood in stool.

➤ Monitor blood urea nitrogen (BUN) level, serum creatinine level, liver function tests, complete blood count (CBC) and differential, and platelet count.

➤ Palpate the fontanelles of infants every 4 hours; report bulging to the physician.

➤ Do not administer tetracyclines to children younger than 8 years of age unless absolutely necessary.

➤ Warn the patient that IM injections are painful.

➤ Administer IV doses slowly, and well diluted, to lessen the chance of venous irritation and phlebitis. Make certain IV infusion is patent before administering drug to avoid extravasation.

Intravenous doxycycline

➤ Check expiration date. Dilute each 100 mg with 10 ml sterile water for injection or normal saline. Further dilute as directed in drug insert with 100 to 1000 ml of compatible fluid. Administer at a rate of 100 mg over 1 to 4 hours.

Intravenous minocycline

➤ Dilute as directed in drug insert. Final dilution is in a volume of 500 to 1000 ml. Administer at an appropriate rate for the volume and the patient's age and size.

Intravenous oxytetracycline

➤ Dilute as directed in drug insert. Administer at a rate of 100 mg or less over at least 5 minutes.

Nursing in the Community

➤ See Nursing Implications Summary in Chapter 43.

➤ Instruct the patient to take oral doses with a full glass (8 ounces) of water.

➤ Usually the patient should take oral tetracyclines on an empty stomach 1 hour before or 2 hours after meals. However, if the drug causes stomach upset, the physician may permit it to be taken with meals or a snack. Doxycycline and minocycline may be taken on a full or empty stomach.

➤ Instruct the patient not to take oral tetracyclines within 1 to 2 hours of having milk, milk products, or formula. Instruct the patient not to take any tetracycline within 1 to 2 hours of taking any of the following medications: antacids, calcium supplements, choline and magnesium salicylate combinations, magnesium salicylate, magnesium-containing laxatives, or sodium bicarbonate. Review other prescribed medications with the patient to clarify these instructions.

➤ Instruct the patient not to take iron or vitamin preparations containing iron within 2 to 3 hours of taking a tetracycline.

➤ Warn the patient that tetracyclines may cause the tongue to become darkened or discolored. This effect is not significant and clears when the drug is stopped.

➤ Contraceptive pills containing estrogen may not be effective while patients are taking tetracyclines; other forms of birth control should be used. Discuss this effect with the physician or pharmacist.

➤ This drug may cause photosensitivity (see the Patient Problems box in Chapter 58 on photosensitivity).

➤ Demeclocycline may be used to treat the syndrome of inappropriate antidiuretic hormone (SIADH) and, when used for this, functions as a diuretic. This diuretic action is effective in patients with SIADH but is not satisfactory in other patients who may require diuresis.

➤ When tetracyclines are used in children younger than 8 years of age, discoloration of the teeth may occur. Notify the physician if this happens.

Continued

Nursing Implications Summary—cont'd

➤ Instruct the patient to observe expiration dates on all medications but especially on tetracyclines. Use of outdated preparations or those that have deteriorated or changed color may cause severe adverse reactions.

➤ Warn the patient taking minocycline to avoid driving or operating hazardous equipment if vertigo or dizziness occurs and to notify the physician.

➤ Teach proper injection technique to a patient who will self-administer IM forms.

➤ Instruct the patient to swallow the capsule form of doxycycline whole, without crushing or breaking.

➤ Topical tetracyclines: Read the manufacturer's patient instruction leaflet. The cream, ointment, and topical liquid forms may stain clothing. Instruct the patient to notify the physician if skin condition does not improve in 4 to 6 weeks or if skin irritation or excessive dryness develops.

➤ Tetracyclines are also available in eye ointment and eye drop forms. See Chapter 5 for information about administering these drug forms. Teach the patient the appropriate administration technique.

chloramphenicol
Drug Administration

➤ See Nursing Implications Summary in Chapter 43.

➤ Assess for history of allergy before administering the drug.

➤ Assess visual acuity before beginning therapy and at regular intervals. Assess for GI tract side effects, skin changes, and signs of hematologic side effects.

➤ Monitor infants for appearance of gray syndrome. Assess for failure to feed, abdominal distension, progressive pallid cyanosis, and irregular respiration. Note that gray syndrome can develop in infants of women who received chloramphenicol during labor or the last few days of pregnancy.

➤ Monitor serum drug levels, CBC and differential, platelet count, BUN level, serum creatinine level, and liver function tests.

Intravenous chloramphenicol

➤ Dilute 1 g with 10 ml of sterile water or D5W. Chloramphenicol may be further diluted with 50 to 100 ml of compatible solution; see the drug insert.

➤ Administer IV push at a rate of 1 g over 3 to 5 minutes. For infusion, administer a volume of 50 to 100 ml over 30 to 60 minutes.

➤ Warn the patient that chloramphenicol may cause a bitter taste in the mouth after IV administration but that it should resolve after a few minutes.

Nursing in the Community

➤ See Nursing Implications Summary in Chapter 43.

➤ Instruct the patient to report unexplained bruising or bleeding, nosebleed, bleeding gums, blood in stools and fever, sore throat, malaise, fatigue, or symptoms of infection. Instruct the patient to report these symptoms even if they develop after the drug has been stopped.

➤ Instruct the patient to take oral doses with a full glass (8 ounces) of water on an empty stomach 1 hour before or 2 hours after meals for best effect. Caution the patient to avoid driving or operating hazardous equipment if confusion or visual changes occur.

➤ Warn diabetic patients that chloramphenicol may cause false results with urine glucose tests. Instruct these patients to consult the physician before changing diet or diabetes medications and to monitor blood glucose levels.

➤ Chloramphenicol is also available in eye ointment, eyedrop, topical cream, and eardrop forms. See Chapter 5 for information about administering these drug forms. Teach the patient the appropriate administration technique.

CHAPTER REVIEW

Application

1. What is the mechanism of action of tetracycline antibiotics?

2. How do bacteria become resistant to tetracyclines?

3. How does the absorption of minocycline and doxycycline differ from that of other tetracyclines?

4. What factors limit the IM use of tetracyclines?

5. What precautions are necessary for using tetracyclines by IV routes?

6. What are the three main routes of excretion for tetracyclines?

7. Are minocycline and doxycycline eliminated in the same way as other tetracyclines?

8. What are the main toxic reactions common to all tetracycline antibiotics?

9. What toxic reaction is especially associated with demeclocycline?

10. What toxic reaction is especially associated with minocycline?

11. What toxicity is associated with outdated tetracycline preparations?

12. What is the effect of administering tetracyclines with antacids? What is the education implication?

13. Why do tetracyclines interfere with the antimicrobial action of penicillins?

14. Name three groups of organisms against which the tetracyclines are effective.

15. What is the mechanism of action of chloramphenicol?

16. What is the mechanism by which bacteria become resistant to chloramphenicol?

17. Which routes of administration give the most rapid and complete absorption of chloramphenicol?

18. Does chloramphenicol efficiently enter CSF?
19. What is the primary route of elimination of chloramphenicol?
20. What is the most dangerous toxic reaction associated with chloramphenicol?
21. What is the gray syndrome?
22. Name a clinical indication for chloramphenicol.

Critical Thinking

1. What factors influence the oral absorption of tetracycline antibiotics? What are some patient education implications?
2. Develop a nursing care plan for a patient receiving one of the drugs discussed in this chapter.

Reference

Degnan R: Pharmacology in practice: antibiotics, *RN* 60(10):49-55, 1997.

Chapter

48

Aminoglycosides

OBJECTIVES

After studying this chapter, you should be able to do the following:

- *Explain why aminoglycosides are administered only by parenteral routes.*
- *Describe the toxicity associated with aminoglycoside use.*
- *Explain why aminoglycosides are sometimes used along with penicillins for serious infections.*
- *Develop a nursing care plan for a patient receiving an aminoglycoside.*

CHAPTER OVERVIEW

This chapter introduces a group of antibiotics with primary usefulness for infections caused by gram-negative aerobic bacteria. **Aminoglycoside** antibiotics are composed of three or four amino sugars held together in glycosidic linkage. Great variability in structure is possible in these component sugars, and as a result several antibiotics of this type exist.

THERAPEUTIC RATIONALE: BACTERIAL INFECTIONS

Diseases caused by aerobic gram-negative bacteria include pneumonias, urinary tract infections, septicemia, and central nervous system (CNS) infections. Because aminoglycosides have serious dose-limiting toxicity, they are used only in serious or life-threatening infections caused by aerobic gram-negative organisms.

THERAPEUTIC AGENTS: DRUGS TO TREAT BACTERIAL INFECTIONS

▼ Aminoglycosides: amikacin, gentamicin, kanamycin, netilmicin, streptomycin, and tobramycin

Mechanism of Action and Bacterial Resistance

Aminoglycosides inhibit early steps in bacterial protein synthesis by binding to bacterial ribosomes. Bacterial protein synthesis may continue in the presence of aminoglycosides but with a greatly increased error rate. Defective proteins formed may damage the bacterial cell. Aminoglycosides also affect bacterial cell membranes. Aminoglycosides are bactericidal, unlike many other antibiotics that inhibit bacterial protein synthesis.

Aminoglycosides must be pumped into bacterial cells to reach their site of action. The pump mechanism requires energy and oxygen in order to function. Thus, in anaerobic sites, aminoglycosides do not enter bacteria in sufficient amounts to inhibit protein synthesis. For this reason, aminoglycosides are used only for aerobic bacteria.

Resistance to aminoglycosides occurs as a result of decreased antibiotic uptake, changes in antibiotic binding to ribosomes, or enzymatic destruction of the aminoglycosides. By far the most common mechanism for resistance involves antibiotic destruction. Many sites for enzymatic attack exist on the amino sugars in aminoglycosides. Bacterial enzymes modify aminoglycosides in several ways. The primary sites of attack are amino and hydroxyl groups on the sugars. Amino groups may be acetylated, and hydroxyl groups may have a phosphate or an adenylate group added. Any of these substitutions inactivates the aminoglycoside. At least 13 separate enzymes catalyzing these reactions have been identified. Aminoglycosides differ in susceptibility to degradation, ranging from kanamycin, which is destroyed by at least six different enzymes, to **amikacin,** which is sensitive to only two enzymes.

Pharmacokinetics

Aminoglycosides are polycationic molecules at physiologic pH. As a result of being charged, these drugs do not readily penetrate mammalian membranes and are not absorbed orally. Therapy with aminoglycosides is therefore by intramuscular (IM) or intravenous (IV) routes and usually involves hospitalized patients who have moderate to severe infections. Absorption of aminoglycosides from IM injection sites is rapid, and peak serum concentrations occur within 60 to 90 minutes.

Aminoglycosides do not enter the CNS to any significant extent in normal persons, but some drug does appear in cerebrospinal fluid when meningitis is present. **Gentamicin** may be given by intralumbar or intraventricular injection to improve drug levels in the CNS. Aminoglycosides enter most other body fluids and tissues. These drugs cross the placenta and achieve significant concentrations in fetuses.

Aminoglycosides are excreted by glomerular filtration in the kidney. Active drug is concentrated in urine. Because the kidneys are the primary site for elimination of these drugs, any reduction in renal function may lower excretion sufficiently to cause aminoglycoside accumulation. The approximate half-time for elimination of these drugs is 2 to 4 hours, but in renal failure it may be greatly prolonged. Excretion is also lower in neonates, who have immature kidneys, and in older adult patients, whose renal function is diminished simply as a function of age (see Geriatric Considerations box).

Uses

The clinical use of these drugs is limited by their toxic potential. In general the aminoglycosides are reserved for serious infections caused by aerobic gram-negative bacteria or by mycobacteria (see Chapter 50). Individual drugs in this family differ in specific uses as a result of differences in relative toxicity and antibacterial activity. Table 48-1 lists the most important clinical uses of individual aminoglycosides.

Streptomycin is most useful today in combination with other agents to treat infections in which strict bactericidal action is required for most effective therapy. Examples of these infections are bacterial endocarditis and tuberculosis (see Chapter 50).

One difference among aminoglycosides is their different degree of activity against *Pseudomonas aeruginosa.* Amikacin, gentamicin, **netilmicin,** and **tobramycin** are most effective against this pathogen. Kanamycin usually is not effective. Amikacin differs from other aminoglycosides in being less sensitive to common aminoglycoside-degrading enzymes. Amikacin is therefore active against some bacterial strains that are resistant to other aminoglycosides. Table 48-1 lists common dosages for aminoglycosides used in patients with normal renal function.

Adverse Reactions and Contraindications

Because aminoglycosides may be nephrotoxic, renal function must be monitored in patients receiving aminoglycosides (see next section). Serum levels of these drugs are monitored to prevent intoxication.

Aminoglycosides must be used with caution in patients with any condition that impairs transmission at the neuromuscular junction or otherwise weakens muscular function. Therefore patients with myasthenia gravis, Parkinson's disease, or infant botulism would normally not receive aminoglycosides; if they receive aminoglycosides, they must be watched carefully for excessive muscle weakness during therapy.

Patients with preexisting renal, auditory, or vestibular damage would ordinarily not be given an aminoglycoside if an alternative drug was available. These patients may be more at risk for the dose-related toxicity described in the next section.

Less common adverse reactions include effects on a variety of organ systems. Blood dyscrasias, although rare, may occur with any aminoglycoside. Rare neurotoxicity causes headaches, paresthesias, tremor, confusion, and disorientation. The aminoglycosides are also somewhat irritating and may cause pain at the injection site. Allergies to aminoglycosides are possible, and a prior allergic reaction to any aminoglycoside is a contraindication to receiving the drugs again.

Toxicity

The aminoglycosides exert significant dose-dependent toxicity of three major types: ototoxicity, renal toxicity, and neuromuscular blockade. **Ototoxicity** may cause hearing loss, loss of equilibrium control, or both. Hearing loss in some patients continues even after the drug is discontinued. Loss of equilibrium may be less obvious than hearing loss but can usually be revealed by appropriate tests. Nausea or dizziness

GERIATRIC CONSIDERATIONS

Aminoglycosides

THE PROBLEM

Patients older than 60 years of age have reduced renal function and therefore may excrete aminoglycosides more slowly than younger adults. In older adults aminoglycosides may accumulate because alternative paths of elimination are limited. Older adults also have some hearing loss because of their age and may therefore be more susceptible to drug-induced hearing loss.

SOLUTIONS
- Lower dosages to avoid accumulation.
- Monitor serum aminoglycoside concentrations.
- Monitor renal function tests.
- Perform baseline auditory function tests; repeat during therapy.

Table 48-1   Aminoglycosides

Generic Name	Trade Name	Administration/Dosage	Comments
amikacin	Amikin*	INTRAMUSCULAR, INTRAVENOUS: *Adults and children*—5 mg/kg body weight every 8 hr. Do not exceed 1.5 g/day. Give intravenous doses by slow infusion. FDA pregnancy category D. *Neonates*—10 mg/kg initially, then 7.5 mg/kg every 12-24 hr.	Serious infections caused by aerobic gram-negative bacteria, including *P. aeruginosa*.
gentamicin	Cidomycin† Garamycin*	INTRAMUSCULAR, INTRAVENOUS: *Adults*—1-1.7 mg/kg every 8 hr. Do not exceed 8 mg/kg/day. FDA pregnancy category C. *Children*—2.5 mg/kg every 8-24 hr. *Neonates*—2.5 mg/kg every 12-24 hr.	Serious infections caused by aerobic gram-negative bacteria, including *P. aeruginosa*.
kanamycin	Kantrex	INTRAMUSCULAR, INTRAVENOUS: *Adults and children*—5 mg/kg body weight every 8 hr. FDA pregnancy category D. INTRAPERITONEAL: *Adults*—500 mg. INHALATION: 250 mg 2-4 times/day.	Serious infections caused by aerobic gram-negative bacteria, *not* including *P. aeruginosa*.
neomycin		TOPICAL: *Adults and children*—Commonly used as 0.35% creams and ointments. Also used in many combinations with other antibiotics.	Topical use only.
netilmicin	Netromycin*	INTRAMUSCULAR, INTRAVENOUS: *Adults*—1.3-2.2 mg/kg every 8 hr. FDA pregnancy category D. *Children*—2.75-4 mg/kg every 12 hr. *Neonates*—2-3.25 mg/kg every 12 hr.	Serious infections caused by aerobic gram-negative bacteria, including *P. aeruginosa*.
streptomycin		INTRAMUSCULAR: *Adults*—250 mg-1 g every 6-24 hr. FDA pregnancy category D. *Children*—Up to 20 mg/kg every 12 hr. *Geriatric dose*—500-750 mg once daily.	Used alone to treat tularemia or plague. Combined with other antibiotics to treat tuberculosis (with isoniazid or other drugs), endocarditis (with penicillin G), or brucellosis (with tetracyclines).
tobramycin	Nebcin*	INTRAMUSCULAR, INTRAVENOUS: *Adults*—1-1.7 mg/kg every 8 hr. FDA pregnancy category D. *Children >1 wk*—1.5-1.9 mg/kg every 6 hr. *Neonates*—Up to 2 mg/kg every 12-24 hr.	Serious infections caused by aerobic gram-negative bacteria, including *P. aeruginosa*.

NOTE: These dosages are guidelines only. Dosages must be individualized based on the patient's renal function.
*Available in Canada and the United States.
†Available in Canada only.

may signal disturbance of equilibrium. Ototoxicity is more severe when serum concentrations of aminoglycosides exceed 8 to 10 μg/ml. The total dose administered may also be a factor because some patients treated over long periods may display these symptoms despite never having excessively high serum levels of the drug.

Aminoglycosides may damage both tubules and glomeruli in the kidney, especially when high dosages are given. This toxic potential can cause a rapid clinical deterioration because renal damage can cause drug accumulation, which causes further damage to the kidney. This cycle of accumulation and increasing renal damage can destroy kidney function. Patients who accumulate the drug because of renal dysfunction are also more prone to ototoxicity.

The third characteristic toxic reaction to aminoglycosides is neuromuscular blockade. This reaction is usually observed in surgical patients when an aminoglycoside is used in peritoneal lavage. Neuromuscular blockade usually is manifested by respiratory paralysis because the muscles of the chest involved in breathing are prevented from functioning. Some of the aminoglycosides produce a competitive neuromuscular blockade, which may be reversed by neostigmine. Others, such as kanamycin, produce an irreversible blockade, which neostigmine does not affect, although calcium may relieve the blockade in some cases. Patients who have recently received muscle relaxants are more prone to experience neuromuscular blockade with aminoglycosides. Patients with myasthenia gravis are also more sensitive to this effect.

Interactions

The ototoxicity and nephrotoxicity of aminoglycoside antibiotics may be enhanced by a variety of agents. For example, if a patient who is receiving an aminoglycoside is also given a nephrotoxic drug such as a cephalosporin or methoxyflurane, the risk of kidney damage is increased. Likewise, ototoxic drugs such as ethacrynic acid may enhance ototoxicity in a patient receiving an aminoglycoside antibiotic. All aminoglycosides possess neuromuscular-blocking activity. This action has led to enhancement of agents used for neuromuscular-blocking action during surgery.

Gentamicin is commonly combined with an anti-*Pseudomonas* penicillin to treat *P. aeruginosa* infections. Although these drugs may be used in the same patient, they should never be physically mixed because penicillins chemically inactivate gentamicin in solution.

Aminoglycosides are many times more effective at the slightly alkaline pH of normal serum (pH 7.4) than at the acidic pH of normal urine (pH 5). Therefore, in the treatment of urinary tract infections with these drugs, a therapeutic advantage may be gained by alkalinizing urine.

Nursing Process Overview

Aminoglycosides

Refer to Chapter 43 for general guidelines on the nursing process with antibiotic therapy. The additional material in this chapter relates specifically to the aminoglycosides.

Assessment

Perform a full assessment focusing on the signs and symptoms of infection. Assess renal function, hearing acuity, and vestibular function. Note other medications the patient is receiving.

Nursing Diagnoses

- Potential complication: ototoxicity related to aminoglycoside therapy
- Potential complication: renal damage or failure related to aminoglycoside therapy

Patient Outcomes

The patient's infection will resolve without serious drug side effects. If ototoxicity or renal failure develops, the nurse will manage and minimize these side effects.

Planning/Implementation

Once the decision is made to administer aminoglycosides, gather the proper supplies for proper administration by the parenteral route chosen. Note whether the patient has received any other neuromuscular-blocking agents or whether the patient has any other condition such as myasthenia gravis that would predispose the patient to respiratory paralysis. Have available equipment to deal with respiratory paralysis if it occurs. Ensure that the medications are administered at the times prescribed. If samples are being taken for the measurement of blood levels of these drugs, obtain samples as ordered because the timing is critical for proper interpretation of the information.

Evaluation

Monitor vital signs closely, and assess objective and subjective signs and symptoms. Hearing loss caused by aminoglycosides may progress during and after therapy. Continue to evaluate the patient for this symptom and for any loss of control of equilibrium as evidenced by difficulty in walking or by staggering or dizziness.

Nursing Implications Summary

Aminoglycosides
Drug Administration

- See Nursing Implications Summary in Chapter 43.
- Assess for history of allergy before administering drug.
- Review discussion of toxicity observed with these drugs. Assess for changes in hearing and balance and for development of tinnitus and buzzing.
- Monitor intake and output and weight. Assess for increased thirst, nausea, vomiting, loss of appetite, and increase or decrease in frequency of urination.
- Monitor vital signs and auscultate lung sounds.
- Monitor serum creatinine level, blood urea nitrogen (BUN) level, urinalysis, liver function tests, serum electrolyte level, complete blood count (CBC) and white blood cell (WBC) differential, and platelet count.
- Monitor serum drug levels. Peak and trough levels may be available. Peak levels indicate serum levels after a dose is given and reflect the highest serum level for that patient at that dose. Trough levels are drawn shortly before a dose is given and reflect the lowest serum level for that patient at that dose. If peak and trough levels are ordered, notify the laboratory of the time a dose will be given so that blood specimens can be obtained at the proper times for drug level calculations.
- Have available neostigmine and calcium chloride when aminoglycosides are used with high-risk patients (e.g., in the operating room, recovery room, and intensive care units).

- Monitor respiratory status. Have available a suction machine at the bedside.
- Use gentamicin without preservatives for intrathecal administration.
- Do not mix aminoglycosides in a syringe with other medications.
- For pediatric doses and dilutions, consult the manufacturer's literature.
- Because of the possibility of hypotension or vertigo, keep siderails up. Supervise ambulation.
- Neomycin may be ordered orally or via enema to inhibit ammonia-forming bacteria in the gastrointestinal tract of patients with hepatic encephalopathy.
- Streptomycin may cause peripheral neuritis. Assess for burning of face, numbness, and tingling.

Intramuscular streptomycin

- Dilute as directed on the label of the vial. Use a large muscle mass. This drug is not administered by the IV route. Teach IM administration technique to patients who will self-administer at home.

Intravenous amikacin

- Dilute 500 mg in 100 to 200 ml of normal saline or D5W; administer to adults over 30 to 60 minutes. Administer doses to infants over 1 to 2 hours.

Intravenous gentamicin

- Dilute a single dose in 50 to 200 ml of normal saline or D5W.

Continued

Nursing Implications Summary—cont'd

The concentration should not exceed 0.1% (1 mg/ml). Administer each dose over 30 to 60 minutes in adults or up to 2 hours in children. Prepared dilutions are available.

Intravenous kanamycin

➤ Dilute the prescribed dose in normal saline, D5NS or D5W to a concentration of 500 mg in 100 to 200 ml. Administer over 30 to 60 minutes.

Intravenous netilmicin

➤ Dilute a single dose in 50 to 200 ml of diluent; see the drug insert. Administer over 30 minutes to 2 hours.

Intravenous tobramycin

➤ Dilute the dose in 50 to 100 ml of D5W or normal saline and administer over 20 to 60 minutes.

Nursing in the Community

➤ See Nursing Implication Summary in Chapter 43.

➤ Instruct the patient to report hearing loss, nausea, dizziness or vertigo, decreased urinary output, nausea, vomiting, loss

of appetite, and increased thirst.

➤ Streptomycin is often given in combination with other drugs in long-term therapy for tuberculosis.

➤ Streptomycin may cause peripheral neuritis. Caution the patient to report changes in vision, burning, numbness, or tingling.

➤ With topical preparations, systemic side effects are rare but can occur. Factors that influence the likelihood of toxicity include the frequency of application, the size of the area to which the preparation is being applied, whether the skin surface was intact, and the amount and kind of other ototoxic or nephrotoxic drugs the patient might be receiving concomitantly.

➤ Photosensitivity has been reported with topical preparations (see the Patient Problems box in Chapter 58 on photosensitivity).

CHAPTER REVIEW

Application

1. What is the mechanism of action of aminoglycoside antibiotics?

2. What is the most common mechanism for bacterial resistance to aminoglycosides?

3. Which routes of administration are appropriate for aminoglycosides?

4. What is the primary route of excretion of aminoglycosides?

5. What effects may aminoglycoside antibiotics have on the ears?

6. What groups of patients might be more prone to aminoglycoside ototoxicity and nephrotoxicity?

7. How do aminoglycosides affect the neuromuscular junction?

8. What special precautions must be taken when gentamicin and carbenicillin are used together?

9. Name three clinical uses of streptomycin.

10. How does the clinical indication for the use of kanamycin differ from the indications for gentamicin, tobramycin, netilmicin, and amikacin?

Critical Thinking

1. How do aminoglycoside antibiotics affect the kidneys? How should you assess for these effects?

2. What groups of patients are most likely to develop respiratory paralysis after therapeutic use of aminoglycoside antibiotics? How should you monitor these patients?

3. Develop a nursing care plan for a patient receiving gentamicin.

Reference

Degnan R: Pharmacology in practice: antibiotics, *RN* 60(10):49-55, 1997.

Chapter 49

Sulfonamides, Trimethoprim, and Drugs to Treat Urinary Tract Infections

OBJECTIVES

After studying this chapter, you should be able to do the following:

- *Explain why sulfonamides are especially useful for treating urinary tract infections.*
- *Explain why trimethoprim is given in fixed combination with a sulfonamide.*
- *Discuss the limited indications for nitrofurantoins.*
- *Develop a nursing care plan for patients receiving drugs that are discussed in this chapter.*

CHAPTER OVERVIEW

This chapter focuses on drugs that are used mainly to treat urinary tract infections (see Patient Problems box). Sulfonamides and trimethoprim have antimicrobial mechanisms and pharmacokinetic properties that make these drugs useful in certain systemic infections as well, but nitrofurantoins are used only in urinary tract infections.

THERAPEUTIC RATIONALE: URINARY TRACT INFECTIONS

Bacterial infections of the urinary tract are one of the most common complaints seen by physicians. The organisms that cause these infections are mostly gram-negative bacteria. The agents that are covered in this chapter are effective because they act against the organisms most likely to cause **urinary tract infections (UTIs)** and because the drugs are concentrated in the urinary tract.

THERAPEUTIC AGENTS: DRUGS TO TREAT URINARY TRACT INFECTIONS

▼ Sulfonamides: sulfadiazine, sulfamethizole, sulfamethoxazole, sulfapyridine, sulfasalazine, and sulfisoxazole

Mechanism of Action and Bacterial Resistance

Sulfonamides are metabolic inhibitors that block bacterial synthesis of folic acid, a vitamin required for the synthesis of

543

PATIENT PROBLEMS

Urinary Tract Infection

THE PROBLEM

Urinary tract infections (UTIs) are more common in females than in males because the urethra is shorter in females. UTIs are also more common in patients wearing urinary retention catheters (Foley catheters) and in patients requiring intermittent catheterization or urinary tract manipulation. Drugs may be prescribed when an infection develops, prophylactically when genitourinary examination or manipulation is planned, or when a history of chronic UTI exists.

SIGNS AND SYMPTOMS

- Burning on urination, frequent urination, itching in the area of the urinary meatus, fever, and malaise

NURSING IN THE COMMUNITY

- Instruct the patient to drink sufficient fluids to ensure a daily urine output of 1500 to 2000 ml. Usually, this means drinking at least 6 to 8 full glasses (8 ounces each) glasses of fluid for adults.
- Instruct the female patient to always wipe from front to back after voiding or defecating to avoid accidental contamination of the urinary meatus with bacteria from the anal region.
- Instruct the patient to avoid bubble baths. Some patients may have to eliminate all baths and shower only.
- Wash soap off the perineal region completely to avoid irritation from the soap. Some patients may have to wash with water only.

- Teach women to avoid feminine hygiene sprays and perfumed hygiene products; to wear loose-fitting clothing, including underwear with a cotton crotch; and to avoid wearing pantyhose and pants at the same time. Tell women to remove wet or damp clothes (e.g., bathing suits) as quickly as possible.
- Instruct the patient to void immediately after sexual intercourse.
- Some drugs for UTIs are most effective if urinary pH is changed. This is difficult to do through diet alone, so other drugs may be prescribed by the physician. If sodium bicarbonate or other drugs are prescribed, instruct the patient to take as ordered for best treatment of the UTI.
- Instruct the patient to take drugs for the full prescribed dose (often 7 to 10 days) and not stop when symptoms begin to subside.

FOR PATIENTS WITH URINARY CATHETERS

- Secure catheter well so that there is minimal pulling on the meatal area.
- Wash the catheter insertion area with soap and water, but avoid rough scrubbing. Rinse well.
- Avoid opening the drainage system unless necessary.
- Clean the tubing and bag as directed (unless replacing them with a new device), usually with a dilute bleach solution or as instructed by the discharge nurse.
- In the hospital, use sterile technique to insert catheters. In the home, use clean technique as instructed.
- Maintain a good fluid intake.

---

amino acids and nucleic acids (Figure 49-1). The metabolically active form of folic acid, tetrahydrofolic acid (THFA), is synthesized in bacteria from simple precursor molecules. Two of the enzymes involved in these conversions have been exploited as targets of antibacterial drugs. Dihydropteroate synthase, which converts paraaminobenzoic acid (PABA) and other small molecules to dihydropteroate, is the target for sulfonamides. Sulfonamides competitively inhibit this enzyme. The second target in this pathway is dihydrofolic acid reductase, the enzyme that forms THFA (see trimethoprim).

Sulfonamides are selectively toxic to organisms that must form folic acid from PABA and the other precursors. Fortunately, humans are not sensitive to this action because we cannot synthesize folic acid but must absorb it preformed in our diet. Sulfonamides are primarily bacteriostatic against those organisms they affect.

Bacterial resistance to sulfonamides has become widespread and has reduced the clinical usefulness of these drugs. Some bacteria such as pneumococci acquire an altered dihydropteroate synthase, which is less sensitive to sulfonamides. Overproduction of PABA is a common mechanism of resistance for several pathogens, including staphylococci, pneu-

mococci, and gonococci. Because sulfonamides are only competitive inhibitors of PABA incorporation into folic acid, excess PABA overcomes the sulfonamide inhibition.

Pharmacokinetics

Sulfonamide antibacterial agents with a wide variety of pharmacokinetic properties are available (Tables 49-1 to 49-3, on pp. 545, 546, and 547, respectively). For example, sulfasalazine is poorly absorbed from the gastrointestinal (GI) tract but is cleaved within the bowel to release sulfapyridine and mesalamine. This preparation is useful for ulcerative colitis because active material is released at the site of infection. The released sulfapyridine acts as an antimicrobial agent, and the mesalamine has direct antiinflammatory actions by blocking formation of prostaglandins (see Chapter 31), and perhaps by scavenging oxygen free radicals, which are increased in inflammatory bowel disease.

Topical sulfonamides such as mafenide and silver sulfadiazine are used to treat or prevent infections on burned or abraded skin. Systemic absorption is not expected by this route but can occur when the drugs are used on extensive areas of burned skin.

Table 49-1   Summary of Sulfonamides: Single-Component Formulations

Generic Name	Trade Name	Administration/Dosage	Clinical Use
sulfadiazine		ORAL: *Adults*—Single loading dose of 2-4 g, then 1 g every 4-6 hr. FDA pregnancy category C. *Children >2 mo*—75 mg/kg body weight to load, then 25 mg/kg every 4 hr, or 37.5 mg/kg every 6 hr.	Used with pyrimethamine for toxoplasmosis and malaria.
sulfamethizole	Thiosulfil Forte	ORAL: *Adults*—0.5-1 g every 6-8 hr. FDA pregnancy category C. *Children >2 mo*—7.5-11.25 mg/kg every 6 hr.	For urinary tract infections only.
sulfamethoxazole	Gantanol	ORAL: *Adults*—Single 2 g loading dose, then 1 g 2 or 3 times/day. FDA pregnancy category C. *Children >2 mo*—50-60 mg/kg loading dose, then 25-30 mg/kg twice daily, not to exceed 75 mg/kg/day.	For urinary tract infections, nocardiosis, otitis media, malaria, and toxoplasmosis.
sulfapyridine	Dagenan†	ORAL: *Adults*—500 mg 4 times/day. Reduce dosage as improvement allows.	For dematitis herpetiformis.
sulfasalazine	Azulfidine Salazopyrin*	ORAL: *Adults*—1 g every 6-8 hr. FDA pregnancy category B. Children >2 yr—10 mg/kg every 4 hr initially, then 7.5 mg/kg every 6 hr.	For ulcerative colitis.
sulfisoxazole	Gantrisin Sulfizole†	ORAL: *Adults*—2-4 g loading dose, then 1-2 g every 6 hr. FDA pregnancy category C. *Children >2 mo*—75 mg/kg loading dose, then 25 mg/kg every 4 hr, or 37.5 mg/kg every 6 hr.	For urinary tract infections and systemic infections caused by sensitive organisms.

*Available in Canada and the United States.
†Available in Canada only.

The sulfonamides used to treat systemic infections are well absorbed orally. Distribution of these drugs to body tissues including the brain is good. Concentrations of sulfonamides in cerebrospinal and other body fluids may approach those of serum. Sulfonamides also pass the placental barrier and enter fetuses. Elimination of sulfonamides involves both the liver and kidneys. The liver converts a portion of the sulfonamide in blood to an acetylated derivative, which is usually bacteriologically inactive. Acetylated as well as free drug are eliminated by the kidneys, primarily by glomerular filtration. Tubular reabsorption is significant for some sulfonamides. Excretion of sulfonamides is favored by alkalinizing urine. This procedure increases the solubility of these drugs in urine and also converts the drugs to a charged form that does not undergo renal tubular reabsorption.

Uses

Sulfonamides are potentially active against a wide range of gram-positive and gram-negative organisms, as well as *Nocardia, Chlamydia,* and *Actinomyces,* but bacterial resistance has limited use for many bacterial infections requiring systemic therapy. **Sulfamethoxazole** is the most widely used sulfonamide for general infections.

Sulfonamides may be combined with phenazopyridine to treat UTIs (see Table 49-2). The sulfonamide component supplies antibacterial activity and the phenazopyridine, which is excreted in urine, exerts an analgesic effect on the mucosa of the urinary tract. The added phenazopyridine therefore relieves the pain, burning, and itching associated with the UTI.

Sulfonamide preparations are available for vaginal application, but no evidence of effectiveness exists. Moreover, sensitization may be produced.

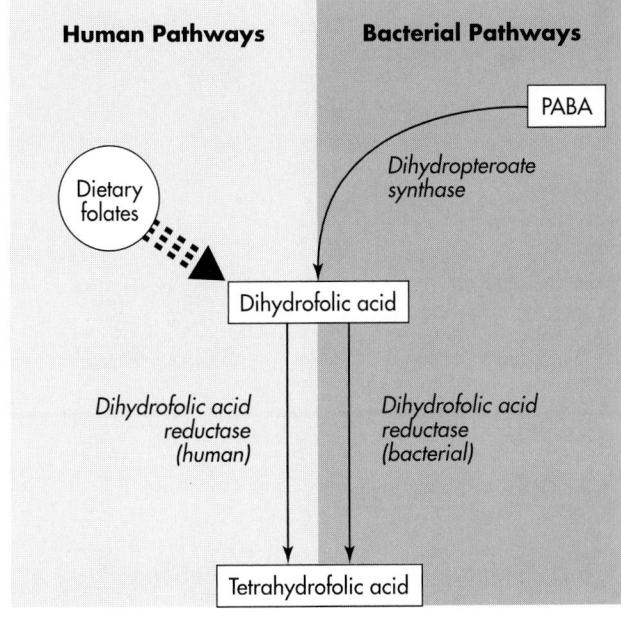

Figure 49-1 Synthesis of tetrahydrofolic acid (THFA) in bacteria and humans. THFA is vitamin required for nucleic acid and amino acid synthesis. Many bacteria form this vitamin from paraaminobenzoic acid *(PABA)* and other small molecules. Two enzymes involved in this synthesis have proved useful in chemotherapy: dihydropteroate synthase and dihydrofolic acid reductase. Sulfonamides inhibit dihydropteroate synthase, thereby blocking THFA synthesis in bacteria. Humans are immune from this action because preformed folate and dihydrofolic acid are supplied in diet. Dihydrofolic acid reductase in bacteria is inhibited by trimethoprim, but the human form of the enzyme is relatively resistant.

Table 49-2 Summary of Sulfonamides: Fixed Combinations for Oral and Intravenous Use

Components of Combination	Drug Form	Trade Name	Dosage	Clinical Use
sulfamethoxazole: 400 mg trimethoprim: 80 mg	Tablet	Bactrim* Cotrim Roubac† Septra*	*Adults*—800 mg sulfamethoxazole and 160 mg trimethoprim every 12 hr. *For pneumocystis pneumonia:* 25 mg/kg sulfamethoxazole and 5 mg/kg trimethoprim every 6 hr. FDA pregnancy category C. *Children >2 mo*—4-6 mg/kg trimethoprim and 20-30 mg/kg sulfamethoxazole every 12 hr.	For urinary tract infections, otitis media, bronchitis enteritis caused by sensitive *Shigella*, pneumocystis pneumonia.
sulfamethoxazole: 200 mg/5 ml trimethoprim: 40 mg/5 ml	Oral suspension	Bactrim* Septra*	*Adults and children*—As for tablet form.	As for tablet form.
sulfamethoxazole: 400 mg/5 ml trimethoprim: 80 mg/5 ml	IV injection	Bactrim IV Septra IV	*Adults, children >2 mo*—10-12.5 mg sulfamethoxazole and 2-2.5 mg trimethoprim every 6 hr. Dosage doubled for pneumocystis pneumonia.	As for tablet form.
sulfadiazine: 410 mg trimethoprim: 90 mg	Tablet	Coptin†	*Adults*—820 mg sulfadiazine and 180 mg trimethoprim once daily.	For urinary tract infections.
sulfadiazine: 205 mg/5 ml trimethoprim: 45 mg/5 ml	Oral suspension	Coptin†	*Children 3 mo-12 yr*—7 mg sulfadiazine and 1.5 mg trimethoprim per kg every 12 hr.	For urinary tract infections.
sulfadoxine: 500 mg pyrimethamine: 25 mg	Tablet	Fansidar*	*Adults—For malaria:* 3 tablets as single dose on third day of quinine treatment; or 1 tablet every 7 days for chemoprophylaxis. FDA pregnancy category C. *Children >2 mo—For malaria treatment:* 1.25 mg/kg pyrimethamine with 25 mg/kg sulfadoxine on day 3 of quinine therapy. *Children—For chemoprophylaxis: Age 2 mo-4 yr*—¼ tablet every 7 days; *4-8 yr*—½ tablet once every 7 days; *9-14 yr*—¾ tablet once every 7 days.	For malaria, chloroquine-resistant.
sulfamethoxazole: 500 mg phenazopyridine: 100 mg	Tablet	Azo Gantanol	*Adults*—4 tablets to load, then 2 tablets every 12 hr for 2 days.	For urinary tract infections only.
sulfisoxazole: 500 mg phenazopyridine: 500 mg	Tablet	Azo Gantrisin*	*Adults*—4-6 tablets to load, then 2 tablets every 6 hr for 2 days.	For urinary tract infections only.

IV, Intravenous.
*Available in Canada and the United States.
†Available in Canada only.

Adverse Reactions and Contraindications

Sulfonamides induce allergic reactions in a significant proportion of patients receiving the drugs. The most common reactions are skin rashes and itching, but drug fever and other more serious reactions such as Stevens-Johnson syndrome may occur. Anaphylaxis has been reported. Because sulfonamides are chemically related to the thiazide diuretics, acetazolamide, and oral hypoglycemic agents, a patient who becomes allergic to a sulfonamide may also become allergic to one or more of these agents. Photosensitivity to sulfonamides may also be a problem. The redness of the skin may be confused with an allergic reaction, but photosensitivity is localized to skin exposed to sun or sunlamps.

GI tract disturbances are common with sulfonamides. In addition to nausea, vomiting, and diarrhea, more serious reactions such as pancreatitis, hepatitis, and stomatitis may occur. Central

nervous system (CNS) alterations have also been observed, including headache, ataxia, hallucinations, and convulsions.

Deaths from aplastic anemia and other blood dyscrasias, although rare, have been connected with sulfonamide therapy. Sore throat, fever, or pallor may signal a serious blood dyscrasia (see Geriatric Considerations box).

Patients with preexisting renal or hepatic disease are more prone to develop side effects because these organs remove sulfonamides from the body. Patients with a genetic deficiency of glucose-6-phosphate dehydrogenase (G6PD) have greater risk for hemolytic anemia induced by sulfonamides. The highest frequency of G6PD deficiency is observed among African-Americans and Mediterranean populations; patients from these groups should be watched carefully for signs of anemia. Sulfonamides may also worsen anemias caused by folate deficiency.

Table 49-3   Summary of Sulfonamides: Topical Agents

Generic Name	Trade Name	Application Form	Clinical Use	Comments
mafenide acetate	Sulfamylon	Cream: 85 mg mafenide acetate/g	Treatment of second- and third-degree burns.	Effective against broad spectrum of pathogens, including *Pseudomonas aeruginosa.*
silver sulfadiazine	Silvadene Flamazine† Thermazene	Cream: 10 mg/g	Treatment of second- and third-degree burns.	Effective against broad spectrum of pathogens, including *P. aeruginosa* and certain yeasts.
sulfacetamide	Bleph* Sulamyd*	Solution: 10%, 15%, or 30% Ointment: 10%	Ophthalmic only. For conjunctivitis, corneal ulcer, and trachoma.	Drug allergy may develop in sensitive patients.
sulfisoxazole diolamine	Gantrisin	Solution: 4% Ointment: 4%	Ophthalmic only. For conjunctivitis, corneal ulcer, and trachoma.	Drug allergy may develop in sensitive patients.

*Available in Canada and the United States.
†Available in Canada only.

GERIATRIC CONSIDERATIONS

Sulfonamides

THE PROBLEM
Older adult patients are more likely than younger adults to experience severe blood and skin reactions to sulfonamides. Diuretics, commonly taken by older adult patients for high blood pressure, compound the risk.

SOLUTIONS
- Monitor blood tests for signs of bone marrow depression.
- Watch for bleeding or reduced platelet counts.
- Inspect carefully for rash or purpura.
- Ascertain whether the patient is taking a thiazide diuretic, either alone or as a component of other preparations.

PEDIATRIC CONSIDERATIONS

Sulfonamides

THE PROBLEM
Sulfonamides displace bilirubin from serum proteins. In neonates, who typically have elevated bilirubin, this displacement may be sufficient to produce kernicterus.

SOLUTIONS
- Avoid sulfonamides in pregnancy near term.
- Avoid sulfonamides in infants younger than 1 month of age.

Toxicity

Renal toxicity was common with sulfonamides in use before 1960. Most of the renal damage associated with these older agents was produced by drug crystallization in urine or tubular fluid, a condition called **crystalluria.** These drugs precipitated because of their low solubility in normal acidic urine. Newer sulfonamides are more soluble under these conditions, and drug precipitation is seldom a problem. The least soluble sulfonamides in use today are sulfadiazine and the acetylated metabolite of sulfamethoxazole. Patients receiving any sulfonamide should receive sufficient fluids to produce at least 1 L of urine daily. If there is a problem, solubility of sulfonamides in urine may be increased by alkalinizing urine. Sulfamethizole and sulfasalazine produce a yellow-orange coloration in alkaline urine. This coloration, also observable in skin, is not harmful.

Interactions

Sulfonamides are highly bound to serum proteins and therefore may displace other drugs from protein-binding sites. This displacement can occur with oral anticoagulants, sul-

fonylureas, the anticonvulsant phenytoin, the antiinflammatory agents phenylbutazone and sulfinpyrazone, and the antineoplastic agent methotrexate. In newborns displacement of bilirubin by sulfonamides may place the patient at risk (see Pediatric Considerations box).

Hemolytic agents such as sulfonylureas, primaquine, procainamide, and quinidine increase the risk of hemolysis with sulfonamides.

The urinary antiseptic methenamine releases formaldehyde in acidic urine for antibacterial effect. Sulfonamides can form insoluble complexes with formaldehyde and thus lead to crystalluria.

Dihydrofolate Reductase Inhibitors

trimethoprim

Mechanism of Action and Bacterial Resistance

Trimethoprim inhibits bacterial dihydrofolic acid reductase, thus preventing THFA formation in bacteria (see Figure 49-1). Dihydrofolic acid reductase functions both in humans and in bacteria because much of the folate in mammalian diets is dihydrofolic acid that must be converted to THFA. Fortunately, dihydrofolic acid reductase in humans is relatively resistant to the action of trimethoprim, and the drug may be given at dosages that inhibit this enzyme in bacteria but not in humans; thus the conversion of dietary folates to THFA in patients can proceed normally in the presence of antibacterial concentrations of trimethoprim.

Pharmacokinetics

Trimethoprim is most often used in fixed combination with sulfamethoxazole (see Table 49-2). This combination repre-

---

CASE STUDY
Urinary Tract Infection

Carla Jones is a 28-year-old African-American woman who is being seen in a primary care clinic with complaints of pain and burning on urination and urinary frequency. She has had these symptoms for about 36 hours. Her vital signs are within normal limits, she has no known allergies, and she is otherwise healthy. The nursing history also reveals that Carla has had this problem twice before within the last 8 months. She was given prescriptions for antibiotics for both of these episodes. Her social history reveals that she was married 9 months ago and uses a diaphragm with contraceptive jelly for birth control. She works as a computer operator and describes her job as "very demanding." As the nurse is finishing his assessment, Carla tells him "I'm so frustrated that I'm having this problem again! My husband and I have plans to go on a vacation to Mexico and we're leaving in four days." The physician examines Carla and orders a clean catch urine specimen for a stat Gram stain followed by culture and sensitivity tests. The Gram stain results reveal more than 100,000 colonies of gram-negative bacteria per milliliter of urine. The physician makes the diagnosis of "cystitis" and prescribes the following medications for Carla: trimethoprim 160 mg with sulfamethoxazole 800 mg orally every 12 hours for 10 days, and phenazopyridine 200 mg orally three times a day for 2 days.

1. Why are trimethoprim and sulfamethoxazole, a sulfonamide, especially useful drugs for treatment of urinary tract infections such as the cystitis that Carla is experiencing?
2. Why are the trimethoprim and sulfamethoxazole used together?
3. What common side effects of trimethoprim-sulfamethoxazole (TMP-SMX) should be included in Carla's teaching?
4. What serious hematologic adverse effects of the sulfamethoxazole (SMX) is Carla at risk for?
5. As the nurse continues his teaching about the TMP-SMX, he also advises Carla to drink 8 to 10 large glasses of water each day and to wear sunscreen or protective clothing. Why are these two points important?
6. Why has the physician prescribed the phenazopyridine in addition to the other two medications? What common side effect of this medication should Carla be alerted about?
7. Before Carla leaves the clinic, the nurse gives her an educational pamphlet with recommendations for preventing urinary tract infections. What key points would you expect the nurse to cover with Carla?

---

sents an exploitation of drug properties for therapeutic effect. These drugs are administered at a 1:5 ratio of trimethoprim/sulfamethoxazole ratio. Both drugs are well absorbed from the GI tract. Serum concentrations of the free drug not bound to serum proteins are usually in a 1:20 trimethoprim/sulfamethoxazole ratio. At this concentration ratio, the drugs have maximum antibacterial activity. The combination is **synergistic,** or more effective in combination than would be expected from the action of either drug alone. Synergy may result because both drugs starve sensitive bacteria for THFA, but the drugs work on two different enzymes in the sequence of reactions leading to THFA. Sequential blockade of this metabolic pathway is much more effective than blockade of a single step by one drug at high concentrations.

Trimethoprim penetrates body tissues better than sulfamethoxazole. Trimethoprim concentrations in breast milk, bile, prostatic fluid, vaginal fluids, liver, spleen, skin, and kidneys may exceed plasma concentrations of the drug. Penetration into other tissues, including the CNS, is adequate.

Trimethoprim appears in urine at a concentration approximately 100 times the plasma concentration, with most of the drug in the active form. The urinary concentration of sulfamethoxazole is about five times the plasma concentration.

Uses

Trimethoprim has a spectrum of antimicrobial activity similar to that of sulfonamides, with some exceptions. Trimethoprim is more active against the gram-negative bacteria *Proteus* and *Klebsiella* but is not useful alone against *Chlamydia* or *Nocardia*. Trimethoprim resistance has not yet become widespread. Although trimethoprim is used in the United States most commonly in combination with a sulfonamide, a preparation of trimethoprim alone is available for use in UTIs.

Adverse Reactions and Contraindications

Serious reactions to trimethoprim are rare, but anorexia, diarrhea, headache, nausea, and vomiting sometimes occur.

Toxicity

Toxicity from trimethoprim is expected only with large overdoses. Treatment may include acidifying the urine to hasten excretion of trimethoprim and giving leucovorin to overcome its antifolate effects.

Trimethoprim may be less toxic than sulfonamides, but when it is combined with sulfamethoxazole, patients should be observed for all signs of sulfonamide toxicity.

Interactions

Trimethoprim is synergistic with any systemically effective sulfonamide. Sulfamethoxazole was chosen for use in the fixed combination with trimethoprim because the kinetics of elimination of the two drugs are similar, as discussed previously. Sulfadiazine is also used with trimethoprim in fixed concentrations for the same reasons.

Trimethoprim should not be combined with methotrexate, pyrimethamine, or trimetrexate because these drugs have potent antifolate activity. The result could be megaloblastic anemia.

nitrofurantoin

Mechanism of Action and Bacterial Resistance

Nitrofurantoin is activated in bacteria to compounds that attack bacterial proteins. It is effective against some gram-positive and gram-negative organisms, including many common pathogens of the urinary tract. *Pseudomonas* species, however, are usually intrinsically resistant. Development of resistance to nitrofurantoin therapy is not a significant problem.

Pharmacokinetics

Many compounds that are effective antibacterial agents in the laboratory are ineffective when used to treat systemic infections because of their unfavorable pharmacokinetics. One example of such a compound is nitrofurantoin (Table 49-4). This drug, despite being adequately absorbed from the small intestine, never achieves satisfactory blood levels. Low blood levels result from a rapid excretion of the drug by the kidneys. Removal of the drug occurs so quickly that it fails to accumulate in blood. Therefore, despite its broad antibacterial spectrum, it is ineffective against systemic infections. Nitrofurantoin is concentrated in the kidneys and achieves bactericidal concentrations in urine. The drug diffuses from renal tubules into renal tissues, so final renal concentrations are much greater than would be expected from the very low blood concentrations of the drug. These properties make nitrofurantoin effective against UTIs.

Uses

Nitrofurantoin is effective against UTIs caused by susceptible strains of *Escherichia coli*, *Enterobacter* species, enterococci, *Klebsiella* species, *Proteus* species, and staphylococci.

Adverse Reactions and Contraindications

Gastric irritation with anorexia, nausea, and emesis is common with nitrofurantoin. The large crystal form (Macrodantin, see Table 49-4) may be less irritating than the microcrystalline form. Gastric irritation is lessened by taking the drug with milk or food; milk or food also increases absorption of nitrofurantoin.

Another common side effect with nitrofurantoin is lung injury. Patients receiving nitrofurantoin for long periods should be observed for pneumonitis or pulmonary fibrosis, which may develop gradually or may appear as an acute illness.

Rashes, allergies, and reversible blood dyscrasias have been observed with nitrofurantoin. Hemolytic anemia similar to that seen with sulfonamides may also be seen. Infants less than 1 month of age have undeveloped enzyme systems that make them especially susceptible to hemolytic anemia induced by nitrofurantoin; therefore the drug is avoided in neonates. Nitrofurantoin should be used with care in pregnant patients and never at term. Persons with G6PD deficiency are also at risk for hemolysis.

Nitrofurantoin causes urine to turn brown, but this reaction is harmless. As with any drug that is excreted primarily by the kidneys, nitrofurantoin may accumulate in patients with renal failure. Therefore patients with renal failure are more likely to have significant side effects of nitrofurantoin therapy. Vitamin B deficiency, common in individuals with alcoholism, may also predispose a patient to peripheral neuropathy. Diabetes mellitus, a disease that may cause peripheral neuropathy, may produce added risk of neural complications.

Toxicity

Peripheral neuropathy is one of the most serious toxic effects of nitrofurantoin. If detected early, the condition disappears after discontinuation of the drug. Damage may be permanent if the drug is continued after signs of peripheral neuropathy have developed.

Interactions

To avoid excessive risk of hemolysis, nitrofurantoin should not be used with hemolytic agents. To avoid excessive neurotoxicity, nitrofurantoin should not be combined with neurotoxic medications. If nitrofurantoin is used with probenecid or sulfinpyrazone, the effectiveness of nitrofurantoin may be impaired because these drugs block renal secretion of nitrofurantoin. As a result, lower concentrations of the antibacterial agent are achieved in urine.

Table 49-4	**Nitrofurantoin and Trimethoprim**			
Generic Name	**Trade Name**	**Administration/Dosage**		**Comments**
nitrofurantoin	Furadantin Furalan	ORAL: *Adults*—50-100 mg every 6 hr. *Children >1 mo*— 0.75-1.75 mg/kg every 6 hr.		Take with food or milk.
nitrofurantoin	Macrobid	ORAL (extended-release): *Adults*—100 mg every 12 hr for 7 days.		Take with food or milk.
nitrofurantoin macrocrystals trimethoprim	Macrodantin* Proloprim* Trimex	As for nitrofurantoin. ORAL: *Adults*—100 mg every 12 hr. FDA pregnancy category C.		Take with food or milk. For urinary tract infections only, unless combined with sulfonamide.

*Available in Canada and the United States.

Nursing Process Overview

Sulfonamides, Trimethoprim, and Nitrofurantoin

Refer to Chapter 43 for general guidelines on the nursing process with antibiotic therapy. The additional material in this chapter relates specifically to drugs used mainly to treat UTIs.

Assessment

The drugs described in this chapter are used mainly to treat UTIs. Focus assessment on renal function. Monitor other clinical signs of infection. Include objective data such as blood tests, history of allergies, and mental function.

Nursing Diagnoses

- Potential altered home maintenance management related to the need to increase fluid intake to 2500 ml/day or more
- Potential complication: blood dyscrasias

Patient Outcomes

The patient's infection will resolve without side effects. The patient will increase fluid intake while taking a sulfonamide.

The nurse will manage and minimize any blood dyscrasias that develop.

Planning/Implementation

Monitor the progress of treatment for UTIs by assessing clinical signs such as relief of pain and itching and by culturing urine. Ascertain that urine samples are appropriately collected to prevent trivial contamination, which renders the culture results meaningless. Blood tests may be required for patients receiving sulfonamides. Encourage adequate fluid intake to maintain good urine flow. Teach patients receiving sulfonamides about the signs of blood dyscrasias, and teach patients receiving nitrofurantoin about the signs of pulmonary distress and peripheral neuropathy. These side effects are usually sufficient cause for the physician to discontinue medication.

Evaluation

Ascertain that the patient can explain how to take the prescribed medication and can point out which side effects are sufficient reason to call the physician.

Nursing Implications Summary

Sulfonamides and Trimethoprim

Drug Administration

➤ Review the Nursing Implications Summary in Chapter 43.

➤ Assess for history of allergy to other sulfonamides, thiazide diuretics, acetazolamide, or oral hypoglycemic agents before administering sulfonamides.

➤ Inspect for rashes or skin changes and GI tract distress. Monitor temperature.

➤ Monitor complete blood count (CBC) and differential, platelet count, blood urea nitrogen (BUN) level, serum creatinine level, liver function tests, and urinalysis.

➤ Topical sulfonamide preparations are used to treat burns (see Table 49-3). Wear sterile gloves when applying medication. The drugs are most effective when the area is cleaned of debris and pus. Dressings are not necessary but may be used. Medicate for pain before redressing the wound. Monitor serum drug and serum electrolyte levels in addition to blood work noted previously.

Intravenous trimethoprim and sulfamethoxazole

➤ Dilute each 5 ml ampule in 125 ml D5W. Administer diluted dose over 60 to 90 minutes. Flush tubing well after administration. For patients who must restrict their fluid intake, see the package insert.

Nursing in the Community

➤ Review the Nursing Implications Summary in Chapter 43.

➤ Review the benefits and possible side effects of drug therapy. Instruct the patient to report fever, sore throat, unexplained

bleeding or bruising, malaise, jaundice, rashes, and skin changes.

➤ Review the Patient Problems box on UTIs earlier in this chapter. Even if drug is not used to treat UTIs, instruct the patient to increase daily fluid intake to 2500 to 3000 ml/day.

➤ Inform the patient receiving sulfasalazine that this drug may turn urine or skin yellow-orange.

➤ Instruct diabetic patients that sulfonamides may produce false-positive results with Benedict's test for urine glucose. Monitor blood glucose.

➤ Instruct diabetic patients not to change insulin dosage or diet without discussing this with the physician. Monitor blood glucose level.

➤ Instruct the patient to take doses with a full glass (8 ounces) of water or other liquid.

➤ Instruct the patient and family not to give sulfonamide drugs to children younger than 12 years of age unless specifically prescribed for the child by a physician.

➤ Review with the patient the Patient Problems box in Chapter 58 on photosensitivity.

➤ Caution the patient to avoid driving or operating hazardous equipment until the effects of this medication are known and to report dizziness to the physician.

➤ Sulfonamides are available for ophthalmic use. See Chapter 5 for a discussion of application of drops and ointment.

➤ Sulfonamides are available for intravaginal use. Make certain that the patient can apply the ordered dose correctly.

Nursing Implications Summary—cont'd

(Review the Patient Problems box in Chapter 51 on treatment of vaginal infections.)

➤ Remind the patient to inform all health care providers of all drugs being used.

phenazopyridine
Nursing in the Community

➤ This urinary analgesic may be prescribed concurrently with an antiinfective or may be a part of a combination drug for treatment of UTIs.

➤ Inform the patient taking phenazopyridine that this drug turns urine reddish orange and may stain clothing. The drug may also cause soft contact lenses to be permanently stained.

➤ Instruct diabetic patients that phenazopyridine dye may produce false results with urine glucose and ketone tests.

➤ Side effects are rare, but instruct the patient to notify the physician if skin changes, jaundice, shortness of breath, excessive fatigue, dizziness, headache, or indigestion develops.

nitrofurantoin
Drug Administration

➤ See the Nursing Implications Summary in Chapter 43.

➤ Assess for GI tract disturbance, skin changes, and peripheral neuropathy. Assess lung sounds and respiratory rate. Monitor weight.

➤ Monitor CBC and differential and liver function tests.

Nursing in the Community

➤ See the Nursing Implications Summary in Chapter 43.

➤ Nitrofurantoin may cause false results with urine glucose tests. Instruct diabetic patients to monitor blood glucose. Caution the patient not to change diet or insulin dosage without checking with the physician.

➤ Review the anticipated benefits and possible side effects of drug therapy with the patient. Instruct the patient to report any new sign or symptom.

➤ Review the Patient Problems box on UTIs earlier in this chapter.

➤ Instruct the patient to take oral doses with meals or a snack to reduce gastric irritation. Warn the patient that oral suspensions may stain teeth. Instruct the patient to dilute doses of suspension with milk, formula, water, or juice before taking.

➤ Inform the patient that nitrofurantoin may cause urine to turn rusty-yellow to brown.

CHAPTER REVIEW

Application

1. What is the mechanism for the antibacterial effect of sulfonamides?
2. Why are sulfonamides not equally toxic to humans and bacteria?
3. By what routes may sulfonamides be administered?
4. Do sulfonamides enter the cerebrospinal fluid?
5. How are sulfonamides eliminated from the body?
6. What are the major toxic reactions to sulfonamides?
7. Why should patients be cautioned to drink several liters of water each day they receive sulfonamides?
8. What is the mechanism for the antibacterial effect of trimethoprim?
9. Why is trimethoprim not equally toxic to humans and bacteria?
10. Why are trimethoprim and sulfamethoxazole combined to treat UTIs and other infections?
11. Why is nitrofurantoin not effective for systemic infections?
12. By what route is nitrofurantoin administered?
13. What reactions to nitrofurantoin are commonly encountered with short-term therapy?
14. What reactions to nitrofurantoin are associated with long-term therapy?

Critical Thinking

1. What is the purpose of combining sulfonamides with phenazopyridine to treat UTIs? What should you teach patients about this?
2. Develop a nursing plan for a patient receiving one of the drugs discussed in this chapter.

References

Degnan R: Pharmacology in practice: antibiotics, *RN* 60(10):49-55, 1997.

Marchiondo K: A new look at urinary tract infection, *Am J Nurs* 98(3):34-39, 1998.

Newland JA: Cystitis in women, *Am J Nurs* 98(1):16AAA, 1998.

O'Hanlon-Nichols T: Lower urinary tract infections: treatment and prevention, *J Urol Nurs* 14(3):1120-1131, 1995.

Chapter 50

Drugs to Treat Tuberculosis and Other Mycobacterial Infections

KEY TERMS

leprosy, p. 558
Mycobacterium avium complex (MAC), p. 560
tuberculosis, p. 553

KEY DRUGS ▼

dapsone, p. 559
isoniazid, p. 553
rifabutin, p. 560
rifampin, p. 559

OBJECTIVES

After studying this chapter, you should be able to do the following:

- *Explain why therapy of mycobacterial diseases must continue for years.*
- *Describe the use of isoniazid and identify the types of patients most at risk for severe reactions to the drug.*
- *Describe the use of dapsone.*
- *Discuss why drug combinations are commonly used for tuberculosis and leprosy.*
- *Develop a nursing care plan for a patient receiving drug therapy for tuberculosis, leprosy, or Mycobacterium avium complex.*

CHAPTER OVERVIEW

Tuberculosis and leprosy are diseases produced by *Mycobacterium*. Both diseases have been known since ancient times and are among the earliest examples of diseases that were recognized as infectious. Tuberculosis was a major cause of death in Europe and Asia until recent times. Leprosy, although less common, was greatly feared because of the disfigurement it caused. This grim picture changed in the early 1940s, when the first effective antituberculosis agent was discovered. Around the same time a sulfone was discovered to be effective for leprosy. With these and more recently discovered agents, both diseases were effectively treated in many patients.

The acquired immunodeficiency syndrome (AIDS) epidemic has led to a renewed interest in mycobacterial diseases. Newly reported cases of tuberculosis in the United States currently number about 20,000 per year, especially in urban populations where the incidence of human immunodeficiency virus (HIV) infection, intravenous (IV) drug abuse, and homelessness is high. Other mycobacterial diseases that are insignificant in persons with intact immune systems may add significantly to morbidity and mortality in AIDS patients. For example, patients with AIDS who also have *M. avium* complex face a poor prognosis. This chapter covers the clinical features of mycobacterial infections that make treatment more difficult than that of most other bacterial diseases and the properties of the drugs that are used to treat these diseases.

THERAPEUTIC RATIONALE: TUBERCULOSIS

Tuberculosis is produced by *Mycobacterium tuberculosis* or less commonly by other mycobacteria harbored by cattle or birds. Three features of *M. tuberculosis* are especially important for understanding how disease is produced in humans by these organisms. First, mycobacteria are strict aerobes, which means that they must live in an oxygen-rich environment and may explain why the first site of infection in humans is usually the alveoli in lungs. Second, mycobacteria induce activity of macrophages, causing these cellular immunity factors to phagocytize *M. tuberculosis*. This action actually may enhance survival and spread of the disease-causing organisms because *M. tuberculosis* resists the acids and enzymes that usually destroy bacteria within macrophages. Third, mycobacteria are slow-growing organisms relative to other bacteria. This slow growth contributes to the difficulty encountered in treating the disease because it is during active growth that an organism is most susceptible to metabolic interference.

Tuberculosis may pass through several phases. The initial or primary infection usually occurs in the lungs as a result of inhaling droplets containing live *M. tuberculosis*. These infective aerosols are generated when a patient with an active infection coughs or sneezes. Once in alveoli, *M. tuberculosis* is phagocytized and reproduces within macrophages at near normal rates. Infected macrophages may remain in the lungs, but many enter the lymphatic system or the blood and are carried throughout the body. In response to the increasing number of tubercle bacilli in the lungs, a pneumonia-like condition may develop within a few weeks. This inflammatory response to the infection may continue for a few weeks, but in most people this process is finally halted by the delayed immune reaction provoked by the infection. Lesions within the lungs resolve when infective loci become calcified. Living tubercle bacilli no longer appear in sputum at this stage, and the disease is said to be inactive. Living *M. tuberculosis* remain within the body, however, and relapses may occur months or years after the initial infection. When relapse occurs, localized areas again become sites of active multiplication of tubercle bacilli. Local necrosis develops while the cellular immunity factors attempt to isolate the infection. Necrosis may spread as a result of this inflammatory response and may cause large cavities within the lungs or other tissues.

M. tuberculosis, like most bacteria, can acquire resistance to drugs. Development of resistance is common when patients are treated with a single drug. To minimize this complication, multiple drug therapy is used. The rationale for this therapy is simple: when two drugs with different mechanisms of action are administered together, the organism must acquire two independent mutations to become resistant to both drugs. Because mutations are rare, the likelihood of simultaneously acquiring two specific mutations is small. Using three or more drugs lowers the probability of developing resistance even further. The options for treating tuberculosis use three to six drugs initially, with therapy continuing 6 to 24 months (Box 50-1). Treated patients rapidly cease to be infectious, but chemotherapy must be continued for long periods to eliminate most of the dormant tubercle bacilli.

The properties and uses of antituberculosis agents are considered in the following sections, with the drugs considered in order of their clinical importance.

THERAPEUTIC AGENTS: DRUGS TO TREAT TUBERCULOSIS (Box 50-2)

Primary Drugs for Tuberculosis

▼ isoniazid

Mechanism of Action and Bacterial Resistance

Isoniazid is a potent inhibitor of mycolic acids involved in cell wall synthesis and also blocks pyridoxine (vitamin B_6) use in a number of intracellular enzymes. Isoniazid is bactericidal and affects both intracellular (within macrophages) and extracellular mycobacteria.

Mycobacteria rapidly acquires resistance to isoniazid. In early trials when isoniazid was used alone to treat active pulmonary tuberculosis, 11% of the patients carried isoniazid-resistant strains at the end of 1 month of therapy. At the end of 3 months, 71% of these patients harbored resistant *Mycobacterium*. Observations such as these have led to the clinical practice of combining isoniazid therapy with one or more drugs. Currently isoniazid resistance varies greatly with geographic location. If the local incidence of isoniazid resistance exceeds 4%, additional drugs must be added to the regimen to insure effectiveness (see Box 50-1).

Pharmacokinetics

Isoniazid is well absorbed after oral administration, achieving peak serum levels in 1 to 2 hours. Bactericidal concentrations are found in most tissues, including pleural fluids and caseous exudates surrounding active loci of infection in lungs.

Isoniazid undergoes several metabolic conversions in liver, most resulting in inactive drug, which is excreted primarily by the kidneys. The major metabolite is an acetylated form of isoniazid. The rate of drug acetylation differs significantly among populations, and two genetically determined types may be distinguished. Rapid acetylators inactivate isoniazid two to three times as rapidly as slow acetylators. As would be expected, rapid acetylators have lower blood concentrations of active drug than slow acetylators, but both types of patients respond well to standard therapeutic doses given once daily. Increasing the drug dose or frequency of administration in slow acetylators is not wise because these patients tend to be more prone to side effects. Slow acetylators include 45% to 65% of Northern European and African-American or Caucasian populations.

Box 50-1 Treatment Regimens for Tuberculosis

Patient Criteria	Treatment Schedule
Option 1 ■ Born in United States ■ Never treated for tuberculosis ■ Low risk of drug-resistant *Mycobacterium*	Isoniazid, rifampin, and pyrazinamide daily for 2 months; then isoniazid and rifampin daily or twice weekly for 4-22 months
Option 2 ■ Born in the United States ■ Never treated for tuberculosis ■ Risk of drug-resistant *Mycobacterium*	Isoniazid, rifampin, ethambutol, and pyrazinamide daily for 6-24 months
Option 3 ■ Non–HIV-infected patients ■ Isoniazid resistance ≥4% in locality ■ Medications taken under direct observation	Isoniazid, rifampin, pyrazinamide, and streptomycin for 8 weeks; isoniazid and rifampin daily or 2-3 times weekly for 16 weeks if organism is susceptible
Option 4 ■ Non–HIV-infected patients ■ Medications taken under direct observation	Isoniazid, rifampin, pyrazinamide, and streptomycin daily for 2 weeks, then twice weekly for 6 weeks; isoniazid and rifampin twice weekly for an additional 16 weeks
Option 5 ■ Non–HIV-infected patients ■ Medications taken under direct observation	Isoniazid, rifampin, pyrazinamide, and streptomycin or ethambutol 3 times weekly for 6 months
Option 6 ■ HIV infected patients ■ Medications taken under direct observation	Options 3, 4, or 5, but continued for at least 9 months and at least 6 months beyond culture conversion
Option 7 ■ Known drug-resistant *Mycobacterium* ■ Retreatment (received drugs before)	Option 5 plus one or two other drugs to include at least 3 drugs demonstrated effective in culture

HIV, Human immunodeficiency virus.

Box 50-2 What Is DOT and Why Are Antituberculosis Drugs Given DOT?

DOT stands for "directly observed therapy." Many published protocols for antituberculosis drugs call for giving the drugs by DOT. DOT is used for two purposes. First, therapeutic compliance is ensured. The populations at risk for tuberculosis include intravenous drug abusers, homeless people, and foreign-born individuals. In these populations, as well as others, compliance may be a problem. DOT ensures that the drugs are taken as prescribed and that the patient receives maximum benefit. The second reason for DOT has to do with public health. Continuous, effective therapy reduces the period of infectiousness in active cases of tuberculosis, thus lowering the risk of spreading the disease. Noncompliance, or early cessation of therapy, also fosters the appearance of drug-resistant strains of *Mycobacterium tuberculosis*. Currently multidrug-resistant *M. tuberculosis* accounts for a little more than 1% of the cases nationwide, but nearly half of these are concentrated in the heavily urban areas of New York and California. Effective programs to identify active cases early and to treat by DOT with effective drug combinations may prevent tuberculosis from becoming an ever greater danger to immunocompromised as well as immunocompetent individuals.

Oriental and Eskimo populations contain predominantly rapid acetylators.

Uses

Isoniazid is considered to be the most useful antituberculosis agent. The drug is available as a single agent formulation and in combination with other antituberculosis agents (Table 50-1).

Isoniazid may be used alone for prophylaxis. The drug is prescribed for patients with known exposure to tuberculosis or patients who have recently converted from negative to positive reactions in the skin test for tuberculosis. These people usually have smaller numbers of mycobacteria than would be found in an active, symptomatic case of tuberculosis, and for them the use of isoniazid alone is usually successful.

Adverse Reactions and Contraindications

Isoniazid reactions occur in a small percentage of patients. The most commonly encountered adverse reaction is pe-

Table 50-1 Antituberculosis Drugs

Generic Name	Trade Name	Administration/Dosage	Comments
aminosalicylate sodium	Nemasol† Tubasal	ORAL: *Adults*—5-6 g every 12 hr. *Children*—50-75 mg/kg every 6 hr, not to exceed 12 g/day.	Alternative drug. Patients with congestive heart failure may be unable to tolerate sodium load with this drug.
capreomycin	Capastat*	INTRAMUSCULAR: *Adults*—1 g/day in single dose. FDA pregnancy category C.	Alternative drug. Hearing impairment, renal function impairment, or muscle weakness may be worsened.
cycloserine	Seromycin	ORAL: *Adults*—250 mg every 12 hr for 2 wk, then 250 mg every 6-8 hr up to maximum daily dose of 1 g. FDA pregnancy category C. *Children*—5-20 mg/kg in divided doses.	Alternative drug. Central nervous system toxicity, including seizures, is more likely in alcoholic patients or patients with prior seizure disorders.
ethambutol	Etibi† Myambutol*	ORAL: *Adults*—15-25 mg/kg once daily or 50 mg/kg twice weekly. Single dose should not exceed 2.5 g. *Children <13 yr*—Should not receive drug, if avoidable.	Primary drug. Patients with reduced renal function require reduced drug dosages. Patients with preexisting visual defects may be difficult to evaluate for drug-induced visual changes.
ethionamide	Trecator SC	ORAL: *Adults*—250 mg every 8-12 hr. *Children*—4-5 mg/kg every 8 hr.	Alternative drug. Patients also receiving cycloserine are at greater risk for seizures.
isoniazid (INH)	Isotamine† Laniazid Nydrazid	ORAL: *Adults*—300 mg/day maximum. FDA pregnancy category C. *Children*—10-20 mg/kg/day up to 300 mg maximum. INTRAMUSCULAR: As for oral.	Primary drug. Older adult patients, alcoholic patients with liver impairment, or patients also receiving rifampin have increased risk of drug-induced hepatitis.
pyrazinamide	Pyrazinamide* Tebrazid†	ORAL: *Adults*—15-30 mg/kg/day up to 2 g or 50-70 mg/kg 2 or 3 times weekly. FDA pregnancy category C. *Children*—15-30 mg/kg body weight/day, up to 2 g maximum dose.	Primary drug. Hepatotoxicity; increased blood concentration of uric acid (hyperuricemia).
rifampin	Rifadin* Rimactane* Rofact†	ORAL: *Adults*—600 mg once daily. FDA pregnancy category C. *Geriatric dose*—10 mg/kg once daily. *Children*—10-20 mg/kg up to 600 mg/day. INTRAVENOUS: *Adults*—As for oral.	Primary drug. Patients with prior liver disease and alcoholic patients are more likely to experience drug-induced hepatotoxicity. Patients also receiving isoniazid have increased risk of drug-induced hepatitis.
rifampin and isoniazid	Rifamate	ORAL: *Adults*—600 mg of rifampin and 300 mg of isoniazid (2 tablets) once daily.	Treatment of pulmonary tuberculosis after dosage of separate drugs has been established.
rifampin, isoniazid, and pyrazinamide	Rifater	ORAL: *Adults*—As for individual components.	Short-course treatment of tuberculosis.
streptomycin	Streptomycin	INTRAMUSCULAR: *Adults*—1 g/day for 2-4 mo or longer. Dosage may then be reduced to 1 g 2 or 3 times weekly. FDA pregnancy category D. *Children*—20 mg/kg once daily, not to exceed 1 g.	Primary drug. Patients with renal insufficiency or older adult patients are more prone to accumulate streptomycin and to develop ototoxicity.

*Available in Canada and the United States.
†Available in Canada only.

ripheral neuropathy. Diabetic patients, alcoholic patients, and malnourished persons are more prone to this complication than the general population. At least some of these reactions are related to low vitamin B_6 levels and may be prevented by taking 5 mg of the vitamin daily. Peripheral neuropathies are more likely to occur in slow acetylators.

Various other reactions, including allergies, blood dyscrasias, gastric distress, and metabolic acidosis, have occasionally been reported with isoniazid.

Toxicity

Hepatotoxicity is the most serious side effect associated with isoniazid. Fatal liver failure has occurred even among patients receiving the drug prophylactically. Hepatitis caused by isoniazid is rare among patients younger than 20 years of age and occurs in patients 20 to 34 years of age at a rate of approximately 3 cases per 1000 patients. After age 50 years, the incidence increases to 23 cases per 1000 patients. Patients also have an increased risk of hepatitis if they are rapid acetylators of isoniazid, if they ingest ethanol daily, or if they also receive the drug rifampin. Liver function should be monitored in all patients receiving isoniazid. Symptoms of hepatitis include anorexia, dark urine, jaundice, nausea, tiredness, or weakness.

Interactions

Isoniazid may enhance metabolism, thus lowering the effectiveness, of the antifungal drug ketoconazole. In contrast, metabolism of alfentanil, carbamazepine, and phenytoin is inhibited by isoniazid, and serum concentrations of these drugs may increase when isoniazid is given. Isoniazid should never be given with other hepatotoxic drugs because of the greatly increased risk of hepatic failure.

▼ rifampin

Mechanism of Action and Bacterial Resistance

Rifampin inhibits DNA-dependent RNA polymerase in sensitive organisms. As a result, gene transcription halts, and protein synthesis ceases. Metabolic activity in the bacteria stops, and the bacteria ultimately die or are eliminated by host defenses.

Resistance to rifampin can occur when the drug is used alone against *M. tuberculosis*. Resistant strains have an altered DNA-dependent RNA polymerase that is no longer inhibited by the drug.

Pharmacokinetics

Rifampin is adequately absorbed orally in the presence or absence of food. Rifampin is a relatively lipid-soluble agent. This property explains why it is found in higher concentrations in body tissues than in serum. Lipid solubility also explains its ability to penetrate white blood cells (WBCs) and to attack mycobacteria living there.

About 40% of a dose of rifampin is excreted in bile, with less in urine. The drug is also deacetylated by the liver to an active metabolite that is excreted via bile into feces.

Uses

Rifampin is used as prophylaxis for *Neisseria meningitidis* and as therapy for tuberculosis. Rifampin is as potent as isoniazid against mycobacteria and distributes well to many sites where mycobacteria survive. These advantages have made rifampin a primary drug for tuberculosis.

Rifampin is available as a single-ingredient formulation and in fixed combination with other antituberculosis drugs (see Table 50-1).

Adverse Reactions and Contraindications

Rifampin can cause a variety of mild reactions such as gastrointestinal (GI) tract upset and rashes. The drug also turns body fluids such as tears, sweat, saliva, and urine an orange-red color, which might be mistaken for blood. This coloration is harmless.

Liver abnormalities may occur with rifampin. Mild abnormalities in liver function may return to normal without discontinuing the drug, but increases in alkaline phosphatase or the appearance of jaundice signals that the drug should be discontinued.

Intermittent doses of rifampin may cause an immune reaction that is associated with a variety of symptoms. This flulike syndrome may progress from chills, fever, vomiting, diarrhea, and myalgia to acute renal failure. Deaths have occurred. Because these symptoms occur when therapy is resumed, patients should be advised not to miss doses of rifampin, especially if they are receiving relatively high dosages. Some treatment centers have significantly lowered rifampin dosages for intermittent therapeutic programs and have reduced these immune reactions.

Toxicity

Overdoses of rifampin can produce serious reactions, including generalized itching, facial edema, and mental changes. Activated charcoal may be used orally as a slurry to remove unabsorbed or recirculated rifampin from the system.

Interactions

Rifampin induces liver enzymes involved in drug and hormone metabolism in humans. This action leads to several drug interactions. Patients receiving coumarin anticoagulants, oral hypoglycemic agents, theophylline, phenytoin, methadone, various antiarrhythmics, verapamil, or digitalis may require dosage adjustment of these agents because rifampin induces liver microsomal enzymes that degrade these drugs. Patients receiving oral contraceptives or replacement doses of cortisol may lose the effectiveness of these agents because rifampin accelerates breakdown of the steroids. Patients receiving isoniazid along with rifampin or patients who regularly use alcohol have an increased risk of drug-induced hepatitis.

pyrazinamide

Mechanism of Action and Bacterial Resistance

Pyrazinamide may be bacteriostatic or bactericidal, depending on the site of infection and the strain of mycobacteria. The mechanism of action or resistance is unknown.

Pharmacokinetics

Pyrazinamide is rapidly and completely absorbed orally. The drug distributes freely to most tissues, including the brain. In the liver, pyrazinamide is converted in part to pyrazinoic acid, which is also active. Renal elimination half-times for these compounds are 10 to 12 hours in normal persons, but 22 to 26 hours when renal function is impaired.

Uses

Pyrazinamide is effective only against mycobacteria and is a primary drug for treatment of tuberculosis (see Table 50-1).

Adverse Reactions and Contraindications

Pyrazinamide often causes joint pain, which may arise from hyperuricemia. Rarely, the drug may cause gouty arthritis or jaundice.

There are no contraindications to pyrazinamide, but the drug should be used cautiously in patients with impaired hepatic function or allergies to ethionamide, isoniazid, or niacin.

Toxicity

Dosages of 40 to 50 mg/kg/day, if sustained for prolonged periods, may cause hepatotoxicity.

Interactions

Drugs such as allopurinol, colchicine, probenecid, and sulfinpyrazone may be less effective when pyrazinamide is given because pyrazinamide tends to elevate blood levels of uric acid.

ethambutol

Mechanism of Action and Bacterial Resistance

Ethambutol is most effective against actively dividing mycobacteria but the precise antibacterial action is unknown. The drug is bacteriostatic. Resistance to ethambutol develops if the drug is used alone in therapy. Ethambutol does not induce cross-resistance to other antituberculosis agents.

Pharmacokinetics

Ethambutol is well absorbed from the GI tract in the presence or the absence of food. Peak serum concentrations are observed 2 to 4 hours after an oral dose. Ethambutol is less extensively metabolized than isoniazid or rifampin, and up to 50% of the drug excreted in urine is in the unaltered active form. Fecal concentrations of the drug represent unabsorbed material.

Ethambutol has been detected in cerebrospinal fluid after oral therapy, although the levels are below those found in plasma. The drug also concentrates in erythrocytes.

Uses

Ethambutol is a primary antituberculosis drug that is chemically unrelated to other antituberculosis drugs or antibiotics. It is effective only against mycobacteria and no other bacteria, viruses, or fungi. It has become a first-line antituberculosis drug because of its relatively wide spectrum of activity against species of *Mycobacterium* and its relatively low toxicity.

Adverse Reactions and Contraindications

Elevated uric acid levels have been reported in patients receiving ethambutol. Gouty arthritis may occur. The drug also causes confusion and headaches, as well as GI tract disturbances.

Other reactions to ethambutol appear rarely. Allergic reactions have occasionally been reported. Peripheral neuritis can occur with higher dosages.

Toxicity

A serious adverse reaction to ethambutol is visual disturbance. Some patients report changes in color vision, whereas others experience a more prominent loss of visual acuity. These signs are cause to terminate ethambutol use. If the drug is discontinued when these visual signs appear, the changes are reversible, although full recovery may take months. These visual changes are caused by optic neuritis and are more common with doses of 25 mg/kg given for 2 months or longer. The drug should not be used in patients with preexisting optic neuritis.

Interactions

Ethambutol has been associated with few significant interactions but should not be used with other neurotoxic drugs.

streptomycin

Mechanism of Action and Bacterial Resistance

Streptomycin inhibits protein synthesis in sensitive bacteria (see Chapter 48) and in mycobacteria. The drug is highly effective against most types of pathogenic mycobacteria with the exception of *M. avium*. Resistance to streptomycin develops quickly when the drug is used alone.

Pharmacokinetics

Streptomycin is not absorbed orally and must be administered by intramuscular (IM) injection for routine clinical use. This property restricts its use to the hospital or to a well-supervised outpatient program.

Streptomycin is well distributed in the body and may be used to treat nonpulmonary tuberculosis. Streptomycin is excreted almost exclusively by renal mechanisms.

Uses

The first antituberculosis drug to be discovered, streptomycin is still a reliable agent for initial therapy in multidrug regimens (see Box 50-1). It is usually discontinued after the number of infective organisms has been greatly reduced, usually after 2 to 4 months, but other drugs continue. Other aminoglycosides such as kanamycin or amikacin (see Chapter 48) have also been used for tuberculosis.

Adverse Reactions and Contraindications

Streptomycin can produce any reaction seen with other aminoglycoside antibiotics (see Chapter 48). Patients with renal insufficiency, older adult patients, and patients receiving long-term streptomycin therapy are more prone to develop side effects or toxic reactions.

Toxicity

Ototoxicity is the most common reaction in patients with tuberculosis. Careful attention to maintaining dosage within safe limits (see Table 50-1) prevents the reaction in most patients.

Interactions

Because streptomycin causes ototoxicity, it should not be combined with other ototoxic drugs such as the diuretic ethacrynic acid. Patients receiving muscle relaxants along with streptomycin may experience excessive muscle relaxation because streptomycin is a weak neuromuscular-blocking agent.

Alternative Drugs for Tuberculosis

aminosalicylate, capreomycin, cycloserine, and ethionamide

Mechanism of Action

Aminosalicylate inhibits folic acid metabolism in mycobacteria. Cycloserine interferes with cell wall biosynthesis. The mechanism of capreomycin and ethionamide are unknown.

Pharmacokinetics

Aminosalicylate, cycloserine, and ethionamide are efficiently absorbed orally, but capreomycin must be given intramuscularly. Distribution is adequate to most tissues, but only cycloserine and ethionamide achieve significant concentrations in the central nervous system (CNS). Excretion is primarily renal for all four drugs, but hepatic metabolism of ethionamide forms mostly inactive products.

Uses

These drugs are included in multidrug regimens when significant resistance to other drugs is expected.

Adverse Reactions and Contraindications

Most patients receiving aminosalicylate report GI tract irritation, which may be relieved by taking the drug with food or antacids. Allergic symptoms, including exfoliative dermatitis and severe organ damage, have also been reported.

Nephrotoxicity is the most common side effect with capreomycin. The characteristic reactions to cycloserine are CNS reactions, including anxiety, confusion, depression, dizziness, irritability, nervousness, mood changes, and thoughts of suicide.

Ethionamide commonly causes anorexia, nausea, vomiting, and a metallic taste in the mouth. The drug also causes orthostatic hypotension. Jaundice, mental changes, and peripheral neuritis are less common.

Toxicity

High dosages or prolonged therapy with aminosalicylate may cause crystalluria or changes in thyroid function. High dosages of capreomycin increase the risk of ototoxicity or nephrotoxicity. High dosages of cycloserine (500 mg or 1 g daily) increase the risk and severity of CNS reactions. Neurotoxicity from ethionamide may be reduced by giving pyridoxine.

Interactions

Aminobenzoates may block absorption of aminosalicylate. Risk of nephrotoxicity, ototoxicity, and neuromuscular blockade with capreomycin is increased by aminoglycosides or loop diuretics. Use of cycloserine with alcohol or ethionamide increases the risk of seizures.

THERAPEUTIC RATIONALE: LEPROSY

Leprosy is currently found primarily in developing countries and is rarely encountered in the United States or Canada. Leprosy is curable with appropriate drug therapy. Patients are usually treated for at least 6 months, and some must be treated for life. Long-term treatment is required because *Mycobacterium leprae*, the causative agent of leprosy, is a slow-growing organism and may remain dormant for long periods in humans.

Nursing Process Overview

Treatment of Tuberculosis

Assessment

Antituberculosis therapy is used in patients diagnosed with active tuberculosis, those whose tuberculosis skin tests convert from negative to positive, or in some instances in those receiving high dosages of adrenocortical steroids. In the latter group of patients, the concern is that high dosages of steroids will alter the patient's ability to resist infection from tuberculosis or will cause reactivation of earlier tubercular infections. Perform a thorough total assessment, emphasizing subjective complaints, possible history of tuberculosis in the patient and family, and recent activities such as travel or moving that might have influenced exposure to the disease. Tuberculosis can appear in other organs besides the lungs (e.g., tuberculosis meningitis). The focus of the assessment would be different if the patient had a nonpulmonary form of tuberculosis.

Nursing Diagnoses

- Anxiety related to diagnosis and long-term drug therapy
- Potential altered home maintenance management related to lack of knowledge about how to incorporate drug therapy into daily activities

Patient Outcomes

The patient will take medication as ordered, and tuberculosis will resolve. Side effects will be reported early and will be treated, or drug therapy will be modified. The patient will state a decrease in anxiety and will describe the risk, transmission, and course of tuberculosis.

Planning/Implementation

As soon as diagnosis is made, begin patient education. If unsure of the local standards regarding care of patients with tuberculosis, contact the local health department or hospital infection control department. Place hospitalized patients in isolation until no longer infectious. Remember that many patients with tuberculosis are diagnosed and treated entirely on an outpatient basis.

Evaluation

Noncompliance is a major cause of treatment failure. Before a patient begins self-management, ascertain that the patient understands why and how to take the drugs ordered, possible side effects, ways to treat minor side effects such as nausea associated with taking medication, and side effects that require notification of the physician. Verify that the patient knows when and why to return for evaluation of laboratory work and other patient data. Also ensure that the patient can demonstrate measures to decrease the possibility of spreading the disease to others. Because exposure to tuberculosis may occur any time the nurse provides care for a patient, nurses should have regular tuberculosis skin tests.

THERAPEUTIC AGENTS: DRUGS TO TREAT LEPROSY

Primary Drugs for Leprosy

▼dapsone

Mechanism of Action and Bacterial Resistance

Dapsone is an antifolate with actions much like sulfonamides. The drug is bacteriostatic, and resistance can develop.

Pharmacokinetics

Dapsone is slowly but nearly completely absorbed orally. The drug distributes well to tissues. Dapsone is metabolized in the liver and excreted in urine. The half-life for elimination of the drug is very long, ranging from 10 to 50 hours.

Uses

Dapsone is the first choice for treating leprosy in the United States. It is also used for dermatitis herpetiformis. Combined with trimethoprim, the drug may be used for prophylaxis of *Pneumocystis carinii* pneumonia in AIDS patients.

Resistance to dapsone appears more often today than in previous years; therefore combination therapy has become accepted in the United States. Combining drugs lessens the likelihood that resistance will occur and increases the likelihood that all mycobacteria will be eradicated to achieve a permanent cure. Rifampin or clofazimine is combined with dapsone for the first 6 months to 3 years, after which dapsone alone may be continued for as long as is necessary. A gluten-free diet (see Dietary Considerations box) may be prescribed for patients with dermatitis herpetiformis. The properties of drugs used to treat leprosy are summarized in Table 50-2.

Adverse Reactions and Contraindications

Dapsone often causes rashes and potentially serious blood dyscrasias such as methemoglobinemia and hemolytic anemia. Symptoms include cyanosis, shortness of breath, bluish coloration to fingernails or lips, anorexia, paleness, and unusual tiredness and weakness. Dapsone is usually avoided if possible in patients with preexisting anemia or glucose-6-phosphate dehydrogenase (G6PD) deficiency, which would increase the risk of hemolytic anemia.

Toxicity

At higher dosages, dapsone may cause GI tract disturbances and CNS toxicity, characterized by headache, insomnia, and restlessness. Overdoses can lead to death by methemoglobin accumulation. Treatment may include IV infusion of methylene blue to preserve oxygenation of tissues.

Interactions

Dapsone requires an acidic environment for good oral absorption. Didanosine may block dapsone absorption because preparations of didanosine include strong buffers to reduce gastric acidity. Dapsone should not be combined with other hemolytic agents to avoid unacceptable risk of hemolysis.

▼rifampin

Rifampin is used in the recommended combination with dapsone for initial therapy of leprosy in the United States. The properties of rifampin are covered in the section on tuberculosis.

 DIETARY CONSIDERATIONS

Gluten-Free Diet

Gluten, which is found in many grains, is restricted in the management of several health problems, including celiac disease (nontropical sprue) and dermatitis herpetiformis. Food items to avoid in a gluten-free diet include cereal grains such as wheat, barley, oats, rye, bran, graham, millet, wheat germ, bulgur, malt, and products containing these grains. Products made with gluten-containing grains include prepared meats, thickened stew, breaded vegetables, root beer, pasta, macaroni products, gluten stabilizer, brewer's yeast, flour (when the source is not indicated), and pizza.

The following foods are permitted: rice, corn, flours made from soybeans, buckwheat, lima beans, gluten-free wheat starch, cornmeal, and hominy.

- Encourage patients to read food labels carefully.
- Refer patients as needed to the dietitian.

Table 50-2	**Drugs to Treat Leprosy**		
Generic Name	Trade Name	Administration/Dosage	Clinical Use
dapsone	Avlosulfon† Dapsone*	ORAL: *Adults*—100 mg/day for 4 yr to life, with rifampin for first 6-36 mo. FDA pregnancy category C. *Children*—1.4 mg/kg/day.	Primary therapy.
clofazimine	Lamprene	ORAL: *Adults*—Up to 300 mg/day for 4 yr to life, with rifampin and dapsone for first 6-36 mo. FDA pregnancy category C.	Alternative or combination therapy. Gastrointestinal distress; discoloration of the skin is an expected, reversible side effect.

*Available in Canada and the United States.
†Available in Canada only.

Alternative Drugs for Leprosy

clofazimine, ethionamide, and thalidomide

The primary drug used to treat leprosy is the sulfone dapsone, but alternatives are now available. Clofazimine has a different mechanism of action from dapsone, and strains of *M. leprae* that acquire resistance to dapsone remain sensitive to clofazimine. The antituberculosis drugs rifampin and more rarely ethionamide have also been used to treat leprosy. Thalidomide is an orphan drug (see Chapter 3) that may be used for leprosy.

Nursing Process Overview

Treatment of Leprosy

Assessment

In the United States the diagnosis of leprosy is unusual. Perform a thorough total assessment, with special emphasis on subjective and objective deviations from normal.

Nursing Diagnoses

- Anxiety related to diagnosis and long-term drug therapy
- Potential complication: depression related to change in skin color related to drug side effect

Patient Outcomes

The patient will state a decrease in anxiety. The patient will take the drug therapy as ordered. If clofazimine is prescribed, the patient will report the development of depression if it occurs, and symptoms will be managed or drug therapy will be changed.

Planning/Implementation

The diagnosis of leprosy causes a great deal of fear and anxiety in patients. Refer the patient to appropriate agencies for education and support and begin Nursing in the Community. Appropriate agencies include the local health department and the Centers for Disease Control and Prevention in Atlanta. Continue regular total patient assessment, with a focus on identifying possible toxic and side effects of the drugs prescribed.

Evaluation

Therapy for leprosy often continues for years. Before discharging patients, ascertain that they understand why and how to take the drugs prescribed, possible side effects, side effects that require notification of the physician, and possible ways to treat more common side effects. Any additional measures that may be prescribed related to the stage of the disease as it was diagnosed should be discussed. Report the diagnosis of leprosy to the local health department for family follow-up.

THERAPEUTIC RATIONALE: *MYCOBACTERIUM AVIUM* COMPLEX

Patients in the latter stages of AIDS are increasingly debilitated from infections not seen in persons with intact immune systems. *Mycobacterium avium* complex (MAC) is one of those infections. *M. avium* and *Mycobacterium intracellulare* are the causative organisms. This infection will occur in most, if not all, AIDS patients as the disease progresses. MAC causes affected patients to require prolonged nursing care and medical support.

THERAPEUTIC AGENTS: DRUGS TO TREAT *MYCOBACTERIUM AVIUM* COMPLEX

▼rifabutin

Mechanism of Action and Bacterial Resistance

Rifabutin has a mechanism similar to rifampin against most bacteria, but the mechanism against *M. avium* and *M. intracellulare* has not been established. Cross-resistance can develop with rifampin.

Pharmacokinetics

Rifabutin is a highly lipophilic drug that is adequately absorbed orally and distributes well to tissues, including the brain. Elimination is mostly by hepatic metabolism to inactive products that appear in feces and urine.

Uses

Rifabutin is used only to prevent MAC in patients with advanced HIV disease. The drug is given for life, at a dose of 300 mg by mouth once daily.

Adverse Reactions and Contraindications

Rifabutin often causes skin rashes, nausea, and vomiting. The drug also produces a red discoloration of body fluids such as urine, tears, sweat, and saliva; this effect is harmless.

Rifabutin is avoided in patients with active tuberculosis because single-drug therapy is likely to cause development of resistance of *M. tuberculosis* to rifampin, one of the primary drugs for treating tuberculosis.

Toxicity

Overdoses of rifabutin may cause uveitis, with loss of vision and pain in the eye.

Interactions

Rifabutin may decrease plasma concentrations of zidovudine, but clinical trials have not consistently shown this effect.

clarithromycin

Clarithromycin, a macrolide covered in Chapter 46, is active against MAC; because resistance develops easily, clarithromycin is best used in combinations.

Nursing Process Overview

Treatment of Mycobacterium avium *Complex*

Assessment

Assess vital signs. Assess weight and history of weight loss, persistent fever, diarrhea, and night sweats. Assess hemoglobin and hematocrit and alkaline-25-phosphatase. If the patient has AIDS, obtain a history of AIDS progression. Monitor CD4 cell count and culture reports. Assess the patient for activity level, general sense of well-being, and other subjective symptoms.

Nursing Diagnoses

- Potential complication: septicemia

Patient Outcomes

The patient will report subjective improvement. The nurse will manage and minimize complications of septicemia.

Planning/Implementation

The clinical picture may vary from a patient mildly ill to a patient critically ill. After assessing the patient, determine the priorities for the patient. Emphasize the importance of taking all medications as prescribed. Work with the dietitian to increase nutritional intake. Continue to monitor vital signs, intake and output, and laboratory work. Patients with MAC may be severely debilitated. Work with the health care team to develop a long-range plan to provide comfort and physical care.

Evaluation

The goal is to treat the infection so it resolves. In fact, the patient's general condition may make cure impossible. Provide physical and emotional support to patient and family. Success may be in the form of slowing deterioration and helping the patient and family cope with the symptoms and physical care.

Nursing Implications Summary

General Guidelines: Patient with Tuberculosis or Leprosy

➤ Provide emotional support for the patient and the family when a diagnosis of tuberculosis or leprosy is made. Both diseases may be associated with patient fears and misunderstandings. Inform the patient and family about the diagnosis and about drug therapy.

➤ Review anticipated benefits and possible side effects associated with drug therapy.

➤ Emphasize the importance of long-term therapy for best effect, even if the patient feels subjectively better.

➤ Encourage the patient to return as scheduled for follow-up appointments. Blood work must be monitored to rule out side effects.

➤ Refer the patient to the local health department for teaching and for follow-up.

➤ Emphasize the importance of taking drugs regularly. Review guidelines for missed doses, which are to be taken as soon as remembered unless shortly before the next dose. Inform the patient not to double up for missed doses.

➤ Health care personnel should obtain a routine annual tuberculosis screening test.

➤ Instruct the patient to inform all health care providers of all drugs being taken.

➤ Some of these drugs are contraindicated during pregnancy or breast-feeding. Advise female patients to consult with their physicians before getting pregnant, if possible.

➤ Instruct patients taking combination drugs (e.g., Rifamate, which is a combination of rifampin and isoniazid) about each of the drugs in the combination.

aminosalicylate
Drug Administration/Nursing in the Community

➤ See the general guidelines for the patient with tuberculosis or leprosy.

➤ Instruct the patient to take oral doses with meals or a snack to lessen gastric irritation. Provide positive reinforcement. This drug is difficult to take. A 5-g dose requires ten 500-mg tablets.

➤ Instruct the patient to discard discolored tablets and obtain a fresh supply. Aminosalicylates deteriorate rapidly. Caution the patient against storing this drug in the bathroom, in damp areas, or near the kitchen sink. Instruct the patient to observe expiration dates.

➤ Instruct the patient to prevent crystalluria by maintaining a fluid intake of 2000 to 2500 ml/day.

➤ Instruct the patient not to take aminosalicylates within 6 hours of doses of rifampin.

➤ Warn diabetic patients that aminosalicylates may cause false urine glucose results. Instruct these patients not to change diet or insulin dosage without consulting the physician. Monitor blood glucose level if possible.

➤ For missed doses, instruct the patient to take missed dose as soon as remembered, unless almost time for the next dose, then omit missed dose and resume regular dosing schedule. Do not double up for missed doses.

capreomycin
Drug Administration/Nursing in the Community

➤ Review the general guidelines for the patient with tuberculosis or leprosy.

Continued

Nursing Implications Summary—cont'd

➤ Capreomycin is for IM administration only. Reconstitute as directed on label. If for home management, teach the patient proper administration technique.

➤ Give cautiously with other drugs known to cause renal impairment or ototoxicity. Examples include aminoglycosides, furosemide, and cisplatin.

➤ Monitor renal function, including blood urea nitrogen (BUN) level and serum creatinine level.

➤ Assess for ototoxicity, including hearing acuity and balance.

➤ Instruct the patient to avoid driving or operating hazardous equipment if drowsiness or dizziness occurs and to notify the physician if these symptoms occur.

cycloserine
Drug Administration/Nursing in the Community

➤ Review the general guidelines for the patient with tuberculosis or leprosy.

➤ Assess for signs of depression, including malaise, lack of interest in personal appearance, insomnia, withdrawal, and weight gain or loss. Review these symptoms with patient and family. Instruct the patient to notify the physician if depression or suicidal thoughts develop.

➤ Monitor serum drug levels if available.

➤ Instruct the patient to take doses after meals if GI tract irritation develops.

➤ Instruct the patient to avoid driving or operating hazardous equipment if drowsiness or dizziness occurs and to notify the physician if these symptoms occur.

➤ Instruct the patient to avoid alcoholic beverages while taking cycloserine.

ethambutol
Drug Administration

➤ See the general guidelines for the patient with tuberculosis or leprosy and the Nursing Implications Summary in Chapter 43.

➤ Assess for visual changes (blurred vision, loss of vision, red-green color blindness, eye pain) and peripheral neuropathy.

➤ Monitor complete blood count (CBC), and WBC differential, and uric acid levels.

Nursing in the Community

➤ Review the general guidelines for the patient with tuberculosis or leprosy.

➤ Instruct the patient to take oral doses with meals or a snack to lessen gastric irritation. Inform the patient that taking a single daily dose maintains the serum drug level better than two or more smaller daily doses.

➤ Instruct the patient to report changes in vision to the physician.

➤ Instruct the patient to avoid driving or operating hazardous equipment until the effects of this medication are known; it may cause drowsiness or dizziness.

ethionamide
Drug Administration/Nursing in the Community

➤ See the general guidelines for the patient with tuberculosis or leprosy and the Nursing Implications Summary in Chapter 43.

➤ Instruct the patient to take doses with or after meals if gastric irritation develops.

➤ Assess for peripheral neuropathy, including numbness, tingling, paresthesia, and feelings of heaviness of the fingers, arms, and legs.

➤ Pyridoxine may also be prescribed with this drug. Emphasize the importance of taking both drugs. See the Dietary Considerations box in Chapter 17 on vitamins.

➤ Instruct the patient to report changes in vision to the physician.

➤ Instruct the patient to avoid driving or operating hazardous equipment until the effects of ethionamide are known; it may cause drowsiness or dizziness.

➤ Assess for depression, including malaise, lack of interest in personal appearance, insomnia, withdrawal, and weight gain or loss.

isoniazid
Drug Administration

➤ Review Nursing Implications Summary in Chapter 43.

➤ Assess for peripheral neuropathy, including numbness, tingling, paresthesia, and feelings of heaviness of the fingers, arms, and legs; review these symptoms with the patient.

➤ Monitor CBC and WBC differential, platelet count, liver function tests, and blood glucose level.

➤ Warn the patient that IM injection may produce pain at the injection site.

Nursing in the Community

➤ Review the general guidelines for the patient with tuberculosis or leprosy.

➤ Instruct the patient to report any new sign or symptom.

➤ Emphasize to the patient the importance of taking pyridoxine if prescribed. Review the Dietary Considerations box in Chapter 17 for information about dietary sources of pyridoxine.

➤ Instruct the patient to avoid the use of alcohol while taking isoniazid and to notify the physician if any signs of hepatitis develop: anorexia, nausea, vomiting, excessive fatigue, jaundice, dark urine, or malaise.

➤ Instruct the patient to take oral doses with meals to avoid gastric irritation.

➤ See the Patient Problems box in Chapter 23 on dry mouth.

➤ Caution the patient to avoid driving or operating hazardous equipment if dizziness, ataxia, tinnitus, or vision changes occur and to notify the physician if these symptoms do occur.

➤ Ingestion of fish or cheese while taking isoniazid may cause a reaction. Symptoms include headache, flushing, nausea,

Nursing Implications Summary—cont'd

vomiting, tachycardia, itching skin, and light-headedness. Instruct the patient to limit or avoid cheese and fish and to notify the physician if these symptoms develop.

➤ Inform diabetic patients that isoniazid may cause false results in urine glucose tests. Instruct diabetic patients not to change diet or insulin dosage without contacting the physician. Monitor blood glucose level if possible.

➤ Instruct the patient not to take aluminum-containing antacids within 1 hour of taking isoniazid.

pyrazinamide
Drug Administration/Nursing in the Community

➤ Review Nursing Implications Summary in Chapter 43 and the general guidelines for the patient with tuberculosis or leprosy.

➤ Monitor liver function tests and serum uric acid level.

➤ Warn diabetic patients that pyrazinamide may alter results of urine ketone tests; monitor blood sugar level.

rifampin
Drug Administration

➤ See the general guidelines for the patient with tuberculosis or leprosy and the Nursing Implications Summary in Chapter 43.

➤ Assess CBC and WBC differential, platelet count, and liver function tests.

➤ Intravenous rifampin: Dilute 600 mg in 10 ml sterile water for injection and swirl gently to dissolve the drug. Further dilute the solution in 500 ml D5W. Administer dose over 3 hours.

Nursing in the Community

➤ Review the general guidelines for the patient with tuberculosis or leprosy.

➤ Instruct the patient to take rifampin on an empty stomach 1 hour before or 2 hours after meals with a full glass (8 ounces) of water. Instruct the patient to take rifampin with meals if gastric irritation is severe when taken on an empty stomach.

➤ Instruct the patient not to take rifampin within 6 hours of taking a dose of aminosalicylate.

➤ Warn the patient that body fluids (tears, sweat, feces, and urine) may turn orange-red while undergoing rifampin therapy. Soft contact lenses may be permanently stained.

➤ It is especially important not to miss rifampin doses. Encourage the patient to take rifampin regularly, as prescribed, for best results.

➤ Instruct the patient to avoid driving or operating hazardous equipment if drowsiness, dizziness, or visual changes occur and to notify the physician if these symptoms do occur.

➤ Instruct the patient to avoid alcoholic beverages while taking rifampin and to report signs of possible hepatitis to the physician: excessive fatigue, anorexia, nausea, vomiting, jaundice, or dark urine.

➤ Oral contraceptives containing estrogen may not be effective in patients who are also taking rifampin. Instruct the patient to use another means of birth control while taking rifampin and to consult the physician.

➤ Inform the patient that capsules of rifampin may be opened and the contents may be mixed with applesauce or jelly for ease in taking.

➤ A suspension can also be made; the patient should consult the pharmacist.

streptomycin

➤ Streptomycin is discussed in Chapter 48.

dapsone
Drug Administration/Nursing in the Community

➤ See the general guidelines for the patient with tuberculosis or leprosy.

➤ Assess for skin changes and peripheral neuropathy.

➤ Monitor CBC and WBC differential, platelet count, liver function tests, BUN level, and serum creatinine level. Monitor urinalysis.

➤ Instruct the patient to take ordered doses with meals or a snack to lessen gastric irritation.

➤ Instruct the patient to take once-daily doses in the morning if insomnia occurs.

➤ Instruct the patient to avoid driving or operating hazardous equipment if dizziness or light-headedness occurs and to notify the physician if these symptoms do occur.

➤ Patients with dermatitis herpetiformis may be prescribed a gluten-free diet (see Dietary Considerations box earlier in this chapter).

clofazimine
Drug Administration/Nursing in the Community

➤ Instruct the patient to take oral doses with meals or a snack to lessen gastric irritation.

➤ Warn the patient that clofazimine may cause red to brown pigmentation of the skin and eyes. Assess for discoloration. If skin changes produce depression or extreme sadness, notify the physician.

➤ See the Patient Problems box in Chapter 58 on photosensitivity.

➤ Clofazimine may discolor feces, sputum, sweat, tears, and urine. It may also produce black, tarry, or bloody stools; instruct the patient to notify the physician if these symptoms occur.

➤ Instruct the patient to use lotion or skin cream to treat dry, scaly skin.

Continued

Nursing Implications Summary—cont'd

➤ Instruct the patient to avoid driving or operating hazardous equipment if drowsiness or dizziness occurs and to notify the physician if these symptoms occur.

rifabutin
Drug Administration/Nursing in the Community
➤ Review the general guidelines for patients with tuberculosis or leprosy.

➤ Monitor WBC count and platelet count.
➤ Warn the patient that body fluids (tears, sweat, feces, and urine) may turn orange-red while undergoing rifabutin therapy. Soft contact lenses may be permanently stained.
➤ Instruct the patient to take doses on an empty stomach unless gastric irritation develops, then take with meals or snack.
➤ Inform the patient that capsules may be opened and contents mixed with applesauce for ease in swallowing.

CHAPTER REVIEW

Application

1. What properties of mycobacteria make controlling tuberculosis more difficult than many other bacterial diseases?
2. During what phase of tuberculosis is the disease contagious?
3. Why does therapy for tuberculosis last for months to years?
4. What is the mechanism of action of isoniazid?
5. What is the outcome of using isoniazid alone to treat active tuberculosis?
6. When is isoniazid used alone?
7. How is isoniazid administered?
8. What is the fate of isoniazid in the body?
9. What toxicity is associated with isoniazid? What types of patients are most at risk?
10. What is the mechanism of action of rifampin?
11. How is rifampin administered in tuberculosis therapy?
12. What is the route of administration of pyrazinamide?
13. What side effect is characteristic of pyrazinamide?
14. How is ethambutol administered in tuberculosis therapy?
15. What toxicity is associated with ethambutol?
16. How is streptomycin administered?
17. What toxicity is associated with streptomycin?
18. Why are aminosalicylate, capreomycin, cycloserine, and ethionamide classified as alternate drugs in tuberculosis therapy?
19. What drugs are most useful in treating leprosy?
20. How long must therapy continue for control of leprosy?
21. What drugs are most useful for control of MAC?
22. How long must therapy continue for MAC?

Critical Thinking

1. Why is tuberculosis usually treated by multiple drug therapy? Name the implications for patient assessment and teaching.
2. How would you advise a patient receiving multidrug therapy for tuberculosis who confided that he had omitted his rifampin dose for the last week?
3. Develop a nursing care plan for a patient with tuberculosis, leprosy, or MAC.

References

Cohen FL: Adherence to therapy in tuberculosis, *Ann Rev Nurs Res* 15:153, 1997.
Skelskey C, Leshem OA: Tuberculosis surveillance in long-term care, *Am J Nurs* 97(10):16BBBB-16DDDD, 1997.
Tuberculosis morbidity—United States, 1997, *Morbid Mortal Wkly Rep* 47:253-257, 1998.

51

Antifungal Agents

OBJECTIVES

After studying this chapter, you should be able to do the following

- *Explain the mechanism of action of amphotericin B and azole antifungal drugs.*
- *Discuss the dose-limiting toxicity of amphotericin B.*
- *Explain why drugs that are too toxic for systemic use may be used for local fungal infections.*
- *Develop a nursing care plan for the patient receiving one of the parenteral, oral, or topical antifungal agents discussed in this chapter.*

CHAPTER OVERVIEW

Fungal diseases range from mild infections in localized areas of the skin to grave systemic infections. Diseases of various types may be produced by a wide range of fungi, and to a great extent, the seriousness of the infection is determined by the nature of the infecting organism and the immune status of the host. This chapter examines some of the more common and the more serious fungal diseases and considers the drugs used to control these specific infections.

THERAPEUTIC RATIONALE: SYSTEMIC FUNGAL INFECTIONS

Although the **fungi** that cause disease in humans are single-celled organisms, they are eucaryotes (see Chapter 43) and therefore resemble human cells more than bacteria in their biochemical properties. These biochemical similarities to human cells present therapeutic problems. For instance, none of the antibiotics that inhibit bacterial protein synthesis affect that process in fungi because fungal ribosomes resemble those in humans and are sensitive to the same drugs. Therefore selective toxicity cannot be achieved by this mechanism. Moreover, fungal cells do not contain a peptidoglycan cell wall, which renders them resistant to all antibiotics that block peptidoglycan synthesis (e.g., penicillins). For these reasons, the antimicrobial agents discussed in previous chapters cannot be used to treat fungal diseases.

The design of new antifungal agents depends on recognizing biochemical differences between fungal and mammalian cells. The only clinically exploited difference lies in the cellular membrane. Human cells contain cholesterol in their membranes, whereas those of fungi contain **ergosterol**. This feature of membrane structure is the basis of action of polyene antifungal agents that bind to ergosterol, and the azole antifungal agents that inhibit the synthesis of ergosterol. Experimental agents now in development are aimed at a different target, namely the enzyme glucan synthetase, which is involved in synthesis of fungal cell walls.

Fungal cells possess many antigens, which ultimately provoke host immune responses. Most fungal infections resolve in this way, many times without the host ever being aware of an active disease. This pattern is especially common with fungal diseases spread by breathing in spores from contaminated soil. Examples of diseases of this type are histoplasmosis, blastomycosis, cryptococcosis, coccidioidomycosis, and aspergillosis. Several of these diseases are concentrated in specific geographic areas. For example, coccidioidomycosis is most common, or endemic, in the southernmost portions of California, Nevada, Utah, Arizona, New Mexico, and Texas, whereas histoplasmosis is endemic in the states bordering the Mississippi and Ohio rivers. Blastomycosis is endemic in isolated areas along the Mississippi and Ohio Rivers, around the Great Lakes, along the St. Lawrence River, and in the Carolinas.

Some fungal diseases are spread by contact with soil contaminated with bird droppings. For example, histoplasmosis is associated with soil contaminated with chicken or starling droppings or bat guano. Cryptococcosis may occur after exposure to high concentrations of pigeon droppings. Although pulmonary forms of these diseases are usually mild and limited by effective development of immunity in the victim, in rare cases the fungus may become disseminated and invade other body tissues. A notorious example is the yeast *Cryptococcus neoformans,* which can cause meningitis, pulmonary disease, and infections at many other sites. The disseminated, or systemic, fungal diseases are most likely to develop in patients with immune systems depressed by disease or drug therapy, especially with glucocorticoids or immunosuppressant antineoplastic agents.

The yeast *Candida* may cause a range of infections from serious systemic disease to annoying mucous membrane infections. Because *Candida* is normally found on the skin and mucous membranes of healthy persons, the growth of *Candida* to cause disease usually represents an **opportunistic infection.** *Candida* infections are therefore most common in persons receiving broad-spectrum antibacterial drugs such as tetracyclines (see Chapter 47) or in persons with suppressed immune systems. *Candida* infections are very common in patients with acquired immunodeficiency syndrome (AIDS).

THERAPEUTIC AGENTS: DRUGS TO TREAT SYSTEMIC FUNGAL INFECTIONS

Systemic fungal infections pertain to the whole body. Table 51-1 summarizes drugs used to treat systemic fungal infections.

Table 51-1   Drugs to Treat Systemic Fungal Infections

Generic Name	Trade Name	Administration/Dosage	Clinical Use
amphotericin B	Fungizone*	INTRAVENOUS: *Adults*—0.25-0.7 mg/kg once daily. Dilute drug to 0.1 mg/ml in 5% dextrose; infuse at rate of 0.1 mg/kg/hr over 6 hr. Daily dose should not exceed 50 mg. Total drug course usually <4 g. FDA pregnancy category C. *Children*—0.25 mg/kg/day infused as for adults.	Disseminated, symptomatic fungal disease caused by *Histoplasma, Blastomyces, Coccidioides, Cryptococcus, Aspergillus, Candida,* and others. Also used for *Leishmaniasis.*
amphotericin B cholesteryl complex	Amphotec	INTRAVENOUS: *Adults and children*—3-4 mg/kg once daily. Infuse at rate of 1 mg/kg/hr. FDA pregnancy category B.	Currently indicated for disseminated aspergillosis only.
amphotericin B lipid complex	Abelcet	INTRAVENOUS: *Adults and children*—5 mg/kg once daily. Infuse at rate of 2.5 mg/kg/hr. FDA pregnancy category B.	May substitute for amphotericin B (Fungizone).
amphotericin B liposomal complex	AmBisome	INTRAVENOUS: *Adults and children*—3-5 mg/kg once daily. Infuse at rate of 1.5-2.5 mg/kg/hr. FDA pregnancy category B.	May substitute for amphotericin B (Fungizone).
fluconazole	Diflucan*	ORAL, INTRAVENOUS: *Adults*—100-400 mg once daily. FDA pregnancy category C. *Children*—3-12 mg/kg once daily.	Meningitis caused by *C. neoformans*; systemic, esophageal, or oropharyngeal candidiasis.
flucytosine	Ancobon Ancotil†	ORAL: *Adults and children*—12.5-37.5 mg/kg every 6 hr. Lower drug dosages are required when renal function is impaired. FDA pregnancy category C.	Disseminated fungal infections caused by sensitive *Candida* strains, cryptococcal meningitis, and other infections; usually combined with amphotericin B.
itraconazole	Sporanox*	ORAL: *Adults*—100-200 mg/day. FDA pregnancy category C.	Aspergillosis, blastomycosis, and histoplasmosis.
ketoconazole	Nizoral*	ORAL: *Adults*—200-400 mg once daily. FDA pregnancy category C. *Children* >2 yr—3.3-10 mg/kg once daily.	Disseminated infections caused by *Histoplasma, Paracoccidioides,* and *Candida.* Also used topically (see Table 51-2).
miconazole	Monistat IV	INTRAVENOUS: *Adults*—0.2-3.6 g, divided into 3 equal doses, depending on causative organism. FDA pregnancy category C. *Children*—Total daily dose 20-40 mg/kg with no single infusion exceeding 15 mg/kg.	Alternate drug for severe systemic infections caused by susceptible fungi. Primarily used topically (see Table 51-2).

*Available in Canada and the United States.
†Available in Canada only.

▼ amphotericin B

Mechanism of Action

Amphotericin B is the only polyene antifungal agent used for systemic fungal infections. **Polyene antifungal agents** have a greater affinity for ergosterol than for cholesterol and therefore react with ergosterol from fungal cell membranes. This action destroys the integrity of the cell membrane and the cell dies as its cytoplasmic components are lost. This membrane-disruptive effect is not entirely selective, and some of the cholesterol-containing membranes of mammalian cells are also damaged.

Pharmacokinetics

Amphotericin B must be administered intravenously, although the drug irritates vascular tissue and often causes phlebitis. This lipid-soluble agent may be administered as a colloidal suspension stabilized with small amounts of the detergent desoxycholate. Amphotericin B in this form (Fungizone, Table 51-1) must be infused at a concentration of less than 0.1 mg/ml in a 5% dextrose solution; these infusions typically take 6 hours. Higher drug concentrations cause precipitation of the drug in the intravenous (IV) solution and endanger the patient.

Amphotericin B has a high affinity for lipids and thus tends to bind to tissues rather than remain in blood. During long-term therapy, only a fraction of the daily dose can be recovered in urine or feces. The unrecovered drug is held in tissues and continues to appear in urine for long periods after therapy is halted. The tissue-binding properties and the relative water insolubility of amphotericin B prevent the drug from entering body fluids efficiently. Therefore concentrations of the drug in the cerebrospinal fluid or in ocular fluid may be too low to effectively eliminate infections at those sites. To overcome this problem, amphotericin B (Fungizone) may be injected intrathecally (into the cerebrospinal fluid) to treat meningitis.

Recently, other forms of amphotericin have been developed to improve the pharmacokinetics of the drug. Amphotericin B may be complexed with cholesteryl sulfate (Amphotec, Table 51-1) or with two phospholipids (Abelcet, Table 51-1) to improve water solubility of the drug. Likewise, amphotericin B has been inserted into **liposomes,** which are lipid structures that maintain a specific form in solution (AmBisome, Table 51-1). In this case the liposomes consist of a bilayer of phospholipids stabilized with alpha-tocopherol. These structures maintain a *hydrophobic* (i.e., a water-repelling, lipid-attracting) region where amphotericin may concentrate, as well as a hydrophilic (i.e., water-attracting) face that is in contact with the solution and maintains solubility. Each of these lipid-containing preparations allows higher concentrations of drug to be used by improving water solubility. These lipid formulations of amphotericin B have also improved distribution of the drug in the body, while lowering toxicity. Care must be taken not to use doses calculated for the new formulations with the older, more toxic formulation (Fungizone); deaths have resulted (Box 51-1).

Uses

Amphotericin B can be used to treat many different fungal diseases, including those caused by *Histoplasma, Blastomyces, Cryptococcus,* and *Aspergillus* organisms. Amphotericin B may also treat systemic *Candida* and *Coccidioides* infections. Topical use of amphotericin B is not recommended because other topical agents are more effective.

Adverse Reactions and Contraindications

Most patients start on low dosages of amphotericin B, and the dosage is increased as tolerance to ensuing side effects develops. Fever, headache, nausea, and vomiting may occur after the first few injections, but these side effects usually subside as therapy continues. Renal damage progresses with length of therapy and may become irreversible when total doses of amphotericin B approach 4 g. Anemia also develops with time, as do electrolyte disturbances, including acidosis and hypokalemia (low blood potassium).

There are no absolute contraindications to the use of amphotericin B for serious systemic fungal disease, but in patients with renal disease, the risk of increased nephrotoxicity is significant.

Box 51-1   Alert for Amphotericin B

The Problem

Amphotericin B is available in two very different types of formulations. The original formulation (Fungizone) contains amphotericin B solubilized with the detergent deoxycholate. The solubility of this preparation is limited, and it must be extensively diluted before administration. It is also highly toxic, and dosages must be carefully controlled to prevent renal damage, electrolyte imbalances, or death.

The new formulations of amphotericin B complex the drug with lipids (Amphotec, Abelcet) or enclose it in liposomes (AmBisome). This process increases the solubility of the drug, alters its disposition in the body, and reduces toxicity. Thus these new formulations can be administered at higher dosages than Fungizone. This difference in dosage has resulted in fatal medication errors, when Fungizone was used at dosages intended only for the newer formulations.

The Solution

- Carefully note the form of amphotericin B that was ordered for the patient. Question any drug orders outside the following guidelines.
- Fungizone must be diluted to 0.1 mg/ml in 5% dextrose and administered at a rate of 0.1 mg/kg/hr. The daily dose should not exceed 50 mg. Question any concentration, rate of administration, or dosage in excess of these values if the preparation being used is Fungizone.
- Amphotec may be infused at a rate of 1 mg/kg/hr; dosages are 3 to 4 mg/kg once daily.
- Abelcet or AmBisome may be infused at rates up to 2.5 mg/kg/hr for dosages of 5 mg/kg once daily.

Toxicity

Amphotericin B therapy must be continued for long periods to attempt to cure disseminated fungal disease. No firm guidelines for therapy exist, although physicians try to limit the total drug dose to less than 4 g. Even with doses approaching this limit, cures are not always obtained. For many patients therapy must be discontinued early because of toxic effects of the drug.

Interactions

Amphotericin B is incompatible in solution with sodium chloride and with benzyl alcohol. These compounds cause precipitation of the colloidal suspension of amphotericin B used for IV administration.

Because amphotericin B has significant toxicity on its own, it can also cause serious interactions with other agents. Bone marrow depressants and radiation therapy may increase the risk of anemia with amphotericin B. Nephrotoxic drugs increase the risk of renal damage with amphotericin B.

Amphotericin B tends to cause hypokalemia. This action increases the risk of toxicity with digitalis glycosides and with potassium-depleting diuretics. The risk of serious hypokalemia is also increased with corticosteroid use.

flucytosine

Mechanism of Action

Flucytosine is a pyrimidine analog that is converted to the cytotoxic agent 5-fluorouracil in sensitive fungi. Because this metabolite is not freely formed in humans, a degree of selective toxicity is achieved.

Pharmacokinetics

Flucytosine is a water-soluble drug that is well absorbed from the gastrointestinal (GI) tract and well distributed into body fluids. Drug concentration in cerebrospinal fluid may be 50% to 70% of serum levels, in contrast to amphotericin B, for which cerebrospinal fluid levels are less than 5% of serum levels. More than 90% of an oral dose of flucytosine appears unchanged in urine, and high concentrations of the drug are observed in urine. The elimination half-life is about 6 hours.

Uses

A relatively narrow range of fungi are sensitive to flucytosine, including *Cryptococcus, Candida,* and a few other rarely encountered pathogenic fungi. Intrinsic resistance to flucytosine may exist in a significant number of clinically encountered *Candida* strains, and resistance to the drug may be acquired by *Cryptococcus* during therapy. This pattern of resistance has limited the drug's usefulness.

Adverse Reactions and Contraindications

Flucytosine therapy is usually continued for several weeks to months. Nausea and diarrhea appear in roughly one fourth of patients. Blood dyscrasias such as anemia and thrombo-

cytopenia (unusual bruising or bleeding) and transient liver abnormalities have been reported.

The only absolute contraindication to the use of flucytosine is a documented allergy to the drug, but the drug should be used cautiously in patients with impairment of renal function or with bone marrow depression caused by drugs or disease.

Toxicity

High serum concentrations of flucytosine increase the risk of hematologic toxicity. Hemodialysis may be required to remove the drug from the system, especially in patients with poor renal function.

Interactions

Because of its effects on the bone marrow, flucytosine should not be used with other agents that also depress bone marrow function.

Flucytosine is often combined with amphotericin B for treatment of disseminated fungal disease. The rationale for combining these drugs for serious infections is twofold: the combination allows the dose of amphotericin B to be lowered somewhat, thereby reducing toxicity, and resistance to flucytosine is minimized by combination chemotherapy.

▼ Azole Antifungal Agents: fluconazole, itraconazole, ketoconazole, and miconazole

Mechanism of Action

Azole antifungal agents inhibit synthesis of ergosterol. As a result, the function of fungal cell membranes is impaired. Development of invasive hyphae by *Candida* cells may also be retarded, enhancing the ability of the host immune system to eliminate fungal cells.

Pharmacokinetics

Ketoconazole is adequately absorbed orally, but bioavailability depends on sufficient stomach acidity. Ketoconazole should not be administered within 2 hours of a dose of antacids or H_2-histamine receptor blocking drugs such as cimetidine. Ketoconazole is not well distributed to some tissues and is especially low in cerebrospinal fluid. Elimination is primarily by the liver, which forms inactive metabolites and excretes the drug into bile. The half-life of the drug is 8 hours.

Fluconazole is well absorbed orally, with a bioavailability of about 90%; absorption does not depend on stomach acidity as much as with ketoconazole. Fluconazole is well distributed to most body tissues, including the cerebrospinal fluid. Little hepatic metabolism of fluconazole occurs, and most of the drug is excreted unchanged in urine. The half-life of the drug in patients with normal renal function is 30 hours.

Itraconazole is relatively lipid soluble and is absorbed after oral administration. Food increases absorption of oral doses of this drug. Itraconazole concentrates in tissues such as the skin and lungs but does not enter the vitreous humor or the cerebrospinal fluid adequately to treat infections at those sites. Itraconazole metabolites are formed in the liver and excreted in urine.

Miconazole must be administered intravenously in systemic infections. The drug enters vitreous humor but poorly penetrates into the cerebrospinal fluid; therefore intrathecal injections must be used for meningitis.

Uses

Azole antifungal agents are used to treat a variety of fungal infections. Fluconazole is indicated for cryptococcal meningitis and for systemic, esophageal, or oropharyngeal candidiasis. Ketoconazole is used against *Histoplasma* and *Paracoccidioides.* It may also be effective in certain patients with disseminated candidiasis and blastomycosis. Itraconazole is indicated for aspergillosis, blastomycosis, and histoplasmosis. Miconazole may be used against systemic coccidioidomycosis, cryptococcosis, and candidiasis but is primarily used as a topical agent. Clotrimazole, econazole, oxiconazole, sulconazole, and terconazole are used topically for a variety of infections including vaginal infections caused by *Candida* (see Patient Problems box) and tinea (Table 51-2).

Adverse Reactions and Contraindications

Ketoconazole is relatively nontoxic for many patients. Nausea and pruritus occur in less than 5% of treated patients. Dizziness, nervousness, and headache have been reported less often.

Fluconazole may cause side effects in up to 13% of treated patients. GI tract disturbances such as nausea or diarrhea and headaches are the most common complaints. Thrombocytopenia, which produces unusual bleeding or bruising, and hepatotoxicity are more serious rare effects. Rarely, patients may develop dangerous allergic reactions such as Stevens-Johnson syndrome or exfoliative skin disorders.

Miconazole may produce rashes, itching, redness at the injection site, or phlebitis. Reversible platelet dysfunction, anemia, and thrombocytopenia may also occur with systemic administration.

Itraconazole appears to cause less hepatotoxicity than does ketoconazole and alters platelet function less than miconazole does. All azole antifungals are capable of inducing allergic reactions.

Toxicity

Hepatotoxicity is an idiosyncratic reaction that occurs in about 1 in 10,000 patients receiving ketoconazole. High dosages of azole antifungals may inhibit testosterone and cortisol synthesis. This inhibition may produce gynecomastia (excessive development of mammary glands), which has been noted in about 10% of males receiving ketoconazole.

Interactions

Azole antifungal agents are subject to a wide array of drug interactions. Pharmacokinetic interactions include those that block absorption of the azoles. For example, antacids or H₂-receptor blockers that raise gastric pH lower absorption of ketoconazole and itraconazole because these azoles require strong acidity for absorption. Didanosine also lowers absorption of azoles because didanosine preparations contain buffers to raise gastric pH.

PATIENT PROBLEMS

Vaginal Infection

THE PROBLEM

The dark, moist environment of the vagina is prone to infection by a variety of organisms. Some chronic health problems such as diabetes mellitus increase susceptibility to vaginal infection. Treatment with some groups of drugs such as antibiotics may increase susceptibility to fungal superinfection. Finally, some invading organisms are passed as venereal diseases. Treatment of vaginal infections may be messy and difficult. It is difficult to reach all mucosal surfaces. Also, because the woman is upright during most of the day, medications drain out because of gravity.

SOLUTIONS

- Use prescribed agents for the full course of therapy; do not stop when symptoms disappear.
- Do not wear tampons during therapy. Wear sanitary napkins to prevent staining of clothing.
- Continue therapy through the menstrual period.
- Wash hands carefully before and after using prescribed medications.
- Use once-daily doses of vaginal medication in the evening, before retiring. Insert vaginal suppository, ointment, or cream just before going to bed to allow the medication to remain in the vaginal area as long as possible.
- If douching is prescribed, wash douche equipment carefully after each use and dry it.
- Depending on the infecting agent, it may be necessary to treat the sexual partner also; consult the physician.
- Usually, avoid sexual intercourse during the course of therapy. If not possible, the sexual partner should wear a condom.

TO HELP PREVENT VAGINAL INFECTION

- Wear clean underwear daily, preferably of cotton material. Synthetic fabrics do not allow air to circulate as well, and thus they keep the vaginal area more moist than normal. Avoid pantyhose for the same reason. Do not wear pantyhose and slacks at the same time.
- Wipe from front to back after voiding or defecating.
- Do not douche unless prescribed by the physician. Do not douche between doses of vaginal medications.
- Avoid bubble baths and soaps that may irritate vaginal mucosa. Wash the vaginal area gently and rinse soap off well. Some women may need to wash with water only if soap is irritating to the vaginal area.
- Use water-soluble lubricants, if needed, in the vagina. Do not use oil-based products such as petroleum jelly.

Table 51-2 **Drugs to Treat Topical Fungal Infections**

Generic Name	Trade Name	Administration/Dosage	Cautions
butenafine	Mentax	TOPICAL: *Adults—For athlete's foot:* Apply 1% cream once daily for 4 wk.	Avoid contact with eyes.
ciclopirox olamine	Loprox*	TOPICAL: *Adults—For tinea infections, including tinea versicolor and cutaneous candidiasis:* Cream or lotion applied twice daily. FDA pregnancy category B.	Avoid contact with eyes. Do not use occlusive dressing.
clioquinol (iodochlor-hydroxyquin)	Vioform*	TOPICAL: *Adults and children—For localized dermatophytoses:* 3% cream or ointment applied 2 or 3 times/day.	Causes false-positive ferric chloride test for phenylketonuria (PKU); can alter iodine content of blood.
clotrimazole	Canesten† Lotrimin Mycelex	TOPICAL: *Adults and children—For tinea or candidiasis:* Cutaneous, 1% cream, lotion, or solution applied twice daily. FDA pregnancy category B.	Avoid contacting eyes with lotions, creams, and solutions.
	Canesten† Gyne-Lotrimin Myclo† Mycelex	INTRAVAGINAL: *Adults—For vulvovaginal candidiasis:* tablets or creams containing 100 mg inserted once daily. FDA pregnancy category B. ORAL: *Adults and children >5 yr—For oropharyngeal candidiasis:* 10-mg lozenge dissolved in mouth 5 times/day. FDA pregnancy category C.	Single dose of 500 mg intravaginally controls some but not all infections.
econazole	Ecostatin† Spectazole	TOPICAL: *Adults and children—For mucocutaneous Candida or tinea:* 1% cream applied to skin 2 times/day. FDA pregnancy category C.	Avoid eyes; do not use occlusive dressings.
griseofulvin	Fulvicin* Grifulvin Grisactin Grisovin†	ORAL: *Adults—For tinea infections:* 500-mg microcrystalline form in single or divided dose. Avoid during pregnancy. *Children—* 5-10 mg/kg/day.	Headache, gastrointestinal disturbances, neuritis, allergies, and hepatotoxicity may occur.
haloprogin	Halotex*	TOPICAL: *Adults and children—For tinea and other superficial fungal infections:* 1% cream or solution applied twice daily. FDA pregnancy category B.	Local irritation may occur; avoid contact with eyes.
ketoconazole	Nizoral	TOPICAL: *Adults and children—For tinea and cutaneous Candida:* 2% cream applied once daily or shampoo used every 4 days. FDA pregnancy category C.	Avoid contact with eyes.
miconazole nitrate	Micatin* Monistat-Derm* Monistat*	TOPICAL: *Adults and children—For dermatophytoses:* 2% cream, lotion, or aerosol applied twice daily. INTRAVAGINAL: *Adults—For vaginal candidiasis:* 1% cream, tampon, or suppositories applied once daily.	Local irritation occurs; avoid contact with eyes.
naftifine	Naftin*	TOPICAL: *Adults and children—For tinea:* 1% cream or gel applied to skin twice daily. FDA pregnancy category B.	Local irritation may occur. Avoid contact with eyes or mucous membranes.
natamycin	Natacyn	OPHTHALMIC: *Adults and children—For fungal blepharitis, conjunctivitis, or keratitis:* 5% ophthalmic suspension, 1 drop every 2-6 hr.	Eye irritation may occur with this chemical relative of amphotericin B.
nystatin	Mycostatin* Nadostine† Nilstat* Nystex	ORAL: *Adults and children—For oropharyngeal candidiasis:* 0.5-1 million units 3 times/day. *Infants—*0.1-0.2 million units 4 times/day. TOPICAL: *Adults and children—For Candida infections of skin:* Ointments, creams, and powder (0.1 million units/g) applied twice daily. INTRAVAGINAL: *Adults—For Candida infections of vagina:* Cream or tablets, 0.1 million units once or twice daily. FDA pregnancy category A.	Nausea, vomiting, or diarrhea may occur; drug not absorbed orally. Irritation of skin may occur. Irritation is rare.
oxiconazole	Oxistat	TOPICAL: *Adults and children—For tinea infections:* 1% cream or lotion once or twice daily. FDA pregnancy category B.	Rash or burning may occur.
sulconazole	Exelderm	TOPICAL: *Adults—For tinea infections:* 1% cream or solution applied once or twice daily. FDA pregnancy category C.	Solution is not effective for athlete's foot.
terbinafine	Lamisil	TOPICAL: *Adults—For tinea infections:* 1% cream applied twice daily. FDA pregnancy category B.	Rarely causes irritation or sensitization.
terconazole	Terazol*	VAGINAL: *Adults—For vulvovaginal candidiasis :* 5 g 0.4% cream or 80-mg suppository applied once daily. FDA pregnancy category C.	Vaginal burning may occur.
tioconazole	Vagistat GyneCure†	INTRAVAGINAL: *Adults—*300 mg as ointment or suppository as a single dose.	Dose may be repeated 1-2 wk later if needed.
tolnaftate	Aftate Tinactin*	TOPICAL: *Adults and children—For tinea infections:* 1% cream, gel, solution, powder, or aerosol twice daily.	Rarely causes irritation or sensitization. Avoid eyes.

*Available in Canada and the United States.
†Available in Canada only.

Another potentially serious pharmacokinetic interaction arises because the azole antifungals, and especially ketoconazole and itraconazole, can inhibit hepatic metabolism of a variety of drugs. This action leads to a rise in blood concentrations of drugs such as the antihistamines astemizole and terfenadine, cyclosporine, digoxin, phenytoin, warfarin, and the sulfonylurea antidiabetic medications. Increased blood levels of these agents can produce serious or even life-threatening side effects.

A few drugs lower the blood concentrations of the azole antifungal agents and cause failure of therapy. Examples include carbamazepine and the antituberculosis drugs rifampin and isoniazid.

Ketoconazole has been linked to hepatotoxic reactions when given with other hepatotoxic agents or when used in alcoholic patients. Concurrent use of ketoconazole and alcohol has caused a disulfiram-like reaction (facial flushing, tightness in the chest, difficulty breathing).

THERAPEUTIC RATIONALE: TOPICAL FUNGAL INFECTIONS

Dermatophytes are fungi whose growth is almost always restricted to the skin of humans. These fungi cause the annoying infections commonly called ringworm and athlete's foot, as well as several others. This group of infections is often referred to as **tinea**. Many of the drugs used topically are not absorbed extensively through the skin. Therefore more toxic agents may be used than can be used systemically, and selective toxicity is achieved against many dermatophytes.

THERAPEUTIC AGENTS: DRUGS TO TREAT TOPICAL FUNGAL INFECTIONS

In this section, drugs that are used to treat topical fungal infections or those restricted to skin, mucous membranes, or GI tract are considered. The properties of specific drugs are listed in Table 51-2. Most of these agents are used strictly locally, being applied at the site of infection. For example, tolnaftate is used to treat simple cases of tinea, but the effectiveness is limited by the accessibility of locally applied drug to the infective fungi. Therefore tinea infections around nails and heavily keratinized skin are hard to eradicate.

griseofulvin

Griseofulvin is effective against several types of dermatophytic infections, including infections of the scalp. It is used orally rather than topically. The usefulness of this drug as an oral agent depends on its ability to localize in skin after oral absorption. Skin cells containing high concentrations of griseofulvin are resistant to infection by dermatophytes. Ul-

timately, all infected cells will be lost through the natural sloughing off of skin cells, and the disease will be cured. This process takes considerable time, and accordingly griseofulvin therapy may need to be continued for several weeks or months, depending on the site and the severity of the infection. Griseofulvin may stimulate metabolism of anticoagulants such as warfarin or oral contraceptives; the effects of these drugs will be diminished.

nystatin

Nystatin is sometimes given orally to treat intestinal fungal infections. This treatment may be considered topical because nystatin is not absorbed orally and is retained in the intestine. Nystatin is also used to treat vaginal infections such as those caused by *Candida*. This treatment is also topical because the drug is administered intravaginally and is not systemically absorbed. Nystatin is too toxic to be used for systemic infections.

terbinafine

Terbinafine inhibits ergosterol biosynthesis by a different mechanism than the azole antifungal agents. Terbinafine disrupts fungal cell membranes and kills affected fungi. The drug is well absorbed orally with or without food. Because it is highly lipophilic, terbinafine distributes well to tissues and especially to skin, hair follicles, and nail beds. The drug is readily metabolized in liver to inactive forms that are eliminated primarily in urine. Despite relatively effective elimination processes, terbinafine persists in tissues for prolonged periods as a result of its high lipid solubility.

Terbinafine commonly causes anorexia, diarrhea, nausea, stomach pain, or vomiting. The drug may also change the sensation of taste. Allergies are possible and rarely these may be severe, including life-threatening conditions such as Stevens-Johnson syndrome. Terbinafine should be used cautiously, if at all, in patients with a history of alcoholism or hepatic impairment. These patients may be at increased risk of terbinafine-induced hepatotoxicity. Patients with renal impairment may require reduced dosages of the drug.

Terbinafine should not be used along with other hepatotoxic drugs. Therefore patients taking terbinafine should avoid the use of alcohol or high dosages of vitamin A or niacin. Other drugs to avoid include steroids, sulfonamides, phenothiazines, or zidovudine.

Terbinafine is metabolized by hepatic cytochrome P-450 systems. Therefore drugs that affect this system can affect clearance of terbinafine. Barbiturates, griseofulvin, phenytoin, and rifampin are examples of drugs that induce P-450, which increases metabolism of terbinafine and lowers blood levels of the drug. In contrast, cimetidine, clarithromycin, estrogens, erythromycins, azole antifungals, fluorquinolones, and isoniazid inhibit P-450 and therefore block metabolism of terbinafine. The result is higher concentrations of terbinafine, which may increase risk of toxicity.

Nursing Process Overview

Fungal Infections

Assessment

Fungal infections are relatively common and can occur in patients of any age. Perform a thorough total assessment, focusing on the specific subjective complaints or objective signs that indicate possible fungal infection. Include as part of the history recent use of drugs that may alter the patient's immune response and measures the patient has tried for eradication of the problem. Patients most likely to have fungal infections include those receiving cancer chemotherapy, immunotherapy, antibiotic therapy, or drugs that alter the normal pH of areas such as the vagina; those receiving nutritional support via peripheral or central venous catheters; patients with human immunodeficiency virus (HIV) or AIDS; and those taking high dosages of adrenocortical steroids.

Nursing Diagnoses

- Potential altered comfort: nausea and vomiting as a side effect of drug therapy

Patient Outcomes

The patient will not experience nausea and vomiting caused by antifungal drug therapy. The nurse will manage and minimize complications related to renal failure.

Planning/Implementation

Teach the patient about the drugs prescribed, the infection, and possible ways to limit the spread of the infection and to prevent its recurrence. Treatment of systemic fungal infections is more serious. Monitor the vital signs and appropriate laboratory work to evaluate possible side effects.

Evaluation

Before discharge, ascertain that the patient understands why the drug is being used, how it should be used and under what circumstances, what to do if side effects should occur, and which side effects require notification of the physician.

Nursing Implications Summary

amphotericin B

Drug Administration

➤ Assess for side effects such as nausea, vomiting, chills, phlebitis, headache, anemia, and electrolyte imbalances. With amphotericin B cholesteryl complex, assess for unexplained bruising or bleeding.

➤ Monitor temperature, vital signs, intake and output, and weight. Monitor blood glucose levels.

➤ Monitor complete blood count (CBC) and differential, platelet count, and serum creatinine, blood urea nitrogen (BUN), liver function tests, and serum electrolyte levels. With amphotericin B cholesteryl complex, monitor prothrombin time (PT).

➤ Use an infusion monitoring device to assist in regulating the rate. Too rapid infusion may be associated with cardiac toxicity.

➤ To prevent side effects, corticosteroids may be administered before or during therapy or may be added to the infusion.

➤ If ordered, administer antiemetics 30 minutes before starting the infusion to help prevent nausea and vomiting.

➤ If ordered, administer acetaminophen before or during infusion to treat fever or headache. Codeine or other analgesics may also be used to treat headache.

➤ Other drugs may be administered to prevent or treat side effects: Heparin may be added to infusions to help prevent thrombophlebitis, IV meperidine may be used to treat rigors (shaking chill), mannitol may be administered

before and after amphotericin B to reduce nephrotoxic effects, a potassium-sparing diuretic may be administered to limit hypokalemia, and diphenhydramine may be administered to prevent chills.

➤ Disagreement exists about the need to cover the tubing and fluid reservoir containing amphotericin B. Follow agency custom; most agencies still cover the bag with a plastic or paper bag.

➤ Keep siderails up and call bell within easy reach. Do not leave the patient unattended for long periods.

➤ Use of IV filters is controversial. If an IV filter is used, it must be at least 1 micron in diameter.

➤ Read orders and doses carefully. See Box 51-1 on amphotericin B.

➤ Fungizone: Prepare IV doses as directed in the package insert. Dissolve doses in sterile water with no bacteriostatic agent. Further dilute to the desired volume in D5W; no other diluent may be used.

➤ AmBisome: Prepare dose by adding 12 ml of sterile water for injection without bacteriostatic agent to each 50-mg vial to produce a concentration of 4 mg/ml. Shake vial vigorously for 30 seconds until particulate matter is dispersed. Withdraw dose, using a 5-micron filter, and dilute in sufficient 5% dextrose injection to produce a concentration of 1 to 2 mg/ml. More dilute solutions may be used for infants and small children. Administer dose over at least 2 hours until patient's response can be evaluated. After

Nursing Implications Summary—cont'd

several doses, time may be reduced to 1 hour if patient tolerates this.

➤ Abelcet: Gently shake vial until no sediment is visible at the bottom. Withdraw ordered dose from required number of vials using an 18-gauge needle. Replace needle with filter needle supplied by manufacturer and add dose to a bag of 5% dextrose injection to make a final concentration of 1 mg/ml. For infants or patients with cardiovascular disease who cannot tolerate large volumes, concentration may be 2 mg/ml. Administer dose at a rate of 2.5 mg/kg/hr. Do not use an in-line filter of any kind.

➤ Amphotec: Reconstitute by adding sterile water for injection to the correct dosage vial (see manufacturer's instructions). Shake gently by hand, rotating vial until all solids have dissolved. Fluid may be clear or opalescent. Further dilute solution to a final concentration of approximately 0.6 mg/ml, using guidelines provided by manufacturer. A test dose may be ordered before the full dose to assess patient's response. To administer test dose, prepare full dose, then administer 10 ml of the final preparation over 15 to 30 minutes, then monitor the patient for an additional 30 minutes. If patient response is satisfactory, administer full dose at a rate of 1 mg/kg/hr. After several doses, infusion time may be shortened to 2 hours if well-tolerated by patient. Do not use an in-line filter of any kind.

➤ For any brand: Do not administer other IV medications via the amphotericin B line without flushing well before and after the dose with D5W. If other IV medications are to be administered during amphotericin B infusion, start and maintain a separate IV access line.

➤ The diluted drug is a suspension. Gently agitate the bag or bottle regularly during the infusion to promote uniform dilution.

➤ If the course of therapy is interrupted for more than a few days, it may be necessary to resume therapy with low dosages and increase the dosage gradually to the desired dosage.

➤ In addition to IV administration, amphotericin B may be administered via intracavitary instillation, intrathecal administration, or bladder irrigation; see the package insert.

Nursing in the Community

➤ Review anticipated benefits and possible side effects of drug therapy with the patient. The patient may require not only teaching but also continued emotional support because IV therapy is continued for weeks to months. Some patients are suitable candidates for home therapy. Assess the patient and consult the physician. Refer home therapy patients to a community-based nursing care agency.

➤ Instruct the patient to report any new sign or symptom to the physician.

➤ Provide instruction on dietary sources of sodium, potassium, and iron as indicated.

➤ Warn the patient to avoid driving or operating hazardous equipment if visual changes occur and to notify the physician if these changes do occur.

➤ Remind the patient to inform all health care providers of all drugs being used.

➤ Side effects with topical preparations are uncommon. Instruct the patient not to cover affected areas with an occlusive dressing. Instruct the patient to use topical forms regularly, as prescribed. Intermittent use may cause the fungal infection to return. The cream form may stain skin. Fabric discoloration from lotion or cream can be removed with soap and water. Fabric discoloration from ointment can be removed with cleaning fluid.

flucytosine
Drug Administration

➤ Inspect the patient for bruising, bleeding, or other signs and symptoms of blood dyscrasias. Assess for GI tract side effects. Monitor weight.

➤ Monitor BUN and serum creatinine levels, CBC and differential, platelet count, and liver function tests.

➤ Check stools regularly for blood and guaiac.

Nursing in the Community

➤ Review the anticipated benefits and possible side effects of drug therapy with the patient. Instruct the patient to report any new sign or symptom to the physician.

➤ Provide emotional support as needed; weeks to months of therapy may be required for adequate treatment.

➤ Instruct the patient to take oral doses with meals or a snack over a 15-minute period to lessen gastric irritation.

➤ Warn the patient to avoid driving or operating hazardous equipment if vertigo or sleepiness occurs and to notify the physician if these symptoms do occur.

➤ See the Patient Problems boxes on photosensitivity (Chapter 58) and bleeding tendencies (Chapter 54).

Azole Antifungal Agents
Drug Administration

➤ Monitor for side effects such as central nervous system (CNS) effects and GI tract distress.

➤ Monitor liver function tests, BUN and serum creatinine, and potassium levels.

➤ A potentially fatal drug interaction exists between azole antifungal agents and astemizole, cisapride, or terfenadine (see Interactions). Inform all health care providers of all drugs being used.

➤ IV fluconazole: The drug is prepacked in a ready-to-use form. Administer at a rate of 200 mg or less over 1 hour. Monitor for side effects, including exfoliative skin disorders, hepatotoxicity, thrombocytopenia, GI tract distress, and headache. Review the Patient Problems box in Chapter 54 on bleeding tendencies.

➤ IV miconazole: Dilute 200 mg in 200 ml of normal saline or D5W. Administer each 200 mg over 2 hours. Monitor vital signs with IV doses and do not administer too rapidly. Perform neurologic assessment regularly. Monitor vital signs and weight. Inspect injection site for phlebitis and pruritus.

Continued

Nursing Implications Summary—cont'd

Nursing in the Community

➤ Review anticipated benefits and possible side effects of drug therapy with the patient. Instruct the patient to report any new sign or symptom to the physician.

➤ Warn the patient to avoid driving or operating hazardous equipment if dizziness or lethargy develops and to notify the physician if these symptoms occur.

➤ Instruct the patient not to take H_2-receptor blocking drugs (e.g., cimetidine, ranitidine), omeprazole, or antacids within 2 hours of ketoconazole or itraconazole doses.

➤ Instruct the patient to avoid alcoholic beverages while taking ketoconazole.

➤ If photophobia develops (sensitivity of the eyes to light), instruct the patient to wear sunglasses and avoid bright lights and sunlight.

➤ For the patient using the oral liquid form: Use the calibrated measuring device provided by the pharmacist for measuring doses.

➤ Absorption of ketoconazole or itraconazole requires an acid pH in the stomach. For patients with achlorhydria, the physician may recommend that the patient dissolve the dose in cola or seltzer water before taking the dose or that the patient dissolve each dose in 4 ml of 0.2N HCl solution. Instruct the patient to use a straw to avoid contact with the teeth and to follow the dose with another half glass of water. Consult the pharmacist and physician as needed.

➤ Provide emotional support as needed. Weeks to months of therapy may be needed.

terbinafine
Nursing in the Community

➤ Instruct the patient to take doses with meals or on an empty stomach.

➤ Emphasize the importance of taking the drug for the full course of therapy, as prescribed, for best effect. Weeks of therapy may be required to treat specific fungal infections.

➤ Instruct the patient to avoid alcoholic beverages while taking this drug.

➤ There are many significant drug interactions with terbinafine. Remind the patient to keep all health care providers informed of all drugs being used.

➤ Instruct the patient to read drug labels and orders carefully and to not confuse terbinafine with terbutaline.

➤ Instruct the patient to report the development of jaundice, rash, blistering of skin, persistent diarrhea, stomach pain to the physician.

Topical Antifungal Agents
Nursing in the Community

➤ Instruct the patient that for best effect tropical antifungal agents must be used regularly, as prescribed. Instruct the patient to contact the physician if redness, itching, discharge, or other problems develop while using a prescribed topical antifungal agent.

➤ With ointments and creams, instruct the patient to apply the dose as directed and gently rub into the area. The patient should not cover the area with a dressing unless instructed to do so by the physician.

➤ Instruct the patient to shake aerosol powders or solutions well before using, hold the spray opening 6 to 10 inches away from the area to be treated, and spray well. Caution the patient not to inhale powder or solution and to avoid the eyes.

➤ Instruct the patient to sprinkle powder forms liberally on the affected area such as the toes and feet.

➤ When treating toes and feet, the patient should make certain the drug reaches the area between toes and on the bottom of the feet. The patient should sprinkle or spray onto socks or in shoes if directed to do so by the physician.

➤ For vaginal forms, see the Patient Problems box on vaginal infections (earlier in this chapter). Instruct the patient to insert a medicated tampon (e.g., miconazole) at bedtime and remove it in the morning.

➤ Azole vaginal forms may cause the latex in condoms, diaphragms, or cervical caps to weaken and break, so these forms of birth control will be unreliable; use an alternate method of birth control. Drugs in this group include butoconazole, clotrimazole, econazole, miconazole, terconazole, and tioconazole.

➤ Remind women that no medications, even topical ones, should be used during pregnancy or lactation without prior consultation with the physician.

➤ For tinea cruris (jock itch): Instruct the patient to avoid underwear that is tight or made of material that does not breathe well, to wear loose cotton underwear, and to change it daily. Instruct the patient to use an absorbent powder or antifungal powder but to not apply powder at the same time as antifungal creams, lotions, or solutions.

➤ For tinea pedis (athlete's foot): Instruct the patient to carefully dry feet, especially between toes, after bathing or showering. Instruct the patient to avoid wearing socks made of materials that hold moisture and to wear clean cotton socks and change at least daily. Instruct the patient to wear sandals or well-ventilated shoes with air holes and to rotate shoes so that they can dry thoroughly between wearings. Instruct the patient to use an absorbent powder or antifungal powder but not to apply powder at the same time as antifungal creams, lotions, or solutions.

nystatin
Drug Administration/Nursing in the Community

➤ Side effects are uncommon. Instruct the patient to report any new sign or symptom to the physician.

➤ With nystatin suspension, the drug may be dispensed with a dropper; use this to measure the dose. Place half the dose in one side of the mouth and the other half in the other side. Instruct the patient to hold, swish, and gargle for as long as possible before swallowing.

Nursing Implications Summary—cont'd

➤ With nystatin powder, add the dose (about ⅛ teaspoon) to 4 to 5 ounces of water and stir well. Instruct the patient to take a mouthful of the suspension and to hold, swish, and gargle for as long as possible before swallowing. The patient should repeat the process with another mouthful until the entire dose has been taken.

➤ Instruct the patient to allow the lozenge form to dissolve slowly in the mouth, which may take 15 to 30 minutes. The patient should swallow the saliva as needed but should not chew or break the lozenge. Warn the patient not to allow children younger than 5 years to have lozenges because they may choke on them.

➤ For fungus on dentures, instruct the patient to soak dentures in nystatin solution. In rare instances, it may be necessary to have new dentures made.

CHAPTER REVIEW

Application

1. Why are fungi resistant to drugs such as penicillins and tetracyclines?
2. What types of infections are commonly caused by *Candida?* What are signs and symptoms of these infections?
3. What are dermatophytes?
4. What is the mechanism of action for the polyene antifungal agent amphotericin B?
5. By what route is amphotericin B administered? What are nursing care activities associated with administration of amphotericin B?
6. What types of fungal infections are properly treated with amphotericin B?
7. How does the lipid solubility of amphotericin B influence its tissue distribution?
8. What are the characteristic toxic reactions associated with systemic use of amphotericin B?
9. What is the mechanism of action of flucytosine?
10. May flucytosine be used as an oral agent?
11. What is the main route of excretion of flucytosine?
12. What toxic reactions occur with the use of flucytosine?
13. Why are flucytosine and amphotericin B sometimes combined for antifungal therapy?
14. What is the mechanism of action of azole antifungal agents?
15. By what route are azole antifungal agents administered?
16. What side effects may occur with azole antifungal agents? How should you assess for these?
17. What is the mechanism of action of griseofulvin?
18. Is therapy with griseofulvin long or short term?

Critical Thinking

1. A colleague places a filter in the IV line through which a patient is to receive amphotericin B. What should you do?

Chapter

52

Antiviral Agents and Drugs to Treat AIDS

OBJECTIVES

After studying this chapter, you should be able to do the following:

- *Discuss the basis of the anti–human immunodeficiency virus activity of zidovudine.*
- *Explain why acyclovir is selectively active against virus-infected cells.*
- *Develop a nursing care plan for a patient receiving HAART therapy.*
- *Summarize the points that the nurse should teach the patient about topical treatment of genital herpes.*

CHAPTER OVERVIEW

Viral diseases are among the most common infections in humans. Viral reproduction is carried out mostly by host cell enzymes and ribosomes, but basic research has revealed that some key viral enzymes are required for reproduction inside the host cells. These viral enzymes or processes that occur only in virus-infected cells have been the most successful points for attack with selectively toxic agents.

INTRODUCTION

Viruses cause a wide variety of clinical diseases, both chronic and acute. Acute illnesses include the common cold, influenza, and hepatitis A. These illnesses often resolve quickly and leave no latent infections or sequelae. Chronic infections are those in which the disease runs a protracted course with long periods of remission interspersed with reappearance of the disease. For example, herpes infections involve active viral replication in epithelial cells alternating with latent periods during which the virus remains dormant within sensory neurons. Hepatitis B and hepatitis C are also examples of chronic infections, which in this case lead to progressive liver disease.

Viral diseases may appear localized because viruses may interact with receptors or cell surface markers found only on one cell type. For example, influenza viruses affect only the tissues of the respiratory tract, interacting primarily with the ciliated epithelial cells. Likewise, **human immunodeficiency virus (HIV)** shows host cell specificity because it specifically binds to the CD4 receptor of T lymphocytes.

Viruses do not necessarily remain localized in the body as a disease progresses but may be shed into the blood in a process called **viremia**. During viremia, tissues throughout the body may be invaded, as shown in Table 52-1. Clinical symptoms do not appear in most diseases spread in this manner until the secondary viremia occurs. Some viruses produce infections that are self-limiting at this stage and usually resolve even without medical attention, examples being varicella (chicken pox) and measles. These viruses very rarely spread to the brain. A different situation exists with poliovirus. This virus produces few if any symptoms during the early stages of the infection, but in about 1% of infected persons, the virus invades the central nervous system (CNS), causing self-limiting aseptic meningitis or rarely paralytic poliomyelitis.

With infections caused by bacteria, symptoms occur during the period of most active bacterial reproduction;

therefore therapy can begin relatively early in the disease and may include bactericidal agents. With viral diseases, this is not the case. Symptoms occur after most of the virus particles have reproduced, and therapy would be instituted late in the disease. Furthermore, the antiviral drugs currently available inhibit reproduction but do not eradicate latent viruses. The following sections consider antiviral drugs in light of these issues.

Table 52-1 Viremic Spread in Mammalian Body

Site	Symptoms
Primary Site of Infection	
For example, lung in pox, measles, and mumps; gastrointestinal tract in polio	First wave of replication produces no symptoms.
Bloodstream	
Viruses free or bound to blood cells	Primary viremia produces no symptoms.
Secondary Sites of Infection	
For example, liver, spleen, bone marrow, or lymphoid tissue	Second wave of replication may produce mild symptoms for some viral diseases.
Bloodstream	
Viruses free or bound to blood cells	Secondary viremia may produce fever, rashes, or chills; severity depends on number of viruses released.
Central Nervous System	Although rarely involved, infections at this site are serious.

THERAPEUTIC RATIONALE: HIV INFECTION

Unless it is treated, HIV infection rapidly leads to loss of CD4 T lymphocytes and failure of the immune system, a condition called **acquired immunodeficiency syndrome (AIDS)**. These patients experience opportunistic infections, or infections caused by organisms that would be unlikely to cause infections in persons with normal immune systems. Therapy is aimed at arresting or delaying replication of the virus to allow CD4 cells to remain plentiful enough to fight infections.

Currently used anti-HIV agents inhibit the viral protease required for maturation of the virus, or inhibit the enzyme reverse transcriptase (RT), which is found in cells infected by retroviruses like HIV but not in normal mammalian cells. A variety of other approaches, including blocking specific absorption of the virus to its target cells or attacking another unique HIV enzyme called integrase, is being explored. The status of these investigational agents changes quickly. Current information can be obtained by consulting the AIDS section at the National Institutes of Health or by consulting current publications devoted to AIDS research. Drugs approved as of December 1998 are included in the following section. Table 52-2 summarizes specific anti-HIV drugs.

One of the most dramatic changes in anti-HIV therapy has occurred with the use of potent combinations of drugs. This strategy is called **HAART,** which stands for high activity antiretroviral therapy (Box 52-1). This type of treatment commonly uses three and sometimes four anti-HIV drugs in combination, with care taken to include drugs with different mechanisms of action. For example, a nucleoside RT inhibitor might be combined with a protease inhibitor, as well as a nonnucleoside RT inhibitor. A potent antiviral effect may be achieved by attacking through two independent mechanisms and the chance for resistance is lowered. A

Box 52-1 What's at the Heart of HAART?

HAART, or high activity antiretroviral therapy, refers to any one of several combinations of anti–human immunodeficiency virus (HIV) drugs that greatly reduce the viral load in patients. HAART reduces viral RNA in blood to below detectable levels in many patients. Other signs of success are weight gain, an elevation in CD4 counts, and clearing of some opportunistic infections.

Each of the drugs used in HAART is flawed when used alone. For example, zidovudine must be given every 4 hours if it is used alone, is toxic, and selects for viral resistance. Protease inhibitors alone quickly select for resistant HIV and lose their effectiveness. The same problem exists for nonnucleoside RT inhibitors used alone. When anti-HIV drugs are used together, many of these problems are lessened. For example, zidovudine is given every 8 hours in combinations, rather than every 4 hours, and combining it with other drugs slows the appearance of drug-resistant mutants. Because the drugs are acting by different mechanisms, there may also be a synergistic antiviral effect.

The bad news is that HAART must be followed exactly to achieve the desired antiviral effect. If doses are missed, especially with the protease in-

hibitors, resistance can develop quickly and the effect of the combinations will be lost. Because these combinations include drugs from all categories of anti-HIV agents, when resistance develops, few other options are available.

Why is HAART hard to follow? The reason is partly that each of the three or four drugs must be taken on its own schedule, with or without food as appropriate. Scheduling these doses is more difficult because an average AIDS patient will be taking more than 10 different medications, such as prophylaxis for *Pneumocystis carinii* pneumonia or for *Mycobacterium avium*. With this many drugs and the serious effects of AIDS itself, adverse reactions are common. These reactions may force discontinuation of one or more medications.

All these factors point out the challenge faced by the patient and the health care support team. For best effectiveness, these drugs must be taken continuously as prescribed. Failure for any reason can lead to development of multidrug-resistant HIV, which will not only complicate subsequent therapy for that patient but also may spread to other contacts and compromise the effectiveness of our best drugs in other patients.

Table 52-2		**Drugs to Treat Human Immunodeficiency Virus**	
Generic Name	Trade Name	Administration/Dosage	Comments
delavirdine	Rescriptor	ORAL: *Adult*–400 mg every 8 hr. FDA pregnancy category C.	Nonnucleoside RT inhibitor.
didanosine	Videx*	ORAL: *Adults >60 kg*–250 mg buffered powder, or 200-mg buffered tablet every 12 hr. *Adults <60 kg*–167 mg buffered powder, or 125-mg buffered tablet every 12 hr. FDA pregnancy category B. *Children*–Doses, adjusted based on body surface area, are given every 8-12 hr: up to 0.4 m^2, 31 mg; 0.5-0.7 m^2, 62 mg; 0.8-1 m^2, 94 mg; 1.1-1.4 m^2, 125 mg.	Nucleoside RT inhibitor.
indinavir	Crixivan	ORAL: *Adult*–800 mg every 8 hr on an empty stomach. FDA pregnancy category C.	Protease inhibitor.
lamivudine	Epivir 3TC†	ORAL: *Adults >50 kg*–150 mg twice daily. *Adults <50 kg*–2 mg/kg twice daily; this drug should be given with zidovudine. FDA pregnancy category C. *Children 3 mo to 12 yr*–4 mg/kg twice daily, not to exceed 150 mg.	Nucleoside RT inhibitor.
lamivudine zidovudine	Combivir	ORAL: *Adult*–150 mg of lamivudine and 300 mg of zidovudine twice daily. FDA pregnancy category C.	Nucleoside RT inhibitors.
nelfinavir	Viracept	ORAL: *Adult*–750 mg 3 times/day with food. *Children*–20-30 mg/kg 3 times/day with food. FDA pregnancy category B.	Protease inhibitor.
nevirapine	Viramune	ORAL: *Adult*–200 mg/day for 14 days, then 200 mg twice daily. FDA pregnancy category C. Use with nucleoside RT inhibitors.	Nonnucleoside RT inhibitor.
ritonavir	Norvir	ORAL: *Adult*–600 mg twice daily with food, or 400 mg twice daily when used with saquinavir. FDA pregnancy category B. *Children*–250 mg/m^2 twice daily, increasing over 7-10 days to 400 mg/m^2. Do not exceed 600 mg per dose.	Protease inhibitor.
saquinavir	Invirase	ORAL: *Adult*–600 mg every 8 hr with food, or 600 mg twice daily when used with ritonavir. FDA pregnancy category B.	Protease inhibitor.
stavudine	Zerit*	ORAL: *Adults >60 kg*–40 mg every 12 hr. *Adults <60 kg*–30 mg every 12 hr. FDA pregnancy category C. *Children up to 30 kg*–1 mg/kg twice daily.	Nucleoside RT inhibitor.
zalcitabine	HIVID*	ORAL: *Adult*–0.75 mg every 8 hr. Use with zidovudine. FDA pregnancy category C.	Nucleoside RT inhibitor.
zidovudine	Retrovir*	ORAL: *Adult*–200 mg 3 times/day, or 300 mg twice daily. FDA pregnancy category C. As prophylaxis for the fetus, HIV-positive pregnant women receive 100 mg 5 times/day plus an intravenous infusion at delivery. *Children 3 mo to 12 yr*–90-180 mg/m^2 every 6 hr. *Neonates born to infected mothers*–2 mg/kg every 6 hr has been used for up to 6 weeks after birth.	Nucleoside RT inhibitor.

NOTE: The drugs listed in this table are seldom used alone because combination therapy has been shown to be much more effective. The doses shown in this table give the dose or range of doses to be expected in the various combinations used.
RT, Reverse transcriptase; *HIV*, human immunodeficiency virus.
*Available in Canada and the United States.
†Available in Canada only.

four-drug regimen might include two nucleoside RT inhibitors, along with a protease inhibitor and a nonnucleoside RT inhibitor. The rationale for using two nucleoside RT inhibitors together is that some combinations of nucleoside RT inhibitors seem to limit development of resistance.

With HAART therapy, AIDS patients have shown the disappearance of HIV from the blood and the progressive return of CD4 cells. Despite these great gains in anti-HIV therapy, failure of treatment often occurs as drug-resistant strains of HIV appear or as patients become intolerant of the drugs. If the drugs are discontinued, relapse occurs even in patients who have had no sign of the virus in the blood for prolonged periods, seemingly because the virus can lie dormant in resting T lymphocytes for years and in the dormant state they are not affected by existing antivirals. Studies are currently running to test if HIV can be eradicated from patients if effective combination therapy is given early in the disease, but as of 1998, there is no evidence that eradication has been achieved.

The prototype anti-HIV agent is zidovudine, which was the first and is the widest used antiretroviral agent. The individual agents are considered in the following section, grouped according to their target.

THERAPEUTIC AGENTS: DRUGS TO TREAT HIV INFECTION

Nucleoside Inhibitors of Reverse Transcriptase

▼ zidovudine

Mechanism of Action

HIV is a retrovirus. Retroviruses use RNA as their genetic material and must therefore convert RNA into DNA within the host cell for viral replication to take place. This unusual reaction, which does not normally occur in host cells, is catalyzed by the enzyme reverse transcriptase. **Zidovudine** inhibits reverse transcriptase. In addition, some of the drug may be incorporated into viral DNA, in which it causes premature DNA chain termination. Both actions block viral replication, and the drug is active only on replicating virus. Zidovudine does not cure HIV infection or AIDS, but by slowing replication of HIV, it may delay damage to the immune system and lower the incidence of opportunistic infections in these patients.

Resistance to zidovudine occurs readily if the drug is used alone against HIV. Therefore zidovudine is most commonly combined with at least one other agent or in combinations used in HAART.

Pharmacokinetics

Absorption of zidovudine from the gastrointestinal (GI) tract is rapid and nearly complete, but the drug is quickly metabolized to an inactive glucuronide on first pass through the liver. These factors give zidovudine a half-life of only 1 hour. Therefore, if used alone, 100 mg of zidovudine is taken every 4 hours around the clock to maintain virustatic concentrations. When used in combinations, the dosage of zidovudine can be increased to 200 mg every 8 hours.

Uses

Zidovudine is a primary drug for HIV infections. It may be used in asymptomatic patients to delay onset of the decline in T-cell counts, as well as in patients with more advanced forms of the disease. Zidovudine has been used in HIV-infected children. The drug is also effective in lowering the incidence of transmission of HIV from an infected mother to her fetus.

Adverse Reactions and Contraindications

Nearly all patients experience toxicity from zidovudine. The most common reactions are granulocytopenia and anemia. Routine blood monitoring is extremely important. Withdrawal from zidovudine may be necessary to allow recovery from drug-induced blood dyscrasias. Neurotoxicity has also been reported but may be difficult to distinguish from the neural effects of HIV infection. Other adverse actions include headache, insomnia, muscle pain, and nausea.

There are no absolute contraindications to the use of zidovudine, but patients with bone marrow depression may be at greater risk of anemia or other blood disorders; these patients should be monitored carefully. Patients with hepatic impairment may be prone to increased drug toxicity.

Toxicity

A few patients have taken large overdoses of zidovudine, through accidents or in deliberate suicide attempts. Signs of overdose include anemia, ataxia, fatigue, leukopenia, severe nausea, nystagmus, thrombocytopenia, and vomiting. Seizures are rare. Treatment is supportive only.

Interactions

Drug interactions may occur with zidovudine and other drugs often used in immunosuppressed patients. Ganciclovir and zidovudine combine to produce severe hematologic toxicity. Other bone marrow depressants may also increase zidovudine toxicity. Ribavirin interferes with activation of

CASE STUDY
Acquired Immunodeficiency Syndrome

Cristine is a 22-year-old single mother with a known history of heroin abuse. She was brought to the emergency department by her mother because of pneumonia. She had also been experiencing weight loss, fever, and diarrhea; her mother blamed these symptoms on "those drugs." Further diagnostic testing revealed that she had human immunodeficiency virus (HIV) with *Pneumocystis carinii* pneumonia. She was admitted to the hospital and treated for 2 weeks. Now, by the time of discharge, the symptoms have resolved somewhat and she is asking for help in stopping her heroin use and financial help to afford the "AIDS drugs." The hospital's charity fund can only provide 1 month's supply of the prescriptions.

1. How would you locate community support for Cristine's problems of drug abuse and lack of funding for medications?
2. Explain the HAART anti-HIV therapy.
3. One of the medications in her regimen is zidovudine. What patient teaching is important regarding this medication?
4. After a month of therapy, the physician changes the combination of drugs that Cristine is taking. She says: "I thought I'd be through with these drugs by now. Why did she have to change them?" What teaching do you need to do with Cristine?

zidovudine within the virus-infected cell and thereby blocks the anti-HIV effect of zidovudine.

Clarithromycin lowers the peak of zidovudine in the blood, which may interfere with anti-HIV activity. Probenecid increases the concentration of zidovudine in blood and slows its elimination, which increases the risk of toxicity.

didanosine

Didanosine is a purine analog that is activated by phosphorylation within cells, and in this active form, it blocks synthesis of HIV DNA by inhibiting reverse transcriptase. This mechanism of action is similar to that of zidovudine.

Didanosine has a poor bioavailability in most patients because it is destroyed by stomach acid. Current formulations include buffers to improve absorption by lowering acidity and preserving integrity of the drug. The average plasma half-life of didanosine is between 30 and 80 minutes, but the half-life within cells is longer than 12 hours. Therefore the drug is given every 12 hours. About 20% of each dose appears in urine as active drug.

Didanosine is currently used for treating adults or children older than 6 months of age who have advanced HIV disease and who are intolerant to zidovudine or have failed therapy with zidovudine. Didanosine is also used in combinations with other nucleoside RT inhibitors.

Peripheral neuropathy may occur in many patients receiving didanosine. Signs include tingling or aching in the legs or feet. Reflexes may be diminished. Side effects affecting the

CNS, including anxiety, headache, irritability, and sleeplessness, are also common. Diarrhea, dry mouth, and nausea are common but usually do not require medical attention.

Less common side effects include acute pancreatitis, allergies, blood dyscrasias, and cardiac failure (shortness of breath, swelling of feet and legs). Peripheral neuropathy is more common with higher dosages of didanosine or in patients in whom the drug accumulates. High dosages were associated with atrophy of the retinal pigment epithelium in three children.

The risk for pancreatitis is increased in patients who also have received other drugs causing this reaction. Peripheral neuropathy is more likely when patients also receive other neurotoxic drugs.

The buffers in didanosine preparations impair absorption of dapsone, itraconazole, and ketoconazole. Fluoroquinolone and tetracycline antibiotics are chelated by components of the buffering system in didanosine, decreasing absorption of the antibiotics.

lamivudine

Lamivudine is activated inside cells to the triphosphate form, which inhibits reverse transcriptase and may also cause DNA chain termination. Lamivudine is combined with zidovudine to delay the appearance of zidovudine resistance.

Lamivudine is well absorbed orally, both with or without food. The drug is poorly metabolized and most of it is excreted in urine unchanged. The serum half-life is variable, but the half-life in cells is 11 to 15 hours.

Lamivudine is used against HIV only in combination with zidovudine or another RT inhibitor. Therefore it is difficult to determine which side effects to attribute to lamivudine and which to the other drug. Nevertheless, the limited studies available suggest that lamivudine can cause pancreatitis and peripheral neuropathy.

stavudine

Stavudine is an analog of thymidine, a precursor of DNA. Inside cells, stavudine is activated by phosphorylation to a form that inhibits HIV reverse transcriptase and also may cause termination of DNA chains being synthesized.

Stavudine is well absorbed orally, with or without food. The drug distributes well in the body and enters cells freely. About 40% of the drug administered is excreted unchanged in urine. The remainder is probably metabolized in various tissues.

Stavudine is used for advanced HIV disease in patients who cannot take the primary drugs or who have failed with established therapy. Stavudine is not used as often as other nucleoside RT inhibitors.

Sensory peripheral neuropathy is the most common serious side effect with stavudine. The burning, numbness, or pain in the extremities may resolve if the drug is discontinued. Other side effects, including allergic reactions, anemia, anorexia, diarrhea, headache, insomnia, pain in muscles and joints, pancreatitis, and weakness, may occur.

There are no absolute contraindications to the use of stavudine, but if the drug must be used in patients with peripheral neuropathy or renal function impairment, lower dosages may be required. Stavudine should be avoided in patients also receiving other drugs that cause peripheral neuropathy (see Appendix B).

zalcitabine

Zalcitabine is an analog of deoxycytidine, a precursor of DNA. Zalcitabine is activated inside cells to a form that inhibits HIV reverse transcriptase and may terminate DNA chains being synthesized. These actions prevent successful replication of virus. Zalcitabine is used in advanced HIV disease, in combination with zidovudine.

Oral absorption of zalcitabine is high in adults but may be lower in children. The drug distributes well in the body and freely enters cells. Little metabolic degradation occurs, and about 70% of the drug administered is excreted unchanged in urine.

Pancreatitis has caused death in a few patients receiving zalcitabine. Less serious adverse reactions include abdominal pain, allergic reactions, diarrhea, headache, nausea, pain in muscles and joints, and ulcers in the mouth.

Peripheral neurotoxicity is the most common serious side effect of zalcitabine. Peripheral neurotoxicity is dose related and therefore is more likely to occur and to be more serious in patients receiving high dosages of zalcitabine.

Zalcitabine should be avoided if possible in combination with other drugs that cause pancreatitis (see Appendix B). Drugs such as dapsone, didanosine, ethambutol, ethionamide, isoniazid, metronidazole, and stavudine may increase the risk of peripheral neuropathy. Aminoglycosides, amphotericin B, and foscarnet block renal excretion of zalcitabine. The result may be increased zalcitabine toxicity.

Nonnucleoside Reverse Transcriptase Inhibitors

delavirdine

Unlike nucleoside RT inhibitors, delavirdine does not require activation. The drug binds directly to HIV RT and inhibits the enzyme. The binding is at a different site than that occupied by nucleoside RT inhibitors.

Delavirdine is adequately absorbed orally and extensively biotransformed by the CYP3A enzymes in the liver. The metabolites are excreted in both feces and urine.

Delavirdine is used in combination with nucleoside RT inhibitors and/or protease inhibitors. The drug should not be used alone because of the rapid development of resistance.

The most common adverse reactions to delavirdine include diarrhea, fatigue, headache, nausea, and skin rashes. Severe rashes may indicate a serious reaction and should be reported to the physician. The drug should be avoided if possible in patients with impaired liver function.

Delavirdine inhibits the liver metabolizing enzymes CYP3A and CYP2C9, which may elevate blood levels of drugs that are normally metabolized by those enzymes (see

Appendix A). This interaction affects benzodiazepines, calcium channel blockers, and indinavir. Carbamazepine, phenobarbital, and phenytoin lower delavirdine concentrations in blood; the drugs should not be used together. Cimetidine and related drugs lower gastric pH and thus reduce absorption of delavirdine. Both rifabutin and rifampin lower the absorption of delavirdine, but clarithromycin increases absorption of delavirdine.

nevirapine

Nevirapine acts directly on HIV RT, without prior activation. It binds at a different site than the nucleoside RT inhibitors.

Nevirapine is readily absorbed orally, with or without food, and is extensively biotransformed by the CYP3A liver enzymes. Most of the drug is slowly excreted in urine, primarily as glucuronide conjugates of various metabolites.

Nevirapine is used in combination with nucleoside RT inhibitors. It should never by used alone because of the rapid development of resistance.

Nevirapine often causes rashes, some of which may be serious. The drug also commonly causes diarrhea, headache, nausea, and stomach pain. Mouth ulcers can occur, as can hepatitis. The drug should be avoided if possible in patients with impaired liver function.

Nevirapine induces the CYP3A enzymes in the liver. Therefore drugs such as estrogens, indinavir, rifabutin, rifampin, ritonavir, and saquinavir, which are metabolized by these enzymes, may lose effectiveness because the increased enzyme activity lowers blood levels of these agents.

Protease Inhibitors

indinavir

Mechanism of Action

Indinavir binds to the active site of HIV protease, preventing the natural substrate from binding. As a result, the protease fails to separate the HIV precursor protein into the active enzymes the virus needs to fully mature. Thus, immature noninfective virus is produced. Indinavir and the other protease inhibitors act only during viral replication.

Resistance to protease inhibitors such as indinavir occurs readily and by several different mutations of the HIV protease. Because resistance occurs so easily, indinavir should ordinarily not be used alone.

Pharmacokinetics

Indinavir is readily absorbed orally, but heavy food can significantly impair absorption. The dose is normally taken on an empty stomach, but grapefruit juice or a light snack may be taken with the dose if necessary. Absorption may be slightly reduced but is usually not clinically significant.

Indinavir is extensively metabolized by liver enzymes, particularly CYP3A4. Most of the metabolites are eliminated in feces, with only limited amounts in urine. Little active drug is excreted. The rapid absorption and metabolism of indinavir produce a short half-life of about 2 hours.

Uses

Indinavir is used only for HIV infections, usually in combination with nucleoside RT inhibitors or in other combinations for HAART.

Adverse Reactions and Contraindications

Kidney stones occur in about 4% of patients receiving indinavir. Patients also often report abdominal pain, diarrhea, headache, insomnia, nausea, vomiting, weakness, and an altered sense of taste. Rarely, diabetes has been induced.

There is no absolute contraindication to indinavir, but it should be used with caution in patients with impaired liver function.

Toxicity

Single doses of indinavir much larger than the normal doses have not resulted in deaths. Long-term use of dosages higher than 2.4 g/day is associated with a higher risk of kidney stones.

Interactions

Indinavir may compete for the liver enzyme CYP3A4 and thus interfere with the metabolism of other drugs normally acted on by CYP3A4 (see Appendix A). Therefore drugs that might accumulate to dangerous levels include astemizole, cisapride, midazolam, and triazolam. Rifampin induces CYP3A4 and can thus enhance the metabolism of indinavir; this combination is usually avoided.

Ketoconazole can increase the plasma concentration of indinavir; the dosage of indinavir should be reduced to 600 mg every 8 hours. Rifabutin slightly increases the plasma concentration of indinavir, but more importantly, indinavir increases the plasma concentration of rifabutin by twofold; thus doses of rifabutin must be reduced when the drug is given with indinavir.

Indinavir must not be given at the same time as didanosine because indinavir requires an acid environment for best absorption, but didanosine is given with buffers to elevate gastric pH. If both drugs are being used for the same patient, the doses should be given at least 1 hour apart on an empty stomach.

nelfinavir

Mechanism of Action

Nelfinavir inhibits HIV protease, preventing the enzyme from separating the HIV precursor protein into the active enzymes the virus needs to fully mature. As a result, immature noninfective virus is produced. The protease inhibitors act only during viral replication.

Resistance to protease inhibitors occurs readily and by several different mutations of the HIV protease. Because resistance occurs so easily, nelfinavir should ordinarily not be used alone.

Pharmacokinetics

Nelfinavir is absorbed orally, and the total absorption is improved by taking the drug with food. Nelfinavir is less extensively metabolized than other protease inhibitors, but there is some metabolism by the liver enzyme CYP3A. The most abundant metabolite retains antiviral activity. The half-life of nelfinavir is 3.5 to 5 hours. Most of the drug is eliminated in feces.

Uses

Nelfinavir is used only for HIV infections, usually in combination with nucleoside RT inhibitors or in other combinations for HAART.

Adverse Reactions and Contraindications

Nelfinavir often causes diarrhea and occasionally other signs of GI distress. Diabetes or signs of ketoacidosis may occur and require medical attention.

Nelfinavir should be used with caution in patients with impaired liver function.

Toxicity

The effects of large doses of nelfinavir have not been documented, but in cases of overdose, charcoal has been used, along with emesis or gastric lavage, to reduce absorption of drug.

Interactions

Nelfinavir has many of the same interactions as indinavir and thus should be avoided with astemizole, cisapride, midazolam, quinidine, rifampin, and triazolam. Rifabutin doses must be reduced when given with nelfinavir because the antiviral increases absorption of rifabutin.

Nelfinavir lowers blood levels of components of oral contraceptives, so the contraceptive action may be lost. Alternative methods of contraception should be used while taking nelfinavir.

ritonavir

Mechanism of Action

Ritonavir inhibits the protease from both HIV-1 (the form common in the United States) and HIV-2 (a form prevalent in Africa and other sites). This action prevents the formation of fully mature HIV, and as a result, immature noninfective virus is produced. The protease inhibitors act only during viral replication.

Resistance to protease inhibitors occurs readily and by several different mutations of the HIV protease. Because resistance occurs so easily, ritonavir should ordinarily not be used alone.

Pharmacokinetics

Ritonavir is adequately absorbed orally and absorption is normally not affected by food. Ritonavir is metabolized by liver enzymes, including CYP3A and CYP2D6. Elimination

is primarily in feces, mostly as metabolites. The half-life of the drug in plasma is 3 to 5 hours.

Uses

Ritonavir is used only for HIV infections, usually in combination with nucleoside RT inhibitors or in other combinations for HAART.

Adverse Reactions and Contraindications

Ritonavir often causes GI disturbances and a feeling of general weakness. Paresthesias may also occur, with numbness or tingling in the hands, in the feet, or around the mouth. Diabetes is a rare complication. There are no absolute contraindications to ritonavir, but it should be used with caution in patients with hepatic impairment.

Toxicity

The effects of very large doses of ritonavir have not been documented, but doses of 1.5 g for 2 days in one patient produced paresthesias that resolved when the drug was stopped. In cases of overdose, charcoal may be used, along with emesis or gastric lavage, to reduce absorption of drug.

Interactions

Ritonavir interacts with many cytochrome P-450 enzymes, including CYP3A, CYP2D6, CYP2C9, and CYP2C19 (see Appendix A). Any other drug that would normally be metabolized by these enzymes can show a rise in plasma concentration because metabolism is blocked by ritonavir, with a resulting increase in risk of toxicity. Drugs affected include antiarrhythmics (see Chapter 19), benzodiazepines (see Chapter 57), nonsteroidal antiinflammatory drugs (see Chapter 31), clarithromycin, and rifabutin.

Ritonavir reduces the blood concentrations of estrogens in oral contraceptives by inducing metabolism, which may block the contraceptive action. Theophylline levels may also be reduced by ritonavir in the same way.

saquinavir

Mechanism of Action

Saquinavir inhibits HIV protease, thus preventing formation of the active enzymes the virus needs to fully mature. As a result, immature noninfective virus is produced. The protease inhibitors act only during viral replication.

Resistance to protease inhibitors occurs readily and by several different mutations of the HIV protease. Because resistance occurs so easily, saquinavir should ordinarily not be used alone.

Pharmacokinetics

Oral bioavailability of saquinavir depends on the formulation used. The original saquinavir mesylate capsules yielded only about 4% bioavailability, as a result of poor absorption and an active first pass effect (see Chapter 1). The newer formulation is a soft gelatin capsule, which more than triples absorption, but the total bioavailability is still low.

Metabolism of saquinavir is primarily by the liver enzyme CYP3A4, and elimination is in feces.

Uses

Saquinavir is used only for HIV infections, in combination with nucleoside RT inhibitors or in other combinations for HAART.

Adverse Reactions and Contraindications

Saquinavir, like other protease inhibitors, causes GI upset and a feeling of weakness. Paresthesia, diabetes, and ketoacidosis are rare.

Toxicity

There have been no reports of serious toxicity with patients taking 7.2 g of saquinavir daily for 25 weeks, which is four times the normal daily dose.

Interactions

Saquinavir should not be used with drugs that depend on the CYP3A4 enzyme for metabolism. This interaction may affect astemizole, benzodiazepines, calcium channel blockers, cisapride, and quinidine. Inducers of CYP3A4 must also be avoided because they reduce the blood levels of saquinavir. Drugs in this category include carbamazepine, dexamethasone, phenobarbital, phenytoin, rifabutin, and rifampin.

Delavirdine and ritonavir can greatly increase the blood levels of saquinavir. Dosage adjustments may be required.

THERAPEUTIC AGENTS: DRUGS FOR VIRAL DISEASES OTHER THAN AIDS

Drugs for Systemic Viral Infections

▼ acyclovir

Mechanism of Action

Acyclovir is one of the most highly selective of the antiviral agents. The drug is activated by viral thymidine kinase, an enzyme found only in virus-infected cells. The activated form of the drug preferentially and irreversibly inhibits the viral DNA polymerase present in infected cells, effectively halting virus production. Much higher concentrations of acyclovir are required to halt normal human cell metabolism. Therefore effective doses for antiviral activity are relatively nontoxic to normal host cells.

Pharmacokinetics

Acyclovir is used intravenously to treat mucocutaneous herpes simplex in immunocompromised patients and to treat severe genital herpes or herpes simplex encephalitis. Oral administration of acyclovir leads to incomplete absorption, but this route is effective when used for mild to moderate genital herpes. Oral absorption is increased by using valacyclovir (Table 52-3), a prodrug form that is rapidly converted to acyclovir and L-valine in the body. Once absorbed, acyclovir is widely distributed to tissues. The topical ointment may be useful in mild herpes infections, but parenteral routes are more effective and usually preferred.

Excretion is by renal mechanisms. Acyclovir may be metabolized by the liver. The drug is eliminated with a half-life of about 2.5 hours in patients with normal renal function.

Uses

Acyclovir is used to treat initial lesions or recurrences of genital herpes, mucocutaneous herpes simplex infections in immunocompromised patients, herpes simplex encephalitis, and herpes zoster infections. Acyclovir can also be used for varicella (chicken pox) if started within 24 hours of the appearance of the rash.

Adverse Reactions and Contraindications

Acyclovir generally causes few side effects. Phlebitis at the injection site may occur with intravenous (IV) acyclovir. Rarely, patients receiving parenteral acyclovir may experience coma, confusion, seizures, or tremors. Light-headedness is common. Oral administration can cause GI tract disturbances.

Acyclovir should not be given at full dosage to patients with renal impairment or to dehydrated patients.

Toxicity

Neuropsychiatric reactions and nephrotoxicity are more common with very high dosages of acyclovir or in patients who accumulate the drug because of poor renal function. Nephrotoxicity, including crystallization of drug in the renal tubule, can be minimized by giving the drug as a slow infusion rather than as a rapid bolus. Increasing water intake also helps.

Interactions

Because of the potential for nephrotoxicity, acyclovir should not be given with other nephrotoxic agents.

amantadine

Mechanism of Action

Amantadine blocks early phases of viral replication, but the exact mechanism is unclear. This drug has a narrow antiviral spectrum, being effective only against influenza type A.

Pharmacokinetics

Amantadine is well absorbed orally and distributes well to tissues. The concentrations in lung tissue may exceed serum concentrations. The concentration of amantadine that reaches the epithelial surfaces of lung tissues is the determining factor in protecting against influenza type A infections. Nearly all elimination of the drug is by renal mechanisms. The half-life for elimination is about 15 hours in patients

Table 52-3 **Drugs to Treat Systemic Viral Diseases**

Generic Name	Trade Name	Administration/Dosage	Comments
acyclovir	Zovirax*	ORAL: *Adults*—200 mg 5 times/day. FDA pregnancy category B. INTRAVENOUS: *Adults*—5 mg/kg infused at constant rate over 1 hr, repeated every 8 hr. FDA pregnancy category C. *Children <12 yr*—250 mg/m² infused at constant rate over 1 hr, repeated every 8 hr. TOPICAL: 5% ointment applied directly to initial lesions of genital herpes, every 3 hr 6 times daily for 7 days.	Specific actions on cells infected with herpesvirus.
amantadine	Symadine Symmetrel*	ORAL: *Adults*—100 mg twice daily. *Older adults*—100 mg once daily. FDA pregnancy category C. *Children*—2.2-4.4 mg/kg every 12 hr, up to 150 mg/day.	Prophylaxis of influenza type A infections in high-risk patients.
cidofovir	Vistide	INTRAVENOUS: *Adults*—5 mg/kg infused over 1 hr, on week 1 and 2; then alternate weeks for maintenance. Give 2 g probenecid 3 hr before each dose and 1 g probenecid at 2 and 8 hr after each infusion. FDA pregnancy category C.	Used for CMV retinitis in patients with AIDS.
famciclovir	Famvir*	ORAL: *Adults*—500 mg every 8 hr for 7 days. FDA pregnancy category B.	For control of herpes zoster infections (shingles) in immunocompetent adults.
foscarnet	Foscavir	INTRAVENOUS: *Adults*—60 mg/kg 3 times/day for induction; 90-120 mg/kg/day for maintenance therapy. FDA pregnancy category C.	Treatment of CMV retinitis in patients with AIDS.
ganciclovir	Cytovene*	ORAL: *Adults*—Maintenance, 1000 mg 3 times/day with food. INTRAVENOUS: *Adults*—5 mg/kg infused over at least 1 hr, every 12 hr for 14-21 days. FDA pregnancy category C. INTRAVITREAL IMPLANT: *Adults*—Surgical implant replaces ganciclovir for 5-8 mo; for intraocular infection only.	Treatment of CMV retinitis in immunosuppressed patients, including AIDS patients.
interferon alfa-2b, recombinant	Intron A*	INTRAMUSCULAR, SUBCUTANEOUS: *Adults*—3 million units 3 times/wk. FDA pregnancy category C.	For chronic or active hepatitis (non-A, non-B/C).
interferon alfa-n3	Alferon N	INTRALESIONAL: *Adults*—250,000 units twice weekly for 8 wk. FDA pregnancy category C.	For treatment of external genital warts.
interferon alfacon-1	Infergen	SUBCUTANEOUS: *Adult*—9 µg 3 times/wk. FDA pregnancy category C.	For chronic or active hepatitis C.
ribavirin	Virazole*	INHALATION: *Children*—20 mg/ml in Viratek small particle aerosol generator model SPAG-2 12-18 hr/day. FDA pregnancy category X.	Severe pneumonia caused by respiratory syncytial virus.
rimantadine	Flumadine	ORAL: *Adults and children >10 yr*—100 mg twice daily. FDA pregnancy category C. *Children <10 yr*—5 mg/kg once daily, not to exceed 150 mg/day.	For prophylaxis or therapy of influenza type A.
valacyclovir	Valtrex*	ORAL: *Adult*—0.5-1 g 1-3 times/day. FDA pregnancy category B.	For herpes genitalis or herpes zoster.

CMV, Cytomegalovirus; *AIDS*, acquired immunodeficiency syndrome.
*Available in Canada and the United States.

GERIATRIC CONSIDERATIONS

Amantadine

THE PROBLEM

Older adults are more sensitive to the antimuscarinic side effects of amantadine than are younger adults.

SOLUTIONS
- Cut normal adult dosage by half for older adults.
- Watch carefully for antimuscarinic signs such as confusion or difficulty in urination.

with normal renal function, 24 to 29 hours in older adults, and 7 to 10 days in renally impaired patients.

Uses

Amantadine is effective at preventing influenzae caused by type A virus. Prophylaxis is usually limited to older adult patients or others in whom influenza is likely to lead to life-threatening complications. If used within 24 hours of the onset of symptoms, amantadine may be helpful in treating influenza type A.

Amantadine has also been used to treat parkinsonism (see Chapter 62).

Adverse Reactions and Contraindications

Amantadine can cause amphetamine-like stimulation of the CNS, lethargy, ataxia, slurred speech, and other symptoms. Because of these CNS effects, the drug should be used cautiously, if at all, in older adult patients (see Geriatric Considerations box) with cerebral arteriosclerosis or in patients with a history of epilepsy.

Anorexia and nausea are common side effects with amantadine. Anticholinergic side effects, including constipation, dry mouth, blurred vision, difficulty in urination, and CNS signs, may also be seen.

Side effects are more common when amantadine is used for parkinsonism because the doses of drug are about twice those used for influenza prophylaxis.

Toxicity

Signs of overdose include CNS and cardiopulmonary toxicity. Symptoms may include cardiac arrhythmias, pulmonary edema, toxic psychosis, or convulsions.

Interactions

Alcohol increases the risk of seizure activity with amantadine. Anticholinergics may be dangerously potentiated by the anticholinergic action of amantadine. CNS stimulants increase the risk of CNS irritability or seizures.

famciclovir

Famciclovir is activated only by viral thymidine kinase. Therefore, like acyclovir, famciclovir is converted to an active agent only in virus-infected cells. Famciclovir is used for herpes zoster infection (shingles) in immunocompetent adults.

Famciclovir is a prodrug that is converted to penciclovir in the intestinal wall after oral absorption. Penciclovir is the form that enters cells and is activated by viral thymidine kinase. Oral bioavailability is good. The drug is cleared primarily by the kidneys, but some penciclovir appears in feces. Reduced dosages of famciclovir may be required in patients with renal impairment. Probenecid may block renal excretion of penciclovir.

Headache is a common complaint, but diarrhea, dizziness, fatigue, nausea, and vomiting may also occur.

Little toxicity is noted with famciclovir, presumably because the drug is converted to its cytotoxic form only in virus-infected cells.

interferons, alfa

Mechanism of Action

Interferons inhibit virus replication in infected cells and in general inhibit cell proliferation (see Chapter 56). Interferons are produced by mammals as part of an immune response. Interferons are **host specific** and not virus specific. This property means that interferons induce resistance to several types of viruses at once. Host specificity of interferons determines that only human interferon prevents viral disease in humans. Human interferons are produced as drugs by recombinant DNA technology or are harvested from pooled human leukocytes.

Pharmacokinetics

Interferons are proteins that must be administered parenterally. Uptake is good from intramuscular (IM) or subcutaneous injections.

Uses

Interferon alfa-2b, recombinant, is used to treat non-A, non-B/C hepatitis. Interferon alfa-n3 is used by intralesional injection to treat genital warts, which are induced by papillomavirus. Interferon alfacon-1 is a recombinant protein used by subcutaneous injection to treat chronic hepatitis C.

Adverse Reactions and Contraindications

Adverse reactions are more common when interferon is used systemically to treat hepatitis than when interferon is used locally for genital warts. Possible reactions include anorexia, blood dyscrasias (anemia, leukopenia, thrombocytopenia), diarrhea, fatigue, nausea, and vomiting. A flulike syndrome with fever, chills, and headache is common and may physically stress the patient. Patients with cardiac disease, severe diabetes, or pulmonary disease may be unable to cope with this stress.

Interferons should be avoided in patients with autoimmune disease because the immune reactions may increase. In contrast, chicken pox or herpes zoster may be worsened. The conditions of patients with CNS disease, including psychiatric disorders and seizures, may be worsened by interferons.

Interferon alfa-2b should be avoided in patients with impaired thyroid function because thyroid function may be further worsened.

Toxicity

Cardiotoxicity has been reported; however, this condition is rare.

Interactions

Blood dyscrasias may be worsened by other drugs producing the same side effects as the alfa interferons.

ribavirin

Ribavirin is a synthetic purine nucleoside that interferes with multiple steps leading to synthesis of viral nucleic acids. In the United States, ribavirin is indicated only for therapy of severe respiratory syncytial virus (RSV) in children, but in other parts of the world, the drug has been used to treat various viral-induced hemorrhagic fevers.

Ribavirin is administered as an aerosol to treat respiratory viruses. In this way, drug levels in the lung are maximized, but systemic absorption is low, which minimizes side effects.

Skin rashes can occur. Health care workers exposed during administration of the drug can experience headaches and irritation of the eyes. Oral or IV administration of ribavirin often causes anemia and may cause CNS or GI tract effects. Little systemic toxicity occurs when ribavirin is given by inhalation.

Because ribavirin blocks phosphorylation of nucleosides, it interferes with activation of zidovudine and therefore should not be given to patients receiving zidovudine.

rimantadine

Rimantadine is thought to interfere with uncoating of the influenza type A virus when it enters mammalian cells. This action prevents viral replication because uncoating is required for release of the viral genome in infected cells. Rimantadine is used only for prophylaxis or treatment of infections caused by influenza type A virus. Treatment is approved only for adults, but prophylaxis may be carried out in adults or children.

Rimantadine is well absorbed orally and extensively metabolized in the liver. Metabolites are eliminated in urine. The half-life of the drug ranges from 13 to 38 hours. In general, older adults or those with liver impairment eliminate the drug more slowly.

Rimantadine causes CNS effects less often than the related drug amantadine, but headache, insomnia, and fatigue are possible. Anorexia, dry mouth, nausea, and vomiting are also possible.

Patients with a history of seizures may be at risk of increased frequency of seizures with rimantadine. Patients with reduced hepatic function require reduced dosages of rimantadine to compensate for slower elimination of the drug.

THERAPEUTIC AGENTS: ANTIVIRAL DRUGS FOR OPHTHALMIC DISEASES

Systemically Administered Agents

▼ ganciclovir

Mechanism of Action

Ganciclovir acts similarly to acyclovir, both drugs being readily activated within virus-infected cells to a form that inhibits virus reproduction. Unlike acyclovir, ganciclovir is also activated to a limited degree by normal cells.

Pharmacokinetics

Ganciclovir is poorly absorbed orally, with a bioavailability of less than 5%. Therefore administration is by IV infusion. The drug distributes widely into tissues, including the eye. Ganciclovir is not biotransformed and is excreted unchanged in urine. An implantation form for insertion into the vitreous humor has recently been developed. This form releases drug directly into the eye for 5 to 8 months before it must be surgically replaced.

Uses

Ganciclovir is indicated only for treatment of cytomegalovirus (CMV) retinitis in immunocompromised patients.

Adverse Reactions and Contraindications

Ganciclovir causes granulocytopenia, marked by sore throat and fever, in about 40% of patients receiving the drug. Ganciclovir also causes thrombocytopenia, marked by bruising and unusual bleeding, in 20% of patients. These reactions are usually reversible. Anemia, allergies, and signs of CNS irritability have also been reported less often.

Ganciclovir is used cautiously, if at all, in patients with low neutrophil or platelet counts. Dosages must be reduced in patients with renal failure.

Toxicity

Subcutaneous or IM injection leads to severe tissue damage because ganciclovir preparations have a very high pH. Thus care must be taken with IV administration to avoid infiltration into surrounding tissues.

Interactions

Ganciclovir may cause dangerous blood dyscrasias when combined with zidovudine. Other bone marrow depressants may lead to unacceptable side effects with ganciclovir.

cidofovir

Cidofovir is activated by phosphorylation to a form that selectively inhibits viral DNA polymerase. Thus viral replication can be blocked at concentrations of cidofovir that do not normally affect human DNA polymerase. Cidofovir is used only for CMV retinitis in AIDS patients.

Cidofovir is given only by IV infusion and is combined with probenecid. The drug is rapidly cleared by renal excretion if given alone, but probenecid slows renal excretion.

Nephrotoxicity is a common adverse reaction and is usually dose limiting. Therefore cidofovir should not be used with other nephrotoxic drugs.

Neutropenia, GI upset, and headache also occur.

foscarnet

Foscarnet inhibits viral DNA polymerases and reverse transcriptases. Because foscarnet is a chemical relative of inorganic phosphate, it does not require activation within cells.

Foscarnet is poorly absorbed orally and must be given by IV injection or infusion. The drug distributes to tissues, including brain tissues, although levels are variable. As an analog of inorganic phosphate, foscarnet seems to be incorporated into bone. Most of the remainder of the drug is excreted unchanged in urine.

Foscarnet has shown activity against HIV, herpesviruses, and hepatitis B but is presently indicated only for control of CMV retinitis in HIV-infected patients.

Renal toxicity is the major concern with foscarnet. Signs of serious renal toxicity may occur in up to 25% of patients receiving the drug. Some protection may be afforded by ensuring adequate hydration before administering foscarnet. Other side effects of foscarnet use include nausea, headache, dizziness, and anemia.

Nephrotoxicity may include acute renal tubular necrosis. Other nephrotoxic drugs should be avoided during therapy with foscarnet.

Ophthalmic Agents

Ophthalmic antiviral agents are available for use directly in the eye to treat localized viral infections (Table 52-4). The primary disease is keratitis caused by herpes simplex virus.

Table 52-4 **Drugs to Treat Viral Diseases at Specific Sites**

Generic Name	Trade Name	Administration/Dosage	Comments
idoxuridine	Herplex* Stoxil*	OPHTHALMIC: *Adults and children*—0.1% solution, 0.5 % ointment used 5 times/day.	Local irritation and pitting defects may occur in cornea. Systemic toxicity is possible but rare.
imiquimod	Aldara	TOPICAL: *Adults—For genital warts:* Apply cream once every other day (3 times/wk); wash drug off with mild soap and water 6-10 hr after application. FDA pregnancy category B.	Commonly causes local irritation; remove before sexual intercourse.
podofilox	Condylox	TOPICAL: *Adults—For genital warts:* Apply gel or solution twice daily for 3 days; wait 4 days, then repeat treatment. No more than 4 treatment cycles should be attempted. FDA pregnancy category C.	Local irritation is common; nausea, vomiting, or oral ulcers may signal systemic absorption.
trifluridine	Viroptic*	OPHTHALMIC: *Adults and children*—1% solution applied every 2 hr up to 9 times/day. FDA pregnancy category C.	Local irritation.
vidarabine	Vira-A*	OPHTHALMIC: *Adults and children*—3% ointment used 5 times/day. FDA pregnancy category C.	Local irritation, superficial punctate keratitis, and allergy.

*Available in Canada and the United States.

These drugs have mechanisms similar to other antiviral agents but are not as selective and are therefore much more toxic. For this reason, the use of these drugs is restricted to topical applications.

Idoxuridine, trifluridine, and vidarabine are potentially mutagenic and carcinogenic. It is unclear how important this potential may be when these agents are used topically because these drugs are not well absorbed from the eye into systemic circulation.

idoxuridine

Idoxuridine is incorporated into DNA in place of thymidine, thereby preventing normal DNA replication and halting virus formation. Herpes simplex infections of the cornea, conjunctiva, and eyelids tend to recur, and idoxuridine does not prevent reappearance of the infection or scarring and resultant loss of sight in serious cases.

When used topically in the eye, little idoxuridine enters the systemic circulation. The drug can produce local reactions in the eye, the most serious being corneal defects. It may also interfere with corneal epithelial regeneration and healing. Idoxuridine is potentially mutagenic and carcinogenic.

trifluridine

Trifluridine, like idoxuridine, is activated by viral and host cell thymidine kinase to a form of drug that inhibits DNA polymerase. Trifluridine may be less damaging to the cornea than idoxuridine or vidarabine; nevertheless, conjunctival or corneal burning can occur when the drug is placed in the eye. Swelling of the eyelids (palpebral edema)

has also been noted. Trifluridine is potentially mutagenic and carcinogenic.

vidarabine

Vidarabine inhibits viral DNA synthesis in a variety of DNA viruses. Vidarabine is activated by host cell enzymes to ara-ATP, a potent and selective inhibitor of viral DNA polymerase. Clinically important selectivity of action is achieved against herpesvirus-infected cells.

Ophthalmic use is not usually associated with serious side effects, but local irritation and sensitivity of the eyes to light may occur. Vidarabine is potentially mutagenic and carcinogenic.

THERAPEUTIC AGENTS: TOPICAL ANTIVIRAL DRUGS FOR GENITAL WARTS

imiquimod and podofilox

Imiquimod and podofilox are new drugs intended for use topically against genital warts, which is a sexually transmitted disease caused by papillomaviruses. Podofilox is a potent inhibitor of mitosis and tends to cause the infected cells and surrounding tissues to undergo necrosis as a result of treatment. In contrast, imiquimod seems to induce cytokines, which may aid normal immune processes to destroy the infected tissue, but is not itself cytotoxic.

These topically applied agents cause few systemic effects but are likely to cause redness, peeling, itching, or swelling at the site of application. It is also important to avoid spreading these medications to unaffected tissues or to the eyes.

Nursing Process Overview

Antiviral Agents

Assessment

Antiviral agents are used with patients in whom supportive therapy has not been helpful or in patients with viruses known to be particularly virulent or associated with serious side effects or complications. Perform a thorough total assessment. Emphasize the subjective and objective complaints related to the virus. Assess laboratory work, cultures, and other studies that would help monitor the progress of the disease.

Nursing Diagnoses

- Potential complication: blood dyscrasias, renal failure, or pancreatitis related to drug therapy (varies with drug)

Patient Outcomes

The nurse will manage and minimize blood dyscrasias, renal failure, or pancreatitis.

Planning/Implementation

Monitor appropriate laboratory work, vital signs, and other objective data that help chart the progress of the disease. Moni-

tor for side effects known to occur with the drug used. If the patient will receive antiviral drug therapy after discharge, instruct the patient and family about possible side effects. If the virus is known to be virulent, isolate the patient during hospitalization. For information about specific viruses, consult the infection control department at the local hospital, the local health department, or the Centers for Disease Control and Prevention in Atlanta. Many serious viral illnesses should be reported to the local health department since this information is used for epidemiologic charting of viral spread; examples include polio and rabies. Finally, immunize family members and health care team members if appropriate.

Evaluation

Before discharge, ensure that the patient understands how to take the drug correctly, what side effects may occur, and what situations require consultation with the physician.

Nursing Implications Summary

GENERAL GUIDELINES FOR DRUGS FOR PATIENTS WITH HIV

➤ Routinely check drug insert for current information. Protocols for treatment and prevention of HIV infection change often.

➤ Instruct the patient to take doses as ordered, to not increase dose or frequency without talking with the physician, to not omit doses, and to not discontinue therapy if feeling better or symptoms disappear.

➤ Emphasize the importance or returning to the physician for regular blood work to monitor for side effects and drug effectiveness.

➤ Remind the patient to keep all health care providers informed of all drugs being used. Caution the patient not to take any other medication, whether prescription or over the counter, without checking with physician first.

➤ Inform the patient that taking these drugs will not prevent the spread of HIV. If possible, HIV-positive patients should avoid sexual activity or should always use protection to avoid spreading HIV. Men should use latex condoms, and women may wish to carry condoms with them so that they will always be available. Using a spermicide may help prevent the spread of HIV. The patient should not use lubricants such as oil-based jelly, cold cream, baby oil, or shortening but can use oil-free lubricants such as K-Y Jelly.

➤ Instruct the patient who injects drugs not to share needles with others.

➤ Provide emotional support as needed.

➤ Some of these drugs may be used with individuals who have experienced an occupational exposure to HIV.

delavirdine

Drug Administration/Nursing in the Community

➤ See the general guidelines.

➤ Assess patients for skin rash, blisters, conjunctivitis, fever, oral lesions, difficulty breathing, diarrhea, excessive fatigue, headache, nausea, and vomiting. Instruct the patient to report the development of these problems or any unexpected sign or symptom to the physician.

➤ Instruct the patient to take doses on a full or empty stomach and not to take doses within 1 hour of taking antacids.

➤ Instruct patients with achlorhydria to take doses with an acidic beverage such as orange juice or cranberry juice.

➤ Instruct the patient to take doses whole or disperse in water. To disperse, put dose in at least 3 ounces of water and allow to stand for several minutes. Stir until dispersion is uniform, then drink entire volume. Rinse glass with a little more water, and drink this water also.

didanosine

Drug Administration

➤ Assess patient for severity of symptoms: fever, night sweats, swollen lymph nodes, weight loss, excessive fatigue, diarrhea,

Nursing Implications Summary—cont'd

cough, weakness, anorexia, and yeast infections (oral or vaginal).

➤ Assess for peripheral neuropathy, including numbness or tingling of fingers and extremities. Assess deep tendon reflexes.

➤ Assess for pancreatitis, including epigastric or left upper quadrant abdominal pain, nausea, vomiting, and fever. Monitor white blood cell (WBC) count, serum lipase, serum triglycerides, serum electrolytes, and serum uric acid.

Nursing in the Community

➤ Instruct the patient to take oral doses on an empty stomach 2 hours before or 2 hours after eating.

➤ Instruct the patient taking pediatric oral suspension to measure doses using the calibrated measuring device supplied by the pharmacist.

➤ Instruct the patient using didanosine for oral solution to pour contents of foil packet into 4 ounces of water and not to mix with fruit juice or any acidic beverage. Stir for 2 to 3 minutes to dissolve powder, then drink immediately.

➤ Instruct the patient to chew or crush tablets thoroughly before swallowing or mix with 1 ounce of water until a suspension forms, then swallow the mixture.

➤ Each tablet contains the drug and a buffer. For patients older than 1 year, the prescribed dose should always be 2 tablets. Tablets must be taken together to get enough of the buffer. For children younger than 1 year of age, there is enough buffer in 1 tablet.

➤ Each 2-tablet dose of didanosine contains 529 mg sodium, and each single-dose packet of buffered didanosine for oral solution contains 1380 mg sodium. Inform patients on sodium-restricted diets about the sodium. Teach patients with phenylketonuria that tablets contain phenylalanine.

indinavir

Drug Administration/Nursing in the Community

➤ See the general guidelines.

➤ Assess for generalized weakness, diarrhea, nausea, vomiting, headache, and change in sense of taste.

➤ Instruct the patient to report the development of kidney stones (blood in urine, sharp pain in back) to the physician. To help prevent kidney stones, instruct the patient to increase fluid intake to at least 1.5 L/day (six 8-ounce glasses of liquid).

➤ Instruct the patient to take doses 1 hour before or 2 hours after a large meal. The patient may also take doses with a light meal, such as with dry toast, juice and coffee, or a bowl of cereal with milk.

➤ Monitor blood glucose. Rarely, diabetes or hyperglycemia may develop. Instruct patients to report the development of dry or itchy skin, fatigue, hunger, increased thirst, or unexplained weight loss to the physician.

lamivudine

Drug Administration/Nursing in the Community

➤ See the general guidelines.

➤ Assess the patient for pancreatitis (nausea, vomiting, ab-

dominal pain); tingling, burning, or numbness of the hands, arms, feet, or legs; excessive fatigue; fever; chills; sore throat; skin rash; headache; insomnia; cough; and dizziness. Teach patients to report the development of any of these signs or symptoms to the physician.

➤ Monitor liver function tests, serum amylase, lipase and triglycerides, blood urea nitrogen (BUN), and serum creatinine levels.

nelfinavir

Drug Administration/Nursing in the Community

➤ See the general guidelines.

➤ Assess for diarrhea, nausea, and rash.

➤ Monitor blood glucose. Rarely, diabetes or hyperglycemia may develop. Instruct patients to report the development of dry or itchy skin, fatigue, hunger, increased thirst, or unexplained weight loss to the physician.

➤ Instruct the patient to take doses with food. Nelfinavir should be taken 2 hours before didanosine or 1 hour after doses of didanosine.

➤ Prepare powder form by mixing dose with a small amount of water, milk, formula, soy milk, or dietary supplements. Do not mix with acidic foods or juices such as apple juice or applesauce, orange juice, or grapefruit juice. Do not reconstitute the dose in the original container.

➤ Tell patients with phenylketonuria that nelfinavir oral powder contains 11.2 g phenylalanine per gram of powder.

nevirapine

Drug Administration/Nursing in the Community

➤ See the general guidelines.

➤ Assess for skin rash, fever, jaundice, sores in the mouth, abdominal pain, diarrhea, and headache. Instruct the patient to report the development of these or any other signs or symptoms to the physician.

➤ Monitor liver function tests.

➤ Instruct the patient to take doses with or without food.

➤ Instruct women using estrogen-containing contraceptives to use another form of birth control while taking nevirapine and for several weeks after stopping nevirapine.

ritonavir

Drug Administration/Nursing in the Community

➤ See the general guidelines.

➤ Assess for circumoral paresthesia (numbness around the mouth); numbness or tingling of the fingers, hands, or feet; generalized weakness; anorexia; nausea; vomiting; abdominal pain; headache; and change in sense of taste. Instruct the patient to report the development of these or any unexpected signs or symptoms to the physician.

➤ Monitor blood glucose. Rarely, diabetes or hyperglycemia may develop. Instruct patients to report the development of dry or itchy skin, fatigue, hunger, increased thirst, or unexplained weight loss to the physician.

Continued

Nursing Implications Summary—cont'd

➤ Caution patients to avoid driving or operating hazardous equipment if dizziness or excessive sleepiness develops.

➤ Instruct the patient to take doses with food. Ritonavir oral solution may be mixed with chocolate milk or a dietary supplement such as Ensure to improve taste. Tell the patient to consume dose within 1 hour of mixing.

saquinavir

Drug Administration/Nursing in the Community

➤ See the general guidelines.

➤ Assess for burning or prickling sensations, rash, weakness, abdominal pain, oral ulcers, nausea, and headache. Instruct the patient to report the development of these or any unexpected sign or symptom to the physician.

➤ Instruct the patient to take doses within 2 hours after a full meal.

stavudine

Drug Administration/Nursing in the Community

➤ See the general guidelines.

➤ Assess for peripheral neuropathy: numbness, tingling, or pain of the fingers, hands or feet. Assess for joint pain, fever, skin rash, excessive fatigue, nausea, vomiting, abdominal pain, and headache. Instruct patients to report the development of these signs or symptoms to the physician.

➤ Monitor liver function tests, serum amylase, and lipase.

zalcitabine

Drug Administration/Nursing in the Community

➤ See the General Guidelines.

➤ Assess for peripheral neuropathy: numbness, tingling, or pain of the fingers, hands, or feet. Assess for joint pain, skin rash, fever, muscle pain, ulcers of the mouth or throat, jaundice, sore throat, nausea, vomiting, abdominal pain, and headache. Instruct the patient to report the development of these signs or symptoms to the physician.

➤ Monitor liver function tests, serum lipase and amylase, serum triglycerides, serum creatinine, and BUN.

zidovudine

Drug Administration/Nursing in the Community

➤ See the general guidelines.

➤ Assess for headaches, anxiety, and confusion. Inspect for rashes. Monitor temperature and pulse. Instruct the patient to report the development of any unexpected sign or symptom to the physician.

➤ Monitor complete blood count (CBC), differential, and platelet count, and liver function tests.

➤ See the Patient Problems boxes in Chapter 54 on bleeding tendencies and leukopenia.

Intravenous zidovudine

➤ Review drug package insert for current information about dilution. Administer the diluted dose evenly over 1 hour. May also be administered as a continuous infusion.

DRUGS FOR VIRAL DISEASES OTHER THAN AIDS

acyclovir

Drug Administration

➤ Assess for GI tract symptoms and CNS side effects. Inspect for skin rashes.

➤ Monitor intake and output and weight.

➤ Monitor CBC and differential, platelet count, and BUN and serum creatinine levels.

➤ For best effect in treatment of chicken pox, begin therapy as soon as possible after the rash appears, within 24 hours of onset. For best effect in treatment of recurrent herpes simplex infections, begin therapy as soon as possible after symptoms appear.

Intravenous Administration

➤ Dilute as directed in the drug insert. Administer dose over 1 hour. Use an infusion control device or microdrip tubing to help regulate infusion rate. Inspect the IV site frequently and question the patient regarding symptoms of phlebitis or irritation. Because excretion is via the kidneys and the drug half-life is about 2½ hours, the patient should be well hydrated during IV infusion to prevent precipitation of the drug in the renal tubules.

Nursing in the Community

➤ Review the anticipated benefits and possible side effects of drug therapy with the patient.

➤ Instruct the patient to take oral doses with a full glass (8 ounces) of water. For oral suspension form, instruct the patient to measure doses using the calibrated measuring device supplied by the pharmacist.

➤ Warn the patient to avoid driving or operating hazardous equipment if dizziness, fatigue, or vertigo develops and to notify the physician if these symptoms do occur.

➤ For topical application, instruct the patient to use a glove or finger cot to apply ointment to avoid contamination of the finger. Caution the patient to avoid contact with the eyes and to use the drug regularly, as prescribed, for best effect. Instruct the patient to consult the physician if improvement does not occur within 1 week.

➤ Instruct the patient with genital herpes how to lessen the chance of spreading the virus by avoiding sexual activity when open lesions or scabs are present. Male partners should wear condoms. Acyclovir will not prevent the spread of herpes.

➤ Instruct the patient to keep areas of infection clean and dry and to wear loose-fitting garments. Caution the patient not to use other creams or ointments on viral lesions unless prescribed by the physician.

➤ Encourage women with genital herpes to have regular Pap smears to check for cervical cancer.

amantadine

➤ See the Nursing Implications Summary in Chapter 62.

cidofovir

Drug Administration/Nursing in the Community

➤ Assess visual acuity. Assess for fever, diarrhea, anorexia, nausea, and headache. Monitor intake and output.

Nursing Implications Summary—cont'd

➤ Monitor serum creatinine, CBC and WBC differential, urine protein, and intraocular pressure.

➤ See manufacturer's insert for the recommended protocol. Handle this medication in the same manner as antineoplastic drugs. Prepare IV doses in a laminar flow hood. Wear gloves and a long-sleeve gown. Avoid contact with skin and mucous membranes. Dispose of needles and tubing according to agency guidelines.

➤ Administer correctly diluted doses over 1 hour. Use an infusion monitoring device.

➤ Emphasize the importance of returning for regular follow-up visits to monitor drug effectiveness.

foscarnet
Drug Administration

➤ Check drug insert for current information.

➤ Monitor intake and output and weight. Monitor serum electrolyte level, CBC, BUN level, and serum creatinine level.

➤ Assess for nausea, excessive fatigue, numbness, or tingling around mouth or of fingers, hands, or toes. Instruct the patient to report the development of these problems to the physician.

Intravenous foscarnet

➤ Use undiluted solutions in central lines only. For peripheral IV infusion, dilute drug in an equal volume of D5W or normal saline for a dilution of 12 mg/ml. Discard any excess drug from the IV bottle; to avoid overdose, only the prescribed dose should be in the IV bottle at the start of the infusion. Administer the dose over at least 1 hour. The dose should not exceed 1 mg/kg/min. Use an infusion pump to deliver accurate dose.

Nursing in the Community

➤ Instruct the patient to ensure adequate hydration before administering the drug to lessen the chance of renal toxicity. Encourage the patient to drink several additional 8-ounce glasses of water each day while taking foscarnet.

➤ This drug may cause sores to develop on the genitals. Instruct the patient to wash genitals after urinating to decrease the chance of sores forming.

➤ Encourage the patient with CMV infection of the eyes to have regular ophthalmic examinations to monitor progress.

famciclovir
Drug Administration/Nursing in the Community

➤ Instruct the patient to report the development of persistent or severe headache, diarrhea, dizziness, fatigue, or nausea to the physician.

➤ Instruct the patient to take doses with meals.

➤ For best effect, begin famciclovir at the first sign of rash or symptoms, within 48 hours of the onset of rash. Instruct the patient to continue therapy for the full course and not to stop when symptoms begin to clear.

➤ Instruct the patient to keep the area affected by herpes as clean and dry as possible and to wear loose-fitting clothing.

ganciclovir
Drug Administration/Nursing in the Community

➤ Assess for rash, excessive fatigue, anorexia, nausea, and vomiting.

➤ Monitor CBC and platelet count, liver function tests, and BUN level.

➤ Monitor intake and output.

➤ See the Patient Problems box in Chapter 54 on bleeding tendencies.

➤ Instruct the patient (men and women) to use measures for contraception during treatment and for at least 90 days after treatment.

➤ Encourage the patient to have an ophthalmic examination at the start of therapy and at regular intervals to monitor progress. Encourage the patient to report any changes in vision to the physician.

➤ Ganciclovir shares some properties with antitumor agents (carcinogenicity and mutagenicity). Avoid getting the drug on skin or mucous membranes. Use a laminar air flow hood for preparation of IV doses. Consider wearing gloves when preparing doses. Do not open or crush capsules.

➤ Instruct the patient to take oral doses with food.

➤ IV ganciclovir: See drug insert for preparation guidelines. Administer each dose over 1 hour as an infusion. Use microdrip tubing and an infusion monitoring device.

➤ Intravitreal implants: Review manufacturer's instructions. This form is implanted surgically. Emphasize the importance of regular follow-up visits to monitor for side effects. Instruct the patient that decreased visual acuity is expected in the affected eye for 2 to 4 weeks after implantation. Instruct the patient to contact the physician immediately if any sudden change in vision, pain, or other eye problems develop.

interferons
Drug Administration

➤ Review the manufacturer's instruction leaflet. If the patient is to administer injections at home, teach proper injection technique as well as proper handling and disposal of contaminated syringes and needles.

➤ Assess for development of side effects. Be alert to signs of depression, including insomnia, weight loss, withdrawal, anorexia, and lack of interest in personal appearance.

➤ Monitor pulse and blood pressure. Auscultate lung and heart sounds. Monitor intake, output, and weight.

➤ Monitor hematocrit or hemoglobin level, platelet count, WBC differential, and liver function tests.

Nursing in the Community

➤ Review the anticipated benefits and possible side effects of drug therapy with the patient.

➤ Review the dosing schedule and discuss with the patient what to do if a dose is missed if drugs are to be self-administered. Ensure that the patient can inject the dose correctly.

➤ Instruct the patient to stay well hydrated to lessen symptoms from hypotension.

Continued

Nursing Implications Summary—cont'd

➤ Warn the patient to avoid driving or operating hazardous equipment if fatigue or dizziness develops.

➤ These drugs often cause a flulike reaction, with fever, chills, and headache. The nurse should consult the physician about appropriate instructions for the patient related to notifying the physician and self-medicating with acetaminophen to reduce fever and headache.

➤ Instruct the patient not to change to other brands of interferon without consulting the physician.

➤ Instruct the patient to avoid other drugs that may also cause drowsiness or fatigue unless specifically approved by the physician; this includes alcohol, antihistamines, sedatives, sleeping medications, prescription medication for pain, and medications for seizures. Instruct the patient to keep all health care providers informed of all drugs being used.

➤ Review the Patient Problems boxes in Chapter 54 on leukopenia and bleeding tendencies.

➤ Instruct the patient to take doses at night to lessen daytime fatigue.

ribavirin
Drug Administration/Nursing in the Community

➤ Review the anticipated benefits and possible side effects of drug therapy with the patient and family. Encourage the patient or family to report new signs or symptoms to the physician.

➤ Auscultate lung sounds and assess respiratory status. Monitor temperature and vital signs.

➤ Check drug package insert for current information. Do not give simultaneously with other aerosolized medications. Use only the aerosol generator specified by the manufacturer.

➤ Health care workers should avoid contact with the drug if possible because it may cause eye irritation or headaches.

rimantadine
Drug Administration/Nursing in the Community

➤ Assess for a history of seizures before administering rimantadine.

➤ For best results, drug therapy should be started before exposure to influenza type A or as soon as possible after exposure. Instruct the patient to continue therapy as prescribed for the full course, even if feeling better or symptoms improve.

➤ Instruct the patient to avoid driving or operating hazardous equipment if drowsiness, dizziness, or excessive fatigue develops.

valacyclovir
Drug Administration/Nursing in the Community

➤ Assess for headache, nausea, dizziness, fatigue, and GI disturbances.

➤ Instruct the patient to take doses with meals or on an empty stomach.

➤ Instruct the patient to keep affected areas clean and dry and to wear loose-fitting clothing to avoid irritating lesions.

➤ For best results, valacyclovir should be started within 48 hours of the development of lesions.

Ophthalmic Antiviral Agents
Drug Administration/Nursing in the Community

➤ Review the technique for administration of eye medications with the patient (see Chapter 5).

➤ If photophobia develops, instruct the patient to avoid bright lights and to wear sunglasses.

➤ Caution the patient that vision may be blurry for several minutes after administering eye medications. Instruct the patient to avoid driving or operating hazardous equipment if vision is not clear.

➤ Encourage the patient to have regular ophthalmic examinations to monitor progress. Remind the patient to use medications as ordered for best effect and to use them for the full course of therapy.

➤ Instruct the patient to notify the physician if vision worsens or exudate, itching, or other symptoms develop.

CHAPTER REVIEW

Application

1. Why does HIV specifically attack T lymphocytes?
2. What is the mechanism of action of zidovudine?
3. How is zidovudine used to treat viral disease?
4. What side effects are associated with zidovudine? How should you assess for these?
5. How do nonnucleoside RT inhibitors differ from nucleoside RT inhibitors like zidovudine?
6. What is the mechanism of action of indinavir?
7. What is HAART?
8. What is the mechanism of action of acyclovir?
9. How is acyclovir used to treat viral diseases?
10. What side effects are associated with acyclovir? How should you assess for these?
11. How is amantadine used to treat viral diseases?
12. Explain why famciclovir is called a prodrug.
13. How may interferons be used against viruses?
14. How is ribavirin used to treat viral disease?
15. How are ganciclovir, cidofovir, and foscarnet used as antiviral agents?
16. How are idoxuridine, trifluridine, and vidarabine used as antiviral agents?

Critical Thinking

1. An AIDS patient on HAART confides in you that he has stopped taking one of the medications in his regimen because it made his stomach hurt. What problems can you foresee arising from his action?

2. HIV-positive patients are at greater risk for opportunistic infections. These patients may be treated with zidovudine. Does treatment with this drug lessen the risk of infection for these patients?

3. How would you find out the newest information about AIDS or about new drugs for AIDS? If you have access to the Internet, try contacting the National Institutes of Health. Hint: try http://www.NIH.gov

References

Kenny P: Managing HIV infection, *Nursing* 26(8):26-35, 1996.

Klaus BD, Grodesky MJ: HIV and HAART in 1997. Highly active antiretroviral therapy, *Nurse Pract* 22(8):139-142, 1997.

Lisanti P, Zwolski K: Understanding the devastation of AIDS, *Am J Nurs* 97(7):26-34, 1997.

Williams AB: New horizons: antiretroviral therapy in 1997, *J Assoc Nurses AIDS Care* 8(4):26-38, 1997.

Drugs to Treat Protozoal and Helminthic Infestations

OBJECTIVES

After studying this chapter, you should be able to do the following:

- *Discuss how the site of infestation may affect the success of drug therapy.*
- *Describe the type of patients in whom specific protozoal or helminthic diseases might be more likely.*
- *Explain hygienic measures that should accompany drug therapy in controlling pinworm infestations.*
- *Develop a nursing care plan for the patient receiving one of the drugs in this chapter.*

CHAPTER OVERVIEW

On a worldwide scale, infestations caused by protozoans or worms cause the most common chronic diseases of human beings. Although these diseases flourish primarily in tropical regions, several are encountered in North America. The discussion in this chapter centers on the treatment of diseases that occur in the continental United States and Canada.

Parasitic diseases are caused by eucaryotic organisms against which selective toxicity is sometimes difficult to achieve. The selection of an effective drug involves matching the tissue distribution of the drug with the sites of infestation of the parasite, as well as choosing an agent that possesses intrinsic activity against the parasite.

For the purposes of discussion, parasitic diseases are divided into the following categories in this chapter: amebic disease, malaria, selected parasitic diseases (*Giardiasis,* pneumocystosis, toxoplasmosis, trichomoniasis), and diseases caused by helminths (worms).

THERAPEUTIC RATIONALE: AMEBIC DISEASE

Amebic disease is caused by microscopic, single-celled parasitic organisms. *Entamoeba histolytica* is a common human pathogen, passed from host to host by oral ingestion of fecally contaminated food or water. The organism is ingested as a cyst. Cysts have thick walls that resist the action of stomach acids. In the intestine the nonmotile cyst changes to a motile, sexually active form called a trophozoite. Trophozoites produce active disease as they reproduce and invade tissues.

Amebic disease may be restricted to the intestinal lumen. However, trophozoites invade the intestinal lining in the course of the disease and may penetrate the intestinal wall and create abscesses in other tissues and organs. The liver and lung are most commonly affected in this way.

The choice of drug for treating amebic disease depends on the stage of the disease. For acute colitis that occurs while the disease is limited to the intestinal tract, several drugs are available (Table 53-1). For more extensive intestinal disease or for abscesses in other organs, metronidazole is the safest

Table 53-1 **Drugs to Treat Amebic Infestations**

Generic Name	Trade Name	Administration/Dosage	Comments
chloroquine	Aralen*	ORAL: *Adults—For amebic liver abscesses:* 250 mg 4 times/day for 2 days, then 250 mg twice daily for up to 3 wk. *Children—For amebic liver abscesses:* 10 mg/kg/day for 3 wk.	Alternative drug used in combinations for amebic liver abscesses.
diloxanide	Entamide‡ Furamide‡	ORAL: *Adults*—500 mg 3 times/day for 10 days. *Children >2 yr*—6.7 mg/kg 3 times/day. Maximum daily dose 1.5 g.	Alternative drug for asymptomatic intestinal disease.
iodoquinol	Diodoquin† Diquinol Yodoxin	ORAL: *Adults*—650 mg 3 times/day for 20 days. Maximum daily dose 2 g. *Children*—10-13.3 mg/kg 3 times/day for 20 days. Maximum daily dose 1.95 g.	Primary drug for asymptomatic intestinal disease.
metronidazole	Flagyl* Protostat Trikacide†	ORAL: *Adults—For amebiasis:* 500-750 mg 3 times/day for 5-10 days. *For anaerobic bacterial infections:* 7.5 mg/kg 4 times/day. FDA pregnancy category B. *Children—For amebiasis:* 11.6-16.7 mg/kg 3 times/day for 10 days. For *anaerobic bacterial infections:* 7.5 mg/kg 4 times/day.	Primary drug for intestinal or extraintestinal amebiasis; anaerobic bacteria.

*Available in Canada and the United States.
†Available in Canada only.
‡Available in the United States only through Centers for Disease Control and Prevention (CDC) in Atlanta.

and most effective agent. Metronidazole therapy is usually followed by iodoquinol or diloxanide, drugs that more effectively destroy free amebae within the intestinal lumen.

THERAPEUTIC AGENTS: DRUGS TO TREAT AMEBIC DISEASE

Primary Agents

iodoquinol

Mechanism of Action

Iodoquinol is an effective amebicidal agent (see Table 53-1), but its mechanism of action is unknown.

Pharmacokinetics

Iodoquinol given orally is poorly absorbed from the intestine. Iodine is increased in the blood, which suggests that some drug is absorbed or that iodine is absorbed after breakdown of the drug in the gut.

Uses

Iodoquinol is used alone for intestinal amebiasis or with metronidazole for serious invasive intestinal amebiasis.

Adverse Reactions and Contraindications

Iodoquinol is relatively nontoxic, but nausea and other gastrointestinal (GI) tract symptoms can occur. Allergic reactions, fevers, and chills may also develop.

Iodoquinol can cause the thyroid gland to enlarge because the drug contains significant iodine. This iodine content also makes iodoquinol potentially dangerous for patients with hepatic or renal failure.

Toxicity

Prolonged high dosages of iodoquinol may produce optic neuritis or atrophy and other signs of neuropathy.

Interactions

No documented drug interactions are clinically important, but iodoquinol causes persistent interference with thyroid function tests because iodine levels are high in blood.

▼ metronidazole

Mechanism of Action

Metronidazole is most effective against anaerobic organisms, being reduced in those organisms to a form that directly damages DNA. Metronidazole attacks amebas at intestinal and other tissue sites (see Table 53-1).

Pharmacokinetics

Metronidazole is well absorbed after oral administration. The drug is metabolized by various pathways. Both metabolites and unchanged drug appear in urine. Some patients observe a reddish brown discoloration of urine while taking metronidazole. This harmless discoloration is caused by a colored metabolite of metronidazole.

Uses

Metronidazole is a primary agent for intestinal amebiasis and for tissue abscesses caused by amebae. It has also been used to treat trichomoniasis and *Giardiasis* (see Table 53-3), as well as infections and abscesses caused by anaerobic bacteria.

Adverse Reactions and Contraindications

Metronidazole can produce various GI tract symptoms, including a sharp, metallic taste, as well as nausea, diarrhea, vomiting, epigastric pain, and abdominal cramping. Although annoying, these symptoms rarely require stopping the drug.

Metronidazole commonly causes dizziness or headache, but other central nervous system (CNS) effects such as ataxia (incoordination affecting walking), numbness, and paresthesias are uncommon. These latter symptoms may signal that metronidazole should be withdrawn. Metronidazole may also produce discomfort in the pelvic organs. Dysuria, cystitis, and dryness of the vagina may be experienced.

Because of its action on DNA, metronidazole may be mutagenic or carcinogenic in experimental animals. This potential problem precludes routine use of the drug in pregnant women. Metronidazole is also avoided if possible in patients with significant CNS disease or blood dyscrasias because the drug may worsen both conditions. Patients with hepatic impairment may accumulate the drug because the liver is the primary organ for elimination of metronidazole; reduced dosages may be used.

Toxicity

High dosages of metronidazole may cause seizures.

Interactions

Metronidazole causes an alarming reaction when ethyl alcohol is ingested. Patients experience intense flushing, nausea, headaches, and abdominal cramps. This reaction is similar to that experienced by patients taking both disulfiram and ethyl alcohol.

Metronidazole may potentiate the action of warfarin. Patients receiving both drugs should be observed for signs of bleeding.

Alternative Drugs
diloxanide

Diloxanide is not available commercially in either Canada or the United States, but it may be obtained from the Centers for Disease Control and Prevention in Atlanta. Diloxanide eliminates *E. histolytica* from the intestine of persons mildly infected and who are passing cysts in their stools (see Table 53-1). The mechanism of action of diloxanide is unknown.

Diloxanide is given orally and is well absorbed by that route. Excretion is primarily renal. It is a relatively safe drug, producing few systemic side effects. Flatulence (intestinal gas) is the most common side effect. Other GI tract disturbances such as nausea, diarrhea, and esophagitis may rarely occur.

Table 53-2   Drugs to Treat Malaria

Generic Name	Trade Name	Administration/Dosage	Comments
chloroquine	Aralen*	ORAL: *Adults—For suppression:* 500 mg once every 7 days. *For therapy:* 1 g initially, 500 mg 6-8 hr later, then 500 mg once daily for 2 days. *Children—For suppression:* 8.3 mg/kg once every 7 days, not to exceed 500 mg. *For therapy:* 16.7 mg/kg initially, then 8.3 mg/kg at 6, 24, and 48 hr later. The first dose should not exceed 1 g and later doses should not exceed 500 mg. INTRAMUSCULAR: *Adults—For therapy:* 200-250 mg repeated in 6 hr if needed. INTRAMUSCULAR, SUBCUTANEOUS: *Children—For therapy:* 4.4 mg/kg repeated in 6 hr if needed. INTRAVENOUS: *Children—*16.6 mg/kg infused over 8 hr initially, then 8.3 mg/kg every 6-8 hr (infusion over 4 hr).	Primary drug for therapy or prophylaxis of malaria.
halofantrine	Halfan‡	ORAL: *Adults—*500 mg on empty stomach, repeated at 6 and 12 hr. Repeat schedule 1 wk later. *Children <40 kg—*8 mg/kg, repeated at 6 and 12 hr. Repeat schedule 1 wk later.	Therapy for acute malaria caused by chloroquine-resistant *Plasmodium falciparum.*
hydroxychloroquine	Plaquenil*	ORAL: *Adults—For suppression:* 400 mg once every 7 days. *For therapy:* 800 mg initially, 400 mg 6-8 hr later, then 400 mg once daily for 2 days. *Children—For suppression:* 6.4 mg/kg once every 7 days, not to exceed 400 mg. *For therapy:* 12.9 mg/kg initially (not to exceed 800 mg), then 6.4 mg/kg at 6, 24, and 48 hr later, not to exceed 400 mg/dose.	Primary drug for therapy or prophylaxis of malaria.
mefloquine	Lariam	ORAL: *Adults—For prophylaxis:* 250 mg once a week. *For therapy:* 1250 mg once. FDA pregnancy category C. *Children 15-45 kg body weight—For prophylaxis:* ¼, ½, or ¾ tablet once weekly based on body weight. *For therapy:* 16.5 mg/kg as a single dose.	Prophylaxis or therapy of malaria, including disease caused by chloroquine-resistant *P. falciparum.*
primaquine		ORAL: *Adults—*26.3 mg once daily for 14 days. *Children—*0.68 mg/kg once daily for 14 days.	Primary drug for radical cure of malaria (*P. vivax, P. ovale*); kills gametocytes of *P. falciparum.*
pyrimethamine	Daraprim*	ORAL: *Adults:—*75 mg once with 1.5 g of sulfadoxine. May be combined with quinine or mefloquine. FDA pregnancy category C. *Children—*1.25 mg/kg once with 25 mg/kg sulfadoxine on day 3 of quinine therapy.	Therapy for malaria caused by chloroquine-resistant *P. falciparum.*
quinine		ORAL: *Adults—*600-650 mg every 8 hr for 3-7 days. May be combined with doxycycline, clindamycin, or sulfadoxine/pyrimethamine. FDA pregnancy category X. *Children—*8.3 mg/kg every 8 hr for 3-7 days. May be combined with clindamycin or sulfadoxine/pyrimethamine.	Therapy for malaria caused by chloroquine-resistant *P. falciparum.*

*Available in Canada and the United States.
‡Not commercially available in the United States or Canada.

▼ chloroquine

Chloroquine may be used along with iodoquinol or diloxanide to treat liver abscesses caused by amebic infections. Chloroquine is only an alternative drug for amebic disease (see Table 53-1) but is a primary drug for malaria. Chloroquine is discussed fully under malaria and in Table 53-2.

THERAPEUTIC RATIONALE: MALARIA

Malaria is a serious infectious illness transmitted by the bite of infected mosquitoes. Four species of *Plasmodium* produce human disease: *P. falciparum*, *P. vivax*, *P. ovale*, and *P. malariae*.

Plasmodia have complex life cycles. Sporozoites enter human blood, travel directly to the liver, and may persist there for prolonged periods. Clinical malaria is produced when merozoites, the plasmodial form produced in liver cells, are released into the blood. Merozoites attack red blood cells and ultimately cause them to rupture, thus producing the fever, chills, and sweating characteristic of malaria. A few gametocytes are also formed. Only gametocytes cause a mosquito to become infectious and capable of transmitting the disease. Thus patients at this stage of the disease can transmit parasites to mosquitoes and thence to other human hosts.

Therapy for malaria depends on the stage of the disease and which plasmodial species is involved. *P. falciparum* and *P. malariae* do not produce persistent tissue forms of the parasite; therefore therapy that destroys blood forms of the protozoan will be curative. With *P. vivax* and *P. ovale*, therapy must include a drug that destroys the persistent tissue forms of *Plasmodium*.

Chloroquine has been the leading antimalarial drug for decades, but chloroquine-resistant malaria has developed in several regions of the world. Chloroquine-resistant malaria is treated with combinations of quinine, mefloquine, halofantrine, and pyrimethamine with sulfadoxine. Clindamycin, dapsone, doxycycline, and tetracycline have also been included in treatment regimens for chloroquine-resistant disease.

Several of the drugs used to treat malaria may also be used for prophylaxis. Chloroquine, hydroxychloroquine, mefloquine, and pyrimethamine with sulfadoxine are given in once-weekly doses.

THERAPEUTIC AGENTS: DRUGS TO TREAT MALARIA

Primary Agents

▼chloroquine and hydroxychloroquine

Mechanism of Action

Chloroquine and hydroxychloroquine are both 4-aminoquinolines. This family of drugs has been the mainstay of antimalarial therapy worldwide since the late 1940s. All effective members of this family can bind tightly to double-stranded DNA, thereby altering the physical properties of DNA. These drugs may also inhibit metabolic processes in *Plasmodium*.

Pharmacokinetics

Chloroquine phosphate and hydroxychloroquine sulfate are satisfactorily absorbed from the GI tract. Chloroquine hydrochloride is available for intramuscular (IM) injection when oral dosage is impossible.

Drugs of the 4-aminoquinoline family are strongly concentrated in liver, spleen, kidneys, and lungs. More important to the therapeutic usefulness, the drugs are also concentrated in red blood cells. Infected red blood cells may contain up to 1000-fold higher concentrations than in plasma.

4-Aminoquinolines may be metabolized by hepatic microsomal enzymes; some of the metabolites retain antiplasmodial activity. The drugs and metabolites are eliminated by the kidneys. Renal excretion is enhanced by acidifying urine, which converts the drug to a charged form that is not reabsorbed.

Uses

Chloroquine and hydroxychloroquine are both used for suppressive treatment and treatment of acute malaria caused by *P. falciparum*, *P. malariae*, *P. ovale*, and *P. vivax*. Chloroquine-resistant strains of *P. falciparum* require combinations of drugs. Radical cure of *P. ovale* and *P. vivax* requires addition of primaquine to the drug regimen.

Adverse Reactions and Contraindications

At dosages commonly used in therapy, chloroquine and hydroxychloroquine can produce nausea and other GI tract symptoms. These symptoms may be minimized by taking the drugs with meals.

Visual changes may also occur with 4-aminoquinolines; ciliary muscle impairment may be minor, but persistent or more severe changes in vision may signal overdose (see next section).

Chloroquine and hydroxychloroquine are relatively safe drugs if care is taken to avoid overdose, prolonged use, or use in sensitive patients. Patients with glucose-6-phosphate dehydrogenase (G6PD) deficiency are more likely than normal patients to experience hemolysis when treated with these drugs. Children are also more sensitive to these agents than are adults (see Pediatric Considerations box). Patients with liver disease or retinal damage are also more at risk of severe toxic reactions.

Toxicity

The toxic reactions to 4-aminoquinolines are greatly increased when the drugs are used for prolonged periods, such as with long-term malaria prophylaxis. Signs of overdose include cardiovascular signs (arrhythmias, cardiovascular collapse, hypotension), CNS toxicity (drowsiness, excitability, headache, seizures), and visual disturbances (blurred vision). Blurred vision may signal reversible impairment of accommodation, but retinal or corneal changes are irreversible. Patients reporting misty vision, patchy vision, or foggy patches in the visual field may be developing serious eye damage.

PEDIATRIC CONSIDERATIONS

Chloroquine and Hydroxychloroquine

THE PROBLEM

Infants and children are more sensitive than adults to 4-aminoquinolines. Children have died after swallowing as little as 750 mg of chloroquine. Severe reactions and sudden death have been reported with parenteral use.

SOLUTIONS
- Use minimal effective doses in children.
- Do not give these drugs long term to children.
- Carefully observe children receiving these drugs.
- Keep drugs out of easy reach of children.
- Use childproof caps on medication containers.
- Never refer to medication as candy.

Interactions

The 4-aminoquinolines should not be used with penicillamine because they may cause excessive accumulation and toxicity of penicillamine.

primaquine

Mechanism of Action

Primaquine is an 8-aminoquinoline. The mechanism of action may be different from the related 4-aminoquinolines, but the exact mechanism by which primaquine kills certain forms of plasmodia is unknown (see Table 53-2).

Pharmacokinetics

Primaquine is well absorbed after oral doses. Drug concentrations in plasma peak within 6 hours of taking the dose, but the drug is extensively metabolized and rapidly cleared from blood.

Uses

Primaquine keeps gametocytes of *P. falciparum* from the blood, thereby preventing the transmission of malaria to the mosquito and thence to human hosts. In addition, primaquine is used to produce a radical cure of *P. vivax* and *P. ovale* infections. By destroying the tissue-bound forms of the pathogen, primaquine prevents relapses.

Adverse Reactions and Contraindications

Primaquine given at normal therapeutic dosages causes little toxicity. Abdominal cramps or epigastric distress can occur, but these symptoms can usually be relieved by taking the drug with meals.

Primaquine may damage red blood cells. The drug blocks production of an intracellular-reducing agent, NADPH. In normal cells this deficit is made up by glucose metabolism, and the cell continues to function normally, but patients with reduced levels of G6PD cannot use glucose rapidly enough to make up the deficit. Red blood cells in these pa-

tients accumulate oxidized products such as methemoglobin, which is not an efficient oxygen carrier. Cyanosis may result. Ultimately, these red blood cells may rupture. Hemolysis can be severe and signals that the drug dosage should be reduced or that treatment should be stopped. One sign of hemolysis that may be seen easily is darkening of urine.

Primaquine side effects are more severe in patients lacking G6PD. The lack of G6PD is genetically determined and exists in high proportions of certain populations such as Sardinians, Sephardic Jews, Greeks, and Iranians. African-Americans are less prone to this deficiency than these groups but have a higher incidence than the U.S. Caucasian population. Patients with these increased sensitivities to primaquine may be given lower dosages of the drug.

Toxicity

High dosages of primaquine cause methemoglobinemia, as well as other signs of blood dyscrasias.

Interactions

Primaquine is not routinely used with other bone marrow suppressants because the risk of leukopenia is too great. Quinacrine is also avoided with primaquine because of excessive toxicity with the combination.

Alternative Drugs

halofantrine

Halofantrine is not available commercially in North America but is used elsewhere for acute malaria caused by chloroquine-resistant *P. falciparum*.

Halofantrine may interfere with digestion of hemoglobin by the organism. Oral doses should be taken on an empty stomach; fatty foods may promote a rapid uptake that produces cardiotoxicity. Halofantrine is not excreted renally; drug appears unchanged in feces. GI tract side effects and rashes are the most likely side effects. Cardiovascular toxicity is rare but potentially fatal. Therefore halofantrine is avoided in patients with a history of cardiac arrhythmias. The drug is also avoided in patients receiving mefloquine because the risk of cardiovascular toxicity is increased.

mefloquine

Mefloquine is used for prophylaxis or therapy of malaria caused by chloroquine-resistant *P. falciparum* or for malaria caused by *P. malariae, P. ovale,* or *P. vivax.* For radical cure of *P. ovale* or *P. vivax,* primaquine must be added to the regimen. Mefloquine is often considered as an alternative to its chemical relative quinine. Mefloquine, like quinine, acts only against the bloodborne forms of *Plasmodium* (see Table 53-2). The exact mechanism of action is unknown.

Oral absorption of mefloquine is usually in excess of 85%. The drug distributes well to many tissues, including cerebrospinal fluid and brain. Mefloquine is concentrated in red blood cells, which may contribute to the effect against the organisms harbored there.

Mefloquine is metabolized to a variable degree in liver. Elimination is slow, with drug remaining in the body for up to 1 month. This long elimination half-life allows the drug to be given as a single dose to treat malaria.

Mefloquine may cause GI tract distress, including vomiting. At higher dosages it may also cause CNS effects such as dizziness, headache, anxiety, confusion, and seizures. Visual disturbances have also been noted. Slowing of the heart rate (bradycardia) is a rare side effect. Mefloquine is not combined with chloroquine to avoid excessive CNS toxicity or with quinidine or quinine to avoid excessive cardiovascular toxicity.

pyrimethamine

Pyrimethamine in combination with quinine and sulfadoxine is used to treat chloroquine-resistant *P. falciparum*. It is also a primary agent for toxoplasmosis; see p. 601 for a full discussion of pyrimethamine.

Pyrimethamine, as it is normally used in treating chloroquine-resistant malaria, produces few side effects.

quinine

Quinine may be active against all four forms of *Plasmodium* and is used today primarily for drug-resistant malaria (see Table 53-2). In acute illness when patients require intravenous (IV) medication, the related drug quinidine (see Chapter 19) may substitute for quinine, which is too irritating to be given parenterally. Quinine should be combined with pyrimethamine and sulfadoxine for best effect.

Quinine is rapidly absorbed orally. The drug is generally well distributed throughout the body, although it does not enter the cerebrospinal fluid to a significant degree. Quinine is extensively metabolized and excreted in urine. Excretion is enhanced in acidic urine.

Quinine can produce cinchonism (quinine comes from cinchona bark). Symptoms include ringing in the ears (tinnitus), altered hearing acuity, headache, blurred vision, and diarrhea. At the dosages used today, these symptoms are usually mild. If the dosage is increased or if the patient is hypersensitive, severe cinchonism can arise. Various blood dyscrasias may occur as well.

sulfadoxine

Sulfadoxine is a sulfonamide used in combination with pyrimethamine to treat chloroquine-resistant *P. falciparum* malaria (see Table 53-2). For a full description of the properties of sulfadoxine, see Chapter 49.

THERAPEUTIC RATIONALE: SELECTED PARASITIC DISEASES

The diseases covered in this section ordinarily occur in small numbers of patients. The diseases may be related to travel *(Giardiasis)*, occur as opportunistic infections mostly in immunosuppressed hosts (cryptosporidiosis, pneumocystosis, toxoplasmosis), or be passed from host to host (trichomoniasis).

Cryptosporidiosis and Microsporidiosis

Cryptosporidia and microsporidia are protozoans that infect microvilli of host intestinal cells and cause diarrhea in several species of animals and in humans. The most common infections in humans are caused by *Cryptosporidium parvum*. The disease is passed from host to host by ingestion of thick-walled cysts; but within a single host, thin-walled cysts can release sporozoites that are invasive and invade surrounding host cells. This recycling autoinfection is more common in severely immunocompromised patients.

Cryptosporidium has spread as a waterborne infection when the highly chlorine-resistant thick-walled cysts contaminate water supplies. Runoff from feedlots where large numbers of cattle are maintained may pose a risk of contaminating water supplies unless these facilities are kept well away from the watershed area of the water supply. Animals, including calves, puppies, kittens, and rodents, harbor *Cryptosporidium* and may pass it to humans.

Many patients with acquired immunodeficiency syndrome (AIDS) have chronic, debilitating diarrhea in the late stages of their disease; for many of these patients, infection with *C. parvum* or a microsporidium is a contributing factor to the diarrhea. Patients with intact immune systems generally recover well with only supportive therapy to maintain fluid and electrolyte balance. No effective therapy for these infections exists, although macrolides have been tried. New drugs will be required to aid severely immunosuppressed patients.

Giardiasis

Giardiasis is an intestinal infection caused by the protozoan *Giardia lamblia*. This disease, which is passed between human hosts by ingestion of fecally contaminated food, may be asymptomatic in many patients. For others it may be much more severe, producing diarrhea, GI tract distress, and malabsorption. Quinacrine or metronidazole are primary drugs for *Giardiasis* in adults (Table 53-3).

Pneumocystosis

Pneumocystis carinii has been recognized as an opportunistic pathogen for several decades, but knowledge of the life cycle is incomplete. Although the organism is closely related to fungi, the clinically effective drugs are antiprotozoal agents. *P. carinii* seldom causes disease in healthy humans, but it can produce severe pulmonary disease in patients receiving immunosuppressive drugs or in patients with AIDS. Young, malnourished children are also susceptible. As many as half the patients who acquire this disease may die unless treated. Patients receiving immunosuppressive cancer chemotherapy or those receiving immunosuppressive drugs to prevent rejection of a transplanted organ usually respond well to the fixed combination of sulfamethoxazole and trimethoprim for prophylaxis or therapy (see Chapter 49).

Sulfamethoxazole and trimethoprim may be used to treat *P. carinii* pneumonia in AIDS, but AIDS patients have an unusually high incidence of serious reactions to these drugs. Pentamidine is also effective against *P. carinii* pneumonia

Table 53-3   Drugs to Treat Selected Parasitic Diseases

Generic Name	Trade Name	Administration/Dosage	Comments
atovaquone	Mepron*	ORAL: *Adults*—750 mg 2 or 3 times/day, with high-fat meal. FDA pregnancy category C.	Alternative drug for *Pneumocystis carinii* pneumonia.
furazolidone	Furoxone	ORAL: *Adults*—100 mg 4 times/day for 7-10 days.	Alternative drug for *Giardiasis*.
metronidazole	Flagyl*	ORAL: *Adults—For Giardiasis:* 2 g once daily for 3 days. *For trichomoniasis:* 2 g once, then 250 mg every 8 hr for 7 days. FDA pregnancy category B. *Children—For Giardiasis:* 5 mg/kg 3 times/day for 5-7 days. *For trichomoniasis:* 5 mg/kg every 8 hr for 7 days.	Primary drug for *Giardiosis* and for trichomoniasis.
pentamidine	Pentam Pentacarinat†	INTRAVENOUS: *Adults and children*—4 mg/kg infused over 1-2 hr once daily for up to 21 days. FDA pregnancy category C.	Primary drug for pneumocystosis.
pyrimethamine	Daraprim*	ORAL: *Adults—For toxoplasmosis in patients with acquired immunodeficiency syndrome:* Loading dose: 100-200 mg/day with 0.5-1.5 g sulfadiazine every 6 hr. Therapy continues with 50-100 mg/day with 0.5-1.5 g sulfadiazine every 6 hr. Maintenance dose: 25-50 mg daily with 250 mg-1 g of sulfadiazine every 6 hr for life. FDA pregnancy category C. *Children*—1 mg/kg once daily for 1-3 days, then 0.5 mg/kg once daily for 4-6 wk, with sulfonamide.	Primary drug for toxoplasmosis.
quinacrine	Atabrine*	ORAL: *Adults*—100 mg 3 times/day for 5-7 days. *Children*—2 mg/kg 3 times/day for 5-7 days.	Alternative drug for *Giardiasis*.
trimetrexate	Neutrexin*	INTRAVENOUS: *Adults*—45 mg/m² of body surface once daily for 21 days, with leucovorin 20-40 mg/m² every 6 hr continued throughout therapy and for 72 hr after halting trimetrexate. FDA pregnancy category D.	Alternative drug for *P. carinii* pneumonia.

*Available in Canada and the United States.
†Available in Canada only.
‡Not commercially available in the United States or Canada.

but also causes serious toxicity. Alternative therapy for *P. carinii* pneumonia in AIDS patients includes atovaquone, clindamycin with primaquine, dapsone with trimethoprim, and trimetrexate with leucovorin.

Toxoplasmosis

In the United States, toxoplasmosis is primarily acquired from ingestion of the oocyte of *Toxoplasma gondii*. The most common source of infection is cat feces. In adult humans the disease is usually mild and transitory, with symptoms resembling those of mild mononucleosis. Occasionally, the disease may involve the eyes or nervous system in adults, but congenital toxoplasmosis is usually fatal, causing severe damage to eyes, brain, and other organs of the fetus. Because of the dangers this disease poses to fetuses, many obstetricians suggest that pregnant women not handle used cat litter and avoid close contact with cats. Pyrimethamine and sulfadiazine are used in combination to treat this disease (see Table 53-3).

Toxoplasmosis is common in AIDS patients, with encephalitis causing death. Aggressive therapy with pyrimethamine and sulfonamides is usually attempted; for patients who cannot tolerate sulfonamides, other drugs such as clindamycin may be combined with pyrimethamine. Alternative agents include atovaquone or piritrexim.

Trichomoniasis

Vaginal infections caused by *Trichomonas vaginalis* occur commonly. **Trichomoniasis** is marked by watery discharge from the vagina and signs of tissue irritation. Trichomonas

may be unnoticed in the urinary tract and in the rectum, but these sites can serve as sources of infection.

Vaginal trichomoniasis may be treated with local agents applied as gels or douches. Complete cure of the sites outside the vagina and of infections in the male urinary tract may require a systemic agent. Metronidazole is the drug of choice (see Table 53-3).

THERAPEUTIC AGENTS: DRUGS TO TREAT SELECTED PARASITIC DISEASES

Primary Drugs

▼metronidazole

Metronidazole has become a primary agent for *Giardiasis* and trichomoniasis (see Table 53-3). A full discussion of the drug appears in the section on amebic disease (p. 595), for which it is also a primary agent.

pentamidine

Mechanism of Action

The action of pentamidine against *P. carinii* (see Table 53-3) is not completely understood but involves an interference with DNA function.

Pharmacokinetics

Pentamidine is given intravenously for therapy. For prophylaxis of *P. carinii* pneumonia, pentamidine may be aerosolized. When properly administered by this route, the drug is carried into the lungs in droplets small enough to be deposited into the alveoli, where *P. carinii* lodges. Therefore high concentrations are achieved at the site of infection, but because systemic absorption from lungs is low, whole body toxicity is minimized. Unfortunately, *P. carinii* infections at other sites occur because the systemic concentration of drug is low.

Pentamidine is concentrated in renal tissue and is excreted primarily in urine. Complete elimination from the body is slow, with drug appearing in urine as long as 8 weeks after therapy stops.

Uses

Pentamidine is the primary drug for *Pneumocystis pneumoniae* in patients who cannot tolerate trimethoprim and sulfamethoxazole.

Adverse Reactions and Contraindications

Patients receiving pentamidine intravenously may experience acute hypotension, cardiac arrhythmias, and death. Hypoglycemia may be severe. Long-term effects may include hyperglycemia or diabetes mellitus. Nephrotoxicity and blood dyscrasias can also develop. The incidence of side effects can vary, depending on the patient being treated. In general, AIDS patients experience more of the major and minor reactions to pentamidine than do other patients.

Pentamidine is contraindicated in patients who have had allergic reactions to either parenteral or inhaled pentamidine. Pentamidine worsens bone marrow depression, diabetes mellitus, heart disease, hypoglycemia, and renal impairment.

Toxicity

High dosages of pentamidine given rapidly by IV infusion cause dangerous hypotension.

Interactions

Pentamidine worsens the effects of bone marrow depressants or nephrotoxic drugs. The risk of pancreatitis is worsened with didanosine. Foscarnet and pentamidine significantly alter calcium and magnesium levels in blood.

pyrimethamine
Mechanism of Action

Pyrimethamine inhibits the enzyme dihydrofolate reductase in susceptible organisms, thereby blocking formation of tetrahydrofolic acid (THFA), a cofactor required for several metabolic transformations. The blocked enzyme normally converts dihydrofolic acid (DHA) to THFA. The formation of DHA may be blocked by sulfonamides (see Chapter 49). Combining pyrimethamine and a sulfonamide is an example of synergistic effects produced by two drugs acting in the same metabolic pathway. Another example is trimethoprim and sulfamethoxazole (see Chapter 49).

Pharmacokinetics

Pyrimethamine is well absorbed orally. The drug concentrates in blood cells and tissues, including liver, where it is metabolized. Metabolites are excreted in urine. Pyrimethamine appears in the milk of nursing mothers.

Uses

Pyrimethamine in combination with sulfadiazine is used to treat or suppress toxoplasmosis. Clindamycin may substitute for sulfadiazine if patients cannot tolerate sulfonamides. Pyrimethamine is an alternate agent for malaria, being used with sulfadoxine and quinine for chloroquine-resistant *P. falciparum* malaria.

Adverse Reactions and Contraindications

As it is normally used in treating chloroquine-resistant malaria, pyrimethamine produces few side effects. At higher dosages, such as those used to treat toxoplasmosis, the drug may impair host folic acid metabolism, leading to megaloblastic anemia and various other blood dyscrasias. Treatment with leucovorin (a folinic acid supplement) may be required.

Pyrimethamine is usually avoided if possible in patients with anemia, bone marrow depression, or a history of seizures.

Toxicity

Large doses of pyrimethamine may produce nausea and vomiting. Excitability and signs of CNS overstimulation, including seizures, may occur within 2 hours of taking the dose. Very high dosages may produce respiratory depression or circulatory collapse and death.

Interactions

Pyrimethamine is avoided if possible in persons also receiving other folate antagonists or bone marrow depressants to avoid excessive actions of these agents.

quinacrine
Mechanism of Action

Quinacrine has multiple metabolic effects that may account for its usefulness for *Giardiasis* (see Table 53-3).

Pharmacokinetics

Quinacrine is well absorbed from the GI tract, but when given orally, the drug induces vomiting in many patients because it is very bitter tasting. Quinacrine is well distributed throughout the body and seems to bind strongly to tissues. Patients may notice a yellow discoloration of the skin. The reaction is not a sign of jaundice but simply illustrates the distribution of this yellow-colored drug to the skin.

Uses

Quinacrine is a primary drug only for *Giardiasis*. It has been replaced by safer drugs for malaria and for helminthic infestations.

Adverse Reactions and Contraindications

Quinacrine causes few serious side effects when used for short-term treatment. Dizziness and toxic psychosis are occasionally noted. Psoriasis may be exacerbated. The most common reactions to quinacrine are headache, nausea, and vomiting. Quinacrine crosses the placenta and should not be used in pregnant patients. The drug is also avoided if possible in patients with psychosis or psoriasis because these conditions may be worsened.

Toxicity

Use of high dosages of quinacrine or prolonged use of the drug may cause aplastic anemia, corneal edema, hepatitis, or retinopathy. Life-threatening overdose is characterized by seizures, hypotension, and arrhythmias followed by cardiovascular collapse.

Interactions

Primaquine toxicity may be worsened because quinacrine may increase primaquine concentrations in blood. This rise in blood levels may result from lowered metabolism of primaquine and displacement of primaquine from tissues.

Alternative Drugs
atovaquone

Atovaquone is an oral agent used to treat *P. carinii* pneumonia in patients who cannot tolerate trimethoprim and sulfamethoxazole. The agent is also in trials against *T. gondii* in AIDS patients.

Atovaquone is absorbed poorly, and the amount of drug absorbed varies greatly from patient to patient. The half-life of the drug is between 2 and 3 days. There is little biotransformation, with most of the drug being slowly eliminated in feces.

Side effects of atovaquone observed in AIDS patients include allergic reactions (fever, skin rash) and GI tract symptoms (diarrhea, nausea, vomiting). Coughing, headache, and insomnia were also reported.

furazolidone

Furazolidone is a nitrofuran similar in action to those used to treat urinary tract infections (see Chapter 49). The drug is used orally to treat infections of the bowel. Like other nitrofurans, it does not reach high serum concentrations.

Furazolidone is metabolized by the liver. One of the breakdown products is a potent inhibitor of monoamine oxidase (MAO). Inhibition of this enzyme lowers elimination of catecholamines, which may cause hypertension. In addition, this action makes drugs such as sympathomimetics (e.g., ephedrine, phenylephrine), MAO inhibitors (e.g., pargyline), or foods rich in tyramine (e.g., cheese, beer, wine) unsafe for patients receiving furazolidone.

Furazolidone may produce hemolytic reactions, especially in patients who have G6PD deficiency. Allergies and GI tract symptoms may also occur. Patients receiving furazolidone who also drink alcohol may exhibit a disulfiram-like reaction with flushing, difficulty in breathing, and a feeling of constriction in the chest.

sulfamethoxazole and trimethoprim

Sulfamethoxazole and trimethoprim are used together to treat pneumocystosis. For a full description of these drugs, see Chapter 49.

trimetrexate

Trimetrexate is an alternate drug for *P. carinii* pneumonia. Trimetrexate acts in the same way as pyrimethamine but is a much more potent inhibitor of dihydrofolate reductase and therefore does not require coadministration of a sulfonamide. Trimetrexate requires coadministration of leucovorin, a form of folic acid that rescues mammalian cell from the antifolate effects of trimetrexate.

Trimetrexate is administered intravenously. There is hepatic metabolism of the drug, producing several metabolites, including a glucuronide. The drug and metabolites are eliminated by the kidneys.

The most common side effect with trimetrexate is neutropenia, with fever and sore throat. Other blood dyscrasias, such as thrombocytopenia or anemia, may also occur; signs include unusual bleeding, bruising, or tiredness. Less common side effects are confusion, itching, and GI tract symptoms.

THERAPEUTIC RATIONALE: DISEASES CAUSED BY HELMINTHS

Helminths include flukes, tapeworms, and roundworms that can cause disease. Table 53-4 summarizes antihelminthic agents.

Ascariasis

Ascariasis, also called roundworm infestation, is caused by ingesting the eggs of *Ascaris lumbricoides*. This common disease is spread by fecally contaminated food and water. Larvae and adult worms migrate through lungs, liver, gallbladder, or other organs and may cause severe damage. *Ascaris* infestations may be treated effectively with several agents, including albendazole, mebendazole, piperazine, and pyrantel (see Table 53-4).

Enterobiasis

Enterobiasis is pinworm infestation. Pinworms are freely passed between people living close together. Constant reinfection occurs because huge numbers of eggs are passed and they adhere to clothing, towels, and hands. The disease is usually mild, but some patients may experience pruritus ani, pruritus vulvae, or more serious symptoms.

Because pinworms tend to stay within the intestinal tract, treatment of the disease is relatively simple. Albendazole, mebendazole, and pyrantel are all nearly 100% effective after a single dose. Piperazine is also effective, but therapy continues over several days (see Table 53-4).

Table 53-4   Drugs to Treat Diseases Caused by Helminths

Generic Name	Trade Name	Administration/Dosage	Comments
albendazole	Eskazole‡ Zentel‡	ORAL: *Adults and children >2 yr*—For ascariasis, enterobiasis, hookworm, or whipworm: 400 mg once. *For threadworms or tapeworms:* 400 mg once daily for 3 days. *For trichinosis:* 400 mg twice daily for 15 days.	Alternative drug for helminthic infestations.
ivermectin	Meclizan‡	ORAL: *Adults*—Up to 200 µg/kg as single dose taken with a full glass of water on an empty stomach.	Alternative drug for threadworm infestation.
mebendazole	Vermox*	ORAL: *Adults and children >2 yr*—For enterobiasis: 100 mg once. Repeat in 2-3 wk. *For ascariasis, hookworm, or whipworm:* 100 mg in morning and evening for 3 days. Repeat if needed in 2-3 wk. FDA pregnancy category C.	Primary drug for ascariasis, enterobiasis, and hookworm or shipworm infestations.
niclosamide	Niclocide	ORAL: *Adults*—2 g as single dose or for up to 7 days, depending on kind of tapeworm. FDA pregnancy category B. *Children 11-34 kg*—1 g as single dose; may be followed by 500 mg/day for up to 6 days, depending on kind of tapeworm. *Children >34 kg*—1.5 g as single dose; may be followed by 1 g/day for up to 6 days.	Primary drug for tapeworm infestation.
piperazine	Entacyl† Piperazine	ORAL: *Adults—Tablet form:* for ascariasis: 3.5 g/day for 2 days. *For enterobiasis:* 65 mg/kg/day for 7 days. *Children—Tablet form: For ascariasis:* 75 mg/kg daily for 2 days. *For enterobiasis:* As for adults.	Alternative drug for ascariasis and enterobiasis.
praziquantel	Biltricide	ORAL: *Adults and children >4 yr*—20-25 mg/kg 2 or 3 times/day for 1 day. FDA pregnancy category B.	Alternative drug for infections caused by flatworms; primary drug for schistosomiasis.
pyrantel	Antiminth Combantrin†	ORAL: *Adults and children >2 yr*—For ascariasis or enterobiasis: 11 mg/kg as single dose; repeat in 2-3 wk if needed. Maximum daily dose 1 g.	Primary drug for ascariasis and enterobiasis.
thiabendazole	Mintezol	ORAL: *Adults and children >13.6 kg*—25 mg/kg twice daily for 2-7 days, depending on site and type of infection. FDA pregnancy category C.	Primary drug for hookworm or threadworm infestation and trichinosis.

*Available in Canada and the United States.
†Available in Canada only.
‡Not commercially available in the United States or Canada.

Whipworm Infestation

Whipworm infestation is usually asymptomatic, although large numbers of worms in small children may produce diarrhea, anemia, and cachexia. Whipworm infestations are effectively treated with mebendazole (see Table 53-4).

Threadworm Infestation

Threadworm infestation, also called strongyloidiasis, is more serious than many infestations because the worms may reproduce in humans. Larvae migrate from the intestinal wall into systemic circulation and thence return to the intestine to mature and further increase the numbers of worms in the host. Malabsorption syndrome, diarrhea, and duodenal irritation may occur.

Most drugs used against helminths are ineffective against threadworms because they live within intestinal tissue. Thiabendazole is well distributed to the tissues where this parasite lives and thus eliminates infestation. Ivermectin, a drug developed to treat river blindness and filariasis in tropical regions, is also useful against threadworms (see Table 53-4).

Hookworm Infestation

Hookworm infestation, called necatoriasis, occurs in the southern United States. Although two species of hookworms are known, most infestations encountered in the United States are caused by *Necator*. Therefore most patients may be treated with mebendazole or pyrantel. Another type of hookworm from dogs and cats produces a cutaneous lesion called creeping eruption, or cutaneous larva migrans. Thiabendazole, either topically or orally, may kill the parasites and limit allergic responses, which cause itching, burning, and skin damage (see Table 53-4).

Trichinosis

Trichinosis, or pork roundworm infestation, is uncommon today. Ingested cysts from raw or improperly cooked meat develop into adult worms in the intestine. Larvae are released into the circulation and enter muscle to form cysts. Patients experience GI tract upset, fever, muscle aches, and eosinophilia.

Trichinosis cannot yet be effectively treated. Most patients receive therapy to minimize symptoms rather than produce a cure (most patients survive the disease and carry the quiescent worms encysted in skeletal muscle for the rest of their lives). Thiabendazole, albendazole, and mebendazole have been used in some cases to try to prevent migration of worms to muscles (see Table 53-4).

Tapeworm Infestation

Tapeworms, or **cestodes,** of several types can infest humans. Beef, pork, fish, and dwarf tapeworms are all sensitive to niclosamide. Praziquantel, a drug used primarily in the tropics for schistosomiasis, may also be effective against tapeworms (see Table 53-4). All detected infestations are treated, even though they are mostly asymptomatic. Pork tapeworm infestations may become serious if reflux of eggs from the intestine allows them to reach the stomach and hatch into larvae that invade tissues.

THERAPEUTIC AGENTS: DRUGS TO TREAT DISEASES CAUSED BY HELMINTHS

Primary Agents

▼ mebendazole

Mechanism of Action

Mebendazole is an effective broad-spectrum antihelminthic agent that causes microtubules in helminths to disintegrate (see Table 53-4). This action blocks glucose uptake in sensitive helminths. Because these organisms require externally supplied glucose to maintain energy levels, blockade of glucose absorption destroys the worms.

Pharmacokinetics

Mebendazole is used orally for its action against intestinal helminths. Very little drug is absorbed into systemic circulation. The small amount of drug that enters the blood is metabolized by the liver and excreted in urine. If liver function is impaired, the small amount of drug absorbed may accumulate and cause toxicity. Fatty foods favor absorption of mebendazole.

Uses

Mebendazole is an excellent agent against a variety of helminthic diseases, including ascariasis and enterobiasis, as well as infestations caused by hookworm or whipworm (see Table 53-4).

Adverse Reactions and Contraindications

Mebendazole produces few toxic reactions. Abdominal discomfort and diarrhea may result, especially if large masses of worms are expelled.

Toxicity

High dosages of mebendazole typically cause GI tract disturbances that last for a few hours. Little systemic toxicity is expected.

Interactions

Few interactions with mebendazole exist, but patients taking mebendazole often have higher-than-normal liver enzyme (alanine aminotransferase [ALT], aspartate aminotransferase [AST]) and blood urea nitrogen (BUN) levels.

niclosamide

Mechanism of Action

Niclosamide is effective against tapeworms. These segmented flatworms are killed by a single dose of niclosamide. The dead worm segments are often digested by proteolytic agents in the gut. Therefore a cathartic may be given 1 or 2 hours after the drug has been taken to allow the dead-but-still-intact worm parts to be identified in feces. This purge is required when the tapeworm infestation is caused by the pork tapeworm. With this organism, digestion of the dead worm segments releases living eggs, which can develop in humans and cause more serious, invasive disease. The purge removes the worm segments before they rupture and prevents this complication.

Pharmacokinetics

Niclosamide is not absorbed from the bowel and exerts all of its actions within the lumen of the bowel.

Uses

Niclosamide is a primary drug for a variety of tapeworm infestations that are limited to the intestinal tract. It is not effective for cysticercosis, in which tapeworm larvae live in the intestinal wall.

Adverse Reactions and Contraindications

Niclosamide is almost without side effects because the drug is not absorbed. Some patients have mild GI tract symptoms on the day of therapy. There are no contraindications other than possible history of allergy to the drug.

Toxicity

Niclosamide overdoses are treated with laxatives and enemas to remove the drug. Systemic toxicity is unlikely.

Interactions

Niclosamide interactions with other drugs are unlikely because niclosamide is essentially unabsorbed from the bowel.

pyrantel

Mechanism of Action

Pyrantel is a depolarizing neuromuscular blocker, similar in action to succinylcholine. Pyrantel causes spastic paralysis and contraction of the muscle in worms (see Table 53-4). The parasites are eliminated from the body by normal peristalsis.

Pharmacokinetics

Pyrantel is not absorbed from the GI tract to any great extent. The small amount absorbed is excreted by the kidneys. Pyrantel produces its desired effects entirely within the lumen of the bowel.

Uses

Pyrantel is effective, when given in short courses, against a variety of worms, including roundworms (ascariasis) and pinworms (enterobiasis). Purges are not necessary adjuncts to therapy with this drug.

Adverse Reactions and Contraindications

Because pyrantel is not well absorbed after oral dosage, few systemic effects occur. Headache, muscle twitching, and dizziness may result from CNS effects of this drug. More commonly the drug causes mild GI tract upset and transient changes in liver function tests.

Toxicity

Little toxicity is expected with pyrantel because it is largely contained in the bowel.

Interactions

Piperazine may antagonize the action of pyrantel; they are not used together.

thiabendazole

Mechanism of Action

Thiabendazole is a potent and specific antihelminthic agent (see Table 53-4). Its exact mechanism of action is unknown, but it is believed to attack a metabolic process essential in helminths but not found in humans.

Pharmacokinetics

Thiabendazole is well absorbed orally, and peak blood levels occur within 1 hour of ingestion. Most of the drug is eliminated by hydroxylation and conjugation, these metabolites being the predominant forms of the drug excreted in urine. Very little unchanged drug appears in feces.

Uses

Thiabendazole is used for cutaneous or visceral larva migrans caused by hookworm and other agents, for threadworm infections, and for trichinosis. The drug must be used very soon after infestation of meat infected with *Trichinella spiralis* to lessen subsequent infection in host muscle. Thiabendazole has no effect on larvae encysted in muscle.

Adverse Reactions and Contraindications

Thiabendazole can cause a wide variety of transient, dose-related reactions. The most common effects are anorexia, nausea, vomiting, numbness in the extremities, and dizziness. A few patients experience more severe GI tract symptoms or CNS effects such as drowsiness, headache, or giddiness. Rarely, tinnitus, abnormal sensations in the eyes, or metabolic derangements occur. Although these symptoms may incapacitate a patient, it is rare for the effect to persist beyond 48 hours and most subside much sooner.

Thiabendazole alters liver function in some patients. Therefore patients with preexisting liver disease should be more carefully observed for progressive liver damage.

Patients often report a strong, unpleasant odor to their urine after thiabendazole therapy. The odor is reminiscent of that produced when asparagus is ingested. Patients may be reassured that this odor is caused by a metabolite of thiabendazole and is harmless.

Toxicity

Thiabendazole overdoses can cause significant GI tract and CNS symptoms. No specific antidote exists, but emesis or gastric lavage may help limit reactions.

Interactions

Thiabendazole significantly lowers clearance of theophylline, thereby causing theophylline to accumulate to dangerously high concentrations in blood. Serious CNS toxicity may arise.

Alternative Drugs

ivermectin

Ivermectin seems to act as an agonist at gamma-aminobutyric acid (GABA) receptors, which interferes with function of the nervous system in threadworms and other parasites (see Table 53-4). The paralyzed worms may die.

Ivermectin is given as a single oral dose that is effective for up to 1 year. The drug concentrates in the liver and fatty tissues. Excretion is primarily in feces, with little drug being found in urine.

Ivermectin may cause dizziness, fever, headache, arthralgia, myalgia, and swollen lymph nodes. Postural hypotension is rare.

piperazine

Piperazine is effective against *Ascaris* and pinworm infestations (see Table 53-4). The drug apparently blocks the action of acetylcholine on the muscles of these parasites. As a result, the worms are paralyzed and are eliminated from the bowel by normal peristaltic flow. The eliminated worms are alive.

Piperazine is well absorbed after oral administration. A portion of the drug is metabolized to various inactive products. The kidney is the primary route for excretion. Patients with impaired renal or hepatic function may be more sensitive to piperazine than other patients.

Piperazine produces few toxic effects at dosages routinely used to treat helminthic infestations. GI tract upset and occasional skin rashes have occurred. Transient neurologic signs ranging from headache and dizziness to ataxia, paresthesias, or convulsions have been seen, but severe reactions are more common with overdoses. The more severe reactions also occur in patients with renal dysfunction, who tend to accumulate the drug, and in patients with seizure disorders, who are more sensitive to the CNS effects of the drug.

praziquantel

Praziquantel interferes with muscle function in flukes and other helminths and can cause local destruction of the integument of these organisms.

Praziquantel is well absorbed after oral administration but undergoes extensive first-pass metabolism in the liver (see Chapter 1). The metabolites that are formed are excreted by the kidneys.

Praziquantel often causes mild and transient effects on the CNS. Common signs are headache, dizziness, and malaise. Most patients also report GI tract distress. The medication can cause immediate gagging or vomiting if the tablets are chewed instead of being swallowed whole.

Nursing Process Overview

Protozoal or Helminthic Therapy

Assessment

Perform a baseline assessment of the patient. Include in the patient history questions related to travel within and outside the United States or Canada, recent exposure to new food or water supplies, possible exposure through family members or school or business contacts who have had a similar illness recently, and any previous history of infection with protozoal or helminthic agents. Once drug therapy is ordered, monitor appropriate laboratory work related to potential drug side effects.

Nursing Diagnoses

- Potential knowledge deficit related to transmission of specific protozoal or helminthic infestation

Patient Outcomes

The patient will describe measures to treat and help prevent future infestations.

Planning/Implementation

Monitor the patient's overall condition, with close attention to subjective and objective data related to the infection. It may be appropriate to monitor close family members for the appearance of the infection. Refer the patient to the local health department for follow-up and for the epidemiologic tracking of health problems.

Evaluation

Many of these drugs do not cause side effects when used for a single infestation and for a short period. Before discharge, ascertain that the patient understands why and how to take the drug, what side effects may occur, what side effects require consultation with the physician, what symptoms indicate unsuccessful treatment or reinfestation, and what other measures to use for assistance in eliminating the protozoa or helminthic agent causing the problem.

Nursing Implications Summary

General Guidelines for Drugs to Treat Protozoal and Helminthic Infestations

Nursing in the Community

➤ Encourage the patient to report any unexpected sign or symptom.

➤ Remind the patient to keep these and all medications out of the reach of children. Many of the medications are available in pleasant-tasting syrups or chewable tablets, which may tempt young children.

➤ Many of the problems discussed in this chapter require treatment of an entire family. Dosages of medication for children may be quite different than adult dosages. Emphasize the importance of taking the medication as prescribed.

➤ Remind the patient to keep all health care providers informed of all drugs being used or that have been used in the preceding 6 months.

➤ Most of these drugs are not recommended for use during pregnancy unless absolutely necessary and should not be used during lactation. Question female patients about possible pregnancy before administering the drug.

➤ Reinforce to the patient the need to continue the course of medication for as long as prescribed and to avoid discontinuing medications without notifying the physician.

➤ Remind the patient to use medications only as directed. Many of these drugs are dispensed with patient information leaflets; review these with the patient before discharge.

➤ Review with the patient and family appropriate ways to treat or prevent the problem. Review as appropriate activities such as handwashing, sanitation, and cleaning infected bedding

or clothing. Be nonjudgmental and supportive. Obtain information about diseases caused by protozoa and helminths from the local health department or the Centers for Disease Control and Prevention in Atlanta. Refer the patient as appropriate to the local health department for follow-up.

➤ Suggest that the patient considering international travel contact the Centers for Disease Control and Prevention about health hazards in countries they will be visiting.

➤ If these are drugs to prevent malaria, emphasize the importance of taking the drug on a regular schedule, as prescribed. For example, if ordered once a week, instruct the patient to take doses on the same day each week. The patient should begin therapy at least 2 weeks before exposure to areas where malaria is endemic and for up to 4 weeks after leaving the area.

➤ To help avoid exposure to malaria-carrying mosquitoes, advise the patient to sleep under mosquito netting impregnated with repellent and/or in an air-conditioned room. Instruct the patient to wear long-sleeved shirts, long pants, and socks, especially when outside. Mosquitoes are out from dusk to dawn. Instruct the patient to use mosquito repellent on exposed skin surfaces during this time and limit outdoor activities. Instruct the patient to use mosquito sprays in living quarters during evening and nighttime hours to kill mosquitoes. These same guidelines apply if patients are trying to avoid exposure to sandflies (which carry kala-azar) or tsetse flies (which carry African sleeping sickness).

➤ For treatment of pinworms: Pinworms are easily passed among household members, so the entire family may be

Nursing Implications Summary—cont'd

treated. Instruct the patient(s) to take all doses of medication as ordered. Instruct the patient(s) to wear pajamas and underwear to sleep during treatment and to wash all bedding and pajamas after treatment to prevent reinfection.

➤ For treatment of hookworms: Infection with hookworms may cause anemia. If the patient is to take medication to treat anemia, emphasize the importance of taking the iron preparation as prescribed and continuing it for 3 to 6 months after treatment for hookworms.

➤ For treatment of tapeworms: Review with the patient the importance of inspecting meat carefully and cooking it thoroughly.

➤ For treatment of thread worms: Review the importance of cooking vegetables thoroughly before eating to destroy thread worms.

INDIVIDUAL DRUGS

➤ Any drug not listed in the following is discussed fully in the text or is similar to others in its class.

iodoquinol

Drug Administration

➤ Assess allergy to this drug, chloroxine, clioquinol, iodine, pamaquine, pentaquine, and primaquine.

➤ For treatment of amebiasis, assess signs of dehydration, intake and output, weight, abdominal pain, and diarrhea.

➤ Assess and monitor neurologic function. Assess for visual changes. Inspect for skin changes, rashes, and skin discoloration.

Nursing in the Community

➤ Review anticipated benefits and possible side effects of drug therapy with the patient.

➤ Instruct the patient to take doses after meals. Tablets may be crushed and mixed with applesauce or chocolate syrup. Review with the patient how to crush tablets if necessary.

➤ Because iodoquinol can interfere with thyroid function tests, remind the patient to keep all health care providers informed for at least 6 months after therapy with iodoquinol is completed that this drug has been taken.

➤ Caution the patient to avoid driving or operating hazardous equipment if visual changes occur and to notify the physician if these changes do occur.

metronidazole

Drug Administration

➤ When metronidazole is used for trichomoniasis, assess for vaginal discharge and itching and irritation of the bladder, urethra, or vagina.

➤ When metronidazole is used for amebiasis, assess for signs of dehydration, intake and output, weight, abdominal pain, and diarrhea. Monitor stool examination.

➤ When metronidazole is used for *Giardiasis,* assess diarrhea, characteristics of stool, and abdominal cramping.

➤ Superinfection can occur. Assess for *Candida* overgrowth in mouth or vagina; assess for diarrhea.

Intravenous metronidazole

➤ Review the manufacturer's instructions about reconstitution of IV doses. Do not use syringes with aluminum needles or hubs. Administer prepared dose over at least 1 hour; dose may also be given as a continuous infusion. Instruct the patient to report redness or pain in the extremity to the physician. Monitor serum drug levels if available.

Nursing in the Community

➤ Review anticipated benefits and possible side effects of drug therapy with the patient.

➤ Instruct the patient to take oral doses with meals or a snack to lessen gastric irritation.

➤ Instruct the patient to avoid drinking alcohol while taking oral, IV, or vaginal metronidazole. See the Patient Problems box in Chapter 57 on disulfiram-like reactions.

➤ See the Patient Problems boxes on vaginal infections (Chapter 51) and dry mouth (Chapter 23).

➤ For vaginal dryness, suggest that women use a commercially available lubricant designed for vaginal mucosa.

➤ Warn the patient to avoid driving or operating hazardous equipment if visual changes or dizziness occurs and to notify the physician if these symptoms do occur.

➤ Warn the patient that urine may temporarily turn reddish brown because of the drug.

➤ Tactfully assess changes in libido. Provide emotional support as appropriate. Remind the patient not to discontinue drug therapy without notifying the physician.

➤ Metronidazole is available in vaginal tablet, gel, and cream formulations. Instruct the patient in the correct use of the prescribed medication. The patient should avoid sexual intercourse during treatment.

➤ When metronidazole is used to treat trichomoniasis, the physician may wish to treat the patient and the sexual partner. The physician also may recommend that the patient use a condom during sexual intercourse until the infection clears.

➤ Metronidazole is available in a topical gel form to treat rosacea. Instruct patients to avoid getting gel into the eyes. Instruct patients to wash the affected area with a mild cleanser, rinse well, and pat dry. Apply gel to affected areas with fingertips, then wash hands. The gel may cause slight burning or stinging for a minute or two, but pronounced or persistent discomfort should be reported to the physician. Patients may continue to use cosmetics during treatment but should use "oil-free" brands, apply them lightly, and use them only occasionally.

diloxanide

Drug Administration/Nursing in the Community

➤ When diloxanide is used for amebiasis, assess for signs of dehydration, intake and output, weight, abdominal pain, and diarrhea. Monitor stool examination.

Continued

Nursing Implications Summary—cont'd

➤ Encourage the patient to return for regular follow-up to monitor for drug effectiveness.

➤ Remind the patient to take drugs as prescribed for the full course of therapy.

4-Aminoquinolines (chloroquine and hydroxychloroquine)
Drug Administration

➤ When 4-aminoquinolines are used for malaria, assess myalgia, fatigue, malaise, chills or history of shaking chills, and lung sounds. Monitor blood smear to confirm malaria.

➤ Assess for visual changes; signs of depression such as withdrawal, lack of interest in personal appearance, insomnia, or anorexia; and hearing acuity.

➤ Monitor blood pressure and electrocardiographic (ECG) changes (when patients are receiving long-term therapy), complete blood count (CBC) and differential, platelet count, serum creatinine level, and BUN level.

➤ IV chloroquine: Review manufacturer's insert for instructions about dilution. Administer dose over at least 4 hours.

Nursing in the Community

➤ Review common side effects with the patient. Instruct the patient to report signs of blood dyscrasia, including pallor, malaise, sore throat, fever, and unexplained bleeding or bruising, to the physician.

➤ Because many CNS side effects, including personality changes, have been reported, instruct family members to report any persistent personality changes, apathy, agitation, or irritation.

➤ Instruct the patient to notify the physician if changes in vision or difficulty in reading develop. Caution the patient to avoid driving or operating hazardous equipment if visual changes occur and to notify the physician if these changes do occur. Encourage the patient receiving long-term therapy to have periodic ophthalmic examinations.

➤ Instruct the patient to notify the physician if hearing loss develops.

➤ Instruct the patient to take doses with milk, meals, or a snack to lessen gastric irritation and to report persistent or severe gastric irritation to the physician.

➤ These drugs are especially toxic to children. Remind the patient to keep medication out of the reach of children.

➤ See the general guidelines for information about malaria prophylaxis.

➤ If used to treat arthritis, lupus, or other chronic problems, instruct the patient that weeks of therapy may be necessary to see improvement. Emphasize the importance of returning to the physician regularly for follow-up.

primaquine
Drug Administration/Nursing in the Community

➤ When used for malaria, assess myalgia, fatigue, malaise, chills or history of shaking chills, and lung sounds. Monitor blood smear to confirm malaria.

➤ Monitor CBC and differential and platelet count.

➤ Warn the patient to avoid driving or operating hazardous

equipment if visual changes occur and to notify the physician if these changes do occur.

➤ Instruct the patient to take doses with meals or antacids to reduce gastric distress and to notify the physician if gastric distress is severe or persistent.

➤ Instruct the patient to report the development of fever, dark urine, anorexia, excessive fatigue, and bluish color of fingernails, lips, or skin. Instruct the patient to report any new side effect to the physician.

halofantrine
Drug Administration/Nursing in the Community

➤ When used for malaria, assess myalgia, fatigue, malaise; chills or history of shaking chills, and lung sounds. Monitor blood smear to confirm malaria.

➤ Instruct the patient to take doses on an empty stomach.

➤ See the general guidelines for information about malaria prophylaxis.

mefloquine
Nursing in the Community

➤ When mefloquine is used for malaria, assess myalgia, fatigue, malaise, chills or history of shaking chills, and lung sounds. Monitor blood smear to confirm malaria.

➤ Instruct the patient to take doses with a full glass (8 ounces) of water and with food.

➤ Caution the patient to avoid driving or operating hazardous equipment if visual changes, vertigo, or light-headedness occurs and to notify the physician if these symptoms do occur.

➤ Instruct the patient to take doses of mefloquine at least 12 hours after taking the last dose of quinidine or quinine if both drugs are prescribed.

➤ See the general guidelines for information about malaria prophylaxis.

pyrimethamine
Drug Administration

➤ When pyrimethamine is used for malaria, assess myalgia, fatigue, malaise, chills or history of shaking chills, and lung sounds. Monitor blood smear to confirm malaria.

➤ When pyrimethamine is used for toxoplasmosis, assess rash, jaundice, weakness, and lung sounds.

➤ When pyrimethamine is combined with sulfadoxine (Fansidar), assess for allergy to sulfonamides, furosemide, thiazide diuretics, sulfonylureas, and carbonic anhydrase inhibitors.

➤ Assess and monitor neurologic status; assess for skin changes and visual acuity.

➤ Monitor CBC and differential and platelet count.

Nursing in the Community

➤ Remind the patient to report any new side effects to the physician.

➤ Warn the patient to avoid driving or operating hazardous equipment if excessive fatigue develops and to notify the physician if this symptom develops.

Nursing Implications Summary—cont'd

➤ See the Patient Problems boxes on bleeding tendencies (Chapter 54) and agranulocytosis (Chapter 20).

➤ Instruct the patient to take oral doses with meals if desired. Tablets may be crushed to make a suspension; consult the pharmacist. Instruct the patient to notify the physician if GI symptoms are severe or persistent. Emphasize to the patient the importance of taking doses at regularly spaced intervals and trying not to forget any doses.

➤ Pyrimethamine may cause anemia, which is treated with leucovorin (see Chapter 22).

quinine
Drug Administration

➤ When quinine is used for malaria, assess myalgia, fatigue, malaise, chills or history of shaking chills, and lung sounds. Monitor blood smear to confirm malaria.

➤ Assess and monitor neurologic status; assess for cinchonism (see text). Be alert to symptoms of hypoglycemia, such as pallor, perspiration, tachycardia, palpitations, nervousness, emotional changes, weakness, trembling, hunger, headache, blurred vision, and incoherent speech. Monitor blood glucose levels.

➤ Monitor CBC and differential, platelet count, prothrombin time, partial thromboplastin time, and liver function tests.

Intravenous Administration (quinidine gluconate)

➤ Dilute as directed. Administer a loading dose over 1 to 2 hours, while monitoring for hypotension and widening of the QRS interval. A constant infusion of a smaller dose is administered after the loading dose. Keep the patient supine until blood pressure is stable. Keep siderails up. Monitor ECG changes. See Chapter 19.

Nursing in the Community

➤ Instruct the patient to report any new side effects to the physician.

➤ Warn the patient to avoid driving or operating hazardous equipment if visual changes occur and to notify the physician if these changes do occur.

➤ Instruct the patient to take doses with meals or a snack to reduce gastric irritation. Warn diabetic patients to monitor blood glucose levels carefully.

sulfadoxine
➤ See Chapter 49.

pentamidine
Drug Administration

➤ For *P. carinii* pneumonia, assess vital signs, lung sounds, cough, dyspnea on exertion, and weight loss. Monitor blood gases and/or pulmonary function tests if available.

➤ With aerosolized doses, toxicity is less common. Monitor pulse, blood pressure, and respiratory rate. Auscultate lung sounds.

➤ With systemic administration, assess for signs of hypoglycemia, such as pallor, perspiration, tachycardia, palpitations, nervousness, irritability, weakness, trembling, hunger,

headache, blurred vision, cycloplegia, incoherent speech, emotional changes, and fatigue. Monitor blood glucose levels.

➤ Assess for skin changes. Monitor intake and output and weight.

➤ Monitor serum creatinine and BUN levels, CBC and differential, liver function tests, and serum electrolyte level.

➤ Warn the patient that IM injections may cause a burning sensation and tenderness at the injection site. Use meticulous technique to avoid abscess formation.

Parenteral Administration

➤ Review the manufacturer's insert for current guidelines. Keep the patient in a supine position. Monitor blood pressure before administering pentamidine and at 5- to 15-minute intervals. Monitor ECG changes if the patient's condition warrants it. Administer IV doses over 60 minutes. Monitor IV administration sites and instruct the patient to report pain or irritation.

➤ Have drugs, equipment, and personnel available to treat acute allergic reactions in the setting where pentamidine is administered.

Nursing in the Community

➤ Instruct the patient to report any unexpected side effects.

➤ Review the Patient Problems boxes in Chapter 54 on bleeding tendencies and leukopenia. These problems are more common with the systemic form of pentamidine.

➤ For inhalation pentamidine: If the patient using the inhalation form of pentamidine and is also supposed to use an inhalation bronchodilator, instruct the patient to use the bronchodilator first, then wait 5 to 10 minutes before using the pentamidine unless otherwise instructed by the physician. Instruct the patient not to mix any drugs with the pentamidine for inhalation.

➤ Instruct the patient to avoid smoking while receiving inhalation therapy.

➤ Inhalation pentamidine may cause a metallic or unpleasant taste in the mouth. Instruct the patient to try sucking on hard candy to relieve this side effect.

➤ Instruct the patient to report the development of difficulty breathing or swallowing, skin rash, wheezing, nausea and vomiting, pain in the upper abdomen or chest, chills, cold sweats, headache, shakiness, or unusual fatigue to the physician.

quinacrine
Drug Administration

➤ When quinacrine is used for *Giardiasis,* assess diarrhea, characteristics of stool, and abdominal cramping.

➤ Assess and monitor mental status; assess for skin and vision changes. Monitor weight in patients receiving long-term therapy.

➤ Monitor CBC and differential, platelet count, and liver function tests. Monitor stool examinations for *Giardiasis.*

Nursing in the Community

➤ Remind the patient to report any new side effects to the physician.

Continued

Nursing Implications Summary—cont'd

➤ Warn the patient to avoid driving or operating hazardous equipment if dizziness or confusion develops and to notify the physician if these symptoms occur.

➤ Instruct the patient to notify the physician if GI tract symptoms are severe or persistent.

➤ Encourage the patient to have regular ophthalmic examinations if recommended by the physician.

➤ Warn the patient that this drug may cause a yellowish discoloration of the eyes, skin, or urine. This discoloration is harmless and will clear when the course of drug therapy is over. Review the drug package insert for information about treating tapeworms.

➤ Instruct the patient to take doses after meals with a full glass (8 ounces) of water, juice, or tea. Tablets may be crushed and mixed with jam, honey, chocolate syrup, or other sweet foods to mask the bitter taste. Instruct the patient to mix with only a small amount of food and take all the dose as ordered.

atovaquone
Drug Administration/Nursing in the Community

➤ For *P. carinii* pneumonia, assess vital signs, lung sounds, cough, dyspnea on exertion, and weight loss. Monitor blood gases and/or pulmonary function tests if available. Monitor CBC and liver function tests.

➤ For toxoplasmosis, assess rash, jaundice, lung sounds, and weakness.

➤ Instruct the patient to take doses with a balanced meal. If needed, tablets may be crushed to make them easier to swallow.

➤ Emphasize the importance of taking all doses, as prescribed, even if feeling better. Teach patients that tablets and oral suspension cannot be used interchangeably without a change in dose or frequency. For measuring the oral suspension, instruct the patient to use the calibrated measuring device supplied by the pharmacist.

furazolidone
Drug Administration/Nursing in the Community

➤ Assess for nausea and vomiting. If persistent or severe, notify the physician. For *Giardiasis,* assess diarrhea, abdominal cramping, and characteristics of stool.

➤ Review information on nitrofurans in Chapter 49.

➤ Review the Patient Problems box in Chapter 57 on disulfiram-like reactions. Instruct the patient to avoid alcohol while taking furazolidone and for 4 days after completing therapy.

➤ Review the Dietary Considerations box in Chapter 59 on tyramine. Effects of tyramine may persist for up to 2 weeks after finishing the course of furazolidone.

➤ Instruct patients to limit caffeine-containing foods or drinks, such as chocolate, coffee, tea, and cola, while taking furazolidone and for up to 2 weeks after the drug is discontinued.

➤ Instruct diabetic patients to monitor blood glucose levels carefully; furazolidone may cause hypoglycemia.

➤ Instruct the patient that urine may be dark yellow or brown while taking this drug.

➤ Doses may be taken with food. For measuring the oral suspension, instruct the patient to use the calibrated measuring device supplied by the pharmacist.

➤ There are many drug interactions with furazolidone. Remind the patient to keep all health care providers informed of all drugs being taken.

trimetrexate
Drug Administration/Nursing in the Community

➤ For *P. carinii* pneumonia, assess vital signs, lung sounds, cough, dyspnea on exertion, and weight loss. Monitor blood gases and/or pulmonary function tests if available. Monitor CBC and liver function tests.

➤ Review the manufacturer's insert for current information. Administer a single dose over 60 to 90 minutes. Flush the IV line before and after administration with D5W. Handle with caution, using the same precautions as with cancer chemotherapy drugs: prepare under a laminar flow hood, wear gown and gloves, and dispose of all IV equipment in specially labeled containers.

➤ See Chapter 22 for information about leucovorin.

➤ See the Patient Problems boxes in Chapter 54 on bleeding tendencies and leukopenia.

mebendazole
Drug Administration

➤ For treatment of roundworms (ascariasis), assess lung sounds and cough, fever, anemia, weight loss, vomiting, and abdominal discomfort.

➤ For treatment of hookworms or threadworms, assess rash or vesicular eruption, cough and lung sounds, abdominal pain, diarrhea, and fever.

➤ For treatment of tapeworms, assess abdominal discomfort, anemia, and weight loss.

➤ For treatment of pinworms, assess oral or perianal itching or irritation, especially at night. Monitor laboratory result of cellophane tape swabbing of anal region.

➤ For treatment of whipworms, assess characteristics of diarrhea and stool, anemia, and weight loss.

Nursing in the Community

➤ Instruct the patient to report any unexpected signs or symptoms to the physician.

➤ Warn the patient to avoid driving or operating hazardous equipment if visual changes occur and to notify the physician if these changes occur.

➤ Instruct the patient to notify the physician if severe or persistent GI tract symptoms occur.

➤ Tablets may be chewed, swallowed whole, or crushed and mixed with food. Instruct the patient to take doses with high-fat meals, such as with whole milk or ice cream.

Nursing Implications Summary—cont'd

niclosamide

Drug Administration

➤ For treatment of tapeworms, assess abdominal discomfort, anemia, and weight loss.

Nursing in the Community

➤ Warn the patient to avoid driving or operating hazardous equipment if visual changes occur and to notify the physician if these changes occur.

➤ Instruct the patient to report any unexpected finding to the physician.

➤ Instruct the patient to take doses after a light meal to avoid gastric upset.

➤ Instruct the patient to chew tablets well before swallowing. For small children, instruct the parent to crush the tablet and mix with water to form a paste.

pyrantel

Drug Administration

➤ For treatment of roundworms (ascariasis), assess lung sounds and cough, fever, anemia, weight loss, vomiting, and abdominal discomfort.

➤ For treatment of pinworms, assess anal or perianal itching or irritation, especially at night. Monitor laboratory result of cellophane tape swabbing of anal region.

Nursing in the Community

➤ Instruct the patient to notify the physician if new side effects develop.

➤ To measure doses of the oral suspension, instruct the patient to shake bottle well, then use the calibrated measuring device supplied by the pharmacist.

➤ Instruct the patient to avoid driving or operating hazardous equipment if dizziness or drowsiness develops.

thiabendazole

Drug Administration

➤ For treatment of hookworms or thread worms, assess rash or vesicular eruption, cough and lung sounds, abdominal pain, diarrhea, and fever.

➤ For treatment of tapeworms, assess abdominal discomfort, anemia, and weight loss.

➤ For treatment of whipworms, assess characteristics of diarrhea and stool, anemia, and weight loss.

➤ For treatment of trichinosis, assess rash, periorbital edema, difficulty breathing and lung sounds, abdominal discomfort and diarrhea, photophobia, mental status examination, fever, weakness, headache, edema, and pain in the muscles.

➤ For cutaneous larva migrans, assess rash or vesicular eruption, cough and lung sounds, abdominal pain, diarrhea, and fever.

➤ Monitor pulse and blood pressure.

➤ Monitor CBC and white blood cell differential, serum creatinine and BUN levels, liver function tests, and blood glucose levels.

Nursing in the Community

➤ Instruct the patient to report any new side effects to the physician.

➤ Warn diabetic patients to monitor blood glucose levels carefully.

➤ Warn the patient to avoid driving or operating hazardous equipment if dizziness or visual changes occur and to notify the physician if these symptoms occur.

➤ Instruct the patient to take doses after meals or a snack to lessen gastric irritation. Instruct the patient taking the chewable tablets to chew or crush tablets before swallowing them.

➤ Inform the patient that this drug may cause urine to have a temporary, harmless odor for up to 24 hours.

➤ For topical preparations, instruct the patient to apply the medicine directly to the infected area and in a large circle around the area, up to 2 to 3 inches in each direction.

ivermectin

Drug Administration

➤ For treatment of hookworms or thread worms, assess rash or vesicular eruption, cough and lung sounds, abdominal pain, diarrhea, and fever.

Nursing in the Community

➤ Caution the patient to avoid driving or operating hazardous equipment if visual changes occur and to notify the physician if these changes occur.

➤ Review the Patient Problems box in Chapter 13 on orthostatic hypotension.

➤ Instruct the patient to notify the physician if any unexpected signs or symptoms develop.

piperazine

Drug Administration

➤ For treatment of roundworms (ascariasis), assess lung sounds and cough, fever, anemia, weight loss, vomiting, and abdominal discomfort.

➤ For treatment of pinworms, assess anal or perianal itching or irritation, especially at night. Monitor laboratory result of cellophane tape swabbing of anal region.

Nursing in the Community

➤ Instruct the patient to report any unexpected signs or symptoms to the physician.

➤ Instruct the patient to notify the physician if GI tract symptoms are severe or persistent.

➤ Instruct the patient to take doses after meals or a snack to lessen gastric irritation. Instruct the patient to prepare granules for oral solution by dissolving the contents of 1 packet of granules in 2 ounces of water, milk, or fruit juice. Drink all the liquid to get the full dose.

praziquantel

Drug Administration

➤ For treatment of schistosomiasis, assess rash and fever. Monitor stool and urine examination.

➤ For treatment of tapeworms, assess abdominal discomfort, anemia, and weight loss.

Continued

Nursing Implications Summary—cont'd

Nursing in the Community

➤ Warn the patient to avoid driving or operating hazardous equipment if visual changes occur and to notify the physician if these changes occur.

➤ Instruct the patient not to chew tablets but to swallow them whole. Suggest that the patient take doses during meals to avoid a bitter taste in the mouth.

➤ Instruct the patient to notify the physician if unexpected signs or symptoms develop.

CHAPTER REVIEW

Application

1. Why is metronidazole effective for amebic infections outside the intestine but iodoquinol is not?
2. What parasitic diseases other than amebiasis are treated with metronidazole?
3. Why should patients receiving metronidazole avoid ethyl alcohol?
4. Name two sites where plasmodia exist in the human body.
5. How is the use of the 8-aminoquinoline primaquine different from the uses of chloroquine?
6. What toxicity is associated with primaquine?
7. What drugs may be used for chloroquine-resistant *P. falciparum* malaria?
8. What type of disease is produced by *Giardia lamblia*?
9. What patients are most at risk from toxoplasmosis?
10. What patient group is most likely to contract pneumocystosis?
11. What two routes are used for pentamidine administration? Why?
12. What is the mechanism of action of mebendazole?
13. How does the tissue distribution of mebendazole affect mebendazole use?
14. What is the tissue distribution of orally administered niclosamide?
15. What is the mechanism of action of pyrantel?
16. What patient education is most important to help patients with enterobiasis avoid reinfection?
17. What transient effects follow thiabendazole administration?

Critical Thinking

1. How does the tissue distribution of the 4-aminoquinolines increase the usefulness of the drugs in treating malaria?
2. What toxicity is associated with the 4-aminoquinolines? How should you assess for these?
3. What is the rationale for combining trimethoprim with sulfamethoxazole or combining pyrimethamine with sulfadiazine to treat parasitic infections?
4. What toxicity is associated with pyrimethamine? How should you assess for it?

References

Compton J: Malaria in the emergency department, *J Emerg Nurs* 23(2):120-123, 1997.

Danis DM: Indigenous malaria transmission, *J Emerg Nurs* 23(1):56, 1997.

Finn L: Threadworm infections, *Commun Nurse* 2(7):Nurse Prescriber: 39, 1996.

Selleck CS: Identifying and treating bacterial vaginosis, *Am J Nurs* 97(9):16AAA-16BBB, 16DDD, 1997.

Introduction to Cancer Chemotherapy

OBJECTIVES

After studying this chapter, you should be able to do the following:

- *Explain what is meant by the term cancer.*
- *Explain the difference between tumor promoters and carcinogens.*
- *Explain the cell cycle.*
- *Discuss the principle of selective toxicity as it applies to cancer.*
- *Develop nursing care interventions for the patient with depressed white blood cell production, bleeding tendencies, or stomatitis.*

CHAPTER OVERVIEW

Cancer occurs when normal cells become transformed by chemicals, viruses, or radiation and thereby become resistant to appropriate regulation of cell division. This chapter considers cell proliferation in normal and cancerous tissues. This presentation forms the basis for understanding the principle of selective toxicity as applied to cancer.

THERAPEUTIC RATIONALE: CANCER

Diseases Called Cancer

The public thinks of cancer as a single disease, but it is a large family of related diseases that differ from one another in characteristic disease patterns (Table 54-1). For example, skin cancer runs a different clinical course than lung cancer. Skin cancer, lung cancer, and many other forms of cancer may affect diverse types of patients, but other cancers such as Wilms' tumor, Kaposi's sarcoma, and choriocarcinoma tend to strike a certain age and sex of patient (see Table 54-1).

Cancers may be more formally grouped and categorized according to the cells or tissue of origin (Table 54-2). For example, carcinomas all arise from epithelial cells, but because epithelial cells may be found in many organs or sites in the body, carcinomas likewise can be found in many sites, including lungs, liver, or kidneys. This classification scheme also allows subdivisions within the categories of cancer. For example, leukemias can arise from any of the various cells within bone marrow. Therefore myelogenous leukemias (arising from myeloid tissue in the marrow), lymphocytic leukemias (arising from cells that form lymphocytes), and other forms of the disease exist (see Table 54-2).

One reason for thinking of cancer in terms of its cell of origin is that cancerous cells may retain some properties of the parental cells. For example, carcinomas of the breast or of the prostate may retain some of the hormone receptors normally present in the cell of origin. Chemotherapy may thus be able to be directed to these cancerous cells by using the retained hormone receptors as targets. Likewise lymphomas may retain the receptors that recognize

Table 54-1	Selected Neoplastic Diseases
Disease	**Characteristics**
Burkitt's lymphoma	Rapidly growing tumor of lymphoid tissue; highly responsive to chemotherapy.
Choriocarcinoma (gestational trophoblastic tumors)	Rapidly growing tumor of embryonic cells; seeded in mother during abortion, childbirth, or after hydatidiform mole; highly responsive to chemotherapy.
Ewing's sarcoma	Rapidly growing tumor most often found in children; responsive to combination of surgery, radiation, and chemotherapy in early stages.
Hodgkin's disease	Tumor of lymph nodes, spleen, and other lymphoid tissue; highly responsive to chemotherapy.
Kaposi's sarcoma	Highly malignant, metastasizing tumor usually noted on skin of extremities. Although characteristic of AIDS patients, tumor is also seen in older men without AIDS.
Lymphocytic leukemia	Cancer of lymphoid tissue causes excess lymphocytes or lymphoblasts in blood; response to therapy is best in acute form of disease.
Myelogenous leukemia	Cancer of myeloid tissue leads to excess granular polymorphonuclear leukocytes in blood; response to therapy not as good as in lymphocytic leukemia.
Wilms' tumor	Rapidly growing tumor of children; highly responsive to combination of surgery, radiation, and chemotherapy.

AIDS, Acquired immunodeficiency syndrome.

Table 54-2	Tissue of Origin for Types of Cancer
Cancer	**Tissue of Origin**
Carcinoma	Epithelial cells (e.g., skin and mucous membranes of lung and gastrointestinal tract)
Leukemia	Blood-forming organ (e.g., bone marrow or lymphoid tissue)
Lymphoma	Lymphoid tissue
Melanoma	Pigmented skin cells
Myeloma	Bone marrow
Sarcoma	Connective tissue (e.g., bone, cartilage)

glucocorticoid hormones; thus lymphomas may be suppressed by these hormones in the same way as normal lymphoid tissue.

Common Properties of Cancer

Clinical Observations

The clinical course of many cancers illustrates some unique properties of cancer cells. For example, cancer cells lose the normal property of contact inhibition. **Contact inhibition** prevents normal cells from dividing when they are crowded together, but cancer cells continue to divide even when the pressure of the surrounding cell mass is considerable. In certain tissues, as the cancer proliferates, it forms a solid mass and crowds surrounding normal tissue as the mass, or tumor, grows. In other tissues, such as bone marrow, growth of the neoplastic cells is more diffuse, but ultimately normal tissue is overwhelmed and crowded out by the uncontrolled proliferation of the cancerous tissues.

A second unique property of cancers is their ability to spread far from the original site. In this process, cancer cells separate from the original mass and move directly or are carried by blood or lymph to distant sites. There the cells lodge in healthy tissue and begin to divide, thus producing a **metastasis** (secondary tumor). Tumors have been produced in experimental animals with single cancer cells. This prop-

erty of cancer cells explains why cure of malignancies may require destruction of every cancer cell in the body.

The single defining property of cancer cells is that they are no longer responsive to appropriate signals controlling cell proliferation. Thus an injured liver may regenerate to replace lost tissue but the process is self-limited and stops after a certain amount of tissue is replaced. In contrast, a liver tumor proliferates continuously to the point of crowding out and destroying normal surrounding tissue. The proliferation of these cancerous cells is not self-limited and will continue so long as the host survives. The next section presents normal cell proliferation and explains how cells can escape from normal regulation of this process.

Regulation of Cell Division

The **cell cycle** is the programmed sequence of events that occur during cell division. The cycle is divided into several segments according to the processes that occur during that phase. The first phase of the cycle, termed G_1, involves primarily RNA synthesis (Figure 54-1). This phase is crucial to the fate of the cell and is regulated by extracellular signals. Up to a certain point in G_1, if these external signals are removed, the cell reverts to the resting phase (G_0) and does not divide. At some time late in G_1, cells pass a control point and become committed to cell division, even if the external signals are withdrawn. This transition from G_1 is regulated by proteins called **cyclins,** which act on cyclin-dependent protein kinases (CDKs). The activation of these proteins increases the activity of several enzymes crucial for DNA synthesis. This process sets the stage for the next phase in the cell cycle, the S phase, during which DNA synthesis occurs. DNA is the nucleic acid that contains the genetic information for the cell. When DNA synthesis is complete, the cell contains twice the amount of DNA found in a nondividing cell. At this point RNA and protein synthesis increase, and the cell enters the G_2 phase. At the end of this phase the cell contains enough material to form two complete cells, and mitosis begins.

In **mitosis** DNA condenses to form chromosomes. As mitosis begins the cell has two copies of each chromosome. To separate these pairs so that one copy of each chromosome goes into each daughter cell, the cell forms microtubules that

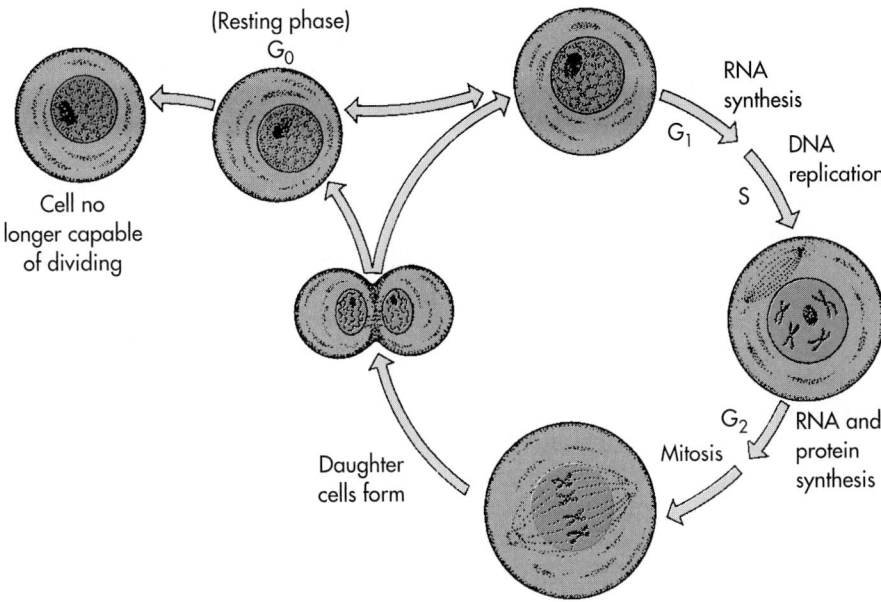

Figure 54-1 Proliferative cycle of mammalian cells. In actively dividing cells, metabolic processes required for cell division take place at different times during cycle. DNA synthesis precedes messenger RNA and protein synthesis; these processes must be complete before mitosis, or cell division, can occur. Because of metabolic differences, cells at different phases of cycle have different sensitivities to many drugs used to control cancer.

are organized into the mitotic spindle. Without the mitotic spindle to pull the chromosomes into opposite ends of the cell, reproduction would halt. Once the chromosomes have been successfully segregated into two complete sets, division is completed by closing the cell membrane to divide the mother cell into two daughter cells.

After cell division a cell may immediately reenter the reproductive cycle or it may become temporarily nonreproductive. In this nonreproductive phase, called G_0, the cell only repairs existing DNA and synthesizes only the RNA and protein needed for maintenance of the cell. A cell in the G_0 phase may become altered so that it is no longer capable of dividing, or after some time, it may enter phase G_1 and divide again.

The control point between G_1 and S phase is regulated by cyclins and CDKs, as noted previously. This transition point is also the focus of another regulatory system that serves as a brake to the cyclin system that drives proliferation. This braking or checkpoint system involves a gene called p53. This gene seems not to be required for cell division but becomes necessary when the cell's DNA is damaged. Under these conditions p53 interferes with the signals that would drive the cell through the G_1-S phase transition point, so the cell becomes arrested at the G_1 phase. This delay gives the cell time to repair its DNA before it is replicated. If DNA is too badly damaged, p53 may induce **apoptosis,** or programmed cell death. Thus the overall action of p53 is to protect the accuracy of gene replication during cell division and ensure that only healthy cells with intact genomes survive and divide. Because of its function to remove genetically damaged

cells, which may of course include cancer cells, the p53 gene is sometimes called a tumor suppressor gene.

Origin and Molecular Basis of Cancer

Carcinogenesis is the process by which a normal cell is transformed into a cancerous cell. Agents called carcinogens may start this transformation by causing mutations or chromosomal translocations. Cells at this stage may divide, die, or remain in the resting state.

Tumor promoters are agents that do not necessarily affect the DNA of a cell but in some other way can influence the fate of a transformed cell. For example, some chemicals can promote division of the altered cell and may cause it to become fully malignant.

Cell division in cancer is perturbed so that cells seem to divide independent of any external signal. Significant genetic changes are associated with this property, including the expression of oncogenes. **Oncogenes** are genes that are activated in human cancers and override normal regulation of gene expression and drive cell proliferation. These genes are very similar to normal genes encoding proteins that transmit growth stimulatory messages. The oncogenes code for altered forms of these regulatory proteins so that the message to divide is powerful and constant in a cancer cell.

More than 100 oncogenes have been recognized in human cancers. Some of these oncogenes involve positive regulators such as Ras and Myc. Ras is a protein that occurs early in the cascade that ultimately increases the formation of cyclin D1, which drives cells through the G_1-S phase transition. Myc is a protein from the latter stages of that same pathway. If Ras or Myc are altered so that the signal to produce cyclins is continuous, the cell may be driven to divide continuously.

Oncogenes may also involve tumor suppressor genes. For example, some disruption of the function of p53 has been noted in up to half of all human cancers, making these mutations the most common in human disease.

How Can Cancer be Controlled?

Host Responses

In theory, one cancer cell left living after therapy can cause recurrence of cancer. In contrast, antibacterial therapy can be successful if bacteria are stopped from growing long enough for the immune system to attack and eliminate the invaders. With cancer the immune system seems much less effective. One reason for this difference is that cancer cells are not easily recognized as foreign by the host immune system. Another factor that seems to lower immune responses to cancer is that as tumors become massive, they produce a specific immune tolerance. Modulation of the immune system is becoming feasible in several clinical situations (see Chapter 40), and there is hope that in the future the immune system can be recruited to combat cancer. Experimental strategies include targeting cytotoxic drugs to tumor cells by linking the drugs to antibodies that would specifically bind to the cancer cells.

Chemotherapy

Chemotherapy of cancer involves the use of **cytotoxic** drugs, drugs that are designed to cause cell death. Obviously, such drugs must be used with caution because normal cells as well as cancer cells can be killed by these agents. The issue with these agents, as with all drugs, is one of selectivity of action.

Chemotherapy of cancer is complicated by the similarities between cancer cells and normal cells. Indeed, for many cancers, the primary difference is a derangement in regulation of growth so that the cancer cells divide continuously. Thus growth rate may be the only obvious difference between normal and cancerous cells. A logical target for chemotherapy is therefore actively dividing cells. This strategy generates some selective drug action because most normal tissues have very few cells actively reproducing at any one time. Most of the cells are either temporarily or permanently incapable of division, but there are exceptions to this rule. For example, bone marrow is the site for formation of blood cells and as a result is constantly undergoing cell division. Lymphoid tissue is the site for formation of lymphocytes and monocytes and therefore has a high rate of cell division. The intestinal lining, testes, ovaries, endometrium, and hair follicles are all additional sites of rapid cell division.

The normal cell types with rapid, noncancerous growth will often be targeted by cytotoxic anticancer drugs, right along with the cancerous tissues. Therefore, when you study the specific drugs in Chapter 55, you should expect to see bone marrow toxicity (see Patient Problems boxes on leukopenia and bleeding tendencies), gastrointestinal (GI) distress (see Patient Problems box on stomatitis) depression of spermatogenesis, and hair loss as common side effects. The action of so many cytotoxic drugs on the bone marrow also explains why chemotherapy for cancers is often followed by autologous bone marrow transplantation to replace the blood-forming cells destroyed by the drugs.

Drugs may also be targeted to specific cells by means of receptors (see Chapter 56). Antiestrogens can thus be directed to cancer cells that carry estrogen receptors; by blocking that receptor antiestrogens may cause the death of cancer cells that depend on estrogen. A similar strategy is used for prostatic cancers by using drugs that deprive the tumor of the androgens it needs to survive.

ALTERNATIVE THERAPIES

Antioxidant and Anticancer Activity

GREEN TEA

Tea is traditionally made from the leaves of the oriental plant *Camelia sinesis*. This beverage, which has been made for thousands of years in China, may fall into three categories depending on how the tea leaves are handled both before and after picking. Black tea, which is common in the United States, is made from fermented tea leaves. This tea tends to have a high content of tannins, which accounts for the dark color and the astringency of the brew. Oolong tea is made from semifermented leaves and tends to have less tannin than black tea. Green teas are brewed from leaves that are harvested and dried without any fermentation. Some forms of green tea leaves are taken from plants that are protected from the sun for several days, whereas others come directly from plants growing openly in the field. On average, green teas contain less tannin and more proteins or amino acids than black or oolong tea. The color of green tea is a light green or light tan.

The benefit of tea, and especially green tea, is related to the complex mixtures of chemicals in the leaves that act as antioxidants. This protective effect from the destructive action of oxygen can be demonstrated in laboratory tests with isolated cells. In animal trials, green tea seems as effective as vitamin E as an antioxidant under many conditions. One of the most interesting claims for green tea is that its antioxidant effects may protect against development of cancer. Such action has been seen in several animal trials and tests in humans are under way.

No matter what the outcome of the trials for anticancer effects, green tea with its low tannin and moderate caffeine content is a beverage that has comforted people for thousands of years and no doubt will continue to be enjoyed throughout the world.

Gene therapy or therapy aimed at reversing the effects of oncogenes are in the future for cancer. However, the rapid pace of research in the area of cell cycle regulations suggests that trials with some of these strategies will not be very long in coming.

Classifications of Drugs Used Against Cancer

Scientists and clinicians have classified anticancer drugs in a variety of ways. One widely used scheme is based on the chemical properties and origins of the drugs (Table 54-3). In this scheme, an antibiotic is a chemical made by a fungus, bacteria, or streptomycete and has an action on other organisms—in this case mammalian cells. Alkylating agents are synthetic highly reactive chemicals that change DNA and other substances by adding a carbon-containing substituent to certain sites. Antimetabolites interfere with normal metabolic pathways by mimicking normal metabolites and blocking one or more enzymes in the pathway.

One drawback of the classification scheme just described is that it is based on properties distant from clinical experience, and because the system is quite old, it does not reflect the current level of understanding of mechanisms of the drugs. Therefore, in this text the drugs are grouped according to the site in the cell cycle where the drug acts (Figure 54-2, on p. 620).

Table 54-3	Classification of Anticancer Drugs Based on Source and Chemistry

Alkylating Agents	**Antimetabolites**
busulphan	cytosine arabinoside
chlorambucil	fludarabine
cyclophosphamide	5-fluorouracil
dacarbazine	gemcitabine
nitrogen mustards	6-mercaptopurine
nitrosoureas	methotrexate
procarbazine	
	Mitotic Inhibitors
Antibiotics	paclitaxel
bleomycin	vincristine
dactinomycin	vinblastine
daunorubicin	
doxorubicin	

PATIENT PROBLEMS

Leukopenia

THE PROBLEM

Some drugs suppress the bone marrow, resulting in decreased production of white blood cells (WBCs). With some drugs, this is a common side effect and is anticipated, as with many cancer chemotherapy drugs. With other drugs, this side effect is unexpected and occurs only occasionally. Several medical terms may be used to describe this effect: agranulocytosis or granulocytopenia (severe reduction in granulocytes—basophils, eosinophils, and neutrophils) or neutropenia (reduction in neutrophils). The danger to the patient is the increased susceptibility to infection that results from a decreased supply of granulocytes.

SIGNS AND SYMPTOMS

Signs and symptoms include fever, sore throat, rash, malaise, chills, urinary frequency, dysuria, and altered level of consciousness. If the situation is untreated or unrecognized, the patient may develop a serious bacterial infection requiring intravenous drug therapy and hospitalization. The first line of treatment is to discontinue the drug causing the problem.

NURSING CARE

- Wash hands meticulously before caring for patients with suppressed WBC counts.
- Avoid putting patients with low white cell counts into multibed rooms where other patients have diagnoses of infection. If possible, admit the patient to a private room.
- Use protective isolation only if necessary because this environment isolates the patient from family and friends; rather, screen visitors, and do not permit visits from individuals with obvious colds, bronchitis, chicken pox, herpes simplex or herpes zoster, childhood infectious diseases, or any other infections.
- Avoid the use of rectal thermometers.
- Carefully assess patients who are also receiving steroids because steroids may mask the symptoms of infection.
- Monitor the complete blood count (CBC), WBC differential, and hematocrit, hemoglobin, and platelet counts.

NURSING IN THE COMMUNITY

- Notify the physician if symptoms develop.
- Monitor and record the body temperature (if the patient is able).
- If a period of bone marrow suppression is anticipated with each course or dose of drug, find out when the nadir of bone marrow suppression will occur. The nadir is the period of greatest bone marrow suppression or the period of lowest WBC count.
- If a period of suppressed WBC production is anticipated, as with cancer chemotherapy drugs, avoid contact with persons with colds or infections during periods of greatest susceptibility.
- Wash hands carefully after using the bathroom and after contact with other persons. Ask family members and friends to wash hands carefully before coming in contact with the patient.
- Instruct patients to avoid touching their eyes or the inside of the nose unless they have just washed their hands.
- Instruct patients to avoid immunizations.
- Do not bring cut flowers or fresh fruits and vegetables (unless washed carefully) to patients.

PATIENT PROBLEMS

Bleeding Tendencies

May be caused by anticoagulant therapy or low platelet count (thrombocytopenia).

THE PROBLEM
The platelet level is low, so the patient bleeds easily, or the patient is receiving anticoagulant therapy.

SIGNS AND SYMPTOMS
Bruising; petechiae (minute, pinhead-size hemorrhagic spots on the skin; seen only with reduced platelets); bleeding such as bleeding gums or nose bleeds (epistaxis); change in the color of urine, which might indicate bleeding in the kidney; anal bleeding; and bleeding in stools.

NURSING IN THE COMMUNITY
- Notify the physician if unexplained or excessive bleeding or bruising develops.
- Avoid using a razor with a blade; use an electric shaver.
- If gums are bleeding, stop flossing teeth until gums no longer bleed. Use a soft-bristle toothbrush. If brushing causes bleeding, stop brushing and use a water-spraying oral-care device if available.
- Permit only experienced professionals to draw blood.
- Do not go barefoot because foot injuries may be associated with excessive bruising or bleeding.
- Do not permit intramuscular injections if you are receiving anticoagulants or know your platelet count is below 60,000.
- Avoid getting constipated; drink plenty of fluids, stay active within the guidelines, drink fruit juices, and eat fruit and fiber. Do not use enemas unless told to do so by the physician.

- If you develop a headache or stiff neck, notify the physician.
- Wear a medical identification tag or bracelet identifying the medications you are receiving or that you have a low platelet count.
- Avoid using aspirin and over-the-counter medications unless approved by the physician.

SPECIFICALLY FOR PATIENTS WITH LOW PLATELET COUNTS
- Keep track of platelet counts by maintaining close contact with the physician. When the platelet count is below 10,000 to 15,000, stop flossing teeth and use water-spraying oral-care devices on low only. When the platelet count drops to 5000 to 10,000, stop brushing teeth and clean the mouth with a swab or 4×4 gauze pad using a mild mouthwash or saline solution. Avoid mouthwashes containing alcohol and lemon-glycerin swabs.
- Consider limiting activities. The following is one regimen prepared by the American Cancer Society:
  For platelet counts of 50,000 to 100,000, continue with moderate activity, including walking, swimming, and usual activities of daily living.
  For platelet counts below 50,000, only mild activities are permitted such as walking, light housework, or yard work.

ADDITIONAL GUIDELINES FOR THE NURSE
- Check stools for occult blood, and monitor urinalysis.
- Inspect venipuncture sites for hematoma; apply pressure for at least 10 minutes after venipuncture to limit hematoma formation at venipuncture sites.
- Handle patients gently. Avoid restraints; if used, pad and inspect under restraints every 2 hours. Keep siderails padded.

To illustrate the differences in these two systems, consider the drugs bleomycin and dactinomycin. Both drugs are antibiotics and are grouped together on this basis in the old system, but the drugs have different mechanisms of action. Dactinomycin binds to DNA and prevents DNA-dependent RNA synthesis, whereas bleomycin binds to DNA and induces cross-linking or breaks in the DNA strands (see Chapter 55). Because of these differences in mechanism, dactinomycin is classified with drugs that block RNA synthesis and bleomycin is classified with drugs that chemically change DNA.

Combinations of Anticancer Drugs

Few of the anticancer drugs discussed in this chapter are used alone. Experience has demonstrated that combinations of these drugs are much more effective than single agents. Several reasons for this increased success exist. First, combinations of drugs acting by different mechanisms are less likely to cause drug resistance. Like microbial cells, cancer cells can adapt and become drug resistant. This process oc-

curs easily if only a single drug is used. If several are used, the cancer cell has greater difficulty in developing simultaneous resistance. Simultaneous resistance is not impossible, however, if the cancer cells acquire the multidrug resistance pump, a system that effectively removes many drugs from inside cells.

Second, drug combinations allow the physician to select agents that produce different patterns of toxicity and thereby reduce the damage directed at any one organ system. Many anticancer drugs produce bone marrow suppression. Combining these suppressive drugs with drugs such as bleomycin or vincristine, which do not damage bone marrow, allows more anticancer effect to be achieved with no added damage to bone marrow.

Third, combining anticancer agents that act at different stages of the cell cycle allows for more tumor cells to be killed than would occur with the use of only one drug. For example, a drug like procarbazine is specific for the S phase of the cell cycle. Therefore tumor cells that pass into that

PATIENT PROBLEMS

Stomatitis

THE PROBLEM

Mucosal cells lining the gastrointestinal (GI) tract are sensitive to some drugs, especially many of the cytotoxic drugs used in cancer chemotherapy and gold preparations in rheumatoid arthritis. As the mucosal cells are destroyed, there may be pain and inflammation along the entire GI tract, which is called stomatitis.

SIGNS AND SYMPTOMS

Included are inflamed oral mucous membranes, oral ulcers, areas of irritation in the mouth, pain on chewing and swallowing, anal discomfort, and pain on defecation.

NURSING IN THE COMMUNITY

- If possible, have teeth professionally cleaned and dental caries repaired before the start of drug therapy.
- If chewing and swallowing are painful, switch to a liquid diet, including milkshakes and ice cream. If discomfort is severe, try to maintain an intake of clear fluids of at least 2000 ml (approximately eight 8-ounce glasses) per day to prevent dehydration.
- Try chilling food before eating it.
- If tooth brushing is irritating, try using swabs to clean the mouth. Avoid flossing when stomatitis is severe. Use water-spraying oral-care devices on low setting only. Rinse the mouth after each meal with a mild solution of baking soda and water; baking soda, salt and water; or hydrogen peroxide and water.
- Try painting the inside of the mouth with substrate of magnesia up to four times a day. Allow the milk of magnesia to settle to the bottom of the bottle. Pour off the liquid portion at the top of the bottle, and paint the mouth with the white pasty portion remaining.

- If a special mouthwash has been prescribed, use it as ordered. Many mouthwashes are effective only when used regularly throughout the day. Over-the-counter mouthwashes may be irritating because many contain alcohol; avoid them unless the physician has prescribed them.
- Avoid spicy foods and foods with hard crusts or edges.
- Try keeping a humidifier running to keep the room air moist.
- Wear dentures or bridgework only while eating, and remove them at other times to decrease irritation.
- Keep the lips moist with a lip balm or moisturizer.
- For anal irritation, avoid suppositories, enemas, rectal thermometers. Try sitting in a tub of warm water several times daily. After bowel movements, clean the anal area completely; some patients find a babywipe to be cooling for this purpose.
- If vaginal irritation is a problem, keep the vaginal area clean and dry, wipe from front to back, avoid soaps in the vaginal area, and pat dry. Avoid douching or using tampons. Notify the physician if vaginal discharge develops or a change in the color, consistency, odor, or amount occurs. To decrease irritation during intercourse, use a commercially available, water-soluble lubricant; avoid hand lotion or petroleum jelly.

ADDITIONAL NURSING CARE MEASURES

- Assess the mouth of patients at high risk for stomatitis at least once each shift. In addition, inspect for development of oral fungal infections (thrush).
- Monitor intake and output.
- Some physicians suggest that patients suck on ice or iced pops during intravenous administration of drugs known to cause stomatitis. The local vasoconstriction caused by the cold may decrease the severity of stomatitis.

---

phase while exposed to procarbazine die, but cells in resting phase survive. If an alkylating agent is added to the treatment regimen, a percentage of the cells that survive procarbazine treatment are expected to be killed by the second drug. Adding a third drug with yet a different mechanism of action such as vincristine further reduces the number of surviving cancer cells.

Finally, if it is possible to add a tissue-specific drug to the regimen, even more anticancer effect may be gained (see Chapter 56). An established and effective treatment regimen such as has just been described exists for the lymphoma known as Hodgkin's disease. The regimen includes the alkylating agent mechlorethamine (Mustargen), the mitotic poison vincristine (Oncovin), the DNA synthesis inhibitor procarbazine (Matulane), and prednisone, a steroid that specifically suppresses lymphoid tissue. This particular regimen is abbreviated MOPP. Many other established combination therapies exist for various types of cancer (Table 54-4).

Why Don't Drugs Cure All Cancers?

A primary difficulty in treating neoplastic diseases is that cancer cells offer fewer targets for selective toxicity than do bacterial cells, for example. This similarity in structure and metabolic processes reminds us that cancer cells are derived from host cells. Some differences between normal and cancerous cells can be identified, but they are mostly quantitative rather than qualitative. Thus nearly all the effective drugs have a **dose-limiting toxicity,** which is a side effect that limits the dose of drug that can be given. If the drugs were given at high enough concentrations to kill all the cancer cells, so many normal cells would also be killed that the patient could not survive. Thus most anticancer drugs have a low therapeutic index and a narrow safety margin (see Chapter 1).

Another difficulty with cancer chemotherapy arises because diagnosis cannot be expected until late in the course of the disease. A single transformed cell after 10 cycles of cell division can produce at most 1024 cells, a mass far too small

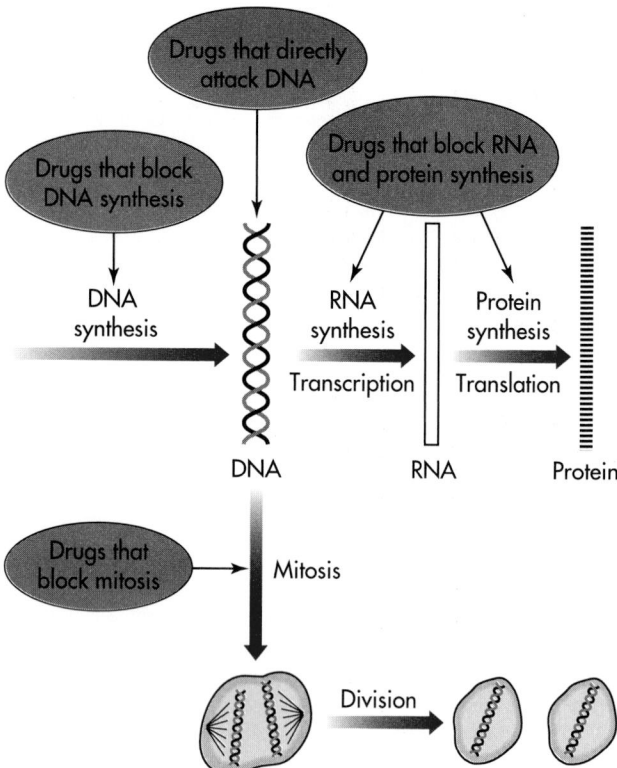

Figure 54-2 Molecular processes targeted by anticancer drugs. RNA and protein synthesis take place in every cell, although the processes will be stimulated in cell division. Likewise, the DNA is used for transcription in resting as well as dividing cells. Drugs targeted at these processes can therefore affect resting or dividing cells. Drugs that target DNA synthesis or mitosis tend to be most effective against dividing cells.

Table 54-4	**Combination Chemotherapeutic Regimens**	
Regimens	**Drugs Included**	**Disease**
ABVD	doxorubicin (Adriamycin) bleomycin vinblastine dacarbazine	Hodgkin's disease
BCVPP	carmustine (BiCNU) cyclophosphamide vinblastine procarbazine prednisone	Advanced Hodgkin's disease
CHOP	cyclophosphamide doxorubicin vincristine (Oncovin) prednisone	Non-Hodgkin's lymphoma
CMF	cyclophosphamide methotrexate fluorouracil	Breast carcinoma
CVP	cyclophosphamide vincristine prednisone	Non-Hodgkin's lymphoma
MOPP	mechlorethamine vincristine (Oncovin) procarbazine prednisone	Hodgkin's disease
POMP	prednisone vincristine (Oncovin) methotrexate mercaptopurine	Acute lymphocytic leukemia
TAD	thioguanine cytarabine (Ara-C) daunorubicin	Acute myeloid leukemia
VeIP	vinblastine (Velban) ifosfamide cisplatin (Platinol)	Testicular cancer
VIP	etoposide (VePesid) ifosfamide cisplatin (Platinol)	Testicular cancer

to be noticed. By the time the tumor weighs about 1 g, it will have gone through about 30 division cycles. A 1-g tumor is approximately the size of a small grape. In many locations within the body, a tumor this size may easily escape detection, yet in just 10 more cell divisions this tumor could exceed a mass of 1 kg (2.2 lb). Most tumors do not grow nearly as rapidly as the theoretical example just cited, in which it was assumed that every cell formed immediately reentered the reproductive cycle, but no matter how long it takes, the result of this process is a large mass containing more than 1 billion cells. Treatment at this stage with a drug that killed 99.99% of these cells, which would be an exceptionally effective drug, would still leave 100,000 cells that could eventually regrow.

The example in the preceding paragraph reminds us that earlier detection could give a therapeutic advantage for chemotherapy in that there would be fewer cancer cells to deal with. For several diseases, early detection is being made possible by the use of molecular markers of disease. For example, prostatic cancer can be detected in a blood test far earlier than it might be detected in a physical examination because this type of cancer releases into the blood a protein called prostate-specific antigen (PSA).

THERAPEUTIC AGENTS: DRUGS USED IN SUPPORTIVE THERAPY OF CANCER PATIENTS

Cancer patients require many drugs during the course of their disease. The drugs discussed in Chapters 55 and 56 attack the cancer directly. In addition to these agents, cancer patients often require other drugs to relieve symptoms of the disease or to ease the side effects of the highly toxic antineoplastic drugs. A brief summary of drugs used in supportive care of cancer patients follows.

allopurinol

Allopurinol may be needed when large tumor masses are quickly destroyed by chemotherapy, releasing many breakdown products, including uric acid. Uric acid can severely damage kidney cells if it is allowed to increase unchecked. Allopurinol inhibits the formation of uric acid and therefore can prevent this complication. Allopurinol is also used to treat gout (see Chapter 31).

Analgesics

Because pain associated with advanced cancer can be severe, hospitals and hospices specializing in care for dying cancer patients have a policy of liberal use of narcotic analgesics (see Chapter 32). Frequent dosing and large doses may be needed to control pain. Fear of addiction should not prevent adequate pain control in terminal cancer.

Antiemetics

Many drugs used to attack cancer cells also attack the GI mucosa. Therefore nausea or vomiting are common side effects of chemotherapy. Some anticancer drugs cause such severe vomiting that it must be treated to prevent electrolyte imbalance. In other cases it is transient and less severe. Nevertheless, control of nausea and vomiting can improve a patient's sense of well-being and aid in maintaining good nutrition.

Many antiemetic agents are available (see Chapter 25). The severe nausea and vomiting encountered in cancer patients who receive cytotoxic drugs often requires the strong antiemetic action of phenothiazines. Patients may also be sedated to control nausea.

Drugs to Control Direct Drug Toxicity

A few agents that have been designed to directly offset a specific toxicity of a cytotoxic drug are now available. For example, ifosfamide and cyclophosphamide produce toxic metabolites, including acrolein, that cause bladder damage (hemorrhagic cystitis). Mesna binds these toxic metabolites and protects the bladder from injury. Likewise, amifostine is metabolized to a thiol, which protects the kidneys by binding toxic free radicals produced by cisplatin.

Drugs to Control Hypercalcemia

Hypercalcemia can be a dangerous side effect of cancer chemotherapy, especially when tumor metastases exist in bone. Several agents are available to protect patients from this complication. Etidronate, pamidronate, and gallium nitrate block overproduction of calcium (see Chapter 68). Plicamycin helps with this symptom and in addition has anticancer activity (see Chapter 55).

Nursing Process Overview

Antineoplastic Chemotherapy

Assessment

Patients requiring chemotherapy may be of any age. Perform a thorough total assessment. Include as areas of focus drugs likely to be used and their known side effects. Obtain a detailed health history, especially if the patient has previously received chemotherapy. Previous response to chemotherapy will be a guide to anticipating response to a repeated dose of chemotherapeutic drugs. Assess laboratory work, including the hematocrit, hemoglobin, and blood count; liver function and renal function studies; and bone, liver, and other scans.

Nursing Diagnoses
- Altered comfort: nausea and vomiting as drug side effect
- Self-concept disturbance related to alopecia as side effect of drug therapy
- Fatigue

Patient Outcomes

The patient will not experience nausea and vomiting or will experience minimal nausea and vomiting. The patient will discuss feelings about alopecia. The patient will establish priorities for daily and weekly activities to lessen fatigue.

Planning/Implementation

Continue to monitor vital signs, body weight, and progress of anticipated side effects. When a side effect occurs with regularity, begin preventive or prophylactic measures as soon as possible. Monitor fluid intake and output. Monitor appropriate laboratory work, and institute nursing interventions based on that information. If medications are being administered via constant infusion, use an infusion control device. Ensure that intravenous (IV) infusion lines are patent, and avoid extravasation. Investigate thoroughly any new signs or symptoms.

Evaluation

A few drugs for cancer treatment can be used by the patient in the home. For many patients cancer chemotherapy is administered in the hospital or in the physician's office because many of these drugs must be administered intravenously. Before discharge, ascertain that the patient understands how to take medications correctly, what side effects may occur, how to treat side effects, what side effects require notification of the physician, and what measures should be used to prevent complications caused by side effects. Because the nadir or most profound bone marrow suppression often occurs days to weeks after the drug is administered, the patient should know when to anticipate the side effects and what actions to take to deal with them. Teach all patients which situations require immediate notification of the physician.

Nursing Implications Summary

General Guidelines: Patient Receiving Cancer Chemotherapy

Drug Administration

➤ See the Patient Problems boxes earlier in this chapter on stomatitis, bleeding tendencies, and leukopenia (decreased white blood cell count), as well as Patient Problems box in Chapter 24 on constipation.

➤ Many patients receiving cancer chemotherapy develop anemia, which may be caused in part by anorexia, poor nutrition, the effects of chronic disease, and/or bone marrow depression. The anemia may be caused by the drugs or by the cancer.

Nursing Measures to Decrease Anemia

➤ Assess for malaise, fatigability, and pale skin color. Monitor hematocrit and hemoglobin counts, and check stools for occult blood.

➤ Obtain a dietary history. Teach the patient about diet and counsel as appropriate. Iron-rich foods may be unappealing if anorexia or nausea is present; see the Dietary Considerations box in Chapter 22 on iron.

➤ Encourage frequent, small feedings. See interventions under anorexia.

➤ Suggest that patients eat their largest meal in the morning, before increasing fatigue makes them too tired to eat late in the day.

➤ Encourage the use of iron preparations, if prescribed, although they may have limited value until chemotherapy is completed. Fluoxymesterone (Halotestin), an androgen, or other drugs may also be prescribed to reverse anemia.

Nursing Measures to Decrease Anorexia

➤ Anorexia may arise from drug therapy or may be caused by the underlying disease.

➤ Assess dietary intake; monitor weight.

➤ Avoid foods having a strong odor. Cool or cold foods may be more appealing than hot foods. Red meat may be less appealing than fish or chicken.

➤ Encourage small frequent feedings. Instruct caregivers to fix small portions in an attractive manner.

➤ If the patient craves a specific food item, it is usually permissible for the patient to have it. The alternative may be a completely skipped meal.

➤ If food preparation is tiring to patients, suggest that they prepare and freeze small portions of food on days they feel better so that when not feeling well, it is necessary only to thaw and eat the food. Encourage interested friends and family members to prepare individual servings for the patient also. Encourage snacking and nibbling during the day. Encourage the patient to keep available in the refrigerator high-protein beverages or snacks that may be appealing (e.g., milk shakes, eggnogs, frozen yogurt, ice cream). Obtain recipes for high-protein snacks from dietitians, the American Cancer Society, or the oncologist's office. Some patients may wish to purchase commercially prepared high-protein supplements that can be consumed as a drink or frozen and eaten as ice cream.

➤ Although a microwave oven is not a necessity, the patient may find it helpful to have one to quickly heat food. Explore this possibility with the patient and family and community resources.

➤ Some patients may find that a small glass of sherry or wine before dinner will stimulate their appetite. Consult the physician and the patient.

Nursing Measures to Decrease Diarrhea

➤ Certain drugs used for cancer chemotherapy cause diarrhea. This symptom may appear within 24 to 48 hours of receiving the drug or may be delayed for 5 to 10 days.

➤ Instruct the patient to switch to a clear-liquid diet or a low-residue diet high in protein and calories. The goal is to maintain a fluid intake of at least 2000 to 2500 ml/day. Caution the patient to avoid foods known to be irritating to the GI tract, such as fruit, fruit juices, spicy foods, raw vegetables, corn, and coffee.

➤ Review possible clear-liquid food the patient may like, such as broth, gelatin, tea, iced pops, soft drinks, and water. The patient may be able to tolerate chicken noodle soup. Although electrolyte-containing drinks such as Gatorade are not required, they may provide a pleasant-tasting alternative less irritating than fruit juice.

➤ Instruct the patient to notify the physician if diarrhea is severe or persists longer than 2 to 4 days.

➤ Teach the patient that diarrhea can lead to electrolyte imbalance. When possible, monitor serum electrolyte level. In severe cases the patient may need to be admitted to the hospital for IV replacement of fluids and electrolytes.

➤ Instruct the patient not to use enemas, rectal suppositories, or rectal thermometers.

➤ If anal irritation occurs, suggest that the patient shower or sit in a warm tub of water several times per day. Wash the anal area with mild soap and water, and pat the area dry gently after each loose bowel movement.

➤ Some patients may find it easier or more comfortable to wash the area with prepackaged towelettes such as those used to clean infants during diaper changes or with preparations such as Tucks.

Nursing Measures to Decrease Nausea and Vomiting

➤ Nausea and vomiting may occur within hours of receiving a dose of chemotherapy or may be delayed for 5 to 10 days.

➤ Monitor response to chemotherapy. Record on the care plan actions that seem to contribute to or lessen the incidence of nausea and vomiting.

➤ Administer antiemetics, sedatives, and other drugs as ordered to decrease nausea. They are usually more effective if administered ahead of chemotherapy or at least before severe nausea and vomiting occur, rather than afterward.

➤ Consider the following interventions: Reschedule chemotherapy time in relation to meal times, either closer to or further from usual mealtimes. Limit oral intake to clear liquids on the day of or the evening before chemotherapy. Keep the environment odor free; do not wear perfume. Have the patient

Nursing Implications Summary—cont'd

avoid spicy, fatty, or greasy foods the day of or before chemotherapy.

➤ Instruct the patient and family in relaxation techniques, hypnotism, guided imagery, or distraction techniques if they are interested.

➤ Instruct the patient to report severe or persistent vomiting occurring at home to the physician because dehydration and electrolyte imbalance may develop.

Nursing Measures to Decrease Alopecia

➤ Alopecia (hair loss) occurs when sensitive cells in the hair follicle are damaged by chemotherapy or radiation.

➤ Before starting chemotherapy, inform patients about the possibility of alopecia. Some patients may wish to invest in a wig resembling their own hair color and style before hair loss begins. In some communities the American Cancer Society has a "wig bank" from which cancer patients can borrow wigs during periods of alopecia. Explore this possibility. In addition, some insurance companies may reimburse patients for the cost of wigs.

➤ Point out that alopecia may involve eyebrows, eyelashes, nasal hair, and pubic hair, although hair loss may be patchy rather than total in these areas.

➤ Some drugs, including cyclophosphamide, daunorubicin, docetaxol, doxorubicin, ifosfamide, paclitaxel, teniposide, vinblastine, and vincristine, typically cause complete baldness. Some drugs cause a moderate degree of alopecia. Examples include etoposide, floxuridine, irinotecan, methotrexate, and mitomycin. Finally, some drugs cause only mild alopecia or sporadic thinning of hair. These drugs include bleomycin, carmustine, fluorouracil, lomustine, and melphalan.

➤ Reassure the patient that in most cases hair will grow back after the course of chemotherapy is finished. Some patients will begin to have hair growth before the course of chemotherapy is completed; this is variable from person to person. Usually, new hair is the same color and texture as the hair that was lost, but occasionally it is different.

➤ During alopecia, instruct the patient to wash hair every 2 to 4 days. Use a mild shampoo but not necessarily "baby shampoo," which may be a little harsh. The patient's barber or hairdresser may be able to recommend a specific product. Instruct the patient to use a cream rinse or conditioner. If the scalp is dry, tell the patient to apply a thin layer of baby oil, mineral oil, or A and D ointment. Brush and comb hair gently. Instruct the patient not to use dyes, tints, rinses, or any unnecessary chemicals on remaining hair.

➤ Suggest that patients use satin pillow covers.

➤ Caution the patient to avoid direct exposure to the sun either by wearing a hat or by using a maximum-protection sunscreen when out of doors (SPF 15 or greater). During cold weather, tell the patient to wear a hat when out of doors.

➤ Sometimes, the patient's head may be cooled with cold compresses before IV chemotherapy. This approach is used to cause vasoconstriction to the area, with the hope that less of the medication will reach the scalp, so alopecia will be less severe. Inform patients that hair loss will probably occur even with the use of cold compresses.

Nursing Measures to Decrease Extravasation

➤ Many cytotoxic agents are highly irritating to normal tissues. When these drugs are administered intravenously, great care must be taken to prevent them from escaping into tissues surrounding the injection site. Pain, tissue damage, and necrosis can result.

➤ Assess for signs of extravasation when administering IV chemotherapy such as redness or swelling at the insertion site, decreased infusion rate, inability to obtain return of blood, pain, or resistance during injection of medication.

➤ Signs of extravasation may not be evident at the time a drug is administered or may be subtle. The patient may note simply that the infusion feels different than previously. If extravasation of a vesicant has occurred and ulceration is going to develop, it may take several weeks for the full damage to appear.

➤ Try to avoid extravasation of any IV drugs, but be especially alert when the following drugs are administered because of tissue necrosis and sloughing that may occur: dactinomycin, mitomycin, carmustine, cisplatin, dacarbazine, daunorubicin, plicamycin, streptozocin, mitoxantrone, vincristine, and vinblastine.

➤ In the ideal situation, perform a fresh venipuncture for administering chemotherapy. Otherwise, ascertain that the infusion line to be used is patent.

➤ Use a forearm infusion site rather than the dorsum of the hand for infusion of drugs that may cause necrosis and sloughing if extravasation occurs. Extravasation in the forearm may be less severe than in the dorsum of the hand, where muscles and tendons that control hand movement and function may be affected. Remain with the patient during the infusion.

➤ If extravasation occurs, discontinue the infusion but leave the needle or catheter in place. Attempt to aspirate any drug that can be retrieved. Follow agency procedures for managing the situation. A typical procedure would be to administer a corticosteroid subcutaneously in the area of extravasation or via the infusion catheter that is still in place, cover the area with a topical steroid, then cover with an occlusive dressing. Finally, apply ice compresses for 15 minutes four times a day, and keep the extremity elevated for 48 hours. Notify the physician. Use a fresh venipuncture site for infusion of any remaining chemotherapy drug.

➤ Medical orders for treatment of extravasation should be written before infusion is begun. These orders should be readily available to all persons who administer chemotherapy. Keep drugs ordered for treatment of extravasation readily available.

Safe Handling of Intravenous Chemotherapeutic Drugs

➤ See the manufacturer's literature for current information about preparation and administration of IV drugs.

Continued

Nursing Implications Summary—cont'd

➤ Avoid direct contact with chemotherapeutic agents because the nurse may be exposed to drug toxicity through repeated skin or aerosolization contact; see the Research Highlights box in Chapter 55.

➤ Prepare IV medications with a laminar airflow hood. Wash hands before and after handling chemotherapy drugs.

➤ Wear disposable gloves and long-sleeved gown during drug preparation. Wear gloves during drug administration.

➤ Use correct technique to avoid skin contact with prepared dosages. Use Luer-Lok fittings when possible to avoid inadvertent separation of syringe and needle. Establish and follow procedures for disposal of drug containers, contaminated gloves, syringes, and IV tubing. For additional information and guidelines, contact the Centers for Disease Control and Prevention in Atlanta, or the Occupational Safety and Health Administration.

➤ After drawing up dosages into the syringe, discard the needle, and attach a new sterile needle to avoid skin contact with any traces of medication that might be on the outside of the first needle.

➤ Check ordered doses carefully. Several drugs have similar names.

➤ Consult the manufacturer's literature for information about dilution and rate of administration.

➤ These drugs are highly toxic. Many agencies limit the number of persons who can administer these drugs to a few nurses who have had experience and additional training in their use.

➤ Allergic reactions have been reported with many of these drugs. Question patients about drug allergy before administering the drug. Have drugs, equipment, and personnel available to treat an acute allergic reaction in the setting in which these drugs are administered. Assess patients frequently during IV administration. Do not leave patients unattended for prolonged periods during treatment.

➤ Monitor laboratory work, including complete blood cell count (CBC) and differential, platelet count, blood urea nitrogen (BUN) and serum creatinine serum uric acid level, and liver function tests, on an ongoing basis.

➤ These drugs are contraindicated during pregnancy. Counsel the patient about contraceptive measures as appropriate. Menstrual irregularities are common in women receiving chemotherapy. Instruct women to keep a record of menstrual periods and to consult a physician immediately if pregnancy is suspected.

➤ Chemotherapy may cause diminished production or viability of sperm. Male patients may wish to arrange for deposit of sperm in a sperm bank before beginning chemotherapy.

Nursing Measures to Reduce Uric Acid Levels

➤ Elevation of uric acid levels often accompanies administration of chemotherapy to patients with leukemia or some lymphomas. This is caused by the release of large quantities of breakdown products in these rapidly dividing forms of cancer. Therefore chemotherapy orders may routinely be accompanied by orders for allopurinol. Monitor the uric acid levels. Keep the patient well hydrated (see Chapter 31).

Nursing in the Community

➤ Review with the patient and family the anticipated benefits and possible side effects of drug therapy. Provide support to these patients who may be facing a difficult diagnosis and anticipating serious drug side effects.

➤ Encourage the patient to notify the physician if any new side effects develop.

➤ Encourage the patient to return for follow-up visits as directed. Point out that many side effects may not become evident for 2 to 3 weeks after the final dose of therapy.

➤ Remind the patient to inform all health care providers of all medications being taken. This is especially important because bone marrow suppression, stomatitis, and other side effects may not appear until days to weeks after the drug has been administered.

➤ Remind the patient not to use over-the-counter (OTC) preparations without first consulting the physician. Emphasize the importance of keeping these and all drugs out of the reach of children.

➤ Warn the patient not to receive immunizations while taking cytotoxic drugs unless first approved by the physician. Instruct persons living with the patient to avoid oral polio vaccine while the patient is receiving chemotherapy. Also have the patient avoid contact with others who have recently had oral polio vaccine; if contact is necessary, have the patient wear a mask over the nose and mouth. Before starting chemotherapy, some physicians recommend that patients receive flu shots or update immunizations; consult the physician.

➤ Inform the patient that ridges in the fingernails may appear during chemotherapy; these reflect the effect of the drugs on the dividing cells of the nails.

➤ For information about the drugs, drug protocols, protocols to treat extravasation, oral gargles, mouthwashes, dietary supplements, snack recipes, patient teaching aids, and other information for patients, families, and health care providers, contact the chemotherapy department of local medical centers; the American Cancer Society; the Office of Cancer Communications at the National Cancer Institute, Bethesda, MD 20892, Telephone 1-800-4-CANCER (Spanish-speaking staff members are also available); the Department of Health and Human Services; or local oncologists' offices. Refer patients as appropriate to the local visiting nurse agencies or hospice.

➤ Unless additional teaching points are listed, points on Nursing in the Community about the drugs discussed in this chapter are the same.

➤ Teach the patient to take prescribed medications as ordered, even if not feeling well. Before discharge, review what to do if the patient vomits shortly after taking oral doses.

CHAPTER REVIEW

Application

1. What is the single most definitive property of cancer cells that distinguishes them from normal cells?
2. What properties of cancer cells allow them to spread through the body?
3. What are the phases of the cell cycle, and what events take place during each phase?
4. What are cyclins? How do they relate to p53?
5. What is apoptosis?
6. What is carcinogenesis?
7. On what property of cancer cells does most cancer chemotherapy depend?
8. What is the rationale behind combination chemotherapy in the treatment of cancer?
9. Why is allopurinol commonly used in cancer treatment programs?
10. What principle governs the use of analgesics in treating cancer patients?
11. Why are antiemetics commonly used as adjuncts to cancer chemotherapy?
12. Why are drugs to lower blood calcium levels often required in cancer patients?

Critical Thinking

1. How does apoptosis protect the body from cancer?
2. Why are anticancer drugs cytotoxic, unlike most other therapeutic agents?
3. How would you explain to patients why they are taking some drugs that do not directly attack their cancer (e.g., allopurinol, etidronate)?

References

Held-Warmkessel J: Chemotherapy complications, *Nursing* 28(4): 41-46, 1998.

Krontiris TG: Oncogenes, *N Engl J Med* 333(5):303-330, 1995.

Labuhn K, et al: Nurses' and pharmacists' exposure to antineoplastic drugs: findings from industrial hygiene scans and urine mutagenicity tests, *Cancer Nurs* 21(2):79-89, 1998.

Madeya ML: Oral complications from cancer therapy. Part 2: nursing implications for assessment and treatment, *Oncol Nurs Forum* 23(5):808-821, 1996.

Chapter 55

Cytotoxic Drugs to Treat Cancer

OBJECTIVES

After studying this chapter, you should be able to do the following:

- *Discuss the side effects common to cytotoxic agents.*

- *Discuss the risks anticancer drugs may pose to health care personnel and how these risks can be minimized.*

- *Discuss the reasons for precautions taken to protect patients who are receiving anticancer drugs from exposure to infectious agents.*

- *Develop a nursing care plan for the patient receiving one or more of the drugs discussed in this chapter.*

CHAPTER OVERVIEW

This chapter addresses specific cytotoxic agents used in cancer therapy. In addition, the rationale behind successful therapeutic regimens is highlighted with the individual agents involved.

THERAPEUTIC RATIONALE: CANCER CHEMOTHERAPY

In a variety of ways, the cytotoxic drugs used for cancer chemotherapy cause the death of cells. Specificity of action is difficult to achieve because the drugs are usually most effective against rapidly dividing cells, which includes not only cancerous cells but also many normal tissues (see Chapter 54). The drug attack on cancer cells can involve direct damage to DNA, inhibition of DNA synthesis, blockade of RNA and protein synthesis, or arrest of the cell in mitosis. These specific mechanisms are discussed in the following sections, with each class of therapeutic agents.

THERAPEUTIC AGENTS: CYTOTOXIC DRUGS

Agents That Directly Attack DNA

Properties common to this class of drugs are presented next; properties unique to individual drugs are covered with each agent.

Mechanism of Action

The genetic information necessary for cell reproduction resides in DNA. Nucleated cells contain all the genetic information required to form new cells, but information is seldom expressed in normal cells in most tissues because they rarely divide, and they have effective mechanisms for DNA repair. Therefore damage to the DNA of many normal cells is undetectable; in contrast, cancer cells with their rapid rates of replication and more limited DNA repair mechanisms may be killed by damage to their DNA. This rationale explains the use of a large group of anticancer drugs called **alkylating agents,** which chemically modify DNA.

Alkylating agents may attack DNA in its double-stranded form, attaching various compounds to one strand or the other. Other agents may form cross-links, or chemical bonds, between the strands. Because the strands must unwind and separate during replication, **cross-linking** effectively blocks replication.

Pharmacokinetics

Many drugs of this type are rapidly destroyed in the body. A few drugs like cisplatin, mechlorethamine, and melphalan are hydrolyzed or destroyed by nonenzymatic mechanisms in many fluids and tissues. Other drugs like altretamine, bleomycin, busulfan, carmustine, chlorambucil, and lomustine are rapidly metabolized in liver. A few drugs such as bleomycin are degraded by enzymes in many tissues.

Metabolism lowers activity of most of these drugs, but altretamine, chlorambucil, ifosfamide, and lomustine are activated by metabolism or the metabolites retain significant activity.

The duration of action of this class of agents is variable and does not always match the kinetics of elimination. For example, drugs like mechlorethamine are destroyed within seconds of administration, but the biologic effect may persist for weeks.

Renal excretion is the most common route of elimination with these drugs. Some, such as chlorambucil and lomustine, are eliminated as metabolites; others, such as ifosfamide and bleomycin, are excreted largely unchanged.

Uses

The clinical uses of antineoplastic drugs that directly attack DNA are summarized in Table 55-1.

Adverse Reactions and Contraindications

The specificity of agents that destroy nucleic acid is not great. All cells will undergo attack by these chemicals, although the action is lethal primarily when cells attempt division. Therefore tissues with high growth fractions are most sensitive. Clinical symptoms to be expected when these agents attack normal rapidly dividing tissues include bone marrow suppression that produces leukopenia (low white cell counts) (see Patient Problems box in Chapter 54 on leukopenia), thrombocytopenia (low platelet counts) (see Patient Problems box in Chapter 54 on bleeding tendencies), or other blood dyscrasias; mucocutaneous reactions, including stomatitis (see Patient Problems box in Chapter 54 on stomatitis) or other signs; and gastrointestinal (GI) toxicity, including acute or delayed nausea and vomiting.

The alkylating agents chemically alter DNA and are thus mutagenic. Therefore this class of agents can induce cancers of various types that may show up years after exposure to the drug. Not every patient will develop a second cancer as a result of chemotherapy, but for patients exposed to alkylating agents, the risk is increased many times over the normal low incidence rate.

Some of these drugs have immunosuppressive activity. This action is especially strong with cyclophosphamide but is also observed with chlorambucil and melphalan. Mechlorethamine is weakly immunosuppressive.

Toxicity

The dose-limiting toxicity with many of these agents is bone marrow suppression, which increases as doses increase. In addition to these expected effects on bone marrow, which are reflected in lower numbers of various cells in the blood, some of these drugs also have dose-related effects on other organs. For example, bleomycin and carmustine cause pulmonary toxicity, whereas cyclophosphamide causes cardiotoxicity.

Interactions

All drugs of this class except bleomycin may have significant interactions with bone marrow suppressants or radiation because the combinations can profoundly depress production of blood cells. Live virus vaccines are avoided in patients who receive any of these drugs because generalized viral infections may occur as a result of the immunosuppression these drugs produce. Oral polio vaccines may also be contraindicated for family members of patients who receive these drugs.

altretamine

Altretamine is similar to alkylating agents, but its exact mechanism is unknown. This highly lipid-soluble drug is rapidly absorbed orally and must be activated by liver metabolism.

In addition to anemia, leukopenia, and thrombocytopenia, side effects such as neurotoxicity that affects both the central and peripheral nervous systems are common. Patients may express anxiety or show awkwardness, confusion, dizziness, depression, numbness in limbs, or weakness. Seizures are less common.

Nausea and vomiting occur commonly with altretamine. This reaction usually appears several days after the start of therapy.

In addition to the expected interactions with bone marrow depressants and live virus vaccines, altretamine also interacts with monoamine oxidase (MAO) inhibitors. Severe orthostatic hypotension can result from this combination.

bleomycin

Bleomycin is a glycopeptide antibiotic that produces breaks in DNA strands and may also inhibit enzymes that normally repair damaged DNA. Most tissues rapidly inactivate

Table 55-1   **Anticancer Drugs That Directly Attack DNA**

Generic Name	Trade Name	Administration/Dosage	Comments/Uses
altretamine	Hexalen Hexastat†	ORAL: *Adults*—65 mg/m² 4 times/day after meals and at bedtime for 14-21 consecutive days/month. FDA pregnancy category D.	Used for ovarian carcinomas.
bleomycin	Blenoxane*	INTRAMUSCULAR, INTRAVENOUS, SUBCUTANEOUS: *Adults and children*—0.25-0.5 unit/kg once or twice weekly initially; 1 unit/day or 5 units/wk for maintenance. FDA pregnancy category D.	Palliative therapy for lymphomas, squamous cell carcinomas, and testicular or ovarian carcinomas.
busulfan	Myleran*	ORAL: *Adults and children*—60-120 μg/kg/day or 1.8-4.6 mg/m²/day. FDA pregnancy category D.	May prolong survival in chronic myelocytic leukemia.
carboplatin	Paraplatin*	INTRAVENOUS: *Adults*—300 mg/m² once every 4 wk. FDA pregnancy category D.	Palliative therapy for recurrent ovarian carcinoma.
carmustine	BiCNU*	INTRAVENOUS: *Adults*—150-200 mg/m² as single dose, repeated no more often than every 6 wk. FDA pregnancy category D.	Palliative therapy for central nervous system tumors, lymphomas, and myelomas.
chlorambucil	Leukeran*	ORAL: *Adults and children*—0.1-0.2 mg/kg/day for treatment; smaller doses for maintenance. FDA pregnancy category D.	Effective against lymphocytic leukemias and lymphomas.
cisplatin	Platinol*	INTRAVENOUS: *Adults*—Up to 100 mg/m² once every 4 wk after heavy hydration to protect kidneys; dosages are lower in combinations. FDA pregnancy category D.	Used to treat testicular cancer and carcinomas in many tissues.
cyclophosphamide	Cytoxan*	ORAL: *Adults*—1-5 mg/kg/day. *Children*—2-8 mg/kg, various schedules. INTRAVENOUS: *Adults*—1.5-3 mg/kg/day. *Children*—2-8 mg/kg on various schedules. FDA pregnancy category D.	Effective for lymphomas, solid tumors, leukemias, and myelomas.
dacarbazine	DTIC† DTIC-Dome	INTRAVENOUS: *Adults*—2-4.5 mg/kg for 10 days every month or 150-250 mg/m² for 5 days every 21 days. FDA pregnancy category C.	Used to treat malignant melanoma and lymphomas.
etoposide	Etopophos Toposar VePesid*	ORAL: *Adults*—70-100 mg/m²/day for 5 days. Repeat every 3-4 wk. INTRAVENOUS: *Adults*—50-100 mg/m²/day for 3-5 days. Repeat at 3-4 wk. FDA pregnancy category D.	Used for refractory testicular tumors and small-cell lung carcinoma.
ifosfamide	IFEX*	INTRAVENOUS: *Adults*—1.2 g/m²/day for 5 days. FDA pregnancy category D.	Used for germ cell testicular tumors.
irinotecan	Camptosar	INTRAVENOUS: *Adults*—125 mg/m² infused over 90 min once weekly for 4 wk. FDA pregnancy category D.	Colorectal carcinoma refractory to first-line drugs.
lomustine	CeeNU*	ORAL: *Adults*—Up to 130 mg/m² in single dose; repeat in 6 wk. FDA pregnancy category D.	Similar to carmustine in use and properties.
mechlorethamine	Mustargen*	INTRAVENOUS: *Adults and children*—0.4 mg/kg total dose in single or several doses. FDA pregnancy category D. INTRACAVITARY: *Adults*—0.3-0.4 mg/kg.	Used to treat Hodgkin's disease and other lymphomas; may be palliative for solid tumors or their effusions.
melphalan	Alkeran*	ORAL: *Adults*—0.15 mg/kg/day for 2-3 wk or 0.25 mg/kg/day for 4 days. After recovery of bone marrow, 2-4 mg/day. FDA pregnancy category D.	Used to treat multiple myeloma and ovarian carcinomas.
mitomycin	Mutamycin*	INTRAVENOUS: *Adults and children*—Up to 20 mg/m² as single dose, repeated no more often than every 6 wk.	Used to treat gastrointestinal tumors.
procarbazine	Matulane Natulan†	ORAL: *Adults*—2-4 mg/kg day for 1 wk; then 4-6 mg/kg/day until bone marrow toxicity occurs. On recovery of marrow, dosages are 50-100 mg/day. FDA pregnancy category D. *Children*—50 mg/m²/day.	Palliative for Hodgkin's lymphoma.
teniposide	Vumon	INTRAVENOUS: *Children*—Up to 250 mg/m² once weekly for 6-8 wk, with other agents. FDA pregnancy category D.	Used in childhood acute lymphocytic leukemia and neuroblastoma.
thiotepa	Thiotepa*	INTRAVENOUS: *Adults*—0.3-0.4 mg/kg every 1-4 wk. TOPICAL: *Adults*—30-60 mg in 30-60 ml for application to bladder for bladder carcinoma. FDA pregnancy category D.	Palliative therapy for lymphomas, carcinomas, and malignant effusions.
topotecan	Hycamtin*	INTRAVENOUS: *Adults*—1.5 mg/m² daily for 5 days; repeat every 21 days. FDA pregnancy category D.	Ovarian carcinoma after first-line drugs fail.

NOTE: Doses are representative and may not include doses used in various combinations or specific protocols.
*Available in Canada and the United States.
†Available in Canada only.

bleomycin, but skin and lungs are exceptions; therefore the drug tends to concentrate at those sites and produce toxic reactions. Tumors tend not to inactivate bleomycin, so the drug is also concentrated there.

Bleomycin often produces skin and mucous membrane changes, fever, chills, anorexia, and vomiting. Pulmonary re-actions occur in 10% to 40% of treated patients, and 1% may die. Lung toxicity begins as pneumonitis and progresses to pulmonary fibrosis. Pulmonary toxicity is both age and dose dependent.

Bleomycin usually does not suppress the bone marrow and therefore need not be avoided in patients who receive bone marrow suppressants or live virus vaccines. Bleomycin makes lung tissues more susceptible to damage by oxygen. As a result, general anesthetics may provoke a rapid deterioration in pulmonary function.

Bleomycin is often used in combinations for lymphomas (see Table 54-4). The benefit of bleomycin in combinations is that bleomycin gives added effects on the DNA target without contributing to bone marrow suppression, which is often dose-limiting for other drugs in the combinations.

busulfan

Busulfan is an alkylating agent capable of cross-linking DNA. For reasons that are unclear, busulfan possesses a degree of selectivity that is unique among this class of drugs. Busulfan is a myelosuppressant at doses that do not significantly lower the levels of other blood cells, although platelets may be reduced. Because of this selectivity, busulfan is used in chronic myelocytic leukemia.

Busulfan is well absorbed orally and is used by this route in chronic intermittent therapy. The drug is highly reactive in blood and tissues and is rapidly broken down in the body to a variety of products that are excreted by the kidneys and other routes.

Busulfan may cause leukopenia, usually beginning 10 days after therapy. Hemorrhage may result if the drug is not discontinued. With long-term therapy, many body systems may show signs of toxicity. Busulfan may destroy large numbers of granulocytes during therapy. These dying cells release chemicals that may be converted to uric acid, excessively elevating blood levels of uric acid. To avoid the nephrotoxicity produced by uric acid, allopurinol may be given during busulfan therapy.

In addition to the expected interactions with bone marrow depressants and live virus vaccines, busulfan interacts with probenecid and sulfinpyrazone. This interaction is based on the high levels of uric acid that may be released by busulfan.

carboplatin and cisplatin

Cisplatin and carboplatin are platinum-containing complexes that act like alkylating agents. These drugs cross-link DNA and are not specific for cell cycle. Both drugs must be given by intravenous (IV) injection and are hydrolyzed in solution to the form that reacts with DNA; cisplatin is rapidly inactivated following hydrolysis. The effects of single doses last for weeks.

Cisplatin is a toxic drug that almost always causes severe nausea and vomiting. The drug is also toxic to renal tubules and may cause serious damage with high dosages or too frequent administration. A drug called amifostine is used to protect the kidneys from damage by cisplatin. Amifostine generates free thiols that concentrate in tissues and protect against free radicals and other damaging by-products of cisplatin.

Cisplatin causes hearing loss in the upper frequency ranges and ringing in the ears (tinnitus). Ototoxicity tends to progress with repeated doses. Myelosuppression shown by lowered leukocyte and platelet counts persists for 3 to 4 weeks after a single injection of cisplatin.

In addition to anemia, leukopenia, neutropenia, and thrombocytopenia, carboplatin causes pain at the site of injection. Extreme tiredness or weakness is also common. Nausea and vomiting usually start 6 to 12 hours after a dose and last for 24 hours. About 65% of treated patients experience vomiting. Carboplatin causes less renal toxicity than does cisplatin.

Peripheral neuropathies may occur with either drug. Loss of taste has also been reported. Both drugs show the expected interactions with bone marrow depressants or live virus vaccines. Cisplatin shows additive nephrotoxicity or ototoxicity with other drugs sharing these side effects.

Cisplatin is often used in combinations with anticancer drugs having different mechanisms of action (see Table 54-4).

carmustine and lomustine

Carmustine is a rapidly acting alkylating agent that affects numerous enzymes and nucleic acids. Lomustine is chemically related to carmustine and similarly alkylates DNA and has widespread metabolic effects. One advantage carmustine and lomustine have over many other alkylating agents is that they penetrate the blood-brain barrier well.

Carmustine is given by IV infusion. The drug is rapidly degraded, so only metabolites are detectable in blood or in tissues a few minutes after the dose is administered, but the metabolites are active. Metabolites are excreted in urine for several days after therapy. Carmustine is also used as an implant for insertion into the cavity left by surgical removal of a brain tumor called glioblastoma multiforme. This implant, which is made from a biodegradable polymer, raises the concentration of drug at the site and prolongs the action.

Lomustine is used orally and is well absorbed by that route. Once absorbed, it is metabolized and excreted similarly to carmustine.

Carmustine and lomustine cause delayed bone marrow suppression. After a single dose of drug, bone marrow function may reach its lowest point 4 to 6 weeks after therapy. Therefore doses are given every 6 weeks or less often if the bone marrow does not promptly recover.

Pulmonary fibrosis may be an insidious side effect with these drugs. Shortness of breath or cough should be investigated quickly for cause. Nausea and vomiting are dose-related toxic reactions to carmustine and lomustine. Carmustine is highly irritating and may cause hyperpigmentation if it touches the skin. Pain during infusion is common. Patient discomfort can be reduced by slowing the rate of infusion of the drug and by properly diluting it before use.

Carmustine is often combined with agents having a different mechanism of action and/or a different toxicity profile to treat various cancers (see Table 54-4).

chlorambucil

Chlorambucil is chemically related to mechlorethamine and, like that drug, kills cells by cross-linking DNA. Chlorambucil is distinguished by being the slowest acting and the least toxic of the nitrogen mustard alkylating agents. In addition to its cell cycle nonspecific cytotoxicity, chlorambucil displays a somewhat selective lympholytic action.

Chlorambucil is administered orally. Large doses (20 mg or more) may produce nausea and vomiting, but more common doses are well tolerated and reliably absorbed. The drug is rapidly metabolized by the liver, and the major metabolite is active.

Chlorambucil commonly suppresses the bone marrow, although at normal doses the effects are usually mild and reversible. Chlorambucil can produce central nervous system (CNS) stimulation, GI irritation, pulmonary fibrosis, liver toxicity, and skin reactions at high dosages, but these responses are not commonly seen with normal clinical dosages. Chlorambucil is often well tolerated when used at low dosages for maintenance therapy. Uric acid in the blood can reach dangerous levels after chlorambucil treatment. Allopurinol should be used, rather than probenecid or sulfinpyrazone, to avoid nephrotoxicity.

Chlorambucil causes the expected interactions with bone marrow depressants and live virus vaccines.

▼ cyclophosphamide

Cyclophosphamide is a noncytotoxic form of nitrogen mustard that must be activated by liver microsomal enzymes. Several metabolites of cyclophosphamide are formed in the liver, and at least one of these metabolites is a potent alkylating agent with activity similar to that of nitrogen mustard. Because the drug as administered is not active, it does not possess the strong vesicant activity (direct blistering and damage of tissues) seen with other nitrogen mustards.

Cyclophosphamide may be used either orally or parenterally, which is a distinct advantage over most alkylating agents. Oral absorption is good; the absorbed drug passes through portal circulation directly to the liver where the drug is activated.

Cyclophosphamide produces all the expected side effects of nonspecific alkylating agents. Bone marrow suppression occurs and is often used to guide the physician in adjusting dosages. In most patients the bone marrow begins to recover 7 to 10 days after the drug is discontinued.

GI toxicity with cyclophosphamide is common and usually consists of nausea and vomiting although more severe reactions can occur. Hair loss (alopecia) occurs with cyclophosphamide therapy much more commonly than with other drugs of this class. Most patients report regrowth of hair after therapy.

Immunosuppression is an expected side effect. Cyclophosphamide suppresses gonadal tissue; complete suppression of the menstrual cycles and of sperm formation have been reported.

Cyclophosphamide and its metabolites are excreted predominantly through the kidneys. The accumulation of these cytotoxic compounds in the bladder can produce hemorrhagic cystitis. Bladder fibrosis and carcinoma occur more often in patients who receive long-term therapy with cyclophosphamide.

High-dose or long-term therapy is associated with increased risk of cardiotoxicity, pneumonitis, renal toxicity, and uric acid accumulation.

In addition to the expected interactions with bone marrow depressants and live virus vaccines, cyclophosphamide may produce excessive uric acid levels; this latter action may cause interactions with probenecid or sulfinpyrazone. Immunosuppressants contribute to the risk of infection with cyclophosphamide. Cytarabine increases the risk of cardiotoxicity with cyclophosphamide.

Cyclophosphamide is commonly used in three-, four-, or five-drug combinations for lymphomas or other cancers (see Table 54-4).

dacarbazine

Dacarbazine apparently acts as an alkylating agent and is cell cycle nonspecific. The drug must be given intravenously. It is secreted by renal tubules, with about half the dose excreted by this route; the remaining drug appears in blood as a metabolite.

Dacarbazine causes delayed bone marrow toxicity (16 to 20 days after therapy). Most patients report nausea and vomiting within a few hours after therapy. Tolerance to this symptom develops. Dacarbazine can cause severe pain and tissue damage if it seeps from the vein into surrounding tissues.

Dacarbazine causes the expected interactions with bone marrow depressants and live virus vaccines. The drug is used for Hodgkin's disease in the combination called ABVD, along with another DNA cross-linking agent (bleomycin), an RNA synthesis inhibitor (doxorubicin) and a mitotic inhibitor (vincristine) (see Table 54-4).

etoposide and teniposide

Etoposide (VP-16) and teniposide (VM-26) are inhibitors of topoisomerase II, an enzyme involved with maintaining DNA structure. Inhibition of this enzyme causes DNA strands to break and go unrepaired, which leads to the death of the cell.

Although about 50% of a dose may be absorbed orally, etoposide is usually administered intravenously; teniposide is used only intravenously. Both drugs are highly protein bound and slowly eliminated renally, mostly as unchanged drug. Neither drug distributes well to the CNS.

Etoposide and teniposide produce similar adverse reactions, mostly consisting of bone marrow suppression with anemia and thrombocytopenia. Anorexia, nausea, vomiting, and alopecia also occur. Interactions with bone marrow depressants and live virus vaccines occur with etoposide, but teniposide primarily interacts with other drugs that are tightly bound to plasma proteins; thus, drugs like salicylates, sulfonamides, and tolbutamide may displace teniposide from plasma proteins and increase toxicity of the anticancer drug.

ifosfamide

Ifosfamide is metabolically activated to a form that acts as an alkylating agent. The drug must be given by IV infusion. Unchanged drug as well as active and inactive metabolites are excreted by the kidneys.

In addition to leukopenia and thrombocytopenia, ifosfamide also causes dose-related CNS effects and hemorrhagic cystitis. Cystitis can be controlled by administering the drug mesna at 20% of the ifosfamide dosage; mesna is given by IV injection at the time ifosfamide is administered and 4 and 8 hours later. Nausea, vomiting, and alopecia are also common side effects.

Ifosfamide causes the expected interactions with bone marrow depressants and live virus vaccines.

irinotecan

Irinotecan binds to **topoisomerase** I, an enzyme required for DNA replication. The drug allows topoisomerase I to make a break in a single strand of double-strand DNA, which is a normal part of replication, but the drug prevents repair of those breaks. As a result, DNA is progressively damaged and the cell dies.

Irinotecan is used by IV infusion and is widely distributed in the body. Liver metabolism forms both active and inactive metabolites; metabolites and unchanged drug are eliminated by biliary and renal mechanisms.

Side effects of irinotecan commonly include anemia, leukopenia, neutropenia, diarrhea or other GI effects, stomatitis, edema, or difficulty breathing. Weakness is also common. Hair loss occurs in many patients.

The diarrhea caused by irinotecan raises the potential for dangerous interactions with diuretics, which can lead to severe dehydration. Pelvic or abdominal irradiation and other bone marrow suppressants are avoided with irinotecan because of the greatly increased risk of bone marrow suppression.

mechlorethamine

Mechlorethamine (nitrogen mustard) is a potent alkylating agent that cross-links DNA. Mechlorethamine is so highly unstable that it must be administered intravenously immediately after the solution is prepared. The drug is so highly reactive that it is destroyed within minutes of its injection. No active drug appears in urine or is excreted by any other route.

Mechlorethamine may induce various malignancies. The drug is also an immunosuppressant and predisposes the patient to infections.

Mechlorethamine is an extremely toxic agent with a very narrow margin of safety. Significant toxicity is to be expected in every treated patient. Bone marrow suppression usually appears within a day, but suppression is most profound 1 to 3 weeks later. Platelet counts may decrease enough to cause bleeding gums and subcutaneous hemorrhages. Nausea and vomiting are common acute toxic reactions.

Germinal tissue may be severely damaged by mechlorethamine. Men may have complete arrest of spermatogenesis. Women may have menstrual irregularities. Fetuses of treated mothers are damaged by mechlorethamine.

Mechlorethamine is a potent vesicant. Patients and medical personnel must be rigorously protected from improper contact with the drug. Because of its instability the drug must be dissolved immediately before use and injected directly into a free-flowing IV line. This procedure avoids the danger of extravasation (leakage into tissues around the vein), which produces extreme pain and tissue destruction.

In addition to the expected interactions with bone marrow depressants and live virus vaccines, mechlorethamine may cause excessive uric acid levels, which leads to interactions with probenecid or sulfinpyrazone. Mechlorethamine is combined with other anticancer agents in MOPP, a widely used combination regimen for Hodgkin's disease (see Table 54-4).

melphalan

Melphalan (L-PAM, or phenylalanine mustard) is a derivative of nitrogen mustard that acts as an alkylating agent. Melphalan is adequately absorbed orally in most patients. The drug persists in blood longer than most alkylating agents; it is detectable for up to 6 hours after a single dose.

Melphalan produces bone marrow suppression, commonly occurring 2 to 3 weeks after the drug is started. Dosages are usually adjusted to produce mild leukopenia but no further damage. High dosages can produce severe bone marrow depression, bleeding, and nausea and vomiting.

In addition to the expected interactions with bone marrow depressants and live virus vaccines, melphalan may raise uric acid levels, which leads to interactions with probenecid or sulfinpyrazone.

mitomycin

Mitomycin is an antibiotic that is activated by enzymes in the body, so it becomes capable of alkylating DNA. Like other alkylating agents, mitomycin is nonspecific for cell cycle. Mitomycin must be given intravenously because it is not absorbed orally and is highly irritating to skin and muscle. The drug does not distribute to the brain.

Mitomycin produces severe and progressive myelosuppression. Leukopenia and thrombocytopenia occur within 3 to 8 weeks and may persist for up to 10 weeks or longer after therapy. Mitomycin should not be readministered until platelet and white blood cell (WBC) counts show the bone marrow has recovered. Mitomycin also commonly causes nausea and vomiting, skin rashes, and alopecia. A few patients may also experience renal failure with hemolysis, liver toxicity, and lung damage. Mitomycin also causes local necrosis if allowed to escape into cutaneous tissues during IV injection.

Mitomycin causes the expected interactions with bone marrow depressants and live virus vaccines.

procarbazine

Procarbazine has multiple effects on cellular enzyme systems and nucleic acids, including causing chemical changes in DNA. These changes have their greatest effect in the S-phase of the cell cycle (see Chapter 54).

Procarbazine is well absorbed after oral administration. The drug rapidly equilibrates between plasma and cerebrospinal fluid. Procarbazine is converted to an active metabolite by the liver and is excreted as the metabolite primarily by the kidneys.

Procarbazine often produces bone marrow depression and immune suppression. CNS stimulation and pneumonitis are also common. Menstrual periods are typically suppressed. Nausea, vomiting, and excessive tiredness are common.

Procarbazine causes the expected interactions with bone marrow suppressants and live virus vaccines. The drug also causes many other interactions because it inhibits monoamine oxidase. Therefore patients should not receive both procarbazine and drugs that elevate biogenic amine levels (e.g., sympathomimetics, tricyclic antidepressants, phenothiazines, tyramine-containing food).

Ethyl alcohol can produce a disulfiram-like reaction with procarbazine. Procarbazine can also produce significant interactions with anesthetics, agents with anticholinergic effects, antidiabetic agents, MAO inhibitors, CNS depressants, dextromethorphan, fluoxetine, levodopa, meperidine, methyldopa, and methylphenidate.

Procarbazine is used in combinations such as BCVPP and MOPP for Hodgkin's disease (see Table 54-4).

thiotepa

Thiotepa, also called triethylenethiophosphoramide, is a nonspecific alkylating agent. Because it is so nonselective, the drug is applied directly to the tumor when possible. This therapy allows large doses to be achieved at the tumor site, with smaller doses escaping into systemic circulation. Because toxicity is dose related, such a treatment regimen minimizes systemic toxicity.

Thiotepa is primarily toxic to bone marrow. Because the drug produces its effects slowly, care must be taken not to excessively damage the bone marrow by too high a dosage in the early stages of therapy. WBC counts may be used as an index of toxicity. The drug may also produce nausea and anorexia. Thiotepa is relatively nonirritating and can be administered rapidly through IV lines.

In addition to the expected interactions with bone marrow depressants and live virus vaccines, thiotepa may raise uric acid levels, which leads to interactions with probenecid or sulfinpyrazone.

topotecan

Topotecan inhibits topoisomerase I, an enzyme required for DNA replication. As a result of this inhibition, DNA strands are broken and the affected cell dies.

Topotecan is used by IV infusion. The drug distributes to many sites, including blood cells and the CNS. Metabolism of this drug occurs, with most of an administered dose being excreted renally or by biliary routes.

Neutropenia is the dose-limiting toxicity with topotecan. Serious anemia may be seen in more than half of the patients treated. Various GI symptoms are also common, as are loss of hair, muscle weakness, tingling of the hands or feet, and sores in the mouth.

Topotecan may increase the risk of infection if given with immunosuppressants (see Chapter 40). The drug also produces the expected interactions with bone marrow depressants and live virus vaccines.

Agents That Block DNA Synthesis (S-Phase Inhibitors)

Properties common to this class of drugs are presented next; properties unique to individual drugs are covered with each agent.

Mechanism of Action

The uncontrolled proliferation of cancerous cells is often expressed as rapid cell division or as a high growth fraction. Because only cells in the S phase of the cell cycle synthesize DNA, they are most sensitive to agents that block DNA synthesis.

Drugs may block DNA synthesis in several ways. Some of the drugs discussed in this section are specific enzyme inhibitors and prevent the action of an enzyme that is required for DNA synthesis. Other drugs that are chemically very similar to the natural purines and pyrimidines used to form DNA may be incorporated into DNA but make the DNA unstable and nonfunctional. The enzyme **DNA polymerase** is a common target of agents of this type, being inhibited by various activated forms of these drugs. The enzyme may also contribute to instability of formed DNA by recognizing these activated drugs as substrate and inserting them into DNA in place of the normal bases.

A cell that is not forming DNA will not be damaged by a drug that inhibits DNA synthesis. Therefore nonproliferating cells or cells in resting phase are relatively insensitive to these drugs. These drugs are called cycle-specific or phase-specific agents because they affect primarily cells in S phase.

The property of phase specificity explains why S-phase inhibitors must be given on a repeating schedule. In a single treatment, only the growing fraction of cells in the tumor will be affected. A recovery period with no drug given allows normal tissues with high growth fractions such as bone marrow to return to normal function. During this recovery period, many cells in the cancerous tissue will move from G_0 phase into the reproductive cycle. Other cells that were not in S phase during treatment continue to proliferate, and the tumor continues to grow. Repeated widely spaced doses of the drug give the maximum opportunity for the drug to catch the dividing cells in S phase when they will be sensitive.

Pharmacokinetics

Many S-phase inhibitors must be activated before they exhibit anticancer activity. Some are activated in liver, but others are activated in cells of many types.

Uses

The clinical uses of antineoplastic drugs that block DNA synthesis are summarized in Table 55-2.

Table 55-2 Anticancer Drugs That Block DNA Synthesis

Generic Name	Trade Name	Administration/Dosage	Comments/Uses
cladribine	Leustatin*	INTRAVENOUS: *Adults*—0.1 mg/kg/day for 7 days. FDA pregnancy category D.	Used for hairy cell leukemia.
cytarabine	Cytosar*	INTRAVENOUS: *Adults and children*—100-200 mg/m²/day for 5-10 days. FDA pregnancy category D. SUBCUTANEOUS: *Adults and children*—1 mg/kg once or twice per week.	Used to induce and maintain remission in leukemia patients and lymphomas.
floxuridine	FUDR	INTRAARTERIAL: *Adults*—0.1-0.6 mg/kg over 24 hr. FDA pregnancy category D.	Palliative for solid tumors not treatable by other means.
fludarabine	Fludara*	INTRAVENOUS: *Adults*—25 mg/m²/day for 5 days; repeat monthly. FDA pregnancy category D.	Used for chronic lymphocytic leukemia.
fluorouracil, or 5-FU	Adrucil*	INTRAVENOUS: *Adults*—7-12 mg/kg for 4 days as initial therapy. Less frequent dosing is used for maintenance therapy. FDA pregnancy category D.	Palliative for solid tumors incurable by surgery or other means.
	Efudex* Fluoroplex*	TOPICAL: *Adults*—Used as 1%, 2%, or 5% solution or cream.	Topical fluorouracil is used to treat multiple actinic (solar) keratoses.
gemcitabine	Gemzar*	INTRAVENOUS: *Adults*—1000 mg/m² infused over 30 min once a week for up to 7 doses. FDA pregnancy category D.	Palliative therapy for pancreatic carcinoma.
hydroxyurea	Hydrea*	ORAL: *Adults*—Dosages range from 20-30 mg/kg/day up to 80 mg/kg every 3 days.	Used to treat melanoma, myelocytic leukemia, and carcinomas.
mercaptopurine	Purinethol*	ORAL: *Adults and children*—2.5 mg/kg/day initially. May continue for weeks if toxicity does not supervene. FDA pregnancy category D.	Produces remissions in leukemias.
methotrexate	Folex Mexate	ORAL: *Adults and children*—From 2.5 mg/day to 40 mg/m² once weekly, depending on disease. FDA pregnancy category X. INTRAMUSCULAR: *Adults and children*—15-30 mg/day for 5 days, or 3.3 mg/m² in combinations. INTRAVENOUS: *Adults*—2.5 mg/kg every 14 days. INTRATHECAL: *Adults and children*—0.2-0.5 mg/kg up to 12 mg total.	Methotrexate can cure choriocarcinoma; maintains remissions in lymphocytic leukemia; is palliative for lymphomas and carcinomas.
mitoxantrone	Novantrone*	INTRAVENOUS: *Adults*—12 mg/m²/day for up to 3 days, with other drugs. FDA pregnancy category D.	Used for nonlymphocytic leukemias.
thioguanine	Lanvis†	ORAL: *Adults*—2 mg/kg/day initially. May continue for weeks if toxicity does not supervene.	Used for myelocytic leukemia.

NOTE: The doses listed are representative. Very different doses and schedules may be indicated in specific diseases or protocols.
*Available in Canada and the United States.
†Available in Canada only.

Adverse Reactions and Contraindications

Because the specificity of S-phase inhibitors is toward any active DNA synthesis, many normal cells will be sensitive. At highest risk of toxicity are tissues with a high growth fraction. Bone marrow depression and suppression of lymphocyte formation are characteristic side effects of these drugs. Lowered lymphocyte formation reduces the ability of the patient to fight infection (immunosuppression), which may reduce the patient's chance for survival. GI mucosa also has a high growth fraction and is a target of serious toxic reactions to the drugs of this family. Nausea, vomiting, and stomatitis are observed.

Toxicity

Bone marrow suppression is often a dose-related side effect. Therefore very high dosages may have profound effects on the bone marrow.

Interactions

S-phase inhibitors all may produce serious interactions with bone marrow suppressants or radiation because the combinations significantly depress production of blood cells. The immunosuppression these drugs produce also puts patients at risk of generalized viral infections if they are given a live virus vaccine during or shortly after receiving an S-phase inhibitor. Oral polio vaccines for family members may also put these patients at risk.

In addition to these expected interactions, a wide variety of other interactions are also possible; these are noted with the individual drugs in the next section.

cladribine

Cladribine is an analog of adenosine, a normal component of DNA. The drug is activated in cells and accumulates in monocytes and lymphocytes, where it impairs DNA repair. Although the primary action is this antimetabolite activity, cladribine is unlike most antimetabolites in affecting not only S-phase cells but also cells in other phases of the cell cycle. Cladribine is used by IV injection for a single course of therapy. The effect on lymphocytes is noted within 1 week, but the antileukemic effect may take up to 4 months to become evident.

In addition to the expected effects of anemia, neutropenia, and thrombocytopenia, cladribine also causes skin rashes, fever, infections, nausea, anorexia, vomiting, headache, and excessive tiredness in significant numbers of patients.

Cladribine causes the expected interactions with bone marrow depressants and live virus vaccines. In addition, cladribine elevates uric acid concentrations and may change the dosage of probenecid or sulfinpyrazone needed to control hyperuricemia.

▼ cytarabine

Cytarabine is a chemical analog of cytidine, a normal component of DNA. Cytarabine interferes with the function of the enzyme DNA polymerase, which inserts cytidine into DNA but cannot insert cytarabine; therefore cytarabine slows or stops DNA synthesis. Cytarabine is rapidly inactivated by enzymes that deaminate the molecule. Blood and liver enzymes apparently contribute to this process.

Cytarabine must be injected, either subcutaneously, intrathecally, or intravenously. Subcutaneous injections are used only to maintain remissions and are given once or twice a week. Cytarabine does not easily pass into the cerebrospinal fluid. If it is administered intrathecally, it may persist in cerebrospinal fluid for several hours because that fluid has little of the deaminating enzyme that inactivates cytarabine.

Cytarabine is a potent bone marrow suppressant, acting on that tissue by the same mechanism effective in cancer cells. Bone marrow depression is most profound 1 to 3 weeks after the drug is stopped. Recovery of marrow function takes at least 1 month for most patients and longer for those receiving the drug for extended periods. Cytarabine may also cause significant GI toxicity. Some patients may experience perforation or necrosis of the bowel. CNS toxicity is reported in up to 10% of treated patients.

Cytarabine causes the expected interactions with bone marrow depressants and live virus vaccines. The drug may also have additive effects with other immunosuppressants, which can increase the risk of infections. In addition, cytarabine elevates uric acid concentrations and may change the dosage of probenecid or sulfinpyrazone needed to control hyperuricemia. Cytarabine with cyclophosphamide increases the risk of cardiotoxicity.

Cytarabine is used in many chemotherapeutic combinations for leukemias and lymphomas, including a combination with thioguanine and daunorubicin used for acute myeloid leukemia (see Table 54-4).

floxuridine and fluorouracil

Fluorouracil and floxuridine are synthetic pyrimidine bases that may be converted in the body to an active agent (floxuridine monophosphate). This active form of fluorouracil resembles the pyrimidine that is directly incorporated into RNA or that is converted to thymidylate for DNA synthesis.

Fluorouracil and floxuridine disrupt these pathways in at least two ways. First, the activated drug may enter RNA, creating a defective form of that nucleic acid that does not allow normal protein synthesis. Second, thymidylate synthase, the enzyme required to form thymidylate for DNA synthesis, is inhibited. With thymidylate synthase blocked, DNA synthesis halts.

Oral absorption of fluorouracil is erratic, and the drug is commonly given intravenously. For most patients, best results seem to be produced by giving loading doses intravenously for 4 consecutive days and then tapering to weekly maintenance doses.

Fluorouracil is extensively metabolized by the liver and other tissues. Less than 15% of the drug dose appears as active drug in the urine. Fluorouracil is cleared from the blood within 3 hours of an IV injection, but the effects persist longer.

The route of administration of floxuridine determines its metabolic fate and its effectiveness. Floxuridine given intravenously by rapid injection is broken down to fluorouracil and thence to the normal breakdown products of fluorouracil. When floxuridine is given slowly by intraarterial infusion, metabolism to fluorouracil is reduced and most of the drug is converted to floxuridine monophosphate. The intraarterial route requires a lower dose yet is more effective than IV administration.

Fluorouracil and floxuridine are highly toxic to the GI tract. Inflammation of the membranes of the mouth and pharynx may be an early sign of such toxicity. Nausea, vomiting, and diarrhea almost always occur, and if the drug is not discontinued, duodenal ulcers may occur and the bowel may perforate. Patients with preexisting poor nutritional status are at much greater risk with these drugs.

Blood dyscrasias also occur with fluorouracil and floxuridine and may limit therapy. Leukopenia continues for 1 or 2 weeks after therapy is stopped. Various skin reactions and alopecia also occur but usually do not cause the drug to be discontinued.

Both fluorouracil and floxuridine cause the expected interactions with bone marrow depressants and live virus vaccines.

Fluorouracil has been used in many combinations for various cancers, including CMF, a combination with cyclophosphamide and methotrexate used for breast carcinoma (see Table 54-4).

fludarabine

Fludarabine is an analog of adenine, but it resists inactivation by adenosine deaminase. The drug is activated to the triphosphate inside cells. The drug is given by IV injection and is rapidly altered in the blood to a form better able to enter cells.

In addition to the expected side effects of anemia, leukopenia, and thrombocytopenia, fludarabine also causes diarrhea, nausea, pain, pneumonia, skin rash, vomiting, and excessive tiredness.

Interactions with fludarabine include those expected with bone marrow depressants and live virus vaccines. In addition, fludarabine elevates uric acid concentrations and may change the dosage of probenecid or sulfinpyrazone needed to control hyperuricemia. The use of fludarabine with pentostatin increases the risk of potentially fatal pulmonary damage.

gemcitabine

Gemcitabine is chemically related to pyrimidines used for nucleic acid synthesis. The drug must be activated by forming the diphosphate, which inhibits various DNA synthetic enzymes, and the triphosphate, which is incorporated into DNA by DNA polymerase and impairs reading of the DNA. The result of both actions is a strong blockade of DNA synthesis and function.

Gemcitabine must be given by IV infusion. Distribution of the drug in the body is influenced by the rate of infusion and the patient's age and gender. Slow infusion favors distribution of drug into the tissues. Because gemcitabine is eliminated almost entirely by the kidneys, the normal age-related decline in renal function causes an age-related decline in clearance of the drug. Females of all ages eliminate gemcitabine less efficiently than males of the same age.

Bone marrow suppression, leading to anemia, thrombocytopenia, and leukopenia, is the dose-limiting toxicity with gemcitabine. The drug can also cause shortness of breath, hypertension, stroke, cardiac arrhythmias, and hemorrhage. Less serious reactions include various GI toxicity and a flu-like syndrome.

Gemcitabine causes the expected interactions with other bone marrow depressants or with live virus vaccines. In addition, the strong immunosuppressant action of gemcitabine is increased if the drug is given with other immunosuppressants.

hydroxyurea

Hydroxyurea inhibits the enzyme that converts ribonucleotide precursors of RNA to deoxyribonucleotides, which form DNA; thus DNA synthesis is inhibited.

Hydroxyurea is well absorbed when given orally and distributes well to many tissues, including the brain. The drug is excreted by the kidneys.

Hydroxyurea produces bone marrow suppression as the most common side effect. This reaction is reversible. GI disturbances, renal impairment, and skin reactions are reported less often.

Interactions with hydroxyurea include those expected with bone marrow depressants and live virus vaccines. Hydroxyurea may also elevate uric acid concentrations and change the dosage of probenecid or sulfinpyrazone needed to control hyperuricemia.

mercaptopurine and thioguanine

Mercaptopurine (6-Mercaptopurine or 6-MP) resembles adenine and guanine and blocks several points in the synthesis of these nucleic acid precursors. Thioguanine (TG or 6-TG) blocks two reactions, which are also sensitive to mercaptopurine. As a result of the blockade of purine synthesis, DNA synthesis is blocked by either drug; therefore both mercaptopurine and thioguanine are S-phase–specific inhibitors. Both drugs are activated in tissues.

Mercaptopurine is adequately absorbed orally. Part of the dose is excreted renally, but significant metabolic degradation also occurs. The properties of thioguanine are similar to those of mercaptopurine. These drugs do not readily cross the blood-brain barrier.

Bone marrow suppression may occur with mercaptopurine or thioguanine. Anemia may contribute to weakness and to fatigue. Immunosuppression contributes to increased risk of infection in treated patients.

Mercaptopurine toxicity may be greatly increased by concomitant treatment with allopurinol. Allopurinol blocks uric acid synthesis and is often used to prevent toxic accumulation of that substance after extensive tumor cell destruction by chemotherapy, but allopurinol also inhibits the metabolism of mercaptopurine. Therefore, when the drugs are combined, more mercaptopurine persists in blood and in tissues for longer periods and greater toxicity results. Thioguanine metabolism is not greatly affected by allopurinol.

Both mercaptopurine and thioguanine have significant interactions with bone marrow suppressants and live virus vaccines. Mercaptopurine also interacts with immunosuppressants and hepatotoxic agents. Both drugs are widely used in combinations for leukemias (see Table 54-4).

▼ methotrexate

Methotrexate is commonly described as a folic acid antagonist because it prevents the regeneration of the metabolically active form of folic acid, tetrahydrofolate (THF). Without THF, cells cannot carry out carbon-transfer reactions, and normal metabolism is blocked at several points. One of these blockades prevents the formation of thymidylic acid, and another arrests adenine and guanine nucleotide synthesis at an early stage. Without these precursors, DNA synthesis halts. Methotrexate is therefore specific for the S phase of the cell cycle.

Methotrexate may be administered by oral, intramuscular (IM), IV, intraarterial, or intrathecal routes. For many patients the oral route is satisfactory because effective serum concentrations are reached within 1 hour. Parenteral administration results in a slightly faster absorption rate. The intrathecal route is required to treat patients with leukemias that have penetrated the CNS. Methotrexate does not pass from the blood into cerebrospinal fluid in useful amounts.

Methotrexate is well distributed in the body and may accumulate in some tissues. Liver cells seem especially able to bind the drug for long periods. It also persists in the kidneys. These tissue sites of drug accumulation normally account for a small fraction of the total dose of methotrexate. Most of the drug is excreted directly in urine. Little degradation of methotrexate occurs, and the excreted drug is unchanged.

Methotrexate produces toxicity typical for drugs of this class. The rapidly dividing tissues of the GI mucosal lining are severely damaged. Stomatitis and diarrhea are common signs of toxicity that call for discontinuation of the drug. If therapy continues after these symptoms arise, severe GI damage, including perforation, can result.

Bone marrow function is also compromised with methotrexate. The result, as with other drugs of this class, is leukopenia. Other blood changes may occur and may produce uncontrolled bleeding. Methotrexate is an immunosuppressant and may damage the body's ability to fight infection.

The effectiveness and toxicity of methotrexate may be affected by a variety of other drugs. Bone marrow suppressants and live virus vaccines produce the expected interactions. In addition, salicylates (e.g., aspirin) tend to increase methotrexate toxicity by displacing methotrexate from plasma proteins. The increase in free plasma methotrexate often produces toxicity.

Acyclovir may increase the risk of CNS effects when methotrexate is injected intrathecally. Alcohol or other hepatotoxic drugs increase the risk of liver damage. Asparaginase may block the action of methotrexate. Nonsteroidal antiinflammatory drugs (NSAIDs) may increase bone marrow effects of methotrexate.

Methotrexate produces cytotoxicity by blocking regeneration of THF. Thus it is possible to prevent the action of the drug by supplying the body with THF. This use has been exploited for treating methotrexate overdose. Tumors such as osteosarcoma are treated with massive doses of methotrexate. Under ordinary circumstances, these doses would destroy the bone marrow and would be lethal, but if the patient receives IV leucovorin, an agent containing THF and other forms of folic acid, the bone marrow can be protected. This type of therapy is called leucovorin rescue.

mitoxantrone

Mitoxantrone reacts with DNA probably by tight binding to the nucleic acid, which blocks RNA synthesis and ultimately protein synthesis. Mitoxantrone is available for IV use only. The drug is metabolized in the liver and excreted to some degree in bile. The small amount of drug or its metabolic products in urine add a blue-green color to urine for 24 hours after each dose.

Mitoxantrone is an extremely potent myelosuppressant. Most patients also experience GI irritation or distress. Approximately one third of patients experience cough or dyspnea. Cardiovascular toxicity is a risk, especially as the total dose exceeds 140 mg/kg.

In addition to the expected interactions with bone marrow depressants and live virus vaccines, mitoxantrone may raise uric acid levels, which leads to interactions with probenecid or sulfinpyrazone.

Agents That Block RNA or Protein Synthesis

Properties common to this class of drugs are presented next; properties unique to individual drugs are covered with each agent.

Mechanism of Action

The rapid proliferation of cancer cells can be inhibited by agents that block RNA formation or interfere with the use of RNA as a template for protein synthesis. Many of these drugs have this action because they bind very tightly to DNA and prevent reading of genes. These agents are not highly specific for cancer cells but rather interfere with RNA and protein synthesis in any rapidly dividing tissue. The exception to this rule is asparaginase, a drug with some selectivity for cancer cells.

Pharmacokinetics

The pharmacokinetics of these drugs is varied. Many persist for some time inside cells. The effects of the drugs persist for days to weeks.

Uses

The clinical uses of these drugs are summarized in Table 55-3.

Adverse Reactions and Contraindications

These inhibitors of RNA and protein synthesis attack all rapidly dividing tissues and therefore produce the expected array of side effects: bone marrow suppression, leading to lower production of various blood cells; damage to the epithelial layer of the GI tract, producing symptoms ranging from nausea to stomatitis; and damage to the hair follicles, causing hair loss. The exception is asparaginase, a drug whose different mechanism for inhibiting protein synthesis leads to a different array of side effects.

Toxicity

Bone marrow suppression tends to be a dose-dependent side effect. Therefore high dosages cause more profound suppression in more patients.

Interactions

Inhibitors of RNA and protein synthesis, with the exception of asparaginase, may produce serious interactions with bone marrow suppressants or radiation because the combinations significantly depress production of blood cells. The immunosuppression these drugs produce also puts patients at risk of generalized viral infections if they are given a live virus vaccine during or shortly after receiving one of these agents. Oral polio vaccines for family members may also put these patients at risk.

Treatment with an inhibitor of RNA and protein synthesis often causes an elevation in uric acid in the blood. Therefore dosages of drugs like probenecid or sulfinpyrazone may need to be changed to prevent hyperuricemia or gout.

In addition to these expected interactions, a wide variety of other interactions are also possible; these are noted with the individual drugs in the section that follows.

asparaginase and pegaspargase

Asparaginase is an enzyme that converts the amino acid asparagine to aspartic acid; pegaspargase is a chemically modified form of asparaginase. The therapeutic effect of these agents arises because many types of cancer cells cannot form asparagine fast enough to support their growth. The enzyme destroys circulating asparagine, starving the cancer cells for asparagine. Normal cells are spared because they can form asparagine internally.

Table 55-3 **Anticancer Drugs That Block RNA and/or Protein Synthesis**

Generic Name	Trade Name	Administration/Dosage‡	Comments/Uses
asparaginase	Elspar Kidrolase†	INTRAMUSCULAR: *Children*—6000 IU/m^2 on a specific schedule with other drugs. INTRAVENOUS: *Adults*—200 IU/kg/day for 28 days. FDA pregnancy category C. *Children*—1000 IU/kg/day for 10 days.	Induces remissions in acute lymphocytic leukemia in children. Used with other drugs.
dactinomycin	Cosmegen*	INTRAVENOUS: *Adults*—0.5 mg/m^2 once weekly for 3 wk. FDA pregnancy category C. *Children*—0.015 mg/kg or 0.45 mg/m^2 for 5 days.	Used to treat choriocarcinoma, Wilms' tumor, sarcomas, and carcinomas.
daunorubicin	Cerubidine*	INTRAVENOUS: *Adults*—45 mg/m^2/day for 3 days. Lifetime dose should not exceed 550 mg/m^2. FDA pregnancy category D. *Adults* >60 yr—30 mg/m^2/day for 3 days. *Children*—25 mg/m^2 once weekly, with vincristine and prednisone.	Used primarily for leukemias. Heart toxicity occurs especially when total doses approach 500 mg/m^2.
daunorubicin, liposomal	DaunoXome	INTRAVENOUS: *Adult*—40 mg/m^2 infused over 60 min; repeat in 2-wk intervals. FDA pregnancy category D.	Kaposi's sarcoma.
doxorubicin	Adriamycin* Rubex	INTRAVENOUS: *Adults*—60-75 mg,^{2} as single injection repeated no more often than every 3 wk. Lifetime dose should not exceed 500 mg/m^2. *Children*—30 mg/m^2/day for 3 days; repeat every 4 wk.	Effective against leukemias, lymphomas, sarcomas, and carcinomas. Heart toxicity occurs especially when total doses approach 500 mg/m^2.
doxorubicin, liposomal	Doxil	INTRAVENOUS: *Adult*—20 mg/m^2 infused over 30 min; repeat in 3-wk intervals.	Kaposi's sarcoma.
epirubicin	Pharmorubicin†	INTRAVENOUS: *Adults*—75-90 mg/m^2; repeat every 3 wk.	Used for carcinomas and lymphomas.
idarubicin	Idamycin*	INTRAVENOUS: *Adults*—12 mg/m^2/day for 3 days with other drugs. FDA pregnancy category D.	Used for acute myelocytic leukemia.
pegaspargase	Oncaspar	INTRAMUSCULAR: *Adults up to 21 yr and children*—2500 IU/m^2 every 2 wk. FDA pregnancy category C. *Children* <0.6 m^2—82.5/m^2 every 2 wk.	Used for acute lymphoblastic leukemia.
plicamycin	Mithracin	INTRAVENOUS: *Adults*—0.025-0.050 mg/kg every other day for 8 doses. FDA pregnancy category X.	Used to treat testicular carcinoma and metastatic bone tumors associated with hypercalcemia.

NOTE: The doses listed are representative. Very different doses and schedules may be indicated in specific diseases or protocols.
*Available in Canada and the United States.
†Available in Canada only.

To be most effective, asparagine starvation should occur in the G$_1$ phase of the cell cycle. If asparagine levels are kept low during that period, the asparagine-dependent cancer cell will be unable to carry out protein synthesis, and ultimately, RNA and DNA synthesis will cease. If asparagine starvation occurs later in the cell cycle after many critical proteins and nucleic acids have been formed, the cell may not die.

Asparaginase is a protein and must therefore be administered by parenteral routes. The original form of asparaginase persists in blood for 1 to 2 days; the modified form (pegaspargase) persists much longer, allowing this form of the drug to be used every 2 weeks. Neither form enters cerebrospinal fluid in useful amounts. Excretion is mostly by nonrenal mechanisms.

Asparaginase produces a wide range of toxic reactions. Because the drug is a protein, it is an effective antigen and may provoke severe allergic reactions. The modified version of the protein in pegaspargase is less antigenic. Renal and hepatic function may be impaired, and some patients have bleeding episodes because the drug suppresses various clotting factors. Hyperglycemia or hypoglycemia has also been observed. Many patients show signs of CNS toxicity, including depression, lowered consciousness, and coma. Asparaginase toxicity is increased by vincristine or prednisone. Nevertheless, these drugs are cautiously used together in certain combination treatment regimens. The anticancer effects of methotrexate may be diminished by asparaginase or pegaspargase. Pegaspargase interferes with normal clotting mechanisms and thus may have dangerous interactions with anticoagulants, aspirin and other salicylates, or NSAIDs (see Chapter 31).

In addition to the interactions noted previously, asparaginase has the expected interactions with probenecid, sulfinpyrazone, and live virus vaccines.

▼ dactinomycin

Dactinomycin (actinomycin D) is an antibiotic derived from *Streptomyces*. The drug binds strongly to double-stranded DNA and prevents the DNA from serving as a template for RNA synthesis. The cell, unable to form messenger RNA, is thus unable to synthesize proteins or complete cell division.

Dactinomycin is not well absorbed orally. The drug is also extremely corrosive to soft tissues and must therefore be given only by the IV route. Dactinomycin is rapidly cleared from blood, entering the liver and other tissues. The drug does not cross the blood-brain barrier in effective amounts. Excretion of dactinomycin is mainly into bile, with smaller amounts of unchanged drug also appearing in urine.

Dactinomycin is very toxic and must be administered with great care. The highly corrosive nature of the compound makes it imperative that IV injection be given properly, with no leakage of drug into tissues that surround the vein. Such extravasation can cause extensive tissue damage.

Dactinomycin causes significant hematologic changes, which may include aplastic anemia. These blood changes are most pronounced several days after therapy. GI toxicity is severe with dactinomycin. Patients may experience extreme nausea and vomiting within hours of drug administration. Phenothiazine antiemetics may be required to control vomiting. Dactinomycin also irritates the lining of the entire GI tract. Patients commonly report lip inflammation (cheilitis), difficulty in swallowing (dysphagia), mouth sores (ulcerative stomatitis), inflammation of the pharynx (pharyngitis), abdominal pain, and anal inflammation (proctitis).

Dactinomycin also severely damages hair follicles, causing alopecia. The drug may cause reddening of the skin (erythema) and signs of inflammation, especially in an area also receiving irradiation.

Dactinomycin has the expected interactions with bone marrow suppressants, probenecid, sulfinpyrazone, and live virus vaccines.

daunorubicin, doxorubicin, epirubicin, and idarubicin

These drugs bind strongly to double-stranded DNA and thus stop the formation of RNA. Cells are most significantly affected during S and G_2 phases of the cell cycle.

Doxorubicin has a wide range of antitumor activity, including leukemias, lymphomas, sarcomas, genitourinary carcinomas, squamous cell carcinomas of the head and neck, and lung cancer. Daunorubicin has been used primarily in patients with leukemias. Idarubicin, which has very similar properties to doxorubicin and daunorubicin, is used primarily for patients with acute myelocytic leukemia. A related compound, epirubicin, has been used for patients with carcinoma of the breast or lymphomas.

These drugs are not well absorbed orally and are highly irritating to skin and soft tissues; therefore they must be given intravenously. The drugs are widely distributed to many tissues and organs, but rapid and extensive metabolism occurs in the liver. Active and inactive metabolites are formed. Most drug elimination occurs through the liver. These drugs do not readily enter the CNS.

Liposomal preparations with rather different pharmacokinetics than the standard preparations are available for both daunorubicin and doxorubicin. In the liposomal formulations the drugs tend to stay in the blood rather than enter normal tissues and are protected from metabolic breakdown. The liposomal preparations do enter tumors, where the active drug is slowly released.

Doxorubicin causes delayed leukopenia and other blood changes. Damage to bone marrow limits the amount of drug that may be used and the frequency of administration. Ordinarily, 21 days will be required for the bone marrow to recover. Toxicity to the heart also limits the total amount of drug that can be administered. Total doses of more than 550 mg/m^2 may produce irreversible toxicity to the heart, including electrocardiographic (ECG) changes and congestive heart failure. Preexisting heart disease, prior irradiation to the region of the heart, or prior use of the cardiotoxic drugs cyclophosphamide, mitomycin, or dactinomycin may greatly increase the likelihood for heart damage with these drugs.

Because these drugs are metabolized and eliminated by the liver, patients with impaired liver function may have drug accumulation and increased toxicity unless doses are appropriately reduced. Some metabolites of doxorubicin and daunorubicin appear in urine of all treated patients and produce a harmless red coloration of urine. These drugs can cause severe tissue necrosis if allowed to escape from the vein during drug administration. Damage to veins may occur if the same vein is used repeatedly. Alopecia and GI irritation also occur commonly.

These drugs have the expected interactions with bone marrow suppressants, probenecid, sulfinpyrazone, and live virus vaccines. Doxorubicin and daunorubicin are often used in combinations for various types of cancers (see Table 54-4).

plicamycin

Plicamycin binds DNA, thereby preventing RNA synthesis. Plicamycin also blocks parathyroid hormone activity on osteoclasts, thereby lowering the release of calcium into the blood. This ability to lower blood calcium levels may be useful in patients with hypercalcemia as a result of metastatic cancer of the bone. Plicamycin must be given intravenously because oral absorption is poor. It damages skin and muscle tissues.

Plicamycin produces anorexia, nausea, vomiting, skin changes, and lowered blood concentrations of calcium, potassium, and phosphorus. High dosages increase the risk of bleeding and the risk of renal or hepatic damage.

The tendency of plicamycin to cause bleeding establishes the cause of several important interactions. Risk of hemorrhage is increased when plicamycin is used with anticoagulants, antiinflammatory drugs, dipyridamole, heparin, sulfinpyrazone, or valproic acid. Hepatotoxic or nephrotoxic medications may be more toxic in the presence of plicamycin. Plicamycin also produces the expected reactions with bone marrow suppressants and live virus vaccines.

Agents That Prevent or Arrest Mitosis

Properties common to this class of drugs are presented next; properties unique to individual drugs are covered with each agent.

Mechanism of Action

To segregate chromosomes, a dividing cell must form a mitotic spindle composed of microtubules. Microtubules normally function as part of the cytoplasmic transport systems in cells and are required for certain types of cell movement. The major component of microtubules is the protein tubulin.

The structure of microtubules can be disrupted by substances that bind to tubulin and cause it to be released from microtubules or cause the tubulin to be held in nonfunctional aggregates. These alterations of microtubular structure may not be lethal to a cell unless it is in the process of forming the mitotic spindle. Cells exposed at this stage of division are arrested at that point, and reproduction cannot proceed. Ultimately, these cells die. Substances that act in this way are called **mitotic inhibitors.**

Pharmacokinetics

Most of the compounds in this class have relatively long half-lives that range from a few hours to longer than 2 days. Most of the compounds are biotransformed by the liver and excreted in bile, but renal mechanisms may also operate.

Uses

The clinical properties of mitotic poisons and related compounds used to treat cancer are summarized in Table 55-4.

Adverse Reactions and Contraindications

The effects of these drugs are most pronounced on actively dividing cells; therefore side effects can be expected to be related to normal rapidly dividing tissues. Bone marrow suppression with altered production of blood cells is a common feature with these drugs, resulting in immunosuppression. Alopecia is especially common with this group of drugs. GI symptoms, including nausea and vomiting, also occur.

Toxicity

Each drug in this category has specific dose-limiting toxicity. For example, for vincristine it is neurotoxicity, but for vinblastine it is bone marrow suppression.

Interactions

All drugs of this class increase the risk of severe generalized viral disease if the patient receives a live virus vaccine. Bone marrow suppressants also cause excessive depression of the bone marrow if used with most of these agents. Specific interactions are noted with each individual drug below.

docetaxel and paclitaxel

Paclitaxel and docetaxel alter microtubule function inside cells and prevent normal cell division. These drugs must be used intravenously. They are eliminated through metabolism in the liver by CYP3A enzymes (see Chapter 1).

Adverse reactions of paclitaxel include the expected effects on bone marrow, with anemia, leukopenia, neutropenia, and thrombocytopenia. Diarrhea, nausea, vomiting, and hair loss also occur commonly. Peripheral neuropathies with numbness or tingling in the limbs are also common. Both drugs less often cause pain in muscles and joints.

Interactions with paclitaxel and docetaxel are those expected with bone marrow depressants and live virus vaccines. In addition, inhibitors of CYP3A, such as erythromycin, ketoconazole, and androgens (see Appendix A), can block metabolism of docetaxel and lead to increased toxicity.

vinblastine, vincristine, vindesine, and vinorelbine

Vinblastine, vincristine, vindesine, and vinorelbine are all **vinca alkaloids** with similar mechanisms of action. These drugs interfere with microtubule assembly, preventing the formation of a functional mitotic spindle, ultimately arresting the cell in mitosis. Microtubules also function in neurotransmission; thus the action of vinca alkaloids in nerve cells may cause toxicity.

These drugs must be administered intravenously. They do not cross the blood-brain barrier well enough to combat CNS spread of leukemia but are well distributed to other tissues. They are rapidly cleared from blood and concentrated in the liver. The drugs are excreted primarily in bile, with

---

Table 55-4 Anticancer Drugs That Prevent or Block Mitosis

Generic Name	Trade Name	Administration/Dosage‡	Comments/Uses
docetaxel	Taxotere*	INTRAVENOUS: *Adults*—60-100 mg/m², given as 1-hr infusion; may repeat in 3 wk. FDA pregnancy category D.	Used for breast carcinoma.
paclitaxel	Taxol*	INTRAVENOUS: *Adults*—135 mg/m² as 24-hr infusion; repeat every 21 days. FDA pregnancy category D.	Used for ovarian or breast carcinoma.
vinblastine (VLB)	Velban Velbe† Velsar	INTRAVENOUS: *Adults*—Dosages must start at 0.1 mg/kg/wk and increase gradually. Range is usually 0.15-0.2 mg/kg/wk. FDA pregnancy category D. *Children*—2.5 mg/m²/wk, increased gradually to maximum dosage allowed by bone marrow toxicity.	Palliative for lymphomas, carcinomas, and sarcomas.
vincristine (VCR)	Oncovin* Vincasar	INTRAVENOUS: *Adults*—Up to 1.4 mg/m²/wk as single dose. FDA pregnancy category D. *Children*—Up to 2 mg/m²/wk as single dose.	Used in acute leukemia, lymphomas, sarcomas, and Wilms' tumor.
vindesine	Eldisine†	INTRAVENOUS: *Adults*—3 mg/m² every 7-10 days for 8 doses.	Indicated for acute lymphocytic leukemia.
vinorelbine	Navelbine*	INTRAVENOUS: *Adults*—30 mg/m² over 6-10 min once weekly. FDA pregnancy category D.	Used for non-small-cell lung carcinoma.

NOTE: Doses listed are representative. Very different doses and schedules may be indicated in specific diseases or protocols.
*Available in Canada and the United States.
†Available in Canada only.

little drug appearing in urine. Biliary obstruction or liver impairment can dangerously impede elimination of these agents and doses need to be adjusted.

Vincristine dosages are usually limited by the peripheral neuropathy it produces. Mental depression and headache may accompany signs of peripheral neuritis or other peripheral neurologic disorders.

Many symptoms of nerve dysfunction may be observed, but loss of the Achilles tendon reflex is viewed as the first sign of neuropathy. Vinblastine produces neurologic toxicity similar to that produced by vincristine. Vinorelbine has the lowest affinity for tubulin in nerve cells within this group of drugs and thus at normal dosages causes less neurotoxicity than other vinca alkaloids.

The vinca alkaloids may be extremely irritating if they are allowed to escape from the vein into surrounding tissues during administration. Severe pain is produced, and necrosis may develop in the exposed tissue.

Vincristine produces alopecia in approximately 20% of treated patients. Many patients complain of constipation and abdominal pain, but these symptoms can usually be re-

lieved with enemas and laxatives. Unlike other members of this class, vincristine usually does not produce significant bone marrow depression.

Vinblastine produces significant bone marrow suppression, primarily leukopenia. Leukopenia normally progresses to a low point 4 to 10 days after the dose, but recovery usually occurs within 7 to 14 days. Nausea and vomiting are common. Stomatitis, diarrhea, and constipation can also occur.

Alopecia is common but often reverses even while the drug therapy is continued.

Vinorelbine also suppresses bone marrow function, leading to granulocytopenia, anemia, or leukopenia. Like other vinca alkaloids, vinorelbine can cause GI side effects such as anorexia, nausea, or vomiting.

All live virus vaccines should be avoided in patients receiving vinca alkaloids. Probenecid and sulfinpyrazone should also be avoided in patients receiving vincristine or vinblastine. Because of their effects on bone marrow function, vinblastine and vinorelbine can cause additive suppression of the bone marrow if used with other drugs acting on the bone marrow.

RESEARCH HIGHLIGHTS

Nurses' and Pharmacists' Exposure to Antineoplastic Drugs: Findings from Industrial Hygiene Scans and Urine Mutagenicity Tests

—Labuhn K, Valanis B, Schoeny R, Loveday K, Vollmer WM: Cancer Nursing *21(2):79-89, 1998.*

PURPOSE
In recent years there has been increased development and use of antineoplastic drugs. These drugs are known to be carcinogenic, mutagenic, and teratogenic. The U.S. Occupational Safety and Health Administration (OSHA) first issued guidelines for personal protection of drug handlers in 1986, but adherence to these standards is variable. The purpose of this study was to document the degree of drug exposure to antineoplastic drugs by nurses and pharmacists.

METHODS
Subjects included 23 pharmacists who prepared antineoplastic drugs (ANDs), 28 nurses who prepared and administered ANDs, 32 nurses who administered ANDs, and 35 nurse and pharmacist controls. All AND handlers prepared or administered more than 25 doses per week during the preceding year. Subjects kept logs of each AND administered and/or prepared and protective equipment used for 1 week. An industrial hygiene scan was performed once on each subject when a dose of Adriamycin was prepared because this drug appears bright orange-red under fluorescent light from the scanning device used. At the end of the target week, a 24-hour urine specimen for mutagenicity tests was collected.

RESULTS
Pharmacists prepared 1 to 50 doses in a week; 70% used adequate respiratory protection, 78% always used gloves and gowns when preparing drugs, and adequate skin protection was used on 86% of all drug-handling occasions. Nurses who administered

ANDs handled only 1 to 33 doses, wore adequate skin protection 27% of the time; 59% never used both gowns and gloves, and 16% of these reported skin contact. Nurses who prepared and administered ANDs prepared 0 to 96 doses during the week and administered 3 to 94 doses. Of these nurses, 79% used adequate respiratory protection, and skin protection was adequate 20% of the time; 64% never had adequate skin protection, and 29% reported skin contact. The scans indicated that 11 (13%) were positive: 3 pharmacists who prepared ANDs, 6 nurses who administered ANDs, and 2 nurses who prepared and administered ANDs; all of these subjects reported less use of protection than colleagues with negative scans. A total of 18 subjects had positive urine mutagenicity tests, but the proportion of positive urine tests was the same for all groups, including controls. Additional information relating positive tests to number of drug handling or administering episodes is also reported in the article.

IMPLICATIONS
Contamination with antineoplastic drugs can easily occur, and in this study most contamination was detected on protective gloves and gowns. Failure to wear personal protective equipment places nurses who prepare and administer ANDs at risk.

CRITICAL THINKING: Who prepares and administers ANDs in your clinical setting? What personal protective equipment is used? Is it used consistently? Are vertical laminar flow hoods and biologic safety cabinets used for drug preparation? Where can you obtain a copy of the OSHA guidelines on this subject?

Because the vinca alkaloids work by different mechanisms than most cytotoxic agents for cancer, the vinca alkaloids are commonly combined with two, three, or four other drugs for a variety of cancers (see Table 54-4). Certain combinations are to be avoided, however. For example, mitomycin seems to predispose patients to pulmonary reactions with vinorelbine. Likewise, doxorubicin is avoided with vincristine because the risk of excessive myelosuppression is increased. Vincristine is used only cautiously with asparaginase because of the risk of excessive neurotoxicity.

Nursing Process Overview

Antineoplastic Chemotherapy

Assessment

Perform a thorough total assessment. Anticipate the side effects of drugs that will be administered. Obtain a detailed health history, especially if the patient has previously received chemotherapy. Previous response to chemotherapy will be a guide to anticipating response to a repeated dose of chemotherapeutic drugs. Assess laboratory work, including the hematocrit, hemoglobin, and blood count; liver function and renal function studies; and bone, liver, and other scans.

Nursing Diagnoses

- Altered comfort: nausea and vomiting as drug side effect
- Self-concept disturbance related to alopecia as side effect of drug therapy
- Fatigue

Patient Outcomes

The patient will not experience nausea and vomiting or will experience minimal nausea and vomiting. The patient will discuss feelings about alopecia. The patient will establish priorities for daily and weekly activities to lessen fatigue.

Planning/Implementation

Continue to monitor vital signs, body weight, and progress of anticipated side effects. When a side effect occurs with regularity, begin preventive or prophylactic measures as soon as possible. Monitor fluid intake and output. Monitor appropriate laboratory work, and institute nursing interventions based on that information. Use care in preparing and administering chemotherapeutic drugs, and dispose of contaminated needles and tubing appropriately (see Research Highlights box). If medications are being administered via constant infusion, use an infusion control device. Ensure that IV infusion lines are patent, and avoid extravasation. Investigate any new signs or symptoms.

Evaluation

A few drugs can be used by the patient in the home for cancer treatment. For many patients cancer chemotherapy is administered in the hospital or in the physician's office because many of these drugs must be administered intravenously. Before discharge, ascertain that the patient understands how to take medications correctly, what side effects may occur, how to treat side effects, what side effects require notification of the physician, and what measures should be used to prevent complications caused by side effects. Because the nadir or most profound bone marrow suppression often occurs days to weeks after the drug is administered, the patient should know when to anticipate the side effects and what actions to take to deal with them. Teach all patients which situations require immediate notification of the physician.

Nursing Implications Summary

ANTICANCER DRUGS THAT DIRECTLY ATTACK DNA
altretamine
Drug Administration/Nursing in the Community

➤ See the general guidelines in Chapter 54 for information about anemia, nausea and vomiting, and diarrhea, and see the Patient Problems boxes in Chapter 54 on leukopenia and thrombocytopenia (bleeding tendencies).

➤ Assess for CNS effects, including clumsiness, confusion, dizziness, weakness, and numbness in the arms and legs.

➤ Assess for depression: depressed mood, lack of interest in personal appearance, insomnia, and weight gain or loss.

➤ Monitor the complete blood count (CBC), WBC differential, and platelet count.

➤ Instruct the patient to take doses after meals.

bleomycin
Drug Administration/Nursing in the Community

➤ The physician may order a test dose of medication to be given before the full dose to test for idiosyncratic reaction. See the manufacturer's literature.

➤ See the general guidelines in Chapter 54 for information about nausea and vomiting, alopecia, and administration of IV chemotherapeutic agents; also see the Patient Problems box in Chapter 54 on stomatitis.

➤ Assess for dyspnea and cough, and auscultate lung sounds. Tell the patient to report cough, shortness of breath, or difficulty breathing, which may develop for up to 1 month after the last dose of medication. Encourage patients to stop smoking.

Continued

Nursing Implications Summary—cont'd

➤ Assess for skin changes; monitor blood pressure and pulse. Monitor weight.

➤ Monitor CBC and differential, platelet count, blood urea nitrogen (BUN), serum creatinine, and urinalysis. Monitor pulmonary function tests if ordered.

➤ The physician may order other medications concurrently to prevent side effects: acetaminophen to reduce fever and antihistamines and/or steroids to decrease allergic responses.

busulfan
Drug Administration/Nursing in the Community

➤ See the general guidelines in Chapter 54 for information about anemia, elevated uric acid levels, nausea and vomiting, and alopecia. See the Patient Problems boxes in Chapter 54 for thrombocytopenia (bleeding tendencies) and depressed WBC count.

➤ Auscultate lung sounds, and assess for dyspnea and cough. Monitor weight and blood pressure. Assess for skin changes.

➤ Monitor CBC and differential, platelet count, serum uric acid, and liver function tests.

carboplatin and cisplatin
Drug Administration/Nursing in the Community

➤ See the general guidelines in Chapter 54 for information about anemia, nausea and vomiting, and with carboplatin, alopecia. See the Patient Problems boxes in Chapter 54 for depressed WBC count and thrombocytopenia (bleeding tendencies). See information about IV chemotherapy.

➤ Assess hearing acuity, and assess for tinnitus and loss of balance. Refer appropriate patients for audiograms; consult the physician.

➤ Assess for metallic taste in the mouth. Because this may affect nutritional intake, monitor weight.

➤ Monitor blood pressure and pulse; auscultate lung sounds.

➤ Monitor CBC and differential, platelet count, liver function tests, BUN and serum creatinine levels, serum electrolyte level, and uric acid levels.

➤ To limit the severe nausea and vomiting that often accompany cisplatin administration, the regimen may include administration of antiemetics, sedative, steroids, and other drugs. In addition, to limit renal toxicity, the drug is often infused with large fluid volumes, such as 250 ml/hr for 4 hours, or with mannitol or furosemide. Monitor intake and output hourly for the first 6 to 8 hours, then every 12 to 24 hours. See information about extravasation in the general guidelines in Chapter 54.

carmustine (BCNU) and lomustine (CCNU)
Drug Administration/Nursing in the Community

➤ See the general guidelines in Chapter 54 for information about anemia, alopecia, and nausea and vomiting. See the Patient Problems boxes in Chapter 54 on depressed WBC count, thrombocytopenia (bleeding tendencies), and stomatitis.

➤ Assess for dyspnea and cough; auscultate lung sounds. Encourage the patient to stop smoking. Monitor weight. Inspect for skin changes and edema.

➤ Monitor CBC and differential, platelet count, liver function tests, serum uric acid, BUN and serum creatinine level. Monitor pulmonary function tests, if available.

➤ Wear gloves when preparing or administering these drugs; hyperpigmentation may occur if the drug touches the skin. See the general guidelines in Chapter 54 about IV chemotherapy.

➤ Teach the patient taking lomustine to take doses on an empty stomach. In addition, when the prescription is filled, the correct dose may be a combination of different kinds of capsules. Instruct the patient to take all the capsules in one container, as ordered. If there are questions, consult the pharmacist or physician.

chlorambucil
Drug Administration/Nursing in the Community

➤ See the general guidelines in Chapter 54 for information about nausea and vomiting, and high uric acid levels. See the Patient Problems boxes in Chapter 54 on depressed WBC count, thrombocytopenia (bleeding tendencies), and stomatitis.

➤ Auscultate lung sounds, and assess for dyspnea and cough. Inspect for jaundice, skin changes, and rash.

➤ Monitor uric acid levels, liver function tests, CBC and differential, and platelet count.

cyclophosphamide
Drug Administration

➤ See the general guidelines in Chapter 54 for information about anemia, nausea and vomiting, diarrhea, high uric acid levels, and alopecia. See the Patient Problems boxes in Chapter 54 for depressed WBC count, thrombocytopenia (bleeding tendencies), and stomatitis.

➤ Auscultate lung sounds; assess for cough and dyspnea. Assess pulse and blood pressure. Monitor weight.

➤ Monitor CBC and differential, platelet count, liver function tests, serum electrolyte levels, uric acid levels, BUN and serum creatinine, urinary specific gravity, and urinalysis.

Nursing in the Community

➤ See the general guidelines in Chapter 54.

➤ Tell the patient to take doses in the morning on an empty stomach, unless otherwise instructed by the physician.

➤ Teach the patient to force fluids, up to eight 8-ounce glasses of water daily, and to notify the physician if blood is in the urine.

➤ Warn the patient to avoid driving or operating hazardous equipment if blurred vision, confusion, or lethargy occurs and to notify the physician.

dacarbazine
Drug Administration

➤ See the general guidelines in Chapter 54 for information about anemia, nausea and vomiting, alopecia, stomatitis (rare), and extravasation. See the Patient Problems boxes in

Nursing Implications Summary—cont'd

Chapter 54 on depressed WBC count and thrombocytopenia (bleeding tendencies).

➤ Assess for skin changes.

➤ Monitor the CBC and differential, platelet count, liver function tests, BUN and serum creatinine level, and serum uric acid.

➤ Monitor the infusion carefully to avoid extravasation. See the general guidelines in Chapter 54 for IV chemotherapy.

Nursing in the Community

➤ See the general guidelines in Chapter 54.

➤ Warn the patient to avoid driving or operating hazardous equipment if blurred vision, confusion, or lethargy occurs and to notify the physician.

etoposide and teniposide

Drug Administration/Nursing in the Community

➤ See the general guidelines in Chapter 54 for information about anemia, anorexia, nausea and vomiting, and alopecia. See the Patient Problems boxes in Chapter 54 on depressed WBC count, thrombocytopenia (bleeding tendencies), and stomatitis.

➤ Monitor pulse, blood pressure, and weight. Auscultate lung sounds; assess for dyspnea. Monitor ECGs at regular intervals. See the Patient Problems box in Chapter 13 on orthostatic hypotension. Assess for skin changes.

➤ See the general guidelines in Chapter 54 for information about IV chemotherapy and extravasation.

➤ Monitor CBC and differential and platelet count.

ifosfamide

Drug Administration

➤ See the general guidelines in Chapter 54 for information about nausea and vomiting and alopecia. See the Patient Problems boxes in Chapter 54 on depressed WBC count, stomatitis (rare), and thrombocytopenia.

➤ Assess for CNS effects: agitation, confusion, dizziness, and hallucinations.

➤ Monitor liver function tests, serum creatinine and BUN, CBC, WBC differential, platelet count, and serum phosphate and potassium. Examine urine for red blood cells (RBCs) before each dose.

➤ See the general guidelines in Chapter 54 about IV chemotherapy.

➤ Mesna: Dilute a single dose in at least 4 ml D5W, D5NS, D5 ½ NS, NS, or lactated Ringer's to make a concentration of 20 mg/ml. May be administered as a bolus, one dose over 1 minute, or infused at the same rate as ifosfamide if given together. Ifosfamide and mesna may be mixed in the same infusion. Mesna may cause a bad taste in the mouth, diarrhea, nausea, vomiting, allergic reactions, headache, or hypotension.

Nursing in the Community

➤ Review side effects with the patient. Instruct the patient to increase fluid intake for the day before therapy and for at least 72 hours after therapy to help prevent hemorrhagic cystitis. Instruct the patient to notify the physician if bladder pain, urinary frequency, blood in the urine, or painful urination develops.

irinotecan

Drug Administration/Nursing in the Community

➤ See the general guidelines in Chapter 54 for information about anemia, diarrhea, and alopecia. See the Patient Problems boxes in Chapter 54 on depressed WBC, stomatitis, and thrombocytopenia (rare).

➤ Assess for dyspnea and headache. Instruct patient that diarrhea may develop up to several days after drug therapy, may be severe, and may contribute to severe dehydration and electrolyte imbalance. Notify physician if diarrhea is severe or persistent.

➤ See the general guidelines in Chapter 54 for information about IV chemotherapy.

➤ Monitor CBC and platelet count.

mechlorethamine

Drug Administration

➤ See the general guidelines in Chapter 54 for information about anemia, nausea and vomiting, elevated uric acid level, amenorrhea, and azoospermia. Alopecia is a rare side effect. See the Patient Problems boxes in Chapter 54 on depressed WBC count and thrombocytopenia (bleeding tendencies).

➤ Assess neurologic function: tinnitus, loss of hearing, and numbness or tingling of fingers, toes, face. Emphasize the importance of audiometric testing, if prescribed.

➤ With IV administration, if extravasation occurs, discontinue the infusion and aspirate any remaining drug. Promptly infiltrate the area with sterile isotonic sodium thiosulfate injection, then apply cold compresses for 6 to 12 hours. See the general guidelines in Chapter 54 about IV chemotherapy.

➤ If the drug comes in contact with the skin, wash immediately with copious amounts of water for 15 minutes, then rinse with a 2% sodium thiosulfate solution. If the drug comes in contact with the eye, irrigate immediately with 0.9% sodium chloride or balanced salt ophthalmic solution, then promptly consult an ophthalmologist.

➤ Prepare the dose just before administration.

➤ Monitor liver function tests, CBC and platelet count, serum bilirubin, and serum uric acid.

➤ For topical administration, wear protective gloves. Assess for rashes. Shower or wash the area before applying the solution or ointment. Make certain the skin surfaces are dry. Apply to the prescribed areas, but apply lightly to the axillary, perineal, inguinal, and inframammary areas to avoid irritation. Do not shower again until before the next dose. Tell patients that topical preparations may cause the skin to darken, but this should disappear when the drug is stopped.

Nursing in the Community

➤ See the general guidelines in Chapter 54.

➤ Warn the patient to avoid driving or operating hazardous equipment if drowsiness, vertigo, weakness, or other neurologic symptoms develop and to consult the physician.

Continued

Nursing Implications Summary—cont'd

melphalan
Drug Administration

➤ See the general guidelines in Chapter 54 for information about nausea and vomiting, elevated uric acid levels, and diarrhea; alopecia is uncommon. See the Patient Problems boxes in Chapter 54 on depressed WBC count, stomatitis, and thrombocytopenia (bleeding tendencies).

➤ Monitor pulmonary function; auscultate lung sounds. Assess for dyspnea and cough. Inspect for skin changes.

➤ Monitor CBC, differential and platelet count, BUN, serum creatinine, and serum uric acid.

mitomycin
Drug Administration/Nursing in the Community

➤ See the general guidelines in Chapter 54 for information about anemia, anorexia, nausea and vomiting, and alopecia. See the Patient Problems boxes in Chapter 54 on depressed WBC count and thrombocytopenia (bleeding tendencies).

➤ Auscultate lung sounds, and assess for dyspnea and cough. Monitor intake and output and weight.

➤ See the general guidelines in Chapter 54 for IV chemotherapy and extravasation.

➤ Monitor CBC and differential, platelet count, serum creatinine level, and BUN level.

procarbazine
Drug Administration

➤ See the general guidelines in Chapter 54 for information about anemia, nausea and vomiting, anorexia, diarrhea, and alopecia. See the Patient Problems boxes in Chapter 54 on depressed WBC count and thrombocytopenia (bleeding tendencies).

➤ Assess mental status, and monitor neurologic status. Anticipate CNS side effects. Keep siderails up, supervise ambulation, and keep a night-light on.

➤ Monitor pulse and blood pressure. See the Patient Problems box in Chapter 13 on orthostatic hypotension.

➤ Auscultate lung sounds. Assess for cough and dyspnea. Inspect for skin changes.

➤ Monitor CBC and differential, platelet count, blood glucose level, and urinalysis.

Nursing in the Community

➤ See the general guidelines in Chapter 54.

➤ Warn the patient to avoid the use of alcohol; see the Patient Problems box in Chapter 57 on disulfiram-like reactions. Warn the patient to avoid foods containing tyramine (see the Dietary Considerations box in Chapter 59 on tyramine). Warn the patient to limit intake of caffeine-containing foods such as chocolate, coffee, tea, and cola drinks. These dietary limitations should continue for at least 2 weeks after the last dose of procarbazine.

➤ Tell diabetic patients to monitor blood glucose levels carefully; an adjustment in diet or insulin dosage may be necessary.

➤ Warn the patient to avoid driving or operating hazardous equipment if disorientation, dizziness, or unsteadiness develops and to notify the physician.

➤ Encourage the patient to wear a medical identification tag or bracelet if taking procarbazine.

thiotepa
Drug Administration/Nursing in the Community

➤ See the general guidelines in Chapter 54 for information about anemia, nausea and vomiting, alopecia, and elevated uric acid. See the Patient Problems boxes in Chapter 54 on stomatitis, depressed WBC count, and thrombocytopenia (bleeding tendencies).

➤ Assess for skin changes. Auscultate lung sounds. Instruct the patient to report wheezing or the development of other respiratory symptoms to the physician. Assess for urinary tract problems such as urgency, frequency, and change in urine color.

➤ Monitor CBC and differential, platelet count, BUN and serum creatinine, liver function tests, and serum uric acid.

topotecan
Drug Administration/Nursing in the Community

➤ See the general guidelines in Chapter 54 for information about anemia, nausea and vomiting, and alopecia. See the Patient Problems boxes in Chapter 54 on stomatitis, depressed WBC count, and thrombocytopenia (bleeding tendencies).

➤ Assess for excessive fatigue, fever, headache, and burning or tingling of the hands or feet.

➤ See the general guidelines in Chapter 54 for information about IV chemotherapy.

➤ Monitor CBC, WBC differential, and platelet count.

ANTICANCER DRUGS THAT BLOCK DNA SYNTHESIS
cladribine
Drug Administration/Nursing in the Community

➤ See the general guidelines in Chapter 54 for information about anemia, anorexia, nausea and vomiting, and elevated uric acid. See the Patient Problems boxes in Chapter 54 on leukopenia and thrombocytopenia (bleeding tendencies).

➤ Assess for fever, skin rash, shortness of breath, and edema in lower extremities.

➤ Monitor CBC, WBC differential, platelet count, CD4 and CD8 T-lymphocyte counts, and serum uric acid.

cytarabine
Drug Administration/Nursing in the Community

➤ See the general guidelines in Chapter 54 for information about anemia, anorexia, nausea and vomiting, diarrhea, elevated uric acid levels, and alopecia. See the Patient Problems boxes in Chapter 54 on depressed WBC count, stomatitis, and thrombocytopenia (bleeding tendencies).

➤ Auscultate lung sounds, and assess for dyspnea and cough. Monitor pulse and blood pressure. Assess for skin changes,

Nursing Implications Summary—cont'd

and inspect for edema. Rarely, ara-C syndrome may occur: bone or muscle pain, chest pain, fever, general feeling of discomfort or weakness, reddened eyes, and skin rash.

➤ Assess for changes in vision, and instruct patients to report changes in vision to the physician.

➤ See the general guidelines in Chapter 54 for information about IV chemotherapy. Use brands and diluents that do not contain benzyl alcohol as a preservative for intrathecal administration or for pediatric administration. Intrathecal administration may be associated with CNS side effects. Keep siderails up. Anticipate CNS effects.

➤ Monitor CBC and differential, platelet count, liver function tests, and serum uric acid level.

floxuridine and fluorouracil
Drug Administration/Nursing in the Community

➤ See the general guidelines in Chapter 54 for information about anemia, nausea and vomiting, diarrhea, and alopecia or thinning of hair. See the Patient Problems boxes in Chapter 54 on stomatitis, depressed WBC count, and thrombocytopenia (bleeding tendencies).

➤ See the general guidelines in Chapter 54 for information about IV chemotherapy.

➤ Assess for ataxia, and assess mental status. Inspect for skin changes.

➤ Monitor CBC and differential, platelet count, and liver function tests.

fludarabine
Drug Administration/Nursing in the Community

➤ See the general guidelines in Chapter 54 for information about anemia, nausea and vomiting, alopecia (rare), and elevated uric acid. See the Patient Problems boxes in Chapter 54 on stomatitis, leukopenia, and thrombocytopenia (bleeding tendencies).

➤ Auscultate lung sounds. Assess for cough and shortness of breath. Assess lower extremities for swelling. Assess for CNS effects, including agitation, confusion, blurred vision, loss of hearing, and numbness or tingling in fingers or toes.

➤ See the general guidelines in Chapter 54 for information about IV chemotherapy.

➤ Monitor the CBC, WBC differential, platelet count, and serum uric acid level.

gemcitabine
Drug Administration/Nursing in the Community

➤ See the general guidelines in Chapter 54 for information about anemia, nausea and vomiting, and alopecia (rare). See the Patient Problems boxes in Chapter 54 on stomatitis, leukopenia, and thrombocytopenia (bleeding tendencies).

➤ Assess for fever, edema of feet and lower extremities, shortness of breath, coughing, noisy respiration, and tightness in the chest. Monitor blood pressure.

➤ See the general guidelines in Chapter 54 for information about IV chemotherapy.

➤ Monitor CBC and WBC differential, platelet count, liver function tests, BUN and serum creatinine, and urinalysis for proteinuria.

hydroxyurea
Drug Administration/Nursing in the Community

➤ See the general guidelines in Chapter 54 for information about anorexia, diarrhea, nausea and vomiting, and elevated uric acid levels. See the Patient Problems boxes in Chapter 54 on stomatitis, depressed WBC count, and thrombocytopenia (bleeding tendencies).

➤ The contents of the capsule may be opened and emptied into water. The powder floating on the top of the water is inert filler.

➤ Assess neurologic and mental status. Monitor weight, and inspect for skin changes and edema.

➤ Monitor CBC and differential, platelet count, serum creatinine, BUN, and uric acid levels.

mercaptopurine and thioguanine
Drug Administration/Nursing in the Community

➤ See the general guidelines in Chapter 54 for information about anemia, anorexia, diarrhea, nausea and vomiting, and elevated uric acid levels. See the Patient Problems boxes in Chapter 54 on stomatitis, depressed WBC count, and thrombocytopenia (bleeding tendencies).

➤ Assess for skin changes.

➤ Monitor CBC and differential, platelet count, serum uric acid, serum creatinine, and BUN levels, and liver function tests.

➤ Instruct patients taking mercaptopurine to avoid alcoholic beverages because they may contribute to increased toxicity.

methotrexate
Drug Administration

➤ See the general guidelines in Chapter 54 for information about anemia, nausea and vomiting, diarrhea, alopecia, and elevated uric acid levels. See the Patient Problems boxes in Chapter 54 on stomatitis, depressed WBC count, and thrombocytopenia (bleeding tendencies).

➤ Monitor weight; inspect for skin changes and edema.

➤ Intrathecal administration is associated with CNS changes. Monitor mental status. Keep siderails up; supervise ambulation.

➤ See the general guidelines in Chapter 54 for information about IV chemotherapy.

➤ Monitor CBC and differential, platelet count, urinalysis, liver function tests, and serum uric acid, serum creatinine, BUN, and blood glucose levels.

➤ See the discussion of leucovorin rescue in Chapter 22.

Nursing in the Community

➤ See the general guidelines in Chapter 54.

Continued

Nursing Implications Summary—cont'd

➤ Warn patients to avoid driving or operating hazardous equipment if blurred vision, drowsiness, dizziness, or ataxia develops and to notify the physician.

➤ Instruct the patient to avoid other medications that contain aspirin or other salicylates or NSAIDs because these drugs in combination with methotrexate may contribute to toxicity.

➤ Review the Patient Problems box in Chapter 58 on photosensitivity.

➤ Instruct the patient to avoid alcoholic beverages because they may increase liver toxicity.

mitoxantrone
Drug Administration/Nursing in the Community

➤ See the general guidelines in Chapter 54 for information about nausea and vomiting, diarrhea, and alopecia. See the Patient Problems boxes in Chapter 54 on stomatitis, depressed WBC count, and thrombocytopenia (bleeding tendencies).

➤ Monitor intake and output and weight. Auscultate lung sounds. Assess for cough or shortness of breath and headache. Inspect for edema. Monitor vital signs.

➤ See the general guidelines in Chapter 54 for information about IV chemotherapy.

➤ Monitor the CBC and differential, platelet count, serum uric acid, and liver function tests.

➤ Tell the patient that urine may be bluish green and sclera may be blue for a day or two after therapy. This effect is not significant and will disappear.

AGENTS THAT BLOCK RNA AND/OR PROTEIN SYNTHESIS

asparaginase and pegaspargase
Drug Administration/Nursing in the Community

➤ See the general guidelines in Chapter 54 for information about anorexia, elevated uric acid, and nausea and vomiting. See the Patient Problems boxes in Chapter 54 on depressed WBC count, stomatitis, and bleeding tendencies.

➤ Assess neurologic and mental status. Monitor blood pressure and pulse. Monitor weight. Assess for skin changes and edema. Check stools for guaiac or occult blood.

➤ Assess for allergic reaction: difficulty breathing, joint pain, puffy face, and skin rash; and for pancreatitis: severe stomach pain with nausea and vomiting.

➤ See the general guidelines in Chapter 54 for information about IV chemotherapy.

➤ Monitor CBC and differential, prothrombin time, partial prothrombin times, liver function tests, and serum creatinine, BUN, blood glucose, and serum amylase levels.

dactinomycin
Drug Administration/Nursing in the Community

➤ See the general guidelines in Chapter 54 for information about anemia, nausea and vomiting, diarrhea, alopecia, and extravasation. See Patient Problems boxes in Chapter 54 on

stomatitis, depressed WBC count, and thrombocytopenia (bleeding tendencies).

➤ Monitor weight, blood pressure, pulse, and intake and output. Assess for edema. Auscultate lung sounds. Inspect for skin changes.

➤ See the general guidelines in Chapter 54 for information about IV chemotherapy.

➤ Monitor CBC and differential, platelet count, serum uric acid, liver function tests, serum bilirubin, and lactate dehydrogenase.

daunorubicin, doxorubicin, epirubicin, and idarubicin
Drug Administration/Nursing in the Community

➤ See the general guidelines in Chapter 54 for information about anemia, elevated uric acid levels, alopecia, nausea and vomiting, diarrhea, and extravasation. See the Patient Problems boxes in Chapter 54 on stomatitis, depressed WBC count, and thrombocytopenia (bleeding tendencies).

➤ Monitor pulse and blood pressure. Assess for signs of congestive heart failure, such as weight gain, edema of dependent areas, dyspnea, and jugular venous distension. Auscultate lung sounds, and monitor respiratory rate. Monitor serial ECGs and results of echocardiographs and radionuclide determination of ejection fraction.

➤ See the general guidelines in Chapter 54 for information about IV chemotherapy. With liposomal formulations, an infusion-related reaction may occur during the first 5 minutes of the infusion and is characterized by rigors (feeling unusually cold, shivering), chest pain, chest tightness, headache, hypotension, and flushing. Monitor vital signs.

➤ Doxorubicin liposomal may produce palmar-plantar erythrodysesthesia, characterized by erythema, scaling of the skin on the hands and feet, and swelling of the skin. In its worst form, blisters may form on the hands and feet, which may interfere with activities of daily living and become infected. Instruct the patient to notify the physician if scaling skin or swelling develops.

➤ Monitor CBC and differential, platelet count, lactate dehydrogenase and liver function tests, serum creatinine, and serum uric acid level.

➤ Inform the patient that urine may be reddish for 1 to 2 days after each dose of daunorubicin, doxorubicin, or idarubicin (not liposomal forms).

plicamycin (Mithramycin)
Drug Administration/Nursing in the Community

➤ See the general guidelines in Chapter 54 for information about anorexia, diarrhea, nausea and vomiting, and extravasation. See the Patient Problems boxes in Chapter 54 on stomatitis, depressed WBC count, and thrombocytopenia (bleeding tendencies).

➤ Monitor mental status. Warn the patient to avoid driving or operating hazardous equipment if drowsiness, dizziness, fatigue, or lethargy develops and to notify the physician.

Nursing Implications Summary—cont'd

➤ Monitor CBC and differential, platelet count, serum creatinine, BUN, serum electrolyte levels, and urinalysis.

➤ Assess for hypercalcemia and hypocalcemia. See Table 17-1 for a description of common electrolyte abnormalities. Some physicians recommend a low-calcium, low–vitamin D diet for patients taking this drug.

➤ Instruct the patient to avoid medications containing aspirin, salicylates, or acetaminophen.

➤ See the general guidelines in Chapter 54 for information about IV chemotherapy.

ANTICANCER DRUGS THAT PREVENT OR BLOCK MITOSIS

docetaxel

Drug Administration/Nursing in the Community

➤ See the general guidelines in Chapter 54 for information about anemia, extravasation, nausea and vomiting, diarrhea, and alopecia. See the Patient Problems boxes in Chapter 54 on leukopenia, thrombocytopenia (bleeding tendencies), and stomatitis.

➤ Monitor vital signs. Assess for CNS effects: numbness and burning or tingling of hands or feet. Assess for hypersensitivity reaction: back pain, flushing of face, skin rash or itching, or shortness of breath. Monitor ECG. Assess for swelling of fingers, hands, feet, or lower extremities; assess for scaly, peeling skin, especially on hands or feet; auscultate lung sounds and monitor weight.

➤ See the general guidelines in Chapter 54 for information about IV chemotherapy.

➤ Monitor the CBC, WBC differential, and platelet count, liver function tests, serum bilirubin and lactate dehydrogenase.

paclitaxel

Drug Administration/Nursing in the Community

➤ See the general guidelines in Chapter 54 for information about anemia, extravasation, nausea and vomiting, diarrhea, and alopecia. See the Patient Problems boxes in Chapter 54 on leukopenia, thrombocytopenia (bleeding tendencies), and stomatitis (rarely).

➤ Monitor vital signs. Assess for CNS effects: numbness and burning or tingling of hands or feet. Assess for hypersensitivity reaction: flushing of face, skin rash or itching, or shortness of breath. Monitor ECG.

➤ See the general guidelines in Chapter 54 for information about IV chemotherapy.

➤ Monitor the CBC, WBC differential, and platelet count.

vinblastine

Drug Administration/Nursing in the Community

➤ See the general guidelines in Chapter 54 for information about anemia, nausea and vomiting, anorexia, diarrhea, elevated uric acid, alopecia, and extravasation. See the Patient Problems boxes in Chapter 54 on stomatitis, depressed WBC count, and thrombocytopenia (bleeding tendencies).

➤ Assess neurologic and mental status. Warn the patient to avoid driving or operating hazardous equipment if dizziness or numbness develops and to notify the physician.

➤ Assess for peripheral neuropathy, including tingling or numbness of extremities. Assess for skin changes.

➤ See the general guidelines in Chapter 54 for information about IV chemotherapy.

➤ Monitor CBC and differential, platelet count, and serum uric acid.

vincristine

Drug Administration/Nursing in the Community

➤ See the general guidelines in Chapter 54 for information about anemia, extravasation, constipation, nausea and vomiting, alopecia, and elevated serum uric acid level. See the Patient Problems boxes in Chapter 54 on stomatitis, depressed WBC count (rare), and thrombocytopenia (rare) (bleeding tendencies).

➤ Assess neurologic and mental status. Assess for peripheral neuropathy, including depressed deep tendon reflexes, changes in gait, tingling of extremities (paresthesias), and other changes in the neurologic assessment.

➤ Monitor intake and output, blood pressure, pulse, and respiratory rate. Auscultate lung and bowel sounds. Monitor reflexes and gait.

➤ See the general guidelines in Chapter 54 for information about IV chemotherapy.

➤ Monitor CBC, serum electrolytes, liver function tests, serum bilirubin, lactate dehydrogenase, and uric acid levels.

 # CHAPTER REVIEW

Application

1. What is the mechanism of action of alkylating agents used as anticancer medications?

2. What type of toxicity is most common with the use of alkylating agents?

3. Which of the alkylating agents is not a strong vesicant as administered because it must be activated by liver microsomal enzymes?

4. Which drugs that directly damage the structure of DNA do not produce bone marrow suppression?

5. What is the mechanism of action of anticancer agents that block purine and pyrimidine formation or use?

Continued

6. Why are inhibitors of purine and pyrimidine formation or utilization considered phase-specific agents?
7. Which anticancer drug inhibits DNA synthesis by preventing regeneration of tetrahydrofolate (THF)?
8. What is the basis of the anticancer effect of drugs that block RNA or protein synthesis?
9. What properties of asparaginase make it unique among anticancer drugs?
10. Which anticancer drugs that inhibit RNA formation have special toxicity toward the heart?
11. What is the basis of the anticancer effects of drugs that disrupt microtubule formation?
12. What toxicity is characteristic of mitotic poisons? How should you assess for these effects?

13. Which of the mitotic poisons is most likely to cause bone marrow suppression?

Critical Thinking

1. What normal cells are especially vulnerable to attack by alkylating agents? How should you assess for these effects?
2. What type of toxicity is most common with drugs that inhibit DNA synthesis? How should you assess for these effects?
3. What toxicity is most common with anticancer drugs that inhibit RNA or protein synthesis? How should you assess for these effects?

References

Armstrong T, Rust D, Kohtz JR: Neurologic, pulmonary, and cutaneous toxicities of high-dose chemotherapy, *Oncol Nurs Forum* 24(1):Suppl:23-33, 1997.

Clayton K: Cancer-related hypercalcemia: how to spot it, how to manage it, *Am J Nurs* 97(5):42-48, 1997.

Eisenberg S: Intravenous drug compatibility: a challenge for the oncology nurse, *Oncol Nurs Forum* 24(5):859, 1997.

Harwood K: Straight talk about breast cancer, *Nursing* 26(10):39-44, 1996.

Meissner JE: Caring for patients with liver cancer, *Nursing* 26(1):51-53, 1996.

Snyder CL, Stocker J: Confronting a tempest: acute leukemia, *Nursing* 27(2):32a-32b, 32d-32e, 1997.

Thompson SD, Szukiewicz-Nugent JM, Walczak JR: When ovarian cancer strikes, *Nursing* 26(10):33-38, 1996.

Warmkessel JH: Caring for a patient with colon cancer, *Nursing* 27(4):34-39, 1997.

Warmkessel JH: Caring for patients with non-Hodgkin's lymphoma, *Nursing* 27(6):48-49, 1997.

Chapter

56

Tissue-Specific Anticancer Agents

KEY TERMS

antiandrogens, p. 650
antiestrogens, p. 652
aromatase, p. 653
LH-RH analogs, p. 651
lympholytic, p. 654

OBJECTIVES

After studying this chapter, you should be able to do the following:

- *Discuss why hormones such as estrogens, androgens, and progestins may have anticancer activity.*
- *Explain the anticancer activity of glucocorticoids.*
- *Name the target organ for mitotane and streptozocin.*
- *Develop a nursing care plan for the patient receiving one or more of the drugs discussed in this chapter.*

CHAPTER OVERVIEW

Most of the anticancer drugs discussed in Chapter 55 are not tissue specific in their cytotoxic action. For example, although chlorambucil is clinically useful because it attacks lymphoid tissue, it also attacks other tissues, especially at higher dosages. This chapter discusses anticancer agents that are effective not because of general cytotoxicity but because they act on specific receptors or other targets associated with specific types of cells.

THERAPEUTIC RATIONALE: CANCER OF SPECIFIC REPRODUCTIVE TISSUES

The sex steroids (androgens, estrogens, and progestins) are used in cancer chemotherapy because the presence (or absence) of these hormones regulates growth and function of many reproductive tissues. These steroid hormones enter sensitive cells and, complexed with specific receptor proteins, are transported to the cell nucleus. Within the nucleus they alter RNA and protein synthesis, thereby changing the function of the cell. The rationale behind all forms of this therapy is that tumors of reproductive tissues tend to retain some dependence on hormones. Thus the use of these agents in cancer chemotherapy depends on a knowledge of the hormone dependence of specific tissues. For example, the prostate gland depends on androgens; without these hormones the gland shrinks and loses function. Carcinoma of

the prostate gland retains a degree of this hormonal control, and tumor regression can often be produced by suppressing androgen production or function. Suppression of production may be with surgical castration to remove the major source of endogenous androgens or may be with a luteinizing hormone–releasing factor (LH-RH) analog that suppresses androgen synthesis. Androgen function may be diminished by antagonists that block binding to androgen receptors; estrogens and drugs like flutamide act in this way.

Suppression of tumor growth can be achieved in many breast carcinomas in women by treating them with estrogens, antiestrogens, or androgens, the choice of drug being determined by the receptor pattern of the particular tumor. For estrogen-responsive tumors, the strategy may be to antagonize estrogen effects with excess androgenic steroids or by the use of antiestrogens such as tamoxifen. Alternatively, compounds may be used that block aromatase,

649

an enzyme required for the conversion of certain adrenal steroids to estrogen. These strategies are most effective in postmenopausal women. In these women estrogens are no longer produced by the ovaries, and most of the estrogen in their bodies is produced by the action of aromatase on steroids from the adrenal glands.

THERAPEUTIC AGENTS: ANTICANCER AGENTS TARGETED TO REPRODUCTIVE TISSUES

Steroids and Related Agents

Androgens and Anabolic Steroids

Mechanism of Action

For estrogen-dependent tissues, androgens often interfere with estrogen function. Androgens can therefore cause involution of these tissues. This action forms the basis for the use of androgen to control some forms of breast cancer in postmenopausal women. Results of this form of therapy usually do not become evident until after 8 weeks of treatment or longer. Anabolic steroids may share this action because of their androgenic activity.

Pharmacokinetics

Androgens are in general not well absorbed orally, but testolactone, a semisynthetic analog of testosterone used for breast cancer (Table 56-1), is an exception. Nandrolone, the anabolic steroid most often used for breast cancer, must be given by injection; this oil-soluble substance is slowly absorbed from intramuscular (IM) sites. Androgens are metabolized by the liver.

Uses

Testolactone is used almost exclusively for breast carcinoma (see Table 56-1). Other androgens, used primarily in replacement therapy, may occasionally be used to treat specific cancers. These drugs include fluoxymesterone, methyltestosterone, testosterone enanthate, and testosterone propionate (see Chapter 72).

Nandrolone, as an anabolic steroid, may be used to treat certain anemias; the androgenic effects are of use in breast cancer. Nandrolone should not be given to males with breast cancer or prostate cancer because these diseases may be promoted by androgenic compounds.

Patients with hypercalcemia should not receive testolactone or nandrolone because of the risk of increasing the already high calcium levels. Patients with hepatic or renal disease may also be at risk.

Adverse Reactions and Contraindications

An advantage of testolactone is that it does not cause as much virilization in women as other androgens. Side effects are minimal; peripheral neuropathy with numbness or tingling in the face or limbs, anorexia, diarrhea, nausea, or vomiting is possible. Water retention with swelling of feet and ankles may also occur.

Nandrolone may cause a degree of virilization in women. Anemia, edema, and varying signs of liver toxicity are also possible.

Toxicity

Hypercalcemia may arise from rapid destruction of tumors; testolactone may need to be withdrawn and the patient may need support with large fluid volumes. Nandrolone at high dosages may cause hepatotoxicity.

Interactions

Anticoagulant effects may be increased; dosage adjustment may be required with either testolactone or nandrolone. Nandrolone may also cause additive liver toxicity when given with other hepatotoxic drugs.

Antiandrogens: bicalutamide, flutamide, and nilutamide

Mechanism of Action

Bicalutamide, flutamide, and nilutamide are not steroids, but they bind to androgen receptors inside cells and prevent the normal action of androgenic steroids. Thus these agents act as receptor antagonists. Because of the effects of their actions, these agents are called **antiandrogens**.

Pharmacokinetics

Bicalutamide, flutamide, and nilutamide are well absorbed orally but undergo extensive metabolism in the liver. Metabolites are excreted both renally and in bile.

Uses

Bicalutamide, flutamide, or nilutamide is combined with one of the LH-RH analogs (see next section) for metastatic carcinoma of the prostate, a tumor that often depends on androgens for its growth. The combination of antiandrogens with two different mechanisms very effectively eliminates any androgen contribution to tumor growth.

Adverse Reactions and Contraindications

When given with an LH-RH analog, bicalutamide, flutamide, and nilutamide reduce testosterone levels to those expected in castrated males. Many of the side effects patients experience are the result of low testosterone levels. Hot flashes are common. Most patients report reduced libido or impotence. Gynecomastia occurs in about 9% of patients. In addition to symptoms arising from testosterone suppression, these agents may also cause gastrointestinal (GI) disturbances, edema, or peripheral neuropathy.

Nilutamide and bicalutamide are usually avoided in patients with liver disease because metabolism of the drugs may be impaired.

Toxicity

Most of the side effects of bicalutamide, flutamide, and nilutamide are related to the very low levels of testosterone they induce. Therefore higher dosages may not produce

Table 56-1 **Drugs Used for Cancers of the Reproductive System**

Generic Name	Trade Name	Administration/Dosage	Comments/Uses
Androgens and Anabolic Steroids			
nandrolone	Durabolin	INTRAMUSCULAR: *Adults*—25-100 mg at 1- to 4-wk intervals. FDA pregnancy category X.	Palliative for metastatic breast cancer.
testolactone	Teslac	ORAL: *Adults*—250 mg 4 times/day. FDA pregnancy category C.	Palliative for carcinomas of breast in postmenopausal women.
Antiandrogens			
bicalutamide	Casodex	ORAL: *Adults*—50 mg once daily. FDA pregnancy category X.	Given with LH-RH analog for advanced prostatic cancer.
buserelin	Suprefact†	SUBCUTANEOUS: *Adults*—0.5 mg 3 times/day for 7 days; then 0.2 mg/day for maintenance. INTRANASAL: *Adults*—0.4 mg every 8 hr for maintenance (replaces subcutaneous maintenance).	Analog of LH-RH lowers follicle-stimulating hormone and luteinizing hormone, thus lowering androgens to castration levels; for prostatic cancer.
flutamide	Euflex† Eulexin	ORAL: *Adults*—250 mg every 8 hr. FDA pregnancy category D.	Blocks androgen actions on cells; use with LH-RH analog.
goserelin	Zoladex*	SUBCUTANEOUS (IMPLANT): *Adults*—3.6-mg base every 28 days. FDA pregnancy category X.	For prostatic carcinoma; action similar to that of buserelin.
leuprolide	Lupron*	SUBCUTANEOUS: *Adults*—1 mg/day. INTRAMUSCULAR: *Adults*—7.5 mg once a month. FDA pregnancy category X.	Suppresses secretion of androgens like buserelin; used with flutamide for prostatic carcinoma.
nilutamide	Nilandron	ORAL: *Adults*—300 mg once daily for 30 days, then 150 mg once daily. FDA pregnancy category C.	Used with castration for prostatic cancer.
Estrogens			
diethylstilbestrol	Stilphostrol Honvol†	INTRAVENOUS: *Adults*—0.5 g/250 ml for 5 days. Maintenance, 250-500 mg once or twice weekly. ORAL: *Adults*—50-200 mg 3 times/day. FDA pregnancy category X.	Palliative for prostatic carcinoma.
estramustine	Emcyt*	ORAL: *Adults*—14 mg/kg/day in 3 or 4 doses.	For prostatic carcinoma.
Antiestrogens			
anastrozole	Arimidex	ORAL: *Adults*—1 mg once daily. FDA pregnancy category D.	Palliative for breast cancer in postmenopausal women.
letrozole	Femara	ORAL: *Adults*—2.5 mg once daily. FDA pregnancy category D.	Used for breast cancer in postmenopausal women.
tamoxifen	Nolvadex* Tamofen†	ORAL: *Adults*—10 or 20 mg twice daily. FDA pregnancy category D.	Palliative for advanced carcinoma of the breast.
toremifene	Fareston	ORAL: *Adults*—60-mg base once daily. FDA pregnancy category D.	Used for estrogen-responsive breast cancer in postmenopausal women.
Progestins			
medroxyprogesterone	Depo-Provera*	INTRAMUSCULAR: *Adults*—0.4-1 g/wk. FDA pregnancy category X.	Palliative for advanced breast cancer.
megestrol	Megace*	ORAL: *Adults*—320 mg/day in divided doses. FDA pregnancy category X.	Palliative for advanced endometrial or breast carcinomas.

LH-RH, Luteinizing hormone–releasing factor.
*Available in Canada and the United States.
†Available in Canada only.

side effects that are significantly worse than with regular dosages.

Interactions

The combination of bicalutamide, flutamide, and nilutamide with one of the LH-RH analogs produces a desired interaction in that these drugs prevent the full activity of androgens and the LH-RH analogs lower the production of androgens. The result is an almost complete abolition of androgen action.

Undesirable interactions with these agents are unusual, but nilutamide may cause a flushing reaction if taken with alcohol. Nilutamide may also interfere with hepatic metabo-

lism of anticoagulants, phenytoin, and theophylline because these drugs are metabolized by the same systems.

Antiandrogens: LH-RH Analogs

Mechanism of Action

Leuprolide, buserelin, and goserelin are synthetic analogs of LH-RH. These **LH-RH analogs** tend to increase testosterone levels during the first week of therapy, but when given continuously, they begin to suppress secretion of gonadotropin-releasing hormone, resulting in lower synthesis and release of testosterone. These agents ultimately produce the same low levels of male sex steroids produced by surgical castration.

Pharmacokinetics

Leuprolide, buserelin, and goserelin are peptides and therefore cannot withstand the acidic environment of the stomach. These drugs are absorbed from subcutaneous or IM injection sites. Buserelin is also available as a nasal spray; the peptide is adequately absorbed across the nasal membranes for use in maintenance therapy.

Uses

LH-RH analogs are used for prostatic cancer to lower circulating androgens that might stimulate the tumor. LH-RH analogs are nearly always combined with bicalutamide, flutamide, or nilutamide (see previous section).

Adverse Reactions and Contraindications

Buserelin and goserelin may cause an initial flare of the disease, with pain and swelling, difficult urination, and possibly weakness. Approximately 10% of patients taking goserelin experience disease flare, but only about 1% of patients taking buserelin have this reaction. These early reactions may be related to the initial increase in testosterone produced by these drugs. Later effects such as hot flashes and decreased sexual desire are symptoms caused by the lowering of testosterone levels. Anorexia, breast tenderness, edema, nausea, and vomiting are also possible. In addition, goserelin may cause cardiovascular effects, including arrhythmias, strokes, or infarctions. Goserelin may also be associated with chronic obstructive pulmonary disease or congestive heart failure.

Leuprolide causes all of the side effects associated with low testosterone levels mentioned previously. In addition, it may be associated with cardiac arrhythmias or other cardiac symptoms, especially in men. In women the drug suppresses menstrual cycles. Both men and women may show blurred vision, dizziness, edema, headache, insomnia, nausea, numbness in hands or feet, or vomiting.

Toxicity

Overdoses of these drugs have not been studied, but because most effects of the drugs are related to changes in testosterone levels, symptoms may be similar to clinical doses.

Interactions

The LH-RH analogs are used with bicalutamide, flutamide, or nilutamide for a desired interaction: greater suppression of androgen effects on tumors. Undesirable interactions with other drugs have not been noted.

Estrogens

Mechanism of Action

For androgen-dependent tissues, estrogens often interfere with androgen function. Estrogens can therefore cause involution of these tissues. This action forms the basis for the use of estrogens to control prostatic carcinoma. Some carcinomas of the breast also respond to exogenous estrogen therapy, especially in postmenopausal women.

Estramustine combines estradiol with a nitrogen mustard. The rationale for the combination is that the drug will be most concentrated in estrogen-sensitive tissues, including tumors. In those tissues the anticancer effects of the estradiol and the nitrogen mustard may be focused. The toxicity of the drug is largely caused by the estrogen component because release of the active nitrogen mustard into blood is low.

Pharmacokinetics

Natural steroid estrogens are not absorbed orally, but several of the synthetic, nonsteroidal estrogens may be given successfully by this route. The estrogen used most often for cancer, diethylstilbestrol, is not a steroid at all and is well absorbed orally (see Table 56-1). Estrogens are metabolized by the liver. Patients with significant liver impairment may accumulate these compounds.

Estramustine is concentrated in the prostate gland because the drug binds to specific protein in that tissue. This concentration of the drug contributes to the tissue-specific action.

Uses

Of the many estrogen preparations available, only one is recommended primarily for use in prostatic carcinoma (see Table 56-1). Many of the estrogens discussed in Chapter 70 may also be used in palliative therapy for prostatic carcinoma. Estramustine is indicated only for prostatic carcinoma because of the cytotoxic component in the preparation.

Adverse Reactions and Contraindications

Estrogens increase the risks of thromboembolytic disease. Estrogens also increase salt and water retention, alter mood in some patients, decrease glucose tolerance, elevate calcium levels, produce nausea and vomiting, and cause breast tenderness and abdominal cramps. Of these reactions, thromboembolytic disease, hypercalcemia, and edema are the most threatening for cancer patients.

Estramustine and estrogens are usually avoided in patients with thrombophlebitis or other thromboembolytic diseases.

Toxicity

When estrogens are used at high dosages in men with prostatic or breast carcinoma, the risk of heart attack, pulmonary embolism, and thrombophlebitis is increased.

Interactions

Neither estramustine nor other estrogens should be used with other potentially hepatotoxic drugs because the risk of liver damage is increased. Cardiovascular side effects are more common in patients who smoke.

Antiestrogens: tamoxifen and toremifene

Mechanism of Action

Tamoxifen and toremifene are called **antiestrogens** because they block estrogen binding at receptor sites in cells. This action prevents estrogens from supporting the growth of estrogen-dependent cells. Therefore these drugs are most useful in palliating symptoms of breast carcinoma in which estrogen dependence of the tumor has been established.

Pharmacokinetics

Tamoxifen and toremifene are administered orally. Both drugs are extensively metabolized and handled similarly by the body. Metabolites enter the blood slowly, with peak concentrations occurring 3 to 7 hours after an oral dose. However, drug and metabolites persist in blood for days as a result of enterohepatic circulation (see Chapter 1). Elimination is primarily in feces. The kidney contributes little to the excretion. The full anticancer effect of antiestrogens may take months to develop.

Uses

Antiestrogens are indicated only for breast carcinoma. They are more likely to benefit women whose tumors contain estrogen receptors.

Adverse Reactions and Contraindications

Tamoxifen and toremifene may produce cancer and birth defects in animals. It is unknown whether they produce these effects in humans. The drugs seem less toxic than the estrogens and androgens used in anticancer therapy. The most common reactions to antiestrogens are nausea, vomiting, and hot flashes.

Patients who begin tamoxifen or toremifene therapy sometimes report an increase in pain at the tumor site and within metastases in bone. Tumor metastases within soft tissue may temporarily increase in size, and the surrounding tissue may become inflamed. This reaction, sometimes called disease flare, may occur even when therapy is effective.

Toxicity

High dosages may increase the incidence of dizziness, headache, or nausea. The antiestrogenic effects such as hot flashes may be more profound. At higher dosages, the weak estrogenic side effects of these drugs may become more noticeable, most commonly as vaginal bleeding.

Interactions

Interactions are generally of minor importance for tamoxifen. Antacids or histamine H_2-receptor blockers may disrupt the enteric coating on tamoxifen tablets, leading to loss of some tamoxifen activity. Estrogens may antagonize the effect of tamoxifen.

Toremifene may block hepatic metabolism of anticoagulants, leading to more profound effects of those drugs. Phenobarbital and phenytoin may increase metabolism of toremifene by inducing CYP3A4 enzymes in the liver (see Chapter 1).

Antiestrogens: Aromatase Inhibitors: anastrozole and letrozole

Mechanism of Action

Anastrozole and letrozole are nonsteroidal compounds that inhibit an enzyme called aromatase. **Aromatase** normally converts androstenedione, a steroid from the adrenal gland, to estrone. Estrone has some estrogenic activity but is further converted by other enzymes to estradiol, a powerful natural estrogen. In postmenopausal women, this pathway produces most of the estrogens that circulate in the blood. If this pathway is blocked with an aromatase inhibitor, the result is a profound lowering of circulating estrogen levels. Withdrawal of estrogen effects from estrogen-dependent tumors causes an involution of that tissue and is the basis of the anticancer effects.

Pharmacokinetics

Letrozole is completely absorbed orally, with or without food, but the oral absorption of anastrozole may be lowered by food. Both drugs are extensively metabolized in liver, primarily by CYP3A4 or CYP2A6 (see Chapter 1). The elimination half-lives of these drugs average about 2 days in most patients. Because of these long half-lives, it takes 1 to 6 weeks for steady-state levels to be reached in blood.

Elimination of anastrozole is almost entirely by biliary routes, whereas for letrozole renal mechanisms account for most of the elimination.

Uses

Anastrozole and letrozole are used only for breast cancer in postmenopausal women, most often after their cancer has failed to respond to tamoxifen.

Adverse Reactions and Contraindications

Common reactions to these drugs include nausea, chest pain, edema, and shortness of breath. A variety of other effects on the GI tract or nervous system may be noted, but the most dangerous other possibility is a thromboembolism.

Toxicity

Anastrozole at very high dosages may show more GI disturbances in animals, but effects in humans are unknown. Letrozole may cause cardiovascular effects at very high dosages in animals, but no effects have been seen in humans.

Interactions

No clinically important interactions have been noted with these relatively new drugs.

Progestins

Mechanism of Action

Progestins normally establish secretory function in the estrogen-primed endometrium (see Chapter 70). When used as anticancer agents, progestins may be effective by blocking tissue responses to other steroid hormones such as estrogens, androgens, or glucocorticoids.

Pharmacokinetics

Progestins are available in various forms suitable for oral or IM administration. The drugs are metabolized primarily in the liver; derivatives of progestins appear in urine.

Uses

The use of progestins as antineoplastic agents has been limited primarily to palliative therapy in endometrial carcinoma, but renal, breast, or prostatic carcinomas may also be susceptible (see Table 56-1).

Adverse Reactions and Contraindications

Progestins usually produce few reactions. Patients should be observed for signs of thromboembolytic disease or sudden changes in vision. Fluid retention and disruption of normal menstrual cycles may also occur. Progestins that are injected may cause pain and tissue changes at the injection site.

Toxicity

High dosages of progestins are associated with greater risk of thromboembolism.

Interactions

Drugs such as carbamazepine, phenobarbital, phenytoin, rifabutin, and rifampin induce liver enzymes that metabolize progestins. As a result, these drugs may interfere with the action of progestins.

THERAPEUTIC RATIONALE: CANCER OF SPECIFIC NONREPRODUCTIVE TISSUES

Tissue-specific anticancer agents may be targeted by designing them to interact with specific receptors on a particular type of cell. For example, glucocorticoids affect lymphoid tissue because that tissue contains specific receptors for glucocorticoids. This action may be helpful in controlling cancers arising from lymphoid tissue. Other agents such as streptozotocin are selectively concentrated in beta cells of the pancreas, so the effects of the drug are mostly limited to those cells.

THERAPEUTIC AGENTS: ANTICANCER AGENTS TARGETED TO SPECIFIC NONREPRODUCTIVE TISSUES

Lympholytic Agents

prednisone

Prednisone is the glucocorticoid most commonly used as an anticancer agent, although several of these agents are used for symptomatic relief (Table 56-2). Prednisone is an effective anticancer agent because it is a **lympholytic** agent; that is, it causes regression of lymphoid tissue (see Chapter 41). Therefore prednisone is effective against lymphoid tumors and lymphoblastic leukemias, especially in children, when used in various combinations (see Table 54-4).

Prednisone is effectively absorbed orally and is metabolized to the active form of the drug, prednisolone. Liver disease may impair this process and thus interfere with the effectiveness of prednisone.

Table 56-2   Anticancer Drugs that Target Specific Nonreproductive Tissues

Generic Name	Trade Name	Administration/Dosage	Comments/Uses
Lympholytic Agents			
prednisone	Deltasone*	ORAL: *Adults*—Up to 250 mg/day. FDA pregnancy category C. *Children*—0.5 mg/kg 4 times/day.	Used in combinations for leukemias and lymphomas.
rituximab	Rituxan	INTRAVENOUS: *Adults*—375 mg/m² 4 times in doses spaced 7 days apart. FDA pregnancy category C.	Used for CD20-positive B-cell non-Hodgkin's lymphoma.
Drugs Targeting Various Blood Cells			
interferon alfa-2a recombinant	Roferon-A*	INTRAMUSCULAR, INTRAVENOUS: *Adults*—Up to 36 million units/day. FDA pregnancy category C.	Used for hairy cell leukemia, Kaposi's sarcoma, and other tumors.
interferon alfa-2b recombinant	Intron-A*	INTRAMUSCULAR, SUBCUTANEOUS: *Adults*—Up to 30 million units/m² 3 times/wk. FDA pregnancy category C.	Used for hairy cell leukemia, Kaposi's sarcoma, and other tumors.
interferon alfa-n1	Wellferon†	INTRAMUSCULAR, SUBCUTANEOUS: *Adults*—Up to 3 million units/day for 16-24 wk. FDA pregnancy category C.	Used for hairy cell leukemia, carcinomas, melanoma, and lymphomas.
tretinoin	Vesanoid	ORAL: *Adults*—22.5 mg/kg every 12 hr for up to 90 days, or for 30 days after remission is achieved. FDA pregnancy category D.	Used for acute promyelocytic leukemia.
Adrenal Antagonist			
mitotane	Lysodren*	ORAL: *Adults*—2 g 4 times/day; maximum 16 g/day. FDA pregnancy category C.	Used for adrenal cortical carcinoma.
Beta-Cell Antagonist			
streptozocin	Zanosar*	INTRAVENOUS: *Adults*—500 mg/m² for 5 days every 6 wk. FDA category C.	Used for pancreatic tumors.
Photosensitizing Agent			
porfimer	Photofrin	INTRAVENOUS: *Adults*—2 mg/kg injected over 3-5 min, followed by laser light illumination.	Used for esophageal or non–small-cell lung tumors.

*Available in Canada and the United States.
†Available in Canada only.

Prednisone may produce all the well-known signs of glucocorticoid excess if given long enough at high dosages. These symptoms are outlined in Chapter 41.

rituximab

Rituximab is a genetically engineered monoclonal antibody that contains part human and part mouse proteins. The antibody was designed to bind to CD20, an antigen found primarily on B lymphocytes and pre–B cells under normal circumstances. B-cell type non-Hodgkin's lymphomas often also express the CD20 antigen. Thus rituximab binds to any normal B cells bearing the CD20 antigen and to the lymphoma cells bearing the antigen. Cells to which the antibody binds will be killed by immune mechanisms or will die by apoptosis (see Chapter 54). Therefore rituximab is used for CD20-positive B-cell non-Hodgkin's lymphoma.

As a protein, rituximab must be given intravenously. The depletion of B cells in blood is not seen until about 2 weeks. Effects on B cells in blood last for 6 to 9 months, and rituximab itself has been detected in blood for up to 6 months after the end of therapy.

Because rituximab is a protein, it may cause acute reactions, including bronchospasm, shortness of breath, edema of the tongue and throat, flushing of the face, and chills. GI disturbances can also occur. Later reactions can include anemia, neutropenia, and thrombocytopenia.

Rituximab contains portions of certain mouse proteins and may thus cause a serious hypersensitivity response in a patient who is allergic to mouse proteins.

Drugs Targeting Various Blood Cells

interferon alfa-2a, alfa-2b, alfa-n1, and alfa-n3

Mechanism of Action

Natural interferons are produced mainly by leukocytes and serve as part of the body's defense system. Interferons modulate the function of macrophages and lymphocytes and generally impede proliferation. Recombinant interferons share these properties. Recombinant interferons are produced by genetic engineering, which uses microorganisms to produce human proteins. Nonrecombinant interferons are produced from cultures of human cells after stimulating interferon production with Sendai virus. The anticancer activity of the interferons is not completely understood.

Pharmacokinetics

As proteins, these interferons cannot be administered orally. Absorption is adequate from IM or subcutaneous sites, producing peak serum concentration in 4 to 7 hours. These proteins are completely metabolized in the kidney and other tissues.

Uses

The recombinant interferons, interferon alfa-2a and interferon alfa-2b, are used in hairy cell leukemia, genital warts, and Kaposi's sarcoma in patients with acquired immunodeficiency syndrome (AIDS). In addition, these drugs are being investigated for their activity in various lymphomas, leukemias, and solid tumors. Interferons alfa-n1 and alfa-n3 in general have the same uses, but not all interferons have been approved for all indications listed.

Adverse Reactions and Contraindications

A flulike syndrome develops in most patients but resolves within 2 to 4 weeks, even when the drug is continued. Signs of neurotoxicity may involve the central nervous system (CNS) (depression, nervousness, and insomnia) or the periphery (numbness or tingling in extremities). Loss of appetite builds during treatment with alfa interferons and may persist for some time after therapy ends. Diarrhea, nausea, vomiting, skin rash, and unusual tiredness are common side effects when interferons are used as anticancer agents.

Toxicity

The flulike syndrome is not dose related, but neurotoxicity, GI tract toxicity, and cardiovascular toxicity are worse at higher dosages.

Interactions

Interactions are usually unimportant with interferons, but the action of CNS depressants or bone marrow depressants may be enhanced by interferons.

tretinoin

Tretinoin is a retinoid, a class of compounds that includes vitamin A. The drug induces maturation or differentiation in primitive promyelocytes, cells that are precursors to blood cells other than lymphocytes. The exact mechanism is unknown. Tretinoin is highly specific, acting only on a subtype of acute promyelocytic leukemia that shows a chromosome translocation called t(15;17). In that type of leukemia, tretinoin causes the leukemic promyelocytes to mature, and gradually normal cells reappear in the bone marrow and blood.

Tretinoin is taken orally and metabolized by the liver. Plasma steady-state levels stabilize in about 1 week after therapy starts, but full clinical remission may take 6 to 7 weeks. Elimination of the drug is by both renal and biliary routes.

Retinoids cause many side effects. Tretinoin causes retinoic acid–acute promyelocytic leukemia (RA-APL) syndrome in more than 10% of treated patients. Symptoms include difficulty breathing, chest pain, bone pain, fever, and weight gain. Other GI, cardiovascular, and pulmonary symptoms are also common. Visual disturbances and CNS effects can also occur.

Inducers or inhibitors of hepatic drug metabolizing enzymes may alter tretinoin metabolism, but the effects of these interactions have not been documented.

Adrenal Antagonists

mitotane

Mitotane is a derivative of the insecticide DDT. Toxicity studies with DDT showed specific effects on the adrenal cortex. Mitotane causes specific atrophy of the zona fasciculata and reticularis, the two inner layers of the adrenal cortex where the glucocorticoid cortisol is formed. Mitotane is not cell cycle specific and is not a general cytotoxic agent. Because of its unusual tissue selectivity, mitotane is used to treat adrenal cortical carcinoma.

Mitotane is satisfactorily absorbed when given orally. The drug is metabolized by the liver before excretion. If liver function is impaired, the drug may accumulate and toxic reactions may increase.

Mitotane causes anorexia, nausea, and vomiting in almost every patient. Nearly half of those treated experience lethargy or dizziness as a result of adrenal insufficiency. Dermatitis occurs in 20% of patients. Less common but serious reactions include abnormalities of the eye, changes in blood pressure, and hemorrhagic cystitis. Higher dosages are associated with more severe side effects.

CNS depressants are usually avoided when patients receive mitotane to prevent excessive depression of CNS function.

Pancreatic Beta-Cell Antagonist

streptozocin

Streptozocin is a specific toxin for the beta cells of the pancreatic islets. Although streptozocin resembles alkylating agents, cells other than pancreatic beta cells are relatively insensitive to the drug. Because of its strong tissue specificity, streptozocin is primarily used to treat insulin-secreting islet cell tumors of the pancreas.

Streptozocin is unstable and must be given intravenously. It is biotransformed by the liver. Both metabolites and unchanged drug are excreted in urine.

Streptozocin can destroy beta cells. Therefore insulin production may cease. Nausea and vomiting occur often. The drug is also toxic to the kidneys, and the toxicity is dose related. At high dosages renal function can be fatally compromised.

Streptozocin should not be combined with other nephrotoxic drugs. Live virus vaccines may cause a generalized disease if used in a patient receiving streptozocin. Phenytoin may interfere with the action of streptozocin in pancreatic cells.

Photosensitizing Agent

porfimer

Porfimer is a polymeric form of the pigment porphyrin. This material is concentrated in skin, liver, and spleen but also concentrates in tumors. The presence of porfimer makes the tissue sensitive to light. By selectively irradiating the tumor with light of 630-nanometer wavelength, selective tumor destruction may be achieved. This technique is used for esophageal cancer and for bronchial invasion by non–small-cell tumors of the lung.

A variety of cardiovascular, GI, and pulmonary side effects occur as a result of inflammation of tissues surrounding the site of therapy. Some of these effects may be serious and include cardiac arrhythmias, pleural effusion, and pneumonia. About 20% of treated patients experience photosensitivity of the skin, with exaggerated sunburn reactions.

Tissue-Directed Isotopes

The use of radioactive isotopes is generally considered palliative therapy for cancer. These agents have their effect by virtue of the ionizing radiation they release. Sodium phosphate P^{32} (^{32}P) enters forming DNA, so it tends to be concentrated where that process is highest. Clinically, the use of this drug is to attempt to control proliferation of blood cells in polycythemia vera or in myelocytic leukemia. The use of sodium I 131 (^{131}I), a radioactive isotope of iodine, to destroy thyroid tissue is discussed in Chapter 67.

Nursing Process Overview

Tissue-Specific Anticancer Agents

Assessment

Perform a complete physical assessment. Monitor vital signs and blood pressure. Obtain a history of the problem being treated.

Nursing Diagnoses

- Activity intolerance related to excessive fatigue caused by interferons
- Pain at tumor site(s) related to drug therapy

Patient Outcomes

The patient will identify measures to reduce activity tolerance and/or set priorities for activities that must be completed each day. The patient will state relief of pain at tumor sites.

Planning/Implementation

The drugs in this chapter vary widely. Monitor vital signs. Monitor the patient receiving interferons for severe and continuing flulike symptoms. Monitor the patient receiving steroid drugs for weight gain, skin changes, and depression. Instruct the patient needing to administer drugs via injection form how to administer the prescribed drugs and dispose of contaminated needles and syringes. Encourage the patient to return for regular follow-up visits to monitor drug effectiveness and the development of side effects. See the general guidelines in the Nursing Implications Summary in Chapter 54 for additional suggestions.

Evaluation

Continue to monitor for expected effects and side effects. Before discharge, verify that the patient can administer the prescribed drugs as needed. Verify that the patient can list side effects and symptoms that would indicate a need to call the physician.

Nursing Implications Summary

STEROIDS AND RELATED AGENTS
Androgens
➤ Androgens are discussed in Chapter 72.
➤ For a discussion of IM administration of oil-based suspensions, see Chapter 5.

ANTIANDROGENS
bicalutamide, flutamide, and nilutamide
Drug Administration/Nursing in the Community
➤ Emphasize the importance of taking both the antiandrogen and the LH-RH analog as prescribed for best effect.
➤ Instruct the patient to take doses on a full or empty stomach.
➤ Monitor vital signs. Assess for dyspnea, chest pain, cough, fever, and shortness of breath; notify the physician if they develop. Assess for common side effects: hot flashes, impotence or decreased sexual desire, gynecomastia, anorexia, nausea, constipation, or diarrhea.
➤ Instruct patients taking nilutamide to avoid alcoholic beverages.
➤ Assess patients taking flutamide for symptoms of methemoglobinemia: bluish-colored lips, fingernails, or palms; dizziness or fainting; or shortness of breath.
➤ Instruct patients taking bicalutamide to take doses at the same time each day.
➤ Assess for liver toxicity: jaundice, abdominal pain, dark urine, anorexia, nausea, or vomiting.
➤ Monitor liver function tests, prostate-specific antigen (PSA), and pulmonary function tests if ordered to evaluate dyspnea.

LH-RH ANALOGS
buserelin, goserelin, and leuprolide
Drug Administration
➤ See the general guidelines in Chapter 54 for information about anorexia, nausea and vomiting, and diarrhea.
➤ Consult the manufacturer's literature for current information.
➤ Assess for tingling of face, fingers, and toes. Assess for numbness and tingling of hands or feet, difficulty urinating, or weakness in legs.
➤ Monitor pulse, blood pressure, and weight. Inspect for edema. Monitor intake and output. Auscultate lung sounds.
➤ Allergic reactions have been reported. Ensure that the patient remains in the health care setting for at least 15 minutes after receiving doses. Have drugs, equipment, and personnel available to treat an acute allergic reaction.
➤ Monitor hematocrit, hemoglobin, serum creatinine, blood urea nitrogen (BUN), and liver function tests.
Nursing in the Community
➤ Review the anticipated benefits and possible side effects of drug therapy with the patient.
➤ When an antiandrogen such as bicalutamide, flutamide, or nilutamide and an LH-RH analog are prescribed, emphasize the importance of taking both medications for best effect.
➤ Assess tactfully for impotence and decreased libido because the patient may not wish to discuss them. Provide emotional support as appropriate. Remind the patient not to discon-

tinue medications without consulting the physician. Reinforce to the patient the importance of taking medications as prescribed for best effect.
➤ Warn the patient that hot flashes may occur as a side effect to the LH-RH analog; provide support as possible.
➤ Warn the patient to avoid driving or operating hazardous equipment if dizziness, blurred vision, lethargy, or memory disorders occur and to notify the physician.
➤ Warn the patient to notify the physician if severe or persistent bone pain develops.
➤ Buserelin (an LH-RH analog) is also available as a nasal spray; review with the patient the instruction sheet provided.
➤ Goserelin is a subcutaneous implant inserted by the physician.
➤ Leuprolide is administered via IM injection. Review the instruction leaflet with the patient and instruct the patient in injection technique. This drug is also used to treat endometriosis (see Chapter 70). This drug is also used to treat central precocious puberty.
➤ Monitor laboratory work appropriate to the drug use: PSA, serum testosterone, and acid phosphatase concentration in treatment of prostate cancer; bone age, height, weight, serum testosterone, and serum estradiol in precocious puberty.

ESTROGENS
Drug Administration/Nursing in the Community
➤ Estrogens are discussed in Chapter 70.
➤ Monitor weight and assess for fluid retention, especially of feet and legs.
➤ See the Patient Problems boxes in Chapter 54 on low white blood cell (WBC) count and thrombocytopenia.
➤ For best results, instruct the patient to take doses of estramustine 1 hour before or 2 hours after meals or milk or milk products.
➤ Review package insert with diethylstilbestrol for instructions about administration of parenteral form. Dilute a single dose in 300 ml of D5W, D5 ½ NS, NS, 0.45 NS, or lactated Ringer's. Administer initially at a rate of 1 ml/min for 10 to 15 minutes, then increase rate of administration to administer dose within 1 hour.

ANTIESTROGENS
tamoxifen and toremifene
Drug Administration
➤ See the general guidelines in Chapter 54 for information about depressed WBC count, thrombocytopenia, nausea and vomiting, and anorexia.
➤ Assess for depression, including withdrawal, change in affect, lack of interest in personal appearance, insomnia, and anorexia.
➤ Assess mental status and neurologic function.
➤ Assess for hypercalcemia; see Table 17-1 for a description of common electrolyte abnormalities.
➤ Monitor weight; assess for edema. Assess visual acuity.
➤ Monitor serum calcium, serum cholesterol and triglycerides, complete blood count (CBC), and liver function tests.

Continued

Nursing Implications Summary—cont'd

Nursing in the Community

➤ Review the anticipated benefits and possible side effects of drug therapy with the patient.

➤ Warn the patient to avoid driving or operating hazardous equipment if confusion, dizziness, lassitude, or lightheadedness develops and to notify the physician.

➤ Instruct the patient to increase fluid intake to 2500 to 3000 ml/day to foster calcium excretion and to help prevent constipation.

➤ Instruct the patient taking the enteric-coated form and an antacid to allow at least 2 hours to elapse between doses of antacid and tamoxifen.

➤ Warn the patient that hot flashes are common; provide support as appropriate.

➤ This drug may cause transient local disease flare, resulting in a temporary increase in bone pain or increase in size of any existing lesions. A flare is temporary; but if it is severe or persistent, instruct the patient to notify the physician.

➤ Instruct a female patient to use birth control measures, although not birth control pills containing estrogen.

anastrozole and letrozole

Drug Administration/Nursing in the Community

➤ See the Patient Problems boxes on low WBC count (Chapter 54) and dry mouth (Chapter 23). See general guidelines in Chapter 54 for information about anemia, nausea, vomiting, and alopecia.

➤ Monitor weight. Assess for edema of feet and legs. Assess for cough, dizziness, skin rash, joint pain, numbness or tingling of hands and feet, and excessive vaginal bleeding.

➤ Instruct the patient to notify the physician if symptoms of thromboembolism develop: pain in chest or legs, especially the calves; severe, sudden headache; slurred speech; unexplained shortness of breath; sudden, severe weakness or numbness of an extremity; or changes in vision.

➤ Monitor liver function tests.

GLUCOCORTICOIDS AND PROGESTINS

➤ Glucocorticoids are discussed in Chapter 41.

➤ Progestins are discussed in Chapter 70.

RITUXIMAB

Drug Administration

➤ See general guidelines in Chapter 54 for information about anemia, anorexia, and diarrhea. See the Patient Problems boxes in Chapter 54 on thrombocytopenia and low WBC count.

➤ Monitor weight and blood pressure. Assess for conjunctivitis, swelling of feet or legs, agitation, joint or muscle pain, cough.

➤ Intravenous rituximab: See manufacturer's insert for latest guidelines about dilution and administration. Most patients experience fever and chills during the first infusion. Infusion-related reactions may occur within 30 minutes to 2 hours of the first infusion and usually diminish with later infusions.

These reactions may include hypotension, bronchospasm, headache, nausea and vomiting, chest pain, and rarely, cardiac arrhythmias. Monitor vital signs and remain with patient. In patients with preexisting heart disease, monitor electrocardiogram (ECG) during infusion.

➤ To counteract infusion reactions, some physicians may prescribe acetaminophen and antihistamine before or at the start of the infusion.

➤ Monitor CBC and platelet count, and ECG if indicated.

INTERFERONS

Drug Administration

➤ Assess for numbness or tingling of fingers, toes, or face. Flu-like symptoms are common after doses. Assess for aching muscles, fever and chills, headache, joint pain, and back pain.

➤ Assess for nausea, vomiting, and diarrhea. Monitor weight.

➤ Monitor vital signs and blood pressure. Monitor periodic ECG changes.

➤ Monitor CBC, WBC differential, platelet count, and liver function tests.

Nursing in the Community

➤ Teach injection technique if the patient is to self-administer at home. See the manufacturer's patient instruction leaflet.

➤ Encourage the patient to increase daily intake of fluids if directed by the physician.

➤ Instruct the patient not to change brands of interferon unless directed to do so by the physician.

➤ Instruct the patient to avoid other drugs that may depress the CNS while taking interferons. Drugs to avoid include alcohol, antihistamines, prescription drugs for pain, tranquilizers, sleeping pills, sedatives, muscle relaxants, and barbiturates. Instruct the patient to keep all health care providers informed of all drugs being used, including over-the-counter drugs.

➤ Caution the patient to avoid driving or operating hazardous equipment if drowsiness, unusual fatigue, or confusion develops.

➤ This drug may cause flulike symptoms. Some physicians recommend that the patient take a dose of acetaminophen before receiving interferons and afterward if the patient develops a fever. Check with the physician and review instructions with the patient.

➤ See the Patient Problems boxes in Chapter 54 on leukopenia, bleeding tendencies (thrombocytopenia), and stomatitis, as well as the Patient Problems box in Chapter 23 on dry mouth. See the general guidelines in Chapter 54 for information about alopecia, which may affect some patients.

TRETINOIN

Drug Administration/Nursing in the Community

➤ See the Patient Problems box in Chapter 54 on stomatitis. Also see the general guidelines in Chapter 54 for information about diarrhea and anorexia.

Nursing Implications Summary—cont'd

➤ Monitor blood pressure and weight. Assess for depression, anxiety, skin changes, earache, difficult or painful urination, decreased urination, abdominal pain, chest pain, and trembling. Auscultate lung sounds. Many side effects occur with this drug; instruct patient to notify physician of unexpected signs or symptoms.

➤ Instruct patients to avoid driving or operating hazardous equipment if vision changes, dizziness, confusion develops and to notify physician.

➤ Notify the physician if symptoms of RA-APL syndrome (see text) develop: bone pain, discomfort or pain in chest, fever, shortness of breath, difficulty breathing, tightness in chest, or weight gain.

➤ Monitor CBC and WBC differential, liver function tests, and serum cholesterol and serum triglycerides levels.

ADRENAL ANTAGONIST
mitotane
Drug Administration

➤ See the general guidelines in Chapter 54 for information about anemia, anorexia, diarrhea, nausea, and vomiting.

➤ Assess for depression, including anorexia, insomnia, lack of interest in personal appearance, and withdrawal.

➤ Monitor blood pressure and pulse. Inspect for skin changes.

➤ Monitor the 8-AM plasma cortisol levels or 24-hour urinary 17-hydroxycorticosteroids.

Nursing in the Community

➤ Review the anticipated benefits and possible side effects of drug therapy with the patient.

➤ Warn the patient to avoid driving or operating hazardous equipment if confusion, somnolence, dizziness, fatigue, or other CNS side effects develop and to notify the physician.

➤ Warn the patient to avoid the use of alcohol or other CNS depressants, including antihistamines, sedatives, sleeping medications, narcotics or prescription drugs for pain, muscle relaxants, and other drugs, unless first discussed with the physician.

➤ Instruct the patient to wear a medical identification tag or bracelet listing medications in use. In the event of trauma or other injury, it is necessary to administer glucocorticoids.

➤ Instruct the patient to contact the physician if sickness or infection develops or an injury occurs because treatment with glucocorticoids may be necessary.

PANCREATIC BETA-CELL ANTAGONIST
streptozocin
Drug Administration

➤ See the general guidelines in Chapter 54 for information about anemia, extravasation, and nausea and vomiting. See the Patient Problems boxes in Chapter 54 on leukopenia and bleeding tendencies (thrombocytopenia).

➤ Monitor intake and output and weight. Assess for swelling of feet and legs.

➤ Monitor CBC, differential, platelet count, serum creatinine level, BUN level, serum electrolyte level, liver function tests, and blood glucose level.

➤ See the general guidelines in Chapter 54 about IV chemotherapy. See manufacturer's instructions for guidelines about dilution and rate of administration.

Nursing in the Community

➤ Review the anticipated benefits and possible side effects of drug therapy with the patient.

➤ Encourage the patient to increase fluid intake to 2500 ml/day.

➤ Inform diabetic patients that streptozocin may alter glucose levels. Instruct these patients to monitor blood glucose and adjust diet or insulin dosage as necessary.

PHOTOSENSITIZING AGENT
porfimer
Drug Administration

➤ See Patient Problems box in Chapter 58 on photosensitivity. However, note that with porfimer, sunscreens are not effective. In addition, the skin and eyes may be sensitive to bright light and sun for up to 30 days after the dose. Before full exposure to bright lights or sun, after the 30-day period, instruct the patient to test a small area of skin (not the face) by exposing it to the sun for up to 10 minutes. If redness, blistering, or edema occurs within 24 hours, instruct the patient to wait an additional 2 weeks before testing skin exposure.

➤ The photosensitivity caused by this drug makes the patient's skin sensitive to bright lights such as unshaded light bulbs, dental and operating room lights, and direct sunlight. Instruct patients to wear dark sunglasses when outside for at least 30 days after drug administration. The sunglasses should transmit less that 4% of white light. Bright lights outside, including car headlights, may be too bright. The patient may not be able to drive if vision is significantly limited with sunglasses.

➤ See manufacturer's instruction about preparation and administration of the dose. Handle as a chemotherapy drug (see the general guidelines in chapter 54). If extravasation occurs, protect area around injection site from light for at least 30 days.

➤ Monitor vital signs and weight. Auscultate lung sounds. Assess for shortness of breath, wheezing, swelling of feet and legs, chest pain, cough, fever, difficulty urinating, bloody urine, changes in vision, abdominal pain, and jaundice.

➤ Caution the patient to avoid driving or operating hazardous equipment if changes in vision, eye pain, or double vision develops.

➤ See the general guidelines in Chapter 54 for information about anemia, constipation, and nausea and vomiting.

➤ Monitor CBC and liver function tests.

CHAPTER REVIEW

Application

1. What is the basis for the anticancer effects of androgens?
2. Why is testolactone the preferred androgen for use in cancer chemotherapy?
3. Why is suppression of androgen action useful for cancer chemotherapy?
4. What is the mechanism of action of flutamide?
5. Buserelin, goserelin, and leuprolide are analogs of what natural peptide?
6. What is the effect of continuous administration of LH-RH analogs?
7. Why are androgen receptor antagonists often combined with an LH-RH analog?
8. What is the cause of most side effects seen with the combination of flutamide and an LH-RH analog?
9. What is the basis for the anticancer effects of estrogens?
10. Why is estramustine used only for cancer and not for estrogen replacement?
11. What is the mechanism of action of tamoxifen and toremifene?
12. What is the effect of inhibiting the enzyme aromatase in postmenopausal women?
13. What is the basis for the anticancer effects of glucocorticoids?
14. What is the basis for the selectivity of rituximab?
15. Why is contraception required during tretinoin therapy?
16. Mitotane is effective against what specific type of cancer?
17. Streptozocin is a specific toxin for what kind of cells?
18. What is the role of natural interferons?

Critical Thinking

1. What side effects of aromatase inhibitors are especially dangerous? How would you assess for these?
2. What side effects are most dangerous with streptozocin? How would you assess for these?
3. A patient receiving an interferon confides to you that he is experiencing tingling in his hands and feet. Is this important information? Why? What should you do?

Reference

Skalla K: The interferons, *Semin Oncol Nurs* 12(2):97-105, 1996.

Chapter

57

Sedative-Hypnotic and Antianxiety Agents

OBJECTIVES

After studying this chapter, you should be able to do the following:

- *Differentiate among sedatives, hypnotics, and anxiolytic agents.*
- *Develop a nursing care plan for patients receiving benzodiazepines, barbiturates, or miscellaneous hypnotics or anxiolytic agents.*
- *Describe the effects of alcohol ingestion on the body.*
- *Develop a teaching plan for the patient receiving disulfiram or a drug that may produce a disulfiram-like reaction when alcohol is ingested.*

CHAPTER OVERVIEW

Sedative-hypnotic drugs and anxiolytic drugs are considered together because they are not different so much in their clinical action as in their historic origin. The term *sedative-hypnotic* is reserved for older drug classes, primarily barbiturates. Barbiturates are a class of chemically related drugs developed in the early 1900s, effective as sedatives and as hypnotics. A small dose to calm an anxious patient is called a **sedative**. A larger dose sufficient to induce sleep is a **hypnotic**.

After the 1950s, drugs were developed specifically as hypnotics. Other drugs were developed as sedatives to treat anxiety. These drugs are called antianxiety drugs or **anxiolytics**, previously called minor tranquilizers. The benzodiazepines are the drug class most used today both to treat anxiety and to induce sleep.

An additional drug appropriate to this chapter is alcohol because it has the pharmacologic actions characteristic of a sedative-hypnotic or an anxiolytic drug. The social use of alcohol is mainly as a self-prescribed anxiolytic agent. Alcohol, when recognized as a drug, is viewed as a major source of drug abuse and dependence.

THERAPEUTIC RATIONALE: ANXIETY AND INSOMNIA

Anxiety Disorders

An **anxiety disorder** is defined as an illness that prevents an individual from coping and that can disrupt daily life. Five types of anxiety disorders are recognized.

Generalized Anxiety Disorder

About 7 million Americans are estimated to have generalized anxiety disorder. This disorder is one of chronic and exaggerated worry and tension without a recognized cause that persists for more than 6 months. People with this disorder are unable to relax and have trouble falling or staying asleep. They may have physical symptoms, such as trembling, twitching, muscle tension, headaches, irritability, sweating, or hot flashes. They are easily startled. They may have to go to the bathroom often or feel nauseated.

The overall impairment associated with generalized anxiety disorder is usually mild. People with this disorder do not feel restricted in social situations or in their jobs. The disorder commonly begins in childhood or adolescence. It is more common in women than in men and tends to run in families. The symptoms tend to diminish with age.

Therapy for generalized anxiety disorder includes cognitive-behavioral therapy, relaxation techniques, and biofeedback. The anxiolytic buspirone is an effective medication, as are benzodiazepines and some antidepressants.

Obsessive-Compulsive Disorder

Obsessive-compulsive disorder is characterized by anxious thoughts and rituals that cannot be controlled. The anxious thoughts include persistent and unwelcome images, and the rituals are driven by an urgent need to perform repetitive acts over and over. Most people have some behavior patterns that are necessary for comfort. However, when rituals become distressing, take 1 hour or more a day, and interfere with daily life, they are viewed as obsessive-compulsive disorder.

Obsessive-compulsive disorder affects about 1 in 50 people and occurs equally in men and women. It usually begins in teens or early adulthood, but about one third of cases begin in childhood. The progression of obsessive-compulsive disorder is highly variable. It can wax and wane or can increase or decrease over time. It may be accompanied by depression or other anxiety disorders.

Exposure and response prevention behavioral therapy can be effective for obsessive-compulsive disorder. The person is exposed to the trigger of the ritual and then through behavioral therapy taught to modify the response. The antidepressants clomipramine and fluoxetine have proved effective as drug therapy for obsessive-compulsive disorder.

Panic Disorder

Panic disorder is a sudden episode of terror that happens repeatedly. The panic attack is characterized by chest pain, heart palpitations, shortness of breath, dizziness, feelings of unreality, and fear of dying. These attacks commonly last from 2 to 10 minutes. The person may develop a phobia based on where the attacks have occurred, for instance an elevator. Depression and alcoholism are other conditions that may accompany panic disorder. Agoraphobia is the extreme condition of panic disorder in which the individual is becomes very restricted in activities that can be tolerated.

It is estimated that between 3 and 6 million Americans have a panic disorder. Agoraphobia occurs in about one third of these cases. Women are more commonly affected that men, and the condition commonly begins in young adults, although it can appear at any age. Many people experience a single panic attack. Treatment is recommended when attacks become common or disabling.

Cognitive-behavioral therapy and or medication are effective in treating 70% to 90% of people with panic disorder. Significant improvement takes about 6 weeks. The cognitive-behavioral therapeutic approach that is most effective is based on teaching how to view the panic situation differently and using breathing and refocusing to reduce anxiety. Benzodiazepines and antidepressants can be useful medications for relieving panic disorder.

Phobias

A phobia is a fear to an intense and irrational degree. It can be specific in which a certain object or situation is feared, such as flying, confining spaces, specific animals, and water. Social phobia is a fear of being painfully embarrassed in a social setting. Agoraphobia, a common part of panic disorder, is a fear of being in any situation that might provoke a panic attack and can leave the individual housebound.

Specific phobias affect about 1 in 10 persons. Childhood phobias are common and usually outgrown. Phobias that persist usually begin in adolescence or adulthood, and only about 20% disappear with time. Cognitive-behavioral therapy involving desensitization through repeated exposure is effective for more than 75% of patients seeking treatment. Drug therapy is effective only in relieving anxiety.

People with social phobia see themselves as incompetent in public. Fear of public speaking is a common social phobia. Some social phobias involve fear of specific public areas, such as restrooms, restaurants, or public phones. Shyness is not the same as social phobia.

Cognitive-behavioral therapy and/or medication can help more than 80% of people seeking help with social phobia. The beta-blocker propranolol is effective in treating performance anxiety in performers such as musicians. The antidepressants of the monoamine oxidase (MAO) inhibitor class are most effective for general social phobia.

Posttraumatic Stress Disorder

Posttraumatic stress disorder is the disabling condition that can follow a terrifying event. Memories of the ordeal come flooding back, with persistent frightening thoughts and nightmares, leaving the individual emotionally numb even to loved ones. Events that lead to posttraumatic stress disorder include war, kidnapping, rape or other violent personal attacks, and serious accidents or natural disasters. Any traumatized person will have flashbacks. Individuals who develop posttraumatic stress syndrome experience the symptoms for more than 1 month beginning within 3 months of the trauma.

Posttraumatic stress disorder can occur at any age, including childhood. Between 5 and 6 million Americans are believed to have posttraumatic stress disorder. Individuals may also abuse alcohol or other substances and be depressed or anxious. Severe symptoms include easy irritability and violent outbursts so that the individual cannot have a normal social life or hold a job.

Treatment for posttraumatic stress syndrome includes group therapy and medications such as antidepressants and anxiolytics.

Insomnia

Insomnia, the inability to sleep, is the most common sleep complaint (see Patient Problems box). Insomnia can be characterized either as difficulty in getting to sleep or as waking up and being unable to get back to sleep. Insomnia is not a disease but a symptom of physical or mental distress.

Causes of Insomnia

Treatment of insomnia involves assessment of physical problems, medications, and sleep habits. People who are depressed often awaken early and cannot go back to sleep. Chronic alcoholism, hyperthyroidism, heart or kidney failure, and pregnancy are commonly accompanied by insomnia. Pain of arthritis or muscle aches can make sleep difficult, as can respiratory problems and urinary tract problems. More than half of people older than 65 years of age have difficulty falling asleep or have excessive sleepiness during the day. Many medications disrupt sleep, including decongestants and beta-blockers and other medications used to treat high blood pressure.

Characteristics of Normal Sleep

Sleep is a normal and necessary cycle of daily living that typically occupies 8 hours, although persons differ in the amount of normal sleep required. Sunlight is a major factor that sets the biologic clock for sleep. Sleep is the result of decreased activity in the reticular-activating system. The *reticular-activating system* refers to neuronal pathways in which incoming signals from the senses (light, sound, smell, touch, taste, and balance) and viscera are collected, processed, and passed on to the higher brain centers.

Normal sleep has two major components: **rapid eye movement (REM) sleep** and non–rapid eye movement (NREM) sleep. REM sleep is characterized by fast brain waves, eye movements, and metabolic and temperature changes. The body is physiologically active during REM sleep, so the heart rate is increased, breathing is irregular, stomach acid is secreted, and the clitoris or penis becomes erect. Muscles lose their tone during REM sleep, however, so only the mind and autonomic nervous system are active during this stage. Because dreaming occurs exclusively during REM sleep, this time is also called dreaming sleep. Many authorities believe that during REM sleep is when we integrate emotionally meaningful experiences. NREM sleep is subdivided into four stages based on brain wave patterns. Individuals cycle between REM and NREM sleep over about a 90- to 100-minute period. During the night an individual will have about four to five NREM periods of sleep. Although REM sleep is associated with dreams, night terrors and sleep walking occur during NREM sleep. Older persons tend to spend less time in stages III and IV of NREM sleep,

PATIENT PROBLEMS

Insomnia

THE PROBLEM
Insomnia strikes most people at some time, often related to stress or worry, travel across several time zones, pain, or injury. If short term in nature, the insomnia will resolve after a few nights. For some people, insomnia is a more persistent or severe problem. These people experience chronic lack of sleep, may be irritable, and may doze off briefly at unanticipated or dangerous times (e.g., while driving).

ASSESSMENT
■ Take a detailed history of usual sleep patterns, including time of retiring, typical patterns of going to sleep and waking at night, and whether the patient snores.
■ Asess all medications the patient is taking and the time of day the doses are taken.
■ Assess diet, especially for caffeine-containing drinks.
■ Assess for depression, which may contribute to insomnia.
■ Perform a physical assessment. Refer to a sleep specialist, nose and throat specialist, or other type of physician if abnormalities are identified.

NURSING IN THE COMMUNITY
Suggest the following changes in lifestyle, if appropriate:
■ Review day-to-day stresses. Can high-stress activities or obligations be modified? Is there anyone to help?
■ Establish a bedtime routine: same time for retiring, same sequence of activities.
■ Try a warm bath and/or backrub before bedtime.
■ Try a drink of milk before bedtime and avoid excessive alcohol intake.
■ Avoid caffeine-containing foods and drinks after 5:00 PM. Limit liquids after 7:00 PM to decrease nocturia.
■ Turn off lights and use a night-light.
■ After review of medications, adjust times of taking final doses of the day of any medications that may cause stimulation or insomnia, if appropriate.
■ Limit afternoon naps. If excessively tired, the patient may want to go to bed early, but many people who go to bed early waken in the middle of the night, unable to go back to sleep. Try to delay going to sleep until 10:00 PM or later.
■ Incorporate regular physical exercise into the daily routine.
■ Make certain that the bedroom temperature is cool and that blankets are sufficient to keep the patient warm. Make certain there are enough pillows for comfortable positioning.
■ Avoid watching scary or anxiety-producing movies or television shows before bedtime.
■ Keep noise to a minimum. Try soft music or "white noise" (e.g., fan, audiotape of rain).
■ Arise at the same time each day, even if not sleeping well. Avoid spending hours in bed when awake. If wakened during the night and unable to go back to sleep, get out of bed and read for 30 minutes in another room.
■ Use sleeping medications as a last resort. Refer to a sleep disorder center if needed.

and they are more easily aroused by sounds. Children spend more total time in stages III and IV of NREM sleep.

Role of the Neurotransmitter GABA

Benzodiazepines and barbiturates are the two major drug classes used clinically as hypnotics and anxiolytics. Benzodiazepines promote the binding of the major inhibitory neurotransmitter, gamma-aminobutyric acid (GABA) to GABA receptors. The nonbenzodiazepine hypnotic zolpidem is a selective inhibitor of one subtype of GABA receptor. GABA receptors are found in neuronal membranes of the central nervous system (CNS). The role of these receptors is to facilitate gating of the chloride channel current through neuronal membranes. Barbiturates also enhance the action of GABA but in a different manner than benzodiazepines. Barbiturates increase the duration of the GABA-gated channel opening. The actions of the older sedative-hypnotics chloral hydrate and ethchlorvynol are similar to barbiturates.

The other major neurotransmitter associated with awareness is serotonin. The new and effective anxiolytic agent buspirone appears to act as a partial agonist at a specific subtype of brain serotonin receptors. The new antidepressants that act as selective serotonin reuptake inhibitors are effective anxiolytic agents for a number of anxiety disorders.

THERAPEUTIC AGENTS: DRUGS TO TREAT ANXIETY AND INSOMNIA

Hypnotic drugs are taken to fall asleep faster or to sleep longer. Studies in sleep laboratories show that most hypnotic drugs suppress REM sleep. When the drug is discontinued, even after a single dose, there is a rebound in REM sleep with vivid dreams and increased awakening. Furthermore, after 3 weeks of continuous therapy, most hypnotic drugs are no longer effective in decreasing the time needed to fall asleep or the duration of sleep. Although a hypnotic may be appropriate for an acute situation, most practitioners believe that chronic insomnia should be handled with nonpharmacologic interventions. These interventions center on improving sleep habits by eliminating napping, recommending warm

baths, reviewing medications, and treating physical impairments that can inhibit sleep.

Use of anxiolytic drugs should also be limited. Patients taking sedative or anxiolytic drugs should be told that drug therapy offers only limited relief. This may be sufficient for anxiety-provoking situations such as surgery or trauma. Cognitive-behavioral therapy is the standard for treating various chronic anxiety disorders. Sedatives or anxiolytic agents decrease the general level of arousal by inhibiting the reticular activating system of the brainstem. This is not a cure for anxiety, although the response is blunted. Rather, authorities agree that drug therapy for anxiety should be limited to a few weeks, and psychotherapy or behavior modification therapy deals directly with the origin of the patient's anxiety. In part, this recommendation is based on tolerance to these drugs developing after a few weeks.

Drugs prescribed for insomnia and anxiety are presented in three sections. The first section discusses benzodiazepines, the most popular drug class today for treating insomnia and anxiety. The second section presents barbiturates, an older class of drugs used for a variety of CNS depressant effects, from sedation to anesthesia. The third section discusses miscellaneous drugs, including two newer and specific drugs, buspirone and zolpidem, as well as older drugs that are seldom used.

Benzodiazepines: General Characteristics

Mechanism of Action

Specific receptors for the benzodiazepines have been identified in the cerebral cortex and limbic system. Because the limbic system is a major integrating system governing emotional behavior associated with self-preservation, the presence of receptors for benzodiazepines in this system may account for their anxiolytic action. Benzodiazepines increase the action of the inhibitory neurotransmitter GABA. Benzodiazepines and barbiturates help GABA open a chloride channel in the postsynaptic membrane of many neurons, which reduces the neuron's excitability.

Pharmacokinetics

The benzodiazepines are readily absorbed after oral administration. Only lorazepam is rapidly and completely absorbed after intramuscular (IM) injection. Chlordiazepoxide and diazepam may be administered by intravenous (IV) or IM routes, but chlordiazepoxide is not reliably absorbed after IM administration. Benzodiazepines are highly lipid soluble and therefore are widely distributed in body tissues. They are also highly bound to plasma protein, usually greater than 80%. No drug interactions have been described for protein binding. However, protein binding is reduced in patients with cirrhosis and renal insufficiency and in newborns, and these patients often have impaired metabolism of benzodiazepines as well, making a reduction in dosage important.

The benzodiazepines are metabolized by the liver. Several benzodiazepines have active metabolites. *N*-desmethyl metabolites are active and have a longer duration of action

ALTERNATIVE THERAPIES

Sedative

VALERIAN

The drug consists of preparations of the dried or fresh root of *Valeriana officinalis* L. Several of the more than 120 components that have been identified in the root and essential oil of valerian exert sedative effects in animals and human beings. Valerian is an approved sleep aid in Germany, but because its active ingredient(s) and their attendant toxicities have not been identified, more extensive clinical trials with the drug are warranted.

than the parent compound. Benzodiazepines with long duration of action based on active metabolites include chlordiazepoxide, clorazepate, diazepam, halazepam, and prazepam. Lorazepam, oxazepam, temazepam, and triazolam do not have active metabolites to prolong their duration of action. These drugs are preferred for older adult patients and for patients with liver disease. Alprazolam is metabolized to weakly active compounds that are eliminated rapidly. The anticonvulsant clonazepam has only weakly active metabolites.

Uses

Benzodiazepines were introduced clinically in the 1960s as anxiolytic drugs. By the early 1970s, diazepam (Valium) was the most widely prescribed drug in the United States. The popularity of the benzodiazepines is caused in part by their high therapeutic index. Overdoses of 1000 times the therapeutic dose have been reported not to result in death. At therapeutic doses, side effects beyond drowsiness and ataxia are uncommon.

In general, benzodiazepines have anxiolytic, hypnotic, muscle relaxing, and anticonvulsant actions. However, each benzodiazepine has its own therapeutic range of uses. All benzodiazepines are schedule IV drugs.

Anxiolytics. Alprazolam (Xanax), chlordiazepoxide (Librium), clorazepate (Tranxene), diazepam (Valium), halazepam (Paxipam), lorazepam (Ativan), oxazepam (Serax), and prazepam (Centrax) are widely prescribed as anxiolytic drugs.

Hypnotics. Estazolam (ProSom), flurazepam (Dalmane), lorazepam (Ativan), quazepam (Doral), temazepam (Restoril), and triazolam (Halcion) are prescribed primarily as hypnotics. Flurazepam undergoes conversion in the liver to a long-acting metabolite and persists in the body the longest. Triazolam has a short half-life and can produce rebound anxiety and confusion, especially in the elderly. Triazolam has also been reported to produce short-term amnesia.

Anticonvulsants. Clonazepam (Klonopin), clorazepate (Tranxene), and diazepam (Valium) have use as anticonvulsants.

Anesthetics. Benzodiazepines are not anesthetics. However, midazolam (Versed) and diazepam (Valium) are used to provide sedation and amnesia for some surgical procedures.

Muscle Relaxant. Diazepam (Valium) is prescribed as a muscle relaxant.

Adverse Reactions and Contraindications

Side effects common with benzodiazepines include daytime sedation, ataxia, dizziness, and headaches. Tolerance commonly develops quickly to these side effects. The older adult is more likely to experience these side effects to a disabling degree. Moreover, older adults do not readily metabolize benzodiazepines, so the drug persists two to three times

longer. Therefore the drug dosage is reduced for older adult patients and for patients who have impaired liver function. However, older adult patients are at risk for falling and injuring themselves while taking these drugs for sleep or anxiety. Less common side effects of benzodiazepines include blurred or double vision, hypotension, tremor, amnesia, slurred speech, urinary incontinence, and constipation.

Patients older than 50 years of age with a history of psychosis are the most likely to develop paradoxical excitement or aggression. Benzodiazepines may worsen glaucoma. Benzodiazepines are contraindicated for women in labor and for nursing mothers because of adverse depression of the infant. An increased incidence of cleft lip has been reported among infants whose mothers took diazepam (Valium) during early pregnancy. In general, benzodiazepines are associated with an increased incidence of congenital abnormalities in children whose mothers used the drugs during pregnancy. Benzodiazepines are distributed into breast milk. Infants do not readily metabolize these drugs and can become lethargic, so benzodiazepines are not recommended for nursing mothers.

Acute Toxicity

An acute overdose of benzodiazepines alone is seldom fatal. Patients often regain consciousness and normal vital signs with a large concentration of drug still in their bodies. Flumazenil (Mazicon), a benzodiazepine antagonist, is available to reverse symptoms of benzodiazepine overdose.

Abuse Potential and Withdrawal

Benzodiazepines are schedule IV drugs because their abuse potential is considered low. Daily use of 30 mg of diazepam in the absence of alcohol or other depressant drugs for 3 months seldom produces dependence. Although tolerance to sedation and ataxia develops rapidly, tolerance to the anxiolytic effect develops slowly. If dependence develops, the appearance of withdrawal symptoms after discontinuance will take several days for those benzodiazepines with active metabolites. An acute phase of chronic withdrawal symptoms, consisting of depression, insomnia, nightmares, agitation, and psychologic distress, can persist for 6 weeks. Withdrawal begins during the first week after discontinuance of the drug, with symptoms of agitation, nausea and vomiting, nervousness, sweating, and muscular cramps. Seizures are seldom seen unless high doses have been abused; however, if seizures do occur, it is at the end of the first week. To lessen withdrawal symptoms, the dosage of benzodiazepines should be tapered gradually over 2 to 16 weeks, adjusted for the specific drug and starting dose.

Interactions

Like the barbiturates, the sedative effect of the benzodiazepines is increased by other drug classes including alcohol and other general CNS depressants, tricyclic antidepressants, opiate analgesics, antipsychotics, and antihistamines. Unlike barbiturates, benzodiazepines have only slight effects on the liver microsomal enzymes.

Specific Benzodiazepines

Specific benzodiazepines are also listed in Table 57-1.

▼ alprazolam

Alprazolam (Xanax) is indicated for the short-term relief of anxiety and may be effective in relieving anxiety associated with depression. Another use is to treat panic disorders. Alprazolam has a potential dependence liability with patients unable to give up use of the drug. Rebound panic, seizures, and delirium have been reported when the drug is rapidly discontinued.

Alprazolam is rapidly absorbed and is effective for about 12 hours. Although the drug is eliminated somewhat more slowly in older than in young adults, the metabolites are only weakly active. Steady-state plasma levels are reached in 2 to 5 days with regular administration.

bromazepam

Bromazepam (Lectopam) is prescribed as an anxiolytic agent. It is available in Canada but not in the United States. Bromazepam has a short to intermediate half-life and does not tend to accumulate with multiple doses. The dose for older adult patients should be half the usual adult dose.

chlordiazepoxide

Chlordiazepoxide (Librium) is prescribed as an anxiolytic drug, as a preanesthetic medication for sedation, and to treat symptoms of alcohol withdrawal. Chlordiazepoxide is absorbed better orally than intramuscularly; care must be used with IV injections. Chlordiazepoxide is metabolized by the liver to an active metabolite to give a persistent effect.

clonazepam

Clonazepam (Klonopin) is mainly used as an anticonvulsant (see Chapter 61). It also treats panic attacks.

clorazepate

Clorazepate (Tranxene) is prescribed for anxiety, for panic attacks, for the symptomatic relief of acute alcohol withdrawal, and as adjunctive therapy in the management of partial seizures. Clorazepate is not absorbed orally until converted by stomach acid to an active metabolite. Any condition or medication such as antacids or cimetidine that reduce stomach acidity significantly interferes with clorazepate absorption. The metabolite persists in the body.

▼ diazepam

Diazepam (Valium) has many clinical uses in addition to treating anxiety and panic attacks. It relieves muscle spasticity in patients with cerebral palsy or other conditions and stops continued convulsions (status epilepticus). Diazepam is also used in the hospital as a preanesthetic medication for sedation. Alcohol withdrawal symptoms may be treated with diazepam.

Diazepam is well absorbed orally and is effective within 1 hour. Absorption from IM injection is erratic, and pain occurs at the injection site, so this route is seldom used. IV injection must be given slowly and carefully into a large vein to minimize irritation and swelling at the injection site, with possible phlebitis or thrombosis.

estazolam

Estazolam (ProSom) is prescribed for insomnia. It has a fast onset of action and is effective for 6 to 8 hours.

flurazepam

Flurazepam (Dalmane) is prescribed as a hypnotic only. It suppresses stage 4 sleep but does not significantly depress REM sleep. Flurazepam is effective for more than 2 weeks. Also, it does not produce rebound insomnia when it is discontinued, probably because of the long half-life of its active metabolites. The persistence of active metabolites accounts for decreased mental alertness during the day, particularly after repeated use of flurazepam by older adult patients and by patients with decreased liver function.

halazepam

Halazepam (Paxipam), an anxiolytic drug, is well absorbed orally and is metabolized to an active metabolite with a long half-life. Accumulation of the drug and its metabolite occurs with repeated doses, particularly in older adult patients or in patients with impaired liver function.

ketazolam

Ketazolam (Loftran) is an anxiolytic agent. It is available in Canada but not in the United States. Ketazolam has a long half-life and accumulates with multiple dosing.

▼ lorazepam

Lorazepam (Ativan) is effective as a hypnotic and an anxiolytic drug. It is well absorbed orally and intramuscularly. Parenteral lorazepam is sometimes given as a preanesthetic medication in adults. Lorazepam produces sedation, relieves anxiety, and decreases ability to recall events that day. The drug does not have active metabolites and therefore has a relatively short duration of action, about 15 hours.

midazolam

Midazolam (Versed) is used as an IV anesthetic and is discussed in Chapter 36.

nitrazepam

Nitrazepam (Mogadon) is a hypnotic. It is also indicated as an anticonvulsant. It is available in Canada but not in the United States. Nitrazepam has a short to intermediate half-life and has minimal accumulation with multiple dosing.

oxazepam

Oxazepam (Serax) is effective as an anxiolytic drug, especially in anxiety associated with depression, tension, agitation, and irritability in older adult patients. Oxazepam also reduces the anxiety associated with alcohol withdrawal.

Table 57-1   Benzodiazepines and Benzodiazepine Antagonist

Generic Name	Trade Name	Administration/Dosage	Comments
Benzodiazepines			
alprazolam	Xanax*	ORAL: *Adults*—0.25-0.5 mg 3 times/day. Maximum daily dose: 4 mg. FDA pregnancy category D. *Older adults*—0.25 mg 2 or 3 times/day.	Used to treat anxiety. Metabolites are only weakly active. Schedule IV substance.
bromazepam	Lectopam†	ORAL: *Adults*—6-30 mg/day in divided doses.	Used to treat anxiety.
chlordiazepoxide	Libritabs Librium* Novopoxide† Various others	ORAL: *Adults—For anxiety:* 5-25 mg 3 or 4 times/day. *Older adults*— 5 mg 2-4 times/day. *Children*—0.5 mg/kg body weight/day in 3-4 doses. May be given intramuscularly. INTRAVENOUS: *Adults—For alcohol withdrawal:* 50-100 mg slowly over at least 1 min, then 25-50 mg every 6-8 hr, with the total dose not more than 300 mg.	Used to treat anxiety and alcohol withdrawal. Half-life is 24-48 hr. Metabolites are active. Hydrochloride salt is used for injection. Schedule IV substance.
clonazepam	Klonopin Rivotril†	ORAL: *Adults*—Initially, 0.5 mg 3 times daily. Increase in increments of 0.5 mg-1 mg every 3 days if necessary. FDA pregnancy category D.	Primarily used as an anticonvulsant. Use to treat panic disorders is under investigation. Schedule IV substance.
clorazepate	Tranxene* Novo-Clopate†	ORAL: 7.5-15 mg 2-4 times/day. *Older adults*—6.5-15 mg/day.	Used to treat anxiety. Half-life is 30-200 hr. Metabolites are active. Schedule IV substance.
diazepam	Apo-Diazepam† Valium* Various others	ORAL: *Adults*—2-10 mg 2-4 times/day. *Older adults*—2-2.5 mg 1-2 times/day. *Children*—0.12-0.8 mg/kg/day in 3-4 doses. ORAL (EXTENDED-RELEASE): *Adults*—15 or 30 mg once a day. INTRAVENOUS: Administer no more than 5 mg/min. *For severe anxiety, severe muscle spasm, status epilepticus, or recurrent seizures: Adults*—5-10 mg initially, repeated in 3-4 hr if needed. *Children*— 0.04-0.2 mg/kg initially, repeat in 3-4 hr if necessary. *For basal sedation for cardioversion or endoscopic procedures: Adults*— 10-20 mg as required. *For acute alcohol withdrawal symptoms: Adults*—5-20 mg, then 5-10 mg in 3-4 hr if necessary.	Used to treat anxiety, severe muscle spasm, status epilepticus, and acute alcohol withdrawal symptoms and to provide sedation. Half-life is 48-200 hr. Metabolites are active. Schedule IV substance.
estazolam	ProSom	ORAL: *Adults*—1 mg at bedtime; some patients may require 2 mg. FDA pregnancy category X. *Small or debilitated patients*— 0.5 mg.	Used to treat insomnia. New drug.
flurazepam	Apo-Flurazepam† Dalmane* Novoflupam† Somnol Various others	ORAL: *Adults—As hypnotic:* 15-30 mg at bedtime. *Older adults*— 15 mg. Onset 20-45 min. Duration: 7-8 hr.	Used as hypnotic only. Active metabolite is formed with half-life of 47-100 hr, so repeated use leads to accumulation of this metabolite, which may impair daytime activity. Schedule IV substance.
halazepam	Paxipam	ORAL: *Adults*—20-40 mg 3 or 4 times/day. FDA pregnancy category D. *Older adults*—Reduce dosage to 20 mg 1 or 2 times/day.	Used to treat anxiety. Active metabolite with long half-life. Schedule IV substance.
ketazolam	Loftran†	ORAL: *Adults*—15 mg 1-2 times/day.	Used to treat anxiety.
lorazepam	Ativan* Nu-Loraz† Various others	ORAL: *Adults—For anxiety:* 1-2 mg 2-3 times/day, may increase dose to 10 mg maximum daily. *As hypnotic:* 2-4 mg at bedtime. INTRAVENOUS: *Adults—For anxiety, amnestic:* 0.044 mg/kg body weight up to 2 mg. *For status epilepticus:* 0.05 mg/kg body weight up to 4 mg, administered slowly. If seizures continue or recur after 10-15 min, may administer an additional dose. FDA pregnancy category D. *Older adults*—½ adult dose.	Used to treat anxiety and insomnia. Repeated use for insomnia can cause rebound insomnia. Half-life is 15 hr, so little accumulation occurs. Metabolites are inactive. Schedule IV substance.
nitrazepam	Mogadon†	ORAL: *Adults*—5-10 mg at bedtime. *Children* (anticonvulsant)— 0.3 mg-1 mg/kg body weight in 3 divided doses. May increase gradually if needed and tolerated.	Used as sedative in adults and as anticonvulsant in children.
oxazepam	Apo-Oxazepam† Serax* Novoxapam†	ORAL: *Adults—For anxiety:* 10-30 mg 3-4 times/day. *Older adults*— 30 mg in 3 divided doses, increased if necessary to 45-60 mg.	Used to treat anxiety. Half-life is 3-21 hr, so little accumulation occurs. Metabolites are inactive. Schedule IV substance.
prazepam	Centrax	ORAL: *Adults*—10 mg 3 times/day or 20-40 mg at bedtime. *Older adults*—10-15 mg.	Used to treat anxiety. Half-life is 30-200 hr. Metabolites are active. Schedule IV substance.
quazepam	Doral	ORAL: *Adults*—Initially, 15 mg. Reduce to 7.5 mg as needed.	Used to treat insomnia. Metabolites have long half-life. Schedule IV substance.

*Available in Canada and in the United States.
†Available in Canada only.

Continued

Table 57-1　Benzodiazepines and Benzodiazepine Antagonist—cont'd

Generic Name	Trade Name	Administration/Dosage	Comments
Benzodiazepines—cont'd			
temazepam	Restoril*	ORAL: *Adults*—30 mg at bedtime. FDA pregnancy category X. *Older adults*—Reduce dose to 15 mg.	Used as hypnotic only. Slowly absorbed. Metabolites are not active. Schedule IV substance.
triazolam	Apo-Triazo† Halcion* Novo-Triolam† Various others	ORAL: *Adults*—0.125-0.25 mg at bedtime. FDA pregnancy category X. *Older adults*—Reduce dose to 0.125 mg.	Used as hypnotic. May also be used as antianxiety drug and anticonvulsant. Metabolites are not active. Schedule IV substance.
Benzodiazepine Antagonist			
flumazenil	Anexate† Romazicon	*Reversal of conscious sedation or in general anesthesia:* INTRAVENOUS: *Adults*—0.2 mg administered over 15 sec initially. Wait 45 sec for response. Further doses of 0.2 mg may be repeated at 60 sec intervals if needed to a cumulative dose of 1 mg per treatment. Treatment may be repeated at 20-min intervals, with no more than 3 mg given in 1 hr. FDA pregnancy category C. *Management of suspected benzodiazepine overdose:* INTRAVENOUS: *Adults*—0.2 mg is administered over 30 sec initially. If desired level of consciousness is not seen after waiting 30 sec, further dose of 0.3 mg is administered over another 30 sec. Further doses of 0.5 mg may be administered over 30 sec at 1-min intervals up to cumulative dose of 3 mg. In event of resedation, treatment may be repeated at 20-min intervals, with no more than 1 mg administered at one time and not more than 3 mg given in 1 hr. FDA pregnancy category C.	Benzodiazepine antagonist for reversal of benzodiazepine-induced sedation.

*Available in Canada and in the United States.
†Available in Canada only.

Absorption is slow. The metabolites are not active; thus drug effects are not likely to be cumulative and do not persist for more than 24 hours.

prazepam

Prazepam (Centrax), an anxiolytic drug, is slowly absorbed orally. The metabolites are active; thus cumulative effects are seen with repeated administration.

quazepam

Quazepam (Doral) is a new benzodiazepine used to treat insomnia. Its characteristics are much like flurazepam.

temazepam

Temazepam (Restoril) is a hypnotic. Temazepam is slowly absorbed, and onset of sleep is not improved. The number of awakenings is decreased, however, and overall duration and quality of sleep improve. As with flurazepam, stage 4 sleep is suppressed, but REM sleep is not. Unlike flurazepam, temazepam does not have active metabolites, and accumulation is not generally a problem.

triazolam

Triazolam (Halcion) is prescribed as a hypnotic. It is rapidly absorbed. Its metabolites are not active and are rapidly eliminated. Triazolam and alprazolam are closely related chemically.

The safety of triazolam has been questioned. However, the Food and Drug Administration (FDA) determined that the incidence of severe side effects is not greater for triazolam than for flurazepam and temazepam, two other popular hypnotics, when compared at equivalent doses. Side effects include anxiety, restlessness, amnesia, aggression, and paranoia.

Benzodiazepine Antagonist

flumazenil

Flumazenil (Mazicon) is the first benzodiazepine antagonist to be released for clinical use (see Table 57-1). Flumazenil binds to the benzodiazepine receptor competitively and thereby inhibits the action of benzodiazepines.

Flumazenil has two major clinical uses. First, flumazenil is a diagnostic tool to confirm or exclude benzodiazepine intoxication. Flumazenil, administered intravenously, will reverse benzodiazepine intoxication in 5 minutes. Once benzodiazepine intoxication is confirmed, flumazenil can be given repeatedly to reverse the depression of the respiratory drive caused by benzodiazepine intoxication so that the need for endotracheal intubation and artificial ventilation is avoided or decreased. Second, flumazenil is used to reverse the sedative effects of benzodiazepines given during surgical procedures to induce conscious sedation or general anesthesia. Flumazenil is also being tested as an agent to induce remission of functional CNS impairment, especially that of hepatic encephalopathy.

Flumazenil is generally well tolerated. Surgical patients are more likely to experience nausea and vomiting. Patients being treated for an overdose of benzodiazepines may experience agitation, restlessness, discomfort, and anxiety.

Barbiturates: General Characteristics

Mechanism of Action

Barbiturates depress the reticular activating system, probably by promoting the inhibitory synaptic action of the neurotransmitter GABA.

Pharmacokinetics

The barbiturates are classified according to their duration of action and have been traditionally divided into four classes: ultrashort-acting, short-acting, intermediate-acting, and long-acting. Although traditional, this classification was derived from animal data and is somewhat arbitrary in the clinical setting, where the variables of dosage and patient expectations can modify the degree and duration of effectiveness. In particular, the contrast between short-acting and intermediate-acting sedative-hypnotics is not as striking in clinical practice.

The ultrashort-acting barbiturates are administered intravenously, but other barbiturates are usually given orally and are well absorbed. Differences in onset and duration of action among barbiturates depend on their lipid solubility and protein binding. These properties are determined by the chemical structure. The ultrashort-acting barbiturates are lipid soluble; on IV administration the concentration of ultrashort-acting barbiturates reaching the brain is large because the brain has a high blood flow and the barbiturates readily cross the blood-brain barrier and depress the reticular-activating system. The action is quickly terminated, however, because the barbiturates are redistributed into organs with a lesser blood flow, so the concentration reaching the brain quickly drops. Ultrashort-acting barbiturates may persist in body fat because of their high lipid solubility and in muscle, reflecting their high degree of protein binding.

Barbiturates are released slowly from muscle and fat into the blood for eventual metabolism by the liver and excretion by the kidney. The persistence of low concentrations of barbiturates in the body is believed to account for the "hangovers" after the therapeutic effect has worn off. Short- and intermediate-acting barbiturates are redistributed less rapidly into body fat and muscle, thus acting longer. The long-acting barbiturate phenobarbital binds even less to protein and is much less lipid soluble than the ultrashort-acting barbiturates. Although ultrashort-, short-, and intermediate-acting barbiturates must be metabolized by the liver to water-soluble metabolites for excretion by the kidney, 30% to 50% of a dose of phenobarbital is excreted unchanged in urine.

Uses

Sedative-hypnotics. Barbiturates have been used for the short-term treatment of insomnia or for sedation to relieve anxiety, tension, and apprehension. However, benzodiazepines have largely replaced barbiturates for these uses.

Anesthestics. The ultrashort-acting barbiturates methohexital and thiopental are used as general anesthetics. Amobarbital, butabarbital, pentobarbital, phenobarbital, and secobarbital are used for preoperative medication.

Anticonvulsants. Phenobarbital, mephobarbital, and metharbital are used in treating epilepsy and convulsions (see Chapter 61).

Adverse Reactions and Contraindications

Side effects are generally mild. Some individuals experience confusion or irritability. Rarely, regular use can cause agranulocytosis, thrombocytopenia purpura, or megaloblastic anemia. Allergic reactions are also a rare reaction but may include angioedema, morbilliform rash, erythema multiforme, or Stevens-Johnson syndrome.

As discussed for hypnotics in general, barbiturates are not effective as hypnotics after 2 weeks of use. Also, even a single dose suppresses REM sleep and leads to REM rebound when the barbiturate is discontinued. Mild withdrawal symptoms from short-term use of barbiturates include nightmares, daytime agitation, and a "shaky" feeling.

An acute overdose of barbiturates causes depression of the medullary centers controlling respiration and the cardiovascular system. The symptoms are a fast heart rate (tachycardia) and a fall in blood pressure (hypotension) that leads to shock. Reflexes disappear, and respiration is significantly depressed. The patient becomes comatose, and death may result from respiratory and cardiovascular collapse. No specific antagonist exists for barbiturates; thus treatment of barbiturate poisoning supports respiration and maintains blood oxygen levels.

Toxicity

Metabolic Tolerance. Administration of barbiturates for a few days activates the liver to synthesize more of the drug-metabolizing enzymes. This activation is called enzyme induction. Because these enzymes are located in the microsomal fraction of broken cell preparations, these drug-metabolizing enzymes usually are referred to as the liver microsomal enzyme system. After induction of the microsomal enzymes, the barbiturates are more rapidly metabolized, decreasing average blood levels after a given dose. This is a classic example of metabolic tolerance. Because many other drugs are also metabolized by the same microsomal enzymes, barbiturates can induce tolerance of other drugs. Examples are the coumarins (anticoagulants) and the anticonvulsant phenytoin (Dilantin).

Pharmacodynamic Tolerance. In addition to drug-induced tolerance, pharmacodynamic tolerance also develops with repeated administration of the barbiturates. This is the tolerance described previously for all general CNS depressants

DRUG ABUSE ALERTS

Barbiturates

BACKGROUND

Barbiturates are abused to bring about a sense of euphoria and a lessening of anxiety. They can be taken orally or injected.

PHARMACOLOGY

Barbiturates are sedative-hypnotics. Slurred speech, staggering gait, poor judgment, and uncertain reflexes are symptoms of barbiturate use.

HEALTH HAZARDS

There is only a fourfold margin between a sedative dose and an overdose of barbiturates. This margin is decreased by the ingestion of alcohol or another central nervous system depressant. A barbiturate overdose causes shallow respiration, cold and clammy skin, dilated pupils, and a weak and rapid pulse. In addition to the dangers of overdose, repeated use of barbiturates leads to dependence. Withdrawal symptoms include anxiety, insomnia, tremors, delirium, and convulsions.

in which the nervous system adapts to the presence of the depressant. However, the medullary centers controlling respiration and the cardiovascular system do not adapt to general CNS depressants because they are not affected at the usual doses taken. The lethal dose for barbiturates therefore does not increase with drug dependence; this accounts for the accidental death of individuals dependent on high dosages of barbiturates because these doses can be lethal. The lethal dose for barbiturates in nontolerant individuals is about 15 times the hypnotic dose.

Abuse Potential and Withdrawal

Barbiturates are a class of widely abused drugs (see Drug Abuse Alerts box). As with other abused classes of drugs, individual drugs with the most rapid onset are the most abused. This is because the euphoric feeling, or "rush," depends on a rapid rate of altering perception. Among the barbiturates, secobarbital, pentobarbital, and amobarbital are schedule II drugs (drugs having a high potential for abuse). Butabarbital is a schedule III drug (lesser abuse potential), whereas phenobarbital and mephobarbital are schedule IV (low abuse potential) drugs (see Chapter 3 for a discussion of schedules). With the schedule II barbiturates, a daily consumption of 400 mg leads to severe drug dependence in about 6 weeks. With larger doses, the time decreases.

Severe withdrawal symptoms begin within 24 hours after the drug is discontinued in an individual with severe drug dependence. Grand mal convulsions and delirium are common symptoms; elevated temperature, coma, and death are less common. Because of the danger associated with barbiturate withdrawal, gradual withdrawal is used to detoxify a dependent person. Withdrawal is achieved by reducing the dosage of the barbiturate to zero over 10 to 20 days. Some-

times the long-acting barbiturate phenobarbital is substituted for a short-acting barbiturate for once-a-day administration. Phenobarbital (30 mg) is substituted for 100 mg of secobarbital, pentobarbital, or amobarbital.

Interactions

The depressant effect of barbiturates not only is additive with the other general CNS depressants but also is potentiated by antipsychotics and narcotic analgesics. These interactions are important to remember for the patient scheduled to undergo surgery. If secobarbital or pentobarbital is prescribed as the night-before sleeping pill, it should be given at least 8 hours before any of the major tranquilizers, narcotic analgesics, or general anesthetics are administered to avoid undue depression of the medullary control of respiration and the cardiovascular system.

Specific Barbiturates

Specific barbiturates are also listed in Table 57-2.

thiopental and methohexital

Thiopental (Pentothal) and methohexital (Brevital) are ultrashort-acting barbiturates administered intravenously for the induction or maintenance of anesthesia. These barbiturates are discussed with the general anesthetics in Chapter 36.

amobarbital, aprobarbital, pentobarbital, and secobarbital

Amobarbital (Amytal), aprobarbital (Alurate), pentobarbital (Nembutal), and secobarbital (Seconal) are used most commonly as hypnotic drugs. The combination of secobarbital and amobarbital is sold under the name *Tuinal* as a hypnotic. Although these barbiturates are effective hypnotics for a few days, they lose their effectiveness by the second week of use. Because barbiturates depress REM sleep, REM rebound occurs when they are discontinued. This REM rebound can lead to insomnia. Also drug dependence can develop with the usual hypnotic dosages within 2 months, although this does not lead to severe withdrawal symptoms unless the dosage has been raised to more than 400 mg/day.

butabarbital

Butabarbital (Butisol) is an intermediate-acting barbiturate prescribed for daytime sedation and less commonly for inducing sleep at night. It often is combined in sedative doses with other drugs used to treat conditions with psychogenic overtones such as allergies, ulcers, and inflammatory bowel disease.

phenobarbital

Phenobarbital (Luminal) is the longest acting and most widely used of the barbiturates. Phenobarbital and mephobarbital (Mebaral) control some kinds of epilepsy (see Chapter 61). Phenobarbital is rarely abused because it is slower in onset of action and it does not give a rush. Peak blood levels occur 6 to 18 hours after an oral dose, and the half-life is 3 to 4 days.

Table 57-2 Barbiturates

Generic Name	Trade Name	Administration/Dosage	Comments
amobarbital‡	Amytal*	ORAL: *Adults—As sedative:* 50-300 mg/day in divided doses. *As hypnotic:* 65-200 mg at bedtime. *Children—As sedative:* 6 mg/kg body weight in 3 divided doses. INTRAMUSCULAR INTRAVENOUS: *Adults—As hypnotic:* 65-200 mg. *As sedative:* 30-50 mg. FDA pregnancy category D. *Children—As hypnotic:* 2-3 mg/kg body weight. *As sedative:* 3-5 mg/kg body weight.	Intermediate-acting barbiturate that acts similarly to short-acting barbiturate in humans. Used for daytime sedation, preanesthetic sedation, and hypnosis. Precautions are same as for secobarbital. Schedule II substance.
aprobarbital	Alurate	ORAL: *Adults—*40-160 mg at bedtime. FDA pregnancy category D.	Intermediate-acting barbiturate. Used as hypnotic. Reduce dosages for older adult patients. Schedule III substance. Not available in Canada.
butabarbital	Butisol Sarisol No. 2	ORAL: *Adults—As sedative:* 15-30 mg 3 or 4 times/day. *As hypnotic:* 50-100 mg at bedtime. FDA pregnancy category D. *Children—As sedative:* 6 mg/kg in 3 divided doses daily.	Intermediate-acting barbiturate used for sedation or for insomnia when need is to prolong sleep rather than to induce sleep. Schedule III substance.
pentobarbital‡	Nembutal* Novopentobarb†	ORAL: *Adults—As sedative:* 30 mg 3 or 4 times/day or 100 mg in timed-release form in morning. *As hypnotic:* 100 mg at bedtime. FDA pregnancy category D. *Children—As sedative:* 6 mg/kg in 3 divided doses daily. RECTAL: *Adults—*120-200 mg as required for sedation or hypnosis. *Children—As sedative:* 30-120 mg/day. INTRAMUSCULAR: *Adults—As hypnotic:* 150-200 mg. INTRAVENOUS: *Adults—As hypnotic:* 100 mg. After 1 min, can administer small increments, but no more than 500 mg total.	Short-acting barbiturate used principally for insomnia and preanesthetic sedation and occasionally for daytime sedation. Precautions are same as for secobarbital. Schedule II substance.
phenobarbital‡	Luminal* Solfoton	ORAL: *Adults—As sedative:* 30-120 mg daily in 2 or 3 divided doses. *As hypnotic:* 100-320 mg at bedtime. FDA pregnancy category D. *Children—As sedative:* 6 mg/kg/day in 4 divided doses. INTRAMUSCULAR, INTRAVENOUS: *Adults—As sedative:* 30-120 mg. *As hypnotic:* 100-320 mg, with no more than 100 mg (2 ml of 5% solution)/min intravenously. Full effect lasts 15 min. RECTAL: *Children—As sedative:* 6 mg/kg divided in 3 doses.	Long-acting barbiturate used principally as sedative. (For use as anticonvulsant, see Chapter 61.) Not readily addictive. Schedule IV substance.
secobarbital	Seconal* Novosecobarb†	ORAL: *Adults—As sedative:* 30-50 mg. *As hypnotic:* 100-200 mg at bedtime. *For preoperative sedation:* 200-300 mg 1-2 hr before surgery. FDA pregnancy category D. *Children—As sedative:* 6 mg/kg in 3 divided doses. *For preoperative sedation:* 50-100 mg. RECTAL: *Adults—*120-200 mg as required for sedation or hypnosis. *Children—*15-120 mg. INTRAMUSCULAR: *Adults—As hypnotic:* 100-200 mg. *Children—As hypnotic:* 3-5 mg/kg, up to 100 mg.	Short-acting barbiturate used principally for insomnia and as preanesthetic sedative. Not indicated for repeated use because tolerance develops, rebound insomnia becomes significant, and addiction potential is high. Schedule II substance.

*Available in Canada and the United States.
†Available in Canada only.
‡Also available as the sodium salt. Only the sodium salt is suitable for administration as a solution by the rectal, intramuscular, or intravenous route.

Phenobarbital is the barbiturate that most readily induces the liver microsomal enzyme system, thereby enhancing its own metabolism and those of many other drugs. Phenobarbital treatment enhances the degradation of bilirubin and is used in infants and children to lower elevated plasma bilirubin levels.

Phenobarbital may be substituted for other barbiturates or nonbenzodiazepine hypnotics when decreasing drug levels for withdrawal. Its longer action allows once-a-day therapy.

Other Hypnotic and Anxiolytic Drugs

The miscellaneous hypnotic and anxiolytic drugs listed in Table 57-3 are more similar to the barbiturates than the benzodiazepines in that they are generally shorter acting, which makes them more readily abused. Discontinuance produces withdrawal symptoms resembling those described for the barbiturates. The degree of dependence is sometimes determined by giving 200 mg of pentobarbital every 2 hours until signs of intoxication appear. The patient is then detoxified with divided doses (4 to 6 doses/day) of pentobarbital, and the total daily dose is decreased by 100 mg/day. This approach is possible because pentobarbital is cross-tolerant with these other drugs. Alternatively, the abused drug is decreased daily over a 10- to 20-day period, or phenobarbital is administered in decreasing daily doses.

In addition to these drugs, several antihistamines have a pronounced sedative effect, for which they are sometimes used (see Chapter 29).

▼ buspirone

Buspirone (BuSpar) is a new anxiolytic drug that is not a benzodiazepine or barbiturate. Buspirone may act through serotonin or dopamine receptors. Buspirone does not cause the CNS depression characteristic of barbiturates and benzodiazepines. A lag time of 1 to 2 weeks is usual before a decrease in anxiety is noted, so the major clinical use of buspirone is to treat generalized anxiety disorders. Little sedation or mental impairment is noted. However, at higher dosages, patients may experience sedation or a bad mood. Side effects are uncommon but include headaches, dizziness, nervousness, and light-headedness. Buspirone reportedly has little abuse potential. It is metabolized and excreted in urine.

chloral hydrate

Chloral hydrate (Noctec) is the oldest of the currently used hypnotic drugs, introduced in the nineteenth century. Although it is effective for only 2 weeks, it does not suppress REM sleep and therefore does not cause REM rebound. Chloral hydrate and its active metabolite trichloroethanol have a half-life of only 8 hours, so no persistent effect occurs as with flurazepam.

Chloral hydrate has an unpleasant taste and odor, which can be masked by taking the drug in capsules, as a chilled elixir or syrup, or as a suppository. The drug produces fewer side effects (particularly paradoxical excitement) among children or older adults than other hypnotics, but it causes gastric irritation in some patients and displaces the coumarin anticoagulants from plasma protein. Drug dependence is produced by long-term use; an acute overdose can result in coma, with the patient having pinpoint pupils. In folklore,

chloral hydrate added to an alcoholic beverage produces a "knockout" drink, the Mickey Finn, resulting from the additive effect of the two general CNS depressants.

ethchlorvynol

Ethchlorvynol (Placidyl) was introduced in the 1950s as a hypnotic. The most common patient complaint is an aftertaste. Patients occasionally show exaggerated depression, with deep sleep and muscular weakness. Some individuals have an idiosyncratic response of CNS stimulation that may be mild or hysteric. Ethchlorvynol is a schedule IV drug with a duration of action similar to that of the short-acting barbiturates.

hydroxyzine

Hydroxyzine (Atarax, Vistaril), an antihistamine with sedative properties, is used as an anxiolytic agent when it is desirable to have the antiemetic and antihistaminic properties for motion sickness or allergic skin reactions. Hydroxyzine is also used as a preanesthetic medication.

meprobamate

Meprobamate (Equanil, Miltown) was introduced in the 1950s as the first widely prescribed anxiolytic drug. Although physical dependence readily develops with abuse, meprobamate is a schedule IV drug. Withdrawal symptoms range from insomnia and anxiety to hallucinations and grand mal seizures. Meprobamate is sometimes used as a centrally acting skeletal muscle relaxant, although its effectiveness in this role is questionable.

Table 57-3 Miscellaneous Sedative-Hypnotic and Anxiolytic Drugs

Generic Name	Trade Name	Administration/Dosage	Comments
buspirone	BuSpar*	ORAL: *Adults*—Initially, 5 mg 3 times/day. May increase by 5 mg/day every 2-3 days until desired response is obtained. Maximum daily dose: 60 mg. FDA pregnancy category B.	Nonbenzodiazepine anxiolytic drug with minimal sedation. Does not interact with alcohol or antidepressants.
chloral hydrate	Aquachloral Supprettes Generic Novochlorhydrate†	ORAL, RECTAL: *Adults*—*As sedative:* 250 mg 3 times/day after meals. *As hypnotic:* 500 mg-1 g 15-30 min before bedtime. FDA pregnancy category C. *Children*—*As sedative:* 25 mg/kg body weight in 3-4 doses/day. *As hypnotic:* 50 mg/kg as bedtime dose, not to exceed 500 mg.	Generally safe hypnotic. Unpleasant taste and odor can be masked by chilling drug or using capsule form. Schedule IV substance.
ethchlorvynol	Placidyl*	ORAL: *Adults only*—*As hypnotic:* 500 mg-1 g at bedtime. FDA pregnancy category C.	Physical and psychological dependence may occur. Schedule IV substance.
hydroxyzine hydrochloride hydroxyzine pamoate	Atarax* Vistaril Various others	ORAL: *Adults*—*For anxiety:* 50-100 mg.	Antihistamine that has antiemetic and antianxiety properties. Used for motion sickness and as preanesthetic medication. Usual doses of barbiturates or narcotics must be cut by 50% if given concurrently.
meprobamate	Equanil* Meprospan* Miltown*	ORAL: *Adults*—*For anxiety:* 400 mg 3 or 4 times/day. *Children >6 yr*—*For anxiety:* 25 mg/kg/day in 2 or 3 divided doses.	Physical and psychological dependence may occur. Schedule IV substance.
zolpidem tartrate	Ambien	ORAL: *Adults*—10 mg at bedtime. *Older adults*—5 mg at bedtime. FDA pregnancy category B.	Nonbenzodiazepine hypnotic drug with short half-life and negligible hangover side effects. Schedule IV drug.

*Available in Canada and the United States.
†Available in Canada only.

zolpidem

Zolpidem (Ambien) is a new nonbenzodiazepine hypnotic. However, like barbiturates and benzodiazepines, zolpidem depresses the reticular-activating system, probably by promoting the inhibitory synaptic action of the neurotransmitter GABA. Zolpidem appears to act at a selected receptor subtype for GABA. It has short half-life and therefore does not accumulate to cause drowsiness or dizziness the next day. Older adult patients should receive half the normal adult dose.

THERAPEUTIC RATIONALE: ALCOHOL AND ALCOHOLISM

Alcohol: General Characteristics

Alcohol is a widely used and abused drug. This section reviews the important actions of alcohol and its interactions with other drugs.

Mechanism of Action

Alcohol causes all the behavioral changes associated with general CNS depressants: sedation, disinhibition, sleep, and anesthesia. As summarized in Table 57-4, the amount of alcohol in the blood, which can be predicted from the amount consumed, produces characteristic behavioral effects. Alcohol also enhances the sedative-hypnotic effects of other drug classes, including all the general CNS depressants discussed in this chapter and other drug classes with sedative side effects, including the antihistamines, the phenothiazines, the narcotic analgesics, the tricyclic antidepressants, and the MAO inhibitors. This enhancement of CNS depression means that irreversible coma or death can occur when alcohol is taken concurrently with other drugs, a fact not widely enough appreciated in our society.

Acute ingestion of alcohol has effects in addition to those attributed to its general CNS depression. Rising levels of alcohol may activate the vomiting center. Alcohol acts centrally to produce vasodilation and a feeling of warmth. This vasodilation can produce a significant hypotensive response in persons taking guanethidine or nitroglycerin.

Pharmacokinetics

Alcohol is absorbed more readily from the small intestine than from the stomach. Absorption of alcohol therefore is decreased by food, which dilutes the alcohol and keeps it

Table 57-4	**Alcohol Intake and Its Behavioral Effects**			
Alcohol Content (oz)	Beverage Intake in 1-hr*	Blood Alcohol Level (mg/dl) in 150-lb man	Behavioral Effects	
½	1 oz 100-proof spirits 1 glass wine 1 can beer	0.025	No noticeable effect.	
1	2 oz 100-proof spirits 2 glasses wine 2 cans beer	0.050	Lowered alertness, impaired judgment, good feeling, less inhibition.	
2	4 oz 100-proof spirits 4 glasses wine 4 cans beer	0.100	Slow reaction time, impaired motor function, less cautious; should not drive; may activate vomiting reflex.	
3	6 oz 100-proof spirits 6 glasses wine 6 cans beer	0.150	Reaction times markedly slowed.	
4	8 oz 100-proof spirits 8 glasses wine 8 cans beer	0.200	Significant depression of sensory and motor abilities.	
5	10 oz 100-proof spirits 10 glasses wine 10 cans beer	0.250	Severe depression of sensory and motor abilities.	
6	12 oz 100-proof spirits 12 glasses wine 12 cans beer	0.300	Stuporous and unconscious of surroundings.	
7	14 oz 100-proof spirits 14 glasses wine 14 cans beer	0.350	Unconscious.	
8	16 oz 100-proof spirits 16 glasses wine 16 cans beer	0.400	Lethal dose in 50% of the population.	
12	24 oz 100-proof spirits 24 glasses wine 24 cans beer	0.600	Lethal dose in 95% of the population.	

*Because only ¼ to ⅓ oz of alcohol is metabolized each hour, alcohol will rapidly accumulate.

in the stomach longer. Alcohol in concentrations of 10% or less will stimulate gastric secretions, thereby aiding digestion, but larger concentrations inhibit gastric secretions and damage the cells lining the stomach. This irritation may make some people nauseated the day after heavy drinking and accounts for the inflammation of the stomach (gastritis) and ulcers often seen in alcoholic patients. Aspirin is another drug that readily damages the stomach lining. The combination of aspirin and alcohol can produce bleeding in the stomach.

More than 90% of ingested alcohol is oxidized by the liver, with the remainder being excreted in the breath and urine. The oxidation of alcohol to carbon dioxide and water means that alcohol is a source of calories. Alcoholics may get most of their calories from alcohol but may be malnourished because alcoholic beverages lack vitamins, minerals, and protein. Two enzyme systems in the liver transform alcohol. The major enzyme for alcohol metabolism is alcohol dehydrogenase, which is also the enzyme that limits the rate of alcohol metabolism. In the average adult, the liver alcohol dehydrogenase can metabolize only about 10 ml of alcohol in 1 hour. This means that no matter how much someone has drunk, only 10 ml of alcohol can be metabolized in 1 hour, and alcohol readily accumulates in the body when this amount is exceeded. Neither coffee, fresh air, nor exercise will speed up alcohol metabolism to help someone "sober up."

ALTERNATIVE THERAPIES

Central Nervous System Depressant

KAVA-KAVA

The name *kava-kava* usually refers to a beverage prepared from the root of the pepper plant, *Piper mesthysicum,* which grows in Polynesia and Micronesia. Kava-kava serves the same purposes in these regions as alcoholic drinks serve elsewhere. In small quantities, kava-kava produces a relaxed mood, reduces anxiety, and relaxes muscles. Larger amounts cause intoxication, significant drowsiness, nausea, and blurred vision. Chronic use reddens the eyes and may discolor the skin (from accumulation of plant pigments). The active principles in kava-kava are pyrone derivatives known as kava lactones.

Because kava-kava depresses the central nervous system (CNS), it should be treated with the same precautions encouraged for any other CNS depressant (i.e., users should not drive automobiles or operate machinery while under its influence). Likewise, kava-kava should not be used in combination with other CNS depressants (alcohol, antihistamines, prescription medications for anxiety or insomnia). There has been at least one published report of a possible adverse interaction between kava-kava and a benzodiazepine, apparently with normal doses of each.

The product of alcohol metabolism by alcohol dehydrogenase is acetaldehyde, a highly toxic compound. Ordinarily, acetaldehyde does not accumulate because it is metabolized further by aldehyde dehydrogenase. Disulfiram (Antabuse) and other drugs can inhibit this enzyme so that acetaldehyde accumulates and produces unpleasant symptoms, which include headache, nausea, and vomiting.

The liver microsomal enzyme system described for the barbiturates also can degrade alcohol but ordinarily with a very limited capacity. As with phenobarbital, alcohol can induce this enzyme system so that the liver can metabolize not only more alcohol but more of other drugs as well, and this is one source of drug interactions. Alcoholics are able to metabolize twice as much alcohol as those who do not have chronic alcoholism.

An elevated value of serum gamma-glutamyl transpeptidase (GGTP) in the absence of other elevated enzymes is a good predictor of long-term alcohol or drug consumption. This enzyme is induced in the liver by alcohol and drugs and secreted into the circulation. An elevated GGTP is often the first biochemical sign of alcoholism and may occur before overt clinical signs and symptoms develop.

Acute Toxicity

Unless a large amount of concentrated alcohol has been rapidly swallowed on an empty stomach or ingested with another CNS depressant drug, an acute overdose of alcohol commonly causes an individual to pass out before lethal doses can be drunk. However, note that a pint of 100-proof liquor is a lethal dose in 50% of the population (LD_{50}) for a small man (see Table 57-4). With rapid drinking of straight liquor, someone can drink enough to die. The greatest danger of acute alcohol intoxication to nonalcoholic individuals is that they may involve themselves or others in traffic accidents (30,000 alcohol-related traffic deaths per year) or that they may fall and injure themselves.

A hangover is common on recovery from an acute alcohol intoxication and includes such symptoms as an upset stomach, thirst, fatigue, headache, depression, anxiety, and generally feeling out of sorts. Many of these symptoms are caused by congeners, the natural byproducts of fermentation and aging. Vodka, which is a mixture of pure alcohol and water and contains a few congeners, also produces few hangover symptoms compared with wines and aged spirits, which have higher congener contents.

Chronic Toxicity

Long-term drinking can produce characteristic degenerative changes in the body, as listed in Table 57-5. These changes are seen after about 10 years of drinking 150 ml of alcohol daily. In addition to these degenerative changes, some alcoholic persons may have blackout spells, periods in which they are awake and functioning but of which they have no memory. Heavy drinking during pregnancy is associated with a 63% incidence of neurologic abnormalities in the offspring.

Fetal alcohol syndrome is now recognized in the offspring of alcoholic mothers, a syndrome characterized by a flat face with widely spaced, small eyes and mental retardation.

Withdrawal

Long-term drinking also leads to withdrawal symptoms when the person stops drinking. The severity of the withdrawal symptoms depends on the individual's drinking history, but the symptoms are most common when a long-term drinker stays intoxicated for 2 weeks or more and then stops drinking. The first symptoms, which appear within a few hours, are tremors and anxiety. As the first stage progresses, bradycardia occurs, the blood pressure increases, and there is heavy sweating, loss of appetite, nausea and vomiting, and insomnia. The second stage of withdrawal is characterized by hallucinations, usually visual, but sometimes involving hearing or feeling things. The patient is still oriented and only mildly confused despite these hallucinations.

About 10% of untreated patients have seizures within the first 48 hours of withdrawal. **Delirium tremens** is a stage of withdrawal that occurs in about 10% of untreated alcoholic persons 2 to 7 days after the start of withdrawal. Delirium tremens lasts about 2 days, during which time the person is completely disoriented, is extremely agitated, sweats, and has a fever and a changing pulse and blood pressure. The person usually has no memory of this condition.

Withdrawal Treatment

A patient undergoing alcohol withdrawal may be treated with one of the long half-life benzodiazepines, most commonly diazepam or chlordiazepoxide, but occasionally clorazepate or flurazepam. Older alcoholics or those with severe liver disease may be treated with a short half-life benzodiazepine, oxazepam, lorazepam, or temazepam. This treatment is effective because alcohol is cross-tolerant with the benzodiazepines. Benzodiazepines are also used to treat the anxiety and tremors of alcohol withdrawal and to reduce the risk of seizures and delirium.

Additional therapy during withdrawal is designed to restore normal metabolic parameters and overcome the thiamin, vitamin B_{12}, and folic acid deficiencies. This supportive therapy relieves neurologic symptoms related to hypoglycemia, ketosis, and vitamin deficiency.

Naltrexone to Prevent Relapse. Naltrexone (ReVia) is sometimes prescribed to help prevent relapse and reduce alcohol cravings in those who drink. Naltrexone is an opioid antagonist originally developed to reduce opioid craving. A study of alcoholic men receiving naltrexone demonstrated that the relapse rate was reduced by 50% and of those who relapsed, only 50% returned to heavy drinking.

Disulfiram to Prevent Relapse. Disulfram (Antabuse) is occasionally prescribed for the detoxified patient who wishes to avoid drinking again (see Patient Problems box on alcohol use and disulfiram). Disulfiram blocks the oxidation of acetaldehyde. The accumulation of acetaldehyde causes unpleasant reactions, which include flushing, throbbing in the head and neck, throbbing headache, respiratory difficulty, nausea, copious vomiting, sweating, thirst, chest pain, rapid breathing, tachycardia, fainting, weakness, vertigo, blurred vision, and confusion. These effects can be elicited by alcohol for 1 to 2 weeks after disulfiram is discontinued. The reaction lasts from 30 minutes to 1 to 3 hours. Severe reactions can cause death from cardiovascular collapse or respiratory failure. Because of the severity of the reactions, only well-informed, motivated patients are considered for disulfiram therapy, which is at best a supportive treatment when

Table 57-5	Degenerative Changes Common with Chronic Alcohol Consumption
System	**Comments**
Brain	Lack of vitamin B_1 (thiamine) common to alcoholic persons produces Wernicke's disease: brain lesions manifested as inability to learn or recall. Korsakoff's psychosis describes alcoholic persons who are confused and disoriented as to time or place. Wernicke's disease and Korsakoff's psychosis are considered variations of same brain disease. Replacement of vitamin B_1 helps reverse symptoms in early stages but will not restore lost function later.
Liver	Chronic drinking produces fatty liver because in presence of alcohol, fatty acids are stored in liver rather than being metabolized. About 75% of alcoholic persons show some cirrhosis after 10 years. In cirrhosis, fibrous tissue replaces liver cells. Severe cases result in liver failure and death. Hepatitis (inflammation of liver) is also common among alcoholic persons.
Stomach and gastrointestinal tract	Alcohol causes gastritis, which leads to ulcers and blood loss. Nonspecific diarrhea is common. Inflammation of pancreas (pancreatitis) is common.
Heart	Some alcoholic individuals develop an enlarged heart that functions poorly (cardiomyopathy).
Blood	Because of blood loss and lack of folic acid, alcoholic persons can have both iron deficiency (microcytic) anemia and folate deficiency (macrocytic) anemia. Liver disease may result in clotting factor deficiency. White blood cells and platelets are decreased.
Metabolic	Alcoholic persons are often hypoglycemic because alcohol inhibits glucose production by liver. Because alcohol is converted to substrate for carbohydrate and fat metabolism, high levels of lipids, lactic acid, uric acid, and ketone bodies may appear in blood. Plasma magnesium, plasma phosphate, and plasma albumin concentration are low.
Skin	Vasodilation caused by alcohol eventually produces permanent rosy nose and cheeks. Skin ulcers are common.

supplemented by psychiatric therapy. Patients whose drinking problem is lack of moderation after the first drink are considered the best candidates for disulfiram therapy. However, studies have not shown the treatment with disulfiram to be more effective than counseling alone.

By itself, disulfiram produces transient effects such as drowsiness, fatigue, impotence, headache, acne, and a metallic or garliclike aftertaste. These effects usually disappear within 2 weeks. Drug interactions with disulfiram are numerous because of the role of the liver in drug metabolism.

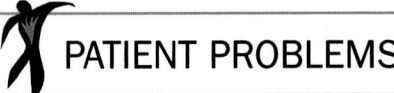

PATIENT PROBLEMS

Alcohol Use and Disulfiram

THE PROBLEM

Disulfiram is prescribed to patients who want to avoid drinking alcohol again. When a patient taking disulfiram consumes alcohol, a serious physiologic reaction occurs. Other drugs also are associated with disulfiram-like reactions in combination with alcohol. Examples are furazolidone, metronidazole, chlorpropamide, and the antibiotic moxalactam.

SIGNS AND SYMPTOMS

The combination of alcohol and disulfiram produces flushing, throbbing in the head and neck, throbbing headache, respiratory difficulty, nausea, copious vomiting, sweating, thirst, chest pain, rapid breathing, tachycardia, fainting, weakness, vertigo, blurred vision, and confusion. Severe reactions can cause death.

NURSING IN THE COMMUNITY

- Review the signs and symptoms of disulfiram-like reactions. Instruct the patient to seek medical help for a severe reaction.

- Review sources of alcohol. An obvious source includes ingestion of beer, liquor, or wine. Other dietary sources include sauces that may contain wine, cooking sherry, or liquors; wine vinegars; and some liquid medications such as cough syrups and elixirs. In patients sensitive to this reaction, topical contact with aftershave lotion or colognes, alcohol-containing liniments, or after-bath lotions may produce symptoms. Instruct the patient to avoid inhalation of the vapors of any chemical that may contain alcohol such as shellac, varnish, or paint.
- Instruct the patient to read the labels on food items, medicines, and cooking ingredients. If in doubt about a drug, have the patient consult the pharmacist.
- Encourage the patient to wear a medical identification tag or bracelet indicating that disulfiram is being taken.
- Instruct the patient to avoid alcohol-containing products for up to 2 weeks after stopping disulfiram or a drug associated with disulfiram-like reactions.

Table 57-6 Drug Interactions with Alcohol

Effect	Interacting Drugs	Comments
Increased central nervous system depression	Barbiturates meprobamate Hypnotics Antihistamines Narcotic analgesics Monoamine oxidase inhibitors Tricyclic antidepressants Benzodiazepines chlorpromazine and other sedating phenothiazines	Any drug causing sedation or drowsiness is potentiated by alcohol. Most of these drugs carry warnings stating not to drive or operate dangerous equipment and stating that situation worsens if alcohol is ingested. Alcohol can cause coma or death by respiratory depression when combined with central nervous system depressants even when the dose of either drug is not lethal by itself.
Increased liver metabolism	Barbiturates phenytoin tolbutamide warfarin	When taken over a long period, alcohol induces liver microsomal enzyme system for drug degradation. This speeds up metabolism of drugs metabolized by these enzymes, so the effective therapeutic dose must be increased. Alternatively, if an alcoholic person receiving one of these drugs becomes detoxified, drug dosage may need to be lowered.
Gastric and mucosal irritation	aspirin nicotine	Aspirin and alcohol act synergistically to irritate stomach and to cause bleeding. Alcoholic smokers have up to a 15-fold greater incidence of oral cancer.
Hypoglycemia	insulin	Alcohol acts to lower blood glucose levels independently of insulin and may cause significant hypoglycemia when taken with insulin.
Disulfiram-like reaction	disulfiram Sulfonylureas (oral hypoglycemic agents) nitroglycerin	Disulfiram inhibits degradation of acetaldehyde, which then accumulates and causes hypotension, gastrointestinal distress, and headache.
Vasodilation	guanethidine nitroglycerin	Alcohol acts centrally to produce vasodilation, which can potentiate action of these drugs.

Drugs whose metabolism is slowed by disulfiram, leading to a potentiation of drug effect, include benzodiazepines, coumarins, and phenytoin. Tricyclic antidepressants enhance the action of disulfiram. Isoniazid and metronidazole may cause neuropsychiatric symptoms in the presence of disulfiram.

Psychosocial Treatment to Prevent Relapse. Three psychosocial treatments have been tested and found equally effective in alcohol treatment: 12-step facilitation therapy based on the principles of Alcoholics Anonymous, cognitive behavioral coping-skills therapy, and motivational-enhancement therapy. The 12-step facilitation was superior for patients with few or no psychological problems. Otherwise, all therapies worked equally well, with an overall 50% reduction in heavy drinking.

Interactions

Alcohol is a major source of drug interactions because it is so widely consumed. Alcohol particularly influences other CNS depressants, drug metabolism, gastric mucosal integrity, blood glucose levels, and vasodilation. Table 57-6 summarizes drug interactions with alcohol. The importance of alcohol as a source of drug interactions can be appreciated by considering the estimate that 5% of adults in the United States are alcoholic and that 30% to 60% of hospitalized individuals are alcoholic.

Nursing Process Overview

Sedative-Hypnotic and Anxiolytic Drugs

Assessment

Perform a systematic assessment, with attention to vital signs, level of consciousness, and emotional affect. Investigate fully any subjective complaints and other health problems.

Nursing Diagnoses

- Potential complication: drug dependence or addiction
- Risk for depressed level of consciousness

Patient Outcomes

The patient will use sedatives or hypnotics for a short period, with no accompanying side effects. The patient will state relief of insomnia or anxiety. Other outcomes are appropriate for other uses of these drugs.

Planning/Implementation

The common denominator of the drugs discussed in this chapter is that they produce CNS depression. Assess level of consciousness, affect, vital signs, and blood pressure. Work with the patient to identify nonmedicinal treatments that may help. For example, patients being treated with sedative-hypnotics to produce sleep may be aided by bedtime remedies such as drinking warm milk, relaxing in a warm bath, or reading briefly. Monitor the ability of hospitalized patients to ambulate safely, and keep siderails up at night. If these drugs are being used by IV routes, have appropriate equipment for resuscitation and a suction machine available.

Evaluation

The success of these drugs depends on the original purpose for which they were being used. Before discharge, verify that the patient understands how to take the prescribed medication correctly, what symptoms may indicate too high a dosage of medication, what to do if the medication is no longer effective, and when to return to the physician for follow-up. Determine that the patient can list other drugs to avoid such as alcohol or other anxiolytic drugs. Use judgment in indicating to the patient that continued prolonged use of these drugs or use in increasing amounts can lead to drug dependence or addiction.

Nursing Implications Summary

General Guidelines: Use of Anxiolytic Agents and Sedative-Hypnotics

Drug Administration

▶ In the institutional setting, keep siderails up after administering anxiolytic and sedative-hypnotic agents. Supervise ambulation and smoking. Keep a night-light on.

▶ Use "sleeping pills" judiciously. Do not deprive patients of needed medication, but use medications as an adjunct to nursing measures such as a backrub, repositioning, a small snack, or a glass of warm milk.

▶ Tactfully assess side effects. Some drugs cause changes in libido or sexual activity. Provide emotional support as appropriate. Consult with the physician about changes in drug or dosage.

▶ Be alert in the outpatient setting to patients who return for prescription refills on an increasingly frequent basis; this may indicate improper use or abuse or lack of knowledge about the hazards of continued use of the drugs. Evaluate patients carefully for possible depression and suicidal tendencies.

Continued

Nursing Implications Summary—cont'd

Nursing in the Community

➤ Remind the patient to take these drugs only as directed and not to increase the dose or frequency without consulting the physician. Stress the importance of returning for regular follow-up visits if these drugs are used for long-term treatment.

➤ Warn the patient to avoid driving or operating hazardous equipment if drowsiness, dizziness, unsteadiness, or clumsiness develops. Tell parents to supervise the play of children taking these drugs.

➤ Warn the patient to avoid ingestion of alcohol. Instruct the patient to avoid the use of other drugs that may depress the CNS, unless they are specifically prescribed by the physician. Examples include antiemetics, narcotic analgesics, and antihistamines.

➤ For insomnia, instruct the patient to take doses 30 minutes before bedtime.

➤ Instruct the patient that the commonly encountered hangover effect in the morning after use of a sedative-hypnotic is a side effect of the medication and not a sign that the patient needs a larger dose of medication the next evening.

➤ Caution the patient taking anticonvulsant medication that drowsiness may continue for several days to weeks but should gradually diminish. Emphasize the importance of taking the drug as ordered and not discontinuing the drug without consultation with the physician. Encourage the patient with a history of seizures to wear a medical identification tag or bracelet.

➤ Instruct the patient to inform all health care providers of all drugs being used, even occasional sleeping pills.

➤ Instruct the patient to keep these and all drugs out of the reach of children, to use childproof caps in settings where small children are present, and to keep drugs in clearly labeled containers.

➤ Remind the patient not to share drugs with friends or relatives.

➤ Refer the patient who is having continuing problems with insomnia or anxiety to appropriate resources for counseling or evaluation.

➤ After long-term use, the patient may have difficulty discontinuing the medication abruptly. Instruct the patient to consult the physician before discontinuing medications.

➤ See the Patient Problems box in Chapter 23 on dry mouth.

Benzodiazepines

Drug Administration

➤ See the general guidelines.

➤ Monitor blood pressure and pulse, intake and output, and weight. Monitor the respiratory rate and auscultate breath sounds. Inspect for skin changes.

➤ Monitor complete blood count (CBC) and platelets, liver function tests, blood urea nitrogen (BUN), and serum creatinine levels.

➤ Instruct the patient taking flurazepam that several weeks of therapy may be needed to see the full effects of therapy.

➤ Lorazepam oral solution may be diluted with liquid or semisolid food such as applesauce or pudding. Teach patients to let sublingual lorazepam dissolve slowly under the tongue and not to swallow for at least 2 minutes to allow for drug absorption.

➤ Excessive or prolonged use of benzodiazepines may result in physical or psychological dependence. Caution patients to use the medications only as prescribed.

Intravenous Benzodiazepines

➤ Have a suction machine and equipment for intubation and ventilatory support available. Have available resuscitative drugs, including flumazenil. Too rapid administration may cause apnea, hypotension, or respiratory or cardiac arrest. Monitor respiratory rate and blood pressure. Do not leave the patient unattended unless the individual is sufficiently alert to handle secretions and to call for assistance.

➤ Keep siderails up.

➤ Have the patient rest in bed for 2 to 8 hours after IV doses. Monitor vital signs, mental status, and balance.

Intravenous chlordiazepoxide

➤ Dilute each 100 mg of chlordiazepoxide with at least 5 ml 0.9% sodium chloride injection or sterile water for injection; do not use the diluent provided for IM injection for IV administration. Administer 100 mg diluted over at least 1 minute.

Intravenous diazepam

➤ Administer diazepam undiluted, at a rate of 5 mg (1 ml) or less over 1 minute in adults. Administer the dose over 3 minutes in children and infants. Do not mix with any other drugs.

Intravenous lorazepam

➤ Dilute lorazepam just before administering with an equal volume of compatible IV fluid such as 0.9% sodium chloride or 5% D5W. Administer at a rate of 2 mg or less over 1 minute.

Intravenous midazolam

➤ Read labels carefully: two dosage strengths are available. Midazolam may be diluted with normal saline, D5W, or lactated Ringer's solution. Concentrations should not exceed 0.5 mg/ml. Rate of administration is often determined by the patient's response (e.g., 1 mg/4 ml, administered over at least 2 minutes until speech is slurred). For conscious sedation, evaluate carefully to avoid overmedication; wait 2 minutes between increments. Because of the risk of respiratory depression, use this drug only in settings where personnel are trained in the use of the drug and trained in the ability to intubate and provide ventilatory support. Have oxygen, a suction machine, and resuscitation equipment nearby. Monitor vital signs. Use lower dosages in older adults or debilitated patients.

Nursing in the Community

➤ See the general guidelines.

➤ Instruct the patient to report any new side effects.

Nursing Implications Summary—cont'd

➤ See the Patient Problem boxes on dry mouth (Chapter 23) and photosensitivity (Chapter 58).

➤ Instruct the patient to take doses with meals or a snack to lessen gastric irritation.

➤ Diazepam is available for rectal administration for control of seizures. Review administration procedure with physician and pharmacist, then instruct patient and family.

flumazenil

Drug Administration

➤ Consult the manufacturer's literature for current guidelines about dilution. Administer doses to reverse conscious sedation over 15 seconds. For management of suspected benzodiazepine overdose, administer each dose over 30 seconds.

➤ Monitor vital signs, blood pressure, and level of consciousness. Monitor electrocardiogram and pulse oximetry. Have a suction machine at the bedside. Keep siderails up. Do not leave the patient unattended. Observe for resedation and respiratory depression.

➤ Administration of this drug to patients who have used benzodiazepines on a long-term basis may precipitate withdrawal symptoms.

➤ Keep the patient and family informed of the patient's condition.

Barbiturates

Drug Administration

➤ See the general guidelines.

➤ Monitor blood pressure and pulse, intake and output, and weight. Monitor the respiratory rate and auscultate breath sounds. Inspect for skin changes.

➤ Monitor CBC, platelet count, and liver function tests.

➤ With IV administration, monitor vital signs and respiratory rate. Have a suction machine and equipment for intubation and ventilatory assistance available. The patient should rest in bed until the condition is stable.

➤ No more than 5 ml should be injected into any single injection site because of possible tissue irritation.

➤ Phenobarbital is also discussed in Chapter 61.

Intravenous amobarbital

➤ Dilute each 125 mg of amobarbital with at least 1.25 ml sterile water for injection to make a 10% solution. Administer each 100 mg or less over 1 minute in adults and each 60 mg or less over 1 minute in infants or children. Too rapid injection may cause symptoms of overdose (serious respiratory depression).

Intravenous pentobarbital

➤ Pentobarbital may be administered undiluted or may be diluted in sterile water, normal saline for injection, or Ringer's injection. Add 1 ml (50 mg) of pentobarbital to 9 ml diluent to make a dilution of 5 mg/ml. Administer at a rate of 50 mg or less over 1 minute. Too rapid administration may cause symptoms of overdose (serious respiratory depression).

Intravenous secobarbital

➤ Secobarbital may be administered undiluted or diluted with sterile water for injection, 0.9% sodium chloride injection, or Ringer's injection. Reconstitute powder form by adding 9 ml diluent to 1 ml (50 mg) of drug to make a 5% solution. Administer at a rate of 50 mg or less over 1 minute. Too rapid administration may cause symptoms of overdose (serious respiratory depression).

Nursing in the Community

➤ See the general guidelines.

➤ Instruct the patient to report any new side effects.

➤ Instruct the patient to take doses with meals or a snack to lessen gastric irritation.

buspirone

Drug Administration/Nursing in the Community

➤ Monitor liver function tests, BUN, and serum creatinine. Monitor blood pressure and pulse.

➤ Caution patients to avoid driving or operating hazardous equipment if dizziness, light-headedness, blurred vision, or excessive drowsiness occurs and to notify the physician.

➤ Teach patients that 1 to 2 weeks of therapy may be required to see full effects of therapy.

➤ Caution patients to avoid alcohol and other drugs that depress the CNS. Review the patient's other drugs.

MISCELLANEOUS AGENTS

Drug Administration

➤ See the general guidelines.

➤ Monitor blood pressure and pulse and intake and output.

➤ When used in the doses ordered, side effects are rare

➤ For chloral hydrate: Take capsule form with a full glass (8 ounces) of water, fruit juice, or ginger ale to decrease gastric irritation.

➤ For chloral hydrate syrup: Dilute dose in up to 4 ounces (120 ml) of clear liquid such as water, apple juice, or ginger ale to improve taste and decrease gastric irritation.

➤ For oral chloral hydrate: Drug may be dissolved in olive oil or cottonseed oil to administer as a retention enema if needed; consult pharmacist.

➤ For ethchlorvynol: Instruct the patient to take doses with snack or milk to lessen dizziness caused by rapid absorption.

zolpidem

Drug Administration/Nursing in the Community

➤ See the general guidelines.

➤ Assess for nightmares, depression, and hypotension. The elderly are at greater risk for side effects and may be at risk for falling.

➤ For best effect, instruct the patient to take doses on an empty stomach, just before retiring.

naltrexone

Drug Administration/Nursing in the Community

➤ Naltrexone is also discussed in Chapter 32.

Continued

Nursing Implications Summary—cont'd

➤ When used for treatment of alcoholism, this drug is one part of a therapeutic plan that includes counseling and/or support group meetings.

➤ Remind patients to keep all health care providers informed of all drugs being used. Instruct patients to wear a medical identification tag or bracelet or to carry an identification card indicating that naltrexone is being used.

➤ Remind patients to return as directed to have blood work monitored.

disulfiram
Drug Administration/Nursing in the Community

➤ See the Patient Problems box earlier in this chapter on disulfiram-like reactions, and review the side effects discussed in the text.

➤ Treatment with disulfiram is not a cure for alcoholism and should be used only with other forms of supportive therapy. Assess the patient carefully before administering this drug.

➤ Treatment of severe disulfiram reaction may require hospitalization. Instruct the patient's family about the effects of concomitant alcohol consumption and disulfiram use.

➤ Caution patient to avoid driving or operating hazardous equipment if drowsiness develops after disulfiram administration. The physician may suggest administering the dose at bedtime to lessen daytime drowsiness.

➤ Do not administer disulfiram until the patient has been alcohol free for at least 12 hours and the blood alcohol level is 0.

➤ The effects of disulfiram may persist for up to 2 weeks after disulfiram therapy is discontinued.

CHAPTER REVIEW

Application

1. Define sedative, hypnotic, and anxiolytic drugs.
2. Name the stages of sleep and describe which stages are affected by hypnotics.
3. What are the common chronic anxiety disorders? What symptoms would you observe?
4. What major advantages do benzodiazepines have over barbiturates?
5. Describe the uses of benzodiazepines. For what conditions are these drugs used?
6. Describe the four categories of barbiturates and list which drugs belong in each category.
7. Describe withdrawal symptoms from barbiturates. What symptoms might you observe?
8. Differentiate between metabolic tolerance and pharmacodynamic tolerance.
9. What are the uses of barbiturates?
10. Are hypnotics more similar to barbiturates or to benzodiazepines?

11. What drug interactions are seen with alcohol?
12. What factors affect alcohol absorption?
13. Describe alcohol metabolism. How does disulfiram interfere with alcohol metabolism?
14. What are the side effects of alcohol ingestion with disulfiram?
15. What physiologic changes are associated with long-term drinking?
16. How is alcohol withdrawal treated? What interventions might you take?

Critical Thinking

1. What drug interactions are seen with benzodiazepines? What steps in patient education would you take?
2. What are some of the resources in your community for patients who express an interest in stopping alcohol consumption?
3. As a home health nurse, what would you assess in the home to provide information about the level of alcohol consumption of your patients?

Reference

Woodin LM: Resting easy: how to care for patients receiving I.V. conscious sedation, *Nursing* 26(6):33-40, 1996.

Antipsychotic Drugs

OBJECTIVES

After studying this chapter, you should be able to do the following:

- *Outline the kinds of psychoses discussed.*

- *Discuss the role of the neurotransmitters dopamine, norepinephrine, and acetylcholine in the actions of the antipsychotics.*

- *Describe the signs and symptoms of extrapyramidal reactions to antipsychotic drugs.*

- *Develop a nursing care plan for a patient receiving one of the antipsychotic drugs discussed.*

- *Develop a care plan for a patient receiving a drug that may cause photosensitivity.*

CHAPTER OVERVIEW

One of the remarkable advances in pharmacology in recent decades has been the discovery and application of drugs effective in treating the major mental illnesses: schizophrenia and depression. This chapter discusses the antipsychotic or antischizophrenic drugs, also called neuroleptic drugs. **Neuroleptic** refers to the ability of these drugs to cause a general quiescence and a state of psychic indifference to the surroundings, quieting a severely agitated patient. New agents have been released that are successful in treating schizophrenia not responsive to the older antipsychotic drugs.

THERAPEUTIC RATIONALE: SCHIZOPHRENIA AND PSYCHOSES

Schizophrenia

Schizophrenia is a chronic mental illness with psychotic episodes and is the most disabling of the major mental illnesses. About 1% of Americans will develop schizophrenia during their lives. Men and women are affected equally. Men typically experience their first psychotic episode in their teens or twenties, women in their twenties or early thirties. Symptoms may develop gradually or may appear abruptly.

Before the advent of the antipsychotic drugs in the 1950s, schizophrenia accounted for most of the patient population in mental hospitals. Today, with continued advances in antipsychotic drug therapy, patients with schizophrenia do not usually require the degree of supervision found in mental hospitals.

About 14% to 30% of patients with a single psychotic episode have total recovery. For others, treatment is lifelong, although patients may not require medication for several weeks or months during a disease remission. About 75% will relapse within 18 months after discontinuation of antipsychotic drug therapy. Many individuals with schizophrenia can live in the community with strong family or group support and vocational training. However, about 5% to 15% of patients have relatively severe continuous psychosis. About 40% of patients in long-term hospitals have schizophrenia. Studies indicate that 30% to 40% of America's homeless have severe mental illness, including schizophrenia. The appropriate societal oversight of individuals with remitting or severe schizophrenia has not been resolved.

Psychoses

Psychotic symptoms are a hallmark of schizophrenia. A **psychosis** is a major emotional disorder with an impairment of mental function great enough to prevent the individual from participating in everyday life. The hallmark of a psychosis is the loss of contact with reality.

Psychotic Symptoms

There is no one symptom of a psychosis. Symptoms may include agitation, hostility, combativeness, hyperactivity, delusions, hallucinations, disordered thought and perception, emotional and social withdrawal, paranoid symptoms, and personal neglect. The older antipsychotic drugs specifically reduce the "positive symptoms," such as delusions, hallucinations, bizarre behavior, catatonia, and thought disorder so that patients can think and function more coherently. The new "atypical" antipsychotics are also effective in treating the "negative symptoms," such as low levels of emotional arousal, mental activity, and social drive. These negative symptoms tend to be debilitating for persons with chronic schizophrenia.

Functional Psychoses

A functional psychosis may be an isolated "breakdown" caused by a major traumatic event. This psychosis is usually amenable to treatment with an antipsychotic drug. The acute manic phase of manic-depressive illness is treated with an antipsychotic drug or lithium (see Chapter 59 for lithium).

Organic Psychoses

An organic psychosis results from damage to the brain by infectious diseases, deficiency diseases, lead poisoning, tumors, and injury through trauma or interrupted blood supply such as in cerebrovascular accidents (stroke) and Alzheimer's disease. Organic psychoses are not treated with antipsychotic drugs as successfully as functional psychoses.

Toxic Psychoses

A toxic psychosis can arise during withdrawal from alcohol or other drugs. Some toxic psychoses are treated with diazepam, an antianxiety drug, rather than with antipsychotic drugs. Amphetamine can cause a toxic psychosis because it releases dopamine in the central nervous system (CNS), and therefore the blockade of dopamine receptors by antipsychotic drugs provides specific therapy for an amphetamine-induced psychosis.

Defects Underlying Schizophrenia

No single cause of schizophrenia has been identified. New imaging techniques may highlight abnormalities in brain structure or function associated with schizophrenia. Evidence exists for hereditary, fetal development, and environmental bases of schizophrenia.

The neurotransmitter dopamine has long been associated with theories of schizophrenia. Alterations in the dopamine system, particularly in the projection of dopamine neurons from the limbic to cortical area, are key to the pathogenesis of schizophrenia. Five subtypes of dopamine receptors have been characterized in the brain. The clinical potency of the older antipsychotic drugs such as chlorpromazine and haloperidol correlates well with their potency to inhibit the D_2 dopamine receptor, although the older antipsychotics inhibit other subtypes of dopamine receptors as well. Inhibition of the D_2 receptor also correlates with appearance of extrapyramidal side effects. The new atypical antipsychotics such as clozapine and olanzapine are weaker blockers of dopamine D_2 receptors. However, they do block the serotonin 5-HT2A receptor effectively. The new atypical antipsychotics do not produce extrapyramidal symptoms and are effective in treating the negative symptoms of schizophrenia such as apathy and social withdrawal.

In addition to dopamine and serotonin, the inhibitory neurotransmitter gamma-aminobutyric acid (GABA) may be important in the pathology of schizophrenia. Studies indicate that GABA levels may be low in brains of schizophrenic patients as a result of a depletion in the synthesis and uptake of GABA.

With new brain imaging techniques and an explosion of knowledge based on the molecular subtypes of neurotransmitter receptors and functions, therapies for schizophrenia are improving rapidly.

THERAPEUTIC AGENTS: ANTIPSYCHOTIC DRUGS

The antipsychotic drugs are presented in two sections: the classic antipsychotic drugs and the new atypical antipsychotic drugs.

Classic Antipsychotic Drugs: General Characteristics

Chemical Classes

The classic antipsychotic drugs are presented in Table 58-1. The prototype drugs are **chlorpromazine** and **haloperidol**.

The largest antipsychotic drug class is the phenothiazines. The phenothiazines are subdivided into three subgroups based on chemical differences in side groups on the three-ringed main structure. These subgroups are the aliphatic, the piperidine, and the piperazine phenothiazines. The three subgroups differ in potency and in the incidence of key side effects, as summarized in Table 58-2 on p. 687.

Chlorpromazine was the first phenothiazine introduced in the United States and is still the most widely used drug in this class. Chlorpromazine originally was licensed as an antiemetic drug, later as a drug to potentiate anesthesia, and finally as an antipsychotic drug. The other major class of antipsychotic drugs, the thioxanthenes, have a three-ringed main structure that differs by only one atom from that of the phenothiazines. The remaining drug classes are chemically different from the phenothiazines and from each other. However, all these classes behave the same pharmacologically with respect to potency and side effects.

Table 58-1 Antipsychotic Drugs

Generic Name	Trade Name	Administration/Dosage	Comments
Phenothiazines			
acetophenazine maleate	Tindal	ORAL: *Adults*—60 mg/day in divided doses that can be increased in 20-mg increments. Optimum level is usually 80-120 mg. Occasionally, severe symptoms require 400-600 mg. *Older adult patients*—⅓-½ adult dose. *Children*—0.8-1.6 mg/kg body weight in divided doses. Maximum: 80 mg/day.	Management of psychotic disorders.
chlorpromazine hydrochloride	Chlorpromanyl† Largactil† Novo-Chlorpromazine† Thorazine Thor-Prom Various others	*Psychiatric outpatients:* ORAL: *Adults 12-40 yr*—Average dose, 400-800 mg/day. *Adults >40 yr*—Limit of 300 mg/day is suggested. *Acutely psychotic hospitalized patients:* INTRAMUSCULAR: *Adults*—25-100 mg every 1-4 hr until symptoms are controlled. *Older adult or debilitated patients*—10 mg every 6-8 hr to control acute symptoms. *Children*—0.5 mg/kg body weight every 6-8 hr, gradually increasing dose to maximum of 40 mg for children <5 yr and 75 mg for those between 5-12 yr. INTRAVENOUS: Not recommended because it is highly irritating. Drug must be diluted to at least 1 mg/ml and no more than 1 mg/min given. ORAL: *Adults*—200-600 mg/day in divided doses, increased every 2-3 days by 100 mg, up to 2 g if needed. *Older adult or debilitated patients*—⅓-½ adult dose with 20- to 25-mg increments. *Children*—0.5 mg/kg every 4-6 hr. *To control nausea and vomiting:* ORAL: 10-25 mg every 4-6 hr. INTRAMUSCULAR: 25 mg initially, then 25-50 mg every 3-4 hr to stop vomiting. *Other uses:* ORAL: *Adults*—25-50 mg 3 or 4 times/day. INTRAMUSCULAR: 25 mg every 3 or 4 hr.	Control of initial acute psychotic episodes is achieved with high dosages, which are then tapered to lowest maintenance dosage when patient's condition stabilizes. Best tolerated by patients <40 yr of age and those hospitalized less than 10 yr. Sedation is pronounced at start of therapy, which may be desired for highly agitated patients. Incidence of hypotension, ophthalmic changes, and dyskinesias is high in older adult patients. Antiadrenergic and anticholinergic side effects usually diminish after first week. Not for seizure-prone patients. Severe nausea and vomiting can be controlled by low dosages. Other uses include intractable hiccups, tetanus, and acute intermittent porphyria.
fluphenazine decanoate	Prolixin Decanoate Modecate†	INTRAMUSCULAR, SUBCUTANEOUS: *Adults <50 yr*—12.5 mg initially, then 25 mg every 2 wk. Increase by 12.5-mg increments if needed. Treatment rarely requires more than 100 mg every 2-6 wk.	Long-acting depot forms last at least 2 wk. Dosage should be stabilized in hospital because severe episodes of parkinsonism can appear. Not recommended for older adult patients or patients who have had difficulty with extrapyramidal reactions.
fluphenazine enanthate	Prolixin Moditen Enanthate†	INTRAMUSCULAR, SUBCUTANEOUS: *Adults*—25 mg; repeat or increase every 1-3 wk as needed and tolerated.	Most potent of phenothiazines used for management of psychotic disorders.
fluphenazine hydrochloride	Moditen† Permitil Prolixin	ORAL: *Adults*—2.5-10 mg initially, reduced to 1-5 mg/day for maintenance. *Older adult patients*—⅓-½ adult dose. INTRAMUSCULAR: *Adults*—1.25 mg increased gradually to 2.5-10 mg/day in 3-4 doses. *Older adult patients*—⅓-½ adult dose.	See above.
mesoridazine besylate	Serentil†	ORAL: *Adults*—150 mg/day initially. Increased by 50-mg increments until symptoms are controlled. *Older adult patients*—⅓-½ adult dose. INTRAMUSCULAR: *Adults and children >12 yr*—25-175 mg/day in divided doses (irritating).	Management of psychotic disorders. Metabolite of thioridazine with antiemetic activity and no reported retinopathy.
methotrimeprazine hydrochloride	Nozinan Oral Drops† Nozinan Liquid†	ORAL: *Adults—For psychotic disorders or presurgical sedation:* 6-25 mg/day in 3 divided doses with meals. *For severe psychosis:* 50-75 mg/day in divided doses with meals. *Children*—0.25 mg/kg body weight/day in 2 or 3 divided doses with meals. Increase gradually as needed, but no more than 40 mg/day in children <12 yr old.	Used as antipsychotic, analgesic, antianxiety agent, and sedative. For moderate to severe pain of bedridden patients; obstetric pain and sedation; anxiety before surgery; and adjunctive therapy in general anesthesia to increase effects of anesthetics.
methotrimeprazine maleate	Nozinan†	ORAL: *Adults and children*—Same dosages as for hydrochloride.	For pain relief.

*Available in Canada and the United States.
†Available in Canada only.

Continued

Table 58-1	**Antipsychotic Drugs—cont'd**		
Generic Name	**Trade Name**	**Administration/Dosage**	**Comments**
Phenothiazines—cont'd			
methotrimeprazine	Levoprome* Nozinan†	INTRAMUSCULAR: *Adults—For acute pain:* 10-20 mg at 4- to 6-hr intervals; *For obstetric pain:* 15-20 mg, repeat if needed. *For postoperative pain:* 2.5-7.5 mg immediately after surgery, repeated every 3-4 hr as needed.	When intramuscular route is used, take precautions for postural hypotension. Syrup is available for oral administration; dilute concentrate in fruit juice or chocolate-flavored drinks.
pericyazine	Neuleptil†	ORAL: *Adults—*Initially, 5-20 mg in morning and 10-40 mg in evening as needed and tolerated. Maintenance: 2.5-15 mg in morning and 5-30 mg in evening.	To treat psychotic disorders.
perphenazine	Apo- Perphenazine† Phenazine† Trilafon*	ORAL: *Adults—*16-64 mg/day in divided doses. *Older adult patients—*⅓-½ adult dose. *Children >12 yr—*6-12 mg/day. INTRAMUSCULAR: *Adults—*5-10 mg initially, then 5 mg every 6 hr with 15 mg maximum daily in ambulatory and 30 mg/day in hospitalized patients. *Older adult patients—*⅓-½ adult dose. *Children >12 yr—*Lowest adult dosage.	For acute psychotic disorders. Lower dosages needed when used as an antiemetic.
pipotiazine palmitate	Piportil L₄†	INTRAMUSCULAR: *Adults—*Initially, 50-100 mg, dosage increased in increments of 25 mg every 2 or 3 wk as needed and tolerated, usually up to maintenance dose of 75-150 mg every 4 wk.	To treat psychotic disorders.

prochlorperazine
 	
prochlorperazine
  edisylate
 	
prochlorperazine
  maleate
	Compazine
	
	Compazine
	Edisylate
	
	Compazine
	Maleate
	PMS-Prochlorper-
	  azine†
	Prorazin†
	Stemetil†
		Psychiatric disorders:
		ORAL: *Adults—*5-10 mg 3-4 times/day.
		Raise dosage every 2-3 days as required. From 50-75 mg/day is common range for mild cases and 100-150 mg for severe cases. *Older adult patients—*⅓-½ adult dose. *Children >2 yr—*2.5 mg 2-3 times/day up to total dose of 20-25 mg. Same dosage used rectally.
		INTRAMUSCULAR: *Adults—*10-20 mg in buttock; repeat every 2-4 hr up to 80 mg total. *Older adult patients—*⅓-½ adult dose. *Children >2 yr—*0.13 mg/kg body weight initial dose only, then switch to oral.
		Nausea and vomiting:
		ORAL: *Adults—*5-10 mg 3 or 4 times/day. *Children 20-29 lb—*2.5 mg 1-2 times/day. *Children 30-39 lb—*2.5 mg 2-3 times/day. *Children 40-85 lb—*2.5 mg 3 times/day or 5 mg 2 times/day.
		INTRAMUSCULAR: *Adults—*5-10 mg every 3-4 hr. *Children—*0.06 mg/lb.
		RECTAL: *Adults—*25 mg twice daily. *Children—*Same as oral dosage.
			More widely used to control severe nausea and vomiting than for psychiatric treatment. Hypotension is seen when given intravenously for surgery.

promazine hydrochloride	Primazine Prozine-50 Sparine*	*Severely agitated patients:* INTRAMUSCULAR: *Adults—*50-150 mg initially; if no calming effect in 30 min, additional doses may be given to total of 300 mg. ORAL: *Adults—*10-200 mg every 4-6 hr (may also be given intramuscularly).	Total daily dose for adults should not exceed 1000 mg.
thiopropazate hydrochloride	Dartal†	ORAL: *Adults—*10 mg 3 times/day, adjusting gradually by 10 mg every 3 or 4 days as needed and tolerated. Maintenance dose: 10-20 mg 2-4 times/day. Reduce dosage for older adult, emaciated, or debilitated patients.	To treat psychotic disorders.
thioproperazine mesylate	Majeptil†	ORAL: *Adults—*Initially, 5 mg/day, adjusted gradually by 5 mg every 2 or 3 days as needed and tolerated. Usual effective dose is 30-40 mg/day.	To treat psychotic disorders.
trifluoperazine	Stelazine Terfluzine† Various others	ORAL: *Adults—*2-4 mg/day in divided doses (outpatient), 4-10 mg/day (hospitalized). *Older adult or debilitated patients—*⅓-½ adult dosage. *Children >6 yr—*1 mg 1-2 times/day, gradually raised to maximum of 15 mg. INTRAMUSCULAR: *Adults—*1-2 mg every 4-6 hr, maximum 10 mg/day. *Older adult or debilitated patients—*⅓-½ adult dose. *Children >6 yr—*Same as oral dosage.	Management of psychotic disorders.

*Available in Canada and the United States.
†Available in Canada only.

Table 58-1 Antipsychotic Drugs—cont'd

Generic Name	Trade Name	Administration/Dosage	Comments
Phenothiazines—cont'd			
triflupromazine hydrochloride	Vesprin	ORAL, INTRAMUSCULAR: *Children >12 yr*—10-25 mg every 4-6 hr. *Psychotic disorders:* ORAL: *Adults*—50-150 mg/day. *Older adult patients*—20-30 mg/day orally. *Children >2½ yr*—0.5 mg/kg body weight, up to 150 mg maximum. INTRAMUSCULAR: *Adults*—50-150 mg/day. *Older adult patients*—10-75 mg/day. *Children >2½ yr*—0.2-0.25 mg/kg up to 10 mg maximum. All daily doses for children should be divided. *Nausea and vomiting:* INTRAVENOUS: *Adults*—1 mg up to 3 mg. INTRAMUSCULAR: *Adults*—5-15 mg every 4 hr up to 60 mg/day. ORAL: *Adults*—20-30 mg total daily. ORAL, INTRAMUSCULAR: *Children >2½ yr*—0.2 mg/kg up to 10 mg in 3 doses daily.	Management of psychotic disorders. Control of nausea and vomiting.
thioridazine hydrochloride	Apo-Thiorid-azine† Mellaril* Novo-Ridazine†	*Psychotic disorders:* ORAL: *Adults*—50-100 mg 3 times/day, increasing up to 800 mg. *Older adult patients*—⅓-½ adult dose. *Children >2 yr*—1 mg/kg body weight in divided doses. *Depressive neurosis, alcohol withdrawal syndrome, intractable pain, and senility:* 10-50 mg 2-4 times/day.	Management of psychotic disorders. Little antiemetic activity. Safe for patients with epilepsy. Possibly effective in alcohol withdrawal syndrome, intractable pain, and senility. Pronounced sedative and hypotensive side effects initially. One of the least likely of antipsychotic drugs to cause extrapyramidal reactions because of pronounced anticholinergic action. Photosensitivity has not been reported. Dosages higher than 800 mg/day have produced serious pigmentary retinopathy.
Thioxanthenes§			
chlorprothixene	Taractan Tarasan†	ORAL: *Adults and children >12 yr*—75-200 mg/day in divided doses. Gradually increase if necessary, with total optimum dose usually <600 mg/day. *Older adult patients*—½ adult dose. INTRAMUSCULAR: *Adults and children >12 yr*—75-200 mg/day in divided doses. *Older adult patients*—½ adult dose.	Management of psychotic disorders. Incidence of side effects is same as for aliphatic phenothiazines, including high sedation, autonomic effects, and low extrapyramidal effects.
flupenthixol† decanoate	Fluanxol Depot†	INTRAMUSCULAR: *Adults*—Initially, 20-40 mg every 4-10 days. May increase in 20-mg increments.	Management of psychotic disorders.
flupenthixol hydrochloride	Fluanxol†	ORAL: *Adults*—1 mg 3 times/day initially, increasing by 1 mg every 2-3 days as needed. Maintenance dosages: 3-6 mg, up to 12 mg maximum daily in divided doses. *Older adult patients*—Should be given lower dosage.	See above.
thiothixene	Navane*	ORAL: *Adults and children >12 yr*—6-10 mg/day in divided doses. Gradually increase, with usual optimal dose 20-30 mg/day, rarely as high as 60 mg/day. *Older adult patients*—⅓-½ adult dose. INTRAMUSCULAR: *Adults and children >12 yr*—4 mg 2-4 times/day; gradually increase if necessary to maximum of 30 mg. *Older adult patients*—⅓-½ adult dose.	Management of psychotic disorders. Incidence of side effects same as for piperazine phenothiazines, including low incidence of sedation and autonomic effects and high incidence of extrapyramidal effects.
Drugs of Other Classes			
haloperidol	Apo-Haloperidol† Haldol Novo-Peridol† Peridol†	*Acute psychotic management:* ORAL: *Adults and children >12 yr*—1-15 mg in divided doses initially, which can be increased gradually up to 100 mg to bring symptoms under control. Dosage is then gradually reduced. Maintenance dose: usually 2-8 mg/day. FDA pregnancy category C. *Older adult patients and children <12 yr*—0.5-1.5 mg daily initially.	Management of psychotic disorders. Likely to produce extrapyramidal reactions in patients prone to neurologic reactions. In severe cases of hyperkinetic, retarded patients, large doses may bring improvement in social behavior and concentration. Drug of choice for treatment of Gilles

*Available in Canada and the United States.
†Available in Canada only.
§Chemically related to the phenothiazines.

Continued

Table 58-1 Antipsychotic Drugs—cont'd

Generic Name	Trade Name	Administration/Dosage	Comments
Drugs of Other Classes—cont'd			
haloperidol—cont'd		Dosage increased by 0.5-mg increments if necessary. Usual maintenance dose: 2-4 mg/day. INTRAMUSCULAR: *Adults and children >12 yr*—2-5 mg every 4-8 hr or every hour if acute state requires. Acute symptoms are usually under control in 72 hr, and 15 mg/day is usually sufficient. *Chronic schizophrenia:* ORAL: *Adults and children >12 yr*—6-16 mg in divided doses, gradually increased to achieve control. Dosages as high as 100 mg may be necessary to achieve control. Dosages then are gradually reduced to achieve maintenance of control, usually 15-20 mg/day. *Older adult patients*—0.5-1.5 mg initially, increased very gradually. Maintenance dosage: usually 2-8 mg/day. *Gilles de la Tourette's syndrome:* Initial dosages to achieve control are same as for chronic schizophrenia. Maintenance dosages: *Adults and children >12 yr*—9 mg/day; *Children <12 yr*—1.5 mg/daily. FDA pregnancy category C.	de la Tourette's syndrome. Spectrum of side effects is similar to that of piperazine phenothiazines: low incidence of sedation and autonomic effects but high incidence of extrapyramidal reactions. Also indicated for Tourette's disorder.
haloperidol decanoate	Haldol Decanoate Haldol LA†	INTRAMUSCULAR: *Adults and children >12 yr*—Initially, 10-15 times previous daily oral dose of haloperidol, up to 100 mg. Begin with monthly doses, adjusting interval and amount as needed.	Depot form of haloperidol for severe chronic schizophrenics not compliant with oral medication.
loxapine succinate	Loxitane Loxapac†	ORAL: *Adults and children >16 yr*—10-25 mg twice daily initially, with dosage increased rapidly over 7-10 days to achieve control. Dosage reduced for maintenance to 60-100 mg/day; maximum: 250 mg/day. FDA pregnancy category C. *Older adult patients*—⅓-½ dose just listed.	Effective for schizophrenia and acute psychoses.
molindone hydrochloride	Moban	ORAL: *Adults*—50-75 mg/day in 3-4 doses initially, with increased dosage to control symptoms, up to 100 mg/day. Dosage should then be reduced for maintenance. Severe psychosis may require 225 mg daily. *Older adult patients*—⅓-½ adult dose.	Effective for schizophrenia and acute psychoses.
pimozide	Orap*	ORAL: *Adults and children >12 yr*—1-2 mg/day in divided doses, increasing gradually every other day as needed and tolerated. Usual daily dose is 10 mg or 0.2 mg/kg body weight. FDA pregnancy category C.	Indicated for control of Tourette's disorder.

*Available in Canada and the United States.
†Available in Canada only.

Mechanism of Action

Antipsychotic Drugs as Dopamine Receptor Antagonists. Four effects of antipsychotic drugs have been linked to the blockade of dopamine receptors in various parts of the brain. The antipsychotic effect arises from receptor blockade in the limbic system and the antiemetic effect from receptor blockade in the chemoreceptor trigger zone. These effects are used therapeutically. Extrapyramidal effects arise from blockade in the corpus striatum of neurons from the basal ganglia and endocrine effects from blockade in the pituitary gland. These two effects are undesired actions of antipsychotic drugs.

Antipsychotic Drugs as Adrenergic and Cholinergic Receptor Antagonists. The phenothiazines and thioxanthenes block receptors for norepinephrine and dopamine. At one time the antipsychotic action was believed to be the blockade of CNS norepinephrine receptors. The finding that the butyrophenone haloperidol blocked only dopamine and not norepinephrine receptors, however, solidified the data implicating the major role of dopamine rather than norepinephrine in psychotic disorders.

CNS Effects and Adrenergic Receptor Blockade. Norepinephrine is a neurotransmitter associated with specific neurons in the CNS, just as it is associated with the postganglionic neurons of the sympathetic nervous system. Neurons containing norepinephrine in the reticular-activating system of the brain are associated with alertness. The sedative effect of the phenothiazines and the thioxanthenes may result from their blockade of these receptors for norepinephrine. The blockade of norepinephrine receptors in the vasomotor center inhibits peripheral sympathetic tone and causes orthostatic hypotension.

Table 58-2 Classic Antipsychotic Drugs: Drug Class, Potency, and Major Side Effects

Drug	Equipotent Dose	Sedative Effect	Orthostatic Hypotension	Anticholinergic Effects	Extrapyramidal Symptoms
		Relative Incidence of Side Effects			
Phenothiazines					
Aliphatic					
chlorpromazine	100	High	Moderate	Moderate/high	Moderate
methotrimeprazine	75	High	High	Moderate	Low/moderate
promazine	200	Moderate	Moderate	High	Moderate
triflupromazine	25	High	Moderate	Moderate/high	Moderate/high
Piperidine					
mesoridazine	50	High	Moderate	Moderate	Low
pericyazine	10	High	Moderate	High	Moderate
pipotiazine	100	Low	Low	Low	Low
thioridazine	100	High	Moderate	Moderate/high	Low
Piperazine					
acetophenazine	20	Moderate	Low	Low	High
fluphenazine	2	Low/moderate	Low	Low	High
perphenazine	8	Low/moderate	Low	Low	High
prochlorperazine	10	Moderate	Low	Low	High
thiopropazate	20	Low	Low	Low	High
thioproperazine	10	Low	Low	Low	High
trifluoperazine	4	Moderate	Low	Low	High
Thioxanthenes					
chlorprothixene	100	High	Moderate/high	Moderate/high	Low/moderate
thiothixene	4	Low	Low/moderate	Low	Moderate/high
Drugs of Other Classes					
haloperidol	2	Low	Low/moderate	Low	High
loxapine	10	Moderate	Low/moderate	Low/moderate	Moderate/high
molindone	10	Moderate	Low/moderate	Moderate	Moderate
pimozide	2	Low	Low	Moderate	Moderate/high

Pharmacokinetics

The antipsychotic drugs are administered orally in tablet or syrup form. The syrup form is preferred for patients who hide or do not swallow pills. Many antipsychotic drugs are also available in injectable form. Only haloperidol and fluphenazine are available in depot forms for intramuscular (IM) injection, which require administration only every 3 to 6 weeks. Normally, antipsychotic drugs are given in divided daily doses initially and in daily doses when the patient's condition has stabilized. Peak plasma levels of the drug are reached 2 to 3 hours after oral administration. Up to 90% of the drug may be bound to plasma proteins. The drugs are metabolized in the liver and excreted in urine and feces. Excretion is slow, however, and metabolites may be found in urine as long as 6 months after the drug is discontinued. Apparently some metabolites are active. Improvement can last as long as 3 months after medication is halted; whether this reflects remission or presence of persistent active metabolites is unclear.

Uses

Dopamine Theory of Psychosis. Current ideas on the neurochemical origin of psychotic behavior come from an under-standing of the action of the antipsychotic drugs. These drugs block receptors in the CNS for the neurotransmitter dopamine. The hypothesis is that too much of this neurotransmitter in the limbic system produces psychotic symptoms. The limbic system is that area of the brain that regulates emotional behavior. Blocking the receptors for dopamine in the limbic system reverses psychotic symptoms.

Antipsychotic effects may not be seen for 7 to 10 days after the start of therapy, and 4 to 6 weeks are needed to see the full effect of a given dosage regimen. Dosages must be adjusted for individual patients.

Gilles de la Tourette's Syndrome. Haloperidol and pimozide are indicated for the control of tics and vocalizations of Tourette's disorder in children and adults.

Emesis and Dopamine. Dopamine is the neurotransmitter, located in the medullary chemoreceptor trigger zone, involved in vomiting (emesis). Antipsychotic drugs are effective in preventing vomiting by blocking these dopamine receptors.

Several antipsychotic drugs are prescribed to control vomiting. Chlorpromazine, triflupromazine, perphenazine, and prochlorperazine in particular are widely used as antiemetics. Chlorpromazine is also prescribed for intractable hiccups. Because of the numerous side effects of these drugs, their use as antiemetics is restricted to management of postoperative nausea and vomiting, radiation and chemotherapy sickness, nausea and vomiting caused by toxins, and intractable vomiting. Antipsychotic drugs commonly used as antiemetic drugs are listed in Chapter 25.

The antiemetic dosage is much smaller than for the antipsychotic dosage. The antiemetic effect is seen within 1 hour of administration.

Adverse Reactions, Contraindications, and Toxicity

Extrapyramidal Reactions and Dopamine Deficiency. The most important side effects of the antipsychotic drugs are the extrapyramidal reactions described in Table 58-3. Extrapyramidal reactions are most common with the piperazine phenothiazines and least common with the aliphatic phenothiazines. Extrapyramidal reactions arise from the blockade of dopamine receptors in certain nuclei of the basal ganglia of the brain. This area of the brain is responsible for coordination of movement. A common extrapyramidal reaction is drug-induced parkinsonism. In parkinsonism, degeneration of dopamine neurons going to the basal ganglia occurs, resulting in a local deficiency of dopamine (see Chapter 62). Blockade of dopamine receptors in this area of the brain produces the same symptoms as dopamine deficiency.

Four extrapyramidal syndromes are associated with antipsychotic drugs: acute dystonia, akathisia, pseudoparkin-

sonism, and tardive dyskinesia. It is important to recognize these bizarre reactions as side effects of drug therapy that require palliative medication or reduction or discontinuance of therapy. These reactions should not be treated as manifestations of the psychotic disease being treated, and the drug dosage should not be increased.

Acute dystonia is a spasm of muscles of the tongue, face, neck, or back and may mimic seizures. Dystonia is usually seen in the first 5 days of antipsychotic therapy. It may be treated with an antihistaminic or anticholinergic antiparkinsonian drug (see Chapter 62). Injection of one of these drugs usually dramatically relieves the dystonia. Dystonia reactions are most common in patients younger than 25 years of age and rarely persist after treatment of the acute reaction. Some of the classic reactions seen in dystonia include neck twisting (torticollis), upward gaze paralysis (oculogyric crisis), stereotyped motions of the jaw, and a spasm in which the head and feet create a horseshoe (∩) configuration (opisthotonos).

Akathisia is a motor restlessness and may be mistaken for psychotic restlessness or agitation. Akathisia commonly appears after the first few days of therapy, and if not recognized, the antipsychotic drug dosage may again be mistakenly increased to relieve the agitation. Patients experiencing akathisia have difficulty sitting still and may pace about, fidget, or constantly move their legs. Anticholinergic drugs or a muscle relaxant such as diazepam may treat these symptoms. If these treatments are not effective, a different antipsychotic drug may have to be tried. Tolerance does not quickly develop to akathisia, but akathisia disappears when the drug is discontinued.

Table 58-3	**Side Effects of Classic Antipsychotic Drugs**	
Type of Effect	**Signs and Symptoms**	**Comments**
Adrenergic blockade (central nervous system)	Sedation Postural (orthostatic) hypotension	Usually transient.
Cholinergic blockade	Atropine-like effects: dry mouth, blurred vision, constipation, and delayed micturition	Usually transient.
Endocrine—dopamine blockade	Men: erection problems Women: menstrual irregularities and unexpected lactation	Usually transient.
Extrapyramidal—dopamine blockade	Acute dystonia: neck twisting, facial grimacing, abnormal eye movements, and involuntary muscle movements	Most common during first few days of therapy; usually disappears after brief treatment with antiparkinsonian drugs.
	Akathisia: restlessness, difficulty in sitting still, and strong urge to move about	Most common after first week of therapy; control with antiparkinsonian drugs or diazepam.
	Parkinsonism: motor retardation, masklike face, tremor, rigidity, salivation, and shuffling gait	Most common after first week of therapy; control with antiparkinsonian drugs.
	Tardive dyskinesia: protrusion of tongue, puffing of cheeks, chewing movements, involuntary movements of extremities, and involuntary movements of trunk	Most common when dosage is lowered after prolonged therapy; older adult female patients at greatest risk; may not be reversible.
Allergic reactions	Photosensitivity	Common.
	Cholestatic hepatitis	Rare.
	Agranulocytosis	Rare.

Pseudoparkinsonism is marked by motor retardation and rigidity. Patients find it difficult to initiate movements or to carry them out. The face resembles a mask because emotions do not register on it. The patient has a shuffling gait and hypersalivates. Tremor is seen in the hands and legs. These parkinsonian symptoms commonly appear after 1 week of therapy and are treated with antiparkinsonian drugs. Tolerance does not develop to the parkinsonian symptoms. If they cannot be controlled with drug therapy, the antipsychotic drug must be changed.

Neuroleptic malignant syndrome is a rare side effect but has a mortality of 10% (see Patient Problems box on neuroleptic malignant syndrome). It resembles a severe form of parkinsonism.

Tardive dyskinesia is associated with long-term, high-dose antipsychotic therapy. It is most common in older adult women and in patients who have had a stroke. Tardive dyskinesia is the worst of the extrapyramidal reactions because it cannot be readily treated, is persistent, and may not altogether disappear when the drug therapy is discontinued. It usually appears some months after therapy has been started, when the drug dosage is reduced or discontinued. Tardive dyskinesia may represent the development of receptors that are supersensitive to dopamine after prolonged blockade by the antipsychotic drugs. Thus removing the antipsychotic drug worsens the condition because dopamine then has ready access to these supersensitive receptors. Antiparkinsonian drugs also worsen the condition because they either increase dopamine or block the acetylcholine opposing the dopamine. Some common symptoms of tardive dyskinesia are protrusion of the tongue (fly-catcher sign), puffing of the cheeks or the tongue in a cheek (bonbon sign), chewing movements, and involuntary movements of the extremities and trunk. Recent recognition that tardive dyskinesia is a common reaction in up to 50% of patients treated for a long time with high dosages of antipsychotic drugs has prompted reevaluation of long-term therapy with these drugs. The current choice is to use as low a dosage as possible and to put the patient on a "drug holiday" during periods of remission.

Sedation and orthostatic hypotension are most often seen early in treatment with the aliphatic phenothiazines, the class of phenothiazines with the most prominent adrenergic blocking activity. These side effects are most likely to be prominent in older adults or debilitated patients. If sedation and hypotension are not severe, the dosage can be reduced and then gradually increased to produce tolerance to these effects, or another drug can be tried. Antipsychotic drugs are not addicting.

Anticholinergic Actions. All of the antipsychotic drugs have some anticholinergic action. The atropine-like effects of dry mouth, blurred vision, delayed micturition, and constipation are common side effects. However, a central anticholinergic action is beneficial in controlling some extrapyramidal reactions. Extrapyramidal reactions such as parkinsonian symptoms are believed to reflect a relative lack of dopamine and a relative abundance of acetylcholine in neuronal areas controlling movement coordination (see Chapter 62). Because antipsychotic drugs produce extrapyramidal reactions by blocking the action of dopamine, drugs that also have substantial ability to block the action of acetylcholine have less tendency to cause extrapyramidal reactions.

Electrocardiographic Changes. The aliphatic phenothiazines are also the most likely to produce nonspecific changes in the T wave of the electrocardiogram (ECG). This change has no particular meaning but is undesirable in a patient with concurrent heart disease who is being monitored for ECG changes.

Seizure Potential. Antipsychotic drugs must be used with caution in patients with epilepsy because the drugs can

---

PATIENT PROBLEMS

Neuroleptic Malignant Syndrome

THE PROBLEM
Neuroleptic malignant syndrome (NMS), a potentially fatal syndrome, may occur at any time during therapy with neuroleptics. Although rare, NMS is more commonly seen at the start of therapy, after patients are switched from one drug to another, after a dosage increase, or when a combination of drugs is used.

SIGNS AND SYMPTOMS
The patient may have convulsions, difficult or fast breathing, tachycardia or irregular pulse rate, fever, high or low blood pressure, increased sweating, loss of bladder control, skeletal muscle rigidity, pale skin, excessive weakness or fatigue, and an altered level of consciousness. There may be severe extrapyramidal side effects such as difficulty swallowing, excessive salivation, oculogyric crisis, and dyskinesia. The white blood cell count may be elevated in the range of 9500 to 26,000 cells/mm³, and elevated liver function tests and creatine phosphokinase (CPK) level.

TREATMENT
The patient will require intensive care. Monitor vital signs, notify the physician, discontinue neuroleptic therapy. Monitor electrocardiographic changes. Administer antipyretics and use a cooling blanket to lower temperature. Monitor electrolytes and administer intravenous fluids. Drug treatment for NMS includes dantrolene and/or bromocriptine (experimental).

NURSING IN THE COMMUNITY
NMS is rare. Instruct the patient and family to notify the physician of any sudden change in the patient's condition or of any unexpected sign or symptom.

precipitate convulsions. Because antipsychotic drugs lower the convulsive threshold, the drugs are unsuitable to treat drug withdrawal that is likely to produce seizures such as withdrawal from alcohol, barbiturates, and other sedative-hypnotic drugs.

Endocrine Disturbances. Dopamine inhibits the release of the hormone prolactin by the pituitary gland. Blockade of dopamine leads to hypersecretion of prolactin and secondarily to endocrine disturbances of the reproductive system by mechanisms not yet understood. Women may experience delayed ovulation and menstruation, lack of menstruation (amenorrhea), milk production (galactorrhea), or weight gain. Men may experience impotence, decreased libido, retrograde ejaculation, or moderate breast growth (gynecomastia).

Allergic Reactions. Photosensitivity and cholestatic hepatitis occasionally develop during therapy. Photosensitivity is fairly common and represents an allergic reaction to a metabolite produced not by the body but by reaction with sunlight (see

Patient Problems box on photosensitivity). The long half-life of the antipsychotic drugs and their metabolites has been discussed. These metabolites accumulate in the skin, where exposure to sun causes chemical changes that can cause skin allergies. Patients taking antipsychotic drugs should not sunbathe because they risk a painful skin rash. Some patients develop slate-blue patches on their skin. This is an accumulation of drug metabolites, not an allergy, and is not dangerous.

Cholestatic hepatitis can develop with antipsychotic therapy. Jaundice develops when the bile duct becomes blocked by an allergic inflammation caused by metabolites excreted in the bile. It is commonly seen in the first month of therapy with one of the aliphatic phenothiazines. It is normally mild and self-limiting; but if jaundice is detected, the drug should be stopped and an antipsychotic drug from a different chemical class used.

Blood Dyscrasias. A blood dyscrasia, the depression of the synthesis of one of the blood elements, occasionally occurs with antipsychotic therapy. Depression of leukocytes is common with antipsychotic therapy but is usually transient and not serious. However, agranulocytosis, in which leukocytes are no longer produced, is serious and often fatal. Agranulocytosis is most common within 3 months of the start of therapy. Therefore blood counts should be done early in the therapy. Any sign of fever or sore throat indicates the possible onset of agranulocytosis and should be checked immediately.

Interactions

Antipsychotic drugs potentiate the action of drugs that depress the CNS, including sedative-hypnotic drugs, narcotic analgesics, and anesthetic agents. The potentiation of sedative-hypnotic drugs, including alcohol, is an important drug interaction. The effects of an alcoholic drink or a sleeping pill are greatly exaggerated in patients taking an antipsychotic drug. A toxic overdose of the alcohol or sedative hypnotic drug therefore becomes possible at a lower dosage.

Clinical use is made of the potentiation of narcotic-analgesic drugs by antipsychotic drugs. The chronic pain of terminal cancer patients can be relieved by receiving lower dosages of a narcotic-analgesic drug when an antipsychotic drug is also given. This greatly slows the development of tolerance to the narcotics. The antipsychotic drug has the further advantage of controlling the emesis produced by radiation therapy or chemotherapy.

Finally, droperidol, a drug related to the antipsychotic drug haloperidol, is widely used with a narcotic to produce a state of quiescence and indifference to stimuli, which allows bronchoscopy, x-ray studies, burn dressing, and cytoscopy to be performed. Nitrous oxide can be added to this neuroleptic-narcotic combination to produce general anesthesia for surgery, called neuroleptanesthesia. The anesthesia results

PATIENT PROBLEMS

Photosensitivity

THE PROBLEM
Some drugs can cause the skin to become especially sensitive to the effects of ultraviolet rays, so patients become sunburned with minimal exposure to the sun.

SIGNS AND SYMPTOMS
Sunburn develops after relatively brief exposure to the sun or other sources of ultraviolet light. Blisters, red skin, pain, or discomfort over skin surfaces may also occur.

NURSING IN THE COMMUNITY
- Avoid sunbathing or tanning at tanning salons.
- Limit outdoor activities during the middle part of the day (10 AM to 2 PM) as much as possible.
- If outside, wear a wide-brimmed hat, long-sleeved shirt or jacket, long pants, and socks or other foot covering.
- Use a sunblock lipstick of at least SPF 15 and reapply regularly.
- Use a maximum strength sunblock on exposed skin surfaces (SPF 15 or higher). Read label carefully and choose a product that blocks both ultraviolet rays A and B. Apply liberally to exposed skin surfaces, and repeat application every 1 to 2 hours. If you suspect that the sunblocking agent is causing skin irritation or rashes, try another agent or a product labeled hypoallergenic, which may be less irritating.
- If you experience moderate to severe sunburn, notify the physician.

from the synergistic effect of the drugs with nitrous oxide because nitrous oxide alone is not potent enough to produce surgical anesthesia (see Chapter 36).

Atypical Antipsychotic Drugs: General Characteristics

The atypical antipsychotic drugs are the new agents for treatment of severe schizophrenia (Table 58-4). They have minimal extrapyramidal side effects that complicate therapy with traditional antipsychotics. The atypical antipsychotics are effective in treating the negative symptoms of schizophrenia—apathy, social withdrawal, blunted affect—symptoms not relieved by traditional antipsychotics.

Mechanism of Action

Atypical antipsychotics typically block the dopamine D_2 receptor but not as effectively as the traditional antipsychotics. In addition, atypical antipsychotics also block the serotonin 5-HT2A receptor effectively. This combination is believed to account for their effectiveness in blocking the positive symptoms of psychosis with minimal extrapyramidal effects and in relieving the negative symptoms of schizophrenia.

Atypical antipsychotics also inhibit other classes of dopamine and serotonin receptors, as well as central cholinergic, histaminergic, and adrenergic alpha-receptors.

Pharmacokinetics

Atypical antipsychotics are available only for oral administration. They are metabolized by the liver. Metabolites of clozapine and olanzapine are inactive, but risperidone has an active metabolite that has parameters like the parent compound. These drugs are highly bound to plasma protein. They are primarily eliminated in the urine with some elimination in the feces.

Uses

At present, the atypical antipsychotics are indicated for schizophrenic patients unresponsive to traditional antipsychotics, especially patients with pronounced negative schizophrenic symptoms. However, with increased experience using these agents, they are being more widely prescribed. The advantage is the low risk of the disabling extrapyramidal side effects. These side effects of traditional antipsychotics inhibit doctors from prescribing these drugs long term and patients from taking the medication.

RESEARCH HIGHLIGHTS

Noncompliance with Medication Regimens in Severely and Persistently Mentally Ill Schizophrenic Patients
—*Mulaik CJS:* Iss Mental Health Nurs *13(3):219, 1992.*

PURPOSE

Relapse requiring rehospitalization of schizophrenic patients is a major problem for the patients, the family, and the health care team. Noncompliance (taking significantly less than the prescribed amount of medication over time) with medication regimens is one of many causes of relapse. This study was designed to explore the reasons for noncompliance.

SAMPLE

A convenience sample of 11 "triads" was used. Each triad was composed of a patient, the patient's caretaker or family member, and the primary nurse assigned to the patient. All of the patients had a diagnosis of schizophrenia, a history of several admissions, and two or more documented episodes of medication noncompliance. Characteristics of the patients included seven men and four women, with ages from 19 to 58 years; one patient was employed. Family members included six mothers, one grandmother, one daughter, one wife, one sister, and one father.

METHODOLOGY

A structured interview was used to interview the 11 patients, 11 caretaker/family members, and 5 nurses, for a total of 33 interviews (some nurses care for more than one of the patients). Questions on the interview form were developed based on the Health Belief Model.

FINDINGS

Patients reported various reasons for not taking medicines, including "I don't need medicine," and "I'm tired of taking medicine." Half the patients believed that they did not need the full dose of medication. There were few side effects; one patient each reported sleepiness, dizziness, impotence, weight gain, and heartburn.

Families and nurses agreed about potential problems patients faced in going home, namely potential for patient violence, refusal to take medication, and problems with drug or alcohol use. Other findings included patients' low self-esteem, lack of knowledge about their medications, inability to identify early symptoms of relapse, and families' stress from patients' abusive, unpredictable behavior.

IMPLICATIONS

Schizophrenic patients and their families require continued support from the health care team. Knowledge of the disease and medications must be provided and reviewed frequently. Patients, families, and the health care team must work together to problem solve when noncompliance is an issue. In this study, drug side effects were not a major reason for noncompliance, but the sample in this study was small. Nurses must continue to assess patients thoroughly for causes of noncompliance when it exists.

Table 58-4   Atypical Antipsychotic Agents

Generic Name	Trade Name	Administration/Dosage	Comments
clozapine	Clozaril*	ORAL: *Adults*—Initially, 25 mg 1-2 times/day, increasing in increments of 25-60 mg/day, as tolerated, to achieve dose of 300-450 mg/day by end of 2 wk. Subsequent dosage increments should not exceed 100 mg 1 or 2 times/wk. FDA pregnancy category B.	Indicated only in management of severely ill schizophrenic patients failing to respond to other drugs. Monitor for agranulocytosis and seizures.
olanzapine	Zyprexa	ORAL: *Adults*—Initially, 5-10 mg once daily. Usual daily dose is 10 mg. May increase dose if necessary by 5 mg at weekly intervals. FDA pregnancy category C.	Risk of orthostatic hypotension minimized by starting with 5 mg/day.
risperidone	Risperdal*	ORAL: *Adults*—Day 1: 1 mg twice a day, then 2 mg twice a day on day 2, and 3 mg twice a day on day 3, then increasing by 0.5-1 mg at weekly intervals. Total daily dose is usually 4-16 mg. Decrease by half for elderly or patients with impaired hepatic function. FDA pregnancy category C.	Skin may be more sensitive to sunlight.

*Available in Canada and the United States.

Adverse Reactions and Contraindications

Clozapine may cause cardiovascular side effects such as tachycardia and hypotension or orthostatic hypotension. Drowsiness, headaches, and weight gain are common side effects. Clozapine carries a risk of agranulocytosis at the rate of 1% to 2% per year, a fact that delayed its introduction and requires weekly monitoring of the white blood cell (WBC) count. Risperidone and olanzapine do not carry this risk.

The most common side effects of olanzapine include headache, sleepiness, dizziness, weight gain, and dry mouth.

Risperidone is more likely than the other atypical antipsychotics to cause extrapyramidal side effects. It also raises prolactin levels. Other side effects include dizziness, sexual dysfunction, and mood or mental changes.

All atypical antipsychotics are associated with an increased risk of seizures, especially at high dosages, and should be used with caution for patients with a history of seizures. Although rare, atypical antipsychotics may be associated with neuroleptic malignant syndrome (see Patient Problems box earlier in chapter). Caution should also be used in administering these medications to patients with tardive dyskinesia, orthostatic hypotension, hyperprolactinemia, or hepatic or renal impairment. Patients with cardiovascular disease and breast cancer may be at increased risk for worsening of these conditions.

Toxicity

Treatment of overdose is supportive, with administration of activated charcoal to remove unabsorbed drug.

Interactions

Drugs that increase or decrease the P-450 system will alter the metabolism of these drugs. The hypotensive effects may be potentiated by antihypertensive agents. Atypical antipsychotics will antagonize the effects of levodopa and other dopamine agonists.

Specific Atypical Antipsychotic Drugs

Drugs available include clozapine, olanzapine, and risperidone. Quetiapine (Seroquel) has been approved by the Food and Drug Administration (FDA). Other agents in the pipeline include sertindole (Serlect) and zipradisone (Zeldoz).

▼ clozapine

In 1990, **clozapine** (Clozaril) was the first atypical antipsychotic released in the United States for the treatment of schizophrenia not responsive to the classic antipsychotic drugs. Clozapine quickly became widely used because it relieved the negative symptoms of schizophrenia and did not cause the extrapyramidal side effects that compromise therapy with traditional antipsychotics. Nevertheless, clozapine has a risk of agranulocytosis that requires weekly monitoring of white blood cell levels.

olanzapine

Olanzapine (Zyprexa) was released in the United States in 1996. Olanzapine has minimal risks for seizures and extrapyramidal side effects and has no association with agranulocytosis.

risperidone

Risperidone (Risperdal) was released in the United States in 1994. Risperidone has minimal risks for seizures and agranulocytosis. However, risperidone has a higher incidence of extrapyramidal side effects than the other atypical antipsychotics.

Nursing Process Overview

Antipsychotic Drugs

Assessment

Perform a complete assessment, with a focus on the behavioral component. Assess the patient's emotional affect, ability to interact with others, and ability to initiate appropriate conversation. Assess for abnormal thought processes such as hallucinations or delusions, and observe any unusual mannerisms or conversely the lack of any objective activity. Evaluate judgment, decision making, and overall thought processes. Obtain baseline vital signs and weight. Assess for abnormal movements using the abnormal involuntary movement scale (AIMS). Assess serum drug levels if available.

Nursing Diagnoses

- Altered bowel elimination: constipation related to drug side effects
- Potential impaired physical mobility related to extrapyramidal side effects of antipsychotic therapy

Patient Outcomes

The patient will not experience constipation related to drug side effects. If extrapyramidal side effects develop, the nurse will manage and minimize the severity and effect of these side effects.

Planning/Implementation

Patients requiring antipsychotic drug therapy also require psychiatric care, at least during initial drug therapy. Observe the patient closely for changes in overall affect and behavior. Monitor vital signs, level of consciousness, blood pressure, and signs of drug toxicity. Serious side effects include extrapyramidal reactions or acute dystonia. Continue to monitor serum drug levels and to assess for involuntary movements.

Evaluation

Most patients require continued use of these medications, with brief drug-free periods, for the rest of their lives. Before discharge, verify that the patient or family can understands to take the medication correctly, what symptoms or side effects should be reported immediately to the physician, what situations indicating overdosage or underdosage should be reported to the physician, and what symptoms of disease exacerbation should be reported to the physician. If other medications are used to treat the underlying condition or side effects of the antipsychotic drugs, ascertain that the patient or family can explain the necessary information about these drugs (see Table 58-3).

Nursing Implications Summary

General Guidelines: Care of Patient Receiving Antipsychotic Drugs

Drug Administration

➤ Review the common side effects listed in Tables 58-2, 58-3, and 58-4; these effects will be commonly encountered. Assess the patient on a regular, ongoing basis for these side effects. Assess thoughtfully: what may appear to be increased agitation may be akathisia, or what may resemble anxiety may be early parkinsonian side effects. Review the Patient Problems box on neuroleptic malignant syndrome earlier in this chapter.

➤ Monitor blood pressure every 4 hours until the patient is stable; this may require several days to 2 weeks. Some physicians prefer that blood pressure be monitored with the patient in lying, sitting, and standing positions.

➤ Side effects may make the patient unsteady when ambulating. Supervise ambulation and assist when appropriate.

➤ Monitor fluid intake and output until the patient is stabilized. Weigh the patient weekly. Monitor blood glucose levels.

➤ Supervise the patient carefully to ascertain that medication is swallowed and is not hidden in the mouth to be discarded or stored for later use. Some antipsychotic drugs are available in syrup, injection, or depot injection forms to ensure that the patient receives the prescribed dose. On an outpatient basis, it may be necessary for a responsible family member to supervise medication taking.

➤ Concentrated oral forms of many antipsychotic drugs are available for institutional use. Dilute the dose in 60 to 120 ml in one of the diluents suggested by the manufacturer.

➤ Monitor the patient with a history of seizures carefully because antipsychotics may alter the seizure threshold.

➤ For IM injection, choose a large muscle mass. Aspirate before injecting to avoid inadvertent intravenous (IV) administration. Warn the patient that the drug may cause a burning sensation while being injected. Record and rotate injection sites.

➤ The care of the mentally ill is complex and involves the use of many treatment modalities. See texts and articles appropriate to the care of psychiatric patients.

Nursing in the Community

➤ Review the anticipated benefits and possible side effects of drug therapy with the patient and family. Review extrapyramidal side effects listed in Table 58-3. Because there is no effective treatment for tardive dyskinesia, its appearance should be reported immediately. Fine vermicular (wormlike) movements of the tongue may be the first sign of this

Continued

Nursing Implications Summary—cont'd

side effect. Instruct the patient and family to report any new signs or symptoms.

➤ See the Patient Problems boxes on dry mouth (Chapter 23), constipation (Chapter 24), photosensitivity (earlier in this chapter), and orthostatic hypotension (Chapter 13).

➤ Inform the patient that several weeks of therapy may be necessary before full benefit can be seen. Encourage the patient to return for follow-up visits to monitor drug effectiveness and to check for the development of side effects.

➤ Warn the patient to avoid driving or operating hazardous equipment if vision changes, drowsiness, or sedation occurs and to notify the physician if these symptoms do occur.

➤ For missed doses, if the drug is ordered once a day, advise the patient to take the missed dose as soon as remembered on the day it was due; otherwise, omit the missed dose and resume the regular dosage schedule the next day. If drug is ordered more than once a day, advise the patient to take the missed dose as soon as remembered, if within 1 hour of when scheduled; otherwise omit the missed dose and resume regular dosing schedule. The patient should not double up for missed doses and should check with the physician if he or she has questions.

➤ Caution the patient to inform all health care providers of all drugs being taken. Warn the patient to avoid over-the-counter drugs unless first approved by the physician.

➤ Caution the patient to avoid alcoholic beverages while taking antipsychotics.

➤ Warn diabetic patients that antipsychotics may alter blood glucose levels. Instruct patients to monitor blood glucose levels carefully and to consult the physician about changes in dietary or drug treatment for diabetes.

➤ Instruct the patient not to discontinue therapy abruptly or without consultation with the physician. Instruct the patient to keep these and all drugs out of the reach of children.

➤ Instruct female patients to keep a record of menstrual periods. Some of these drugs may cause amenorrhea or other changes in the cycle. If pregnancy is suspected, instruct the patient to notify physician immediately.

➤ Assess tactfully for changes in libido, gynecomastia, galactorrhea, and other endocrine problems that may develop in some patients. If priapism (prolonged, painful, inappropriate erection of the penis) develops, notify physician.

➤ If additional drugs are prescribed to treat side effects of antipsychotic agents, review their use and side effects with the patient and family.

Phenothiazines
Drug Administration

➤ Contact dermatitis caused by the phenothiazines has been reported. Avoid getting the drugs on the skin, and wash hands carefully after preparing these drugs. If working with these drugs frequently, wear gloves. Caution the patient to avoid getting medication on the skin and to wash spilled drug off hands immediately.

➤ IM injections of nondepot forms of phenothiazines may cause significant hypotension. Keep the patient supine for 30 minutes to 1 hour after the injection, monitor blood pressure, and supervise ambulation. For rare severe reactions, levarterenol and phenylephrine are the vasoconstrictors of choice; do not use epinephrine.

➤ Read orders and labels carefully. Some drugs are available in an aqueous form and an oil-based depot form. Administer oil-based depot forms intramuscularly, never intravenously.

➤ When antipsychotics are used as antiemetics, the dosages are usually lower. Side effects are milder and include sedation, hypotension, and dry mouth. However, any side effect listed can occur in a patient who is extremely sensitive to the drug. When antipsychotic drugs are given as antiemetics with narcotic analgesics, they may potentiate CNS-depressive effects of the analgesics, including hypotension and sedation.

Nursing in the Community

➤ Instruct the patient to take oral doses of loxapine, molindone, phenothiazines, or thioxanthenes, with food or a full glass (8 ounces) of water or milk.

➤ Liquid doses of molindone may be taken undiluted or further diluted in milk, water, fruit juice, or carbonated beverages.

➤ Instruct the patient to dilute thiothixene oral solution just before taking dose with a full glass of water, milk, tomato or fruit juice, soup, or carbonated beverages.

➤ Instruct the patient not to take oral doses of loxapine, molindone, thioxanthenes, or phenothiazines within 2 hours of taking doses of antacids or medicine for diarrhea.

➤ Instruct the patient to swallow extended-release forms whole and not to crush or chew them.

➤ Review with the patient how to measure the correct dose if the drug is dispensed with a dropper. Teach correct administration technique if suppositories or injections are ordered.

➤ Instruct the patient to report signs of agranulocytosis, including sore throat, fever, and malaise. Instruct the patient to report signs of liver dysfunction, including jaundice, malaise, fever, and right upper quadrant abdominal pain.

➤ These drugs may interfere with the body's ability to regulate temperature. Warn the patient to avoid prolonged exposure to extremes of temperature, to allow for frequent cooling off periods when exercising or in hot environments, and to dress warmly for exposure to the cold.

➤ Review possible endocrine side effects (see text) with patient and family. Assess carefully and tactfully for these side effects. Provide emotional support as appropriate. If endocrine side effects are intolerable, consult the physician for possible drug or dosage change.

➤ Phenothiazines may cause the eyes to be more sensitive to light. Instruct the patient to wear sunglasses that block ultraviolet light, even on cloudy days.

➤ Instruct the patient to monitor weight (if appropriate to ability and resources). If weight gain is a problem, counsel about low-calorie diets. Refer to a dietitian as needed.

Nursing Implications Summary—cont'd

➤ The phenothiazines may produce false-positive pregnancy results. Female patients who suspect they are pregnant should consult the physician. Female patients may desire to use contraceptive measures while taking these drugs; counsel as appropriate. As always, pregnant or lactating women should avoid all drugs unless first approved by the physician.

chlorpromazine

➤ IV administration: For direct IV push, dilute chlorpromazine in 0.9% sodium chloride to make a dilution of 1 mg/ml. Administer at a rate of 0.5 mg/min. For infusion, further dilute and infuse slowly. Monitor blood pressure. Keep siderails up. Supervise ambulation after dose.

droperidol

➤ Droperidol is used as an antiemetic, as a preoperative medication, or during anesthesia (see Chapter 36).

➤ For IV administration, droperidol may be given undiluted or may be further diluted. Administer undiluted drug at a rate of 10 mg or less per 1 minute. Monitor blood pressure. Keep siderails up. Supervise ambulation. Titrate diluted doses to patient response.

flupenthixol

➤ Read orders and labels carefully. The decanoate form is a depot, in which the drug is suspended in sesame oil. Use a 21-gauge needle. See information on administering oil-based suspensions in Chapter 5.

fluphenazine

➤ Read orders and labels carefully. The decanoate and enanthate forms are depots, with the drug suspended in sesame oil. Use a dry needle and syringe. A wet needle or syringe causes the drug to turn cloudy. Use a 21-gauge needle. See information on administering oil-based suspensions in Chapter 5.

haloperidol

➤ Read orders and labels carefully. The decanoate form is a depot, with the drug suspended in sesame oil. Use a 21-gauge needle. See information on administering oil-based suspensions in Chapter 5.

➤ Oral doses are best taken alone but may be mixed with water immediately before taking dose. Do not mix with or take with tea or coffee.

perphenazine

➤ IV administration: Read label carefully. Use only single-dose 5-mg ampules for IV use. Dilute each 5 mg (1 ml) with 9 ml of normal saline for injection. Administer at a rate of 0.5 mg (1 ml)/min. Monitor blood pressure. Keep siderails up. Supervise ambulation.

prochlorperazine

➤ IV administration: Dilute each 5 mg (1 ml) with 9 ml of normal saline for injection. Administer at a rate of 5 mg or less over 1 minute. Prochlorperazine may also be further diluted and given as an infusion.

promazine

➤ IV administration: Dilute to 25 mg or less per 1 ml with 0.9% sodium chloride injection. Administer at a rate of 25 mg or less over 1 minute. Monitor blood pressure. Keep siderails up. Supervise ambulation.

triflupromazine

➤ IV administration: Dilute 10 mg with 9 ml of normal saline for injection. Administer at a rate of 1 mg (1 ml) over 2 minutes. Monitor blood pressure. Keep siderails up. Supervise ambulation.

clozapine
Drug Administration/Nursing in the Community

➤ See the general guidelines above.

➤ Monitor blood pressure, vital signs, and weight. Monitor complete blood count (CBC) and WBC differential.

➤ See the Patient Problems boxes for dry mouth (Chapter 23), orthostatic hypotension (Chapter 13), and agranulocytosis (Chapter 20). Extrapyramidal symptoms may develop with clozapine, as well as neuroleptic malignant syndrome (see Patient Problems box earlier in this chapter).

➤ Caution patient to avoid driving or operating hazardous equipment if drowsiness or dizziness develops.

➤ Instruct patients to report the development of any unexpected sign or symptom.

➤ Starting or stopping smoking may necessitate a change in dosage.

olanzapine
Drug Administration/Nursing in the Community

➤ See the general guidelines above.

➤ Monitor liver function tests. Monitor blood pressure, weight, and vital signs.

➤ See the Patient Problems boxes for orthostatic hypotension (Chapter 13), photosensitivity (earlier in this chapter), dry mouth (Chapter 23), and constipation (Chapter 24). Extrapyramidal symptoms may develop with olanzapine, as well as neuroleptic malignant syndrome (see Patient Problems box earlier in this chapter).

➤ Caution the patient to avoid driving or operating hazardous equipment if problems with vision, double vision, dizziness, or drowsiness develops.

➤ Instruct the patient to take doses on a full or empty stomach.

➤ This drug may interfere with the body's ability to regulate temperature. Warn the patient to avoid prolonged exposure to extremes of temperature, to allow for frequent cooling off periods when exercising or in hot environments, and to dress warmly for exposure to the cold.

➤ Starting or stopping smoking may necessitate a change in dosage.

risperidone
Drug Administration/Nursing in the Community

➤ See the general guidelines above.

➤ Monitor liver function tests. Monitor blood pressure, weight, and vital signs.

Continued

Nursing Implications Summary—cont'd

➤ See the Patient Problems boxes for orthostatic hypotension (Chapter 13), photosensitivity (earlier in this chapter), dry mouth (Chapter 23), and constipation (Chapter 24). Extrapyramidal symptoms, as well as neuroleptic malignant syndrome (see the Patient Problems box earlier in this chapter), may develop with risperidone.

➤ Caution the patient to avoid driving or operating hazardous equipment if problems with vision, double vision, dizziness, or drowsiness develops.

➤ These drugs may interfere with the body's ability to regulate temperature. Warn the patient to avoid prolonged exposure to extremes of temperature, to allow for frequent cooling off periods when exercising or in hot environments, and to dress warmly for exposure to the cold.

CHAPTER REVIEW

Application

1. What is the major chemical class of antipsychotic drugs? List the three subclasses.
2. What are the four actions of antipsychotic drugs attributable to blockade of dopaminergic receptors? What symptoms might you see as a result of this blockade?
3. What are two actions of antipsychotic drugs attributable to blockade of receptors for norepinephrine? What symptoms might you see that may be caused by this blockade?
4. What are two actions of antipsychotic drugs attributable to blockade of cholinergic receptors? What symptoms might you see that may be caused by this blockade?
5. List the four types of extrapyramidal reactions, the key features of each type, and when each type is likely to occur during antipsychotic drug therapy. How can you recognize these reactions?
6. Describe allergic reactions attributed to antipsychotic drugs.
7. For which types of psychoses are antipsychotic drugs generally effective?
8. Name the two clinical uses of antipsychotic drugs other than the treatment of psychoses.

Critical Thinking

1. What would you tell a patient taking an antipsychotic drug (and his or her family) about photosensitivity? What points would you emphasize?
2. Describe the potential side effects of antipsychotic therapy and how you would monitor for these in a care plan.

References

Bailey KP: Pharmacologic agents for the treatment of schizophrenia: similarities and differences, *J Am Psychiatr Nurses Assoc* 2(5):181-185, 1996.

Bennett J, Done J, Hunt B: Assessing the side-effects of antipsychotic drugs: a survey of CPN practice, *J Psych Mental Health Nurs* 2:177-182, 1995.

Bihm B: Nursing pharmacology. Psychotropic medications and the elderly. *Medsurg Nurs* 5(3):191-193, 208, 1996.

Kennedy M, Mion LC: Neuroleptic therapy: how much do nurses know? *J Gerontol Nurs* 22(12):7-13, 48-49, 1996.

Chapter
59

Antidepressant and Antimanic Agents

KEY TERMS

bipolar disorder, p. 698

dysthymia, p. 698

heterocyclic (atypical) antidepressants, p. 698, 705

major depression, p. 698

monoamine oxidase (MAO) inhibitors, p. 698, 705

selective serotonin reuptake inhibitors (SSRIs), p. 698, 700

serotonin syndrome, p. 706

tricyclic antidepressants, p. 698, 702

KEY DRUGS ▼

amitriptyline, p. 704

fluoxetine, p. 702

lithium, p. 706

OBJECTIVES

After studying this chapter, you should be able to do the following:

- *Briefly describe the symptoms of depression and of mania.*
- *Develop a nursing care plan for patients receiving a selective serotonin reuptake inhibitor, a tricyclic antidepressant, a heterocyclic antidepressant, a monoamine oxidase inhibitor, or lithium.*
- *Describe the toxic symptoms of lithium and the corresponding blood level.*
- *Develop a teaching plan for a patient on a tyramine-restricted diet.*

CHAPTER OVERVIEW

Drugs covered in this chapter are used for severe disturbances of mood, from depression to manic-depressive disorders. Antidepressants, monoamine oxidase inhibitors, and lithium are presented.

THERAPEUTIC RATIONALE: DEPRESSIVE DISORDERS

Depression

Depression is a disorder of mood (affect) that occurs in an estimated 15% to 30% of all adults at some time during their lives. In any 1 year, it is estimated that 10% of the population experiences depressive illness. Women have twice the risk as men for an episode of major depression. Depressive episodes are often associated with hormonal status, such as with premenstrual tension, during the postpartum period, or after a miscarriage. However, studies have not found that menopause is associated with depression. Although men are not as prone to depression as women, men with depression or bipolar illness are more likely to commit suicide.

Depression is not a single entity; rather it is a syndrome that can include various symptoms, as detailed in Box 59-1. Although there are genetic components predisposing to depression, stressful situations and environments may play a strong triggering role. Changes in life patterns, especially serious losses, a difficult relationship, and financial problems, may underlie a depressive episode. Depression becomes a medical problem when normal functioning is significantly hampered. The three most prevalent forms of depression are major depression, dysthymia, and bipolar disorder.

Box 59-1 **Symptoms of Depression and Mania**

Not everyone who is depressed or manic experiences every symptom. Some people experience a few symptoms, some many. The severity of symptoms varies with individuals.

Depression

- Persistent sad, anxious, or "empty" mood
- Feelings of hopelessness, pessimism
- Feelings of guilt, worthlessness, helplessness
- Loss of interest or pleasure in hobbies and activities that were once enjoyed, including sex
- Insomnia, early-morning awakening, or oversleeping
- Appetite and/or weight loss or overeating and weight gain
- Decreased energy, fatigue, being "slowed down"
- Thought of death or suicide; suicide attempts
- Restlessness, irritability
- Difficulty concentrating, remembering, making decisions
- Persistent physical symptoms that do not respond to treatment, such as headaches, digestive disorders, and chronic pain

Mania

- Inappropriate elation
- Inappropriate irritability
- Severe insomnia
- Grandiose notions
- Increased talking
- Disconnected and racing thought
- Increased sexual desire
- Dramatically increased energy
- Poor judgment
- Inappropriate social behavior

From *Depression*, NIH Publication No. 94-3561, National Institutes of Health, 1994.

Major Depression

Major depression is characterized by a depressed mood most of the day, nearly every day, and a greatly diminished interest or pleasure in most daily activities. In addition, there may be weight changes, sleep problems, anxiety or lethargy, fatigue, feelings of worthlessness or guilt, inability to concentrate or make decisions, and thoughts of death or suicide. Although major depression can occur at any age, the midtwenties is the most common time of development. Episodes typically last about 1 year. Eighty percent of patients will experience more than one episode in their lifetimes, typically two or three.

Dysthymia

Dysthymia is a depression lasting more than 2 years that is not disabling but keeps the patient from functioning fully. Common symptoms include self-criticism, low self-esteem, difficulty in making decisions, and feelings of hopelessness. In any 1 year, about 10% of dysthymic patients will have an episode of major depression.

Atypical depression is characterized by a depressed mood relieved by remissions. Patients typically have symptoms of fatigue and anxiety and require much sleep.

Seasonal affective disorder is characterized by depression in late fall and winter, with remission in spring and fall.

Bipolar Disorder

Bipolar disorder (manic-depressive illness) involves cycles of depression and elation or mania (see Box 59-1). In type I bipolar disorder, hypomania is more common than depressive episodes; in type II bipolar disorder, depressive episodes are more significant than mania. Bipolar disorder appears to have a strong genetic component. At least 2 million Americans have bipolar disorder.

Cyclothymia is characterized by chronic cycles of hypomania with periods of depressed mood. However, the symptoms are not as pronounced as in bipolar disorder. Patients may be described as moody, temperamental, and unpredictable.

Depression as a Side Effect

Depression can be the side effect of some drugs, especially the antihypertensive drugs reserpine, methyldopa, guanethidine, and propranolol. Alcohol and antianxiety drugs often unmask depression by alleviating the anxiety that commonly accompanies depression. Steroids, particularly glucocorticoids and oral contraceptives, can cause depression. Drug-induced depression mimics endogenous depression but is treated by removing the drug or lowering the dosage.

Neurochemical Basis of Mood Disorders

Current views are that depression is a neurochemical disorder that can be treated with appropriate drug therapy. This concept arose from the observation in the 1950s that reserpine caused depression in patients treated for hypertension. Reserpine depleted the neurotransmitter norepinephrine. About the same time, iproniazid, a drug then used to treat tuberculosis, was found to relieve depression in patients, inhibiting the degradation of norepinephrine by inhibiting the enzyme monoamine oxidase (MAO). These two observations suggested that a deficiency in the brain neurotransmitter norepinephrine is associated with depression.

Current evidence favors a biogenic amine theory of depression, in which a deficiency in brain levels of the amine transmitters norepinephrine and serotonin is associated with depression. Tricyclic antidepressants, heterocyclic antidepressants, and MAO inhibitors restore both norepinephrine and serotonin in the brain, whereas selective serotonin reuptake inhibitors target restoration of serotonin.

THERAPEUTIC AGENTS: ANTIDEPRESSANTS

Antidepressants elevate mood, counteracting the extreme sadness characteristic of major depression. Physical activity and activities of daily living are increased, overcoming the sense of despair and lack of interest in living. Appetite and sleep patterns are improved.

Antidepressants can be described in four categories: **selective serotonin reuptake inhibitors (SSRIs), tricyclic antidepressants, heterocyclic (atypical) antidepressants,** and **monoamine oxidase (MAO) inhibitors.** These antidepressants are listed in Table 59-1. The botanical St. John's Wort

Table 59-1 Antidepressant Drugs

Generic Name	Trade Name	Administration/Dosage	Comments
Selective Serotonin Reuptake Inhibitors			
citalopram	Celexa	ORAL: *Adults*—20 mg/day in the morning or evening. May increase dose by 20 mg if needed.	For major depression.
fluoxetine	Prozac*	ORAL: *Adults*—20 mg as single morning dose; may increase dosage by 20 mg/day if needed, with second dose at noon. FDA pregnancy category C.	For mild to moderate depression and obsessive-compulsive disorders. Being evaluated for eating disorders (obesity, bulimia).
fluvoxamine	Luvox*	ORAL: *Adults*—50 mg at bedtime; increase by 50 mg every 4-7 days if needed. Maximum daily dose is 300 mg. Divide 100 mg or larger doses into 2 doses. FDA pregnancy category C.	For obsessive-compulsive disorder and mild to moderate depression.
paroxetine hydrochloride	Paxil*	ORAL: *Adults*—20 mg as single morning dose; may increase weekly by 10 mg/day, up to 50 mg/day. *Older adults*—10 mg/day, increased if necessary. Maximum daily dose is 40 mg/day. FDA pregnancy category C.	For obsessive-compulsive disorder, panic attacks, and mild to moderate depression.
sertraline hydrochloride	Zoloft*	ORAL: *Adults*—50 mg/day as morning or evening dose; may increase by 50 mg at weekly intervals if needed. Maximum daily dose is 200 mg. FDA pregnancy category C.	For mild to moderate depression.
venlafaxine	Effexor	ORAL: *Adults*—18.75 mg 2 times/day to minimize nausea; then 75 mg a day in 2 or 3 divided doses. Maximum daily dose is 375 mg. FDA pregnancy category C.	For mild to moderate depression. Inhibits both serotonin and norepinephrine reuptake.
Tricyclic Antidepressants			
amitriptyline hydrochloride	Apo-Amitriptyline† Elavil* Endep Levate† Novotriptyn†	ORAL: *Adults*—Begin with 50 mg at bedtime; increase dosage by 25-50 mg if necessary to 150 mg. Alternately, start with 25 mg 3 times/day and increase to 50 mg 3 times/day. Total dosage should not exceed 300 mg/day. Maintenance doses are usually 50-100 mg at bedtime. These are outpatient dosages; inpatient dosages may be twice as much. FDA pregnancy category C. *Adolescents and older adults*—10 mg 3 times/day plus 20 mg at bedtime (50 mg total) is usually sufficient. INTRAMUSCULAR: 20-30 mg 4 times/day.	Bedtime administration is preferred to lessen discomfort of sedation and anticholinergic effects prominent with this drug.
amoxapine	Asendin*	ORAL: *Adults*—50 mg 2 or 3 times/day initially; increase to 100 mg 2 or 3 times/day within the first week as needed. If no improvement in 3 wk, increase dosage 50 mg/day every other week to maximum of 400 mg for outpatients, 600 mg for inpatients. FDA pregnancy category C.	Related to tricyclic antidepressants. Low incidence of anticholinergic, sedative, and cardiovascular effects. May be taken at bedtime to lessen daytime sedation or to treat insomnia.
clomipramine	Anafranil*	ORAL: *Adults*—Initially 25 mg 3 times/day; then up to 200 mg for outpatients, 300 mg for inpatients. *Older adults*—20-30 mg/day in divided doses. FDA pregnancy category C.	Used for obsessive-compulsive disorders, for blocking panic attacks, and to treat cataplexy associated with narcolepsy.
desipramine hydrochloride	Norpramin* Pertofrane†	ORAL: *Adults*—100-200 mg/day in divided doses or as a single dose, up to 300 mg/day. FDA pregnancy category C. *Adolescents and older adults*—25-50 mg/day; increase to 100 mg in divided doses if necessary. *Children 6-12 yr*—10-30 mg, or 1-5 mg/kg body weight, daily in divided doses.	Sedation and anticholinergic effects are not prominent. Metabolite of imipramine.
doxepin hydrochloride	Novo-Doxepin† Sinequan* Triadapin†	ORAL: *Adults*—75 mg, increased to 150 mg in divided doses or at bedtime; maintenance dose usually 25-150 mg/day (maximum: 150 mg/day).	Bedtime administration is preferred to lessen discomfort of sedation and anticholinergic effects prominent with this drug. Doxepin is reported to have much less effect on heart compared with other tricyclic antidepressants.
imipramine hydrochloride, imipramine pamoate	Apo-Imipramine† Novopramine† Tipramine Tofranil* Tofranil-PM	ORAL: *Adults*—75 mg/day in divided doses or at bedtime. Dosage may be increased up to 200 mg/day if required. These are outpatient dosages; inpatient dosages are one-third higher. *Adolescents and older adults*—30-40 mg/day, increased to maximum of 100 mg/day. *Children >6 yr*—25 mg, 1 hr before bedtime; if no response in 1 wk, increase to 50 mg. *Children >12 yr*—May receive up to 75 mg.	Imipramine is prototype tricyclic antidepressant. Sedative and anticholinergic effects are moderate. Can be taken at bedtime.

*Available in Canada and the United States.
†Available in Canada only.

Continued

Table 59-1   Antidepressant Drugs—cont'd

Generic Name	Trade Name	Administration/Dosage	Comments
Tricyclic Antidepressants—cont'd			
maprotiline	Ludiomil*	ORAL: *Adults*—25-75 mg/day in divided doses for 2 wk. If no improvement, adjust by 25 mg/day. Maximum daily dose is 150 mg. FDA pregnancy category B. *Older adults and adolescents—⅓ adult dose.*	Tetracyclic antidepressant. Low incidence of anticholinergic, sedative, and cardio-vascular effects. May be taken at bed-time to lessen daytime sedation or to treat insomnia.
nortriptyline hydrochloride	Aventyl* Pamelor	ORAL: *Adults*—25 mg 3 or 4 times/day; maximum dose is 100-150 mg/day. FDA pregnancy category C. *Children >12 yr*—25-50 mg or 1-3 mg/kg body weight in divided doses. *Children 6-12 yr*—10-20 mg or 1-3 mg/kg body weight in divided doses.	Metabolite of amitriptyline. Sedative effect is moderate; anticholinergic effect is mild. Can be taken at bedtime.
protriptyline hydrochloride	Triptil† Vivactil	ORAL: *Adults*—5-10 mg 3 or 4 times/day. *Children >12 yr*—5 mg 3 times/day, increase if necessary.	This is the only tricyclic antidepressant that has little sedative action and can cause insomnia if given at bedtime. Preferred for patients who have been immobile and sleepy.
trimipramine maleate	Apo-Trimip† Novo-Tripramine† Rhotrimine† Surmontil	ORAL: *Adults*—75 mg/day increased to 150 mg in divided doses or at bedtime. These are outpatient dosages; inpatient dosages are 100 mg/day, increased to 200 mg/day with a maximum of 300 mg/day. FDA pregnancy category C. *Adolescents and older adults*—50 mg/day, increased to no more than 100 mg/day as required.	Sedation is high, but anticholinergic effect is moderate.
Heterocyclic (Atypical) Antidepressants			
bupropion	Wellbutrin Zyban*	*Depression:* ORAL: *Adults*—Initially 100 mg 2 times/day; increase dosage gradually after 3 days of therapy, to 100 mg 3 times/day as needed and tolerated. *Smoking cessation:* ORAL: *Adults*—150 mg/day for 3 days, then 150 mg 2 times/day for 7-12 wk. FDA pregnancy category B.	Seizures may occur at high dosages.
mirtazapine	Remeron*	ORAL: *Adults*—15 mg at bedtime. FDA pregnancy category B.	Sedating; minimal anticholinergic effects.
nefazodone	Serzone*	ORAL: *Adults*—Initially, 100 mg twice daily; increase as needed and tolerated up to 600 mg/day in divided doses. FDA pregnancy category C.	Confusion, dizziness, dry mouth, hypotension, and nausea. Elevates prolactin and growth hormone levels.
trazodone	Desyrel* Trazon Trialodine	ORAL: *Adults*—150 mg in divided doses initially; increase by 50 mg/day every 3 or 4 days. Maximum daily dose is 400 mg. FDA pregnancy category C.	Sedation may be noted. Low incidence of anticholinergic and cardiovascular effects. May be taken at bedtime to lessen daytime sedation or to treat insomnia.
Monoamine Oxidase (MAO) Inhibitors			
isocarboxazid	Marplan*	ORAL: *Adults*—20-30 mg/day in divided doses; maintenance dose is usually 10-20 mg/day.	Patient should be instructed in food and drug interactions with MAO inhibitors.
phenelzine sulfate	Nardil*	ORAL: *Adults*—45-75 mg/day in 3 doses or 1 mg/kg body weight in divided doses. Daily dosage should not exceed 75 mg. *Geriatric patients*—15 mg in the morning, increasing gradually to maximum 60 mg/day. FDA pregnancy category C.	Patient should be instructed in food and drug interactions with MAO inhibitors.
tranylcypromine sulfate	Parnate*	ORAL: *Adults*—20-40 mg/day in 2 doses for 2 wk. Dosage is reduced after response is obtained. Usually maintenance dose is less than 30 mg. *Geriatric patients*—2.5-5 mg/day initially, increasing gradually as needed.	Patient should be instructed in food and drug interactions with MAO inhibitors. Has some psychomotor stimulant activity characteristic of amphetamine.

*Available in Canada and the United States.
†Available in Canada only.

is often taken as an antidepressant (see Alternative Therapies box).

Selective Serotonin Reuptake Inhibitors: General Characteristics

The newest category of antidepressant drugs is the SSRIs. This drug class has a greater pharmacologic specificity, fewer side effects, and minimal potential for fatal overdose compared with the tricyclic antidepressants. By 1996, the SSRIs accounted for 70% of all antidepressant prescriptions.

Mechanism of Action

The SSRIs block the neuronal reuptake of serotonin but have little effect on the uptake of norepinephrine or dopamine

CNS presynaptic
neuron

CNS postsynaptic
neuron

Figure 59-1   Depression results from amine concentration too low to activate sufficient receptors; mania results from overabundance of amine acting at receptor. Biogenic amine theory of depression is applied to actions of antidepressant drugs, tricyclic antidepressants, and monoamine oxidase *(MAO)* inhibitors, and to action of lithium, used to treat mania (opposite of depression). *1,* Lithium inhibits release of norepinephrine *(NE)* and serotonin *(SE).* *2,* Tricyclic antidepressants and MAO inhibitors increase receptor sensitivity to norepinephrine and serotonin. *3,* Tricyclic antidepressants block reuptake of norepinephrine and serotonin. Lithium enhances reuptake of norepinephrine and serotonin. Selective serotonin reuptake inhibitors block reuptake of serotonin. *4,* MAO inhibitors prevent degradation of norepinephrine and serotonin. *CNS,* Central nervous system.

(Figure 59-1). In addition to having an antidepressant effect, this activity may also lessen obsessive-compulsive disorder and eating disorders.

Pharmacokinetics

The SSRIs are taken orally once a day. They are well absorbed. They bind to plasma protein and may displace other drugs. The SSRIs are metabolized by the liver and metabolites are also pharmacologically active. Metabolites are excreted in the urine.

Uses

The approved use of SSRIs is the treatment of depression, especially mild to moderate depression. The antidepressant effect is usually seen faster than with the tricyclic antidepressants but may still take up to 4 weeks. Therapy is continued for 6 to 12 months. The SSRIs are also being tested for their efficacy in treating obsessive-compulsive disorders and eating disorders, including obesity and bulimia.

Adverse Reactions and Contraindications

The side effects of the SSRIs are less pronounced than with the tricyclic antidepressants because of the lack of anticholinergic effects or cardiac conduction disturbances characteristic of the tricyclic antidepressants. Overdoses of the SSRIs are not fatal, so they are safer than the tricyclic antidepressants. Side effects of SSRIs include nausea, nervousness, and insomnia. Less commonly reported side effects include headaches, tremor, anxiety, drowsiness, dry mouth, sweat-

 ALTERNATIVE THERAPIES

Antidepressant

ST. JOHN'S WORT

St. John's Wort consists of the dried flowering tops of *Hypericum perforatum* L. Hypericin, which is one of the many constituents of this herb, is generally considered the active ingredient. Although hypericum extract inhibits uptake of serotonin, norepinephrine, and dopamine and binds to GABA receptors in vitro, in vivo evidence that it crosses the blood-brain barrier has not been reported. Details of the disposition of hypericum in vivo (metabolism, excretion) are unknown. Clinical trials of hypericum in the treatment of mild to moderate depression suggest that the drug is about as effective as conventional antidepressants (*BMJ* 313:253, 1996) and is associated only with minor side effects (dry mouth, constipation, and confusion).

ing, and diarrhea. Sexual dysfunction may include lack of orgasm in women and ejaculatory delay in men.

Individuals with severe liver or kidney disease may have impaired ability to metabolize and excrete SSRIs, and dosages should be reduced and monitored. Because these drugs are excreted in breast milk and are poorly metabolized by infants, they are not recommended for nursing mothers. SSRIs should be used with caution for patients with seizure disorders.

Interactions

The SSRIs are bound to plasma protein and may displace other drugs, especially oral anticoagulants and phenytoin. The central nervous system (CNS) depression of other drugs can be potentiated by the SSRIs. Tryptophan and MAO inhibitors should not be taken concurrently with SSRIs because these also affect serotonin levels. The SSRIs are potent inhibitors of liver metabolizing enzymes and may potentiate the effect of other drugs metabolized by the liver.

Specific Selective Serotonin Reuptake Inhibitors

citalopram

Citalopram (Celexa) is a new SSRI that is chemically different from other SSRIs and other antidepressants. It is effective in treating major depression and is being tested for diabetic neuropathy and as a deterrent to alcohol consumption. Dosage reductions may be required in patients with renal or hepatic insufficiency, as well as in the elderly. Maximal antidepressant effects of citalopram may not be seen for 5 to 6 weeks. Side effects can include headache, restlessness, anxiety, dizziness, insomnia, tremor, nausea/vomiting, constipation, dry mouth, sweating, and visual disturbances.

▼ fluoxetine

Fluoxetine (Prozac) is the first widely used SSRI in the United States. It is well tolerated and effective in treating mild and moderate depression and symptoms of obsessive-compulsive disorder. Antidepressant effects may be apparent in 1 to 4 weeks. The most common side effects are nausea, nervousness, agitation, insomnia, and sexual dysfunction. These effects are generally mild. There has been concern that patients receiving fluoxetine are at increased risk for developing serious suicidal thoughts, but the data do not support this concern. Fluoxetine has a long elimination half-life but has been well tolerated by elderly individuals.

fluvoxamine

Fluvoxamine (Luvox) is an SSRI for treating obsessive-compulsive disorders and depression. The most common side effects are anorexia, nausea, nervousness, agitation, insomnia, and sexual dysfunction. These effects are generally mild.

paroxetine

Paroxetine (Paxil) is used to treat mild to moderate depression, obsessive-compulsive disorder, and panic disorder. It has mild sedating effects. Antidepressant effects and improvement in sleep patterns usually occur in 1 to 2 weeks. Effects on obsessive-compulsive disorder and panic disorder may require several weeks. The most common side effects are anorexia, nausea, and sexual dysfunction. These effects are generally mild.

sertraline

Sertraline (Zoloft) is used to treat mild to moderate depression. Effects are usually seen in 2 to 4 weeks. The most common side effects are anorexia, nausea, nervousness, agitation, insomnia, and sexual dysfunction. These effects are generally mild.

venlafaxine

Venlafaxine (Effexor) is used to treat mild to moderate depression. It is not selective for serotonin reuptake, but it inhibits norepinephrine reuptake. Effects are usually seen in 2 weeks, although overall improvement may take several weeks. Venlafaxine has fewer anticholinergic and CNS side effects than tricyclic agents. However, venlafaxine is associated with dose-dependent hypertension. The most common side effects are anorexia and nausea. It does not inhibit the liver metabolizing enzymes.

Tricyclic Antidepressants: General Characteristics

Mechanism of Action

The tricyclic antidepressants (see Table 59-1) block the reuptake of norepinephrine or serotonin into the presynaptic neurons, as depicted in Figure 59-1. This causes an increase in the synaptic concentration of these neurotransmitters, which is an early effect of the drug. However, clinically no antidepressant response is seen for 2 weeks. Recent research suggests that the tricyclic antidepressants also alter the sensitivity of brain tissue to the action of norepinephrine and serotonin. Because this effect takes 2 weeks to be established, it more closely correlates with the onset of the clinical antidepressant action.

Pharmacokinetics

The tricyclic antidepressants usually are administered orally, although amitriptyline and imipramine are available in injectable forms. Metabolites of the tricyclic antidepressants are active, so an active form of the drug persists despite the drug being well absorbed and readily metabolized by the intestine and liver. The rate of tricyclic metabolism decreases with age, and people older than 55 years of age generally are started at half the regular adult dose.

Uses

Tricyclic antidepressants are indicated for the treatment of depression, including depressive episodes of major depression, bipolar disorder, dysthymia, and atypical depression. Lifting of depression can take 2 to 3 weeks. Because side effects may be troublesome, dosages are usually started low and titrated up during the first week to allow patients to develop tolerance. After 2 weeks of drug therapy, the dosage is reviewed in light of side effects and therapeutic response. The final dosage is individualized for the patient. Therapy is discontinued if no response occurs after 1 month. Therapy is continued for 6 to 12 months, depending on the severity of the depression.

Clomipramine is used to relieve obsessive-compulsive disorder.

Imipramine hydrochloride is used as an adjunct in treating enuresis in children older than 6 years of age.

Adverse Reactions and Contraindications

The major side effects of the tricyclic antidepressants are an atropine-like (anticholinergic) effect and sedation. The relative incidence of these side effects among the tricyclics is listed in Table 59-2. Because of these side effects, the drug is usually given before bedtime so that the patient is asleep when the side effects are at their peak. The more sedating tricyclics, amitriptyline and doxepin, are particularly effective in relieving the insomnia of depression when given as a bedtime dose. These drugs do not interfere with normal sleep patterns.

Anticholinergic side effects include dry mouth, blurred vision, and constipation. Some patients may experience temporary confusion or speech blockage. Patients with glaucoma or those disposed toward glaucoma must have this condition checked when taking tricyclic antidepressants because the anticholinergic effect may worsen this condition. Anticholinergic action also may adversely affect patients, particularly older adult patients, with urinary retention or obstruction.

Cardiac effects have been a major limitation of tricyclic antidepressants. Tricyclic antidepressants have three separate pharmacologic actions on the heart: anticholinergic, adrenolytic, and a quinidine-like action. Therefore the final cardiac effect is complex and depends on dosage. The anticholinergic action increases the heart rate. The adrenolytic action prevents the reuptake of norepinephrine into neurons, an action that tends to deplete norepinephrine stores in peripheral neurons. The most common adrenolytic side effect is orthostatic (postural) hypotension. This decrease in

CASE STUDY
Depression

Mr. Brown is a 76-year-old retired accountant who has been hospitalized with depression. He has a history of coronary artery disease, confirmed by a recent cardiac catheterization, which has been managed pharmacologically with Procardia 10 mg three times daily, Transderm-Nitro patch once daily, and 1 aspirin daily. His daughter suspects he is depressed because his wife recently died after 55 years of marriage and his health has kept him from working part-time with his former partners. Mr. Brown had been losing weight, refusing to eat, and not sleeping well for more than 2 months.

1. The physician prescribed Elavil, 50 mg at bedtime last month, and increased his dosage to 100 mg last week when he was first hospitalized. Today the physician wrote an order to increase the dosage to 150 mg. Are there any concerns about this medication and Mr. Brown's medical history?
2. You call the physician with your concerns, and he changes the order to sertraline HCl (Zoloft) 50 mg at bedtime. Are there any advantages to this switch?
3. What potential drug interactions may occur with sertraline therapy?
4. After 1 week of therapy with sertraline, Mr. Brown's daughter calls you aside and seems very upset: "He's just not any better! I expected him to be more cheerful by now! What is going on?" How should you respond to her?

Table 59-2 Incidence of Side Effects of Antidepressant Drugs

| | Side Effects | | | | | | |
| | Autonomic | Central Nervous System | | Cardiovascular | | Other | |
Drug	Anticholinergic	Drowsiness	Insomnia Agitation	Orthostatic Hypotension	Cardiac Arrhythmias	Gastrointestinal Distress	Weight Gain (>6 kg)
Tricylic Antidepressants							
amitriptyline	++++	++++	0	++++	+++	0	++++
amoxapine	++	++	++	++	+++	0	+
desipramine	+	+	+	++	++	0	+
doxepin	+++	++++	0	++	++	0	+++
imipramine	+++	+++	+	++++	+++	+	+++
maprotiline	++	++++	0	0	+	0	++
nortriptyline	+	+	0	++	++	0	+
protriptyline	++	+	+	++	++	0	0
trimipramine	+	++++	0	++	++	0	+++
Atypical Antidepressants							
bupropion	0	0	++	0	+	+	0
trazodone	0	++++	0	+	+	+	+
SSRIs	0	0	++	0	0	+++	0
MAOIs	+	+	++	++	0	+	++

Modified from *Clinical practice guideline: depression in primary care.* US Department of Health and Human Services. Agency for Health Care Policy and Research. Pub No 93-0552, April, 1993.
SSRIs, Selective serotonin reuptake inhibitors (fluoxetine, fluvoxamine, paroxetine, sertraline); *MAOIs,* monoamine oxidase inhibitors (isocarboxid, phenelzine, tranylcypromine).

blood pressure affects the heart by lowering the workload. The quinidine-like side effects are seen at high concentrations of the tricyclic antidepressants. This decreases heart rate, myocardial contractility, and coronary blood flow. Therefore tricyclic antidepressants are contraindicated for patients with a recent myocardial infarction and present special concern for the patient with cardiac disease. Patients who have hyperthyroidism and are at risk for developing cardiac arrhythmias have this risk potentiated by the tricyclic antidepressants. Doxepin is a tricyclic antidepressant that has minimum cardiac effects.

Toxicity

Tricyclic antidepressants are not addicting, and their abuse potential appears limited. A major problem is their acute toxicity when depressed patients overdose on a tricyclic antidepressant drug in a suicide attempt. Doses of 1 g of the sedating tricyclics are toxic, and doses of 2 g are often fatal. Those doses represent only a 5- and 10-fold margin, respectively, over the therapeutic dose.

The toxic effects of tricyclic antidepressant overdose are anticholinergic poisoning. The early symptoms are confusion, inability to concentrate, and perhaps visual hallucinations. More severe signs include delirium, seizures, and coma. Respiration may be depressed. The patient may have a low body temperature early but an elevated body temperature later. The pupils are dilated, the eyeballs are restless, the reflexes are hyperactive, and motor coordination is compromised. Depending on the patient's cardiac status and the degree of overdose, the overall cardiac effect may range from quickening of the heart rate (tachycardia) to slowing of the heart rate (bradycardia) to various arrhythmias related to an atrioventricular block. Especially serious is the slowing of conduction in the atrioventricular node by the quinidine-like action, which can result in heart block. Sudden death from cardiac arrhythmias may occur several days after an overdose.

Physostigmine (Antilirium), a peripherally and centrally active anticholinesterase agent, reverses the anticholinergic toxic symptoms of tricyclic overdose. Physostigmine, 2 mg, is administered every 1 to 2 hours as necessary. This drug must be administered frequently because it is short acting, whereas tricyclics are long acting.

Tricyclic antidepressants do not decrease the suicide potential among depressed patients during the early weeks of therapy. Depressed patients with suicidal thoughts are best hospitalized to begin drug therapy rather than being given quantities of drugs that may be used in a suicide attempt. Patients who have attempted or threatened suicide often are treated initially with electroconvulsive shock therapy. Because tricyclic antidepressants can increase the seizure potential, they are not administered concurrently with electroconvulsive shock therapy.

Interactions

The tricyclic antidepressants can potentiate CNS depression, anticholinergic effects, and sympathomimetic effects of a number of drug classes, including antihistamines, pheno-

thiazines, thioxanthenes, and sympathomimetics. Cimetidine and methylphenidate can inhibit the metabolism of tricyclic antidepressants, potentially leading to an overdose. Metrizamide may increase the risk of seizures, whereas antithyroid agents increase the risk of agranulocytosis.

The interaction of guanethidine and a tricyclic antidepressant is classic; the tricyclic antidepressant inhibits the uptake of guanethidine by the neurons so that guanethidine cannot reach its site of action and is therefore ineffective in lowering blood pressure. Clonidine and guanadrel are also blocked by the tricyclic antidepressants and may become ineffective antihypertensives.

MAO inhibitors and antiarrhythmics have potentially fatal drug interactions with the tricyclic antidepressants and should not be administered concurrently.

Specific Tricyclic Antidepressants and Related Antidepressants

Amoxapine and maprotiline are not tricyclic antidepressants but have many similar actions and side effects.

▼ amitriptyline

Amitriptyline (Elavil) is associated with a high incidence of sedation and anticholinergic effects. These properties are more pronounced than with other tricyclic antidepressants and can cause confusion in the older adult patient. Weight gain sometimes occurs. Amitriptyline has a plasma half-life of 10 to 26 hours and is metabolized to nortriptyline, an active tricyclic antidepressant.

amoxapine

Amoxapine (Asendin) inhibits amine uptake and is a more potent inhibitor of norepinephrine than of serotonin uptake. It is not a true tricyclic but is chemically related to the tricyclic antidepressants. Amoxapine is a chemical metabolite of the antipsychotic drug loxapine and, as with the antipsychotic drugs, blocks dopamine receptors. Overall, amoxapine treats major depression and relieves anxiety and agitation associated with depression.

Amoxapine has minimum anticholinergic and sedative effects and a lesser incidence of cardiac effects than the tricyclics. Drug interactions are similar to those of the tricyclics.

clomipramine

Clomipramine (Anafranil) is used to treat obsessive-compulsive disorder and to block panic attacks. This drug has a low incidence of sedation but a moderate incidence of anticholinergic and cardiac effects.

desipramine

Desipramine (Norpramin, Pertofrane) has a low incidence of sedation and anticholinergic effects. It is a metabolite of imipramine and has a plasma half-life of 12 to 27 hours.

doxepin

Doxepin (Sinequan) has a high incidence of sedative and anticholinergic side effects. Doxepin does not have the quinidine-like cardiac effect to the degree characteristic of the other tricyclic drugs and therefore is indicated when cardiac function must be considered.

imipramine

Imipramine (Tofranil) has a moderate degree of sedative and anticholinergic side effects. It is metabolized to desipramine, which is also an active tricyclic antidepressant. Imipramine has a plasma half-life of 11 to 25 hours. Imipramine is used to treat enuresis (bed-wetting) in older children or adults.

maprotiline

Maprotiline (Ludiomil) is a tetracyclic antidepressant that inhibits norepinephrine but not serotonin uptake. Drug interactions and side effects are similar to those of the tricyclic antidepressants. Incidence of drowsiness, anticholinergic effects, and cardiac effects is less than with amitriptyline or doxepin.

nortriptyline

Nortriptyline (Aventyl, Pamelor) is moderately sedating and has minimum anticholinergic side effects. It is a metabolite of amitriptyline.

protriptyline

Protriptyline (Vivactil) is the one tricyclic antidepressant with minimum sedating effect and is therefore most useful in depressed patients who seem physically immobilized by their depression or who sleep excessively. The plasma half-life of protriptyline is 4 to 9 days.

trimipramine

Trimipramine (Surmontil) is a tricyclic antidepressant with a high incidence of sedation and a moderate incidence of anticholinergic effects.

Atypical Antidepressants

Antidepressant drugs have been introduced that are neither tricyclics nor MAO inhibitors. The new antidepressant drugs have, to a varying degree, a lesser incidence of anticholinergic side effects, less cardiotoxicity, and a faster onset of action than the tricyclics.

bupropion

Bupropion (Wellbutrin, Zyban) is used to treat depressive episodes. The onset of action is 1 to 3 weeks. An extended-release form of bupropion is indicated as an aid to smoking cessation treatment.

Bupropion differs from tricyclic antidepressants in having a stimulant rather than a sedative effect. It weakly blocks norepinephrine and serotonin. Patients may experience restlessness, agitation, anxiety, and insomnia. Cardiac effects are uncommon.

Bupropion should be used with caution for patients with a history of seizures, heart disease, and hepatic or renal impairment. Bupropion should not be combined with alcohol, MAO inhibitors, or medications that lower the seizure threshold.

mirtazapine

Mirtazapine (Remeron) is used to treat depression. It increases central norepinephrine and serotonin activity. Side effects may include dizziness, drowsiness, and weight gain. Mirtazapine can increase liver function enzymes. It should not be combined with alcohol or other agents acting as CNS depressants or with MAO inhibitors.

nefazodone

Nefazodone (Serzone) is available in Canada to treat depression. It is structurally related to trazodone.

trazodone

Trazodone (Desyrel) is chemically unrelated to other antidepressant drugs. It inhibits serotonin uptake but also inhibits alpha-adrenergic receptors. Drowsiness is a side effect, but minimum anticholinergic and cardiac effects occur. Like the tricyclic drugs, trazodone can cause orthostatic hypotension, but taking the drug with food lessens the effect. Rarely, males experience priapism, which may require surgery. Dilute (1:100,000) epinephrine should be administered quickly into the corpus cavernosa to minimize permanent damage.

Monoamine Oxidase Inhibitors: General Characteristics

MAO inhibitors are less commonly used because of the poor safety profile that requires strict adherence to dietary limitations and potential for drug interactions. However, they may be the only drugs effective for atypical depression. These drugs are listed in Table 59-1.

Mechanism of Action

The MAO inhibitors were in use before the tricyclic antidepressants were discovered. MAO inhibitors irreversibly inhibit the enzyme MAO. According to the biogenic amine hypothesis of depression, MAO inhibitors are effective because they prevent the degradation of norepinephrine and serotonin so that the concentration of these CNS neurotransmitters is increased (see Figure 59-1).

Pharmacokinetics

MAO inhibitors are well absorbed orally. They are metabolized in the liver to inactive forms and excreted in urine. The onset of action requires 2 to 3 weeks. MAO inhibitors act by irreversible inhibition; removal of enough enzyme to produce clinical effectiveness takes time. Similarly, the effect persists for 2 to 3 weeks after MAO inhibitors have been discontinued, reflecting the time to synthesize adequate MAO.

Uses

MAO inhibitors are not as effective as the tricyclic antidepressants in treating common endogenous depression, but they are more effective in treating depressions exhibited as phobias.

DIETARY CONSIDERATIONS

Monoamine Oxidase Inhibitors and Tyramine

Patients taking monoamine oxidase inhibitors may experience a hypertensive crisis (characterized by severe chest pain, severe headache, photophobia, clammy skin, nausea, and palpitations) if they ingest foods containing a large amount of tyramine. Food high in tyramine include the following:

- Avocados
- Bananas
- Beer
- Bologna
- Canned figs
- Chocolate
- Cheese (except cottage cheese)
- Cheese-containing food (e.g., pizza, macaroni and cheese)
- Liver
- Meat extracts (e.g., Marmite, Bovril)
- Offal
- Papaya products, including meat tenderizers
- Paté
- Pickled and kippered herring
- Pepperoni
- Pods or broad beans (fava beans)
- Raisins
- Raw yeast or yeast extracts
- Salami
- Sausage
- Sour cream
- Soy sauce
- Wine and Chianti
- Yogurt

Adverse Reactions and Contraindications

Sedation and anticholinergic effects are common side effects associated with MAO inhibitors, but these drugs usually are administered in divided doses during the day because of their tendency to cause insomnia if given in the evening. Orthostatic hypotension is sometimes a side effect. At one time, MAO inhibitors were used as antihypertensive drugs. As with the tricyclic antidepressants, MAO inhibitors are not addicting.

Toxicity

After ingestion of an overdose of an MAO inhibitor, symptoms appear within 12 hours and reflect increased adrenergic activity such as restlessness, anxiety, and insomnia, progressing to include tachycardia and sometimes convulsions. Dizziness and hypotension may occur, whereas some patients have severe headaches and develop high blood pressure. Some patients develop a high fever, which should be reduced with a sponge bath and external cooling. Treatment is supportive to maintain respiration and circulation. Because the effect of the MAO inhibitor is persistent, patients must be watched for at least 1 week.

Interactions

Several clinically significant problems arise from the interaction of MAO inhibitors with other drugs and certain foods containing tyramine. A hypertensive crisis may be precipitated when a food containing tyramine or a sympathomimetic drug is ingested (see Dietary Considerations box). Sympathomimetic drugs and tyramine are normally degraded rapidly by MAO of the liver. When MAO is inhibited, tyramine remains undegraded and triggers the release of accumulated norepinephrine, which causes a hypertensive episode. The earliest symptom of such a hypertensive response may be a severe headache. The necessity of avoiding these substances to avert a life-threatening hypertensive crisis is the major limitation of MAO inhibitors. Phentolamine, the alpha-receptor antagonist, may be given to lower blood pressure during a hypertensive crisis.

A **serotonin syndrome** consists of altered mental status with confusion, agitation, disorientation, poor concentration, and restlessness along with muscle spasms and exaggerated reflexes, shivering and sweating. This syndrome can develop when MAO inhibitors are combined with any agents that promote increased serotonin, especially tryptophan, meperidine, the SSRIs, or the tricyclic antidepressants.

Specific Monoamine Oxidase Inhibitors

isocarboxazid

Isocarboxazid (Marplan) is not considered as effective as other MAO inhibitors but is prescribed for depressed patients who are unresponsive to tricyclic antidepressants and electroconvulsive shock therapy.

phenelzine

Phenelzine (Nardil) is the safest MAO inhibitor. Patients with a high level of anxiety who do not respond to a tricyclic antidepressant may respond to phenelzine. Dosages must be individualized because wide variability exists in its metabolism.

tranylcypromine

Tranylcypromine (Parnate) can have a stimulatory action similar to amphetamine, and the antidepressant activity is seen more rapidly than with other MAO inhibitors.

THERAPEUTIC AGENTS: ANTIMANIC DRUGS

Lithium has been the mainstay for treating manic episodes in bipolar disorder. More recently, the anticonvulsants carbamazepine and valproic acid have been shown effective in preventing recurrence of manic episodes. These drugs are listed in Table 59-3.

▼ lithium

Mechanism of Action

Lithium affects cellular transport mechanisms, second messenger pathways, and the dynamics of neurotransmitter processing. Lithium alters both the presynaptic and postsynap-

Table 59-3 **Antimanic Drugs**			
Generic Name	**Trade Name**	**Administration/Dosage**	**Comments**
lithium			
lithium carbonate	Eskalith	ORAL: *Adults*—Initially 0.6-2.1 g/day divided	Blood should not be drawn for determination of
	Lithane*	into 3 doses. Increase or decrease dosage	lithium levels earlier than 8 hr after last dose. Lev-
	Lithizine†	by 0.3 g/day to obtain blood level of	els above 2 mEq/L are toxic. Patients should be
	Lithonate	0.8-1.2 mEq/L. FDA pregnancy category D.	instructed not to make up missed dose of lithium.
	Lithotabs	Maintenance dosage is usually 0.9-1.2 g/day	
lithium citrate	Cibalith-Si	in divided doses.	
Other Agents			
carbamazepine	Apo-Carbamazepine†	ORAL: *Adults*—200-400 mg/day in divided doses;	Investigational for treating manic symptoms not re-
	Atretol	may increase by 100 mg/day at weekly inter-	sponsive to lithium.
	Tegretol	vals as needed and tolerated. FDA pregnancy	
	Various others	category C.	
divalproex sodium	Depakote	ORAL: *Adults*—250 mg 2-3 times/day, up to	For treating acute manic symptoms. Delayed-release
	Epival†	1000 mg. FDA pregnancy category D.	tablets lessen gastrointestinal side effects.

*Available in Canada and the United States.
†Available in Canada only.

tic events affecting serotonin, with a net effect of enhancing central serotonin function. The net effect of lithium is to decrease noradrenergic transmission.

Pharmacokinetics

Lithium is administered orally as the carbonate or citrate salt. Because lithium is an element, related in the atomic table to sodium and potassium, it is not metabolized but is excreted by mechanisms similar to those for sodium and potassium. Of the lithium filtered in the kidney, 80% is reabsorbed in the proximal tubule, and 20% is excreted in urine. The half-life of lithium in the plasma is 24 hours and is increased to 36 hours in older adult patients, so the relative dosage of lithium must be decreased to avoid the accumulation to toxic doses. Other factors that decrease lithium excretion include sodium deficiency, extreme exercise, diarrhea, and postpartum status. Factors that increase lithium excretion include high sodium intake and pregnancy.

Uses

Lithium is the drug of choice for treating the manic phase of a manic-depressive disorder. Lithium does not cause CNS depression, excitation, or euphoria. It stabilizes mood, preventing the dramatic mood swings characteristic of the manic-depressive disorder.

If the patient is severely manic, an antipsychotic drug or electroconvulsive shock therapy may be used initially to subdue behavior. Lithium therapy alone usually reverses mild to moderate manic symptoms in 1 to 3 weeks. The duration of lithium therapy depends on the individual. Patients with occasional manic periods may be treated only during those periods.

Continuous lithium therapy is indicated for patients in whom lithium reduces the frequency and intensity of their manic-depressive disorder. Evidence shows that lithium may be effective in treating the depression of the manic-depressive disorder and even endogenous depression. However, lithium is approved only for treating acute mania and as prophylaxis for recurrent mania. In research studies, lithium is being tested for its effectiveness in treating various psychiatric and neurologic brain disorders.

Adverse Reactions and Contraindications

Lithium therapy is contraindicated in early pregnancy because an increased incidence of congenital malformations in infants of treated mothers has been noted. Secretion of the thyroid hormone thyroxine is inhibited by lithium, and a few patients develop an enlarged thyroid gland and may become hypothyroid. A few patients receiving lithium therapy develop nephrogenic diabetes insipidus (see Chapter 65), which is reversed when the lithium dosage is lowered or discontinued. Paradoxically, administration of a thiazide diuretic may reverse polyuria. A more serious consequence is permanent renal damage (initially without symptoms), which may develop with long-term lithium therapy. Renal function should be evaluated periodically for patients receiving long-term therapy.

Toxicity

The therapeutic index for lithium is relatively small, and at the start of treatment, patients are tested at least weekly to ensure that the plasma level is in the therapeutic range. The therapeutic range is 0.6 to 1.2 mEq/L but as low as 0.2 mEq/L in older adult patients. Common side effects early in therapy include mild nausea, dry mouth, increased thirst, increased urination (polyuria), and fine tremor of the hands. Toxic symptoms begin to appear at 1.5 to 2 mEq/L and by 4 mEq/L may be fatal. The toxic symptoms are listed in Table 59-4.

Acute lithium toxicity is treated by hastening lithium excretion while maintaining fluid and electrolyte balance. Lithium excretion is increased by administration of an os-motic diuretic such as urea or mannitol. The drugs aminophylline and acetazolamide increase lithium excretion, and one may be given concurrently with the osmotic diuresis. Peritoneal dialysis, or preferably hemodialysis, may be used for severe toxicity or when renal failure occurs.

Interactions

Several drug interactions occur with lithium. Lithium potentiates haloperidol, tricyclic antidepressants, phenothiazines, benzodiazepines, and neuromuscular-blocking drugs. Lithium is potentiated by methyldopa, sodium-depleting diuretics, and the phenothiazines.

Other Antimanic Agents

carbamazepine

Carbamazepine (Tegretol) is still an experimental agent for the treatment of bipolar disorder in patients who do not respond well to lithium. The role of carbamazepine is still being evaluated. The major use of carbamazepine is to treat epilepsy (see Chapter 61). Side effects include nausea, blurred vision, and ataxia. There are also cases of leukopenia and aplastic anemia. Patients must be monitored for renal, liver, and bone marrow functions.

divalproex

Divalproex (Depakote, Epival) in a delayed-release form is indicated for the treatment of acute manic episodes in bipolar disorder. Divalproex is a complex of valproic acid and its sodium salt. Valproate increases the concentration of the inhibitory transmitter, gamma-aminobutyric acid (GABA). The primary use of valproic acid is to treat epilepsy (see Chapter 61).

Table 59-4	Toxic Symptoms of Lithium
Blood Level (mEq/L)	**Symptoms**
<1.5	Fine tremor of hands
	Dry mouth
	Increased thirst
	Increase urination
	Nausea
1.5-2	Vomiting
	Diarrhea
	Muscle weakness
	Incoordination (ataxia)
	Dizziness
	Confusion
	Slurred speech
2-2.5	Persistent nausea and vomiting
	Blurred vision
	Muscle twitching (fasciculations)
	Hyperactive deep tendon reflexes
2.5-3	Myoclonic twitches or movements of an entire limb
	Choreoathetoid movements
	Urinary and fecal incontinence
>3	Seizures
	Cardiac arrhythmias
	Hypotension
	Peripheral vascular collapse
	Death

Nursing Process Overview

Antidepressants

Assessment

Antidepressants are used for patients with pronounced, prolonged depression or manic-depressive disease. Perform a thorough physiologic assessment and assess mental status, focusing on objective signs of depression. Monitor vital signs, weight, and blood pressure.

Nursing Diagnoses

- Potential body image disturbance related to weight gain as drug side effect
- Risk for self-harm
- Altered bowel elimination: constipation

Patient Outcomes

The patient will not harm himself or herself. The patient will have no constipation or will carry out dietary or other measures to reduce the incidence of constipation. The patient will dis-cuss feelings about self. The patient will assume responsibility for managing weight.

Planning/Implementation

Monitor fluid intake and output, weight, and blood pressure. Review serum drug levels if available. Assess the patient's level of consciousness, with attention to excessive sedation. Assess for possible suicidal tendencies. Monitor for side effects of the drugs such as the dry mouth and constipation that may occur with tricyclic antidepressants.

Evaluation

Before discharging a patient for self-management, ascertain that the patient or family understands what drug is being taken, how to take it correctly, the side effects that may occur and those that should be reported immediately to the physician, dietary restrictions associated with the medication being used, and ways in which the success of the drug will be monitored. Verify that patients understand why follow-up is necessary and when to return for it.

Nursing Implications Summary

General Guidelines: Antidepressants
Drug Administration
➤ The risk of suicide may exist in seriously depressed patients and may persist for several weeks after they begin antidepressant therapy. Some patients who were not suicidal may become so during initial therapy with antidepressants. Assess patients carefully.

➤ Monitor vital signs and weight.

➤ As mood improves, appetite may improve. In addition, some antidepressants contribute to weight gain. If weight gain is significant, counsel patients about weight-reduction diets and increased exercise. Provide emotional support as needed. Consult the physician about possible changes in dosage or drug.

➤ Many antidepressants alter the seizure threshold. In patients with a history of seizures, pad siderails and supervise carefully until effects of the medications can be evaluated.

Nursing in the Community
➤ Inform the patient and family that several weeks of therapy may be necessary before full effects of a drug regimen can be evaluated. Some side effects may lessen with continued drug use.

➤ Common side effects are noted in this text, but encourage the patient to consult the physician when any new side effect develops.

➤ Inform the patient that antidepressants must be taken as ordered, regularly, even if he or she begins to feel better. Instruct the patient to consult the physician before changing the prescribed drug regimen or discontinuing medications.

➤ Warn the patient to inform all health care providers of all drugs being taken.

➤ Instruct the patient to avoid over-the-counter drugs unless first approved by the physician.

➤ Instruct the patient to avoid alcohol unless approved in moderation by the physician.

➤ Warn the patient to avoid driving or operating hazardous equipment if drowsiness or dizziness occurs.

➤ Encourage the patient and family to stay in touch with the physician and to seek assistance from appropriate health care personnel, including physicians, psychologists, nurses, and therapists.

➤ Remind the patient to keep these and all drugs out of the reach of children.

Selective Serotonin Reuptake Inhibitors
Drug Administration
➤ See the general guidelines for antidepressants.
Nursing in the Community
➤ Review the general guidelines for antidepressants with the patient.

➤ Assess for chills or fever, rash or skin changes, anxiety, nervousness, nausea, diarrhea, insomnia, and changes in sexual function or ability.

➤ Instruct the patient to take doses with food or snack to lessen gastric irritation.

➤ For a patient taking fluoxetine: Instruct the patient to stop the drug and notify the physician if rash or hives develop.

➤ Caution the patient to avoid driving or operating hazardous equipment if dizziness, drowsiness, or light-headedness develops.

➤ See the Patient Problems box in Chapter 23 on dry mouth.

➤ Tell the patient to take one-a-day doses in the morning.

Tricyclic and Heterocyclic Antidepressants
Drug Administration
➤ See the general guidelines for antidepressants.

➤ Monitor vital signs and blood pressure.

➤ Assess for skin changes. Auscultate bowel sounds and keep a record of stools.

➤ Monitor complete blood count (CBC) and platelet count, liver function tests, serum creatinine, and blood urea nitrogen (BUN). Monitor serum drug levels if available and needed for dosage adjustment.

➤ Concentrated solutions are available for some of the antidepressants; consult the manufacturer's literature for appropriate diluents.

➤ For amoxapine, see the Patient Problems box on neuroleptic malignant syndrome (Chapter 58), and assess for tardive dyskinesia (see Table 58-3).

➤ Supervise the patient carefully to ascertain that the medication is swallowed and not hidden in the mouth to be discarded or stored for later use.

➤ Imipramine may be used in the treatment of enuresis in children older than 6 years of age. The most common side effects are nervousness, sleep disorders, and gastrointestinal (GI) tract upset, although any side effects listed may occur. Treatment is continued for as short a period as possible to obtain relief, then the dosage is tapered. The drug should be taken about 1 hour before bedtime, although early night bed wetters may have a better response if part of the dose is given in the afternoon and part at bedtime; check with the physician. The treatment of enuresis can be complex. Provide emotional support as needed.

Nursing in the Community
➤ Review the general guidelines for antidepressants with the patient.

➤ See the Patient Problems boxes on orthostatic hypotension (Chapter 13), dry mouth (Chapter 23), constipation (Chapter 24), bleeding tendencies (Chapter 54), and photosensitivity (Chapter 58).

➤ If sedation is a problem, suggest that the patient take daily doses at bedtime.

➤ Instruct the patient to take doses with meals or a snack to lessen gastric irritation.

➤ Advise diabetic patients to monitor blood glucose levels because antidepressants may alter them. A change in diet or insulin dosage may be necessary.

Continued

Nursing Implications Summary—cont'd

➤ For doses usually taken at bedtime but missed, instruct the patient not to take the dose the next morning and to check with physician. For missed doses taken more than once a day, tell the patient to take the missed dose as soon as remembered, unless almost time for the next dose, then omit missed dose and resume regular dosage schedule. Do not double up for missed doses.

➤ Encourage the patient to have regular dental checkups, at least twice a year.

➤ Encourage the patient to avoid driving or operating hazardous equipment if drowsiness is a problem.

➤ For doxepin: Use dropper provided by the manufacturer to measure dose. Dilute dose in 4 ounces of recommended liquid (water, milk, or fruit juice, but not grape juice or carbonated beverages) before taking.

Monoamine Oxidase Inhibitors
Drug Administration
➤ See the general guidelines for antidepressants.

➤ Monitor vital signs and blood pressure.

➤ Auscultate bowel sounds and keep record of stools.

➤ Monitor CBC, platelet count, and liver function tests.

➤ Supervise the patient carefully to ascertain that the medication is swallowed and not hidden in the mouth to be discarded or stored for later use.

Nursing in the Community
➤ Review the general guidelines for antidepressants with the patient.

➤ See the Patient Problems boxes on orthostatic hypotension (Chapter 13), dry mouth (Chapter 23), and constipation (Chapter 24).

➤ Review dietary restrictions with the patient and family. See the Dietary Considerations box on MAO inhibitors and tyramine (earlier in this chapter).

➤ Instruct the patient to avoid excessive caffeine intake, although small amounts are acceptable.

➤ Tell diabetic patients to monitor blood glucose levels because antidepressants may alter them. A change in diet or insulin dosage may be necessary.

➤ Review drug interactions with the patient.

➤ Caution patients to observe the guidelines outlined here for 2 weeks after MAO inhibitors are discontinued (to allow all of the medication to be excreted).

lithium
Drug Administration
➤ See the general guidelines for antidepressants.

➤ Monitor vital signs. Inspect for edema.

➤ Assess for symptoms of toxicity (see Table 59-4).

➤ Monitor serum drug levels. Monitor CBC and white blood cell differential, serum electrolytes, BUN, and serum creatinine.

➤ Monitor weight and height in children.

➤ If urinary output is excessive, assess for diabetes insipidus (dilute, high-volume urine with a specific gravity of 1.000 to 1.003).

➤ Supervise the patient carefully to ascertain that the medication is swallowed and not hidden in the mouth to be discarded or stored for later use.

Nursing in the Community
➤ Review the general guidelines for antidepressants with the patient.

➤ Emphasize the importance of returning for follow-up care to have serum drug levels monitored.

➤ Review the signs and symptoms of lithium toxicity, and teach the patient to report them. Provide emotional support as needed for side effects such as fine hand tremor, polyuria, and metallic taste in the mouth. Remind the patient not to discontinue medications without consulting the physician.

➤ Inform the patient to take lithium at same time daily and to take doses with meals or a snack to lessen gastric irritation.

➤ Instruct the patient to maintain sodium intake. Tell the patient not to diet or change sodium intake significantly without talking with physician.

➤ Instruct the patient to maintain a fluid intake of 2.5 to 3 L/day. Instruct the patient to drink limited amounts of coffee, tea, or colas to prevent significant diuresis. Caution patients to drink plenty of fluids during hot weather and periods of exercise.

➤ Instruct the patient to dilute syrup form in fruit juice or other flavored beverage before taking dose.

➤ See the Patient Problems box in Chapter 23 on dry mouth. Instruct the patient to notify the physician if fever or severe or persistent diarrhea or vomiting occurs because any of these may contribute to electrolyte disturbance, which may contribute to lithium toxicity.

➤ Teach patient to swallow extended-release or slow-release forms whole, without crushing or chewing them.

CHAPTER REVIEW

Application
1. What is the biogenic amine theory of depression?
2. How are the actions of the tricyclic and heterocyclic antidepressants, MAO inhibitors, and lithium consistent with the biogenic amine theory of depression?
3. How can drugs cause depression? How would you determine drug-induced depression?
4. What are the major side effects of the tricyclic antidepressants?
5. How do the heterocyclic antidepressants compare with tricyclic antidepressants?
6. What are the common side effects of MAO inhibitors?
7. What are the symptoms of lithium toxicity?

Critical Thinking

1. Describe the acute toxicity of the tricyclic antidepressants. What are the symptoms?
2. What are the major drug interactions of the tricyclic antidepressants? How should you educate patients?
3. What are the major drug interactions of the heterocyclic antidepressants? How should you educate patients?
4. How can a hypertensive crisis be precipitated in a patient taking an MAO inhibitor? What would you teach a patient to help avoid a hypertensive crisis?

References

Flowers EM: Recognition and psychopharmacologic treatment of geriatric depression, *J Am Psychiatr Nurses Assoc* 3(2):32-41, 1997.

Glod CA: Recent advances in the pharmacotherapy of major depression, *Arch Psychiatr Nurs* 10(6):355-364, 1996.

Isaacs A: Depression & your patient, *Am J Nurs* 98(7):26-31, 1998.

Laraia MT: Current approaches to the psychopharmacologic treatment of depression in children and adolescents, *J Child Adolesc Psychiatr Nurs* 9(1):15-26, 1996.

Masters JC: When lithium does not help: the use of anticonvulsants and calcium channel blockers in the treatment of bipolar disorder in the older person, *Geriatr Nurs* 17(2):75-78, 1996.

Vallone DC: SSRIs: when comforting words aren't enough, *Nursing* 27(12):50-52, 1997.

Central Nervous System Stimulants

OBJECTIVES

After studying this chapter, you should be able to do the following:

- *Name the appropriate clinical uses of central nervous system stimulants.*
- *Discuss the side effects of these agents.*
- *Develop a nursing care plan for a patient who is receiving a central nervous system stimulant.*

CHAPTER OVERVIEW

The central nervous system (CNS) regulates its level of activity by maintaining excitatory and inhibitory systems. Therefore excessive stimulation of the CNS may be produced by excessive activity of excitatory neurons or by blockade of inhibitory neurons. Many types of chemicals at some dose produce a degree of CNS stimulation by one of these mechanisms. CNS stimulants currently are medically accepted only for the treatment of narcolepsy, attention-deficit hyperactivity disorder in children, and obesity. This chapter examines the mechanism of action of CNS stimulants used for these disorders. The properties that make them drugs of abuse are discussed fully in Chapter 8.

THERAPEUTIC RATIONALE: NARCOLEPSY AND ATTENTION-DEFICIT HYPERACTIVITY DISORDER

Narcolepsy is a condition in which patients unexpectedly fall asleep during normal activity such as while typing, driving a car, or talking. During an attack, patients experience paralysis of voluntary muscles similar to that experienced while dreaming and may abruptly collapse and fall. Patients with this sleep disorder should be advised to avoid operating cars or dangerous machinery.

The treatment of narcolepsy usually includes the use of CNS stimulants during active daytime periods. Drugs that have been used include amphetamines, methylphenidate, and ephedrine (see Chapter 16). These agents have alerting effects and reduce the sleeping episodes. Although drug therapy may be beneficial for many narcoleptic patients,

most also require other therapy such as scheduled daytime naps. Psychological counseling may help patients reconcile their living patterns with the constraints imposed by the disease.

Children with **attention-deficit hyperactivity disorder** (ADHD) display a variety of symptoms that impair their ability to learn or to maintain appropriate social interactions. The characteristics that separate these children from ordinarily active youngsters are that the symptoms significantly impair function, that the symptoms occur both at home and at school, and that the symptoms persist for 6 months or longer. To be diagnosed with ADHD, the child's behavior must match six of nine defined criteria for both inattentiveness and hyperactivity/impulsivity (see reference by Goldman et al. at the end of the chapter). A relatively new insight into this disease is the discovery that it persists into adolescence and adulthood for many patients. ADHD also occurs alongside other disorders such as bipolar disorder or anxiety in many patients, and control of both conditions is necessary to improve function.

Children with ADHD may require drug therapy to reduce hyperactive behavior and to lengthen their attention span. The drugs most effective in controlling this disorder are CNS stimulants. These agents, which increase agitation and activity in adults, have a calming effect on these children. Methylphenidate is currently the preferred drug; pemoline may be used but in general is less effective. The recognition that therapy for ADHD may need to be considered for many years, or even for a lifetime, has led to a search for less dangerous drugs. Buspirone (see Chapter 57), desipramine (see Chapter 59), and other newer drugs with similar actions are under investigation for ADHD.

Controversy has surrounded the diagnosis and treatment of children with ADHD. Some authorities have claimed the syndrome is diagnosed more often than it exists and suggest that thousands of children may be receiving CNS stimulants unnecessarily, pointing to the lower rate of drug use for this condition in Europe and England. The adoption of more rigorous criteria for diagnosis has reduced the risk of inappropriate diagnosis. At the same time, numerous clinical trials have shown the efficacy of CNS stimulants at reducing hyperactivity, impulsivity, and inattentiveness in children with ADHD. Dietary manipulation for ADHD has failed to control these symptoms in parallel clinical trials.

THERAPEUTIC AGENTS: DRUGS TO TREAT NARCOLEPSY AND ATTENTION-DEFICIT HYPERACTIVITY DISORDER

Central Nervous System Stimulants

amphetamine, dextroamphetamine, and methamphetamine

Mechanism of Action

Amphetamines increase the effectiveness of catecholamine neurotransmitters in the brain and in peripheral nerves by several mechanisms. These drugs may increase release of neurotransmitters during normal nervous system activity. In addition, amphetamines block specific reuptake of catecholamine neurotransmitters into presynaptic neurons. Because this reuptake system normally terminates the action of neurotransmitters, blockade of the reuptake system produces prolonged and enhanced stimulation of postsynaptic nerves. Norepinephrine and dopamine are thought to be the catecholamines whose actions are most enhanced by amphetamines.

Amphetamines may affect many sites in the brain, but the clinically observed actions of amphetamines may be related to two particular regions. One is the reticular-activating system, which regulates sensory input to the brain and thus controls the level of arousal. Amphetamines stimulate the reticular-activating system, increasing alertness and sensitivity to stimuli. The second area of the brain stimulated by amphetamines is the reward center. Actions affecting dopamine at this site are thought to be the source of the addictive potential of amphetamines.

Pharmacokinetics

Amphetamines for medical uses are given orally. These drugs are well absorbed from the gastrointestinal (GI) tract and produce peak serum concentrations within 2 to 3 hours after ingestion. The half-lives of the various amphetamines in blood range from 4 to 30 hours. These compounds easily penetrate the blood-brain barrier to produce their CNS effects. Amphetamines are excreted primarily by the kidneys. The rate of excretion is highly dependent on urinary pH. Excretion can be greatly enhanced by acidifying urine.

Uses

Amphetamines may be used to control narcolepsy or ADHD, but the high potential for abuse of these drugs limits their usefulness (see Chapter 8). Uses for individual amphetamines are shown in Table 60-1.

Adverse Reactions and Contraindications

Amphetamines stimulate adrenergic systems in both the CNS and cardiovascular system, so patients commonly experience insomnia, irritability, restlessness, and irregular heartbeat.

Children receiving amphetamines may experience growth retardation. This effect can be minimized by giving holidays during which drug therapy is suspended. These drugs may worsen behavior or thought disorders other than ADHD.

Amphetamines should be used with caution in patients with cardiovascular disease, glaucoma, hyperthyroidism, or psychoses because these conditions may be worsened by amphetamines. These drugs should be avoided in patients with a history of drug abuse.

Toxicity

Most CNS toxicity of amphetamines is an extension of effects observed at therapeutic dosages. At high dosages, amphetamines cause restless behavior, tremor, irritability, talkativeness, insomnia, and mood changes. Excessive aggressiveness, confusion, panic, and increased libido also may occur. With long-term use, patients sometimes experience toxic psychosis, which resembles schizophrenia, with hallucinations or delirium.

The sympathomimetic effects of amphetamines can cause various cardiovascular reactions. Patients report headache, chilliness, and palpitations. Pallor or facial flushing may be present. Angina and various cardiac arrhythmias may arise. Hypertension or hypotension may be observed at various stages during intoxication. Severely intoxicated patients may die in circulatory collapse.

Symptoms of withdrawal seen after prolonged use at high dosages include nausea, stomach cramps, vomiting, depression, trembling, and unusual tiredness or weakness.

Table 60-1   Central Nervous System Stimulants for Narcolepsy and Attention-Deficit Hyperactivity Disorder

Generic Name	Trade Name	Administration/Dosage	Comments
amphetamine (also called racemic or *dl*-amphetamine sulfate)		*For narcolepsy:* ORAL: *Adults*—5-20 mg 1-3 times/day. FDA pregnancy category C. *Children >6 yr*—2.5 mg twice daily; gradually increase to adult dose if needed. *For attention-deficit hyperactivity disorder:* ORAL: *Children 3-6 yr*—2.5 mg/day; increase by 2.5-mg increments weekly to achieve desired effect. *Children >6 yr*—initially 5 mg/day; increase by 5-mg increments weekly to achieve desired effect.	Schedule II substance (United States). Dosage is adjusted according to patient's needs and tolerance to side effects. Dosage should be minimum required for control of symptoms.
dextroamphetamine	Dexedrine* Dextrostat	*For narcolepsy:* ORAL: *Adults*—5-60 mg once daily (extended-release capsules) or in divided doses (tablets). FDA pregnancy category C. *For attention-deficit hyperactivity disorder:* ORAL: *Children 3-6 yr*—2.5 mg/day; increase by 2.5-mg increments weekly to achieve desired effect. *Children ≥6 yr*—Initially 5 mg/day; increase by 5-mg increments weekly to achieve desired effect.	Schedule II substance (United States). Class C (Canada). Dosage should be minimum required for control of symptoms.
methamphetamine	Desoxyn	*For attention-deficit hyperactivity disorder:* ORAL: *Children ≥6 yr*—5 mg once or twice daily; increase by 5 mg at weekly intervals; or 20-25 mg (extended-release tablets) once daily.	Schedule II substance (United States). Dosage should be minimum required for control of symptoms.
methylphenidate	Ritalin*	*For attention-deficit hyperactivity disorder:* ORAL: *Children ≥6 yr*—5 mg with breakfast and lunch; increase by 5 or 10 mg weekly; maximum daily dose: 60 mg. Extended-release tablets: 20 mg every 8 hr. *For narcolepsy:* ORAL: *Adults*—5-20 mg 2 or 3 times/day with meals; extended-release tablets: 20 mg every 8 hr.	Schedule II substance (United States). Class C (Canada). Drug of choice for most children with attention-deficit hyperactivity disorder.
pemoline	Cylert*	*For attention-deficit hyperactivity disorder:* ORAL: *Children ≥6 yr*—37.5 mg/day in single dose; increase weekly by 18.75 mg until response is obtained. Do not exceed 112.5 mg/day.	Schedule IV substance (United States). Clinical effects develop over 3-4 wk.

*Available in Canada and the United States.

Interactions

Most of the dangerous interactions with amphetamines involve cardiovascular symptoms. For example, amphetamines with tricyclic antidepressants increases the risk of arrhythmias and hypertension. Use of amphetamines with beta-adrenergic blockers may cause hypertension and slow heart rate as a result of unopposed alpha-adrenergic activity. Use of amphetamines with meperidine may lead to hypotension, respiratory depression, and vascular collapse. Digitalis glycosides or thyroid hormones may increase the risk of cardiac arrhythmias or coronary insufficiency with amphetamines.

Sympathomimetic drugs can increase the effects of amphetamines. Monoamine oxidase (MAO) inhibitors also increase catecholamine levels and potentiate effects of amphetamines; these drugs should not be given within 14 days of one another.

▼ methylphenidate

Mechanism of Action

Methylphenidate is a mild CNS stimulant. Its exact biochemical mechanism of action is unknown but may involve blockade of dopamine uptake in specific regions of the brain.

Pharmacokinetics

Methylphenidate is adequately absorbed orally when taken with meals. Orally administered methylphenidate is extensively metabolized during the first pass through the liver. Metabolites of methylphenidate do not stimulate the CNS or sympathetic peripheral neurons. The drug is excreted in urine mostly as these inactive metabolites.

Uses

Methylphenidate may be useful in the management of narcolepsy because of its mild CNS stimulatory effects on the cortex and other portions of the brain. Methylphenidate is currently the preferred drug for the management of ADHD because blocking dopamine reuptake reduces symptoms.

Adverse Reactions and Contraindications

Methylphenidate often causes nervousness and insomnia. Insomnia may be minimized by not taking the drug in the evening. Nervousness may be controlled by reducing overall drug dosage. Cardiovascular effects such as those produced by amphetamines are also seen and include hypertension and tachycardia.

Methylphenidate causes a temporary slowing of growth in prepubertal children. Most children overcome the deficit and ultimately gain normal stature. Slow growth can be minimized by giving the child a drug-free period during therapy. Anorexia, nausea, and abdominal pain may occur with methylphenidate, which can reduce the appetite.

Methylphenidate is avoided in patients with severe anxiety, depression, motor tics, or glaucoma because these conditions may be worsened by the drug (see Drug Abuse Alerts box on methylphenidate).

Toxicity

Very high dosages cause dangerous CNS effects (agitation, confusion, delirium, seizures, and coma) and cardiovascular effects (arrhythmias and hypertension). Symptoms of withdrawal seen after prolonged use at high dosages include bizarre behavior, depression, and unusual tiredness or weakness.

Interactions

Methylphenidate, like the amphetamines, can interact with many other medications. Because methylphenidate causes its effects by release of catecholamines, the effects may be increased by MAO inhibitors, sympathomimetic agents, or vasopressors. Pimozide should be avoided in patients receiving methylphenidate because the risk of tics is increased.

pemoline
Mechanism of Action

Pemoline stimulates the CNS by actions on dopaminergic systems, but the exact biochemical mechanism for the action of pemoline is unknown.

Pharmacokinetics

Pemoline is well absorbed orally, producing peak serum levels 2 to 4 hours after a dose. The serum half-life for the drug is about 12 hours. Therefore the drug may be given once daily. The kidneys excrete most of the administered pemoline, as unchanged drug and as metabolites.

Although the blood levels reach a plateau within a few days after therapy is begun, the therapeutic effects of pemoline are not immediately evident in hyperkinetic children. Dosage is gradually increased over 2 to 4 weeks after therapy is started. Significant clinical response may not be seen until the third or fourth week.

DRUG ABUSE ALERTS
Methylphenidate
THE PROBLEM
Methylphenidate rarely causes toxic psychosis but may cause psychological drug dependence. Both effects are observed after long-term use of doses in excess of therapeutic dosages. The primary patient is obviously most at risk of developing dependence, but health care personnel must also be alert to the problem among caregivers. For example, adult guardians of children receiving methylphenidate may divert the drug from the child and use it themselves. Adolescents being treated with methylphenidate may also share the drug with acquaintances.

SOLUTIONS
- Confirm that doses are not being extemporaneously increased by the patient or caregiver.
- Be alert for signs that the drug is being diverted from the patient to inappropriate recipients.
- Advise the patient to seek medical advice if drug seems to become less effective after several weeks.
- See that dosage reduction is gradual so that withdrawal symptoms are minimized.

Uses

Pemoline is indicated only for the management of ADHD.

Adverse Reactions and Contraindications

Pemoline often causes insomnia, anorexia, and weight loss. CNS signs such as irritability, mild depression, dizziness, headache, and hallucinations are rare. Pemoline causes anorexia, stomachache, and nausea, which may slow normal weight gain. Children do not seem to experience permanent growth retardation, but careful records of the child's growth should be maintained to allow assessment during therapy.

Pemoline is avoided in patients with hepatic function impairment because the drug may cause liver failure. Pemoline has been associated with at least 13 cases of liver failure that required transplantation or caused the death of the child, many of whom seemed to have normal liver function before therapy.

Toxicity

High dosages of pemoline cause CNS effects (agitation, confusion, convulsions, hallucinations, and restlessness) and cardiovascular effects (severe headache, hypertension, and tachycardia). Symptoms of withdrawal seen after prolonged use at high dosages include bizarre behavior, depression, and unusual tiredness or weakness.

Interactions

Although pemoline may cause additive stimulation if used with other CNS stimulants, most interactions with pemoline are of limited clinical significance.

THERAPEUTIC RATIONALE: OBESITY

Obesity is a complex problem with psychological as well as medical components. Persons seeking to lose weight must develop appropriate eating habits and an exercise plan adjusted to their age and physical limitations. For individuals who find it difficult to limit food intake on their own, drugs may be used for short-term suppression of appetite. As a group, these drugs are called **anorexiants** or appetite suppressants (Table 60-2).

THERAPEUTIC AGENTS: ANOREXIANTS TO TREAT OBESITY

benzphetamine, diethylpropion, mazindol, phendimetrazine, phentermine, phenylpropanolamine, and sibutramine

Mechanism of Action

Many CNS stimulants suppress appetite by effects on the hypothalamus in the brain, even while stimulating other CNS functions. Amphetamines were the original CNS stimulants used to control obesity, but because of the risk of addiction, they are no longer used for this purpose. Currently used anorexiants are listed in Table 60-2.

Tolerance develops to all appetite-suppressing drugs in clinical use. Drugs to suppress appetite may help a patient during the initial stages of a weight-reduction program, but these agents are not the key to a successful long-term program.

Pharmacokinetics

Anorexiants are well absorbed orally and have a duration of anorexiant effect ranging from 4 hours (diethylpropion, phendimetrazine, phentermine) to 15 hours (mazindol). Diethylpropion and phentermine are available in extended-release forms that have a duration of action of 12 to 14 hours.

Uses

The anorexiants are for short-term use in a medically supervised weight-reduction program.

Phenylpropanolamine mildly suppresses appetite and is included in various nonprescription appetite suppressants, alone or with other agents. Phenylpropanolamine also is often used in nonprescription nasal decongestants (see Chapter 7).

Adverse Reactions and Contraindications

Because anorexiants are CNS stimulants, some of these drugs may elevate mood or increase motor activity (Table 60-3). Heart rate and blood pressure may also go up with these drugs.

Because of the effects these agents have on the sympathetic nervous system, they are avoided in patients with hypertension, psychosis, hyperthyroidism, glaucoma, or

---

Table 60-2   Appetite Suppressants

Generic Name	Trade Name	Administration/Dosage	Comments
benzphetamine	Didrex	ORAL: *Adults*—25-50 mg once daily; may increase as needed up to 3 doses daily. FDA pregnancy category X.	Schedule III substance (United States).
diethylpropion	Tenuate* Tepanil	ORAL: *Adults*—25 mg 1 hr before morning, noon, and evening meals and at midevening if needed. Timed-release formulations (75 mg) are taken once daily. FDA pregnancy category B.	Safest anorexiant for use in patients with mild cardiovascular disease. Schedule IV substance (United States). Class C (Canada).
mazindol	Mazanor Sanorex*	ORAL: *Adults*—1 mg/day before breakfast; may increase to 1 mg 3 times/day before meals. Avoid in pregnant patients.	May be used in patients with arteriosclerosis or hyperthyroidism. Schedule IV substance (United States).
phendimetrazine	Anorex Bontril Melfiat Obalan	ORAL: *Adults*—35 mg 2 or 3 times/day taken before meals. Sustained-release: 105 mg taken once in morning.	Schedule III substance (United States).
phentermine	Adipex Fastin* Zantryl	ORAL: *Adults*—Single dose of 15-37.5 mg may be taken 2 hr after breakfast. FDA pregnancy category C.	Schedule IV substance (United States). Class C (Canada).
phenylpropanolamine	Acutrim Dexatrim Phenyldrine	ORAL: *Adults*—25 mg 3 times/day before meals or 50-75 mg of sustained-action formulation once daily at midmorning.	These diet preparations should not be used with cold or allergy medications. Nonprescription drug.
sibutramine	Meridia	ORAL: *Adults*—10 mg once daily, in morning. Maximum daily dose: 15 mg. FDA pregnancy category C.	Schedule IV substance (United States).

*Available in Canada and the United States.

agitated states. Most are also avoided in patients with cardiovascular disease, the exception being diethylpropion. Mazindol is contraindicated in patients with cerebral edema.

Many of the available effective appetite suppressants have a high potential for abuse, and many patients experience some level of dependence on these medications (see Table 60-3 and Drug Abuse Alerts box on appetite suppressants). Therefore appetite suppressants are avoided in patients with a history of drug or alcohol abuse.

The anorexiants have not been proved safe during pregnancy; benzphetamine is rated as Food and Drug Administration (FDA) pregnancy category X. None of these drugs are intended for use in children.

DRUG ABUSE ALERTS

Appetite Suppressants

THE PROBLEM

Many patients experience some level of dependence on the central nervous system stimulants used as appetite suppressants. Patients may seek them from several physicians rather than follow the advice of a single physician who may limit the use of the drugs to 2 to 3 months. Many appetite suppressants also carry the risk of causing psychotic reactions, as a result of either overdosage or prolonged use.

SOLUTIONS
- Warn the patient that the anorectic effect will wear off in 6 to 12 weeks.
- Warn the patient not to increase dosage to prolong the anorectic effect.
- Observe for signs of dependence.
- Offer counseling about healthy dietary limitations and good eating practices.

Toxicity

Overdoses with anorexiants can produce dangerous cardiovascular and CNS effects. Symptoms of overdose include GI tract effects (e.g., abdominal cramping, diarrhea, nausea, vomiting), as well as CNS effects (e.g., aggressiveness, convulsions, coma, hallucinations, hostility, panic, restlessness, tremors), and cardiovascular effects that can be fatal (e.g., arrhythmias, fluctuating blood pressure, cardiovascular collapse).

Symptoms of withdrawal seen after prolonged use at high dosages include GI tract difficulties, insomnia, depression, trembling, and unusual tiredness or weakness.

Interactions

Anorexiants can interact with many other medications. For example, sympathomimetic drugs may have a much greater effect in patients receiving appetite suppressants because the appetite-suppressing drugs tend to increase the effectiveness of catecholamines. This precaution should be mentioned to patients, and they should be warned to avoid cold remedies, allergy medications, and nasal decongestants that include sympathomimetic agents. For the same reasons, MAO inhibitors should not be used within 14 days of taking an anorexiant.

Thyroid hormones or other drugs that stimulate the CNS are avoided with all anorexiants.

THERAPEUTIC RATIONALE: RESPIRATORY DEPRESSION

Certain CNS stimulants have generalized effects on the brainstem and spinal cord, as well as on higher centers in the brain. These drugs may increase responsiveness to external stimuli and stimulate respiration. As a group, these drugs are called **analeptics** (Table 60-4).

Analeptics have been used to stimulate respiration, but their use has become less common because modern techniques of respiratory therapy allow a patient to be adequately ventilated even when the natural reflex is absent. Respiratory paralysis caused by overdoses of narcotic agents is treated with specific narcotic antagonists (see Chapter 32) and not with analeptics.

Table 60-3	**Systemic Effects of Appetite Suppressants**				
Generic Name	Mood	Motor Activity	Heart Rate	Blood Pressure	Abuse Potential
benzphetamine	Elevated	May increase	May increase	May increase	High
diethylpropion	May be elevated	May increase	Unchanged	Unchanged	Relatively low
mazindol	May be elevated	May increase	Increased	Usually no change	Relatively low
phendimetrazine	Highly elevated	Increased	Usually no change	Usually no change	High
phentermine	Usually no change	May increase	Increased	Increased	Relatively low
phenylpropanolamine	Usually no change	Usually no change	May increase	May increase	Low
sibutramine	May be depressed	Usually no change	Increased	Increased	Relatively low

THERAPEUTIC AGENTS: DRUGS TO TREAT RESPIRATORY DEPRESSION

Methylxanthines

caffeine, aminophylline, and theophylline

Mechanism of Action

Methylxanthines block destruction of cyclic adenosine monophosphate (cAMP), the compound that mediates the effects of beta-adrenergic stimulation (see Chapter 12). As a result, these compounds affect many body systems, including the CNS.

Caffeine may stimulate any level of the CNS, depending on the dosage. Caffeine stimulates the medullary centers controlling respiration, vasomotor tone, and vagal tone only at relatively high dosages. Very high dosages of caffeine may stimulate the spinal cord and produce convulsions. Theophylline also acts as a CNS stimulant but exerts more action on the heart than does caffeine.

Pharmacokinetics

Methylxanthines are well absorbed orally and may be given by nasogastric tube for neonatal apnea. Metabolism and clearance of methylxanthines are affected by age and a variety of medical conditions (see Chapter 28); therefore blood levels of these drugs may need to be monitored.

Uses

Methylxanthines such as aminophylline and theophylline are most often used as bronchodilators (see Chapter 28). These drugs and caffeine are not officially approved as respiratory stimulants in newborn infants.

Adverse Reactions and Contraindications

Two properties of analeptic drugs make them especially hard to control. First, they are nonspecific CNS stimulants and may produce unwanted effects in addition to respiratory stimulation. Second, all of these drugs at a high enough dosage or in a predisposed patient may produce convulsions.

Toxicity

High dosages of methylxanthines may cause arrhythmias or convulsions.

Interactions

The interactions that may occur with these drugs are presented in Chapters 8 and 28.

Analeptic

doxapram

Mechanism of Action

Doxapram stimulates respiration in two ways. At low dosages the drug stimulates carotid chemoreceptors, which increases sensitivity to carbon dioxide and thereby increases the impulse to breathe. At slightly higher dosages, doxapram stimulates CNS medullary centers controlling respiration. The result is that patients breathe more deeply and may breathe slightly more rapidly.

Pharmacokinetics

Doxapram is administered intravenously. The drug is very rapid acting, with effects observed within 1 minute after injection. The duration of respiratory stimulation is usually 5 to 12 minutes. Doxapram may be given repeatedly or by infusion to sustain a patient throughout a period of respiratory depression, but total doses should normally not exceed 300 mg.

Uses

Doxapram is indicated only for postanesthesia respiratory depression or acute respiratory insufficiency in chronic obstructive pulmonary disease.

Adverse Reactions and Contraindications

Doxapram can produce a variety of reactions, including apprehension and disorientation. Restless, involuntary muscle activity, and increased reflexes are often observed. Patients may report a feeling of warmth with flushing, sweating, and

Table 60-4	Central Nervous System Stimulants for Respiratory Stimulation		
Generic Name	**Trade Name**	**Administration/Dosage**	**Comments**
aminophylline		ORAL, NASOGASTRIC TUBE: *Neonates*—5 mg/kg initial dose; then 2 mg/kg/day, divided into 2 or 3 doses. Avoid peak serum concentrations above 10 μg/ml.	Most commonly used to treat asthma but also used to treat neonatal apnea.
caffeine		ORAL, NASOGASTRIC TUBE: *Neonates*—10 mg/kg body weight initially; then 2.5 mg/kg/day.	Used in neonatal apnea.
doxapram	Dopram*	INTRAVENOUS: *Adults*—0.5 mg/kg body weight intermittently as needed; not to exceed 1.5 mg/kg single dose or total dose of 2 mg/kg. *For chronic obstructive pulmonary disease:* 1-2 mg/min infusion for 2 hr. FDA pregnancy category B.	Rapidly acting drug whose action is over within 12 min. Do not use in newborn infants because of benzyl alcohol content.
theophylline		ORAL, NASOGASTRIC TUBE: *Neonates*—5 mg/kg body weight initial dose; then 1 mg/kg every 12 hr.	Most commonly used to treat asthma but also used to treat neonatal apnea.

*Available in Canada and the United States.

increased body temperature. Blood pressure is elevated. Chest pains and cardiac arrhythmias may occur.

The drug should be avoided in patients with stroke, head injury, coronary artery disease, heart failure, hypertension, epilepsy, airway obstruction, asthma, or pulmonary embolism. All of these conditions may be worsened by doxapram.

Toxicity

If doxapram is injected too rapidly, hemolysis may occur. Extreme agitation, hallucinations, or convulsions usually occur only with overdose, but certain patients may be more susceptible to these reactions.

Interactions

Because doxapram increases blood pressure, this drug should not be used in combination with other drugs tending to elevate blood pressure, such as sympathomimetics and MAO inhibitors. Adverse interactions can also occur between doxapram and the inhalation anesthetics that sensitize the heart to catecholamines (e.g., halothane, enflurane). A delay of 10 minutes or more between the end of anesthesia with these drugs and the administration of doxapram is suggested to lessen the possibility of excessive cardiac toxicity.

Nursing Process Overview

Central Nervous System Stimulants
Assessment

Perform a complete assessment, with a focus on the problem under treatment. Assess vital signs and blood pressure. For children with ADHD, assess weight, height, typical behavior, attention span, and history of any problems in school. For patients with narcolepsy, assess weight and difficulty with activities of daily living, driving, working, or school. For patients with obesity, assess weight and exercise patterns and obtain diet history. For respiratory stimulation, auscultate lung sounds. Assess mental status.

Nursing Diagnoses

- Risk for growth retardation in children
- Altered comfort: nausea and GI tract discomfort
- Risk for hypertension
- Risk for toxic psychosis related to drug therapy

Patient Outcomes

For ADHD: The patient will demonstrate less hyperactive behavior, with an increased attention span, improvement in school work, and normal growth patterns. The nurse will manage and minimize growth retardation.

For narcolepsy: The patient will remain awake and alert for longer periods and will be awake for required job or school activities.

For obesity: The patient will lose weight and in the long term will learn behavioral changes to sustain weight loss.

For respiratory stimulation: The patient will breathe spontaneously at a normal rate.

Planning/Implementation

The problems addressed by the drugs in this chapter are varied. Work with the patient and family to set reasonable goals of therapy. Monitor the patient for side effects, ranging from insomnia and weight loss to hypertension and changes in affect. Encourage the patient to return for regular follow-up to monitor progress and to monitor for side effects. Refer the patient to local support groups. For respiratory stimulation, keep a suction machine available, monitor serum drug levels, and assess mental status.

Evaluation

Before discharge, ascertain that the patient understands how to administer prescribed drugs, what side effects should be reported to the physician, what to do about missed doses, and when to return for follow-up. If the patient should keep a weight, height, or blood pressure record at home, check to see that the patient can do this and has the necessary equipment at home.

Nursing Implications Summary

General Guidelines: Patient Receiving Drugs for Narcolepsy, Attention-Deficit Hyperactivity Disorder, or Appetite Suppression

Drug Administration
➤ Assess for CNS side effects; if severe, notify the physician.
➤ In the hospital, pad siderails and keep them up. Have a suction machine nearby.
➤ Monitor vital signs and blood pressure. Assess mental status.
➤ Monitor behavior. Assess for restlessness, irritability, confusion, insomnia, and mood changes.

➤ Assess for GI tract symptoms, including vomiting, diarrhea, and abdominal cramps.

Nursing in the Community
➤ Review the anticipated benefits and possible side effects of drug therapy. Tell the patient to report any new symptoms.
➤ Instruct the patient to take these drugs only as directed and not to change dose or frequency without consulting the physician. Point out that these drugs are habit forming.
➤ Remind the patient to inform all health care providers of all drugs being taken. Warn the patient to avoid ingesting drugs

Continued

Nursing Implications Summary—cont'd

or foods that also contribute to cardiovascular side effects such as caffeine and caffeine-containing beverages or over-the-counter (OTC) cold preparations containing phenyl-propanolamine.

➤ Instruct the patient to avoid OTC drugs unless first approved by the physician.

➤ After long-term use, these drugs should not be discontinued abruptly.

➤ None of these drugs are appropriate to treat general fatigue.

➤ Instruct the patient to take the last dose of the day at least 6 hours before bedtime for regular dosage forms, and at least 14 hours before bedtime for extended-release forms to help prevent insomnia. Instruct the patient to take the last dose of methylphenidate before 6 PM each day. Insomnia may lessen with continued use of a drug but may be better treated by eliminating the final dose of medication during the day; consult the physician.

➤ For missed doses, if the dose is taken once a day, instruct the patient to take the dose as soon as remembered, unless later than the time indicated in the previous guideline, otherwise omit missed dose and resume usual dosing schedule the next day. If two or more doses per day are prescribed, instruct the patient to take the missed dose if remembered within 1 hour of when scheduled, otherwise omit the missed dose and resume the usual dosing schedule. The patient should not double up for missed doses.

➤ Remind patients taking long-acting forms to swallow tablets whole, without chewing or crushing them.

➤ See the Patient Problems boxes on dry mouth (Chapter 23) and constipation (Chapter 24).

➤ Warn diabetic patients to monitor blood glucose levels because these drugs may alter blood glucose, necessitating a change in diet or insulin dosage.

➤ Warn the patient to avoid driving or operating hazardous equipment if dizziness, nervousness, agitation, or other CNS effects are severe and to consult the physician if these symptoms become severe.

➤ Except when specifically prescribed for ADHD, CNS stimulants should not be used in children. Instruct the patient to keep these and all drugs out of their reach.

➤ These drugs should not be used during pregnancy unless specifically prescribed by the obstetrician. Counsel the patient about contraceptives as needed.

➤ Instruct the patient to avoid alcoholic beverages unless approved by the physician.

Drugs to Treat Narcolepsy and Attention-Deficit Hyperactivity Disorder
Drug Administration/Nursing in the Community
➤ See the general guidelines.
➤ Weigh the patient two or three times a week until the effects of the drug can be evaluated. Although not being given for

the purpose of weight reduction, most of these drugs will suppress the appetite.

➤ Instruct parents to keep careful weight and height records of children.

➤ Reinforce to the patient that several weeks of therapy may be necessary until full effects of the drug therapy can be evaluated.

➤ Refer the patient and family for appropriate teaching and counseling for narcolepsy and ADHD.

➤ Instruct the patient taking drugs for ADHD and the parents that drug-free periods may be prescribed periodically to assess whether medication is still needed and to allow growth if the prescribed drug has caused growth retardation.

➤ Review dosage schedule with the patient. Some patients require daily dosage, whereas others may require medication during school or work but can be drug free on the weekends or during summer for children.

➤ For best effect, instruct the patient to take doses of methylphenidate on an empty stomach, 30 to 45 minutes before a meal or snack.

Drugs to Suppress Appetite
Drug Administration/Nursing in the Community
➤ See the general guidelines.
➤ Refer the patient for appropriate counseling and instruction on weight-reduction diets. Encourage a regular exercise program.
➤ Inform the patient that weight reduction will be greatest during the first few weeks of therapy but will slow after that.
➤ Phenylpropanolamine is also discussed in Chapter 30.
➤ Instruct the patient to take the last dose of the day of mazindol 1-mg tablets 4 to 6 hours before bedtime or the 2-mg dose 10 to 14 hours before bedtime.

Central Nervous System Stimulants for Respiration
Drug Administration
➤ Anticipate that seizures may occur. Have a suction machine at the bedside. Keep siderails up and use padding. Do not leave the patient unattended.
➤ Have oxygen and resuscitation equipment available.
➤ Monitor pulse, blood pressure, and respirations. Monitor electrocardiographic tracing.
➤ Monitor temperature.
➤ See the manufacturer's literature for specific guidelines about administration of doxapram.
➤ Theophylline and aminophylline are discussed in Chapter 28.
➤ CNS stimulants are rarely used outside of the intensive care setting to stimulate respiration.
➤ Keep the family informed of the patient's condition.

CHAPTER REVIEW

Application

1. What is narcolepsy and how is it treated?
2. What are potential hazards of untreated narcolepsy? As a community health nurse, what would you assess in the home environment of a patient with narcolepsy?
3. What is ADHD? What are some possible signs and symptoms of this problem?
4. How is ADHD treated?
5. What is the mechanism of action of amphetamines in the CNS?
6. What is the route of administration of amphetamines used in clinical medicine?
7. What side effects are common with amphetamines? How should you assess for these? What signs may signal overdose?
8. Why might MAO inhibitors potentiate effects of amphetamines, leading to serious overstimulation of various systems?
9. What are the clinical uses of methylphenidate?
10. What toxicity is associated with use of methylphenidate?
11. How does the action of pemoline differ from that of methylphenidate?
12. What rare but serious side effect should be watched for in a child receiving pemoline?
13. Why are CNS stimulants used to treat obesity?
14. Which appetite suppressant produces CNS depression?
15. Which appetite suppressant is most often found in OTC obesity medications?
16. What toxic reactions may develop during therapy with appetite suppressants?
17. Which methylxanthines are sometimes used to stimulate respiration?
18. What reactions are observed when methylxanthines are used to stimulate respiration?
19. How is doxapram administered, and what is its duration of action?
20. What toxicity is observed with doxapram?

Critical Thinking

1. Should parents keep the school health nurse informed about drug treatment for children with ADHD? Why? What are the responsibilities of the school health nurse with children with this diagnosis who are taking medication?
2. If appetite suppressants contribute to weight loss, why not use them with all obese patients?
3. The chart for a 10-year-old child receiving methylphenidate includes a note instructing that the child's height should be carefully measured and recorded at each visit. Why is that information especially relevant for this child?

References

Goldman LS, Myron G, Bezman RJ, Slanetz PJ: Diagnosis and treatment of attention-deficit/hyperactivity disorder in children and adolescents, *JAMA* 279:1100-1107, 1998.

Ludwikowski K, De Valk M: Attention-deficit hyperactivity disorder. The psychostimulants and beyond, *Adv Nurse Pract* 6:55-60, 1998.

Scahill L, French PT: Nonstimulant medications in the treatment of attention deficit hyperactivity disorder, *J Child Adolesc Psychiatr Nurs* 9(2):39-43, 1996.

Anticonvulsants

OBJECTIVES

After studying this chapter, you should be able to do the following:

■ *Define epilepsy and describe the characteristics of simple and complex partial (focal) seizures and generalized seizures, characterizing the major syndromes: tonic-clonic seizures, absence seizures, myoclonus epilepsy, psychomotor epilepsy, focal motor seizures, and status epilepticus.*

■ *Discuss the principles of drug therapy for epilepsy.*

■ *Develop a nursing care plan for patients receiving valproate, carbamazepine, phenytoin, ethosuximide, or phenobarbital.*

■ *Explain the use of diazepam or lorazepam for the control of status epilepticus.*

■ *Develop a teaching plan for a patient receiving drug therapy for control of seizures.*

CHAPTER OVERVIEW

Anticonvulsants are used to control seizures. The objective of drug therapy is to control seizures as completely as possible without causing intolerable side effects. Therapy is individualized for the drug or drug combinations used and for their doses.

THERAPEUTIC RATIONALE: EPILEPSY

Epilepsy is a neurologic disorder characterized by a recurrent pattern of abnormal neuronal discharges within the brain, resulting in a sudden loss or disturbance of consciousness, sometimes in association with motor activity, sensory phenomena, or inappropriate behavior. The seizure may be preceded by an aura. An **aura** is a sensation peculiar for that patient; it can be a visual disturbance or a certain dizziness or numbness that warns the patient of an impending seizure.

Between 1% and 2% of the population is estimated to have epilepsy. The cause of epilepsy may be unknown (idiopathic) or may be traced to a known brain lesion. In general, epilepsy appearing in childhood or adolescence is likely to be

idiopathic, whereas epilepsy appearing in adulthood is likely to relate to a definable cause such as a head injury, cerebrovascular accident (stroke), or brain tumor.

An appropriate choice of drugs, taken on a long-term basis, can control the seizures of epilepsy in about 80% of patients. The choice of drugs depends on a careful diagnosis of the seizure pattern, which ideally is made from the observation of a seizure and the recording of the brain wave pattern with an electroencephalogram (EEG) during the seizure. The diagnosis is critical to the selection of a drug or drugs because different seizure patterns are controlled by different drugs. Other causes of seizures must be ruled out because seizures may be a result of an organic disorder such as a brain tumor, poisoning, fever, hypoglycemia, and hypocalcemia. Overdose of certain drugs such as local anesthetics and ketamine causes seizures. Abrupt withdrawal of some drugs such as the barbiturates and most other sedative-hypnotic drugs, including alcohol, can precipitate seizures.

Classification of Epilepsy

Epilepsy is described most commonly by the classification published by the International League Against Epilepsy. This classification is presented in Box 61-1. It describes the seizure pattern by the area of the brain involved.

The two major categories of epilepsy are partial seizures and generalized seizures. These are pictured in Figure 61-1. Partial seizures arise from a focal lesion on one side of the brain. The location of the lesion determines the type of

---

Box 61-1   International Classification of Seizures

I. Partial seizures
  A. Simple partial seizures
    1. Motor: most common in older children and adults; consciousness not lost
    2. Somatosensory or special sensory: odor, taste most common
    3. Autonomic
    4. Psychic
  B. Complex partial seizures
    1. Simple partial onset followed by impairment of consciousness
    2. Impairment of consciousness at onset
  C. Partial seizures evolving to secondarily generalized seizures
    1. Simple partial seizures evolving to generalized seizures
    2. Complex partial seizures evolving to generalized seizures
    3. Simple partial seizures evolving to complex partial seizures evolving to generalized seizures
II. Generalized seizures (convulsive or nonconvulsive)
  A. Absence seizures
    1. Typical absence seizures (petit mal seizures)
    2. Atypical absence seizures
  B. Myoclonic seizures
  C. Clonic seizures
  D. Tonic seizures
  E. Tonic-clonic seizures (grand mal)
  F. Atonic seizures
III. Unclassified epileptic seizures

Modified from Commission on Classification and Terminology of the International League Against Epilepsy: Proposal for revised classification of epilepsies and epileptic syndromes, *Epilepsia* 30:389-399, 1989.

---

seizure observed: motor, cognitive, behavioral, or sensory. Consciousness is usually not lost, but patients may not remember seizure episodes when cognitive or behavioral function is involved. Focal and psychomotor seizures are examples of partial seizures that are discussed more fully. **Generalized seizures** result from the discharge of cells over both sides of the brain. Tonic-clonic seizures, absence seizures, and myoclonic seizures are examples of generalized seizures. The patient loses consciousness during generalized seizures.

Partial Seizures

Simple Partial Seizures

Simple **partial seizures** begin with a specific symptom that reflects the particular part of the brain in which the seizure originates. These seizures may be visual, such as flashes of light, or tactile, such as a feeling of numbness or tingling. The patient does not lose consciousness; the patient is aware but not in control of what is happening. **Focal motor seizures** can involve just a finite motion such as turning of the head. Motor seizures of the jacksonian type begin with clonic seizures of a few muscles on half of the face or in one extremity; the seizures then progresses (march) to include more body musculature (e.g., finger, hand, arm).

Psychomotor Epilepsy

Psychomotor epilepsy is a complex partial seizure with complex symptoms that include an aura, automatism, and motor seizures, independently or in combination. These seizures usually last about 5 minutes. The patient remembers the aura but not the automatism or motor seizure. The automatism may consist of chewing or swallowing motions, temperamental changes, confusion, feelings of unreality, or unexplained bizarre behavior. A detailed neurologic examination may be required to differentiate psychomotor epilepsy from psychotic mental illness.

Generalized Seizures

Tonic-Clonic Epilepsy

Tonic-clonic epilepsy (formerly called grand mal) involves the contraction of all skeletal muscles. Before the seizure begins, the patient may experience an aura. The patient then suddenly loses consciousness and may utter a cry as the diaphragm contracts and expels air from the lungs. The seizure

Figure 61-1   Schematic representation of how seizures spread. **A,** Focal seizure with spread to adjacent areas, giving rise to partial seizures. **B,** Focal seizure that gives rise to generalized seizure. **C,** Primary generalized seizure.

consists of sustained (tonic) contractions or intermittent (clonic) contractions of the muscles. The patient may become incontinent. When the contractions cease, the patient regains consciousness. Usually, the patient is confused and drowsy and lapses into prolonged sleep (postictal depression).

Atonic Seizures

An atonic (drop) seizure is characterized by a sudden loss of tone in postural muscles. Consciousness is impaired. In severe cases the patient may suddenly collapse to the floor.

Absence Epilepsy

Absence epilepsy (formerly petit mal) occurs mainly in children 4 to 12 years of age. The child suddenly loses consciousness for a few seconds, although body tone is seldom lost and consciousness is regained with no confusion. The appearance is one of inattention or daydreaming and may be accompanied by slight blinking or hand movements. Attacks usually occur several times a day. The EEG shows a 3-second spike wave pattern. Absence epilepsy does not generally continue into adulthood, but many patients with absence epilepsy subsequently develop other types of epilepsy, particularly tonic-clonic epilepsy. Thus many physicians treat children prophylactically for tonic-clonic epilepsy in addition to treating absence epilepsy. Some evidence suggests that this prophylactic treatment reduces the incidence of subsequent tonic-clonic epilepsy.

Myoclonus Epilepsy

Myoclonus epilepsy is a generalized seizure pattern that develops as a result of anoxic brain damage (intentional myoclonus) or as a genetic disorder (progressive myoclonic epilepsy). Intentional myoclonus is a neurologic symptom consisting of sudden involuntary contractions of skeletal muscles, which are aggravated by purposeful activity (hence the term *intentional*) and by visual, auditory, tactile, and emotional activity. Progressive myoclonic epilepsy is a particular form of intentional myoclonus that appears in childhood and becomes progressively worse. When untreated, the genetic disease leads to death after 15 to 20 years.

Status Epilepticus

Status epilepticus refers to seizures that last 30 minutes or longer or that are repeated for 30 minutes or longer and during which consciousness is not regained. Status epilepticus of the generalized tonic-clonic type is a medical emergency. In about 80% of patients, seizures are a result of a disease, often associated with a low blood concentration of calcium or glucose, or a result of withdrawal from drugs such as the barbiturates or other sedative-hypnotics. The immediate goals are to establish an airway, to stop the seizures, and then to identify their cause.

Molecular Mechanisms Underlying Seizures

The basis of seizures is a regional imbalance of inhibitory and excitatory neuronal inputs and alterations of membrane stability. Three general molecular mechanisms have been identified for antiepileptic drugs. These mechanisms have not been correlated with specific types of seizures.

The GABA$_A$ receptor mediates the inhibitory activity of gamma-aminobutyric acid (GABA), a major inhibitory neurotransmitter of the brain. Drugs that enhance this activity have an anticonvulsant effect. Such drugs include benzodiazepines, barbiturates, and valproate. Tiagabine, a new anticonvulsant, was specifically designed to inhibit GABA reuptake. Gabapentin and topiramate also act to increase GABA levels.

The amino acid glutamate is a major excitatory neurotransmitter of the brain, regulating ion channels. One of these receptor-gated calcium ion channels is identified by stimulation with the agent N-methyl-D-aspartate (NMDA). Drugs that inhibit NMDA receptors or activity are anticonvulsants. Lamotrigine decreases glutamate release. Felbamate and topiramate have some activity to decrease glutamate levels.

Neuronal membrane excitability is largely determined by voltage-dependent calcium, potassium, and sodium channels. The antiepileptic drugs carbamazepine and phenytoin modulate sodium channels to decrease cellular excitability. This activity is also found with felbamate, lamotrigine, topiramate, and valproate.

New Drug Development

The understanding of the molecular mechanisms just described is still incomplete and rapidly evolving. The classic route for identifying new antiepileptic drugs relied on the use of mouse and rat animal models for screening. The identification of new drugs was slow. Now drugs are being developed to act at specific receptor sites. Several new drugs, including felbamate, fosphenytoin, gabapentin, lamotrigine, tiagabine, and topiramate, have been released recently. Other new agents, including clobazam, levetiracetam, oxcarbazepine, zonisamide, and vigabatrin, are expected to be released.

THERAPEUTIC AGENTS: DRUG THERAPY FOR SEIZURES

Therapeutic Principles

Several drugs are available for control of epileptic seizures. The drug choice depends on diagnosis of the seizure patterns and on the patient's tolerance and response to the drug prescribed. Drugs most often effective for various seizure patterns are listed in Table 61-1.

One of the first-line drugs for the seizure pattern diagnosed is started in small doses to allow the patient to develop a tolerance to the drowsiness and motor incoordination (ataxia) associated with most of the anticonvulsant drugs. The dose is increased until the seizures are stopped or until toxic effects of the drug appear. If the drug is ineffective or only partly effective in controlling seizures, another first-line drug is tried. A second drug is added only if three antiepilep-

Table 61-1   Drug Choice by Seizure Type

Seizure Type	First-Choice Drugs	Second-Choice Drugs	Refractory Cases
Partial (includes secondarily generalized tonic-clonic)	carbamazepine phenytoin	gabapentin lamotrigine topiramate valproate	ethotoin mephenytoin methsuximide phenobarbital primidone tiagabine
Generalized absence	ethosuximide valproate	clonazepam lamotrigine	clorazepate methsuximide phensuximide trimethadione
Tonic-clonic	carbamazepine phenytoin valproate	gabapentin lamotrigine topiramate	ethotoin mephenytoin mephobarbital phenobarbital primidone
Myoclonic, atonic	valproate	clonazepam felbamate lamotrigine	carbamazepine clorazepate ethosuximide methsuximide phenobarbital phenytoin

tic drugs have failed to control seizures with an acceptable level of side effects.

Because the most common cause of drug failure is the failure of the patient to take the prescribed drugs, the plasma concentration of drug may be determined before deciding that the drug is ineffective. Patients must be warned not to discontinue medication when the seizures are under control or when the side effects are disturbing. The sudden discontinuance of medication greatly increases the incidence of seizures. Blood and urine analyses often are routinely carried out because many anticonvulsant drugs can occasionally produce blood dyscrasias or renal damage.

Many patients with epilepsy require drug therapy throughout their lives to control seizures. However, patients who are reaching adulthood after childhood treatment for absence epilepsy and patients who have had several seizure-free years may be able to discontinue medication. If the EEG of such a patient appears normal, medication can be gradually discontinued. Seizures recur in 25% to 50% of such patients.

Ketogenic Diet

The ketogenic diet consists of a high-fat diet. The ratio of fat to the combined carbohydrates plus protein content is 4:1 by weight. The caloric requirement is calculated at 75 to 100 kcal/kg body weight, with a protein content of 1 to 2 g/kg body weight. The diet was designed to mimic the favorable effect of starvation on seizures. This diet has proved useful for children who continue to have disabling seizures despite treatment with anticonvulsants or who have unacceptable side effects from anticonvulsants. With the keto-genic diet, about one third to two thirds of children are able to reduce or eliminate anticonvulsant medications.

Therapy and Pregnancy

Pregnancy influences the epilepsy itself as well as the metabolism of many anticonvulsant drugs. In general, the plasma concentration of anticonvulsant drugs decreases in pregnancy, so the concentrations need to be monitored closely. Infants of mothers with epilepsy as a whole are at increased risk for prematurity, low birth weight, low Apgar scores, hypoxia, hemorrhage, and congenital malformations. However, the risk of seizures to the fetus is regarded as greater than the risk of anticonvulsant drugs.

A pattern of congenital abnormalities, the fetal antiepileptic drug syndrome, is characterized by prenatal and postnatal growth deficiencies, microencephaly, developmental delay, short nose, hypoplastic fingernails and distal phalanges, and congenital heart defects. Originally described for phenytoin, this syndrome has also been linked with phenobarbital, carbamazepine, and valproate. The highest rate of this syndrome is associated with phenobarbital; an intermediate rate is associated with phenytoin, and the lowest rate with carbamazepine. Both valproate and carbamazepine also increase the risk of spina bifida or neural tube defect. Pregnancies during which the mother took trimethadione (Tridione) were associated with an 80% incidence of spontaneous abortions or birth defects.

Phenobarbital, primidone, and phenytoin can cause a deficiency in vitamin K–dependent clotting factors in the newborn. This effect is transient and reversible. Infants should be treated promptly with vitamin K.

The effectiveness of oral contraceptives may be impaired for women taking phenytoin, phenobarbital, primidone, carbamazepine, and ethosuximide. These anticonvulsants induce the drug metabolizing enzymes of the liver, which also metabolize sex steroids and can reduce the blood levels of oral contraceptives by 40%. The contraceptive failure rate is estimated at 6% for women taking low-dose oral contraceptives with the enzyme-inducing antiepileptic drugs. A high estrogen formulation may be necessary for effective contraception.

FIRST-LINE ANTICONVULSANTS

A summary of first-line anticonvulsant drugs is presented in Table 61-2.

▼ carbamazepine

Mechanism of Action

Carbamazepine (Tegretol) is chemically related to the tricyclic antidepressants. It limits seizure propagation at the level of synaptic transmission by reducing excitatory sodium currents.

Pharmacokinetics

The plasma half-life is 12 hours, so the drug must be given in divided doses. Carbamazepine is metabolized by the liver, and one of the metabolites has anticonvulsant activity. Absorption from the gastrointestinal (GI) tract is slow; however, this can be improved if the drug is taken at meals.

Carbamazepine has been formulated in a sustained release capsule for twice a day dosage. Also, this formulation decreases fluctuations in serum concentrations by 50% and thereby reduces side effects.

Uses

Carbamazepine is particularly effective in controlling simple or complex partial seizures, including psychomotor seizures. It is also effective for generalized tonic-clonic seizures. A positive side effect is the increased alertness and improvement of mood in patients. Carbamazepine is a first-choice anticonvulsant because of its low behavioral and psychological toxicity and the rarity of serious side effects.

Carbamazepine is also used for the relief of pain caused by trigeminal neuralgia or glossopharyngeal neuralgia. However, carbamazepine is not an analgesic. Other uses include the treatment of alcohol withdrawal, bipolar depression, and excited psychosis.

Adverse Reactions, Contraindications, and Toxicity

Carbamazepine has relatively low behavioral and toxicologic toxicity. The most common side effects are drowsiness, dizziness, ataxia, visual disturbances (particularly double vision), and GI upset. Carbamazepine occasionally causes rashes, liver damage, and bone marrow depression, which require its discontinuance. Blood counts should be made frequently in the early course of treatment and occasionally thereafter. Serious adverse effects are rare.

Interactions

Drug interactions encountered include decreased plasma concentration in the presence of other anticonvulsants because the other agents induce drug-metabolizing enzymes in the liver. Drugs that tend to lower the plasma concentration of carbamazepine by increasing its metabolism include ethotoin, mephenytoin, phenytoin, ethosuximide, methsuximide, phensuximide, clonazepam, primidone, barbiturates, valproate, tricyclic antidepressants, phenothiazines, haloperidol, loxapine, maprotiline, molindone, pimozide, and thioxanthenes. Other drugs increase the plasma concentration of carbamazepine by inhibiting its degradation. Drugs potentiating the action of carbamazepine by increasing its plasma concentration include cimetidine, propoxyphene, clarithromycin, danazol, diltiazem, verapamil, erythromycin, troleandomycin, and isoniazid.

Carbamazepine can lower the effectiveness of several drugs by increasing their metabolism. Drugs so affected include estrogen, quinidine, glucocorticoids, monoamine oxidase inhibitors, and oral anticoagulants. Prolonged use of carbamazepine with acetaminophen can lead to liver damage.

▼ ethosuximide

Mechanism of Action

Ethosuximide (Zarontin) is one of the succinimides. These drugs elevate the seizure threshold in cortex and basal ganglia through a reduction in specific calcium channel currents. This reduces synaptic response to low-frequency, repetitive stimulation. Related drugs are phensuximide (Milontin), which is sometimes effective in treating psychomotor epilepsy, and methsuximide (Celontin).

Pharmacokinetics

GI absorption is rapid. The plasma half-life is about 30 hours in children and 60 hours in adults. The effective serum concentration is 40 to 80 μg/ml, but serum concentrations of up to 160 μg/ml can be tolerated without excessive toxicity.

Uses

Ethosuximide is a drug of choice for typical absent seizures.

Adverse Reactions and Contraindications

Side effects include dizziness, drowsiness, and GI irritation. Blood counts may be performed because of the occasional occurrence of agranulocytosis. The tendency to cause blood dyscrasia may show up in dental problems: increased mouth infection and gingival bleeding.

Contraindications for ethosuximide include blood dyscrasias, intermittent porphyria, and hepatic or renal disease. Ethosuximide is excreted in breast milk.

Interactions

Ethosuximide enhances the central nervous system (CNS) depressive effects of other drugs. Use with haloperidol can cause changes in the pattern or frequency of seizures, and the dose of either drug may need to be changed.

Table 61-2 **Anticonvulsant Drugs**

Generic Name	Trade Name	Administration/Dosage	Comments

First-Line Anticonvulsants

carbamazepine	Apo-Carbamazepine† Epitol Tegretol* Others	ORAL: *Adults*—200 mg 2 times/day first week; increase by 100 or 200 mg/day at weekly intervals to control seizures. Maintenance: 600-1600 mg/day. FDA pregnancy category C. *Children 6-12 yr*—100 mg 2 times on day 1, increase by up to 100 mg/day at weekly intervals to control seizures. Maintenance: 400-800 mg/day. *Children ≤6 yr*—10-20 mg/kg body weight/day in 2-3 divided doses, increasing by up to 100 mg/day at weekly intervals to control seizures. Maintenance: 250-350 mg/day.	First-line drug because of relative lack of serious side effects and low behavioral and psychologic toxicity. Controls partial seizures with simple or complex symptoms; generalized tonic-clonic seizures; mixed seizure patterns; other partial or generalized seizures. Also indicated for treatment of trigeminal neuralgia and glossopharyngeal neuralgia.
ethosuximide	Zarontin*	ORAL: *Adults and children >6 yr*—15-30 mg/kg body weight/day or initially 250 mg 2 times/day; with dose being increased by 250 mg/day at 4- to 7-day intervals to control seizures. Maximum daily dose: 1.5 g. *Children <6 yr*—15-40 mg/kg body weight or initially 250 mg once a day, with dose being increased by 250 mg/day at 4- to 7-day intervals to control seizures. Maximum daily dose: 1 g.	First-line drug for simple absence seizures.
phenytoin	Dilantin*	ORAL: *Adults*—105 mg 3 times/day initially; adjust at 7- to 10-day intervals to control seizures. FDA pregnancy category C. *Children*—5 mg/kg body weight/day divided into 2 or 3 doses initially; adjust as needed to control seizures. Maximum daily dose: 300 mg. *Older adults*—3 mg/kg body weight/day in divided doses, adjusted according to patient response. INTRAVENOUS: *Adults—For status epilepticus:* 15-20 mg/kg body weight administered at rate not to exceed 50 mg/min. Maintenance: 100 mg every 6-8 hr.	First-line drug for tonic-clonic seizures and simple or complex partial seizures. Used for prophylaxis and treatment of seizures during and after neurosurgery. May be used for sustained control of status epilepticus after diazepam treatment. Used for correction of atrial and ventricular arrhythmias induced by digitalis.
valproic acid divalproex sodium	Depakene* Depakote Epival† Others	ORAL: *Adults—Monotherapy:* 5-15 mg/kg body weight/day in 1-3 doses; increase at weekly intervals by 5-10 mg/kg body weight/day to control seizures. *Polytherapy:* 10-30 mg/kg body weight/day; increase at weekly intervals by 5-10 mg/kg body weight/day to control seizures. If dosage exceeds 250 mg/day, divide into 2 or more doses to lessen gastric irritation. FDA pregnancy category D. *Children 1-12 yr—Monotherapy:* 15-45 mg/kg body weight/day; increase by 5-10 mg/kg body weight weekly to control seizures. *Polytherapy:* 30-100 mg/kg body weight/day.	First-line drug for simple and complex absence seizures. Also effective for partial seizures, tonic-clonic seizures, and myoclonic seizures. Monotherapy is preferred because there are complex drug interactions affecting plasma levels of valproate and many other anticonvulsants.

Alternative or Adjunct Anticonvulsants

clonazepam	Klonopin Rivotril†	ORAL: *Adults*—0.5 mg 3 times/day; increase by 0.5-1 mg every 3 days until seizures are controlled or side effects prevent further increase. Maximum daily dose: 20 mg. *Infants and children ≤10 yr* (or *<30 kg body weight*)—0.01-0.03 mg/kg body weight initially divided into 2 or 3 doses; increase by 0.25-0.5 mg every third day until seizures are controlled or maintenance dose of 0.1-0.2 mg/kg body weight is reached.	Treatment for Lennox-Gastaut syndrome; akinetic seizures, myoclonic seizures, absence seizure pattern; adjunctive therapy for simple partial seizure pattern, complex partial seizure patterns. Long-term use by children may impair physical or mental development, which may not be apparent for many years.
clorazepate	Apo-Clorazepate† Gen-XENE Novoclopate† Tranxene*	ORAL: *Adults and children >12 yr*—7.5 mg 3 times/day initially; increase by no more than 7.5 mg at weekly intervals, not to exceed 90 mg daily. *Children 9-12 yr*—7.5 mg 2 times/day initially; increase by no more than 7.5 mg at weekly intervals, not to exceed 60 mg/day.	Adjunctive therapy for refractory partial or generalized seizures.
felbamate	Felbatol	ORAL: *Adults*—1200 mg/day divided into 3 or 4 doses initially; increase gradually to no more than 3600 mg/day. FDA pregnancy category C. *Children 2-14 yr*—15 mg/kg body weight divided into 3 or 4 doses daily initially; increase gradually to no more than 3600 mg/day.	Adjunctive therapy for children with Lennox-Gastaut syndrome not responsive to other treatment; monotherapy for partial seizures refractory to other drugs. Reports of aplastic anemia and liver failure limit use.

*Available in Canada and the United States.
†Available in Canada only.

Continued

Table 61-2   Anticonvulsant Drugs—cont'd

Generic Name	Trade Name	Administration/Dosage	Comments
Alternative or Adjunct Anticonvulsants—cont'd			
gabapentin	Neurontin*	ORAL: *Adults*—300 mg on day 1; 600 mg divided into 2 doses on day 2; 900 mg divided into 3 doses on day 3; then increase as needed to control seizures. Range: 900-3600 mg/day. FDA pregnancy category C.	Adjunct therapy for treatment of partial seizures. Reduce dosage for patients with reduced renal function (creatinine <60 mg/ml).
lamotrigine	Lamictal*	ORAL: *Adults taking valproate and enzyme-inducing anticonvulsants*—25 mg every other day for 2 wk; then 25 mg/day for 2 wk. If needed and tolerated, may increase to 150 mg divided into 2 doses/day. *Adults taking enzyme-inducing anticonvulsants*—50 mg once a day for 2 wk, then 100 mg/day divided into 2 doses. May increase by 100 mg/day on weekly basis based on response. FDA pregnancy category C.	Adjunct therapy for partial seizures in adults. For patients receiving enzyme-inducing anticonvulsant medications but not valproate, double dose given with valproate.
phenobarbital	Generic Solfoton	ORAL: *Adults*—60-250 mg/day as single dose or in divided doses. FDA pregnancy category D. *Children*—1-6 mg/kg body weight/day as single or divided dose.	Alternative agent for treatment of tonic-clonic seizure pattern and simple partial seizure pattern.
primidone	Apo-Primidone† Mysoline* PMS Primidone† Sertan	ORAL: *Adults and children >8 yr*—100-125 mg once a day at bedtime for first 3 days; 2 times/day for days 4-6; 3 times/day for days 7-9; thereafter adjust as needed; not to exceed 2000 mg/day. *Children ≤8 yr*—50 mg at bedtime days 1-3; 50 mg 2 times/day for days 3-6; 100 mg 2 times/day for days 7-9; thereafter 125-250 mg 3 times/day or 10-25 mg/kg body weight/day.	Adjunct or alternate therapy for generalized tonic-clonic, nocturnal myoclonic, complex partial, and simple partial seizures.
tiagabine	Gabitril	ORAL: *Adults and children >12 yr*—4 mg once a day initially. Increase total daily dose by 4-8 mg at weekly intervals as needed, administering as divided doses. Maximum dose: 32 mg for adolescents, 56 mg for adults. FDA pregnancy category C.	Adjunct therapy for partial seizures in adults and children >12 yr.
topiramate	Topamax	ORAL: *Adults*—50 mg/day initially for 1 wk, then increase by 50 mg at weekly intervals. Usual dosage is 400 mg/day in 2 divided doses. FDA pregnancy category C.	Adjunct therapy for partial seizures.
Miscellaneous Anticonvulsants			
ethotoin	Peganone	ORAL: *Adults*—500 mg-1 g on day 1 divided into 4-6 doses; increase over several days, up to 3 g/day. *Children*—Up to 750 mg/day. FDA pregnancy category C.	Alternative therapy for tonic-clonic and simple or complex partial seizures.
mephenytoin	Mesantoin*	ORAL: *Adults*—50-100 mg once a day, increase by 50-100 mg/day at weekly intervals to control seizures. Maximum daily dose: 1.2 g. *Children*—25-50 mg/day; increase by 25-50 mg/day at weekly intervals to control seizures. Maximum daily dose: 400 mg.	Alternative therapy for simple partial seizures in patients not responsive to other agents.
methsuximide	Celontin*	ORAL: *Adults and children*—300 mg once a day; increase by 300 mg/day at weekly intervals to control seizures. Maximum dose: 1.2 g.	Alternative therapy for absence seizures refractory to other medications.
phensuximide	Milontin	ORAL: *Adults and children*—500 mg 2 or 3 times/day; increase by 500 mg/day at weekly intervals until seizures are controlled. Maximum daily dose: 3 g.	Alternative therapy for absence seizures refractory to other medications.
trimethadione	Tridione	ORAL: *Adults*—300 mg 3 or 4 times/day; increase by 300 mg/day at weekly intervals to control seizures. Maximum dose: 2.4 g. *Children ≤2 yr*—100 mg 3 times/day. *Children 2-6 yr*—200 mg 3 times/day. *Children >6 yr*—300 mg 3 times/day.	Alternative therapy for absence seizures refractory to other medications.
Anticonvulsants for Status Epilepticus			
diazepam	D-val Valium* Zetram	INTRAVENOUS: *Adults*—5-10 mg initially; repeat at 10- to 15-min intervals as needed, up to total dose of 30 mg. Repeat in 2-4 hr if necessary. *Children 5 yr*—1 mg every 2-5 min up to total dose of 10 mg. Repeat in 2-4 hr if necessary. *Infants >30 days and children ≤5 yr*—0.2-0.5 mg every 2-5 min up to total dose of 5 mg. Repeat in 2-4 hr if necessary. Administer over 3 min to infants and children.	For status epilepticus and severe recurrent convulsive seizures.

*Available in Canada and the United States.
†Available in Canada only.

Table 61-2 Anticonvulsant Drugs—cont'd

Generic Name	Trade Name	Administration/Dosage	Comments
Anticonvulsants for Status Epilepticus			
diazepam—cont'd	Diastat Rectal Gel	RECTAL: *Adults and children* >*12 yr*—0.2 mg/kg body weight. *Children 6-12 yr*—0.3 mg/kg body weight. *Children 2-6 yr*—0.5 mg/kg body weight. May give second dose 4-12 hr later if needed.	Rectal formulation is absorbed completely. Instruct caregiver in proper use.
lorazepam	Ativan*	INTRAVENOUS: *Adults*—0.05 mg/kg body weight, up to 4 mg, administered slowly. Repeat twice at 10-15 min if seizures continue or recur, but no more than 8 mg total in 12-hr period. FDA pregnancy category D.	For status epilepticus and severe recurrent convulsive seizures.
fosphenytoin	Cerebyx	INTRAVENOUS: *Adults*—15-20 mg PE/kg body weight, administered at 100-150 mg PE/min. Follow with maintenance doses of fosphenytoin or phenytoin. FDA pregnancy category D.	A soluble prodrug of phenytoin, packaged as phenytoin equivalents. Rapidly converted by blood and liver enzymes to phenytoin.

PE, Phenytoin equivalents.
*Available in Canada and the United States.
†Available in Canada only.

Carbamazepine and phenytoin increase the metabolism of ethosuximide; valproate decreases the metabolism.

▼ phenytoin

Mechanism of Action

Phenytoin (Dilantin) acts to stabilize membranes and raise the threshold for depolarization. This is achieved through the reduction of sustained high-frequency firing of neurons, probably through the inactivation of select sodium channels.

Pharmacokinetics

Because phenytoin has a plasma half-life of 24 hours, it takes 4 days to reach steady plasma levels when initiating therapy. To decrease this time, the initial dose is sometimes given as a loading dose at three times the usual daily dose. At serum concentrations much above therapeutic concentrations, the capacity of the liver to metabolize phenytoin is saturated so that plasma concentrations decrease very slowly. Phenytoin is irregularly absorbed from the intestine. Because absorption depends on formulation, it is best to stay with a particular brand of phenytoin.

An extended-release capsule formulation of phenytoin is available for once-a-day administration. Otherwise, phenytoin is administered three times a day.

Phenytoin should not be given intramuscularly or subcutaneously because it is highly irritating and can precipitate in the tissue. The sodium salt can be administered intravenously, but too rapid administration can produce severe hypotension and cardiac arrest.

Uses

Phenytoin, formerly called diphenylhydantoin, is a drug of choice in controlling tonic-clonic seizures and partial seizures in adults.

Sodium phenytoin has been administered intravenously to control status epilepticus alone or after intravenous (IV) diazepam has controlled the seizures. IV sodium phenytoin is also used to control some cardiac arrhythmias (see Chapter 18). This IV formulation will be phased out because of the introduction of the prodrug fosphenytoin.

Adverse Reactions and Contraindications

Effective serum concentrations are 10 to 20 μg/ml, and side effects are seen at higher serum concentrations. At greater than 20 μg/ml, involuntary movement of the eyeballs (nystagmus) appears; at greater than 30 μg/ml, ataxia and slurred speech arise. Tremors and nervousness or drowsiness and fatigue may be side effects of higher serum concentrations. However, an acute overdose of phenytoin is seldom fatal. Persistence of these side effects requires reducing the dosage or switching to another drug, usually phenobarbital.

About 20% of patients taking phenytoin experience overgrowth of the gums (gingival hyperplasia), which is particularly severe in children. Occasionally, folic acid or vitamin D deficiency can occur because phenytoin interferes with the normal metabolism of these compounds. Phenytoin can also cause an allergic rash that can be mistaken for measles or infectious mononucleosis. Phenytoin also worsens acne, which is especially bothersome to teenagers and can increase growth of body hair (hirsutism), which is undesirable in women. There is a higher incidence of congenital malformations in infants of mothers taking phenytoin. These infants are also at risk for hemorrhage and coagulation deficiencies at birth, which can be corrected with vitamin K.

Interactions

Important drug interactions are noted with phenytoin. Phenobarbital can increase the metabolism of phenytoin in some individuals by inducing liver microsomal enzymes, but in others, phenobarbital decreases the rate of drug metabolism of phenytoin by competing with the enzymes for degradation. The oral anticoagulant dicumarol and the anticonvulsant carbamazepine decrease the metabolism of phenytoin by competing with the enzymes for degradation. The anticonvulsant valproic acid displaces bound phenytoin from protein to increase the free concentration of phenytoin while decreasing its total concentration because more phenytoin is available for metabolism. Phenytoin enhances the rate of estrogen metabolism, which can decrease the effectiveness of some birth control pills.

▼ valproate: valproic acid and divalproex sodium

Mechanism of Action

Valproic acid (Depakene) is an analog of the inhibitory central neurotransmitter GABA, which inhibits neuronal activity. One mechanism by which valproic acid may act is to increase the concentration of this inhibitory neurotransmitter. Divalproex sodium (Depakote Epival) is a combination of the acid and salt forms of valproic acid.

Pharmacokinetics

Divalproex sodium is a combination of valproic acid and sodium valproate with an enteric covering to delay absorption for 1 to 4 hours after ingestion. In the GI tract the complex dissolves into valproate. The plasma half-life of the active drug is variable, from 6 to 16 hours. Patients with hepatic impairment, older adults, and children younger than 18 months have a long life for valproate.

A formulation for IV administration of valproate is available.

At low serum concentrations, valproate is highly bound to protein. At serum concentrations above 50 µg/ml, binding sites become saturated and the fraction of free drug increases, dramatically increasing the incidence of side effects and toxicity. Valproate is metabolized by the liver and some metabolites are active or toxic. Children metabolize the drug more rapidly than adults do. Infants and older adults metabolize the drug more slowly than other age groups. The drug and its metabolites are excreted in the urine as glucuronides.

Uses

Valproate is a first-line drug for the treatment of many generalized seizures, including simple and complex absence seizures, myoclonic seizures, and tonic-clonic seizures. Valproate is also a first-line drug for many partial seizures. Clinical studies have shown that valproate is effective in treating manic depression and prophylaxis for migraine.

Adverse Reactions, Toxicity, and Contraindications

The most common side effect seen with valproic acid is GI distress. Sedation is marked at the beginning of treatment unless doses are gradually raised. A hand tremor occasionally is seen with higher dosages. Overdose has produced coma but with uneventful recovery.

Valproate may raise ammonia concentrations in the blood, but this is not associated with any clinical manifestations. Patients taking valproate occasionally may show confusion.

The most serious toxic effect of valproate is liver failure. This usually appears in the first 6 months of treatment. Children less than 2 years of age or children receiving other anticonvulsants with valproate are at greatest risk for liver failure. Nonspecific symptoms include loss of seizure control, malaise, weakness, lethargy, loss of appetite, vomiting, edema, and a Reye's-like syndrome. The incidence of liver failure is rare but potentially fatal.

Valproate is contraindicated for patients with liver disease because of the potential for liver failure. Valproate also interferes with platelet aggregation. This effect is not a problem for most people, but patients with coagulation disorders or patients taking anticoagulants should be carefully monitored.

Interactions

Drug interactions with valproic acid include its decreased plasma concentration in the presence of other anticonvulsants that induce liver microsomal enzymes, including phenobarbital, primidone, phenytoin, and carbamazepine. Phenytoin also can raise the concentration of free-plasma valproic acid by displacing the fraction bound to plasma proteins.

Drugs that alter coagulation, including oral anticoagulants, heparin, platelet aggregation inhibitors, and thrombolytic agents, increase the risk for bleeding when taking valproate.

Valproate potentiates the CNS depressant effect of other drugs, especially alcohol and CNS depressants.

ALTERNATIVE OR ADJUNCT ANTICONVULSANT DRUGS

A summary of alternative or adjunct anticonvulsant drugs is presented in Table 61-2.

clonazepam

Mechanism of Action

Clonazepam (Klonopin, Rivotril) is a benzodiazepine. These drugs enhance presynaptic inhibition by the inhibitory neurotransmitter GABA an action that suppresses the spread of seizures.

Pharmacokinetics

Clonazepam is well absorbed with peak plasma concentrations occurring 1 to 4 hours after administration. The plasma half-life of clonazepam is 20 to 40 hours. Clonazepam is metabolized in the liver to a compound that probably has little anticonvulsant activity.

Uses

Clonazepam is effective in controlling generalized absence seizures and myoclonic seizures. Tolerance often develops to clonazepam, and seizures recur in about a third of patients. Therefore clonazepam is not a first-line drug for epilepsy.

Clonazepam is also effective as an antipanic agent.

Adverse Reactions and Contraindications

Neurologic side effects are commonly seen during therapy with clonazepam and include drowsiness, ataxia, and personality changes. Children may become hyperactive, irritable, aggressive, violent, or disobedient. Slurred speech, tremors, abnormal eye movements, dizziness, and confusion also may be noticed. These effects are dose related and may subside with time or on lowering the dosage. Increased salivation and bronchial secretions sometimes occur and create respiratory problems in children.

Children who are treated long-term with clonazepam may show adverse effects on physical and mental development. There is an increased risk of birth abnormalities in infants whose mothers took clonazepam.

Interactions

Clonazepam does not alter the activity of other anticonvulsant drugs. This allows clonazepam to be added to anticonvulsant therapy as a second drug more readily than other agents. However, clonazepam enhances CNS depression, especially with barbiturates. When clonazepam is given with primidone, behavioral disorders may be seen. Cimetidine, oral contraceptives, and disulfiram can increase the plasma concentration of clonazepam.

clorazepate

Mechanism of Action

Clorazepate (Gen-Xene, Tranxene) is a benzodiazepine. These drugs enhance presynaptic inhibition by the inhibitory neurotransmitter GABA, an action that suppresses the spread of seizures.

Pharmacokinetics

Clorazepate is rapidly absorbed, but it is inactive until it is metabolized in the stomach or plasma to desmethyldiazepam. This metabolite has a long plasma half-life.

Uses

Clorazepate is mainly used as adjunct therapy in patients with partial or generalized seizures. Tolerance often develops to its anticonvulsant activity.

Adverse Reactions and Contraindications

Adverse reactions include drowsiness, ataxia, and sedation. Occasionally, behavioral and personality changes may be noted, especially when given with primidone. Children taking clorazepate may exhibit hyperactivity.

Interactions

Clorazepate enhances the CNS depression of CNS depressant drugs. Cimetidine may slow the metabolism of desmethyldiazepam, resulting in higher plasma concentrations of the active drug, increasing adverse actions.

felbamate
Mechanism of Action

Felbamate (Felbatol) is chemically related to meprobamate, an anxiolytic agent. Felbamate appears to inhibit indirectly the NMDA receptor and thereby limit excitatory CNS responses.

Pharmacokinetics

Felbamate is well absorbed and has a half-life of 16 to 19 hours. The drug is excreted in the urine unchanged (50%) or as metabolites.

Uses

Felbamate is effective as monotherapy or adjunctive therapy for partial seizures with or without secondary generalization of seizures.

It is also effective as adjunctive therapy in the treatment of partial and generalized seizures associated with the Lennox-Gastaut syndrome. This rare and severe seizure syndrome in children is characterized by frequent absence like seizures and mental retardation.

However, felbamate is recommended only for the most severe and refractory patients. A high incidence of aplastic anemia and liver failure has been reported in patients taking felbamate.

Adverse Reactions, Toxicity, and Contraindications

Potential side effects associated with felbamate include nausea, headache, weight loss, and insomnia. Toxic side effects have emerged to limit the use of felbamate. Aplastic anemia appears in an estimated 1 of 2000 patients on felbamate for more than a few weeks.

In addition, a few cases of acute liver failure have been reported for patients taking felbamate. Patients with liver function abnormalities should not be put on felbamate. Markers of liver function (ALT, AST, and bilirubin) should be monitored weekly for patients on felbamate.

Interactions

Felbamate decreases the plasma levels of carbamazepine, but it also increases phenytoin and valproic acid levels. Carbamazepine and valproic acid both decrease plasma levels of felbamate.

gabapentin
Mechanism of Action

Gabapentin (Neurontin) is an analog of the inhibitory CNS neurotransmitter GABA. However, gabapentin does not interact with GABA receptors, and therefore its mechanism of action is unclear.

Pharmacokinetics

Gabapentin is rapidly absorbed and has a plasma half-life of 5 to 6 hours. About 80% to 100% of the drug is excreted unchanged in the urine. Dosages must be adjusted proportionally when renal function as determined by creatinine clearance falls below 60 ml/min.

Uses

Gabapentin is effective as adjunctive therapy in refractory partial seizures in adults and children older than 12 years of age. It is also being tested in the management of chronic pain syndromes.

Adverse Reactions and Contraindications

Adverse reactions of gabapentin include somnolence, dizziness, ataxia, fatigue, diplopia, blurred vision, amnesia, nystagmus, and tremor. These are not usually pronounced. Weight increase and depression have also been reported. No toxicity has been reported. Because the drug is excreted unchanged in the urine, patients with reduced renal function require smaller dosages.

Interactions

No significant drug interactions have been described with the use of gabapentin.

lamotrigine

Mechanism of Action

Lamotrigine (Lamictal) inhibits voltage-dependent sodium currents and inhibits the release of the excitatory neurotransmitter, glutamate.

Pharmacokinetics

Lamotrigine is well absorbed. The plasma half-life in adults is about 25 hours. Lamotrigine is extensively metabolized by the liver to glucuronides that are excreted in the urine.

Uses

Lamotrigine is effective as adjunctive therapy in adults with partial seizures. This is a new drug and additional uses may be added with further clinical testing.

Adverse Reactions and Contraindications

Adverse reactions include nausea, headache, diplopia, blurred vision, dizziness, ataxia, somnolence, and rash.

Interactions

Enzyme-inducing drugs such as phenytoin and phenobarbital that enhance liver metabolism decrease the plasma concentration of lamotrigine. Valproic acid significantly retards the metabolism of lamotrigine and increases the plasma concentration.

phenobarbital and primidone

Mechanism of Action

Phenobarbital (Solfoton) and primidone (Mysoline) are barbiturates. These act as anticonvulsants by enhancing the activity of the inhibitory neurotransmitter GABA.

Pharmacokinetics

Phenobarbital has a long half-life and can be administered once a day. Phenobarbital is a classic inducer of liver microsomal enzymes and thus can speed its own metabolism and that of other drugs. Primidone is a deoxybarbiturate that is metabolized to phenobarbital and phenylethylmalonamide.

Uses

Phenobarbital has been widely used for 60 years and is an alternative drug for treating patients with partial and generalized seizures. Primidone can substitute for phenobarbital to treat partial and generalized seizures, but it is not used for the treatment of absence seizures.

IV phenobarbital is used to stop seizures of status epilepticus that are unresponsive to benzodiazepines and phenytoin. Respiratory and blood pressure support must be available.

Adverse Reactions and Contraindications

The main side effects of the barbiturates are sedation and drowsiness at the beginning of treatment, but tolerance usually develops to these effects. Phenobarbital tends to impair thinking, mood, and behavior. Sudden withdrawal of the drug can precipitate convulsions. In elderly patients and in children, a paradoxical excitement may be seen that impairs learning ability. Phenobarbital increases the incidence of congenital malformations in the fetus but not to the degree associated with phenytoin and trimethadione. Barbiturates are contraindicated for patients with the metabolic disorder porphyria and for patients who are depressed and might consider suicide.

Primidone has a greater incidence of adverse and toxic effects than does phenobarbital.

Interactions

Barbiturates induce liver metabolizing enzymes and can thereby decrease the levels of other drugs that are metabolized by this system. Barbiturates are CNS depressants and synergize the activity of other CNS agents, including alcohol.

tiagabine

Mechanism of Action

Tiagabine (Gabitril) increases GABA levels by binding irreversibly to the neuronal reuptake carrier for GABA.

Pharmacokinetics

Tiagabine is given orally and is rapidly and rather completely absorbed. It is highly bound to serum proteins. The drug is metabolized in the liver. Patients with liver impairment may require smaller doses.

Uses

Tiagabine is an adjunct to other anticonvulsants in the treatment of partial seizures in adults and children older than 12 years of age. It is being tested as monotherapy for partial seizures.

Adverse Reactions and Contraindications

Tiagabine is generally well tolerated and does not cause withdrawal effects. Patients may have some difficulty in concentrating or paying attention. Occasionally, patients may exhibit clumsiness, confusion, paresthesias, or speech problems.

Interactions

Tiagabine does not displace other drugs or induce liver metabolizing enzymes. Patients taking anticonvulsants that induce the liver metabolizing enzymes (barbiturates, carbamazepine, and phenytoin) may require higher dosages of tiagabine.

topiramate

Mechanism of Action

Topiramate (Topamax) enhances the activity of GABA.

Pharmacokinetics

Topiramate is administered orally in divided doses. It is well absorbed. Protein binding is low and the drug is not extensively metabolized. About 70% of the drug is excreted unchanged in the urine.

Uses

Topiramate is indicated as adjunct therapy in the treatment of partial onset seizures.

Adverse Reactions and Contraindications

Sleepiness and fatigue may be experienced at the start of therapy. Confusion, difficulty with concentration, nervousness, and speech problems sometime appear at higher dosages.

Interactions

The concentration of topiramate may significantly be lowered by carbamazepine, phenytoin, or phenobarbital. Valproate and topiramate mutually lower serum concentrations by 10% when given concurrently.

Miscellaneous Anticonvulsant Drugs

A summary of miscellaneous anticonvulsant drugs is presented in Table 61-2.

ethotoin and mephenytoin

Ethotoin (Peganone) and mephenytoin (Mesantoin) are chemically related to phenytoin. Mephenytoin is associated with a high incidence of agranulocytosis and aplastic anemia. Ethotoin is not widely used, although it does not seem to cause gingival hyperplasia, hirsutism, or ataxia.

methsuximide and phensuximide

Methsuximide (Celontin) and phensuximide (Milontin) are succinimides. Ethosuximide, listed earlier, is the only widely used drug of this group. Phensuximide is not as effective as ethosuximide for childhood absence seizures. Methsuximide is adjunct therapy for refractor partial complex seizures.

trimethadione

Trimethadione (Tridione) was the first drug effective in controlling absence epilepsy, but it is now a third-choice drug for absence seizures because of the high incidence of serious side effects.

Trimethadione can produce serious allergic dermatitis, kidney and liver damage, agranulocytosis, and aplastic anemia. Blood counts and urinalyses are done routinely with trimethadione therapy. In adults the drug often produces an intolerance to light (photophobia). The incidence of spontaneous abortions or congenital anomalies in infants of mothers taking trimethadione is 80%.

ANTICONVULSANTS FOR TREATMENT OF STATUS EPILEPTICUS

diazepam

Diazepam (Valium) administered intravenously terminates the tonic-clonic seizures of status epilepticus within two minutes. IV diazepam can also terminate the seizures of eclampsia. Diazepam has a duration of antiseizure activity of 15 to 30 minutes. A new rectal formulation of diazepam (Diastat) allows patients with status epilepticus to be treated before arrival at the emergency room. This rectal formulation can also be used by caregivers for patients with intractable epilepsies who have frequent clusters of seizures.

Oral diazepam occasionally is used with other anticonvulsants to control myoclonic and absence seizures. Main side effects are drowsiness, dizziness, and ataxia. Respiratory depression must be watched during IV administration. Overall, diazepam is a safe drug. A major use of diazepam is as an antianxiety drug (see Chapter 57).

fosphenytoin

Fosphenytoin (Cerebyx) is a prodrug of phenytoin introduced to replace IV phenytoin in the treatment of status epilepticus or seizures during neurosurgery. Whereas phenytoin is poorly water soluble, fosphenytoin is quite water soluble. It is packaged in phenytoin equivalent to facilitate dosage.

Fosphenytoin is dephosphorylated by phosphatases to phenytoin with a half-life of about 15 minutes. Phenytoin is useful for maintaining a prolonged antiseizure effect after initial administration of benzodiazepines. It can also be used as an initial therapy. Hypotension can be a side effect, so caution should be used when administering this drug to patients with hypotension or myocardial insufficiency.

lorazepam

Lorazepam (Ativan) is the drug of choice for the initial treatment of status epilepticus. Lorazepam usually stops seizures within 3 minutes and has a duration of action against seizures of 12 to 24 hours. Respiratory depression must be monitored during IV administration.

Nursing Process Overview

Anticonvulsants

Assessment

Most patients using anticonvulsant drugs have had a seizure, and drug treatment is needed on a long-term basis. Obtain a baseline assessment, with special emphasis on areas known to be affected by the drugs to be used. For example, because phenytoin can cause gingival hyperplasia, assess mouth, teeth, and gums at the start of and periodically during therapy.

Nursing Diagnoses

- Risk for gingival hyperplasia
- Altered comfort: nausea and GI distress associated with drug ingestion

Patient Outcomes

The patient will demonstrate good oral hygiene and will state the importance of regular dental care. The patient will not experience nausea or GI distress related to medication regimen.

Planning/Implementation

Drug dosages are adjusted until seizures are controlled or toxic effects are noted. Monitor the patient's general condition with an emphasis on known drug side effects. Monitor serum levels of the prescribed drugs if available. If the patient continues to have seizures, observe type, duration, and characteristics of the seizure, and continue nursing measures to prevent injury such as padding siderails or supervising ambulation. Refer the patient to health department, social services, or vocational rehabilitation, if appropriate.

Evaluation

Long-term drug therapy often produces side effects. The health care team then must decide which side effects cannot be permitted and which can be treated or tolerated. Evaluate the patient regularly through observation, reassess known problem areas (e.g., the mouth with phenytoin therapy), and make appropriate referrals.

Before discharge, verify that the patient or family can name the drugs being taken and understands how to take them correctly (including dose, time of day, and correct preparation), what side effects may occur, which of these need to be reported immediately, how to treat or prevent those that are more likely to occur, and what to do if a dose is missed. Determine that the patient can state the importance of wearing a medical identification tag or bracelet.

Nursing Implications Summary

General Guidelines: Anticonvulsant Therapy

Drug Administration

- For seizures, assess frequency, characteristics, previous treatment, and alterations in activities of daily living related to seizure activity.
- Monitor serum drug levels if available.
- Assess for side effects. Tactfully question the patient about compliance with therapy.

Nursing in the Community

- Review with the patient the anticipated benefits and possible side effects of drug therapy.
- Provide emotional support as the patient begins anticonvulsant therapy. Drug side effects are common in the first several months of therapy but often diminish with time. Several months of treatment with a drug regimen may be needed to determine adequate dosage.
- Reinforce to patients the importance of continuing prescribed medications even if they have been seizure free for an extended period. Stress the need to take drugs as ordered and to avoid abruptly discontinuing prescribed medications because this may precipitate seizures. Recent evidence suggests that anticonvulsants can be discontinued in some patients who have been seizure free for a long period. This decision must be made on an individual basis in consultation with the physician.
- Counsel the patient to learn from the physician what actions to take in the event of a missed dose of drug. A typical guideline is as follows: Take missed dose as soon as remembered, unless almost time for the next dose, then omit missed dose and resume regular dosing schedule. Do not double up for missed doses. Contact the physician for guidelines about what to do if two or more consecutive doses are missed.
- Females of childbearing age may wish to use contraceptives while taking these drugs. If females wish to conceive, counsel them to keep physicians informed so that they can be given current information about drug effects during pregnancy. In addition, remind the patient to inform her gynecologist of the anticonvulsant being used. Oral contraceptives are not effective when some of these drugs are taken.
- Encourage patients to wear a medical identification tag or bracelet indicating they have a history of seizures. In addition, suggest that they carry a card listing current drugs and dosages in their wallets.
- Remind the patient to inform all health care providers of all medications being taken. Tell the patient not to use over-the-counter (OTC) preparations unless approved by the physician. There are many drug interactions with many of these medications.
- Warn the patient to avoid driving or operating hazardous equipment if drowsiness or visual difficulties develop. Teach

Nursing Implications Summary—cont'd

the patient that visual disturbances are common with many of these drugs; the patient should report the development of double vision, blurred vision, or nystagmus.

➤ Refer the patient as needed to local or national agencies, including the local visiting nurse agency, vocational rehabilitation, or the Epilepsy Foundation of America.

➤ Instruct the patient to avoid drinking alcoholic beverages unless permitted in small amounts by the physician.

➤ Tell the patient not to switch brands of anticonvulsant because bioavailability may differ between brands; consult the pharmacist and the physician for specific information.

➤ Teach the patient using a suspension form to shake the bottle well before pouring each dose. Failure to adequately resuspend the medication may result the drug settling to the bottom of the bottle, causing inadequate doses when the bottle is nearly full and excessive doses when the bottle is less than half full.

➤ Review the procedure for the prescribed drug form with the patient. Usually, swallow capsules whole, without breaking them open. Chewable tablets should be chewed well and not swallowed whole. Enteric-coated forms should be swallowed whole, without crushing or chewing them. If in doubt, consult the manufacturer's literature and the pharmacist.

carbamazepine
Drug Administration
➤ See the general guidelines.

➤ This drug may be used to treat tic douloureux (trigeminal neuralgia). For this, assess characteristics of pain, aggravating factors, and previous treatments.

➤ Monitor blood pressure and weight. Assess for visual changes and double vision. Assess for possible water intoxication (syndrome of inappropriate antidiuretic hormone, SIADH): weakness, nausea, vomiting, confusion, hostility, stupor, increased seizure frequency, decreased urine production, and edema.

➤ Monitor complete blood cell count (CBC) and differential, platelet count, blood urea nitrogen (BUN), serum iron, serum electrolytes, and liver function tests.

➤ Carbamazepine is usually effective at a serum concentration of 6 to 12 μg/ml.

Nursing in the Community
➤ See the general guidelines. Review side effects discussed in text with the patient and family.

➤ Instruct the patient to take doses with meals.

➤ See the Patient Problems boxes on photosensitivity (Chapter 58), constipation (Chapter 24), dry mouth (Chapter 23), bleeding tendencies (Chapter 54), and leukopenia (Chapter 54).

➤ Tell the patient using this medication for trigeminal neuralgia that it is not an analgesic and should not be used for any condition other than that prescribed.

➤ Tell diabetic patients that this drug may alter urine glucose results. Monitor blood glucose levels.

Succinimides (ethosuximide, methsuximide, and phensuximide)
Drug Administration
➤ See the general guidelines.

➤ Monitor CBC and differential, platelet count, liver function tests, BUN and serum creatinine, and urinalysis.

➤ Ethosuximide and methsuximide are usually effective at a serum concentration of 40 to 100 μg/ml.

Nursing in the Community
➤ See the general guidelines.

➤ Encourage the patient to take doses with meals or a snack to lessen gastric irritation.

➤ Tell the patient taking phensuximide that urine may turn red, pink, or red-brown during therapy with this drug; this effect is harmless.

➤ Tell the patient taking methsuximide not to take capsules that appear to have melted or that are only partly filled.

Hydantoins (ethotoin, fosphenytoin, mephenytoin, and phenytoin)
Drug Administration
➤ See the general guidelines.

➤ Assess gait, nausea and vomiting, nystagmus, dizziness, and GI symptoms.

➤ Therapeutic serum drug levels are as follows: ethotoin, 15 to 50 μg/ml; mephenytoin, 25 to 40 μg/ml; and phenytoin, 10 to 20 μg/ml.

➤ Monitor CBC and differential, platelet count, liver function tests, and blood glucose level.

➤ Remember that even when used as an anticonvulsant, phenytoin also has cardiovascular effects (see Chapter 19).

Intravenous fosphenytoin
➤ Fosphenytoin is a prodrug that is converted to phenytoin in the body. Doses of fosphenytoin are always expressed in terms of phenytoin equivalents (PE). Numerous medication errors have been reported as a result of misunderstanding fosphenytoin dosage. Read orders carefully, and seek clarification if unsure of ordered dose.

➤ Solution supplied as 75 mg/ml. Dilute each ml of drug with 2 ml of D5W or normal saline to make a concentration of 25 mg PE/ml. Dilute a 1500-mg dose in 100 ml diluent to equal 15 mg PE/ml. Dilute 1500-mg dose in 1000 ml diluent to equal 1.5 mg PE/ml. Administer at a rate of 150 mg PE or less over 1 minute. This drug is more soluble than phenytoin in IV solution. Monitor blood pressure, and if possible, have patient connected to electrocardiographic (ECG) monitor to monitor cardiac rhythm during and immediately after IV administration.

➤ Fosphenytoin is better tolerated than phenytoin via intramuscular administration.

Intravenous phenytoin
➤ Prepare dose with diluent supplied by the manufacturer. Slightly yellow-colored solutions may be used, but discard solutions that are not clear. Do not mix with other drugs or

Continued

Nursing Implications Summary—cont'd

many IV solutions because precipitation may occur. Flush tubing before and after administration with 0.9% sodium chloride. Administer at a rate of 50 mg or less per minute. Monitor blood pressure, and if possible, have patient connected to ECG monitor to monitor cardiac rhythm during and immediately after IV administration. Recent studies have involved dilutions in large volumes of normal saline solution (preferred) or lactated Ringer's injection (e.g., 100 mg phenytoin in 50 ml normal saline solution) to administer phenytoin as an infusion. Use a 0.45- to 0.22-micron in-line filter. Consult the manufacturer's literature for current recommendations.

Nursing in the Community
➤ See the general guidelines.
➤ Review common signs of overdose, including ataxia, slurred speech, and nystagmus. Tell the family to report these or any unusual side effects. See Patient Problems boxes in Chapter 54 on bleeding tendencies and leukopenia.
➤ Provide emotional support. Acne or hirsutism may be difficult for some patients. Refer patients to a dermatologist as appropriate.
➤ Encourage the patient to have regular dental checkups and to have a thorough dental care program that includes flossing, brushing, and rinsing. Even with meticulous oral care, gingival hyperplasia develops in some patients taking phenytoin or mephenytoin. Provide emotional support.
➤ Instruct the patient to take oral doses with meals or a snack to lessen gastric irritation.
➤ Chewable tablets may be crushed, chewed, or swallowed whole.
➤ Instruct the patient not to change brands or dosage forms without checking with physician.
➤ Instruct the patient to report signs of folic acid deficiency, including fatigability, weakness, fainting, and headache.
➤ Encourage ingestion of foods high in vitamin D (see the Dietary Considerations box in Chapter 17 on vitamins).
➤ Advise diabetic patients to monitor blood glucose levels because an adjustment in diet or insulin dosage may be necessary.
➤ Tell the patient that these drugs may produce a harmless brownish or pinkish discoloration of urine.
➤ Instruct the patient not to take doses of these anticonvulsants within 2 to 3 hours of taking antacids or drugs for diarrhea.

valproic acid and divalproex sodium
Drug Administration
➤ See the general guidelines.
➤ Monitor CBC and differential, platelet count, serum ammonia concentration, BUN and serum creatinine, and liver function tests.
➤ Valproic acid is usually effective at a serum concentration of 50 to 100 μg/ml.

Nursing in the Community
➤ See the general guidelines. Review side effects discussed in text with patient and family.
➤ See the Patient Problems boxes on constipation (Chapter 24) and bleeding tendencies (Chapter 54).
➤ Instruct the patient to take oral doses with meals or a snack to lessen gastric irritation.
➤ Instruct the patient to take the delayed-release tablet form whole, without chewing or breaking the tablet. Instruct the patient taking the delayed-release capsule form to swallow the capsule whole or to pour the contents on a small amount of cool, soft food such as applesauce or pudding and to swallow this food without chewing. Instruct the patient taking the syrup form that the syrup may be mixed with a small amount of food or liquid. Instruct the patient taking the capsule form to swallow the capsule whole, without chewing or crushing it.
➤ Tell diabetic patients that this drug may alter urine tests for ketones, giving false-positive results. Monitor blood glucose levels.

felbamate
Drug Administration/Nursing in the Community
➤ See the general guidelines.
➤ Assess gait. Assess skin for rash or purpura (small red or purple spots) and changes in affect, including agitation, aggression, or other changes in mood; monitor for fever. See Patient Problems boxes for bleeding tendencies (Chapter 54), leukopenia (Chapter 54), and photosensitivity (Chapter 58). Assess for liver failure: jaundice, headache, stomach pain, vomiting, fatigue, weakness, or dark urine.
➤ Monitor the CBC and white blood cell (WBC) differential, and platelet count, liver function tests, and serum iron concentration.
➤ Encourage the patient to take doses with meals or a snack to lessen gastric irritation.

gabapentin
Drug Administration/Nursing in the Community
➤ See the general guidelines.
➤ Assess for nystagmus, ataxia, depression, irritability, tremor, changes in vision, and excessive fatigue or drowsiness. See the Patient Problems box in Chapter 54 on leukopenia.
➤ Gabapentin may be taken with food or on an empty stomach. However, instruct patients to follow specific guidelines given by the physician.
➤ Instruct patients taking doses three times a day not to allow more than 12 hours to elapse between any two doses.
➤ If patient has difficulty swallowing capsules, they may be opened and contents mixed with a small amount of applesauce or juice. Instruct the patient to prepare and consume a single dose at a time; doses should not be mixed in advance and saved.

Nursing Implications Summary—cont'd

lamotrigine

Drug Administration/Nursing in the Community

➤ See the general guidelines. Assess for ataxia, fever, changes in vision, and changes in affect, including depression, irritability, or anxiety.

➤ See the Patient Problems boxes in Chapter 54 on bleeding tendencies and leukopenia.

➤ Instruct the patient to report the development of skin rash immediately.

➤ Tell the patient that doses may be taken with meals or on an empty stomach.

Long-Acting Barbiturates (phenobarbital and primidone)

Drug Administration/Nursing in the Community

➤ See the general guidelines.

➤ Barbiturates are discussed in Chapter 57.

➤ Phenobarbital is usually effective at a serum concentration of 10 to 40 μg/ml. Primidone is usually effective at a serum concentration of 5 to 12 μg/ml.

➤ Review with families signs of intoxication or overdose, including slurred speech, ataxia, and vertigo. If these develop, instruct the patient to notify the physician.

Intravenous phenobarbital

➤ Dilute sterile powder slowly as directed on the package insert. Drug is also available in solution that must be diluted. Administer diluted dose at a rate of 1 gr (60 to 65 mg) over 1 minute. Monitor vital signs and respiration. Have a suction machine at the bedside and equipment for intubation and ventilatory support available. Do not leave the patient unattended until the patient is stable and alert.

Intramuscular phenobarbital

➤ Observe for respiratory depression 30 to 60 minutes after injection. Monitor blood pressure. Supervise ambulation. Keep siderails up.

tiagabine

Drug Administration/Nursing in the Community

➤ See the general guidelines.

➤ Assess for ataxia, confusion, depression, skin changes or itching, and nystagmus. Assess for paresthesias: burning, numbness, or tingling of the fingers, hands, or toes.

➤ Instruct the patient to take doses with meals or a snack.

topiramate

Drug Administration/Nursing in the Community

➤ See the general guidelines.

➤ Assess for ataxia, changes in vision, excessive weakness or fatigue, anorexia, weight loss, nausea, constipation, heartburn, changes in mood, breast pain in females, impotence, or decreased libido. See Patient Problems boxes in Chapter 54 on anemia and leukopenia.

➤ Instruct the patient to increase fluid intake by three to four 8-ounce glasses of water per day to help prevent kidney stones.

➤ Instruct the patient to swallow tablets whole. Breaking or chewing the tablet will produce a bitter taste in the mouth.

Dione Anticonvulsants (paramethadione and trimethadione)

Drug Administration

➤ See the general guidelines.

➤ Monitor CBC and differential, platelet count, liver function tests, serum creatinine and BUN levels, and urinalysis.

Nursing in the Community

➤ See the general guidelines.

➤ Tell the patient to report skin rashes or changes immediately. Because side effects are common, encourage patients to stay in close contact with the physician.

➤ Encourage patients to have ophthalmologic examinations every 6 months.

➤ See Patient Problems boxes on bleeding tendencies (Chapter 54) and agranulocytosis (Chapter 20).

➤ If photophobia develops, instruct the patient to avoid bright lights and to wear sunglasses when outside during the day.

diazepam

Drug Administration/Nursing in the Community

➤ See the general guidelines.

➤ This drug is discussed in Chapter 57.

➤ The rectal form, Diastat, is dispensed in prefilled applicators for one-time use. Review the manufacturer's patient instruction leaflet.

Treatment of Status Epilepticus

➤ This is a medical emergency.

➤ Maintain a patent airway. Turn patient's head to help prevent aspiration. In the hospital, suction the airway if necessary.

➤ Establish IV access, if possible. Administer IV medications as ordered. Do not leave patient unattended. Assess blood pressure and respirations. Have ventilatory support available. Attach patient to ECG monitor if available, especially if phenytoin or fosphenytoin is ordered.

➤ Pad siderails. Do not try to restrain the patient. If the patient has fallen to the floor, place a pad, small pillow, or even a piece of clothing under the head to keep the patient from injuring the head. Clear the area of sharp objects.

➤ Keep a record of sequence of events. When seizures end, reassure patient and family. Remain calm.

Other Drug Groups

➤ Benzodiazepines (clonazepam, clorazepate, and diazepam) are discussed in Chapter 57.

CHAPTER REVIEW

Application

1. Define epilepsy and list some of the known causes. What other conditions can precipitate seizures?
2. Describe tonic-clonic, absence myoclonic, psychomotor, and focal seizures. List the drug of choice for treating each type of epilepsy.
3. What is status epilepticus and how is it treated?
4. What considerations need to be made in beginning drug administration to control epilepsy?
5. What are the adverse effects and drug interactions of phenytoin?
6. What are the adverse effects of ethosuximide?
7. What are some of the special concerns regarding pregnancy and epilepsy?
8. Which benzodiazepines are used as anticonvulsants? For which seizure types are they effective?
9. What are the uses and side effects of carbamazepine?
10. Why is valproic acid a valuable anticonvulsant?
11. Describe the uses of the newest anticonvulsant drugs, including felbamate, gabapentin, lamotrigine, tiagabine, and topiramate.

Critical Thinking

1. What are some of the factors to monitor when a second anticonvulsant drug is added to the therapy?
2. How would you counsel a patient who has been seizure free for several years and wishes to discontinue medication?

References

Bradbury-Golas K, Carson L: Fosphenytoin: a feasible alternative to phenytoin for seizure therapy, *J Emerg Nurs* 22(5):431-432, 1996.

Cohen MR: New antiseizure medication: tricky dosing method, *Nursing* 27(2):14, 1997.

DiIorio C, Henry M: Self-management in persons with epilepsy, *J Neurosci Nurs* 27(6):338-343, 1995.

Faraji B, Yu P: Serum phenytoin levels of patients on gastrostomy tube feeding, *J Neurosci Nurs* 30(1):55-59, 1998.

McNew CD, Hunt S, Warner LS: How to help your patient with epilepsy, *Nursing* 27(9):56-62, 1997.

St. Dennis D, Synoground G: Anticonvulsant medications: new drug update . . . lamotrigine . . . felbamate . . . gabapentin . . . vigabatrin, *J Sch Nurs* 13(1):22, 1997.

Drugs to Treat Parkinson's Disease and Alzheimer's Disease

KEY TERMS

akinesia, p. 739
Alzheimer's disease, p. 745
bradykinesia, p. 739
dyskinesia, p. 744
Parkinson's disease, p. 739
rigidity, p. 739

KEY DRUGS ▼

levodopa, p. 743
tacrine, p. 746

OBJECTIVES

After studying this chapter, you should be able to do the following:

- *List three classic symptoms of Parkinson's disease, and explain the role of acetylcholine and dopamine in Parkinson's disease.*

- *Develop a nursing care plan for patients receiving anticholinergic drugs, amantadine, bromocriptine, levodopa or carbidopa-levodopa, pergolide, pramipexole, ropinirole, selegiline, or tolcapone to treat Parkinson's disease.*

- *Describe the rationale for administering tacrine or donepezil to patients with Alzheimer's disease.*

CHAPTER OVERVIEW

This chapter covers drug therapy for Parkinson's disease and Alzheimer's disease. Parkinson's disease is a progressive neurologic disorder of the extrapyramidal system caused by the degeneration of the dopaminergic neurons. This degeneration results in motor abnormalities. Alzheimer's disease is a progressive dementia characterized by the loss of short- and long-term memory.

THERAPEUTIC RATIONALE: PARKINSON'S DISEASE

Parkinson's disease is a progressive neurologic disease that results from the degeneration of neurons involved in motor control. This disorder most commonly appears in people in their late fifties and progresses over decades. Approximately 500,000 Americans have Parkinson's disease.

Parkinson's disease manifests as a movement disorder characterized by rigidity, akinesia, and tremor. **Rigidity** means that muscle tone is greatly increased but reflex activity is not. When a limb is passively forced through flexor or extensor movements, the muscular resistance alternately increases and decreases to give a cogwheel effect. **Akinesia** (no motion) refers to the difficulty the patient has in initiating any movement. The face has a masklike, fixed expression devoid of emotion.

Early in the course of Parkinson's disease, the difficulty in initiating movement is not as marked and is termed **bradykinesia** (slow motion). The disease typically starts with weakness in an arm or leg or a slight hand tremor. The tremor of Parkinson's disease is seen mostly in the limbs at rest and decreases with movement of the limbs.

Role of Acetylcholine and Dopamine

For many years, anticholinergic drugs such as atropine were used to decrease the tremor characteristics of Parkinson's disease; acetylcholine therefore seemed important in accounting for some symptoms. When the antipsychotic drugs were introduced in the 1950s, symptoms indistinguishable from those of Parkinson's disease began to appear in patients treated with these drugs. It is now known that this is because these drugs block receptors for the central nervous system (CNS) neurotransmitter dopamine.

Subsequently, patients with Parkinson's disease were shown to have degeneration of crucial dopaminergic neurons projecting from the substantia nigra to certain basal ganglia of the extrapyramidal system in the brain. This system is responsible for maintaining motor coordination at the CNS level.

Neurochemical Basis of Parkinson's Disease

The current understanding of Parkinson's disease is that it represents a deficiency in the neurotransmitter dopamine in certain basal ganglia. Dopamine from these neuronal tracts is believed to exert an inhibitory influence on cholinergic neurons of the extrapyramidal system controlling muscle tone. When dopamine is lacking, muscle tone increases because of the unopposed action of acetylcholine, resulting in muscular rigidity, inhibition of spontaneous movements, and tremor. The lack of dopamine is a result of a progressive degeneration of specific dopaminergic neurons. This degeneration can be caused by encephalitis, carbon-monoxide poisoning, manganese poisoning, cerebrovascular accident (stroke), or more commonly, unknown causes. This degeneration cannot be arrested. Symptoms appear when the dopamine level has dropped to 20% of normal.

Drug-Induced Parkinson's Disease

Certain drugs also can cause symptoms of Parkinson's disease. Reserpine (Serpasil), which depletes neuronal stores of dopamine and norepinephrine, and the antipsychotic drugs, which block dopamine receptors, are the usual causes of drug-induced Parkinson's disease. Symptoms depend on the presence of the drug, so lowering the dosage or discontinuing the drug eliminates the symptoms. Other drugs associated with parkinsonism include the antiemetic metoclopramide, the antiarrhythmic amiodarone, and the antihypertensive methyldopa.

Surgical Management of Parkinson's Disease

Pallidotomy has emerged as a surgical approach for managing severe symptoms of Parkinson's disease. It involves destroying a small portion of neural tissue in the globus pallidus, a paired structure of the brain that coordinates signals from the brain to control movement and sensation. The surgery is performed on one side of the brain and must be repeated for the second side, although many patients have benefits to both sides of the body after a single surgery. Patients continue taking medications for Parkinson's disease but usually require lower dosages.

Thalamotomy is also a surgical procedure for Parkinson's disease that is effective in reducing tremor.

THERAPEUTIC AGENTS: ANTIDYSKINETIC DRUGS TO TREAT PARKINSON'S DISEASE

The current rationale for the pharmacologic treatment of Parkinson's disease is to diminish the severity of motor symptoms by blocking the excessive action of acetylcholine or by replenishing the dopamine to return the balance of excitatory acetylcholine action and inhibitory dopamine action toward normal.

Antidyskinetic Drugs: General Characteristics

Mechanism of Action

Antidyskinetic drugs (Table 62-1) are anticholinergic agents that cross the blood-brain barrier and block central muscarinic cholinergic receptors.

Pharmacokinetics

These agents are given orally. The dosage is started low and increased gradually until the tremor and rigidity decrease or the side effects become prominent. When the drug is discontinued, the dosage should be decreased gradually to lessen a rebound appearance of the parkinsonian symptoms.

Uses

Anticholinergic drugs are administered early in the course of Parkinson's disease to lessen rigidity, bradykinesia, and tremor. Atropine and scopolamine, the classic anticholinergic drugs, were used to treat symptoms of Parkinson's disease for many years. Anticholinergic drugs used today are synthetic drugs that are centrally active and produce fewer peripheral side effects. These drugs include biperiden (Akineton), benztropine (Cogentin), ethopropazine (Parsidol), procyclidine (Kemadrin), and trihexyphenidyl (Artane, others). The antihistamine diphenhydramine (Benadryl) is also used in the treatment of Parkinson's disease for its anticholinergic properties.

An antidyskinetic is also the drug of choice for treatment of extrapyramidal reactions (akathisia, acute dystonia, and parkinsonism) caused by the antipsychotic drugs. Tardive dyskinesia is not reversed by anticholinergic drugs. These extrapyramidal reactions are described in Chapter 58.

Adverse Reactions, Toxicity, and Contraindications

Common side effects of the anticholinergic drugs are dry mouth, constipation, urinary retention, and blurred vision. Common mental effects include impairment of recent memory, confusion, insomnia, and restlessness. Mental effects can become serious, with the development of agitation, disorientation, delirium, paranoid reactions, or hallucinations. Mental problems are more common with elderly patients who have preexisting mental disturbances. Patients who have histories of glaucoma, particularly narrow-angle glaucoma, or some type of urinary or intestinal obstruction or tachycardia are not good candidates because anticholinergic drugs can aggravate any of these conditions. Characteristic actions of anticholinergic drugs are discussed in Chapter 11.

Interactions

The antidyskinetics increase the sedative effect of alcohol and other CNS-depressant drugs. They also have additive anticholinergic action with other drugs.

Table 62-1 Drugs to Treat Parkinsonism

Generic Name	Trade Name	Administration/Dosage	Comments
Anticholinergics			
benztropine mesylate	Cogentin*	ORAL: *Adults*—0.5-1 mg at bedtime initially; increase gradually to 4-6 mg if required. FDA pregnancy category C. *For drug-induced extrapyramidal reactions:* ORAL, INTRAMUSCULAR, INTRAVENOUS: *Adults*—1-4 mg 1 or 2 times/day.	To treat Parkinson's disease and drug-induced extrapyramidal reactions. Particularly effective in reversing acute dystonic reaction to antipsychotic drug.
biperiden hydrochloride	Akineton*	ORAL: *Adults*—2 mg 3 or 4 times/day; may increase dose up to 16 mg/day if required. FDA pregnancy category C. *For drug-induced extrapyramidal reactions:* ORAL: *Adults*—2 mg 1-3 times/day. INTRAMUSCULAR: *Adults*—2 mg repeated as often as every 30 min but no more than 4 doses in 24 hr.	To treat Parkinson's disease and drug-induced extrapyramidal reactions.
ethopropazine hydrochloride	Parsidol Parsitan†	ORAL: *Adults*—50 mg 1 or 2 times/day initially. Mild to moderate cases require 100-400 mg/day. Severe cases may require 500-600 mg/day. FDA pregnancy category C.	To treat Parkinson's disease. Phenothiazine with only anticholinergic effects and devoid of antidopaminergic effects.
procyclidine hydrochloride	Kemadrin* Procyclid†	ORAL: *Adults*—Initially, 2.5 mg 3 times/day after meals. Increase gradually to 5 mg three times daily, up to 20-30 mg/day if required. FDA pregnancy category C. *For drug-induced extrapyramidal reactions:* ORAL: *Adults*—2.5 mg 3 times/day; increase to 10-20 mg/day if required.	To treat Parkinson's disease and drug-induced extrapyramidal reactions.
trihexyphenidyl hydrochloride	Apo-Trihex† Artane* PMS Trihexyphenidyl† Various others	ORAL: *Adults*—2 mg 2 or 3 times/day. Increased to 15-20 mg/day (usually) or 40-50 mg/day (rarely) to control symptoms. Also available in extended-release capsules for twice daily dosage. FDA pregnancy category C. *For drug-induced parkinsonism:* ORAL: *Adults*—1 mg initially. Subsequent doses increased if symptoms do not decrease. Usual daily dose: 5-15 mg.	To treat Parkinson's disease and drug-induced extrapyramidal reactions.
Antihistamines			
diphenhydramine hydrochloride	Benadryl* Various others	ORAL: *Adults*—25 mg 3 times/day; increase to 50 mg 4 times/day if required. *For drug-induced extrapyramidal reactions:* INTRAMUSCULAR, INTRAVENOUS: *Adults*—10-50 mg; maximum: 400 mg/day. *Children*—5 mg/kg body weight intramuscularly daily; maximum: 300 mg in 24 hr.	To treat Parkinson's disease and drug-induced extrapyramidal reactions. Marked sedative effects.
Drugs Affecting Amount of Dopamine in Brain			
amantadine	Symadine Symmetrel*	ORAL: *Adults*—100 mg/day after breakfast for 5-7 days. Additional 100 mg may be added after lunch. Dosage reduced for patients with renal impairment. FDA pregnancy category C.	Antiviral agent that augments release of dopamine. Side effects are similar to those of anticholinergic drugs.
bromocriptine	Alti-Bromocriptine† Apo-Bromocriptine† Parlodel*	ORAL: *Adults*—Initially, 1.25 mg twice daily; increase every other week or monthly by 1.25-2.5 mg until benefits are achieved or adverse effects become intolerable. Maximum daily dose: 40 mg. FDA pregnancy category B.	Dopamine agonist. May be added to levodopa or carbidopa-levodopa therapy; occasionally replaces levodopa therapy.
carbidopa-levodopa	Sinemet*	ORAL: *Adults*—Initial daily dose should be ¼ daily dose of levodopa. Sinemet should be administered 8 hr after last levodopa dose and given in 3 or 4 doses/day. Patients not previously receiving levodopa are started with 10:100 mg (carbidopa:levodopa) 3 times/day; dosage is gradually increased as required. Also available in extended-release tablet for twice daily dosage. FDA pregnancy category C.	Carbidopa inhibits degradation of dopamine outside the central nervous system. Levodopa-carbidopa ratio is 10:1.
levodopa	Dopar Larodopa*	ORAL: *Adults*—Initially, 250 mg 2-4 times/day during waking hours with food. Increase dosage 100-750 mg every 3-7 days or more until desired control is achieved. Usually requires 4-6 g and 6-8 wk to achieve control. After several months to 1 yr, dosage may be lowered.	Levodopa is chemical precursor of dopamine.

*Available in Canada and the United States.
†Available in Canada only.

Continued

Table 62-1   Drugs to Treat Parkinsonism—cont'd

Generic Name	Trade Name	Administration/Dosage	Comments
Drugs Affecting Amount of Dopamine in Brain—cont'd			
pergolide mesylate	Permax*	ORAL: *Adults*—Initially, 0.05 mg/day for first 2 days; increase by 0.1-0.15 mg/day at 3-day intervals for 12 days until antiparkinson effect is optimum or maximum of 5 mg/day is reached. Can be administered in 3 divided doses daily. FDA pregnancy category B.	Pergolide has dopaminergic activity.
pramipexole	Mirapex	ORAL: *Adults*—Initially, 0.125 mg 3 times/day, increase each dose by 0.125 mg at weekly intervals to 1.15 mg 3 times/day.	New dopamine agonist to treat early Parkinson's disease or to add to therapy in advanced disease.
ropinirole	Requip*	ORAL: *Adults*—Initially, 0.25 mg 3 times/day; increase each dose by 0.25 mg at weekly intervals to 1 mg 3 times/day. FDA pregnancy category C.	New dopamine agonist to treat early Parkinson's disease or to add to therapy in advanced disease.
selegiline hydrochloride	Carbex Eldepryl Novo-Selegiline†	ORAL: *Adults*—5 mg 2 times/day, at breakfast and lunch. FDA pregnancy category C.	Inhibits degradation of dopamine by inhibiting monoamine oxidase B. May slow progress of Parkinson's disease. Also used as adjunct for patients who exhibit deterioration in response to carbidopa-levodopa therapy.
tolcapone	Tasmar	ORAL: Adults—100-200 mg 3 times/day, in conjunction with levodopa/carbidopa therapy.	Inhibits degradation of dopamine by inhibiting catechol-*O*-methyltransferase.

*Available in Canada and the United States.
†Available in Canada only.

Specific Antidyskinetic Drugs

benztropine

Benztropin (Cogentin) may be administered orally or by intravenous (IV) or intramuscular (IM) injection. When administered orally, the onset of action is 1 to 2 hours. The drug is active within a few minutes after injection. The duration of action is about 24 hours. Benztropine has slight antihistaminic and local anesthetic effects. It increases the efficacy of levodopa if administered concurrently.

biperiden

Biperiden (Akineton) may be administered orally or by IM or IV injection. The duration of action after IV injection is variable, from 1 to 8 hours. Biperiden has a slight effect on the cardiovascular and respiratory system.

diphenhydramine

Diphenhydramine (Benadryl) is an antihistamine with anticholinergic properties. It can be administered orally or by IM or IV injection. This drug can also be administered to children.

ethopropazine

Ethopropazine (Parsidol) is administered orally and has a duration of action of about 4 hours. Like benztropine, ethopropazine has slight antihistaminic and local anesthetic effect. It is also a phenothiazine derivative, and may cause changes in vision, jaundice, hematologic changes, and abnormalities in an electrocardiogram at high dosages.

procyclidine

Procyclidine (Kemadrin) is administered orally and has a duration of action of about 4 hours. It has a direct antispasmodic effect on smooth muscle. The action of procyclidine is more pronounced in reducing rigidity than in reducing tremor. Procyclidine enhances the effect of levodopa when administered concurrently.

trihexyphenidyl

Trihexyphenidyl (Artane) is administered orally. The onset of action is 1 hour, and the duration of action is 6 to 12 hours. For patients stabilized with the drug, an extended-release capsule formulation (Artane Sequels) is available for twice-a-day administration. Trihexyphenidyl has a direct antispasmodic effect on smooth muscle. Although small doses have a sedative effect, large doses can produce excitement. Trihexyphenidyl enhances the effect of levodopa when administered concurrently.

THERAPEUTIC AGENTS: DRUGS AFFECTING THE AMOUNT OF DOPAMINE IN BRAIN

Several drugs are used in the treatment of Parkinson's disease to maintain or increase the level of dopamine in the brain. These drugs are listed in Table 62-1. Amantadine and selegiline may be used early in the disease, but other drugs are reserved for use after disability has begun because they are effective only for a few years. These drugs treat only the symptoms of the disease but do not alter its course. However, some studies indicate that selegiline may slow the progression of Parkinson's disease. This drug is now commonly started when the diagnosis is made.

New drugs that act as dopamine agonists (pramipexole and ropinirole) or inhibit the degradation of dopamine (tolcapone) have been released. Their role in the management of Parkinson's disease will evolve with experience.

amantadine

Amantadine (Symmetrel) is an antiviral agent that also has been found effective in reducing the severity of symptoms of Parkinson's disease when used alone or with an anticholinergic drug. Amantadine promotes the release and inhibits the reuptake of dopamine from the central neurons, an action unrelated to its antiviral action.

Amantadine is often used in the early stages of the disease to control parkinsonian symptoms. It has the advantages of being effective when administered as a single daily dose and of having few side effects. Side effects seen include dizziness, nervousness, inability to concentrate, ataxia, slurred speech, insomnia, lethargy, blurred vision, dry mouth, gastrointestinal (GI) upset, and rash. Amantadine may also be used with anticholinergic drugs or with levodopa because it enhances the effectiveness of these other drugs and allows a reduction of their dosage.

bromocriptine

Bromocriptine (Parlodel) mimics the action of dopamine in the brain. It is an alternative to levodopa when levodopa is contraindicated, is not well tolerated, or does not produce a response. Bromocriptine has a duration of action similar to that of levodopa and may be added to levodopa or carbidopa-levodopa therapy for patients who show symptoms of fluctuating doses such as dystonia and muscle cramps. Dosages of bromocriptine must be individualized. Transient dizziness and nausea are common. Hypotension, abdominal pain, blurred vision, double vision, and vasospasm of the fingers and toes in response to cold also occasionally occur.

carbidopa-levodopa

Carbidopa (Atamet, Sinemet) inhibits the conversion of levodopa to dopamine. Because carbidopa cannot enter the CNS, only peripheral conversion is inhibited. This means that levodopa is converted to dopamine only in the brain, so the presence of carbidopa lowers the dose of levodopa required by 75%. Because the emetic effects of levodopa reflect peripheral dopamine concentrations, the incidence of nausea and vomiting is reduced greatly with carbidopa-levodopa combination. Carbidopa is available only in a fixed-ratio combination with levodopa.

▼ levodopa

Mechanism of Action

Levodopa (Dopar, Larodopa) is the chemical precursor of dopamine, and unlike dopamine, it readily crosses the blood-brain barrier. It is converted to dopamine by the enzyme dopa decarboxylase.

Pharmacokinetics

About 95% of a dose of levodopa is converted to dopamine in the periphery rather than in the brain, and the high plasma concentration of dopamine is responsible for the nausea and cardiac effects occurring with this therapy. For these reasons, levodopa is almost always given in combination with carbidopa (see previous section).

Levodopa is taken orally, and the peak effect is seen 1 to 2 hours later. Dosage is adjusted up or down gradually every 2 to 3 days to lessen the incidence of nausea and to avoid precipitating side effects.

Uses

Levodopa is prescribed when the drugs used in the early stages of Parkinson's disease—anticholinergics, amantadine, or selegiline—no longer control symptoms. Levodopa therapy does not stop the progression of Parkinson's disease, but it relieves the symptoms and dramatically improves ability to function.

Adverse Reactions, Toxicity, and Contraindications

Emetic Effects. Dopamine is the neurotransmitter for the chemoreceptor trigger zone of the medulla and thus produces nausea, vomiting, and anorexia. To create tolerance to this emetic action, levodopa therapy must be initiated by starting with low dosages that are gradually increased. A snack high in protein also helps prevent nausea. Antiemetics from the phenothiazine class should not be used because they block the therapeutic action of dopamine. Trimethobenzamide (Tigan) may be taken early in the morning to control nausea.

Mental Effects. Additional effects typically noted after the start of levodopa therapy include increased alertness, sense of well-being, and increased libido. These effects are attributed to behavioral roles of dopamine in the brain. Further mental changes may occur with prolonged therapy. Euphoria, restlessness, anxiety, irritability, hyperactivity, insomnia, and vivid dreams often occur. Patients occasionally may become paranoid and may experience psychotic episodes. About 40% of patients become depressed, with or without suicidal tendencies. These mental changes are usually reversed by lowering the dosage. Clozapine may be effective in treating the depression, hallucinations, and confusion of Parkinson's disease.

Cardiovascular Effects. Another side effect sometimes seen at the start of levodopa therapy is orthostatic hypotension. The mechanism is unknown but is believed to be a CNS effect rather than a peripheral effect. This hypotension tends to decrease with time. An increase in heart rate and force of contraction may also be apparent at the start of therapy. These cardiac actions are caused by the direct action of dopamine on the heart. Cardiac arrhythmias may develop and must be controlled by appropriate medication.

Other Side Effects. Additional side effects of levodopa therapy may be GI effects, including bleeding, difficulty in swallowing, and a burning sensation of the tongue. Respiratory effects such as cough, hoarseness, and disturbed breathing may appear. Because of these side effects, levodopa therapy is used cautiously for patients with a history of heart disease, asthma, emphysema, or peptic ulcer. Problems in urination from incontinence to retention may arise. Blurred vision or dilated pupils may be caused by levodopa. Levodopa therapy is not considered for patients with narrow-angle glaucoma and only with careful monitoring for patients with chronic (wide-angle) glaucoma.

Laboratory Tests. Hepatic, hematopoietic, cardiovascular, and renal function tests are performed periodically on patients receiving long-term levodopa therapy because many laboratory test values are high in patients receiving levodopa therapy, and only careful monitoring can determine whether a real problem exists. Hematocrit and white blood cell counts may be lowered by levodopa therapy, but therapy is discontinued only when abnormally low counts are found. Therapy is not initiated in patients with blood disorders.

Dyskinesia. After prolonged therapy with levodopa, abnormal involuntary movements (**dyskinesia**) alternating with a sudden lapse in symptom control (the on-off phenomenon) may appear. Dyskinesia usually comprises abnormal involuntary movements of the mouth, tongue, face, or neck. Dyskinesia usually appears 1 to 2 hours after the latest dose of levodopa and represents a mild levodopa toxicity. "End-of-dose" akinesia also may occur. This means that the akinesia appears just before a new dose is to be taken and usually can be avoided by increasing frequency of administration.

Interactions

Drugs that reduce the effectiveness of levodopa include the antipsychotic drugs, the rauwolfia alkaloids, pheny-

toin, papaverine, methyldopa, metoclopramide, and pyridoxine. A hypertensive crisis may be precipitated when levodopa and monoamine oxidase inhibitors are given concurrently.

pergolide

Pergolide (Permax) has direct dopaminergic action. It is more potent than bromocriptine and has a longer half-life. Overall effectiveness of pergolide with carbidopa-levodopa therapy is similar to bromocriptine. Side effects are similar to those of bromocriptine. The most common reactions are hallucinations, nausea, dry mouth, lightheadedness, and dyskinesia.

pramipexole

Pramipexole (Mirapex) is a new dopamine agonist for the control of Parkinson's disease. It is targeted to patients with early disease as well as for patients receiving levodopa therapy. The concurrent administration of pramipexole lowers the dosage of levodopa required. Pramipexole is administered orally, titrating the dosage upward over 2 months. Patients with renal impairment require reduced dosages.

ropinirole

Ropinirole (Requip) is a new dopamine agonist for the control of Parkinson's disease. It is targeted to patients with early disease as well as for patients receiving levodopa therapy. The concurrent administration of ropinirole lowers the dosage of levodopa required. Ropinirole is administered orally, titrating the dosage upward over 4 weeks. The drug is extensively metabolized by the liver and metabolites excreted in the urine.

selegiline

Selegiline (formerly deprenyl) (Eldepryl) inhibits the enzyme monoamine oxidase B, which degrades dopamine in the brain. Because dopamine is not rapidly degraded in the presence of selegiline, the duration of action and dose of levodopa is reduced. Early morning stiffness and end-of-dose symptoms are decreased.

There are some indications that selegiline may slow the progression of Parkinson's disease. It is often administered in the early stages of the disease as a preventive measure, although early symptoms are in general not well controlled by selegiline alone. In advanced cases of the disease, selegiline lessens the wearing off effects of levodopa or carbidopa-levodopa therapy.

Selegiline should not be administered with meperidine and other opioids or with monoamine oxidase inhibitors or serotonin uptake inhibitors.

tolcapone

Tolcapone (Tasmar) is an inhibitor of the enzyme catecholamine-*O*-methyltransferase (COMT), an enzyme that inactivates catecholamines, including dopamine. Tolcapone is used as an adjunct to levodopa and carbidopa for the treatment of Parkinson's diseases. This drug provides a more sustained level of levodopa in the brain, thereby increasing the "good functioning time" for patients receiving levodopa therapy.

Nursing Process Overview

Drugs to Treat Parkinson's Disease

Assessment

Perform a baseline patient assessment, including vital signs, joint movement, amount of tremor, affect and objective signs of the disease, and ability to ambulate and to perform activities of daily living. Because this is often a disease of the elderly, obtain a baseline view of other known health problems such as hypertension, diabetes, and cardiovascular or renal disease.

Nursing Diagnoses

- Altered bowel elimination: constipation caused by drug side effects
- Risk for urinary retention
- Risk for body image disturbance related to dyskinesia or other drug side effects

Patient Outcomes

The patient will describe methods to prevent constipation. The patient will recognize urinary retention and contact the health care team if it develops. The patient will share feelings about body image changes.

Planning/Implementation

Include the patient in the discussion of the goals of therapy. Monitor for subjective and objective improvement and for drug side effects. Improvement in symptoms should outweigh the discomfort of side effects. Some patients find the side effects from a drug are worse than if the disease is untreated, at least at some stages in its progression. Before discharge, refer the patient to social service, vocational rehabilitation, visiting nurse, and other agencies, if appropriate.

Evaluation

Before discharge and at regular intervals during therapy, ensure that the patient understands the prescribed drugs and dosages being taken, how to take the drugs correctly, what the expected goals of therapy are, what drug side effects may occur, how to treat these effects, and when to notify the physician. Verify that the patient can explain any necessary dietary or vitamin restrictions.

THERAPEUTIC RATIONALE: ALZHEIMER'S DISEASE

Alzheimer's disease is a disease of progressive mental degeneration. It appears primarily in persons older than 65 years of age, although some genetic forms have been identified with early onset. About 5% of persons older than 65 years have Alzheimer's disease—about 4 million Americans. Because the population as a whole is aging, the number of persons with Alzheimer's disease will increase dramatically in coming decades.

The normal progression of Alzheimer's disease is a gradual decline in cognitive abilities over 7 to 10 years. Disturbances in judgment, memory, and language are the earliest manifestations. Alzheimer's disease is the most common cause of dementia, accounting for about 50% of cases. *Dementia* refers to a decline in intellectual functioning severe enough to interfere with a person's normal daily activities and social relationships. The next level of loss is control of the bladder and bowel. Eventually patients are unable to walk, and finally unable to swallow.

At death, brains of those with Alzheimer's disease show abnormal plaques in the affected areas and a shrunken brain. Research has been directed at understanding what causes these abnormal plaques. Although knowledge is incomplete, these plaques are composed of a protein fragment called beta amyloid that folds abnormally into strands that accumulate. Through a process not understood, this induces another protein, tau, to form into abnormal strands in the neuron. Because tau is important to maintaining structures for a normal neuron, this is abnormality is believed to cause neuronal death.

The genetic basis of certain proteins associated with Alzheimer's plaques is being studied. An increased prevalence of the gene for apolipoprotein E_4 has been found in patients with Alzheimer's disease. How this variant of the cholesterol-carrying protein is involved in the pathology of Alzheimer's disease is unclear. Genetic studies of families with early-onset Alzheimer's disease have identified a gene for amyloid precursor protein and two presenilin genes (which may affect amyloid production) as associated with this early-onset form of Alzheimer's disease. In addition, many individuals with Down's syndrome (trisomy 21) develop Alzheimer's disease by the time they are 40 years old. These genetic results identify new paths to investigate for the neuropathology of Alzheimer's disease.

THERAPEUTIC AGENTS: DRUGS TO TREAT ALZHEIMER'S DISEASE

Pharmacologic treatment for Alzheimer's disease is lacking because the cause of the disease is still unknown. Cholinergic drugs have been tried because acetylcholine appears to be the primary neurotransmitter affected by the disease process. Two acetylcholinesterase inhibitors have been specifically approved to improve cognitive functions in the early stages of Alzheimer's disease and are listed in Table 62-2.

Clinical trials are under way to determine whether antiinflammatory therapy with prednisone, antioxidant therapy with vitamin E, or administration of estrogen supplements will slow progress of Alzheimer's disease. Some evidence for the amelioration effects of these agents has been obtained in clinical epidemiologic studies. In addition, patients with Alzheimer's disease are subject to sleep disorders, depression, psychotic behavior, and anxiety. These symptoms are treated with appropriate drugs discussed in other chapters.

donepezil
Mechanism of Action
Donepezil (Aricept) is a reversible inhibitor of acetylcholinesterase.

Pharmacokinetics
Donepezil is well absorbed and highly bound to plasma proteins. It is administered once a day at bedtime to minimize side effects. It is extensively metabolized by the liver, and at least two of the major metabolites are active. Elimination is slow, with a half-life of about 70 hours.

Uses
Donepezil is used to treat the mild to moderate dementia of Alzheimer's disease.

Adverse Reactions, Toxicity, and Contraindications
The most common side effects are nausea and diarrhea. Unlike tacrine, donepezil is not associated with hepatotoxicity or elevated transaminase levels. Donepezil can slow the heart rate through its vagotonic effect.

Interactions
Donepezil has not been shown to affect liver metabolizing enzymes or to displace other protein-bound drugs. Drugs that inhibit liver metabolizing enzymes such as ketoconazole and quinidine can inhibit the metabolism of donepezil.

▼ tacrine
Mechanism of Action
Tacrine (Cognex) is a centrally acting acetylcholinesterase inhibitor that also blocks potassium channels and inhibits the reuptake of norepinephrine, serotonin, and dopamine.

Pharmacokinetics
Tacrine is rapidly absorbed. It is extensively removed by first-pass metabolism in the liver and must be administered four times daily. The major metabolite has central cholinergic activity.

Uses
The major indication for tacrine is for symptomatic treatment of mild to moderate dementia in Alzheimer's disease. Efficacy is limited.

Adverse Reactions, Toxicity, and Contraindications
The side effects of tacrine include ataxia, loss of appetite, nausea, vomiting, and diarrhea. About 20% of patients are unable to tolerate tacrine because of the cholinergic side effects, generally GI distress.

Hepatotoxicity limits the use of tacrine. Up to 50% of patients develop elevated levels of liver enzymes. When the dosage is reduced or the drug discontinued, liver function studies commonly return to normal within 6 weeks.

Interactions
Tacrine interferes with the cytochrome P-450 system, leading to elevated levels of theophylline. Cimetidine can increase the plasma concentrations of tacrine. Because tacrine increases gastric acid secretion, it can increase the gastric irritation and potential for bleeding of nonsteroidal antiinflammatory drugs (NSAIDs). Smoking decreases the plasma level of tacrine by two-thirds.

Table 62-2 Drug Therapy for Alzheimer's Disease

Generic Name	Trade Name	Administration/Dosage	Comments
donepezil	Aricept	ORAL: *Adults*—5 mg once a day at bedtime. FDA pregnancy category C.	Some patients have additional benefit from a 10-mg dose, but the incidence of cholinergic side effects increases.
tacrine	Cognex	ORAL: *Adults*—10 mg 4 times/day initially. If drug is tolerated and transaminase levels do not increase, may increase dose to 20 mg 4 times/day and at 6-wk intervals up to 40 mg 4 times/day. FDA pregnancy category C.	Dose must be stopped if transaminase serum value exceeds 5 times normal. May start again if transaminase levels did not exceed 10 times normal and they return to normal.

Nursing Implications Summary

GENERAL GUIDELINES: PATIENT RECEIVING DRUGS FOR PARKINSON'S DISEASE

➤ Assess severity of symptoms, including muscle control and movement, ability to perform activities of daily living, dysphagia, posture, and gait.

Nursing in the Community

➤ Review the anticipated benefits and possible side effects of drug therapy.

➤ Teach the patient and family that several weeks to months of therapy may be needed in some cases to obtain full benefit of drug therapy. Provide emotional support.

➤ Parkinson's disease is primarily a problem of older adults. However, if a premenopausal female develops Parkinson's disease, counsel as needed about contraceptives. These drugs should not be used during pregnancy without consulting the physician.

➤ Point out to the family that confusion is often a drug side effect in the elderly patient and should not be attributed to Parkinson's disease until fully evaluated.

➤ Warn the patient not to discontinue these drugs suddenly. A patient should inform all health care providers of all drugs being taken. Over-the-counter (OTC) medications should be avoided unless approved by the physician.

➤ Counsel the patient to avoid the use of alcohol unless permitted in small amounts by the physician.

Other Drug Groups

➤ Anticholinergic drugs (benztropine, biperiden, ethopropazine, procyclidine, and trihexyphenidyl) are discussed in Chapters 11 and 23.

➤ Intravenous benztropine: May be given undiluted, at a rate of 1 mg over at least 1 minute.

➤ See the Patient Problems boxes on dry mouth (Chapter 23), constipation (Chapter 24), and orthostatic hypotension (Chapter 13).

➤ Antihistamines (diphenhydramine) are discussed in Chapter 29.

➤ Phenothiazines are discussed in Chapter 58.

amantadine

Drug Administration

➤ Assess mental status regularly. Be alert to signs of increasing depression, including lethargy, apathy, decreased appetite, and loss of interest in personal appearance (see Box 59-1). Be alert to suicidal tendencies.

➤ Monitor intake and output, daily weight, blood pressure (BP), and pulse. Auscultate lung sounds. Inspect for edema and skin changes.

➤ Assess for urinary retention. Suggest patients void before taking drug doses.

➤ Monitor complete blood cell count (CBC) and differential.

Nursing in the Community

➤ See the general guidelines. This drug is also used as an antiviral agent.

➤ See the Patient Problems boxes on orthostatic hypotension (Chapter 13), dry mouth (Chapter 23), and constipation (Chapter 24).

➤ Warn the patient to avoid driving or operating hazardous equipment if drowsiness or dizziness develops and to notify the physician.

➤ Capsules may be opened and contents mixed with a small amount of food or fluid for ease in taking dose, although a liquid preparation is also available.

➤ Instruct patients using the liquid form to measure doses with the measuring device supplied by the pharmacist.

➤ Tell the patient that livedo reticularis (bluish or purplish mottling of the skin) may appear during the first year of therapy and may take several weeks to subside when therapy is discontinued.

➤ Instruct the patient to avoid alcohol unless approved by the physician.

bromocriptine

➤ Bromocriptine is discussed in Chapter 65.

carbidopa-levodopa Combination

Drug Administration/Nursing in the Community

➤ No specific side effects have been attributed to carbidopa.

➤ Review with the patient the information about levodopa.

levodopa

Drug Administration

➤ Monitor neuromuscular, neurologic, and mental status regularly.

➤ Monitor BP and pulse, intake and output, and weight.

➤ Check stools for presence of occult blood. Inspect for skin changes.

➤ Monitor CBC and differential, platelet count, blood urea nitrogen (BUN) and serum creatinine, and liver function tests.

Nursing in the Community

➤ See the general guidelines.

➤ See the Patient Problems boxes on constipation (Chapter 24), orthostatic hypotension (Chapter 13), and dry mouth (Chapter 23).

➤ Warn the male patient that priapism has been reported and to notify the physician if it develops.

➤ Tell the patient that sweat may be darker in color while this drug is taken, and urine may be dark, especially if left standing.

➤ Instruct the patient to take doses shortly after meals or a snack to reduce gastric irritation (15 minutes after).

➤ Instruct the patient to swallow carbidopa/levodopa extended-release tablets whole, without chewing or crushing them. The tablets may be broken in half if approved by the physician. If the patient has difficulty swallowing levodopa capsules or tablets, consult the pharmacist about preparing a liquid form.

Continued

Nursing Implications Summary—cont'd

➤ Tell diabetic patients to monitor blood glucose levels carefully because tests for urinary glucose and ketone levels may be inaccurate.

➤ There are many side effects of levodopa therapy. Encourage the patient and family to report any new or unexpected findings.

➤ Pyridoxine (vitamin B_6) may reduce the effectiveness of levodopa. Instruct the patient not to take any vitamin preparations without consulting the physician. Tell the patient to limit intake of foods high in pyridoxine; see the Dietary Considerations box in Chapter 17 on vitamins.

➤ An on-off phenomenon has been reported with this drug. After long use, some patients report the loss of ability to move. This effect may last for a few minutes to several hours. The patient can then move as before. This problem may occur repeatedly. If it develops, notify the physician.

pergolide
Drug Administration/Nursing in the Community

➤ See the general guidelines.

➤ Assess for common side effects, including hallucinations, nausea, dry mouth, light-headedness, and dyskinesia. Monitor weight. See the Patient Problems box in Chapter 23 on dry mouth.

➤ Encourage the patient to take doses with meals or a snack to lessen gastric irritation.

➤ Assess the patient for worsening symptoms if pergolide and levodopa are administered concurrently.

➤ Monitor the BP. Dosages are increased slowly to lessen the degree of hypotension. Encourage patients to take doses at night or to lie down after taking doses to lessen problems with orthostatic hypotension.

➤ Monitor the patient with a history of cardiac arrhythmias carefully when beginning pergolide therapy; increases in atrial premature contractions and sinus tachycardia have been reported.

pramipexole
Drug Administration/Nursing in the Community

➤ See the general guidelines.

➤ Assess for insomnia, nausea, excessive fatigue, hallucinations, and changes in vision. Monitor weight. See the Patient Problems boxes on orthostatic hypotension (Chapter 13), dry mouth (Chapter 23), and constipation (Chapter 24).

➤ Instruct the patient to take doses with meals or a snack to lessen the chance of nausea.

➤ Caution the patient to avoid driving or operating hazardous equipment if drowsiness, dizziness, or visual changes develop and to notify the physician.

ropinirole
Drug Administration/Nursing in the Community

➤ See the general guidelines.

➤ Assess for confusion or depression, edema, nausea, excessive fatigue, hallucinations, and changes in vision. Monitor weight and vital signs. See the Patient Problems boxes on orthostatic hypotension (Chapter 13), dry mouth (Chapter 23), and constipation (Chapter 24).

➤ Instruct the patient to take doses on a full or empty stomach.

➤ Caution the patient to avoid driving or operating hazardous equipment if drowsiness, dizziness, excessive weakness, or visual changes develop and to notify the physician.

selegiline
Drug Administration/Nursing in the Community

➤ See the Patient Problems boxes on orthostatic hypotension (Chapter 13) and dry mouth (Chapter 23). Assess for confusion, dizziness, and insomnia.

➤ Instruct the patient to avoid driving or operating hazardous equipment if dizziness or syncope develops.

➤ Monitor the BP.

➤ At dosages of 10 mg or less a day, there are no dietary restrictions with this drug. At dosages greater than 20 mg/day, the patient should avoid foods high in tyramine. See the Dietary Considerations box in Chapter 59 on monoamine oxidase inhibitors and tyramine. In addition, instruct the patient taking more than 20 mg/day to avoid alcohol, large quantities of caffeine, and OTC cold and cough medications.

tolcapone
Drug Administration/Nursing in the Community

➤ See the general guidelines.

➤ Monitor liver function tests.

➤ Assess for insomnia, nausea, diarrhea, excessive fatigue, hallucinations, and changes in vision. Monitor weight. See the Patient Problems boxes on orthostatic hypotension (Chapter 13), dry mouth (Chapter 23), and constipation (Chapter 24).

➤ Instruct the patient to take doses with meals or a snack to lessen the chance of nausea.

➤ Caution the patient to avoid driving or operating hazardous equipment if drowsiness, dizziness, or visual changes develop and to notify the physician.

➤ Tolcapone may cause the urine to turn bright yellow.

DRUGS FOR ALZHEIMER'S DISEASE
tacrine
Drug Administration/Nursing in the Community

➤ Assess mental and cognitive status. Monitor vital signs and BP.

➤ Teach the patient to take doses on an empty stomach, 1 hour before or 2 hours after meals.

➤ Emphasize the importance of returning for regular follow-up. Blood work must be monitored frequently and regularly for best effect of this drug.

➤ Tell the patient to avoid driving or operating hazardous equipment if dizziness, clumsiness, or unsteadiness develops.

Nursing Implications Summary—cont'd

➤ Remind the patient to keep all health care providers informed of all drugs being used. Instruct the patient not to take any drugs without first checking with the physician and not to discontinue tacrine without first discussing it with the physician.

➤ For missed doses, instruct the patient to take the dose as soon as remembered, unless within 2 hours of the next dose; then omit. Do not double up missed doses.

➤ Tell the patient to avoid smoking while taking tacrine.

donepezil
Drug Administration/Nursing in the Community

➤ Assess mental and cognitive status. Monitor weight, vital signs, and BP.

➤ Assess for diarrhea, nausea, vomiting, insomnia, muscle cramps, headache, tremor, and skin changes. See the Patient Problems box in Chapter 13 on orthostatic hypotension.

➤ Instruct the patient to take doses in the evening, before going to bed. Doses can be taken on a full or empty stomach.

CHAPTER REVIEW

Application

1. Describe the physical characteristics seen in Parkinson's disease.
2. What is the neurochemical defect in Parkinson's disease? How do some drugs mimic this defect?
3. Why are anticholinergic drugs, antihistaminic drugs, and amantadine effective in treating symptoms of Parkinson's disease? What are major side effects of these drug classes?
4. What is the rationale for administering levodopa to treat the symptoms of Parkinson's disease? What role does carbidopa play?

5. What are the side effects of levodopa?
6. What is the rationale for administering tacrine to patients with Alzheimer's disease?

Critical Thinking

1. Prepare a care plan for the patient with Parkinson's disease who is about to begin levodopa therapy.
2. What would you tell the family of a patient with Alzheimer's disease to expect from therapy with tacrine? How would tacrine help the depressed patient with Alzheimer's disease?

References

Culp K, et al: Screening for acute confusion in elderly long-term care residents, *J Neurosci Nurs* 29(2):86-88, 95-100, 1997.

Lusis SA: Pathophysiology and management of idiopathic Parkinson's disease, *J Neurosci Nurs* 29(1):24-31, 1997.

Centrally Acting Skeletal Muscle Relaxants

OBJECTIVES

After studying this chapter, you should be able to do the following:

- *Develop a nursing care plan for the patient receiving a centrally acting skeletal muscle relaxant such as diazepam, baclofen, or dantrolene.*
- *Develop a nursing care plan for the patient receiving drug therapy for muscle spasms.*

CHAPTER OVERVIEW

This chapter discusses drug therapy for spasticity and muscle spasms. Spasticity is a common symptom of upper motor neuron lesions. Muscle spasm is an involuntary contraction of a muscle or group of muscles. This condition can be alleviated with appropriate drug therapy.

THERAPEUTIC RATIONALE: SPASTICITY

Spasticity results from the loss of inhibitory tone in the polysynaptic pathways of the spinal cord, causing loss of fine control of motor activity.

Because the inhibitory tone is controlled largely by neural pathways from the brain, spasticity is seen in patients in whom these inhibitory pathways have been disrupted through spinal cord injury, strokes, multiple sclerosis, or cerebral palsy. The patient with spasticity demonstrates exaggerated reflexes (spinal spasticity) or inappropriate posture (cerebral spasticity).

THERAPEUTIC AGENTS: DRUGS TO TREAT SPASTICITY

Drugs for the treatment of spasticity are presented in Table 63-1. Drugs found to be effective in relieving some cases of spasticity are diazepam (Valium), baclofen (Lioresal), dantrolene (Dantrium), and tizanidine (Zanaflex). Diazepam and baclofen are believed to act within the spinal cord to restore some inhibitory tone, but dantrolene is unique in acting within the muscle. Tizanidine has a central activity on motor tone.

diazepam

Diazepam (Valium) is a benzodiazepine commonly prescribed as an antianxiety drug (see Chapter 57). Although its action as an antianxiety drug results from depression of the reticular-activating system, diazepam also enhances inhibitory descending pathways in the spinal cord governing muscular activity, apparently by enhancing the activity of the inhibitory neurotransmitter gamma-aminobutyric acid (GABA). Diazepam is effective in relieving spasticity associated with spinal cord injury, multiple sclerosis, and cerebral injury and in treating muscle spasms. Relatively high dosages are required to relieve muscle hyperactivity, and drowsiness and ataxia may be prominent side effects.

▼ baclofen

Baclofen (Lioresal) is an analog of the inhibitory neurotransmitter GABA, and although the effect elicited is that desired of a GABA agonist, this mechanism of action cannot be demonstrated in the laboratory. Baclofen is most effective in relieving spasticity caused by spinal cord injury and is less effective in relieving spasticity from brain damage. Side effects include drowsiness, ataxia, and occasional gastrointestinal (GI) upset.

A new delivery system for baclofen is under development for delivery directly into the spinal fluid. A pump is

Table 63-1   Centrally Acting Skeletal Muscle Relaxants

Generic Name	Trade Name	Administration/Dosage	Comments
Drugs for Spasticity			
baclofen	Apo-Baclofen† Lioresal* PMS-Baclofen†	ORAL: *Adults*—Begin with 5 mg 3 times/day. Increase by 5 mg 3 times/day every 3 days as required; maximum: 80 mg/day.	Diminishes reflex responses by decreasing transmission in spinal cord.
dantrolene	Dantrium*	ORAL: *Adults*—25 mg 1 or 2 times/day. Increase to 25 mg 3-4 times/day, then 50-100 mg 4 times/day as required. Increments are adjusted every 4-7 days. *Children*—0.5 mg/kg body weight 2 times/day, then increase by increments of 0.5 mg/kg every 4-7 days as needed. Maximum: 400 mg/day.	Acts peripherally to inhibit calcium release within muscle.
diazepam	Valium* Various others	ORAL: *Adults*—2-10 mg 3-4 times/day. *Children*—1-2.5 mg or 0.04-0.2 mg/kg body weight 3 or 4 times/day. INTRAVENOUS: *Adults*—2-10 mg injected no faster than 5 mg (1 ml)/min. Do not mix or dilute with other solutions, drugs, or intravenous fluids. *Children*—0.04-0.2 mg/kg body weight. Maximum: 0.6 mg/kg in 8 hr.	Benzodiazepines also used to treat spasticity or muscle spasm.
tizanidine	Zanaflex	ORAL: *Adults*—8 mg every 6-8 hr initially, increasing with 2-mg increments as needed. Maximum single dose is 12 mg and 36 mg/day. FDA pregnancy category C.	New drug for intermittent management of spasticity.
Drugs for Muscle Spasms			
carisoprodol	Soma* Vanadom	ORAL: *Adults*—350 mg 4 times/day. *Children 5-12 yr*—6.25 mg/kg body weight 4 times/day.	Related to meprobamate. May cause drowsiness.
chlorphenesin	Maolate	ORAL: *Adults*—800 mg 3 times/day. Can decrease to 400 mg 4 times/day as improvement is noted.	May cause drowsiness and dizziness.
chlorzoxazone	Paraflex Parafon Forte DSC Relaxone	ORAL: *Adults*—250-750 mg 3 or 4 times/day. *Children*—20 mg/kg body weight in 3 or 4 divided doses.	May cause drowsiness. Watch for signs of liver damage (rare).
cyclobenzaprine	Cycloflex Flexeril*	ORAL: *Adults*—10 mg 3 times/day up to maximum total dose of 60 mg. FDA pregnancy category B.	Related to tricyclic antidepressants. Does not cause drug dependence but may cause changes in liver.
diazepam	Valium*	Same as for diazepam to treat spasticity.	
metaxalone	Skelaxin	ORAL: *Adults*—800 mg 3 or 4 times/day.	Monitor patient for development of liver toxicity.
methocarbamol	Carbacot Robaxin* Skelex	ORAL: *Adults*—1.5-2 g 4 times/day for 2-3 days. Decrease to 1 g 4 times/day for maintenance. INTRAMUSCULAR: *Adults*—500 mg every 8 hr, alternating between gluteal muscles. INTRAVENOUS: *Adults*—1-3 g/day for maximum of 3 days. Inject no faster than 300 mg (3 ml)/min.	Not recommended for patients with epilepsy. Do not administer parenterally to patients with impaired renal function because drug vehicle may worsen kidney function.
orphenadrine	Disipal† Flexoject Norflex* Various others	ORAL: *Adults*—100 mg twice daily. INTRAMUSCULAR, INTRAVENOUS: *Adults*—60 mg twice daily. FDA pregnancy category C.	Anticholinergic effects are common side effects. Not for patients with glaucoma, myasthenia gravis, tachycardia, or urinary retention.

*Available in Canada and the United States.
†Available in Canada only.

implanted into the abdomen to release the drug through a catheter into the spinal fluid. This system allows lower dosages to be effective with fewer side effects. The system is intended for patients with cerebral palsy.

dantrolene

Dantrolene (Dantrium) is not a centrally acting skeletal muscle relaxant but instead affects the muscle directly by interfering with the intracellular release of calcium necessary to initiate contraction. At therapeutic dosages, this effect is limited to skeletal muscle and is not seen in the heart or smooth muscle. Dantrolene causes muscular weakness and can worsen the overall condition if the patient already has marginal strength. Dantrolene is most useful for the patient whose spasticity causes pain, discomfort, or limits functional rehabilitation. In addition to the spasticity caused by spinal cord injury, dantrolene relieves spasticity of stroke, cerebral palsy, and multiple sclerosis, for which the other drugs have limited effectiveness.

The major limitation to the use of dantrolene is liver damage. Baseline liver function studies are done before therapy starts, and regular liver function studies are performed throughout therapy. Dantrolene is discontinued if no relief of spasticity is achieved in 6 weeks.

tizanidine

Tizanidine (Zanaflex) is a new drug for the intermittent management of increased muscle tone associated with spasticity, especially that associated with spinal cord injury or multiple sclerosis. Tizanidine is a centrally acting agonist for alpha$_2$-adrenergic receptors. It increases presynaptic inhibition of motor neurons thereby reducing spasticity caused by motor neuron activity.

The most common side effects are sleepiness, dizziness, and loss of vitality. Dry mouth and hypotension are also common side effects.

THERAPEUTIC RATIONALE: MUSCLE SPASMS

Muscle spasms are local muscle contractions initiated by muscle or tendon injury and inflammation. Muscle spasms occur in sprains, bursitis, arthritis, and lower back pain. The primary treatment includes analgesics, antiinflammatory drugs, immobilization of the affected part (if possible), and physical therapy. If relief is not achieved through these means, a centrally acting skeletal muscle relaxant

may be added. Although the mechanism postulated for the centrally acting skeletal muscle relaxants is depression of the poly-synaptic pathways in the spinal cord modulating muscle tone, drugs used as centrally acting skeletal muscle relaxants are related to various antianxiety drugs. Because anxiety worsens a muscle spasm, treatment of the accompanying anxiety may be the more important mechanism of action.

THERAPEUTIC AGENTS: DRUGS TO TREAT MUSCLE SPASMS

Centrally acting skeletal muscle relaxants commonly prescribed to treat muscle spasms are listed in Table 63-1. They are used as part of an overall program for the relief of muscle spasms, a program that includes rest and physical therapy.

Centrally acting skeletal muscle relaxants include carisoprodol (Soma), chlorphenesin (Maolate), chlorzoxazone (Paraflex), cyclobenzaprine (Flexeril), diazepam (Valium), metaxalone (Skelaxin), methocarbamol (Robaxin, others), and orphenadrine (Norflex, others). With the exception of

---

RESEARCH HIGHLIGHTS

Patients' Use of Health-Teaching Materials at Three Readability Levels

—Dowe MC, Lawrence PA, Carlson J, Keyserling TC: Appl Nurs Res *10(2):86-93, 1997.*

PURPOSE

There is a need for health education materials for patients. Almost 25% of adults older than 25 years of age have not completed high school, and those who have may be unable to read at the high school level. The purpose of this study was to examine the influence of reading difficulty on the extent to which patients use and learn from health education literature.

METHODS

Adult patients at a general medical clinic in a medical center who were taking an H$_2$-receptor blocker or a thiazide diuretic were targeted for inclusion. Potential participants were randomly assigned to a control group or one of three experimental groups. Subjects were mailed no leaflet (control group) or an information sheet about their medication (level 1, 2, or 3). Ten days or more after the first mailing, subjects were contacted for a telephone interview by data collectors who were blind to assigned study group. Level 3 (most difficult) leaflets were the standard leaflets produced by the *US Pharmacopeia (USP)*. Level 2 (intermediate difficulty) were "easy-to-read" leaflets recently developed by the *USP*. Level 1 leaflets were developed by the researchers from the level 2 leaflets (with *USP* permission). The article describes the formatting of the level 1 leaflet. There were 275 subjects in the final sample, of which 211 (77%) were female, and 168 were African-American (61%). More than half (*n* = 167; 52%) had not completed high school, and 39 (14%) had completed 2 years or more of college. Of the 275, 125 (45%) were taking H$_2$-receptor blocker, and the rest were taking a thiazide diuretic. The four study groups contained 64 to 72 subjects, and did not differ significantly by age, race, sex, economic status, education, or type of drug studied.

RESULTS

Only 131 (62%) of the 211 subjects who received leaflets said they had read them, and 40 (19%) could not remember. The likelihood of having read the leaflet did not vary significantly with age, gender, economic status, or drug type. The readability level did not have a statistically significant effect on the likelihood of subjects having read the leaflet. However, when having read the leaflet was predicted by readability level and participant's educational level, the interaction of the two predictors was found to be significant [χ^2 (8, *n* = 170) = 19.1, *p* = .01]. The average knowledge score was 64% correct. Knowledge scores were higher in individuals with less than a 9th grade education if they read the less complex leaflet (level 1 leaflet). In contrast, the subjects with a 9th grade or higher education had higher knowledge scores if they read the level 2 or level 3 leaflets.

IMPLICATIONS

It is of concern in this study that less than two thirds of the subjects read the printed material they received on medications, and those who did read the material could answer less than 65% of the questions correctly. Providing patients with written information about their drugs is a recognized teaching strategy, but more research is needed about the kind and difficulty of written materials, and other factors that influence how much patients learn about their medications.

CRITICAL THINKING: *If you have given your patients written information about their medications, did they read it? How do you know? How do you evaluate their knowledge of their medications?*

cyclobenzaprine, these drugs are similar to sedative-hypnotic or antianxiety drugs with respect to side effects, drug interactions, and drug dependence (see Chapter 57); thus short-term rather than long-term therapy is the rule. Cyclobenzaprine is related to the tricyclic antidepressants and does not cause drug dependence or alter sleep patterns.

Drowsiness and dizziness are common side effects of all the centrally acting skeletal muscle relaxants, and they should not be combined with alcohol or other drugs that depress the central nervous system (CNS).

carisoprodol

Carisoprodol (Soma) has a rapid onset of action, and the effect lasts 4 to 6 hours. It is chemically related to meprobamate, which is the principal metabolite. Carisoprodol is contraindicated for patients with acute intermittent porphyria and for nursing mothers.

chlorphenesin

Chlorphenesin (Maolate) has an onset of action of less than 1 hour and a 3- to 4-hour duration of action. Use for more than 8 weeks is not recommended. Chlorphenesin is contraindicated during pregnancy and for nursing mothers. Patients with liver impairment should be given chlorphenesin with caution. Rare but serious reactions include drug fever and blood dyscrasias.

chlorzoxazone

Chlorzoxazone (Paraflex) has an onset of action of less than 1 hour and a 3- to 4-hour duration of action. Rarely hypersensitivity reactions occur and include agranulocytosis and angioedema. Hepatotoxicity is another rare but serious hazard.

cyclobenzaprine

Cyclobenzaprine (Flexeril) is related to the tricyclic antidepressants (see Chapter 59). Drowsiness, dry mouth, and dizziness are the most common side effects. Cyclobenzaprine is contraindicated for patients with hyperthyroidism, arrhythmias, heart block, conduction disturbances, congestive heart failure, or recent myocardial infarction. Monoamine oxidase inhibitors should not be given concurrently.

metaxalone

Metaxalone (Skelaxin) is active in about 1 hour. Rarely it is associated with hemolytic anemia or hepatotoxicity. This drug is contraindicated for patients with a history of these conditions.

methocarbamol

Methocarbamol (Robaxin, others) is effective within 30 minutes when given orally. It is also available for intravenous (IV) or intramuscular (IM) administration. IV administration is used in the treatment of tetanus. When administered intravenously, methocarbamol may cause convulsions, fainting, slow heartbeat, muscle weakness, nystagmus, and facial flushing, especially if administered rapidly. Blurred or double vision are occasional side effects of methocarbamol.

orphenadrine

Orphenadrine (Norflex, others) is an analog of diphenhydramine, an antihistamine, and has anticholinergic properties that include blurred vision, dry mouth and skin, and excitation. Orphenadrine is contraindicated for patients with closed-angle glaucoma or myasthenia gravis. Caution should be used for older adult patients or those with tachycardia, cardiac failure, or urinary retention.

Nursing Process Overview

Centrally Acting Skeletal Muscle Relaxants

Assessment

Perform a general assessment with an additional focus on spasticity, including degree of spasticity, aggravating factors, associated pain, and degree to which spasticity interferes with the activities of daily living or the activities that could increase independence. If dantrolene is used, monitor baseline liver function studies.

Nursing Diagnoses

- Fatigue related to drug side effects (specify drug)

Patient Outcomes

The patient will discuss the causes of fatigue. The patient will establish priorities for daily activities. If appropriate to the patient's situation, the patient will incorporate exercises or other anxiety-reducing activities into the daily schedule.

Planning/Implementation

During dosage adjustment, monitor the patient for drug effectiveness and side effects. Weeks of therapy may be needed before a lessening of spasticity occurs. These drugs may be used with other therapies, including traction, physical therapy, exercises, bed rest, and application of heat.

Evaluation

Evaluate the continuing degree of spasticity. Not all side effects are undesirable, so decisions related to them should be individualized. For example, a patient who is drowsy when receiving short-term diazepam therapy may be better able to tolerate enforced bed rest because of the drowsiness. Before discharge, verify that the patient understands what drugs to take and how to take them correctly, what side effects may occur and which of them require notification of the physician, how to perform additional therapies such as application of heat and exercises, and when to return for additional help.

Nursing Implications Summary

baclofen

Drug Administration

➤ Assess mental status, and monitor regularly.

➤ Monitor blood pressure every 4 hours until stable. Be alert to hypotension when assisting patients to ambulate, especially if they have been immobilized or mostly sedentary before starting drug therapy.

➤ Monitor intake and output and weight. Monitor respiratory rate, auscultate lung sounds, and assess for dyspnea. Inspect for skin changes and edema.

➤ Monitor complete blood count (CBC) and urinalysis.

➤ Tactfully question the patient regarding impotence. Provide emotional support. Remind the patient not to discontinue medications without consulting the physician.

Nursing in the Community

➤ Inform the patient that several days to weeks of therapy may be necessary before improvement is seen. If improvement is not seen in 6 to 8 weeks, the drug is usually withdrawn. However, teach the patient not to stop the medication without consulting with the physician. Depending on the dosage and length of time the patient has been using the medication, it may be necessary to withdraw the drug slowly.

➤ See the Patient Problems boxes on constipation (Chapter 24) and dry mouth (Chapter 23).

➤ Warn the patient to avoid driving or operating hazardous equipment if drowsiness develops.

➤ Caution diabetic patients to monitor blood glucose levels carefully because an adjustment in diet or insulin dosage may be needed.

➤ Warn the patient to avoid the use of alcohol unless permitted in small amounts by the physician.

➤ Remind the patient to inform all health care providers of all drugs being taken.

➤ Instruct the patient to take dose with meals or a snack to lessen gastric irritation.

dantrolene

Drug Administration

➤ Assess mental status, and monitor regularly. Watch for signs of depression, including withdrawal, lack of interest in personal appearance, insomnia, anorexia, and weight loss.

➤ Monitor blood pressure and pulse. When drug is used for treatment of malignant hyperthermia, attach patient to cardiac monitor.

➤ Be alert to hypotension when assisting the patient to ambulate, especially if the patient has been immobilized or primarily sedentary before receiving drug therapy.

➤ Check stools for occult blood.

➤ Monitor intake and output. Monitor urinalysis, or check urine for blood.

➤ Tactfully assess men regarding difficulty in achieving erection. Provide emotional support.

➤ Caution the patient not to discontinue medications without consulting the physician.

➤ Auscultate lung sounds, and watch for pleural effusion.

➤ Inspect skin for abnormal hair growth or rash.

➤ Monitor CBC and liver function tests.

Intravenous dantrolene

➤ Dilute each 20 mg with 60 ml sterile water for injection that does not contain a bacteriostatic agent. Shake solution until clear. Administer as rapid IV push. Once reconstituted and diluted, solution must be protected from light and used within 6 hours.

Nursing in the Community

➤ Review the anticipated benefits and possible side effects of drug therapy. Tell the patient to notify the physician of any unexpected findings.

➤ See the Patient Problems box in Chapter 24 on constipation.

➤ Inform the patient that several days to weeks of therapy may be necessary before improvement is seen. If improvement is not seen in 6 to 8 weeks, the drug is usually withdrawn.

➤ Warn the patient to avoid driving or operating hazardous equipment if dizziness or drowsiness develops.

➤ Warn the patient to avoid the use of alcohol unless permitted in small amounts by the physician.

➤ Remind the patient to inform all health care providers of all medications being taken.

➤ Instruct patients who develop malignant hyperthermia to wear a medical identification tag or bracelet.

➤ For patients who have difficulty swallowing the capsule: Empty contents of capsule(s) into a small amount of fruit juice or other liquid, stir, and drink all of liquid. Rinse glass with a small amount of additional liquid and drink rinse also.

diazepam

➤ For information on diazepam, see Chapter 57.

tizanidine

Drug Administration/Nursing in the Community

➤ Assess the patient for fever, jaundice, nausea and vomiting, changes in mental status, and skin changes. Monitor weight and pulse.

➤ Monitor liver function tests.

➤ Caution the patient to avoid driving or operating hazardous equipment if drowsiness, light-headedness, dizziness, or vision problems develop.

➤ Warn the patient to avoid the use of alcohol unless permitted in small amounts by the physician.

➤ Remind the patient to inform all health care providers of all medications being taken.

➤ Review the anticipated benefits and possible side effects of drug therapy. Tell the patient to notify the physician of any unexpected findings.

➤ See the Patient Problems boxes on dry mouth (Chapter 23) and orthostatic hypotension (Chapter 13).

➤ Inform the patient that several days to weeks of therapy may be necessary before improvement is seen. Caution the patient not to stop this medication abruptly.

Nursing Implications Summary—cont'd

Drugs for Muscle Spasms

Drug Administration

➤ Assess for CNS side effects, including dizziness, ataxia, and vertigo.

➤ Warn the patient that IM injections may cause a burning sensation at the injection site.

➤ Consult the manufacturer's literature for information about IV administration.

➤ For IV administration, keep the patient supine. Keep siderails up. Monitor vital signs. Keep the patient recumbent until blood pressure is stable. Supervise ambulation.

➤ Monitor CBC and differential and liver function tests.

➤ These drugs may cause allergic reactions. Check the patient frequently when beginning therapy. Have drugs and equipment available to treat acute allergic reactions in settings where these drugs are administered.

Nursing in the Community

➤ Review with the patient the anticipated benefits and possible side effects of drug therapy.

➤ If necessary, chlorzoxazone, metaxalone, or methocarbamol tablets may be crushed and mixed with a little food or liquid to make them easier to swallow.

➤ Warn the patient to avoid driving or operating hazardous equipment if drowsiness, dizziness, or visual changes develop.

➤ See the Patient Problems boxes on orthostatic hypotension (Chapter 13), dry mouth (Chapter 23), and constipation (Chapter 24).

➤ Remind the patient to use medications only as directed and to inform all health care providers of all medications being taken.

➤ Warn the patient to avoid alcohol unless permitted in small amounts by the physician.

➤ Instruct the patient to take oral doses with meals or a snack to lessen gastric irritation.

➤ Teach the patient to take the final dose of the day at bedtime.

➤ Warn the patient taking chlorzoxazone that urine may turn orange or purple-red while the drug is taken.

➤ Warn the patient taking methocarbamol that urine may turn black, brown, or green while the drug is taken.

➤ Warn diabetic patients taking metaxalone to monitor blood sugar level carefully. This drug may cause inaccurate results with urine sugar tests.

CHAPTER REVIEW

Application

1. Define spasticity.
2. How do diazepam, baclofen, and dantrolene reduce spasticity?
3. Describe the origin of muscle spasms.
4. What are the characteristics of the drugs used as centrally acting agents to treat muscle spasms?

Critical Thinking

1. Develop a care plan for the spastic patient beginning therapy with baclofen.
2. Develop a care plan for the spastic patient beginning therapy with dantrolene.

Reference

Gianino JM, York MM, Paice JA, Shott S: Quality of life: effect of reduced spasticity from intrathecal baclofen, *J Neurosci Nurs* 30(1):47-54, 1998.

Chapter

64

Introduction to Endocrinology

KEY TERMS

endocrine glands, p. 756

hormone, p. 756

prohormones, p. 757

receptors, p. 757

recombinant proteins, p. 757

replacement therapy, p. 758

target tissues, p. 756

OBJECTIVES

After studying this chapter, you should be able to do the following:

- *Define a hormone.*
- *Name the three uses of hormones in clinical medicine.*
- *Discuss how hormone action is regulated.*
- *Discuss the role of the nurse in hormone therapy.*

CHAPTER OVERVIEW

This introduction to endocrinology defines important terms, introduces the classes of hormones, and illustrates the concept of hormonal regulation of body processes. Properties of individual hormones are detailed in subsequent chapters, along with the specific function of each gland and the effects of related drugs.

THERAPEUTIC RATIONALE: ENDOCRINE DISEASES

Definition of the Endocrine System

A **hormone** is a substance that is synthesized by a specific cell type, is released into the circulation, and acts on target tissues elsewhere in the body to produce a physiologic or biochemical response. An example is thyrotropin, or thyroid-stimulating hormone (TSH), which is synthesized in the anterior pituitary, released into systemic circulation, and taken up by the thyroid gland, there stimulating production of thyroid hormones (see Chapter 67).

Organs producing hormones that enter systemic circulation are the **endocrine glands**—pancreas, adrenals, thyroid, parathyroids, testes, ovaries, and pituitary. Tissues affected by hormones from endocrine glands are designated **target tissues.** For example, TSH from the anterior pituitary has the thyroid gland as a target tissue. Other tissues do not respond to TSH.

Some compounds that have been called hormones act strictly locally, producing their effect at or near the site where they are synthesized. Prostaglandins, which are formed from

membrane fatty acids at the sites of prostaglandin action, are an example of such compounds. Prostaglandins are considered for their action on the uterus in Chapter 71. These locally acting substances are not discussed further in this chapter.

Types and Sources of Hormones

Hormones are of two types, based on their chemical composition. One type, the steroid hormones derived from cholesterol, includes hormones of the adrenal gland (e.g., cortisol, cortisone, aldosterone, corticosterone) and hormones of the sex glands (androgens, estrogens, and progestins).

Many steroid hormones have been synthesized by organic chemists, so their production for medicinal purposes does not depend entirely on isolating them from such natural sources as bovine or porcine adrenal glands obtained from meat-packing plants. Some clinically useful steroids are obtained from natural sources, however, because the steroids are present in high concentrations and are easily extracted, making the procedure economically feasible. An example of such a preparation is Premarin, a mixture of conjugated estrogens extracted from pregnant mare's urine.

The second type of hormone is formed from amino acids. This type may include amino acid derivatives and proteins.

756

Examples of amino acid derivatives are thyroxine and tri-iodothyronine, formed in the thyroid by iodinating tyrosine. Other examples are catecholamines, produced from tyrosine in various tissues.

Peptides and proteins are different in size, with peptides containing fewer amino acids than proteins. Peptides and proteins are similar chemically in that both are formed by peptide bonds linking carboxyl and amino groups of adjacent amino acids. Examples of peptide hormones are releasing factors produced in the hypothalamus (e.g., thyrotropin-releasing hormone, composed of three amino acids) and the posterior pituitary hormones oxytocin and antidiuretic hormone (ADH), which are each composed of nine amino acids. Protein hormones are larger. For example, insulin has 51 amino acids and a molecular weight of 6000 D; follicle-stimulating hormone (FSH) has a molecular weight of 41,000 D.

The active forms of many protein hormones are derived from larger protein molecules called **prohormones.** For example, insulin is originally released as part of a prohormone containing at least 86 amino acids. Cleavage of 35 amino acids from this larger precursor molecule releases active insulin.

The peptide and protein hormones are usually present in very small quantities in natural sources and may be difficult to isolate. For example, insulin, the protein hormone most often used medically, can be prepared in large quantities from bovine or porcine pancreas glands, but the process requires tedious and expensive extraction procedures. Growth hormone, a protein used to treat a rare endocrine disease, may be extracted from pituitary glands, but the only form that is active in humans is human or primate growth hormone. Therefore the supply of this hormone was restricted by the limited source material. In the past, growth hormone was obtained postmortem from human pituitaries, but the risk of viral contamination has caused this product to be dropped.

A powerful method for producing human protein hormones is based on genetic engineering. Genetic engineering for this purpose involves taking genes from one species and placing them into an unrelated species, thereby creating new characteristics in the recipient. The human genes for insulin, growth hormone, interferons, and other proteins have been inserted into host bacteria. These altered bacteria then may be grown on a large scale to produce unlimited quantities of the human protein. Proteins produced in this way are called **recombinant proteins** because the genes were recombined to make the protein in a new way. Recombinant human insulin, recombinant growth hormone, and recombinant interferons are standard clinical agents.

Genetic engineering is applicable to a variety of proteins and solves the problem of limited supply of clinically useful proteins. In addition, hormones produced by this technique are less likely to be contaminated with viruses. Therefore human growth hormone produced by genetically engineered bacteria is now the standard preparation for human use.

Synthesis, Release, and Clearance of Hormones

Hormones are potent agents capable of exerting profound effects on metabolism. To remain healthy, the body must ensure that hormones act only where and when they are needed and that they be present at the proper concentrations. The time of appearance and the concentration of a hormone in blood may be regulated by controlling its rate of synthesis, release from storage sites, degradation, and clearance from the body. Several hormones are stored after synthesis and are released from storage sites only when the proper stimulus is received. For example, thyroxine and tri-iodothyronine are stored complexed with thyroglobulin in the thyroid gland. Insulin is stored in granules within beta cells of the pancreas. In these cases, when the endocrine gland is stimulated to release hormone, the stored hormone is first released. Then if required, newly synthesized hormone is released into the blood.

Regulation of synthesis and release of many hormones involves interactions between the central nervous system (CNS) and the endocrine glands. For example, the hypothalamus in the brain controls the pituitary gland, which regulates production of hormones by ovaries, testes, thyroid, and adrenal glands. This system is the negative feedback regulation discussed in Chapter 65.

Hormones disappear from the blood when they are taken up by various organs or when they are degraded by enzymes in blood. The kidneys degrade or excrete several hormones, including most steroids. The kidneys and the liver degrade insulin. In contrast, ADH is very rapidly destroyed by enzymes in blood. The half-life of vasopressin (i.e., the time required for half of the injected dose to disappear from the blood) is approximately 15 minutes. Other hormones persist for much longer periods. For example, thyroxine has a plasma half-life of about 7 days.

Localizing Hormone Effects

Distribution Limited to Portal Circulation

Controlling the location of action of a certain hormone is accomplished in one of two ways. The first localization mechanism is to restrict distribution of the hormone. Examples are the releasing factors synthesized in the hypothalamus and released into local portal veins carrying the hormones directly to the anterior pituitary and not into general circulation. The second mechanism is discussed next.

Hormone Receptors

A second mechanism localizes the effect of widely released hormones. These hormones interact with specific **receptors** found only in their target tissues. The specific receptor is required for hormone activity. For example, TSH receptors are found in the thyroid gland but not in most other organs. Therefore, even though TSH is released into general circulation, it acts only on the thyroid.

The receptors for hormones may be within cells. For example, steroids and thyroid hormones affect target cells by interacting with intracellular receptors, such as those discussed in Chapter 1 (see Figure 1-4). Steroid hormones are bound by specific receptors that transport the hormones through the cytoplasm of the cell and into the nucleus, where the final effect of the hormone is produced. Thyroid hormones likewise move to the nucleus, where they bind to specific receptors and ultimately alter protein synthesis in cells.

In contrast to the receptors for steroids and thyroid hormones, receptors for peptide and protein hormones exist on the external surface of cell membranes (see Chapter 1, Figure 1-3). Therefore the peptide and protein hormones need not enter cells to become effective. One mechanism by which these externally bound hormones act is by releasing an internal regulator, or second messenger. Second messengers include cyclic adenosine monophosphate (cAMP), calcium ion, and inositol 1,4,5-trisphosphate (IP3).

One of the best understood second messenger systems is that involving cAMP. Many hormones bind receptors that are associated with an enzyme called adenylate cyclase. When the hormone binds to the receptor, adenylate cyclase is stimulated to release cAMP within the cell; cAMP then alters the internal processes of the cell. Hormones that act through this system include parathyroid hormone and ADH. This second messenger system is also used by beta-adrenergic receptors (see Chapter 12).

Other second messenger systems are also important for endocrine function. For example, the multiple metabolic changes produced by insulin within target cells arise from the action of the enzyme tyrosine kinase and do not depend on cAMP.

Modulating Hormone Responses

The response of a target cell to a hormone depends on how many hormone receptors are available. Therefore regulating the number of receptors is another mechanism by which the body can maintain metabolic balance. An example of this type of regulation is found in obese persons with a high food intake. These persons have chronically high insulin concentrations in the bloodstream. To protect itself from the metabolic effects of this high amount of insulin, the body eliminates a certain percentage of the insulin receptors on cells. The loss of insulin receptors, called downregulation, lowers the responsiveness of the cell to insulin.

Defining Endocrine Diseases

Understanding the role of receptors in fulfilling the metabolic role of hormones allows a clearer understanding of endocrine diseases and how they are classified. An endocrine deficiency can arise from a lack of hormone or from a lack of receptors that enables the tissue to respond to the hormone. An example is diabetes insipidus, which may be produced by a lack of ADH or by a lack of receptors in the kidney that can respond to ADH. Similarly, diabetes mellitus can be characterized by the lack of insulin in the blood or by high levels of insulin in blood but lower-than-normal numbers of active insulin receptors on cells.

THERAPEUTIC AGENTS: HORMONES

Hormones are used clinically in one of three ways: as diagnostic agents, in replacement therapy, or as pharmacologic agents.

The most common diagnostic use of hormones is to assess the function of target organs of the administered hormone. For example, adrenocorticotropic hormone (ACTH) may be given to test the ability of the adrenal glands to produce steroids. Similarly, thyrotropin is used to test the capacity of the thyroid gland to synthesize thyroid hormones.

Replacement therapy is aimed at restoring normal levels of hormones, which, for some reason, a patient's body no longer produces. Physiologic doses are used in an attempt to maintain normal hormone levels without producing toxic effects from hormone excesses. The use of thyroxine to treat hypothyroidism or cortisol to treat chronic adrenal insufficiency are examples of replacement therapy. Insulin use in diabetic patients is also an example of replacement therapy.

The use of hormones as pharmacologic agents, with administered doses far in excess of those required to produce physiologic levels, makes use of some function of the compound other than the one seen at physiologic concentrations. For example, adrenal corticosteroids may be given in large doses to suppress inflammatory responses in certain diseases (see Chapter 41). This antiinflammatory effect is not obvious at physiologic concentrations of the steroid.

The next eight chapters deal with specific hormones and explain how the hormone may be used in one or more of these ways.

Nursing Process Overview

Hormonal Replacement Therapy

Assessment

In newly diagnosed patients, it is important to perform a thorough physical assessment to obtain baseline data, giving attention to both subjective and objective changes that have occurred over what may be a long period as the deficiency was developing. For continuing patients, it is important to assess any objective or subjective changes that may suggest control is no longer adequate or that replacement dosages are too high. Monitor laboratory work appropriate to the problem, for example, thyroid function tests if the patient is hypothyroid.

Nursing Diagnoses

- Knowledge deficit of the long-term nature of the disease and it therapy.
- Risk for altered health maintenance related to insufficient knowledge of specific problem.

Patient Outcomes

The patient will demonstrate mastery of drug administration techniques and how to self-assess for development of symptoms. The patient will describe the endocrine problem, factors contributing to symptoms, and the procedures for disease or symptom control.

Planning/Implementation

Teach the patient about the endocrine problem being treated: symptoms, factors that may contribute to exacerbations, drug control, and so on. Provide emotional support as needed. Many patients will need help accepting a lifelong condition that requires constant attention on their part. Help patients through this process by focusing on how to establish simple routines that fit with their lifestyle. Counsel them about the effects of occasionally missing medication and the effects of stopping their medication. If the condition requires it, have the patient obtain an identification tag or bracelet.

Evaluation

Ascertain that the patient understands what medications are to be taken, the schedule for administration, and the consequences of missed doses. Ask the patient to explain symptoms of underdosage or overdosage. If an identification tag or bracelet is required, the patient should have one upon leaving the hospital or state the need to obtain one.

 # CHAPTER REVIEW

Application

1. What is a hormone?
2. What is a target tissue?
3. Describe the two major chemical types of hormones.
4. What is a prohormone?
5. Name three ways in which large amounts of hormones may be obtained for clinical use.
6. What are the three primary clinical uses of hormones?
7. Describe how the amount of hormone in the body may be regulated.
8. How may the site of action of a hormone be restricted?
9. In what ways may the actions of hormones be terminated?
10. What is a releasing factor?
11. Describe the two general types of endocrine deficiency diseases.

Critical Thinking

1. What are the two main types of hormone receptors? How do these receptors differ in the way they interact with hormones?
2. What features of replacement therapy differ from many other types of drug therapy? Discuss an education plan that might be appropriate to use with a patient receiving replacement therapy.

Drugs Affecting the Pituitary Gland

OBJECTIVES

After studying this chapter, you should be able to do the following:

- *Identify the two parts of the pituitary gland.*
- *Describe the function of the two hormones of the neurohypophysis.*
- *Describe the use of antidiuretic hormone.*
- *Identify the source and use of growth hormones.*
- *Develop a nursing care plan for the patient receiving drug therapy for diabetes insipidus, for growth hormone deficiency, or to suppress excessive release of growth hormone.*

CHAPTER OVERVIEW

The pituitary gland consists of less than 1 g of tissue at the base of the brain, but it is the primary regulator of the endocrine system, controls normal growth, and regulates water balance.

The pituitary gland is divided into two portions with different tissue compositions and embryologic origins: the anterior pituitary (or adenohypophysis) and the posterior pituitary (or neurohypophysis). The function of each of these tissues, the regulation of the various hormones produced, and the pathologic states resulting from abnormalities in hormone production are considered in this chapter.

THERAPEUTIC RATIONALE: NEUROHYPOPHYSIS

The **posterior pituitary,** or neurohypophysis, is composed of nerve fibers that arise from the hypothalamus during fetal development. Close contact between the central nervous system (CNS) and the neurohypophysis is maintained in adulthood by the nerve fibers that run from the hypothalamus through the hypophyseal stalk to the neurohypophysis (Figure 65-1). Two peptide hormones closely related in structure—antidiuretic hormone and oxytocin—are released by the neurohypophysis. These hormones are synthesized in the hypothalamus and transported in secretion granules down the axons to the neurohypophysis. The granules accumulate at the nerve fiber terminals in the neurohypophysis, where their release into systemic circulation is regulated by nerve impulses

from the hypothalamus. Damage to the hypophyseal stalk impairs transport of secretory granules to the neurohypophysis and interferes with appropriate release of the hormones.

Neurohypophyseal Hormones
oxytocin

The target organs of oxytocin are breast myoepithelium and smooth muscle of the uterus, especially during the second and third stages of labor. The effects of oxytocin on these tissues are discussed in Chapter 71. Oxytocin also causes milk ejection by stimulating contraction of the myoepithelium of the breast.

The regulation of oxytocin release is a particularly good example of the close interaction of the CNS with pituitary function. Suckling by the infant induces afferent nerve impulses from the breast to the brain, which causes more oxytocin to be synthesized and stored hormone to be released. A similar reflex loop may operate in parturition when dilation of the cervix is thought to stimulate synthesis and release of oxytocin.

No specific syndrome resulting from abnormalities in oxytocin function has been described.

▼ antidiuretic hormone

Physiologic Action

Antidiuretic hormone (ADH), also called vasopressin, acts primarily on renal tubular epithelium. ADH increases permeability of the renal collecting duct to water by causing a protein called aquaporin-2 to associate with the cell membrane, creating a pore or channel through which water may pass. This action allows water to be reabsorbed and the urine to be concentrated. Other target tissues such as smooth muscle of blood vessels and of the gastrointestinal (GI) tract may respond to concentrations of ADH that are higher than normal. ADH actions on these tissues cause vasoconstriction and increased GI motility, respectively.

Regulation of Secretion

Secretion of ADH is regulated mainly in response to plasma osmolarity, the concentration of solute molecules that increase osmotic pressure (see Chapter 17). In dehydration the effective osmotic pressure of blood increases. Osmoreceptors in the hypothalamus respond to this change by stimulating the neurohypophysis to secrete ADH. In turn, ADH causes the kidney to conserve body water and to prevent or slow further dehydration. Recovery from dehydration is aided further by stimulation of the thirst center, leading to increased intake of fluids. Reduction in the effective plasma volume caused by hemorrhage or reduced cardiac output stimulates ADH release and promotes antidiuresis (water retention).

In addition to these physiologic controls, certain drugs also may influence ADH secretion. Acetylcholine, barbiturates, nicotine, morphine, and bradykinin cause release of ADH in healthy subjects. Ethanol or phenytoin may promote diuresis by inhibiting ADH release.

Effects of Antidiuretic Hormone Deficiency

ADH is significantly reduced or absent when the hypothalamic region responsible for its synthesis is destroyed or when the hypophyseal stalk above the median eminence is separated (see Figure 65-1). In these cases, urinary concentration is impossible, and large volumes of dilute, sugar-free urine are produced. This condition is called **diabetes insipidus** and differs from the disease diabetes mellitus, which arises from the inability to use blood glucose or to release insulin.

Diabetes insipidus is not life-threatening unless severe electrolyte imbalances develop. If the patient has a functional thirst center and can balance excessive fluid losses with high fluid intakes, severe imbalances usually do not occur. When a person is unconscious and unable to take in adequate fluids, however, severe dehydration may set in before the condition is noticed. Thus, after head injuries or surgery

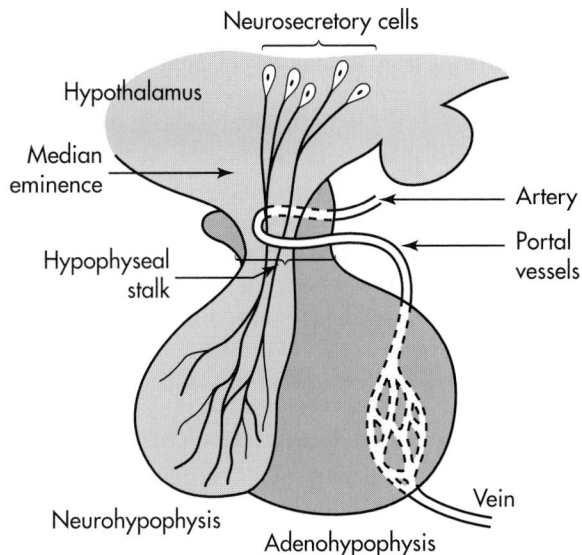

Figure 65-1 Anatomy of pituitary gland.

to the hypothalamic region of the brain, health care personnel must monitor urinary specific gravity and blood sodium levels, along with fluid intake and urinary volumes, to detect excessive diuresis and resultant dehydration.

In many patients with trauma to the hypothalamus or the hypophyseal stalk, the resultant diabetes insipidus may be transitory. In patients whose condition is chronic, reversal of symptoms can be achieved by replacement therapy with a form of ADH or by therapy with pharmacologic agents that relieve the symptoms of the disease.

THERAPEUTIC AGENTS: TREATMENT OF DIABETES INSIPIDUS

Central Diabetes Insipidus

antidiuretic hormone

Mechanism of Action

Central diabetes insipidus is caused by a deficiency in ADH and therefore can be treated by replacement therapy. The administered ADH has the same effect as the natural hormone.

Pharmacokinetics

Because ADH is a peptide hormone, it cannot be administered orally, and all replacement therapy with ADH involves the administration of the hormone parenterally or intranasally (Table 65-1).

Vasopressin, an aqueous preparation of ADH, is not routinely used because the half-life of ADH in the blood is short. This preparation is injected intramuscularly or subcutaneously two or three times daily for short-term management. Lypressin, a synthetic form of ADH that is sprayed onto the mucous membranes of the nasal passages, is usually administered four times daily.

Desmopressin (DDAVP) administered intranasally is the drug of choice in replacement therapy for chronic diabetes insipidus. DDAVP is a chemically altered form of vasopressin, differing from the natural hormone by having a long serum half-life, a more potent antidiuretic effect, and less pressor activity. It is administered only once or twice daily, unlike other ADH preparations.

Uses

The primary use for ADH is as replacement therapy for diabetes insipidus. ADH has been used as a pressor agent but now is not recommended for that use. Occasionally, the vasoconstrictor action of ADH is used to help control massive GI tract bleeding, especially from esophageal varices.

Adverse Reactions and Contraindications

ADH can promote activity of intestinal smooth muscle. During routine therapy of diabetes insipidus this action of ADH may result in nausea, belching, and cramps.

ADH is a vasoconstrictor, which tends to raise blood pressure. This vasoconstrictor action prevents safe use for patients with vascular or coronary artery disease. Even small doses may cause difficulty to a patient prone to angina attacks. Side effects caused by the pressor action of vasopressin are less problematic with desmopressin than with other forms of vasopressin.

Toxicity

Overdose with ADH may produce water intoxication (see Chapter 17).

Interactions

Demeclocycline or lithium may interfere with the effects of ADH on the kidneys, with the result that diuresis continues.

Other Drugs to Treat Diabetes Insipidus

Agents other than ADH preparations have been used to treat diabetes insipidus. Paradoxically, thiazide diuretics (see Chapter 14) are effective in some cases, especially when combined with another oral agent listed in this section. The effectiveness of thiazide diuretics is based on their blockade of electrolyte reabsorption, resulting initially in increased sodium and water excretion. The kidney responds to this change by reabsorbing more water by mechanisms that do not depend on ADH. Moderate salt restriction may enhance the action of these drugs. Doses of thiazides used to treat diabetes insipidus are the same as those used for other indications. The most common side effect is potassium depletion, which in extreme cases may induce cardiac arrhythmias and impair neuromuscular, GI tract, or renal function.

Chlorpropamide, a sulfonylurea used as an oral hypoglycemic agent to treat diabetes mellitus (see Chapter 69), is also used at comparable doses for diabetes insipidus. When chlorpropamide is used to treat diabetes insipidus, the action sought is a direct sensitization of the kidney to ADH so that lower-than-normal levels of ADH cause nearly normal water reabsorption. Alone or with a thiazide diuretic, chlorpropamide usually reduces urine volumes. The major potential toxicity is hypoglycemia. Chlorpropamide is not effective in patients who produce no ADH; the drug may stimulate the pituitary to release ADH.

Clofibrate, an oral agent used to reduce serum triglyceride levels (see Chapter 21), may be effective in treating diabetes insipidus, either alone or combined with a thiazide diuretic. It may produce nausea or rarely muscle cramps and weakness. Clofibrate increases release of ADH from the posterior pituitary.

Nephrogenic Diabetes Insipidus

The form of diabetes insipidus covered in the previous paragraphs is called central diabetes insipidus because it arises from a lack of secretion of ADH from the neurohypophysis. The symptoms of diabetes insipidus may also arise if the neurohypophysis is producing normal amounts of ADH but the kidney is unresponsive or responds poorly to ADH. This syndrome, called nephrogenic diabetes insipidus, may be treated with thiazide diuretics but is resistant to therapy with ADH. Although nephrogenic diabetes insipidus may arise as a genetic disease, it also may be induced by drugs that impair the ability of the kidney to react to ADH. Drugs such as lithium used in treating mental disease (see Chapter 59) and demeclocycline, a tetracycline antibiotic (see Chapter 47), can induce nephrogenic diabetes insipidus by this mechanism.

Table 65-1	**Drugs to Treat Diabetes Insipidus**			
Generic Name	**Trade Name**	**Administration/Dosage**		**Comments**
desmopressin	DDAVP* Stimate	INTRANASAL: *Adults*—10 μg at bedtime initially; up to 40 μg for maintenance. FDA pregnancy category B. *Children 3 mo-12 yr*—5 μg initially at bedtime; up to 4 μg/kg for maintenance. INTRAVENOUS, SUBCUTANEOUS: *Adults*—1-2 μg twice daily.		Synthetic derivative of vasopressin used as replacement therapy.
lypressin	Diapid	INTRANASAL: *Adults*—1-2 sprays in each nostril 4 times/day. FDA pregnancy category C.		Synthetic derivative of vasopressin used as replacement therapy.
vasopressin	Pitressin* Pressyn†	INTRAMUSCULAR, INTRAVENOUS, SUBCUTANEOUS, INTRAARTERIAL: *Adults*-5-10 units 2-3 times/day as needed. May be given intravenously or intraarterially by means of infusion pump. FDA pregnancy category C. *Children*—2.5-10 units 3-4 times/day.		Synthetic vasopressin used as replacement therapy or diagnostic aid.

*Available in Canada and the United States.
†Available in Canada only.

Syndrome of Inappropriate Antidiuretic Hormone

The **syndrome of inappropriate ADH (SIADH)** secretion is a rare condition in which patients show symptoms of water intoxication including hyponatremia, or low sodium levels in the blood (see Chapter 17), and low serum osmolality. Despite these conditions, the kidneys continue to excrete sodium. The symptoms of SIADH are caused by release of more ADH than is appropriate, based on normal osmotic regulatory signals. In most patients with SIADH, the excess ADH is released by a tumor such as a bronchogenic carcinoma. Other less common causes of SIADH are CNS disorders, including head injuries or infections, extreme physical stress such as surgery, or extreme emotional stress. A variety of drugs, including carbamazepine, chlorpropamide, antipsychotics, antidepressants, and thiazide diuretics, occasionally trigger SIADH.

Treatment of SIADH usually is aimed directly at removing the cause of the condition such as removing the tumor or discontinuing the drug thought to precipitate the disorder. Fluid restriction, infusion of hypertonic saline, and use of diuretics all may help control the fluid and electrolyte imbalances associated with SIADH. If the cause of excessive ADH cannot be completely removed, symptoms may be relieved by administering demeclocycline, which renders the kidneys less sensitive to ADH.

THERAPEUTIC RATIONALE: ADENOHYPOPHYSIS

The **anterior pituitary,** or adenohypophysis, is regarded as the master gland of the endocrine system. The adenohypophysis secretes several peptide hormones, most of which directly stimulate secretion by the adrenal glands, the thyroid gland, and the reproductive organs (Table 65-2).

Although the adenohypophysis is true secretory tissue that synthesizes and releases its hormones, control of those secretions lies in the brain. Small polypeptides, called neurohormones, are synthesized in the median eminence of the hypothalamus and are released into the portal venous system (see Figure 65-1) that carries them directly to the adenohypophysis. In the adenohypophysis, these neurohormones act on a specific type of target cell to stimulate or to inhibit synthesis and release of the proper hormone.

Damage to the hypophysis may cause it to produce insufficient amounts of hypophyseal hormones, a condition called panhypopituitarism. Adults who have this syndrome require replacement therapy with thyroid hormones, adrenal steroids, and appropriate sex steroids. Children with panhypopituitarism may also suffer reduced growth because of a lack of growth hormone.

Regulation of Growth

growth hormone

Physiologic Action

Growth hormone regulates the length of the long bones of the skeleton, which determines adult height. In addition, the hormone is a potent anabolic agent that causes many tissues to increase cell size and numbers. This anabolic action results from changes produced in protein, carbohydrate, and fat metabolism. The hormone increases amino acid transport into cells and elevates cellular protein synthesis. Growth hormone also antagonizes the action of insulin; this action tends to decrease glucose uptake and carbohydrate use, thus elevating liver glycogen and blood glucose levels. Finally, growth hormone increases the mobilization of fats for energy, which leads to a rise in blood levels of free fatty acids.

Many actions of growth hormone are mediated by peptides called **insulin-like growth factors** (IGFs), formerly called somatomedins. Growth hormone stimulates production of IGF-I and IGF-II in liver and at the cartilaginous growing plate of bone. In addition to stimulating skeletal growth, these peptides have insulin-like actions on other tissues.

Regulation of Secretion

The secretion of growth hormone is regulated by two hormones from the hypothalamus, one stimulating and one

---

Table 65-2   Physiologic Action of Adenohypophyseal Hormones

Descriptive Name	Other Names	Hypothalamic Factors	Target Tissue	Target Tissue Response
Adrenocorticotropin	ACTH	Corticotropin-releasing hormone (CRH)	Adrenal cortex	Increased steroid synthesis
Follicle-stimulating hormone	FSH	Gonadotropin-releasing hormone (GnRH); FSH-releasing hormone (FRH and FSH-RH)	Ovary / Seminiferous tubules	Increased estrogen production / Maturation
Growth hormone	GH / Somatotropin	Growth hormone–releasing hormone (GHRH); somatostatin or somatotropin-releasing inhibitory hormone (SRIH)	Whole body	Increased anabolism, cell size, and cell numbers
Luteinizing hormone or interstitial cell–stimulating hormone	ICSH / LH	Gonadotropin-releasing hormone (GnRH); luteinizing hormone–releasing hormone (LH-RH)	Ovary / Leydig's cells	Ovulation; formation of corpus luteum / Increased androgen synthesis
Prolactin	PRL	Dopamine	Breast	Milk formation
Thyroid-stimulating hormone	Thyrotropin / TSH	Thyrotropin-releasing hormone (TRH)	Thyroid gland	Increased triiodothyronine (T_3) and thyroxine (T_4) synthesis

inhibiting release. The releasing hormone, GHRH, is a protein containing about 40 amino acids. The inhibitory factor is a smaller, 14–amino acid peptide called somatostatin. In addition to regulating growth hormone release, somatostatin may also influence thyroid-stimulating hormone (TSH) and adrenocorticotropic hormone (ACTH) release from the pituitary. Somatostatin is found in other tissues such as gut and pancreas and can block the release of insulin, glucagon, and gastrin at those sites.

Effects of Growth Hormone Deficiency

Deficiency of growth hormone in childhood results in loss of IGF-I activity, which causes the adult height to be well below average. In addition to the obvious effects on stature, growth hormone deficiency is linked to reduced mass of the left ventricle such as that these patients show poor left ventricular function on exercise. Treatment by replacement therapy with growth hormone corrects both these aspects of the disease.

Effects of Excessive Growth Hormone

Acromegaly and gigantism are produced by excessive growth hormone, but the age of onset causes significant differences in the manifestations of the disease. Excessive growth hormone from an early age produces the rare condition of gigantism, with growth rates up to 3.5 inches per year.

Acromegaly results if excessive growth hormone production starts after puberty (i.e., after the plates of the long bones have joined and normal skeletal growth has halted). In this condition, only those tissues still able to grow and expand respond to growth hormone, resulting in thickened fingers, coarse facial features, and a massive lower jaw. Less obvious changes include myocardial hypertrophy, along with various signs of cellular damage in the heart. Some of these changes can be reversed by lowering growth hormone or IGF-I levels.

Gigantism and acromegaly are both caused by pituitary neoplasms, which secrete excessive amounts of growth hormone. Consequently, therapy is designed to destroy or remove the tumor. Successful treatment arrests progressive symptoms of the disease but does not erase existing deformations. When removal or destruction of the tumor is impossible or is only partially successful, the drug bromocriptine may inhibit release of growth hormone from the hypophysis. Octreotide, an analog of somatostatin, can also help suppress excessive release of growth hormone (Table 65-3).

Regulation of Sexual Development and Function

Gonadotropic Hormones

Physiologic Action

The gonadotropic hormones of the adenohypophysis are follicle-stimulating hormone (FSH), luteinizing hormone (LH), and prolactin. FSH and LH regulate maturation and function of male and female sexual organs. In women, prolactin stimulates milk formation in breast tissue primed by estrogen and progestin.

In the maturing male, FSH causes the seminiferous tubules to mature. LH increases the number of testicular interstitial cells and stimulates their secretion of androgens. These androgens are the steroid hormones that complete the maturation process, leading to the production of viable sperm and the development of secondary male sexual characteristics.

In the maturing female, FSH and LH are produced in greater quantities at puberty and stimulate ovarian estrogen production. Estrogens, the female steroid hormones, cause the female secondary sex characteristics to develop.

Regulation of Gonadotropin Secretion in Adult Females

Release of FSH and LH from the adenohypophysis is controlled by gonadotropin-releasing hormone (GnRH), which

Table 65-3	**Growth Hormone and Related Drugs**		
Generic Name	**Trade Name**	**Administration/Dosage**	**Comments**
bromocriptine	Parlodel*	ORAL: *Adults—For acromegaly:* 1.25-2.5 mg/day for 3 days at bedtime with food; double dose every 3-7 days to maximum of 10-30 mg/day. FDA pregnancy category B.	This derivative of ergot alkaloids suppresses growth hormone secretion.
octreotide	Sandostatin*	SUBCUTANEOUS: *Adults—For acromegaly:* 0.05 mg 2-3 times/day, gradually increased to 0.1 mg 3 times/ day. FDA pregnancy category B. *For diarrhea (gastrointestinal tumor):* 0.05 mg initially, increasing to 0.1-0.6 mg/day. *Children*—0.001-0.01 mg/kg/day in 2-4 doses.	This analog of somatostatin suppresses intestinal hormones, insulin, glucagon, and growth hormone.
sermorelin	Geref	INTRAVENOUS: *Children—For diagnosis of pituitary function:* 1 μg/kg. SUBCUTANEOUS: *Children—For growth hormone deficiency:* 0.03 mg/kg once daily at bedtime.	Form of growth hormone-releasing hormone; stimulates release of growth hormone from intact pituitaries.
somatrem	Protropin*	INTRAMUSCULAR, SUBCUTANEOUS: *Children—For growth failure:* Up to 0.1 mg/kg 3 times/week.	This recombinant protein differs from natural human growth hormone by one amino acid; used as replacement therapy.
somatropin	Humatrope* Nutropin	INTRAMUSCULAR, SUBCUTANEOUS: *Children—For growth failure:* 0.025-0.05 mg/kg 3-6 times/wk.	This recombinant protein is identical to natural human growth hormone; used as replacement therapy.

*Available in Canada and the United States.

is made in the hypothalamus. The clinical uses of GnRH are covered in Chapter 70.

In addition to their role in development, FSH and LH control the menstrual cycle in mature females (Figure 65-2). Regulation of this function involves the hypothalamus, adenohypophysis, ovaries, and endometrium (uterine lining). The first event in the cycle is a rise in the concentration of FSH in blood. In response, one of the hundreds of primordial ovarian follicles begins to develop. As the follicle matures under the influence of FSH, it begins to produce increasing amounts of estrogens, which greatly increase adenohypophyseal secretion of LH. The surge of LH at midcycle is the primary trigger for ovulation, the release of an ovum from the mature follicle.

In the second half of the menstrual cycle, LH causes the follicle from which an ovum was released to develop into a thickened, secretory tissue called corpus luteum. The corpus lu-

teum secretes large quantities of progesterone, another steroid hormone. By day 21 of the cycle, the large quantities of circulating estrogen and progesterone inhibit adenohypophyseal secretion of FSH and LH (see Figure 65-2), and the corpus luteum begins to involute. Steroid hormone production falls rapidly as the corpus luteum fails and brings about the final stage in the cycle, the collapse of the endometrial lining.

During menses the inner uterine surface is denuded, and the endometrium rapidly collapses to about 65% of its former thickness. About 70 ml of blood and serum is lost along with necrotic and dissolving tissue during a typical menstrual period. Normally, this blood does not clot because fibrinolysin is in the fluid. Fibrinolysin is an enzyme that digests the fibrin matrix on which blood clots form. Despite the favorable environment for bacterial growth, the uterus during menstruation is resistant to infection, partly because many leukocytes are present in menstrual fluid.

Figure 65-2 Pituitary regulation of menstrual cycle. Changes in circulating hormone levels are correlated with ovarian follicle and endometrial alterations. *FSH*, Follicle-stimulating hormone; *LH*, luteinizing hormone.

Effects of Gonadotropin Deficiency

Alterations in hypophyseal or ovarian function can upset the interaction of these tissues. Throughout childhood, pituitary secretion of FSH and LH is low, and circulating sex steroid concentrations are also low. At puberty the adenohypophysis greatly increases its secretion of FSH and LH. If this increase does not occur, sexual development does not take place because androgen, estrogen, and progesterone production are not induced.

FSH may be used clinically to help reverse female infertility (see Chapter 70). For long-term replacement therapy in patients with hypogonadism, the androgens and estrogens are usually used (see Chapters 70 and 72).

Regulation of Response to Stress

Adrenocorticotropic Hormone

Physiologic Action

When ACTH is released by the adenohypophysis, it stimulates the adrenal cortex to synthesize and to release cortisol, a major adrenocortical steroid hormone, as well as other glu-

cocorticoids and minor amounts of sex steroids (see Chapter 66).

Regulation of Secretion

Cortisol blood levels are monitored by the hypothalamus, which adjusts the rate of release of corticotropin-releasing hormone (CRH) into the portal venous system to the adenohypophysis, thereby controlling release of ACTH. When cortisol levels become too high, the hypothalamus reduces CRH release. The adenohypophysis, lacking appropriate stimulation, reduces ACTH production, and blood levels of ACTH fall. The adrenocortical production of cortisol then falls because of the lowered ACTH levels. Blood levels of cortisol thus are prevented from exceeding an upper limit. Conversely, when cortisol levels in blood fall too low, the hypothalamus prevents a dangerously low level from developing by releasing CRH into the portal venous system to stimulate release of ACTH from the adenohypophysis. In response to ACTH the adrenal cortex elevates cortisol production. This intricate regulatory sequence is an example of a **negative feedback loop,** a regulatory mechanism in which the prod-

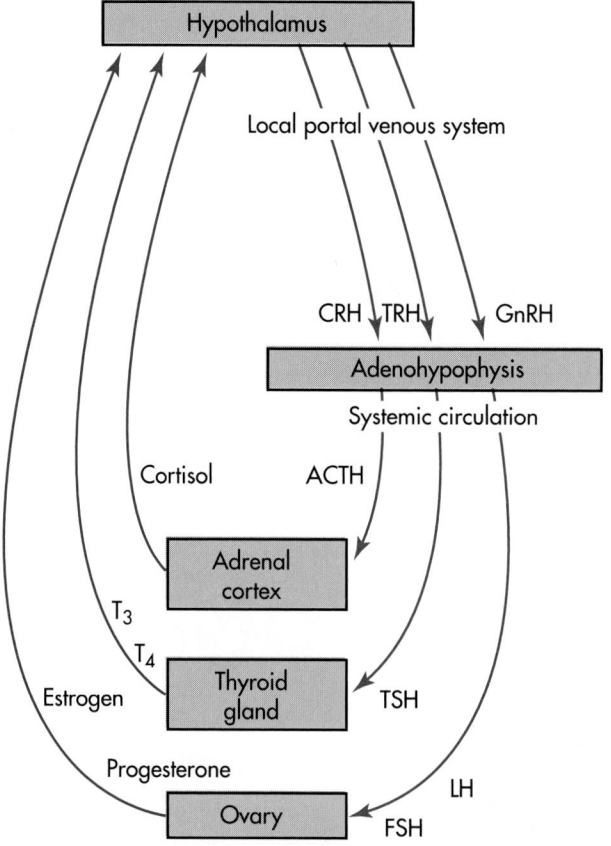

Figure 65-3 Regulation of hormone synthesis by negative feedback loops. Each *arrow* indicates a hormone, its source, and its target tissue. Hypothalamic synthesis of individual releasing factors is suppressed by high blood concentrations of appropriate final hormone. For example, cortisol suppresses corticotropin-releasing hormone *(CRH)* synthesis and release, thereby blocking further cortisol synthesis. Other loops are similarly regulated. *ACTH,* Adrenocorticotropic hormone; *FSH,* follicle-stimulating hormone; *GnRH,* gonadotropin-releasing hormone; *LH,* luteinizing hormone; *T₃,*triiodothyronine; *T₄,* thyroxine; *TRH,* thyrotropin-releasing hormone.

uct of a reaction sequence inhibits operation of the sequence, thereby keeping the concentration of the product between fixed limits (Figure 65-3).

Thyroid-Stimulating Hormone

Negative feedback regulation applies not only to the adrenal cortex and the ovary but also to the thyroid gland (see Figure 65-3). TSH is discussed in Chapter 67.

THERAPEUTIC AGENTS: ADENOHYPOPHYSEAL HORMONES

The diagnostic or therapeutic uses of most adenohypophyseal hormones are covered in the chapters devoted to the target organs. Only growth hormone is considered in this chapter because it targets the whole body.

Growth Hormone

Mechanism of Action

Recombinant growth hormone stimulates growth by the same physiologic mechanisms as natural growth hormone, including stimulating production of IGF-I. Human growth hormone extracted from human pituitaries has not been used since 1985 because of the risk of transmitting Creutzfeldt-Jakob disease.

Pharmacokinetics

Growth hormone, as a peptide, is susceptible to degradation by gastric acid and thus cannot be used orally. When given subcutaneously or intramuscularly, the hormone has a half-life in serum of 5 hours or less, but the duration of measurable metabolic effects may be as long as 2 days. Growth hormone is cleared by hepatic mechanisms.

Uses

Slow or inadequate growth may arise from many causes, but only that form caused by growth hormone deficiency is appropriately treated with growth hormone. The standard preparations for therapy are prepared by recombinant DNA techniques. Recombinant somatotropin has the same amino acid sequence as the natural human hormone (see Table 65-3). Somatrem is a recombinant form that has one more amino acid than natural growth hormone but has the same action as the natural hormone. Children or adolescents with pituitary dwarfism who receive growth hormone typically show an immediate increase in growth and may increase one foot or more in height over several years of treatment. Ultimately, resistance to the protein develops, and growth tapers off.

Adverse Reactions and Contraindications

Growth hormone causes few adverse reactions in most patients. In predisposed individuals, prolonged treatment with growth hormone may precipitate diabetes mellitus because many actions of growth hormone antagonize those of insulin. Hypothyroidism will interfere with the response to growth hormone.

Growth hormone should not be used in adolescents whose epiphyses have sealed because stimulation of further natural growth will not occur. These preparations should not be used to enhance size or bulk in healthy young athletes because the risks outweigh the minimal benefits.

Interactions

Glucocorticoids may antagonize the growth stimulation produced by growth hormone. This effect is more pronounced with long-term dosing of glucocorticoids.

Nursing Process Overview

Pituitary Therapy

Assessment

In most cases patients with pituitary hormone problems have previously had long-term excesses or deficiencies of the hormones. Perform a thorough examination to obtain baseline data, paying particular attention to subjective and objective changes that the patient may indicate have occurred over an extended period.

Nursing Diagnoses
- Knowledge deficit
- Fluid volume excess related to excessive dose of vasopressin

Patient Outcomes

The patient will demonstrate correct administration technique for prescribed medication. The patient will accurately state when and how to use the medication and when to seek medical assistance for side effects. The patient's fluid volume will return to normal.

Planning/Implementation

Monitor the patient for expected drug side effects. Before discharge, begin the teaching and emotional support required to help the patient move to self-management.

Evaluation

Before discharge, ascertain that the patient understands why the prescribed drugs are necessary, how to administer them correctly, what the signs of overdosage or underdosage are, what side effects might occur, and which effects should be reported immediately. If a patient does not have a medical identification tag or bracelet before leaving the hospital, the patient will state the need to obtain one.

Nursing Implications Summary

Care of Patient with Diabetes Insipidus
Drug Administration
➤ Monitor fluid intake and output, serum sodium levels, and urine specific gravity. Diabetes insipidus is characterized by dilute urine, in large volume, with output often exceeding input, and with urine specific gravity of 1.000 to 1.003. This condition is often diagnosed initially by an alert nurse.
➤ Uncontrolled diabetes mellitus may be associated with excessive urine production. Monitor urine and blood glucose levels and urine specific gravity to help differentiate the two.
➤ Monitor blood pressure. Monitor serum electrolyte level.
➤ Read orders carefully. Vasopressin and vasopressin tannate in oil are different and have different requirements for administration. See Box 5-3 for a discussion of administration of oil-based intramuscular (IM) preparations.

Intravenous desmopressin acetate
➤ Desmopressin acetate may be given undiluted in patients with diabetes insipidus. Administer a single dose over 1 minute. Monitor blood pressure and pulse. This drug may also be administered intravenously in patients with hemophilia A and von Willebrand's disease. For these conditions, it is diluted and is administered as an infusion. Consult the manufacturer's literature.

Nursing in the Community
➤ Review with the patient the anticipated benefits and possible side effects of drug therapy.
➤ If appropriate, instruct the patient to measure urine output at home. Most patients will not need to do this because they can usually tell when urine output is increasing and another dose of medication is needed.
➤ In preparing a patient for discharge with a drug for nasal administration, review the manufacturer's instructions. Have the patient give a return demonstration.
➤ Inform the patient that a severe cold, nasal surgery, or anything that interferes with the ability to sniff may necessitate a temporary switch to an injectable drug, and the patient should contact the physician.
➤ If GI tract distress develops, it may indicate too high a dosage. If GI tract distress is severe or persistent, instruct the patient to notify the physician.
➤ Generally, if more than two sprays per nostril of a drug are needed, it is better to increase the frequency of dosage rather than the number of sprays for each dose.
➤ If a dose is missed, instruct the patient to take the dose as soon as it is remembered unless within a few hours of the next dose, in which case the patient should take a dose but omit the next scheduled dose. The patient should not double up for missed doses. Reinforce to the patient the need to consult the physician for questions about doses.
➤ Refer the patient to a community-based nursing agency for follow-up as appropriate.
➤ Instruct the patient with diabetes insipidus to wear a medical identification tag or bracelet indicating his or her diagnosis.
➤ Instruct the patient to avoid ingestion of alcohol unless permitted in small amounts by the physician.

➤ Chlorothiazide and other thiazide diuretics are discussed in Chapter 14.
➤ Chlorpropamide is discussed in Chapter 69.
➤ Clofibrate is discussed in Chapter 21.

oxytocin and bromocriptine
➤ Oxytocin is discussed in Chapter 71.
➤ Bromocriptine is discussed in Chapter 70.

octreotide
Drug Administration
➤ Monitor blood glucose levels.
➤ Preferred sites for subcutaneous administration include the hip, thigh, or abdomen. Rotate sites.
➤ Assess for GI tract symptoms, including abdominal pain, diarrhea, and nausea and vomiting.
➤ Monitor serum glucose levels and thyroid function tests.

Intravenous octreotide
➤ Octreotide may be given undiluted at a rate of one dose over 3 minutes. It may also be diluted in 50 to 200 ml of normal saline or D5W and given over 15 to 30 minutes as an intermittent infusion, or diluted further and given as a continuous infusion. Intravenous (IV) administration is usually reserved for emergency situations; the subcutaneous route is preferred. To lessen local irritation associated with subcutaneous injection, allow solution to reach room temperature before administering dose.

Nursing in the Community
➤ Review administration technique with the patient. See the patient instruction leaflet, which also includes information about proper storage conditions.
➤ Instruct the patient to administer doses between meals and at bedtime to help avoid GI tract symptoms.
➤ Warn diabetic patients to monitor blood glucose levels carefully because changes in diet or insulin dosage may be necessary.
➤ This drug is also used for treatment of severe diarrhea associated with certain intestinal tumors and is being tested for other uses.

sermorelin
Drug Administration
➤ Dilute each 50 μg with at least 0.5 ml of the 2 ml of normal saline provided. Administer a single dose as a bolus and follow with a normal saline flush.
➤ Monitor vital signs. Assess for headache, nausea/vomiting, paleness, strange taste in the mouth, and tightness in chest.

somatrem and somatropin
Drug Administration
➤ Monitor weight and height. Monitor blood glucose levels and thyroid function tests.
➤ Review manufacturer's literature for instruction about dilution of the specific brand.
➤ Encourage the patient to return for regular follow-up visits.

Nursing Implications Summary—cont'd

➤ Warn the patient that pain and swelling at the injection site may occur.

Nursing in the Community

➤ Review with the patient the anticipated benefits and possible side effects of drug therapy. Warn the patient to take the drug only as ordered and not to increase dose unless directed to do so by the physician.

➤ Warn diabetic patients to monitor blood glucose levels carefully because changes in diet or insulin dosage may be necessary.

➤ Consult with the physician, then teach the family to monitor and record the patient's weight, height, and other parameters regularly.

Panhypopituitarism

Drug Administration/Nursing in the Community

➤ The patient who loses all or nearly all pituitary function from trauma, surgery, or disease must be treated with re-placement hormonal therapy to survive. Treatment with ex-ogenous forms of cortisol usually substitutes for ACTH loss. Thyroid hormones usually replace TSH. Growth hormone is not usually replaced, except in children. ADH may or may not be replaced. Gonadotropic hormones are rarely used in replacement therapy. Estrogens and androgens are used as needed for cosmetic and comfort purposes. In females, it is difficult to recreate the monthly cyclic surges of these hor-mones, so this may not be attempted unless requested by the patient; she is usually sterile. Oxytocin is not replaced unless the woman has conceived and the hormone would be needed during labor and delivery. For information about in-dividual hormones, see Chapters 66 to 72.

➤ Instruct the patient requiring hormonal replacement ther-apy to wear a medical identification tag or bracelet.

CHAPTER REVIEW

Application

1. What are the two divisions of the pituitary gland?
2. What is the nature of anterior pituitary tissue?
3. What hormones are released by the posterior pituitary?
4. Where does synthesis of the hormones released by the posterior pituitary take place?
5. What is the target tissue of ADH?
6. What is the mechanism of action of ADH?
7. What physiologic conditions stimulate the release of ADH?
8. What is diabetes insipidus? How should you assess for this?
9. What two types of therapy may be used to treat diabetes insipidus?
10. What advantage does desmopressin (DDAVP) have over other ADH preparations?
11. What are the side effects associated with ADH?
12. How do thiazide diuretics control diuresis in diabetes insipidus?
13. What are the target tissues of oxytocin?
14. What hormones are secreted by the adenohypophysis?
15. Where does synthesis of the hormones secreted by the adenohypophysis take place?

16. What are the target tissues of growth hormone?
17. What are the anabolic effects of growth hormone?
18. What are the antiinsulin effects of growth hormone? What would the manifestations of this be in a patient?
19. What are IGFs?
20. What is the effect of growth hormone deficiency?
21. How is growth hormone deficiency treated?
22. What is the effect of excessive growth hormone?
23. What are the gonadotropic hormones?
24. What roles do FSH and LH play in causing the develop-ment and release of a mature ovum from the ovary?
25. What are the effects of gonadotropin deficiency?
26. What is the target tissue for ACTH?
27. How is the concentration of ACTH in the blood regulated?

Critical Thinking

1. Compare and contrast the symptoms of diabetes in-sipidus and diabetic mellitus. What are the causes of these symptoms?
2. Your preadolescent patient complains that he or she is "too short," and wants medicine "to make me grow." What factors should be considered in deciding if adminis-tration of growth hormone is good for a child?

References

Davies P: Caring for patients with diabetes insipidus, *Nursing* 26(5):62-63, 1996.

Mitchell DH, Owens B: Replacement therapy: arginine vasopressin (AVP), growth hormone (GH), cortisol, thyroxine, testosterone and estrogen, *J Neurosci Nurs* 28(3):140-154, 1996.

Drugs Affecting the Adrenal Gland

OBJECTIVES

After studying this chapter, you should be able to do the following:

- *Describe the two types of hormones produced in the adrenal glands.*
- *Describe the use of corticosteroids as replacement therapy.*
- *Distinguish mineralocorticoid effects from glucocorticoid effects.*
- *Develop a nursing care plan for a patient receiving a corticosteroid.*

CHAPTER OVERVIEW

The human adrenal gland is divided into two functional units: the adrenal medulla and the adrenal cortex. These regions of the gland differ in embryologic origin, type of cells composing the tissue, and hormones produced. The function of these regions of the adrenal gland, the regulation of synthesis of the various hormones produced, and the pathologic states arising from abnormalities in hormone production are discussed in this chapter. The clinical uses of these hormones and their derivatives in diagnosis and replacement therapy are considered in this chapter; the widespread use of glucocorticoids as antiinflammatory agents is covered in Chapter 41.

THERAPEUTIC RATIONALE: ADRENAL CORTEX

The adrenal cortex is composed of lipid-rich secretory tissue. Three distinct layers within the cortex may be distinguished on the basis of histology. These regions differ in cellular arrangement, in the major steroid hormone produced, and in the regulation of steroid synthesis (Figure 66-1).

Adrenal Steroids

Mineralocorticoids

Physiologic Action

The outer layer, or zona glomerulosa, is where the precursor cholesterol is converted to **mineralocorticoids**. These steroids cause the kidneys to retain sodium and associated water but promote potassium loss.

Regulation of Secretion

Regulation of mineralocorticoid synthesis involves the **renin-angiotensin system** (Figure 66-2). The trigger for this feedback system is in the kidneys, where lower blood sodium levels or lower intravascular volume causes release of renin into the blood. The enzyme renin converts angiotensinogen, a protein from liver, to angiotensin I. Another enzyme found in blood and lungs rapidly converts angiotensin I to angiotensin II. Angiotensin II in turn stimulates the adrenocortical zona glomerulosa to secrete mineralocorticoids, especially aldosterone. The result of this regulatory loop is that mineralocorticoid release slows further loss of sodium and water through the kidneys. When sodium and water retention exceeds certain limits, plasma volume expands and renin release decreases. When the concentration of renin falls, production of angiotensin II slows, aldosterone

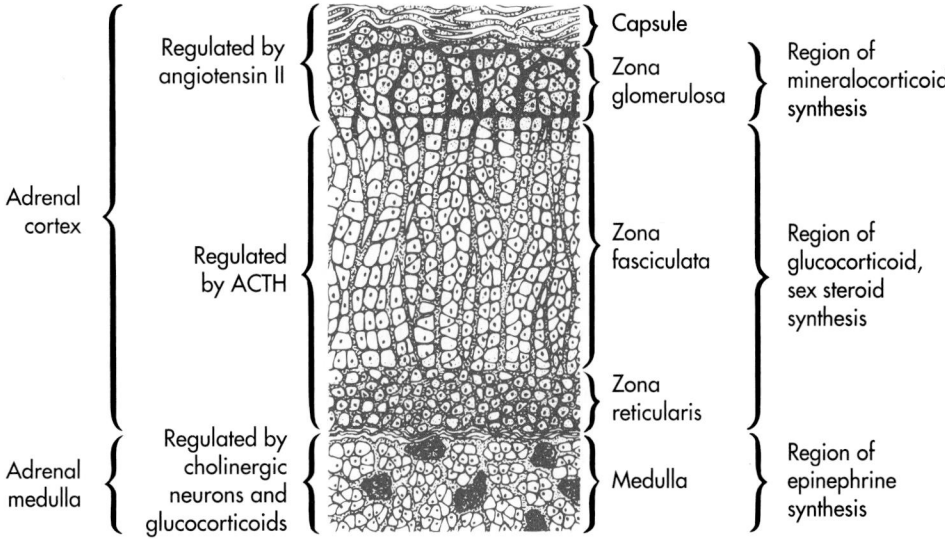

Figure 66-1   Regions of adrenal gland. Each distinct zone of the adrenal gland synthesizes specific hormones and is controlled by specific regulators. Medulla (center of adrenal gland) is thicker than shown in cross section. *ACTH,* Adrenocorticotropic hormone.

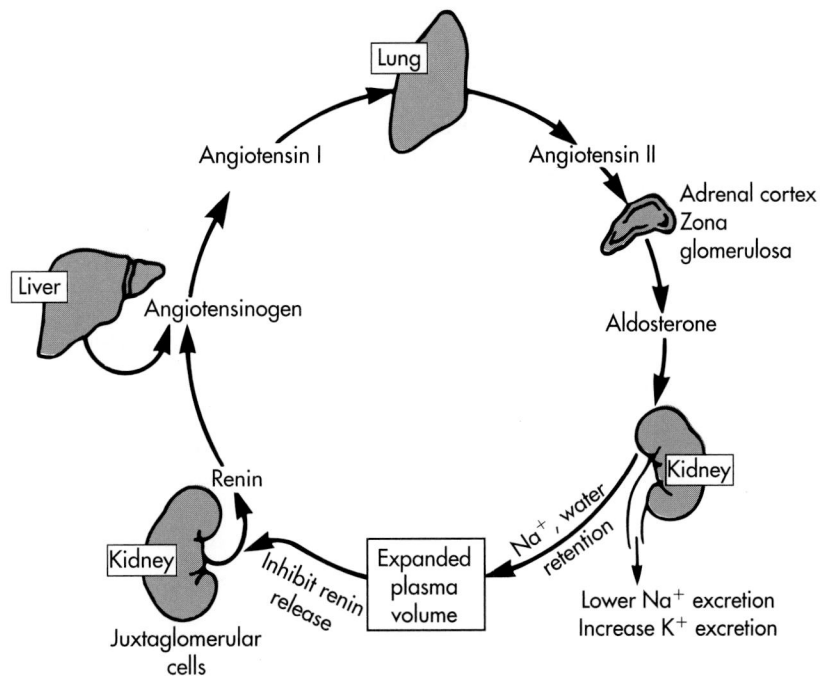

Figure 66-2   Negative feedback loop regulating mineralocorticoid synthesis and release. The kidneys are involved in regulating synthesis and release of aldosterone, the primary natural mineralocorticoid. Renin is released from juxtaglomerular cells of kidneys to set a cascade in motion, and the kidneys are ultimate targets of aldosterone. Expanded plasma volume, which results when the kidneys retain sodium ion *(Na$^+$)* and water, is a regulator that halts renin release. *K$^+$,* Potassium ion.

secretion by the adrenal gland falls, and the kidneys begin to rid the body of accumulated sodium.

Effects of Mineralocorticoid Deficiency

When the adrenal gland fails, mineralocorticoid action is lost. As a result, salt balance becomes deranged. Survival requires replacement of the lost hormone activity.

Effects of Excessive Mineralocorticoids (Hyperaldosteronism)

Tumors of the adrenal gland may produce excessive amounts of aldosterone or less often other mineralocorticoids. In these patients, two types of symptoms appear: those associated with hypertension and those associated with hypokalemia (low blood potassium concentration). Hypertension is caused by sodium and water retention arising from excess aldosterone acting on the kidneys, whereas the muscle weakness associated with hypokalemia is a result of the potassium-wasting action of the steroid in the kidneys. Treatment involves surgical removal of the tumor when possible. Spironolactone, an aldosterone antagonist, may also be used (see Chapter 14).

Corticosteroids

Physiologic Action

The inner two layers of the adrenal cortex convert cholesterol to **corticosteroids,** including glucocorticoids and sex steroids. The primary glucocorticoid is cortisone, and the primary sex steroids are androgens and progestins.

Glucocorticoids produce potent and varied effects on metabolism. The primary metabolic effect is stimulation of gluconeogenesis (the formation of glucose) by actions on peripheral tissues and the liver. In striated muscle, glucocorticoids mobilize amino acids from muscle protein. The result is an increase in circulating levels of amino acids and an overall depletion of muscle protein, which ultimately is expressed as a **negative nitrogen balance** (more nitrogen is excreted than is absorbed in the diet). In the liver, glucocorticoids increase activities of enzymes that convert amino acids to glucose. Much of this excess glucose is then stored in liver as glycogen. In addition, amino acids are the source of precursors for fat synthesis, which is also increased by glucocorticoids.

Glucocorticoids have many direct actions in the body. They maintain water diuresis by antagonizing the effects of antidiuretic hormone (ADH) in the kidney, lower the threshold for electrical excitation in the brain, and reduce the amount of new bone synthesis. In addition, glucocorticoids affect the immune system by suppressing the activity of lymphoid tissue and by reducing the numbers of circulating lymphocytes. These steroids also reduce inflammatory processes by impairing synthesis of prostaglandins and related compounds, an action that has several useful therapeutic applications (see Chapter 41).

In addition to direct effects, glucocorticoids have permissive activities that allow the body to deal successfully with stress or trauma. For example, cortisol sensitizes arterioles to norepinephrine, allowing the catecholamine to increase blood pressure. In the liver, cortisol must be present before epinephrine and glucagon can stimulate breakdown of liver glycogen to glucose, releasing the sugar as an energy source for peripheral muscle.

Regulation of Secretion

The synthesis of these steroids is regulated by the pituitary gland and the hypothalamus via the negative feedback loop (described in Chapter 64). Cortisol is the major glucocorticoid produced, and it is the key to the regulation of steroid synthesis in the zona fasciculata and zona reticularis. Low levels of cortisol in blood stimulate and high levels suppress total steroid synthesis by respectively raising and lowering adrenocorticotropic hormone (ACTH) release from the pituitary.

Effects of Adrenal Insufficiency

Failure of the adrenal cortex is life-threatening. If failure is sudden, which might occur after adrenal injury or thrombosis, death can occur within hours. Early symptoms of acute adrenal insufficiency include confusion, restlessness, nausea, and vomiting. Circulatory collapse, deep shock, and death may follow rapidly.

If synthesis of glucocorticoids is reduced but not halted, patients may not be in immediate danger, in the absence of stress or trauma, but they may still have inadequate amounts of glucocorticoids. This chronic primary adrenal insufficiency is called **Addison's disease.** Symptoms include weakness, weight loss, dehydration, hypotension, hypoglycemia, and anemia. Most patients with Addison's disease also display increased skin pigmentation. This unusual or excessive tanning is caused by a direct effect on melanin-containing skin cells by the long-term excess of ACTH, which is secreted by the hypophysis in response to the elevated corticotropin-releasing hormone (CRH) induced by chronically low blood levels of cortisol.

Symptoms similar to those of Addison's disease are produced when the adenohypophysis is diseased or destroyed and no longer produces adequate ACTH. Without ACTH, the zona reticularis and zona fasciculata do not synthesize cortisol, and over time these adrenal tissues atrophy. This condition is called secondary adrenal insufficiency. One characteristic that often visibly distinguishes these patients from those with Addison's disease is the absence of excessive pigmentation. In secondary adrenal insufficiency, the hypophysis does not release large quantities of ACTH and the skin is not darkened.

Effects of Excessive Glucocorticoids

Overproduction of cortisol, a condition called **Cushing's syndrome,** may be induced by a variety of factors. Some patients have high cortisol production from tumors of the adrenal cortex, which may synthesize massive amounts of the steroid. Other patients have high cortisol synthesis because of increased ACTH release into the blood, which keeps the zona fasciculata and zona reticularis maximally stimulated to produce glucocorticoids. Excess ACTH usually comes from a tumor of the hypophysis, but occasionally it comes from some unusual source, such as a lung tumor, which would not ordinarily be expected to synthesize ACTH. Most often, however, Cushing's syndrome is caused by administration of high dosages of glucocorticoids.

The symptoms of Cushing's syndrome can be predicted from the metabolic actions of cortisol. Certain fat stores, especially those on the face and shoulders, are increased as a result of cortisol stimulation of fat synthesis. The extremities may be weak and, in more advanced cases, may be thin because of the muscle-wasting effects of the hormone. The skin is fragile and easily bruised as a result of protein breakdown in that tissue. Examination of the skin on the trunk may reveal striae, or stretch marks, over areas where fat deposition is most pronounced. Many pa-

ALTERNATIVE THERAPIES

Adaptogen

GINSENG

The state of modern scientific knowledge of the pharmacology and therapeutic usefulness of ginseng deserves to be described as confusing and incomplete. Literally hundreds of books, articles, and scientific reports have been published on ginseng. However, because most of them present primarily anecdotal information or information derived from poorly designed, poorly-controlled scientific studies, little can be said with scientific certainty about the beneficial effects of this interesting drug in human beings.

The drug consists of the dried root of Asian and American ginseng. Asian ginseng is widely cultivated in China and Korea and is relatively available, but American ginseng, which grows wild, has been so massively harvested that it has been declared an endangered species.

Ginseng's medicinal history goes back more than 2000 years. It has been hailed as an aphrodisiac and tonic, and more recently, as an antioxidant, a lipid-lowering drug, and radioprotectant. The currently popular designation for ginseng is as an "adaptogen," an agent that enhances the body's response and resiliency to physical stress. However, neither this therapeutic designation nor any other has been definitively studied and scientifically documented.

The literature spanning centuries contains very few reports of serious toxicity associated with ginseng, although prolonged consumption of high dosages (15 g/day) have been reported, without verification, to cause hypertension and nervousness. Ginseng may reduce the effectiveness of antihypertensive drugs.

Prospective users of commercial ginseng products should purchase them from the most reputable suppliers they can find. High-quality ginseng is very expensive, and unreliable quality control allows commercial ginseng products to vary widely in quality and actual ginseng content. For example, two independent studies of 54 ginseng products showed 60% of them to be substantially substandard. Fully 25% of the products studied contained no ginseng at all.

---

tients also have superficial fungal infections of the skin, related in part to the fragility of the skin and to the reduced host immune response caused by the excess steroid. Bone thinning occurs because of changes in calcium metabolism; compression fractures of the spine may occur relatively easily. Diabetes may be precipitated from the increased insulin demand caused by excess cortisol. Hypertension is common in these patients, and atherosclerosis may occur. Mood changes are also common and may be extreme. Psychosis may be precipitated.

Effects of Excessive Adrenal Production of Sex Steroids

Sex steroids produced in the adrenal cortex are normally of minor importance, the adrenal output being small compared with that of the gonads; however, under certain conditions, sex steroid overproduction in the adrenal glands may cause a devastating endocrine imbalance. For example, a female with an androgen-producing adrenal tumor may undergo masculinization, including development of secondary male sex characteristics and suppression of the menstrual cycle. A male with an estrogen-producing tumor may develop breast tenderness or loss of libido. A child may show precocious sexual development.

THERAPEUTIC AGENTS: ADRENAL STEROIDS AND RELATED COMPOUNDS

Compounds Used in Replacement Therapy

▼ Glucocorticoids: cortisone

Mechanism of Action

Three major activities of the adrenal steroids are metabolic effects on carbohydrate, protein, and fat metabolism; antiinflammatory and immunosuppressive activity; and sodium-retaining activity associated with potassium loss. The first two are classified as glucocorticoid actions and the third as a mineralocorticoid action.

The natural adrenal steroid cortisol possesses both glucocorticoid and mineralocorticoid activity. Therefore treatment with this natural compound produces multiple effects. For example, cortisol at the high dosages required for antiinflammatory action (see Chapter 41) not only changes metabolism as expected from a glucocorticoid but also produces excessive sodium retention and potassium loss, a mineralocorticoid effect. Synthetic glucocorticoids have been designed to have very little mineralocorticoid activity. These drugs include betamethasone, dexamethasone, triamcinolone, and methylprednisolone, which are used primarily as antiinflammatory drugs (see Chapter 41).

To produce their effects, steroids must pass through the membranes of target cells, bind to soluble cytoplasmic receptors, and be carried to the cell nucleus (see Chapter 64). In the nucleus the steroid induces changes in RNA and protein synthesis, which will be expressed as some change in function of the target cell. A considerable delay may occur between uptake of the steroid into the cell and appearance of the effect in the target cell. More time may elapse before the effect ends and the steroid is destroyed.

Pharmacokinetics

The chemical form of a steroid determines the pharmacokinetics of the preparation. Most corticosteroids are relatively insoluble in water and form suspensions that are not suitable for intravenous (IV) administration. In contrast, sodium phosphate and sodium succinate derivatives of several glucocorticoids are quite water soluble; these are the forms that must be used when IV administration of an adrenal steroid is required.

Administered intramuscularly as suspensions, many glucocorticoids are dissolved and absorbed slowly from the injection site, producing a relatively long duration of action, which may be an advantage for control of certain conditions.

Uses

Synthetic glucocorticoids are used primarily for their antiinflammatory and immunosuppressant effects (see Chapter 41). In addition to these indications, corticosteroids have been used in the control of certain types of cancers (see Chapter 56). Corticosteroids used most often for replacement therapy are summarized in Table 66-1.

Examples of replacement therapy include the use of cortisol to treat Addison's disease or secondary adrenal insufficiency. Dosages of adrenal steroids used in replacement therapy are relatively low because they are intended to replace only amounts of the hormone normally present. Because the normal daily production of cortisol is about 15 to 25 mg, the daily replacement dose would be designed to achieve the level of activity produced by that amount of cortisol. Wide variations in dosage exist because stress and other factors affect steroid requirements. The dosage must be adjusted to each patient's needs and monitored to ensure continued success of the therapy.

Successful treatment of adrenal insufficiency often is obtained with hydrocortisone or **cortisone**, natural glucocorticoids with sufficient mineralocorticoid activity to maintain sodium balance for many individuals. Other patients may require additional supplementation with a mineralocorticoid such as fludrocortisone (see Table 66-1).

Adverse Reactions and Contraindications

Adverse reactions are mild when glucocorticoids are used in replacement therapy because dosages are usually low. Higher dosages used for longer than a few days, such as those used to control inflammatory conditions (see Chapter 41), are associated with many more side effects. Patients who receive corticosteroids as replacement therapy would normally continue to receive them for life.

Toxicity

Any glucocorticoid, if given in high enough dosages, will produce Cushing's syndrome. This toxicity is one of the most common reactions seen with glucocorticoid therapy. For these patients the steroid dosage should be reduced, if allowed by the severity of the condition being treated. Although usual replacement doses slightly exceed normal daily production of steroids, these doses would not be expected to cause Cushing's syndrome.

Other common symptoms of glucocorticoid toxicity include euphoria, glucose intolerance, osteoporosis, and muscle wasting. These effects occur after long-term use of glucocorticoids.

Interactions

The effects of many drugs are altered in patients receiving high dosages of glucocorticoids (see Chapter 41). Interactions are unlikely with the low dosages used in replacement therapy.

▼ Mineralocorticoids: fludrocortisone
Mechanism of Action

Any mineralocorticoid could be used for replacement therapy in adrenal insufficiency, but the potent synthetic agent fludrocortisone is preferred. **Fludrocortisone** has the same mechanism of action as natural mineralocorticoids, increasing renal excretion of potassium and hydrogen ions while promoting sodium and water retention.

Pharmacokinetics

Fludrocortisone is the mineralocorticoid of choice because it is well absorbed orally. The duration of action of a single

Table 66-1	**Drugs for Adrenal Replacement Therapy**		
Generic Name	Trade Name	Administration/Dosage	Comments
betamethasone	Celestone*	ORAL: *Adults*—0.6-7.2 mg/day. FDA pregnancy category C. *Children*—5.83 μg/kg 3 times/day.	Synthetic glucocorticoid with little or no mineralocorticoid action; used with mineralocorticoid.
cortisone	Cortone*	ORAL, INTRAMUSCULAR: *Adults*—25-300 mg/day. FDA pregnancy category C. *Children*—0.35 mg/kg twice daily (oral) or once daily (IM).	Natural hormone with both glucocorticoid and mineralocorticoid action.
fludrocortisone	Florinef*	ORAL: *Adults*—0.1 mg/day. FDA pregnancy category C. *Children*—0.05-0.1 mg/day.	Synthetic steroid with strong mineralocorticoid action; used with glucocorticoid for replacement therapy.
hydrocortisone	Cortef*	ORAL, INTRAMUSCULAR: *Adults*—20-240 mg/day. FDA pregnancy category C. *Children*—0.56 mg/kg/day.	Has both glucocorticoid and mineralocorticoid action.
triamcinolone	Aristocort* Kenacort*	ORAL: *Adults*—4-12 mg/day in single or divided doses. FDA pregnancy category C. *Children*—0.117 mg/kg in single or divided doses daily.	Synthetic glucocorticoid with little or no mineralocorticoid action; used with mineralocorticoid.

*Available in Canada and the United States.

dose is 1 to 2 days. The drug is renally eliminated as inactive metabolites.

Uses

Fludrocortisone is used only for its mineralocorticoid action. It is used in the treatment of chronic primary and secondary adrenocortical insufficiency. The drug may also be effective in salt-losing forms of adrenogenital syndrome.

Adverse Reactions and Contraindications

Adverse reactions are rare with fludrocortisone. Allergic reactions are possible. Some patients may be sensitive to the effects of sodium retention caused by the drug, resulting in congestive heart failure or peripheral edema.

There is no contraindication for fludrocortisone when used for replacement therapy. Patients with heart disease or hypertension may require special precautions.

Toxicity

Excessive action of fludrocortisone leads to excessive sodium retention and potassium loss (see Chapter 17).

Interactions

Interactions with fludrocortisone are often associated with the electrolyte changes caused by the drug. For example, the hypokalemia caused by fludrocortisone can increase toxicity of digitalis glycosides and increase the risk with other drugs that cause hypokalemia. Drug preparations or foods that contain large amounts of sodium may cause hypernatremia because kidneys under the influence of fludrocortisone may be unable to clear the excess sodium.

Inducers of hepatic metabolic enzymes may increase metabolism of fludrocortisone, necessitating an increase in dosage of fludrocortisone. Rifampin and phenytoin have been reported to cause this effect.

Compounds Used in Diagnosing Adrenal Disorders

adrenocorticotropic hormone

Adrenocorticotropic hormone (ACTH, corticotropin) is discussed in Chapter 64 as part of the natural feedback regulatory cycle controlling adrenal function. Cosyntropin is a synthetic version of ACTH that contains the first 24 of the 39 amino acids found in natural ACTH. This synthetic form of ACTH (as well as natural ACTH) directly stimulates the adrenal cortex to synthesize adrenal steroids. This action can be used diagnostically to distinguish between Addison's disease and secondary adrenal insufficiency resulting from pituitary dysfunction (Table 66-2). Normal adrenal glands respond to ACTH by synthesizing and releasing cortisol into the bloodstream, where it may be measured. In Addison's disease the adrenal gland cannot respond to ACTH, and no excess cortisol is produced. In patients who have low pituitary function, the adrenal gland may be suppressed and may respond less rapidly to ACTH than would a normal gland.

In the past, ACTH has been used to treat adrenal insufficiency or other diseases responding to glucocorticoids. The rationale for this therapy was that adrenal function was maintained and that a natural balance of steroids was produced. In practice, however, ACTH therapy was not as reliable or convenient as steroid therapy. ACTH must be injected because it is a peptide, whereas oral glucocorticoids are available. In addition, the response of the adrenal gland to ACTH was not easily predictable, making dosage adjustment unreliable. Finally, many patients developed antibodies to ACTH; as a result, they became unresponsive to it. For these reasons and others, ACTH is no longer widely used in therapy. Cosyntropin produces less of an allergic reaction than ACTH but is still inappropriate for conditions that can be treated with steroids.

Table 66-2 Agents Used in Diagnosing Adrenal Gland Dysfunction

Generic Name	Trade Name	Administration/Dosage	Comments
corticorelin ovine	ACTHREL	INTRAVENOUS: *Adults, children*—1 μg/kg given over 30-60 sec. FDA pregnancy category C.	Analog of natural human CRH; stimulates release of ACTH.
corticotropin	Acthar*	INTRAVENOUS: *Adults—For diagnosis of adrenal/pituitary function:* 10-25 units in 500 ml of 5% dextrose, given over 8 hr. FDA pregnancy category C.	Natural ACTH, protein from pituitary glands of animals.
cosyntropin	Cortosyn*	INTRAVENOUS, INTRAMUSCULAR, SUBCUTANEOUS: *Adults*—0.25 mg as single injection or infused over 2 min-6 hr. FDA pregnancy category C. INTRAMUSCULAR: *Children <2 yr*—0.125 mg. *Older children:* Same as adult doses.	Synthetic peptide that matches first 24 amino acids in ACTH.
metyrapone	Metopirone*	ORAL: *Adults—For diagnosis of secondary adrenal insufficiency:* 30 mg/kg at midnight; measure plasma cortisol at 8 AM. FDA pregnancy category C. *Children*—15 mg/kg every 4 hr for 6 doses.	Metyrapone blocks cortisol synthesis in adrenals; acute adrenal insufficiency may occur.

ACTH, Adrenocorticotropic hormone.
*Available in Canada and the United States.

dexamethasone

The highly potent synthetic glucocorticoid dexamethasone may be used diagnostically to test steroid suppression of cortisol synthesis. Relatively small doses of dexamethasone administered over 2 days inhibit cortisol production in a healthy person and, to a lesser extent, in a person with pituitary-induced Cushing's syndrome. Ordinarily, tumor production of cortisol is unaffected.

corticorelin ovine

Corticorelin ovine is a form of CRH that is related to human CRH and has the same ability to cause release of ACTH from the anterior pituitary gland in humans. This form of CRH is used to identify the source of high ACTH levels. Corticorelin ovine induces release of ACTH from the pituitary, but tumors or other ectopic sites of ACTH production usually do not respond. Thus persons with normal pituitary function or with oversecretion from the pituitary show a rise in ACTH and cortisol after administration of corticorelin ovine. Production of ACTH or cortisol is not changed in response to corticorelin ovine when the primary source of ACTH is a tumor.

metyrapone

Metyrapone blocks cortisol synthesis in the adrenal gland and may be used to test the ability of the pituitary gland to increase ACTH release (see Table 66-2). Before the test is run, it should be demonstrated that the patient's adrenal glands respond to ACTH. While metyrapone is being administered, cortisol synthesis falls dramatically. In healthy persons the fall in blood cortisol level stimulates the hypothalamus and in turn the pituitary gland, with the result that ACTH is released into the blood. Under the influence of ACTH, early steps in steroid synthesis proceed, but metyrapone prevents cortisol from being formed in normal amounts. Therefore steroid precursors accumulate and are excreted in urine. If no precursors accumulate under these conditions, it is concluded that the pituitary gland failed to produce ACTH. If the metyrapone test is administered to a person with adrenal insufficiency, a danger exists of precipitating an adrenal crisis because in such a patient metyrapone may stop cortisol synthesis altogether.

THERAPEUTIC RATIONALE: ADRENAL MEDULLA

The adrenal medulla arises from neuroectodermal tissue during embryonic life and remains closely associated with the autonomic nervous system at maturity. The cells (pheochromocytes or chromaffin cells) can synthesize catecholamines by the same series of reactions found in nerve terminals and can release catecholamines into the bloodstream in response to sympathetic cholinergic presynaptic neurons. One major difference between the synthetic pathways is that nerve terminals form norepinephrine as the final product, whereas the adrenal medulla converts norepinephrine to epinephrine. The enzyme for this final conversion is induced by adrenal steroids, indicating that the anatomic closeness of the cortex and medulla may have functional importance.

THERAPEUTIC AGENTS: HORMONES OF THE ADRENAL MEDULLA

The hormones of the adrenal medulla are not essential to survival, but they are useful in adapting to stress. Epinephrine produces widespread effects throughout the body, mediated by the beta- and alpha-adrenergic receptors. The actions of epinephrine are discussed in Chapter 12, and the clinical uses of epinephrine are discussed in Chapter 16.

Nursing Process Overview

Drugs Affecting the Adrenal Gland

Assessment

Monitor vital signs, blood pressure, and weight. Question the patient about history of infections, energy level, and ability to perform activities of daily living.

Nursing Diagnoses

- Potential complication: electrolyte abnormalities

Patient Outcomes

The nurse will manage and minimize electrolyte disturbances.

Planning/Implementation

Many of the drugs discussed in this chapter are used for diagnostic purposes. Keep the patient informed as tests are completed. Provide emotional support as needed. Prepare the patient for self-administration at home, if appropriate. If the drugs are used for a chronic problem, instruct the patient about side effects. Emphasize the importance of continuing therapy as prescribed and not discontinuing drug therapy without talking with physician.

Evaluation

If the drug is used for diagnostic purposes, the drug is effective if the test is completed with no side effects. If used for long-term therapy, make certain the patient can administer the drug correctly, knows the side effects of the drug, and understands when to contact the physician.

Nursing Implications Summary

Glucocorticoids
➤ Glucocorticoids are discussed in detail in Chapter 41.

fludrocortisone and Mineralocorticoids
Drug Administration
➤ All glucocorticoids also have mineralocorticoid activity but in varying amounts (see Table 41-1).
➤ Monitor weight, blood pressure, and pulse. Auscultate lung and heart sounds.
➤ Monitor serum electrolyte levels.
➤ For a discussion of intramuscular (IM) injection of oil-based medications, see Chapter 5.

Nursing in the Community
➤ Review anticipated benefits and possible side effects of drug therapy with the patient.
➤ Counsel the patient about sodium restriction and increasing potassium intake as needed. See the Dietary Considerations boxes on potassium sources (Chapter 14) and sodium and hypertension (Chapter 13).
➤ Encourage the patient to wear a medical identification tag or bracelet.
➤ Remind the patient to inform all health care providers of all drugs being used.

corticorelin ovine
Drug Administration
➤ Obtain baseline vital signs. Warn the patient that flushing of the face, neck, and upper chest may occur. Instruct the patient to report dizziness, feeling faint, or shortness of breath.
➤ Check with laboratory before administering dose for diagnostic purposes to determine schedule for drawing predose and postdose blood work.
➤ Reconstitute immediately before use by adding 2 ml normal saline to each vial. Roll vial to dissolve powder; avoid bubbles and do not shake. Administer dose over 30 to 60 seconds.

corticotropin
Drug Administration/Nursing in the Community
➤ Before IV administration, check that vial states "for IV use." Monitor patient for at least 30 minutes after dose.
➤ Emphasize the importance of continuing this drug as prescribed and not discontinuing this drug without discussing it with the physician.
➤ Review administration technique with the patient.
➤ Reinforce the importance of dietary changes (low-salt or potassium-rich diet) if prescribed.
➤ Review the manufacturer's insert for administration guidelines, depending on use.

cosyntropin
Drug Administration
➤ See the manufacturer's instruction sheet.
➤ For IV administration: Dilute with the diluent provided by manufacturer. Cosyntropin may then be given by direct IV or further diluted in 5% D5W or 0.9% saline and given as an infusion. For a single dose, administer over 2 minutes. For infusion, administer over 4 to 8 hours, depending on the volume of infusion and age and condition of patient.
➤ Monitor vital signs. Assess for dizziness, fever, flushing, rash, and urticaria. Remain with the patient for at least 30 minutes after administration.

metyrapone
Drug Administration/Nursing in the Community
➤ Monitor blood pressure and vital signs.
➤ Instruct the patient that this drug may cause nausea and vomiting and to take doses with food, milk, or meals to lessen this side effect.
➤ Caution the patient to avoid driving or operating hazardous equipment if dizziness, drowsiness, or lightheadedness occurs.
➤ Monitor plasma or urinary cortisol and serum electrolytes.

 # CHAPTER REVIEW

Application
1. What are the two functional units of the adrenal gland?
2. What are mineralocorticoids?
3. In which part of the adrenal cortex are mineralocorticoids synthesized?
4. How is mineralocorticoid synthesis regulated?
5. What is the effect of overproduction of mineralocorticoids?
6. Where are glucocorticoids synthesized?
7. What are the main effects of glucocorticoids on metabolism?
8. What is the result of untreated adrenal insufficiency?
9. What causes Cushing's syndrome?
10. What are the three major actions of corticosteroids?
11. Name three clinical uses of adrenal corticosteroids.
12. What is the aim of replacement therapy in treating adrenal insufficiency?
13. Which mineralocorticoid is most commonly used clinically? Why?
14. How is ACTH used in diagnosis?
15. What forms of ACTH are available and how do they differ?
16. Why is ACTH not commonly used in replacement therapy?

Continued

17. How is metyrapone used for diagnosis of pituitary function?
18. How is corticorelin ovine used for diagnosis?

Critical Thinking

1. What is Addison's disease? How would you assess for this?

2. What are the symptoms of Cushing's syndrome? How would you assess these?
3. What is the effect of long-term overdosage with glucocorticoids? What signs and symptoms would you assess?

Reference

Brenner ZR, Cannito M: Administering steroids, *Nursing* 28(3):34-44, 1998.

Drugs Affecting the Thyroid Gland

OBJECTIVES

After studying this chapter, you should be able to do the following:

- *Discuss the rationale for therapy of hypothyroidism.*
- *Describe the classes of drugs used for hypothyroidism.*
- *Discuss the rationale for therapy of hyperthyroidism.*
- *Describe the classes of drugs used for hyperthyroidism.*
- *Develop a nursing care plan for the patient receiving drug therapy for hypothyroidism or hyperthyroidism.*

CHAPTER OVERVIEW

The thyroid gland is a richly vascularized, horseshoe-shaped organ lying across the trachea in the region of the larynx (Figure 67-1). The gland contains primarily two cell types differing in function and embryologic origin: follicular cells and parafollicular cells. The action of parafollicular cells on calcium metabolism is discussed in Chapter 68. Hormones produced by follicular cells and the drugs commonly used in diagnosing and treating disease states associated with deficient or excessive thyroid function are described in this chapter.

THERAPEUTIC RATIONALE: THYROID GLAND

Follicular Cells

Follicular cells in the thyroid regulate the basal metabolic rate (BMR) for most tissues in the body. This regulation is achieved by the iodine-containing hormones thyroxine (T_4) and triiodothyronine (T_3), which are released by follicular cells into the general circulation and alter oxidative processes in target tissues.

Thyroid Hormones (T_4 and T_3)

Physiologic Action

Thyroid hormones act through a high-affinity receptor in cell nuclei. Thus they regulate expression of genes and modulate the primary function of cells by changing the pattern of protein synthesized. The receptor for thyroid hormones is of the same family of receptors used by adrenal steroids, vitamin D, and vitamin A.

Tissues especially sensitive to thyroid hormones are skeletal muscles, heart, liver, and kidneys. The basal metabolic rate in these tissues is strongly stimulated by thyroid hormones, but other organs, including the brain, are much less responsive. Clinically observed signs of these effects include rapid heartbeat and increased cardiac output.

Regulation of Secretion

Regulation of thyroid hormone levels in the blood is accomplished in part by the negative feedback system described in Chapter 64. Thyroid-stimulating hormone (TSH) from the anterior pituitary (adenohypophysis) stimulates each step in thyroid hormone synthesis described here.

Figure 67-1   Anatomic location of thyroid and parathyroid glands.

The first step in synthesizing T_4 and T_3 is iodine uptake by follicular cells (Figure 67-2). Because iodide ion levels in blood are low, follicular cells must concentrate iodine to carry out the synthetic reactions required. In the normal human body the concentration of iodide ion in the thyroid is 30 to 40 times that found in plasma. In the second step in thyroid hormone synthesis, iodide ion activation is catalyzed by a peroxidase enzyme formed in follicular cells. This activation step takes place on the surface of microvilli that protrude into colloid filling the thyroid follicle.

Once activated, iodine may be attached to thyroglobulin in a process called organification. Thyroglobulin, a large protein synthesized in follicular cells and extruded into follicles, is the major protein component of colloid. Most iodine atoms are attached to tyrosine molecules contained within the peptide chains of thyroglobulin. A tyrosine may contain one (3-monoiodotyrosine, or MIT) or two (3,5-diiodotyrosine, or DIT) atoms of iodine.

After iodination, some tyrosine molecules may undergo a coupling reaction in which two molecules of DIT combine to produce one molecule of thyroglobulin-bound T_4. Coupling may also occur between one molecule each of DIT and MIT to yield one molecule of T_3.

Thyroglobulin is primarily a storage depot for thyroid hormones and the precursors MIT and DIT. In healthy persons, each molecule of thyroglobulin contains about six molecules of MIT, five molecules of DIT, and two molecules of T_4. Less T_3 is stored. A single molecule of T_3 occurs in about one of three molecules of thyroglobulin within the follicles. Thus normal thyroids contain a 30-day supply of T_3 and T_4 and a 20-day supply of iodine stored as MIT and DIT.

When release of thyroid hormones is required, TSH stimulates microvilli of the follicular cells to move droplets of colloid into the cell. The colloid droplets fuse with lysosomes inside the cells to form vesicles called phagolysosomes. The low pH and the protein-digesting enzymes from the lysosomes break thyroglobulin down to amino acids. This process releases T_3, T_4, MIT, and DIT into the cell. T_3 and T_4 are transported to the cell surface and released into the blood. In contrast, MIT and DIT are retained within the cell, and the iodine they contain is reclaimed for use in new hormone synthesis. Patients who lack the salvage pathway lose excessive iodide ion in urine and ultimately fail to produce sufficient thyroid hormones.

Once in blood, thyroid hormones are rapidly and almost completely bound to a special alpha-globulin called thyroid-binding globulin (TBG). A less important carrier is prealbumin..Very little thyroid hormone is bound to plasma albumin in normal persons because the thyroid hormones are so tightly bound to TBG. However, the amount of thyroid hormone that may be bound to TBG is limited. TBG can bind about 2.5 times more hormone than it ordinarily carries. When that limit is reached, the excess hormone is bound to albumin and prealbumin. These proteins are less avid

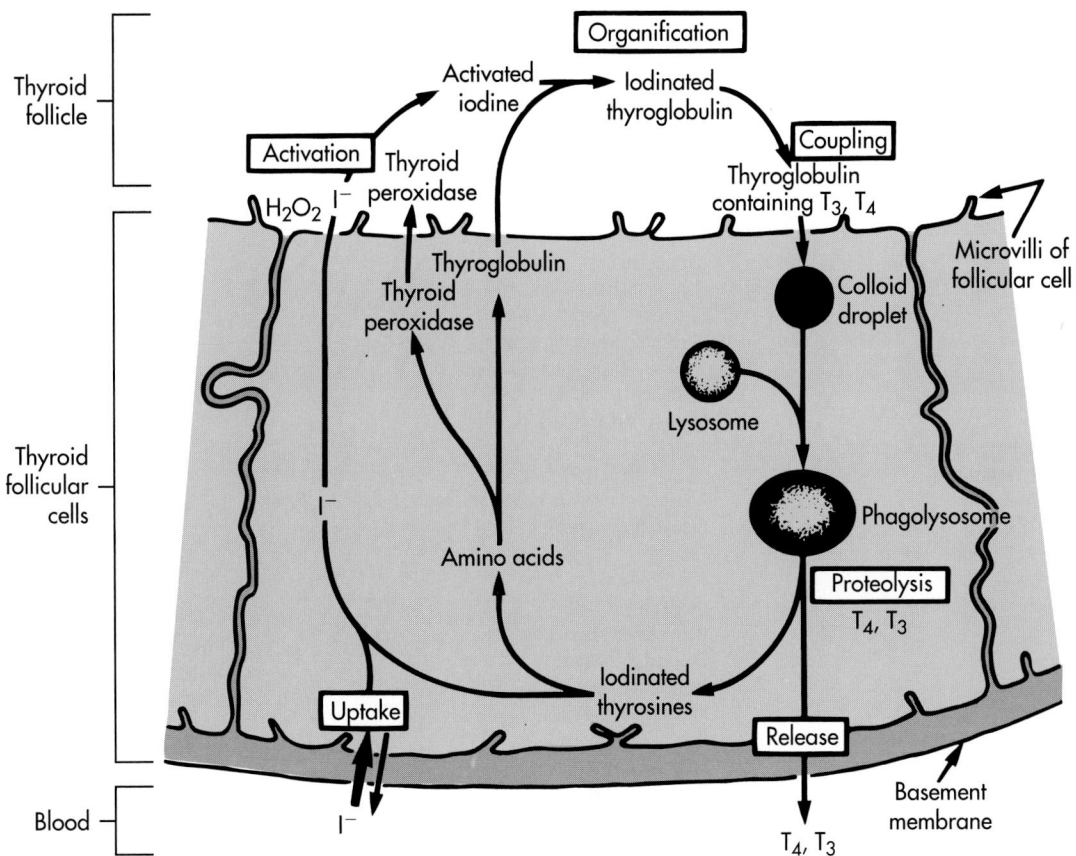

Figure 67-2 Synthesis of triiodothyronine *(T₃)* and thyroxine *(T₄)* by follicular cells within the thyroid gland. Single follicular cell is depicted. Cell base is in close contact with blood, and cell apex is in contact with colloid. These cells surround areas of colloid to form thyroid follicles. Parafollicular cells of thyroid gland do not directly contact colloid.

carriers than TBG but have nearly unlimited capacity for hormones.

The relative distribution of T_3 and T_4 differs within the body. T_4 is much more abundant than T_3 in the thyroid and in blood. The thyroid gland normally releases 70 to 90 μg of T_4 daily and only 1 to 6 μg of T_3, but T_4 is rapidly converted to T_3 in most tissues. Thus the most abundant form of thyroid hormone in target cells is T_3. T_3 is also the primary thyroid hormone that binds to nuclear receptors, setting off the metabolic events characteristic of thyroid action. For these reasons, T_3 is the most important metabolic regulator from the thyroid.

In addition to being converted to T_3, T_4 may be converted to an alternate form called reverse T_3. Reverse T_3 contains a different arrangement of iodine atoms than T_3 and is metabolically inactive.

Effects of Thyroid Hormone Deficiency

Hypothyroidism occurs when the production of thyroid hormones is insufficient to meet the body's demands. Mild hormone deficiencies produce minimum disease with vague symptoms, sometimes making the condition difficult to diagnose. Untreated patients may ultimately develop charac-

teristic signs and symptoms related to slowed metabolic rates and changes in the central nervous system (CNS) (Table 67-1). The severe form of the disease is called **myxedema,** which may progress to a life-threatening coma with profoundly lowered metabolic rate, depressed CNS, and hypoventilation.

Hypothyroidism may develop in newborns because of an embryologic or genetic defect that arrests thyroid development or prevents its function. A child lacking adequate thyroid function during fetal development may appear nearly normal at birth because much of fetal development can be supported by maternal T_4, which readily crosses the placenta and enters the fetal brain. If the disease is not detected soon after birth, however, irreversible brain damage and associated physical signs develop. Congenital hypothyroidism is called cretinism.

Hypothyroidism that develops after the neonatal period but before puberty is called juvenile hypothyroidism. The most prominent early sign of juvenile hypothyroidism is growth stunting. If not treated appropriately, juvenile hypothyroid patients experience not only arrested growth but also other signs and symptoms associated with adult forms of the disease.

Table 67-1 Thyroid Disorders

Condition	Symptoms	Physical Appearance
Hypothyroidism, adult onset (also called myxedema and Gull's disease)	Diminished vigor and muscle weakness Reduced mental acuity Emotional changes, especially depression Slow relaxation of deep tendon reflexes Muscle cramps Constipation Decreased appetite Abnormal menses in females Slow pulse and enlarged heart Tendency to gain weight Lowered basal metabolic rate	Puffy face and eyes Thin, coarse hair and eyebrows Dry, scaly, cold, and slightly yellow skin Enlarged tongue Slow, husky speech Dull or slow-witted appearance

Hypothyroidism, congenital (cretinism)
  At birth
 	
  At 3 months with no treatment
	
	Absence of distal femoral and proximal tibial epiphyses
	Slowed brain development
	Lethargy
	Feeding difficulty
	Constipation
	Neonatal jaundice, persistent
	Respiratory distress
	Hoarse cry
	Intermittent cyanosis
		
		Essentially normal
		Slightly longer and heavier than normal
		Enlarged tongue
		Puffy face and thick neck
		Poor muscle tone
		Depressed nasal bridge with broad, flat nose
		Distended abdomen
		Umbilical hernia
		Short legs

Hyperthyroidism (also called thyrotoxicosis or Graves' disease)	Cardiac arrhythmia Enlarged thyroid gland Rapid pulse rate Increased basal metabolic rate Muscle weakness and wasting Fine tremor Heat intolerance Weight loss in most patients	Restlessness or nervousness Abrupt actions and speech Warm, moist palms Loosening of fingernails from nailbeds Bulging eyes with sclera visible all around iris White, unpigmented patches on skin (vitiligo)

Effects of Excessive Thyroid Hormones

Hyperthyroidism occurs when excess thyroid hormones are released into circulation. The disease ranges from mild forms displaying few of the symptoms shown in Table 67-1 to a severe condition called thyroid storm in which death may result from an abrupt rise in body temperature and vascular collapse. Increased thyroid hormone production may result from hyperfunction of the entire gland or from excessive output of one or more small nodules within the thyroid. A rare cause of hyperthyroidism is excess TSH, either from the pituitary gland or from a tumor.

Hyperthyroidism may exist with or without thyroid nodules. The disease without nodules is the most common form and is called toxic diffuse goiter, thyrotoxicosis, or **Graves' disease.** Many patients with this condition display exophthalmos (bulging eyes). Because many patients also have enlarged thyroid glands, another common name for this condition is exophthalmic goiter. Toxic nodular goiter produces the same general symptoms as Graves' disease, except that eye symptoms are rare in the nodular form.

Hyperthyroidism is rare in children and is most common in adults in the third or fourth decade of life. Women are affected more often than men, but the reasons are unclear.

Graves' disease may be precipitated in women by puberty, pregnancy, or menopause. Subacute thyroiditis can produce a reversible hyperthyroidism. This condition seems to appear sometime after recovery from viral diseases and may be caused by the infectious process.

THERAPEUTIC AGENTS: DRUGS AFFECTING THE THYROID GLAND

Diagnosis of Hypothyroidism

Hypothyroidism is diagnosed by the judicious use of a combination of the thyroid function tests summarized in Table 67-2. An understanding of these tests requires knowledge of normal thyroid physiology and an understanding of the negative feedback regulation of the thyroid (see Chapter 65).

In primary hypothyroidism the thyroid gland is defective. The diagnosis of primary hypothyroidism requires showing that a patient has lower-than-normal thyroid hormone levels and elevated levels of TSH in the blood. Direct TSH determinations are commonly used, along with one of the measures of T_3 or T_4 in serum. Serum T_4 or T_3 uptake may also be measured, although these tests may be affected by

Table 67-2   Tests to Evaluate Thyroid Function

Test	Procedure	Diagnostic Use	Normal Values	Comments
Serum T_4	Total serum T_4 is measured by competitive protein-binding test or radioimmunoassay.	To distinguish hyperthyroid or hypothyroid conditions from euthyroid state.	5-12 $\mu g/100$ ml serum	Conditions that elevate TBG levels (e.g., pregnancy or estrogen use) raise total serum T_4 levels. Lowered TBG levels in cirrhosis or nephrotic syndrome also lower total serum T_4 levels. In both cases free hormone levels are usually normal, and the patient is functionally euthyroid.
Free thyroxine (FT_4)	FT_4 is measured by radioimmunoassay.	Used with other tests.	0.8-2.3 ng/100 ml	Normal values may vary greatly from laboratory to laboratory.
Free T_3	Unbound T_3 is measured by equilibrium dialysis.	Used when protein levels are abnormal to assess for hyperthyroidism.	210-330 pg/100 ml	This test may not be useful if radioisotopes have been used recently in the patient.
Serum T_3	Total serum T_3 is measured by specific radioimmunoassay.	To distinguish hyperthyroid conditions from euthyroid state.	0.08-0.20 $\mu g/100$ ml	Test is not useful in hypothyroidism because T_3 may be more abundant than T_4.
Reverse T_3	Reverse T_3 is measured by radioimmunoassay.	To assess metabolic inactivation of T_4.	80-350 pg/ml	This test may help evaluate thyroid function and metabolism in tissues.
Serum TSH	Serum TSH is measured by specific ELISA.	To monitor therapy for hypothyroidism; to distinguish primary from secondary hypothyroidism.	0.5-5 $\mu U/ml$	Primary hypothyroidism shows elevated TSH levels; secondary hypothyroidism caused by pituitary failure shows little or no TSH.
Thyroid-stimulating immunoglobulin	Specific immunoassay.	To evaluate cause of hyperthyroidism.	Normal is <130% of basal activity.	This test assesses immunoglobulin that overstimulates the thyroid gland.
Protirelin test (TRH test)	Synthetic TRH (500 mg) is given intravenously, causing peak release of TSH 30 min later in patients with normal pituitary glands.	To distinguish hypothyroidism caused by pituitary failure from other forms of hypothyroidism.	Peak levels of TSH seen in normal patients are 5.35 $\mu U/ml$ serum.	No rise is usually observed in serum TSH level in hyperthyroid patients.
Thyroid uptake of radioiodine	Radioactivity in thyroid is measured 4 and/or 24 hr after administration of tracer dose of radioactive iodine.	To distinguish hyperthyroid and hypothyroid conditions from euthyroid state.	Normal glands take up 10%-35% of tracer dose in 24 hr.	This test may be affected by dietary intake of iodine or by use of iodine-containing medications or antithyroid drugs.
TSH test	Bovine TSH is given intramuscularly, after which serum T_3 and T_4 or radioiodine uptake is measured.	To distinguish primary from secondary and tertiary hypothyroidism.	Primary hypothyroidism is indicated if iodine uptake and T_4 release fail to increase.	This test is rarely used when TSH levels are to be measured.

TBG, Thyroid-binding globulin; *TSH*, thyroid-stimulating hormone; *ELISA*, enzyme-linked immunoabsorbent assay; *TRH*, thyroid-releasing hormone.

conditions unrelated to thyroid disease that change the serum concentration of TBG (see Table 67-2).

Thyroidal uptake of iodine is also lowered in hypothyroidism, but this test is seldom useful in diagnosing the disease because thyroidal uptake is affected by intake of iodine, which may come in food or drugs. The patient may be unaware that iodine is being taken. For example, potassium iodide, used as an expectorant, is a constituent of several prescription cough medicines.

Hypothyroidism may arise for reasons other than primary failure of the thyroid gland. For example, if the pituitary fails to release adequate TSH, too little thyroid hormone is made and secondary hypothyroidism develops. Rarely, patients with hypothalamic damage fail to produce thyrotropin-releasing hormone (TRH), which is needed to stimulate TSH production in the pituitary (see Chapter 65); this condition is called tertiary hypothyroidism.

Secondary and tertiary hypothyroidism may be distinguished from primary hypothyroidism by measuring TSH. In primary hypothyroidism, TSH is elevated by the natural action of the negative feedback system attempting to elevate thyroid hormone levels, but TSH levels are low or undetectable in the other two forms of hypothyroidism. If the TSH assay is not available, a TSH test may be performed (see Table 67-2).

Secondary and tertiary hypothyroidism may be distinguished from each other by the protirelin (TRH) test, which measures the ability of the hypophysis to respond to its normal regulatory hormone (see Table 67-2). If TSH rises after TRH is given, the implication is that the hypothalamus is defective, and both the hypophysis and the thyroid could function normally if properly stimulated.

Treatment of Hypothyroidism: Replacement Therapy

Treatment of hypothyroidism requires replacement therapy with the thyroid hormones. The goal of therapy is to produce the **euthyroid** state (normal thyroid hormone levels). Several preparations containing natural or synthetic forms of the hormones are available (Table 67-3).

Thyroid Hormones

Mechanism of Action

Thyroid hormones used in replacement therapy have exactly the same actions as the hormones naturally produced in the body. Basal metabolic rates are increased by actions on nuclear receptors in skeletal muscle, heart, liver, lungs, intestines, and kidneys.

Pharmacokinetics

T_3 and T_4 are metabolized by the liver to glucuronide and sulfate derivatives, which then are eliminated in bile. No significant reuptake of the hormones occurs from the gut.

Table 67-3	**Drugs for Thyroid Replacement Therapy or Diagnosis**		
Generic Name	Trade Name	Administration/Dosage	Comments
Thyroid Hormones			
levothyroxine	Eltroxin† Levothroid Levoxyl Synthroid*	ORAL: *Adults*—Initially 12.5-50 μg/day; gradually increase to maintenance dosage (usually 75-125 μg/day). FDA pregnancy category A. *Children*—Single daily dose: <12 mo, 5-6 μg/kg; 1-5 yr, 3-5 μg/kg; 6-10 yr, 4-5 μg/kg; >10 yr, 2-3 μg/kg up to adult dose. INTRAVENOUS: *Adults*—Up to 500 μg/day. *Children*—Up to 75% of oral dose.	This pure form of T_4 is the preferred therapy for hypothyroidism. Intravenous form is used for myxedema coma.
liothyronine	Cytomel*	ORAL: *Adults*—Initially 2.5-25 μg/day; gradually increase to maintenance dosage (usually 25-50 μg/day). FDA pregnancy category A.	Pure form of T_3; may be used for adult hypothyroidism but not for cretinism because T_3 may not cross the blood-brain barrier as well as T_4.
liotrix	Thyrolar	ORAL: *Adults and children*—Initially 12.5 μg of T_4 with 3.1 μg of T_3 daily; gradually increase to maintenance dosage (usually 50-100 μg T_4 with 12.5-25 μg T_3). FDA pregnancy category A. *Elderly*—Use $\frac{1}{4}$-$\frac{1}{2}$ usual adult dose; double at 6-8 wk until desired effect reached.	This combination of pure T_4 and T_3 in a 4:1 ratio may be used for hypothyroidism.
thyroid	Thyrar	ORAL: *Adults and children*—Initially 15-60 mg/day; gradually increase to maintenance dosage (usually 60-120 mg/day). FDA pregnancy category A. *Elderly*—7.5-15 mg/day; double at 6-8 wk until desired effect reached.	This crude preparation from thyroid glands contains variable amounts of T_4 and T_3. Dosage is difficult to adjust and maintain.
Adenohypophyseal Hormones			
protirelin	Relefact TRH*	INTRAVENOUS: *Adults*—0.5 mg. *Children*—7 mg/kg.	Synthetic tripeptide identical to natural TRH; used for diagnosis (see Table 67-2).
thyrotropin	Thytropar*	INTRAMUSCULAR, SUBCUTANEOUS: *Adults and children*—10 IU/day for 1-7 days. FDA pregnancy category C.	Thyrotropin is natural TSH that is extracted from animals. it is used for diagnosis (see Table 67-2).

*Available in Canada and the United States.
†Available in Canada only.

Other hormone destruction occurs in the target tissues, where the hormones are deiodinated and transformed to reverse T_3 and other inactive products. Elimination of thyroid hormones used for replacement therapy is the same as for the normal hormones.

The protein-binding properties of thyroid hormones explain some clinically important differences between these agents. T_4, being more highly protein bound, leaves the blood more slowly than does T_3. Therefore the onset of action for T_4 is about 2 days, whereas T_3 effects may be expected within 6 hours of administration (Figure 67-3). Moreover, T_4, which is bound to plasma protein, is less available for elimination, excretion, or tissue biotransformation than is T_3. Thus T_4 persists longer in the body than T_3.

The effects of a single equimolar dose (same number of molecules) of T_3 and T_4 are shown in Figure 67-3, in which the basal metabolic rate was followed as an indicator of thyroid hormone action in hypothyroid subjects. When patients are switched from T_4 to T_3, or vice versa, these different time courses must be considered. For example, a patient being switched from a preparation containing primarily T_4 to a preparation containing only T_3 might experience excessive thyroid hormone action if started on full T_3 doses immediately after T_4 administration is terminated. Therefore patients are given small doses of T_3 after T_4 is stopped, and the dose of T_3 is gradually increased as necessary to maintain the euthyroid state.

Uses

Thyroid hormones are primarily used to treat thyroid deficiency. They also have a role in control of goiter and thyroid carcinoma. They may also occasionally be used for diagnosis. Thyroid hormones should never be used in weight-loss programs.

Patients with myxedemic coma must be treated aggressively with thyroid hormones, glucocorticoids, and other supportive measures. Rapid replacement with thyroid hormones is necessary. Because T_3 is well absorbed from the gastrointestinal (GI) tract, T_3 tablets may be crushed and given through a nasogastric tube. Alternatively, T_4 may be injected intravenously.

Adverse Reactions and Contraindications

In patients who have been newly diagnosed as having hypothyroid, thyroid hormones are started at low dosages and increased gradually until the euthyroid state is achieved. Thyroid USP and levothyroxine doses are usually doubled every 2 weeks, but liothyronine doses may be doubled weekly until symptoms are controlled. These gradually increasing doses are used because a sudden return to adequate thyroid hormone levels produces acute stress on several body systems. One dangerous example observed occasionally even with low dosages is angina pectoris, coronary occlusion, or stroke in older adult or predisposed patients (see Geriatric Considerations box). Another difficulty may be

GERIATRIC CONSIDERATIONS

Thyroid Hormones

THE PROBLEM
Adults older than age 60 may be more sensitive than younger adults to the actions of thyroid hormones. This sensitivity may place older adults at risk for angina or strokes when thyroid hormone replacement is started.

THE SOLUTION
Older adults should be started on low dosages of thyroid hormones initially. The dosages should be increased by small amounts every 3 to 4 weeks, unless symptoms of stress appear. The initial doses for older adults may be one fourth to one half the normal dose for mildly hypothyroid younger adults. Maintenance dosages are the minimum required to reverse the signs of hypothyroidism.

Figure 67-3 Time course of thyroid hormone effects. Patient in each test received single oral dose of medication indicated. Dosages of triiodothyronine (*T_3*) and thyroxine (*T_4*) administered are equimolar (contain equal number of molecules).

relative adrenal insufficiency, which arises in patients with inadequate pituitary function who have secondary hypothyroidism and secondary adrenal insufficiency. If thyroid hormone therapy is started in these patients without also restoring adequate glucocorticoid levels, they may experience a dangerous adrenal crisis.

Toxicity

Overdosage with thyroid hormones produces signs of hyperthyroidism (see Table 67-2). There is some evidence that slight overdoses of thyroxine that suppress TSH but cause no overt signs of hyperthyroidism may rise to more cardiovascular side effects or bone loss in older women than doses that allow TSH to remain in the normal range.

Interactions

Catecholamines must sometimes be used to combat the shocklike symptoms found in myxedemic coma. Patients so treated are especially at risk of developing cardiac arrhythmias because catecholamines and thyroid hormones both tend to cause this dangerous side effect.

Cholestyramine or colestipol may impede oral absorption of thyroid hormones; dosages can be adjusted based on thyroid function tests.

Coumarins or other anticoagulants may be influenced by thyroid function; dosages can be adjusted based on prothrombin times.

Specific Thyroid Hormone Preparations

▼ levothyroxine

Levothyroxine is a pure synthetic form of the natural thyroid hormone T_4. Therefore it has a high affinity for serum proteins, has a long half-life in blood, and is converted to T_3 by peripheral tissues. Levothyroxine is the preferred drug for replacement therapy of hypothyroidism.

▼ liothyronine

Liothyronine is a pure synthetic form of the natural thyroid hormone T_3. Therefore it has a shorter half-life in blood than T_4 and is converted to inactive products in peripheral tissues. In addition, T_3 seems to be better absorbed orally than T_4. Liothyronine is the most potent thyroid hormone, with 0.025 mg being equivalent to 1 mg of levothyroxine.

liotrix

Liotrix is a thyroid preparation that contains both pure synthetic T_4 and T_3 in the ratio of 4:1. This mixture was designed to produce normal thyroid function tests when therapy is adequate, but there is little evidence that liotrix has any clinical advantage over levothyroxine. One tablet of liotrix containing 50 μg of T_4 and 12.5 μg of T_3 is equivalent to 1 mg of levothyroxine.

thyroid USP

Thyroid USP is a defatted extract of whole thyroid glands. It contains T_4 and T_3 in the natural ratio of 2.5:1. The iodine content of these preparations is regulated by law in the United States, but thyroid hormone activity is not directly standardized, so variations in strength are possible. Considerable potency also may be lost on long storage or if the powder becomes moist. In terms of biologic activity, 60 mg of thyroid USP is equivalent to approximately 1 mg of levothyroxine.

Diagnosis of Hyperthyroidism

Hyperthyroidism is characterized by elevated serum T_4, serum T_3, free T_4, and free T_3 levels in most patients. Thus diagnostic tests that directly measure one of these parameters (serum T_4 and serum T_3 testing) are often used (see Table 67-2). TSH levels are low for most forms of hyperthyroidism because high circulating levels of T_4 and T_3 suppress the regulatory factors in the hypothalamus and pituitary. Radioactive iodine uptake also may be measured and is useful in distinguishing between various forms of hyperthyroidism. These diagnostic tests form part of a larger clinical picture. Much information is gained by determining the size of the thyroid by palpation, checking for nodules in the thyroid, and conducting a thyroid scan to measure the pattern of radioactive iodine concentration in the gland.

Diagnosis of Graves' disease is based on the realization that the disease has an immunologic basis. In this condition, unusual immunoglobulins bind to the TSH receptor and cause constant stimulation of thyroid hormone synthesis and release; thus these immunoglobulins supplant TSH as the regulator of thyroid function. These immunoglobulins are found in the sera of nearly all patients who have Graves' disease, and the amounts of the immunoglobulins correlate with the severity of the hyperthyroidism observed. Thyroid-stimulating immunoglobulins can be measured to assess presence and degree of Graves' disease (see Table 67-2).

Treatment of Hyperthyroidism

Hyperthyroidism most often is controlled with drugs or radioactive iodine. The drugs fall into two main classes: those that control the symptoms of hyperthyroidism and those that lower the production of T_3 and T_4 by the thyroid.

propranolol

Propranolol, a beta-adrenergic blocking agent discussed in Chapters 12 and 13, represents the class of drugs that controls symptoms of hyperthyroidism but produces no significant long-term change in thyroid hormone levels. Propranolol is effective because it alters the response of peripheral tissues to high circulating levels of thyroid hormones. One action of propranolol is to inhibit conversion of T_4 to T_3 in target tissues. Blockade of beta-receptors reduces palpitation, tremor, sweating, proximal muscle weakness, mental agitation, and cardiac arrhythmias. One advantage of propranolol therapy is that clinical improvement is seen rapidly. With many other drugs, relief of symptoms may be greatly delayed. Propranolol or other blockers of beta-adrenergic receptors may be used to prepare a hyperthyroid patient for surgery.

thioamides

Mechanism of Action

Two thioamides, methimazole and propylthiouracil, are currently used in the United States (Table 67-4). The thioamides inhibit the synthesis of thyroid hormones, blocking each step in synthesis except iodine uptake (see Figure 67-2). Propylthiouracil also inhibits the conversion of T_4 to T_3 in peripheral tissues. Because these compounds are primarily enzyme inhibitors, they do not directly destroy thyroid tissue but only prevent its excessive action.

Thioamide action on the thyroid gland is immediate, and reduced hormone synthesis occurs within hours. However, observable clinical response to the drugs does not appear for days or weeks, the period required for stored thyroid hormones to be depleted. A patient's condition may be maintained for months by thioamide therapy, provided the hyperthyroidism is well controlled during that time. Usually, after about 1 year, the thioamide is withdrawn and thyroid function is reevaluated. Many patients remain euthyroid after thioamides are discontinued. For this 15% to 50% of patients treated, no further therapy may ever be required.

Pharmacokinetics

Thioamides taken orally are rapidly absorbed and concentrated in the thyroid. The drugs also distribute to other tissues and cross the placenta to enter the fetus. Thioamides appear in the milk of nursing mothers, and they are metabolized and excreted in urine.

Uses

Thioamides are used only for control of hyperthyroidism.

Adverse Reactions and Contraindications

Common reactions to thioamides include fever, itching, and skin rash. Blood dyscrasias or peripheral neuropathy may occur. Propylthiouracil is especially associated with pain and swelling of joints or with a lupuslike syndrome. Methimazole may cause dizziness or alterations in taste.

Patients who have had allergic or other severe reactions to thioamides should not receive the drugs again. Patients with impaired hepatic function may require reduced dosages.

Toxicity

Overdosage with thioamides results in hypothyroidism. The signs are the same as for other forms of hypothyroidism (see Table 67-2).

Interactions

Any preparation containing iodine may interfere with the antithyroid action of thioamides. Such agents include amiodarone, iodine solution, potassium iodide, and many contrast imaging dyes.

Coumarins or other anticoagulants may be influenced by thyroid function; dosages can be adjusted based on prothrombin times.

Digitalis dosage may be influenced by thyroid status. Dosages of the cardiac glycoside may require reduction as hyperthyroidism is brought under control.

Table 67-4   Drugs Used to Treat Hyperthyroidism

Generic Name	Trade Name	Administration/Dosage	Comments
Thioamides			
methimazole	Tapazole*	ORAL: *Adults*—Initially 15-60 mg/day in 1 or 2 doses; maintenance: 5-30 mg/day in 1 or 2 doses. FDA pregnancy category D. *Children*—0.4 mg/kg initially in 1 or 2 doses; maintenance: 0.2 mg/kg/day.	Inhibits thyroid hormone synthesis but not release.
propylthiouracil		ORAL: *Adults*—Initially 300-900 mg/day; maintenance: 50-600 mg/day. FDA pregnancy category D. *Children 6-10 yr*—50-150 mg/day. *Children >10 yr*—50-300 mg/day.	Inhibits thyroid hormone synthesis but not release; also inhibits conversion of T_4 to T_3 in peripheral tissues.
Beta-Adrenergic Blocker			
propranolol	Inderal*	ORAL: *Adults*—10-40 mg 3 or 4 times/day. FDA pregnancy category C.	Controls symptoms of hyperthyroidism but does not lower T_4 and T_3 release from thyroid.
Iodine			
potassium iodide	Pima Thyro-Block†	ORAL: *Adults*—250 mg 3 times/day as presurgical medication. 100-150 mg once daily for 1 day before and at least 3 days after exposure to radioactive iodine.	Produces short-term inhibition of thyroid hormone synthesis by direct action on thyroid.
^{131}I as NaI	Iodotope	ORAL: *Adults*—For Graves' disease: 4-10 mCi (148-370 megabecquerels) as single dose. *For thyroid carcinoma:* Single doses of up to 150 mCi (5.5 gigabecquerels) may be used. *For diagnosis:* Smaller doses are used. FDA pregnancy category X.	This radionuclide is concentrated in thyroid and releases radiation, which destroys thyroid tissue.

*Available in Canada and the United States.
†Available in Canada only.

Radioactive iodine uptake may be reduced by thioamides. This action can interfere with diagnostic tests.

iodine

Iodine is required for synthesis of thyroid hormones, but high concentrations of iodine suppress continued uptake of iodine by the thyroid gland and thus slow synthesis of thyroid hormones. Suppression of hormone synthesis is not complete with iodine administration, and many patients return to the hyperthyroid state even with continued high dosages. Iodine is seldom used today for long-term suppression of a hyperactive thyroid gland. The most common current use of iodine is to prepare a hyperthyroid patient for surgery. Iodine not only suppresses thyroid function but also reduces vascularization of the gland, thus reducing surgical risk. Iodine pretreatment is especially important for hyperthyroid patients who have received thioamide therapy because those drugs increase vascularization of the thyroid gland. In addition, iodine may be used as part of emergency therapy for hyperthyroid crisis. In this situation, iodine is given intravenously after a thioamide has been started.

radioactive iodine

Radioactive iodine is used to treat hyperthyroidism and for diagnosis. Therapy depends on the ability of the radioactive iodine to be concentrated in the thyroid gland, where it then destroys surrounding tissue by emitting low-energy radiation. Iodine dosages are small. The use of radioactive iodine allows the thyroid to be functionally destroyed without resorting to surgery. Nearly all patients treated with radioactive iodine ultimately become hypothyroid and require replacement therapy with thyroid hormones. The incidence of hypothyroidism is about 10% of treated patients during the first year after therapy and about 3% per year thereafter. Because of the likelihood of hypothyroidism, patients should be urged to return periodically for thyroid evaluation.

Nursing Process Overview

Thyroid Therapy

Assessment

The nursing process in diseases of the thyroid gland is the same, whether the problem is hyperthyroidism or hypothyroidism. In most cases the original problem develops insidiously. Obtain a complete assessment of the patient, including temperature, pulse, respiration, blood pressure, weight, history of weight changes, level of energy, mood, subjective feeling, and response to temperature. Check the height of children. Question family members to determine onset of symptoms. Check thyroid function test results and blood glucose levels.

Nursing Diagnoses

- Self-concept disturbance
- Activity intolerance related to fatigue related to excessive metabolic rate

Patient Outcomes

The patient will discuss changes in feelings about self. The patient will identify methods to increase activity while medications are being adjusted.

Planning/Implementation

Monitor the temperature, pulse, respiration, blood pressure, weight, height of children, and blood glucose level. Question about the subjective response to therapy. If weight reduction is an additional goal of therapy, teach about diet or refer as needed. If radioactive iodine is used, follow hospital procedures for the handling of radioactive materials.

Evaluation

Before discharge, check that the patient can explain the action of the drug and how to take the prescribed dose. Other parameters the patient should monitor and record at home include pulse, weight, and height. Explain the side effects that may occur and what to do about them, what adjustments may be needed in the treatment of other medical problems (e.g., changes in insulin or anticoagulant dosages), the need for continuing the medication, and the need to wear an identification tag or bracelet. With radioactive iodine, the patient will not receive long-term drug therapy but should be able to explain what symptoms should be reported to the physician.

Nursing Implications Summary

Natural and Synthetic Thyroid Hormones

Drug Administration

➤ The side effects of natural and synthetic thyroid hormones are essentially the same as the symptoms of hyperthyroidism (see Table 67-1).

➤ Assess for headache, insomnia, nervousness, and tremor.

➤ Monitor blood pressure and pulse. If pulse is more than 100 beats/min in an adult, withhold the dose and notify the physician.

➤ Monitor the electrocardiogram before starting therapy and at regular intervals.

➤ Monitor weight. Assess for edema, pallor, and fatigue.

➤ Monitor thyroid function tests. In children, monitor growth, bone age, and psychomotor development.

Intravenous levothyroxine

➤ Read the manufacturer's instructions; different brands permit different diluents. Administer at a rate of 0.1 mg or less over 1 minute. Monitor vital signs.

➤ Monitor thyroid function tests.

Nursing in the Community

➤ Review the anticipated benefits and possible side effects of drug therapy with the patient.

➤ Inform the patient that several weeks to months of therapy may be required before full benefit is seen. Encourage the patient to return for regular follow-up visits and blood tests.

➤ Instruct the patient to take doses in the morning to avoid nighttime insomnia.

➤ Warn diabetic patients to monitor blood glucose levels carefully because an adjustment in diet or insulin dosage may be needed.

➤ Encourage the patient to wear a medical identification tag or bracelet stating that thyroid medication is used regularly.

➤ Instruct the patient not to switch brands of medication without consulting the physician or the pharmacist.

➤ Instruct female patients to keep a record of menstrual periods because menstrual irregularities may occur.

➤ Remind the patient to inform all health care providers of all drugs being used. Regular use of thyroid replacement hormones may contribute to interactions with other drugs.

protirelin

Drug Administration

➤ Have the patient fast for 6 hours before the test, or restrict the diet to low fat before the test.

➤ Have the patient assume the supine position before administering protirelin and maintain the supine position for at least 15 minutes after drug administration. Monitor vital signs.

➤ Protirelin may be administered undiluted, 1 dose over 15 to 30 seconds.

thyrotropin

Drug Administration

➤ Thyrotropin is for intramuscular or subcutaneous use. Reconstitute with the diluent provided by the manufacturer.

➤ Assess for flushing of face, headache, nausea and vomiting, and allergic reaction. Anaphylaxis is rare. Remain with patient for 10 to 15 minutes after administering a dose. Monitor vital signs.

methimazole and propylthiouracil

Drug Administration

➤ Overdose produces clinical hypothyroidism (see Table 67-1).

➤ Assess for tingling of fingers and toes. Monitor weight. Inspect for skin changes or hair loss.

➤ Monitor complete blood count, white blood cell differential, and thyroid and liver function tests.

Nursing in the Community

➤ Review the anticipated benefits and possible side effects of drug therapy with the patient. Side effects may not appear for days to weeks after beginning therapy; remind the patient to report any new side effects. See the Patient Problems box in Chapter 54 on bleeding tendencies.

➤ Instruct the patient to report signs of agranulocytosis, such as fever, chills, sore throat, and unexplained bleeding or bruising.

➤ Instruct the patient to take doses with meals or a snack to lessen gastric irritation.

➤ The patient may take doses without meals; but however doses are taken, they should be taken the same way each time, either always with meals or always on an empty stomach.

➤ Encourage the patient to return as instructed for follow-up visits.

➤ Remind the patient to inform all health care providers of all drugs being used.

➤ If more than 1 dose per day is prescribed, it is best to space doses evenly throughout the day. Work with the patient to develop a satisfactory dosing schedule.

propranolol

➤ Propranolol is discussed on Chapter 13.

potassium iodide

Drug Administration/Nursing in the Community

➤ Teach the patient to take the solution by mouth, even if dispensed with a dropper. Dilute an oral solution well in a full glass (8 ounces) of juice, milk, or beverage of choice.

➤ Teach patients taking the noncoated tablet form to dissolve each tablet in half a glass (4 ounces) of water or milk and to then drink all of the beverage to get the full dose.

➤ Signs of iodism (excessive iodine) include metallic taste in the mouth, sneezing, swollen and tender thyroid gland, vomiting, and bloody diarrhea. Concomitant excessive use of over-the-counter preparations containing iodine (e.g., asthma or cough preparations) may contribute to iodism.

➤ Consult the manufacturer's literature for information about intravenous iodine.

Continued

Nursing Implications Summary—cont'd

radioactive iodine
Drug Administration/Nursing in the Community
➤ The radiation dosage of radioactive iodine is not high, but those preparing or administering the preparation should be careful to avoid spilling the mixture on themselves or on countertops. Wear rubber gloves. Follow agency protocol for handling radioactive substances.

➤ Side effects are rare but include soreness over the thyroid gland and, in rare cases, difficulty in swallowing and breathing because of gland enlargement. Eventually, many patients who take radioactive iodine become hypothyroid.

CHAPTER REVIEW

Application

1. What is the function of the follicular cells of the thyroid gland?
2. What hormones are produced by the follicular cells of the thyroid gland?
3. What is the function of TSH? Where is it produced?
4. What is the function of thyroglobulin?
5. How much T_3 and T_4 is stored in the thyroid gland?
6. How are thyroid hormones transported in blood?
7. How are thyroid hormones eliminated?
8. Which of the thyroid hormones is found most abundantly in target cells and is the primary activator of nuclear receptors?
9. In primary hypothyroidism, how do blood concentrations of TSH and thyroid hormones differ from normal?
10. What is the difference between secondary hypothyroidism and tertiary hypothyroidism?
11. What is the treatment for all forms of hypothyroidism?
12. How do T_3 and T_4 differ in onset and duration of action?
13. Which of the available preparations of thyroid hormones is the most potent?

14. Which preparation of thyroid hormones is preferred for replacement therapy?
15. What general classes of drugs are used to treat hyperthyroidism?
16. To what class of drugs does propranolol belong? Why is it useful in treating hyperthyroidism?
17. What is the mechanism of action of the thioamides?
18. How are the thioamides distributed in the body?
19. How may radioactive iodine be used in the treatment of hyperthyroidism?

Critical Thinking

1. What are the characteristic signs of hypothyroidism? How should you assess for these?
2. What side effects may occur with replacement therapy of thyroid hormones? How should you assess for these?
3. Explain why levothyroxine might be preferred for replacement therapy over other forms of thyroid hormones.
4. Why must replacement therapy begin gradually, rather than with full doses, especially for older patients or patients with cardiac problems?

Reference

Harrell GB, Murray PD: Diagnosis and management of congenital hypothyroidism, *J Perinat Neonat Nurs* 11:75-83, 1998.

Drugs Affecting Calcium Metabolism

OBJECTIVES

After studying this chapter, you should be able to do the following:

- *Describe the hormones that influence calcium metabolism.*
- *Discuss the therapeutic roles for vitamin D.*
- *Describe which patients should receive calcium supplements.*
- *Develop a nursing care plan for a patient receiving dialysis therapy who is taking calcifediol.*
- *Develop a nursing care plan for a patient taking dietary calcium supplements.*

CHAPTER OVERVIEW

Calcium is needed for the proper function of all cells and tissues. Close control of calcium levels is required because very small changes in blood calcium levels can profoundly alter many cellular functions, with effects on many body systems. Because of this fundamental role in maintaining function, calcium uptake, distribution, and elimination are very tightly controlled in the body to maintain a constant concentration of 4.7 to 5.6 mEq/L in plasma or serum. The overall interaction of dietary calcium with parathyroid hormone, calcitonin, and vitamin D allows the body to maintain blood calcium levels within this very narrow margin. This chapter discusses the therapeutic roles of these regulators of calcium metabolism and of calcium itself.

THERAPEUTIC RATIONALE: REGULATION OF CALCIUM METABOLISM

Dietary Calcium

An adult human has two sources of calcium that may be used to meet the daily needs of the body: dietary calcium and calcium deposited in bones. The dietary requirements for calcium have been defined. Children from infants up to 10 years require 400 to 800 mg/day. Adults require 800 to 1200 mg/daily and pregnant or lactating women may require more. These large amounts of calcium can be obtained in a diet rich in dark-green leafy vegetables, seafood, and milk products. Unfortunately, the diets of many Americans do not contain adequate amounts of calcium. If dietary calcium is insufficient, the body will begin to resorb calcium from bones to meet metabolic needs for the element. Over several months or years, this mineral loss can weaken the bones, a process called **osteoporosis.**

Vitamin D

The term **vitamin D** refers to a group of lipid-soluble substances that is formed or interconverted in the body. Cholecalciferol, or vitamin D_3, may be formed from cholesterol in skin when it is exposed to sunlight. The vitamin may also be taken in the diet.

Depending on what form of the vitamin is ingested, various biotransformations are possible. The liver converts vitamin D_3 to the more active 25-hydroxyvitamin D_3. The kidney converts 25-hydroxyvitamin D_3 to calcitriol, the most active metabolite of the vitamin.

Physiologic Action

Vitamin D acts like a hormone in the body, regulating calcium concentrations in concert with parathyroid hormone and calcitonin. Specifically, vitamin D promotes the release of calcium and phosphate from bone, blocks renal excretion of these materials, and promotes their absorption from the gastrointestinal (GI) tract. All of these actions increase calcium concentration in blood.

Vitamin D interacts with receptors in target cells throughout the body to produce its effects on calcium metabolism. The vitamin D receptor, like the receptors for corticosteroids and thyroid hormones, is found in the cytoplasm of cells and moves to cell nuclei where the hormone-receptor complex influences gene expression.

Regulation of Secretion

Synthesis of vitamin D_3 in skin occurs continuously, so long as exposure to sunlight is adequate. Formation of the most active form of vitamin D, calcitriol, is promoted by relative deficiencies of calcium, phosphate, or vitamin D. Active stimulation of the process occurs with parathyroid hormone, whereas very high vitamin D intake can inhibit conversion to the more active metabolite.

Effects of Vitamin D Deficiency

Vitamin D deficiency can occur in persons who are not adequately exposed to sunlight and who ingest a diet poor in the vitamin. A deficiency of the vitamin limits the amount of calcium that can be absorbed from the diet.

In children, vitamin D deficiency leads to a condition called rickets, in which the calcium that would normally be used to build bones is robbed to serve other life-supporting needs. In adults, vitamin D deficiency can contribute to osteoporosis because the inadequate absorption of calcium from the diet leads to bone resorption to supply the necessary element.

Effects of Vitamin D Excess

The most common cause of vitamin D excess is overdosage with dietary supplements. The result is hypercalcemia (Table 68-1).

calcitonin

Physiologic Action

The primary effect of **calcitonin,** when used as a drug, is to prevent the loss of calcium from bone. This action lowers the amount of calcium entering the blood.

Regulation of Secretion

Parafollicular cells of the thyroid synthesize the peptide hormone calcitonin; both synthesis and secretion are stimulated by high concentrations of calcium ion in plasma. The released calcitonin tends to lower plasma calcium concentrations back toward the normal range.

Effects of Calcitonin Deficiency or Excess

Calcitonin deficiency is not a well-documented condition, perhaps because some calcitonin is found in thymus and parathyroid glands, as well as in the thyroid. Calcitonin excess is uncommon but may arise from medullary carcinomas of the thyroid, formed by parafollicular cells.

Parathyroid Hormone

Physiologic Action

The parathyroid glands (see Figure 67-1) synthesize **parathyroid hormone,** a peptide whose major function is to maintain blood calcium levels above the critical threshold required for body function. In many ways, parathyroid hormone acts opposite to calcitonin. For example, parathyroid hormone increases reabsorption of calcium from bones, lowers renal excretion of calcium, and along with vitamin D, increases calcium absorption from the intestine; all of these actions tend to raise calcium concentration in blood.

Regulation of Secretion

Parathyroid hormone secretion is regulated by calcium concentrations in the blood. As the calcium concentration falls, secretion of parathyroid hormone is stimulated and more calcium is mobilized from bone to enter the blood. High calcium concentrations slow secretion of parathyroid hormone.

Table 68-1	Symptoms of Altered Calcium Balance	
Hypercalcemia	**Hypocalcemia**
Early Symptoms	**Early Symptoms**
Central nervous system	Hyperreflexia
Depression	Muscle spasms
Headache	Paresthesias
Irritability	Positive Chvostek's sign
Tiredness or weakness	
Gastrointestinal tract	
Anorexia	
Constipation	
Dry mouth	
Other	
Increased thirst	
Metallic taste	
Late Symptoms	**Late Symptoms**
Central nervous system	Central nervous system
Confusion	Convulsions
Drowsiness	Cardiovascular
Cardiovascular	Arrhythmias
Arrhythmias	Other
Hypertension	Difficulty breathing
Gastrointestinal tract	Laryngeal spasm
Nausea	Tetany
Vomiting	
Other	
Sensitivity to light	
Large urine volume	

Effects of Parathyroid Hormone Deficiency: Hypoparathyroidism

Hypoparathyroidism usually results after thyroid or parathyroid surgery, but idiopathic (unknown cause) forms of the disease exist. Hypoparathyroidism leads to hypocalcemia. This electrolyte imbalance produces symptoms such as paresthesia, muscle spasms, tetany, and convulsions (see Table 68-1). In theory, parathyroid hormone could be used to raise blood calcium levels in conditions in which blood levels are abnormally low; however, administration of one of the forms of vitamin D with or without calcium is the preferred treatment.

A synthetic fragment of parathyroid hormone, teriparatide, retains full biologic activity and is used as a diagnostic agent for hypoparathyroidism. Teriparatide is infused, and urinary cyclic adenosine monophosphate and phosphate are measured to detect the response of a target organ to the hormone. Hypoparathyroidism is a deficiency in parathyroid hormone production, but the target organs respond to exogenous parathyroid hormone. Pseudohypoparathyroidism is a rare condition in which the target organs fail to respond to parathyroid hormone.

Effects of Parathyroid Hormone Excess: Hyperparathyroidism

Hyperparathyroidism usually arises from excess secretion of parathyroid hormone from a tumor. Many patients with this condition show decreases in bone calcification as a result of the action of parathyroid hormone. Large amounts of calcium are excreted by these patients, and renal stones are common. No specific inhibitors of parathyroid release are available for clinical use; thus therapy consists primarily of surgery to remove the source of excess parathyroid hormone synthesis.

THERAPEUTIC AGENTS: DRUGS TO TREAT CALCIUM DEFICIENCY

Calcium Supplements

Mechanism of Action

Calcium present in the diet or in dietary supplements replaces calcium that would otherwise be mobilized from bone to supply the body's metabolic needs. Maintaining an adequate intake of calcium helps prevent loss of calcium from bones and maintains their strength (see Dietary Considerations box). Because the uptake of calcium is regulated by vitamin D, maximum benefit from the dietary calcium supplements is seen when adequate vitamin D uptake is also maintained. For children who drink milk, the requirements for both calcium and vitamin D may be met easily. For elderly adults who do not drink milk, the requirements for calcium and vitamin D may be more difficult; supplements of both the mineral and the vitamin may be needed.

Pharmacokinetics

Calcium is not well absorbed orally, with less than one third of the amount ingested being absorbed. Vitamin D can increase absorption, but certain fiber-rich foods can diminish absorption. Calcium elimination from the body is regulated by the kidneys, under the influence of parathyroid hormone and other factors.

Uses

Oral calcium supplements (Table 68-2) are designed primarily to prevent calcium deficiency and maintain bone strength. These preparations are also often used as antacids.

Adverse Reactions and Contraindications

Systemic effects are uncommon with oral calcium preparations. Constipation and loss of appetite may occur.

Calcium supplements should not be used in patients with symptoms of hypercalcemia, including those with sarcoidosis or renal calculi. Patients with renal impairment should not receive dibasic or tribasic calcium phosphate because the excess phosphate is not easily handled without adequate renal function.

Toxicity

High dosages of calcium supplements can produce signs of hypercalcemia (see Table 68-1).

Interactions

Calcium preparations can diminish absorption of several drugs, including etidronate, phenytoin, and tetracyclines. Calcium also directly antagonizes the effects of drugs such as gallium nitrate and magnesium sulfate.

 DIETARY CONSIDERATIONS

Calcium

Calcium is important for growth and maintenance of healthy bones and for its role in nerve and muscle function and blood clotting. Some medical conditions contribute to hypocalcemia (low blood calcium levels), including hypoparathyroidism, kidney disease, massive cellulitis, burns, and peritonitis. An extremely low level of calcium can result in tetany, a medical emergency that is treated with intravenous calcium. Milder cases of hypocalcemia may be treated in part by having the patient increase dietary intake of calcium. Good dietary sources of calcium include the following:

- Blackstrap molasses
- Calcium-fortified orange juice
- Cheese
- Clams
- Dark-green leafy vegetables (e.g., kale, spinach)
- Ice cream
- Milk products
- Oysters
- Salmon
- Sardines
- Tofu, if made with calcium carbonate
- Yogurt

▼ Vitamin D: calcifediol and ergocalciferol

Mechanism of Action

Vitamin D is required for proper absorption of calcium. Supplemented vitamin D has the same action as the vitamin D normally produced in the body.

Pharmacokinetics

Vitamin D is a highly lipid-soluble material that is readily absorbed orally. Once in the blood, vitamin D is bound to specific alpha-globulins that transport the material to target tissues. This lipid-soluble vitamin is concentrated in liver and other fat stores.

The metabolic fate of vitamin D depends on which form is taken. Vitamin D_3 (cholecalciferol) and vitamin D_2 (**ergocalciferol**) are both converted to calcifediol by the liver. **Calcifediol** and alfacalcidol are both converted by renal tissue to calcitriol (1,25-dihydroxychole-calciferol), the most active vitamin D derivative. Most vitamin D metabolites are excreted in bile.

Uses

All vitamin D derivatives may be used to control hypocalcemia caused by hypoparathyroidism (see Table 68-2). Vitamin D deficiency is usually treated with ergocalciferol. Alfacalcidol or calcitriol may be used to treat vitamin D deficiency in patients with renal failure; calcitriol is identical to the active vitamin D metabolite normally formed in liver but missing in these patients, whereas alfacalcidol is converted to calcitriol by the liver.

Adverse Reactions and Contraindications

Excess of vitamin D produces symptoms that are primarily those expected with high blood calcium concentrations (see Table 68-1).

Table 68-2   Preparations to Correct Calcium Deficiency

Generic Name	Trade Name	Administration/Dosage	Comments
Calcium Supplements‡			
calcium carbonate	BioCal Caltrate 600* Rolaids Tums	ORAL: *Adults–800-1200 mg/day. Children–400-800 mg/day.*	625-mg tablets contain 250 mg calcium; 1500-mg tablets contain 600 mg calcium.
calcium carbonate, oyster-shell derived	Os-Cal 500* Oysco Oyst-Cal	ORAL: *Adults–800-1200 mg/day. Children–400-800 mg/day.*	625-mg tablets contain 250 mg calcium; 1500-mg tablets contain 600 mg calcium.
calcium citrate	Citracal	ORAL: *Adults–800-1200 mg/day. Children–400-800 mg/day.*	950-mg tablets contain 200 mg calcium.
calcium glubionate	Calcionate Neo-Calglucon	ORAL: *Adults–800-1200 mg/day. Children–400-800 mg/day.*	Syrup contains 115 mg calcium in 5 mL.
calcium gluconate	Calcium gluconate	ORAL: *Adults–800-1200 mg/day. Children–400-800 mg/day.*	1000-mg tablets contain 90 mg calcium.
calcium lactate	Calcium lactate	ORAL: *Adults–800-1200 mg/day. Children–400-800 mg/day.*	650-mg tablets contain 84 mg calcium.
dibasic calcium phosphate	Dibasic calcium phosphate	ORAL: *Adults–800-1200 mg/day. Children–400-800 mg/day.*	500-mg tablets contain 115 mg calcium.
tribasic calcium phosphate	Posture	ORAL: *Adults–800-1200 mg/day. Children–400-800 mg/day.*	1600-mg tablets contain 600 mg calcium.
Vitamin D§			
alfacalcidol	One-Alpha†	ORAL: *Adults–1 µg/day initially; maintenance, 0.25-1 µg/day. FDA pregnancy category C.*	For hypoparathyroidism or chronic renal failure.
calcifediol	Calderol	ORAL: *Adults–0.05-0.1 mg/day. FDA pregnancy category C. Children <2 yr–0.02-0.05 mg/day; 2-10 yr, 0.05 mg/day.*	Alternative agent for vitamin D deficiency or rickets.
calcitriol	Calcijex* Rocaltrol*	ORAL: *Adults–0.25 µg slowly increase to maximum of 3 µg/day. FDA pregnancy category C. Children– 0.25 µg/day, gradually increased to 0.08 µg/kg.* INTRAVENOUS: *Adults–0.01 µg/kg by rapid injection 3 times/wk; may increase to 0.05 µg/kg.*	For hypoparathyroidism or chronic renal failure.
dihydrotachysterol	DHT Hytakerol*	ORAL: *Adults–0.1-2.5 mg/day, as needed to maintain normal serum calcium. FDA pregnancy category C. Children–1-5 mg/day for 4 days, then 0.5-1.5 mg/day as needed to normalize serum calcium.*	For hypoparathyroidism or tetany.
ergocalciferol	Calciferol*	ORAL: *Adults and children–For replacement doses: 400 units/day. For rickets or other conditions: 1000- 500,000 units/day. FDA pregnancy category C.*	Used to treat and prevent vitamin D deficiency and hypoparathyroidism.

*Available in Canada and the United States.
†Available in Canada only.
‡Best effects are achieved with adequate intakes of vitamin D.
§Vitamin D preparations should be used with adequate intakes of calcium (1-1.5 g/day).

Toxicity

Large overdosages with vitamin D may be fatal because cardiovascular and renal function is compromised. Chronic overdoses can cause deposits of calcium to appear in blood vessels, kidneys, and other tissues.

Interactions

Antacids or other preparations containing magnesium may be more dangerous when given with vitamin D because high magnesium concentrations in blood may occur.

THERAPEUTIC AGENTS: DRUGS TO TREAT OSTEOPOROSIS AND PAGET'S DISEASE

▼ calcitonin

Mechanism of Action

When calcitonin is used clinically, the effect sought is reduction of calcium release from bone.

Pharmacokinetics

Calcitonin is administered by subcutaneous or intramuscular injection. The absorbed protein is rapidly metabolized in blood, kidneys, and other tissues. The hypercalcemic effect

of the hormone persists for several hours. The protein is also absorbed when given in a nasal spray.

Uses

Calcitonin has been used to treat Paget's disease, in which excessive bone resorption leads to fragile bones. A synthetic form of salmon calcitonin (Table 68-3) is the most potent of the naturally occurring forms of the hormone. Synthetic human calcitonin is also used for treatment of Paget's disease.

Salmon calcitonin has been used to control postmenopausal osteoporosis, along with vitamin D and calcium supplements. A metered spray for intranasal administration makes the use of this agent convenient for chronic use by outpatients.

Adverse Reactions and Contraindications

Many patients experience nausea and vomiting, facial flushing, and occasional inflammatory reactions when calcitonin is injected. Because the hormone is a peptide and is administered in a gelatin solution, allergic reactions may occur. Synthetic human calcitonin may be less likely than salmon calcitonin to cause allergic reactions. Allergic reactions to foreign proteins may increase the risk of reactions to calcitonin.

Table 68-3 Agents for Osteoporosis and Paget's Disease

Generic Name	Trade Name	Administration/Dosage‡	Comments
alendronate	Fosamax*	ORAL: Adults—For prophylaxis of postmenopausal osteoporosis: 5 mg once daily 30 min before breakfast. For treatment of postmenopausal osteoporosis: 10 mg once daily 30 min before breakfast. For Paget's disease: 40 mg once daily 30 min before breakfast for 6 months. FDA pregnancy category C.	Should be used with adequate intakes of calcium (1-1.5 g/day) and vitamin D (400-800 IU/day).
calcitonin human	Cibacalcin	SUBCUTANEOUS: Adults—For Paget's disease: Initially 0.5 mg/day; maintenance: 0.25 mg/day. FDA pregnancy category C.	Lower risk of forming antibodies than with salmon calcitonin.
calcitonin salmon	Calcimar*	INTRAMUSCULAR, SUBCUTANEOUS: Adults—for Paget's disease, 100 IU/day initially; then 50 IU once daily or every other day. For postmenopausal osteoporosis: 100 IU once daily or every other day. For hypercalcemia: 4 IU/kg every 12 hr; increase, if needed, up to 8 IU/kg every 6 hr. FDA pregnancy category C.	Most active form of calcitonin.
	Miacalcin	INTRANASAL: Adults—1 metered spray (200 IU) in one nostril daily. Alternate nostrils.	
etidronate	Didronel*	ORAL: Adults—For Paget's disease: 5 mg/kg/day for up to 6 mo. For heterotropic ossification: 20 mg/kg for 1 mo before and 3 mo after hip replacement. For hypercalcemia: 20 mg/kg/day, for up to 90 days. FDA pregnancy category B.	Interacts directly with bone to slow bone resorption.
pamidronate	Aredia*	INTRAVENOUS: Adults—For hypercalcemia: 60 mg over 4-24 hr. For Paget's disease: 90-180 mg total dose; 30 mg/day infused at 15 mg/hr for 3 days or 60 mg once every 3 wk. FDA pregnancy category C.	Interacts directly with bone to slow bone resorption.
raloxifene	Evista	ORAL: Adults—60 mg once daily, without regard to meals. FDA pregnancy category X.	Mimics estrogen effects on bone, leading to increased mineral deposition in bone.
risedronate	Actonel	ORAL: Adults—for Paget's disease: 30 mg once daily for 2 mo. FDA pregnancy category C.	Slows bone resorption.
tiludronate	Skelid	ORAL: Adults—For Paget's disease: 400 mg taken once daily 2 hr before or after meals. FDA pregnancy category C.	Causes bone-resorbing cells to detach from bone.

*Available in Canada and the United States.
†Available in Canada only.
‡All agents listed in this table should be used with adequate intakes of calcium (1-1.5 g/day) and vitamin D (400-800 IU/day).

Intranasal administration of calcitonin causes few systemic side effects but commonly causes nasal symptoms such as dry membranes, itching, irritation, crusting, or bleeding.

Toxicity

Overdosage of calcitonin may cause hypocalcemia, but the effect is mild and short lived.

Interactions

Calcium or vitamin D preparations may antagonize the actions of calcitonin.

Bisphosphonates: alendronate, etidronate, pamidronate, risedronate, and tiludronate

Mechanism of Action

The bisphosphonates are synthetic analogs of inorganic pyrophosphate that block removal of calcium from bone. These drugs act on **osteoclasts,** the cells that remove calcium from bone to supply metabolic needs and to remodel bone. Alendronate and risedronate inhibit the activity of the osteoclasts, but the cells remain bound to remodeling sites in bone. Etidronate lowers the number of osteoclasts. Pamidronate blocks attachment of osteoclasts to bone. Tiludronate inhibits several processes in osteoclasts and causes them to detach from bone. The effects of all of the agents are to slow bone resorption and to allow calcium to be retained in bone.

Pharmacokinetics

These drugs have a low oral bioavailability that is further impaired by food or beverages other than water. Absorbed drug binds to bone, concentrating at sites where bone is being remodeled. The effects on serum calcium levels develop slowly with oral doses of these drugs. Therapeutic effects on Paget's disease may persist for months after therapy is stopped. This prolonged effect may be related to persistence of drug in bone for months.

Uses

Bisphosphonates are used primarily to control Paget's disease, which promotes excessive remodeling of bone. Etidronate is also used for heterotropic ossification that may follow hip replacement surgery. Alendronate is used for prophylaxis of postmenopausal osteoporosis. Occasionally, etidronate or pamidronate may be used to control hypercalcemia, especially when the condition arises from malignancies of the bone.

Adverse Reactions and Contraindications

Nausea, diarrhea, and allergic reactions are common with these agents. Many patients with Paget's disease experience tenderness or pain weeks or months after therapy is started. The pain localizes at the site of Paget's disease lesions in bones.

Bisphosphonates are avoided in patients with impaired renal function (creatinine clearance of less than 35 ml/min) because their elimination may be limited.

Toxicity

Higher dosages of the drug may cause more severe GI tract symptoms, and possibly hypocalcemia.

Interactions

Foods or drugs that have a high content of metal ions can impair oral absorption of bisphosphonates and prevent their action. Antacids, mineral supplements, multivitamins with added minerals, calcium salts, and calcium-rich dairy products may all be involved.

raloxifene

Mechanism of Action

Raloxifene interacts with estrogen receptors in bone and causes an estrogen-like increase in the accumulation of calcium in bone. Unlike true estrogens, raloxifene causes no proliferation of reproductive tissues and does not block hot flashes and other symptoms of estrogen deficiency.

Pharmacokinetics

Raloxifene is adequately absorbed orally, but the drug is rapidly converted to the glucuronide by a first-pass effect (see Chapter 1). The drug is eliminated primarily in bile.

Uses

Raloxifene is indicated for the prevention of osteoporosis in postmenopausal women. Controlled trials with raloxifene and an anticancer agent tamoxifen showed that raloxifene had a protective effect against breast cancer in women. This latter use is still under study.

Adverse Reactions and Contraindications

A variety of symptoms, including joint or muscle pain, leg cramps, rash, vaginitis, sore throat, painful urination, insomnia, and depression, appear in 3% to 6% of treated patients. About 25% of women treated with raloxifene report hot flashes, caused by the antiestrogen effects of the drug.

Raloxifene should be avoided in women with a history of thromboembolic disorders.

Toxicity

Many of the side effects may be dose related and would be expected to worsen at higher dosages.

Interactions

Cholestyramine should be avoided because it reduces absorption of raloxifene and interferes with enterohepatic recirculation. Estrogens should also be avoided. Warfarin effectiveness is increased by raloxifene, which may lead to bleeding episodes.

THERAPEUTIC AGENTS: DRUGS TO TREAT HYPERCALCEMIA

edetate disodium

Mechanism of Action

Edetate disodium (Table 68-4) is a strong chelator of calcium, forming soluble complexes that are excreted readily by the kidneys. One gram of edetate disodium binds up to 120 mg of calcium. The effect is to rapidly lower blood calcium concentrations.

Pharmacokinetics

Edetate disodium is used by intravenous (IV) infusion with constant monitoring of serum calcium. Up to 95% of a dose appears in urine within 1 day. Edetate is not metabolized in the body.

Uses

Edetate disodium is used for emergency treatment of hypercalcemia. The drug may also be used for treatment of digitalis toxicity, but digoxin immune Fab is the preferred drug.

Adverse Reactions and Contraindications

The most serious side effect with edetate disodium is thrombophlebitis at the site of injection. Dizziness may occur, as well as GI tract signs, including cramps and diarrhea. Nephrotoxicity is also a problem with edetate disodium. The drug is usually avoided in patients with preexisting renal problems.

Toxicity

Acute overdoses of edetate disodium may cause hypocalcemia (see Table 68-1). Calcium ion replacement may occasionally be necessary.

Interactions

Digitalis effects are reduced when serum calcium is lowered.

gallium nitrate

Mechanism of Action

Gallium nitrate blocks removal of calcium from bone, but the exact mechanism is unclear. The effect is to slow bone resorption and lower blood calcium concentrations.

Pharmacokinetics

Gallium nitrate usually shows a half-life of about 1 day, but the effect of the drug persists for up to 6 days.

Uses

Gallium nitrate is used to control hypercalcemia that arises from malignancies of the bone.

Adverse Reactions and Contraindications

Phosphate and calcium are lowered in blood; in some patients this change may cause anorexia or muscle weakness. Nephrotoxicity is also common with gallium nitrate. Nausea, vomiting, and diarrhea are often seen.

Gallium nitrate is avoided in patients with impaired renal function (serum creatinine of more than 2.5 mg/dl) because gallium nitrate elimination may be limited.

Toxicity

Higher dosages of gallium nitrate tend to cause more severe nephrotoxicity.

Interactions

Antacids, mineral supplements, calcium salts, and calcium-rich dairy products can impair the oral absorption of gallium nitrate and prevent its action. Nephrotoxic medications are also avoided because of the risk of additive renal damage.

Table 68-4	Agents for Hypercalcemia			
Generic Name	Trade Name	Administration/Dosage		Comments
edetate disodium	Disotate Endrate	INTRAVENOUS: *Adults—For hypercalcemia:* 50 mg/kg over 24 hr for no more than 5 days; upper limit, 3 g/day. FDA pregnancy category C. *Children*—40 mg/kg in 24 hr.		This strong chelating agent removes excess calcium from system on short-term basis.
gallium nitrate	Ganite	INTRAVENOUS: *Adults*—100-200 mg/m² infused over 24 hr for 5 days. FDA pregnancy category C.		For control of hypercalcemia caused by cancer.

Nursing Process Overview

Drugs Affecting Calcium Metabolism

Assessment

Monitor vital signs. Take dietary history if appropriate. Assess for pain and inability to perform activities of daily living. Assess exercise patterns if appropriate. Monitor serum calcium, phosphorus, blood urea nitrogen (BUN), and serum creatinine levels.

Nursing Diagnoses

- For patients with Paget's disease: risk for bone fractures
- For patients with hypercalcemia: potential complication: arrhythmias

Patient Outcomes

The patient will have no fractures. The nurse will manage and minimize arrhythmic episodes.

Continued

Planning/Implementation

Administer medications as ordered. If concomitant dietary changes are appropriate, instruct the patient as needed or refer to a dietitian. Monitor vital signs and laboratory work. If the patient is at risk for arrhythmias, monitor electrocardiographic (ECG) changes. Work with the physician to develop an appropriate treatment plan if the patient is in pain. Instruct the patient how to take medications at home.

Evaluation

The drugs discussed in this chapter vary in their use. Before discharge, verify that the patient understands how to take medications at home, what symptoms should prompt the patient to contact the physician, and any prescribed dietary changes needed.

Nursing Implications Summary

Calcium Supplements
Drug Administration
➤ See Table 68-1 for symptoms of hypercalcemia and hypocalcemia. Assess patient for hypocalcemia; monitor serum magnesium, phosphate, calcium, potassium, and parathyroid hormone concentrations. Monitor BUN and serum creatinine.

➤ Administer IV calcium slowly. Too rapid administration may contribute to cardiac arrhythmias and cardiac arrest. Monitor vital signs and ECG if possible. Monitor serum calcium levels.

➤ Side effects of IV administration are often related to too rapid administration and include hypotension, dizziness, flushing or sensation of warmth, nausea and vomiting, and tingling sensation. Slow or temporarily halt infusion if the patient displays symptoms or complains of discomfort. Keep the patient recumbent after injection to prevent postural hypotension.

➤ Infiltration of IV calcium may contribute to severe tissue necrosis that requires skin grafting. Ascertain that IV infusion is patent before administering, and check infusion frequently.

➤ IV calcium chloride: May be given undiluted, but it is preferable to dilute with distilled water or normal saline to make a 5% solution. Warm to body temperature before administration. Administer at a rate of 0.5 to 1 ml over 1 minute.

➤ IV calcium gluceptate: May be given undiluted. Warm to body temperature before administration. Administer at a rate of 1 ml or less over 1 minute.

➤ IV calcium gluconate: May be given undiluted or further diluted in up to 1000 ml of normal saline. Warm to body temperature before administration. Inspect solution: it must be free of crystals. To dissolve crystals, heat to 90° C (146° F) in a dry heat oven for at least 1 hour; shake vigorously, and allow to cool. If crystals persist, discard solution and prepare a new one. Administer direct IV, undiluted, at a rate of 0.5 ml over at least 1 minute. For diluted infusion, may be given over 12 to 24 hours. In any case, no infusion should exceed 200 mg/min.

Nursing in the Community
➤ Calcium preparations used as antacids are also discussed in Chapter 26.

➤ Encourage patients to maintain a balanced diet. Take a diet history, if indicated, and refer patients to a dietitian if needed. See the Dietary Considerations box on calcium (earlier in this chapter).

➤ Teach patients the importance of weight-bearing exercises, especially during younger years, to help build and maintain dense bones.

➤ Teach patients the importance of having sufficient vitamin D to help with calcium absorption. Exposure to sunlight for 15 to 30 minutes a day, as a part of daily activities, is sufficient exposure to sunlight for most people to receive adequate vitamin D. However, people who live in extreme northern areas, where sunlight in the winter months may be weak or limited, may need additional vitamin D from other sources, such as diet, multivitamin preparations, or fortified milk.

➤ Instruct patients not to take calcium supplements within 1 to 2 hours of taking other oral medications. Teach patients not to take calcium supplements within 1 to 2 hours of eating large amounts of fiber-containing foods such as bran or whole-grain cereals.

➤ Instruct patients to avoid tobacco and limit alcohol and caffeine intake while taking calcium supplements.

➤ Encourage patients to drink a full glass (8 ounces) of water or juice when taking an oral calcium supplement. Instruct patients to take doses 1 to 1½ hours after meals unless directed to do otherwise by the physician. Patients taking the syrup form should take the syrup before meals. The syrup can be mixed with water or fruit juice for infants or small children.

➤ Calcium carbonate may be used to bind phosphate in patients with renal failure. When used for this purpose, the physician may want it taken with meals. In addition, the patient should usually not take doses with a full glass of liquid.

➤ Calcium supplements may cause constipation. Check to see that patients are taking doses with full glasses (8 ounces) of water. See the Patient Problems boxes on constipation (Chapter 24) and dry mouth (Chapter 23).

➤ Instruct patients to avoid bonemeal or dolomite as a source of calcium; these have been associated with high levels of lead and may contribute to lead poisoning.

Nursing Implications Summary—cont'd

vitamin D Preparations

Drug Administration

➤ The side effects are essentially those of hypercalcemia and are a result of overdosage. Effects include ataxia, fatigue, irritability, seizures, somnolence, tinnitus, hypertension, GI tract distress or constipation, and hypotonia in infants. Other symptoms of overdose include headache, increased thirst, metallic taste in the mouth, nausea or vomiting, and fatigue.

➤ Assess for central nervous system effects. Ongoing assessment is important because some symptoms (e.g., fatigue) may be difficult to distinguish from those accompanying renal failure or chronic disease.

➤ Monitor blood pressure and pulse. Monitor intake and output.

➤ Monitor BUN and serum creatinine levels, serum calcium and phosphorus levels, serum alkaline phosphatase, and urinalysis.

➤ IV calcitriol: May be administered by rapid direct IV push.

Nursing in the Community

➤ Review the anticipated benefits and possible side effects of drug therapy with the patient. Encourage the patient to notify the physician if any new side effects occur.

➤ Remind the patient not to increase or decrease the dosage without consulting the physician.

➤ Warn the patient to avoid driving or operating hazardous equipment if fatigue, somnolence, vertigo, or weakness occurs.

➤ Remind the patient to inform all health care providers of all drugs being used and to avoid taking any medications not previously approved by the physician.

➤ Instruct the patient to avoid antacids containing magnesium.

➤ Instruct the patient to avoid excessive amounts of substances containing vitamin D (see the Dietary Considerations box in Chapter 17 on vitamins).

➤ Instruct the patient to avoid nonprescription medication or dietary supplements containing calcium, phosphorus, or vitamin D unless first discussed with the physician.

➤ Teach the patient that the oral dosage solution form should be taken orally, even if dispensed with a dropper for measuring dose. The dose may be taken undiluted, or dropped into cereal, fruit juice, or other food.

calcitonin

Drug Administration

➤ Monitor weight. If vomiting or diarrhea occurs, monitor intake and output.

➤ Warn the patient that flushing may occur.

➤ Before the first dose of calcitonin salmon, a test dose may be ordered to check for allergic response. Consult the manufacturer's literature. Have drugs, equipment, and personnel available to treat acute allergic reactions in settings where salmon calcitonin is used.

➤ Assess for hypercalcemia or hypocalcemia (see Table 17-1).

➤ Monitor serum electrolyte levels and in patients with Paget's disease, serum alkaline phosphatase, and 24-hour urinary hydroxyproline concentration.

Nursing in the Community

➤ Review the anticipated benefits and possible side effects of drug therapy with the patient.

➤ Encourage the patient to return for regular follow-up visits. For home administration of the injectable form, instruct the patient to administer the drug subcutaneously. Review the injection technique and have the patient give a return demonstration.

➤ For the intranasal form, review manufacturer's instructions with the patient. Skin testing may still be recommended before sending the patient home on the intranasal form.

➤ Store salmon calcitonin in the refrigerator. Store human calcitonin at a temperature below 77° F but do not refrigerate. Store intranasal form in the refrigerator.

➤ Refer the patient to a community-based nursing care agency as needed.

➤ Inform the patient that taking ordered doses in the evening may minimize flushing.

➤ Encourage the patient receiving long-term therapy to wear a medical identification tag or bracelet indicating that calcitonin is being taken regularly.

➤ A low-calcium diet may be prescribed. Review the Dietary Considerations box on calcium (earlier in this chapter) for food items that should be used in limited amounts when trying to restrict calcium intake. Refer the patient to a dietitian as needed.

alendronate

Drug Administration/Nursing in the Community

➤ For Paget's disease, monitor serum alkaline phosphatase and serum calcium, and urinary hydroxyproline and N-telopeptide of type I collagen. For postmenopausal osteoporosis, monitor bone mineral density, serum calcium, and serum creatinine.

➤ Assess for abdominal pain or distension, constipation, gas, headache, and nausea.

➤ Instruct the patient to take doses with 6 to 8 ounces of plain water on an empty stomach, at least 30 minutes before food or beverages or medication each day. Taking doses with coffee, tea, juice, mineral water, or food will decrease absorption of the drug. Instruct the patient to avoid lying down after taking doses.

➤ If calcium and/or vitamin D supplements are also prescribed, emphasize the importance of taking all of the medications ordered. However, the calcium and vitamin D should not be taken at the same time as the alendronate; at least 30 minutes should elapse between doses.

etidronate

Drug Administration

➤ Assess for bone pain, which may occur in patients with Paget's disease.

Continued

Nursing Implications Summary–cont'd

➤ Monitor serum electrolyte levels. Assess for signs of hypocalcemia (see Table 17-1).

➤ Monitor serum creatinine and BUN levels.

➤ IV etidronate: Dilute in 250 ml or more of normal saline. Infuse 250 ml over at least 2 hours.

Nursing in the Community

➤ Review the anticipated benefits and possible side effects of drug therapy with the patient.

➤ Provide emotional support. Weeks to months of therapy may be required to obtain maximum drug effect. Remind the patient not to discontinue therapy without consulting the physician.

➤ Instruct the patient to take doses with black coffee, tea, fruit juice, or water, on an empty stomach, at least 2 hours before or after food. Suggest that patients take doses at midmorning or bedtime.

➤ Tell the patient not to take doses within 2 hours of ingesting milk or milk products, antacids, mineral supplements, or medicines high in calcium, magnesium, iron, or aluminum.

➤ Take a dietary history. Patients should continue following a well-balanced diet with adequate but not excessive amounts of calcium and vitamin D.

➤ Instruct the patient to notify the physician if severe or persistent diarrhea develops or bone pain worsens.

pamidronate

Drug Administration/Nursing in the Community

➤ Assess for symptoms of hypocalcemia (see Table 68-1), fever, chills, sore throat, nausea, and muscle stiffness. See the Patient Problems box in Chapter 54 on leukopenia.

➤ IV pamidronate: Reconstitute each vial with 10 ml sterile water for injection. Further dilute in normal saline, 0.45 normal saline, or D5W. Total volume of diluent may be as little as 250 ml (90 mg/250 ml) or as much as 1000 ml (preferred).

➤ Use microdrip tubing and/or an infusion monitoring device to help ensure even administration. Actual rate of administration depends on total volume, dose, and the patient's condition.

➤ Monitor serum electrolytes and calcium levels, complete blood count with differential, serum phosphate level.

➤ Patient must be adequately hydrated before infusion, yet not overhydrated. It is recommended that patient have a urine output of at least 2 L/day before treatment. Monitor intake and output.

➤ If calcium and/or vitamin D are restricted, emphasize importance of this to the patient and review items to be limited or avoided. Instruct the patient to avoid all other medications unless first approved by the physician.

raloxifene

Drug Administration/Nursing in the Community

➤ Assess the patient for chest pain, urinary tract infection, body aches or pain, fever, sore throat, peripheral edema, skin rash, vaginal itching, GI distress, anorexia, nausea, migraine headaches, joint or muscle pain, hot flashes, and difficulty sleeping.

➤ Instruct the patient to review the manufacturer's leaflet.

➤ Tell the patient to report the occurrence of vaginal bleeding, breast pain, or swelling of hands or feet.

➤ Instruct the patient to discontinue the drug and to seek medical care immediately if pregnancy is suspected.

➤ Stress to patients the importance of weight-bearing exercises in the prevention of osteoporosis.

➤ Instruct the patient to take doses on a full or empty stomach.

➤ There is an increased risk of thromboembolism associated with this drug. Raloxifene should be discontinued at least 72 hours before surgery and during periods of immobility or bed rest, including during long trips when the patient may have limited mobility. Instruct the patient to discuss concerns with the physician in advance of expected travel or elective surgery. Remind the patient to keep all health care providers informed of all medications being used.

risedronate

Drug Administration/Nursing in the Community

➤ See manufacturer's literature for current information.

tiludronate

Drug Administration/Nursing in the Community

➤ Assess for cough, fever, head congestion, voice changes, runny nose, sore throat, changes in vision, edema of face or lower extremities, back or body pain, GI upset, and skin rash. Monitor serum alkaline phosphatase and urinary hydroxyproline.

➤ Instruct the patient to take doses with 6 to 8 ounces of plain water on an empty stomach. Tell the patient not to take doses within 2 hours of consuming other beverages, including mineral water, food, medications, or mineral supplements.

➤ If the patient is also required to take calcium or vitamin D supplements, these should be taken 2 hours before or after tiludronate.

➤ See manufacturer's literature for current information.

edetate disodium

Drug Administration

➤ Read drug labels carefully; do not confuse this drug with edetate calcium disodium.

➤ To prepare dose for an adult, dissolve dose in 500 ml of D5W and administer over at least 3 hours. For a child, dissolve the calculated dose in sufficient diluent (D5W or sodium chloride injection) to make a final concentration no more concentrated than 3% (30 mg/ml). Too concentrated a solution may increase the risk of thrombophlebitis. Administer the dose over at least 3 hours; 4 to 6 hours is preferred. Too rapid infusion may precipitate a sudden drop in serum calcium, resulting in hypocalcemic tetany or cardiac arrhythmias. Have calcium gluconate readily available.

Nursing Implications Summary—cont'd

➤ Monitor vital signs and continuous ECG during the infusion. Keep the patient supine during infusion and for a short time afterward.

➤ Monitor BUN and serum creatinine levels, serum electrolytes, liver function tests, and urinalysis.

➤ Avoid extravasation; can cause tissue necrosis.

gallium nitrate
Drug Administration/Nursing in the Community

➤ Assess for bone pain, loss of appetite, muscle weakness, nausea, vomiting, or diarrhea.

➤ Encourage the patient to have sufficient fluid intake to maintain 24-hour output at 2000 ml or more. Encourage the patient to drink at least eight or nine 8-ounce glasses of liquid a day.

➤ Dilute daily dose in 1 L of 0.9% sodium chloride injection or D5W. Administer over 24 hours. Use an infusion monitoring device and/or microdrip tubing. If the patient is to administer at home, refer to a home care nursing agency.

➤ Monitor BUN and serum creatinine levels, serum albumin, serum calcium, and serum phosphorus.

teriparatide
Drug Administration

➤ Review the pretest instructions with the patient. Usually, the patient may have nothing to drink after 8 PM the night before the test. Instruct the patient to begin drinking 200 ml of water every 30 minutes, beginning 2½ hours before the scheduled time of the test. Urine and blood samples will be drawn periodically during the test.

➤ To prepare teriparatide, use the diluent provided. Administer the dose evenly over 10 minutes.

➤ Allergic reactions are possible, although rare. Have epinephrine, equipment, and personnel available to treat acute allergic reactions.

CHAPTER REVIEW

Application

1. What conditions favor release of calcium from bone?
2. Which metabolite of vitamin D is the most active?
3. What is the metabolic function of vitamin D?
4. What organs form metabolites of vitamin D?
5. What are the signs of vitamin D deficiency?
6. What is the function of parafollicular cells in the thyroid?
7. What are the metabolic effects of calcitonin?
8. What are the metabolic effects of parathyroid hormone?
9. What side effects are common with calcium supplements used orally?
10. What are the dangers associated with high dosages of vitamin D?
11. What two forms of calcitonin are used to treat Paget's disease? How do they differ?

12. How is hypoparathyroidism treated?
13. What effects do bisphosphonates have on osteoclasts?
14. What is the primarily clinical use of bisphosphonates?
15. Why must bisphosphonates not be taken with food or beverages other than water?
16. What is the primary target tissue of raloxifene?
17. With what steroid hormone receptor does raloxifene interact?
18. Why is edetate disodium an effective treatment for hypercalcemia?

Critical Thinking

1. What are the symptoms of hypoparathyroidism? How should you assess for these?
2. What type of patient is likely to benefit most from oral calcium supplements? What other factors should you assess to maximize the potential benefit to the patient?

References

Darovic G: Caring for patients with osteoporosis, *Nursing* 27(5):50-51, 1997.

Lilley LL, Guanci R: Avoiding alendronate-related esophageal irritation, *Am J Nurs* 97(7):12, 14, 1997.

Chapter

69

Drugs to Treat Diabetes Mellitus

OBJECTIVES

After studying this chapter, you should be able to do the following:

- *Discuss the difference between type 1 diabetes mellitus, or insulin-dependent diabetes mellitus, and type 2 diabetes mellitus, or non–insulin-dependent diabetes mellitus.*
- *Explain the advantages of the different forms of insulin.*
- *Explain the clinical uses of oral hypoglycemic agents.*
- *Develop a nursing care plan for a diabetic patient.*
- *Develop a teaching plan for a diabetic patient.*

CHAPTER OVERVIEW

The pancreas is an exocrine gland that supplies digestive juices to the small intestine. Within the gland lie discrete clusters of cells with different functions from those of most pancreatic cells. These cell clusters, called the islets of Langerhans, contain several types of endocrine cells. Three of these cell types release peptide hormones that affect glucose metabolism. Alpha (A) cells synthesize and release the peptide hormone glucagon, beta (B) cells synthesize and release insulin, and D cells synthesize somatostatin. This chapter covers the function of islet cells, a description of diabetes mellitus, and a description of drugs used in the diagnosis and control of that disease.

THERAPEUTIC RATIONALE: DIABETES MELLITUS

Normal Hormonal Regulation of Metabolism

Glucose Metabolism

The body seldom relies on a single mechanism to control an important physiologic function. This rule applies to the regulation of glucose use. The primary hormone regulating glucose metabolism is insulin, a peptide hormone synthesized in beta cells of the pancreas. Insulin stimulates glucose uptake by the glucose transporter GLUT 4 in fat and muscle cells and promotes the conversion of glucose to the storage carbohydrate glycogen in liver and muscle cells.

Insulin does not work alone, and its metabolic actions must always be considered in relation to the actions of other hormones. For example, the elevated blood glucose level after a meal stimulates insulin release from the pancreas. Blood glucose is thereby lowered because insulin stimulates the burning of glucose for energy in fat and muscle cells and the storage of glucose in the liver. As blood glucose levels fall in response to insulin, glucagon release from alpha cells of the pancreas is stimulated. Glucagon in many ways directly opposes the action of insulin in glucose metabolism. Glucagon stimulates the liver to break down glycogen and amino acids so that glucose is released into the blood. Glucagon also inhibits the uptake of glucose by muscle and fat cells. By balancing the action of these hormones, the body protects itself from high blood glucose (**hyperglycemia**) and low blood glucose (**hypoglycemia**).

Even the concept of metabolic balance achieved with two antagonistic hormones does not adequately describe glucose regulation. For example, somatostatin (see Chapter 65) released from D cells of the pancreas inhibits release of insulin and glucagon from islet cells. Other hormones antagonize the peripheral effects of insulin. Cortisol (an adrenocortical glucocorticoid) and epinephrine (a catecholamine from the adrenal medulla), which are elevated during stress, antagonize the actions of insulin in muscle or fat cells (Table 69-1). The overall action of these two hormones is to increase blood glucose levels. Over time, growth hormone (see Chapter 65) also increases blood glucose, primarily by lowering glucose uptake in muscle cells.

Fat and Protein Metabolism

Although insulin is most often considered a regulator of glucose metabolism, it also regulates fat and protein metabolism. Insulin directly stimulates synthesis of storage lipid within fat cells, blocks breakdown and release of stored lipid, and promotes protein synthesis by stimulating amino acid uptake and directly stimulating protein synthetic processes.

As in carbohydrate metabolism, the action of insulin in regulating fat and protein metabolism is opposed by other hormones (see Table 69-1). For example, epinephrine, glucagon, cortisol, and growth hormone stimulate fat breakdown in fat cells, thereby directly opposing the action of insulin in that tissue. Therefore, these hormones tend to raise the blood content of free fatty acids and other breakdown products of lipids. In addition, glucagon and cortisol block protein synthesis in direct opposition to insulin action. Growth hormone differs from the other insulin-opposing hormones in that growth hormone directly stimulates protein synthesis in many body tissues. An understanding of this delicate balance of hormonal actions is important to appreciate the origin of some of the metabolic derangements that occur in diabetes mellitus.

Regulation of Insulin Secretion

The beta cells of the pancreas must respond to changing levels of glucose in the blood and release insulin when it is needed and in the amounts needed to handle the glucose load. The primary glucose sensor is a glucose transporter called GLUT 2. The GLUT 2 transporter has a higher threshold than other glucose transporters in the body, which means that relatively high levels of glucose are needed before this transporter operates. These high glucose levels would be expected after meals.

When the GLUT 2 transporter begins to operate, glucose enters the beta cell of the pancreas and is metabolized to generate energy in the form of adenosine triphosphate (ATP). ATP causes a potassium channel in the cell membrane to close. This closing of the potassium channel leads to depolarization of the cell, a process discussed previously for cardiac cells (see Chapter 18). Depolarization alters the membrane permeability to several ions. The crucial change that triggers insulin release is the opening of a calcium channel, which raises the level of calcium in the beta cell. It is this increase in calcium that finally causes release of the granules that contain insulin. The pancreas stores the equivalent of about 200 units of insulin ready for release on demand. In addition to stimulating release of stored insulin, glucose stimulates synthesis of new insulin.

Diabetes Mellitus

Types and Causes

In **diabetes mellitus,** insulin action is lost. If all insulin production ceases, the disease is called **type 1 diabetes mellitus;** this disease has also been called insulin-dependent diabetes mellitus (IDDM) or juvenile-onset diabetes. As the name implies, diabetes characterized by absence of insulin production primarily affects the young. This form of diabetes

---

Table 69-1   Metabolic Actions of Insulin and Insulin-Opposing Hormones

Tissue and Metabolic Process	Insulin	Glucagon	Epinephrine	Cortisol	Growth Hormone
Liver					
Glycogen formation	Increase	Decrease	Decrease	Increase	—
Glucose formation from amino acids	Decrease	Increase	—	Increase	Decrease
Glucose formation from glycogen	Decrease	Increase	Increase	—	—
Skeletal Muscle					
Glucose uptake or use	Increase	Decrease	Decrease	Decrease	Decrease
Amino acid uptake	Increase	—	—	—	Increase
Protein synthesis	Increase	Decrease	—	Decrease	Increase
Glucose release from glycogen	Decrease	Increase	Increase	—	—
Fat Cells					
Synthesis of storage lipid	Increase	Decrease	Decrease	Decrease	Decrease
Release of free fatty acids from stored lipid	Decrease	Increase	Increase	Increase	Increase
Blood					
Glucose level	Decrease	Increase	Increase	Increase	Increase
Free fatty acid level	Decrease	Increase	Increase	Increase	Increase

accounts for only about 8% of all cases of diabetes mellitus in the United States.

If insulin production continues but is insufficient to meet the body's demands, the disease is called **type 2 diabetes mellitus;** this form of the disease has also been called non–insulin-dependent diabetes mellitus (NIDDM) or adult-onset diabetes. NIDDM is usually a disease of persons who are older than 40 years of age or who are obese. Diabetes in these patients may involve insulin resistance; insulin concentrations in the blood may be normal, but the target tissues are unresponsive to insulin. More than 90% of all cases of diabetes mellitus in the United States are type 2 diabetes.

The exact cause of diabetes mellitus has not been established, but several factors seem to be involved. Viruses and autoimmune mechanisms have been suggested to contribute to development of the disease. Heredity may also play a role in some types of diabetes, especially type 2, but it has never been proved that heredity alone determines who will or will not develop the disease.

Metabolic Derangements

Significant metabolic derangements occur when insulin action is lost. Without insulin, less glucose is used in muscle and fat cells, and more glucose is released into the circulation by the liver. Muscle cells, starved for energy sources, break down protein and release amino acids into the blood. The liver converts a portion of these amino acids into glucose and returns it to the blood. These processes contribute to the persistently elevated levels of glucose in blood. When glucose levels in blood exceed about 160 mg/dl, glucose begins to appear in urine.

The most common early symptoms of diabetes mellitus result directly from osmotic and metabolic changes. Patients often first note a feeling of constant fatigue because energy production in body cells is impaired. Increased frequency of urination (polyuria), often first noticed at night, occurs because excess glucose in urine produces osmotic diuresis (i.e., more water must be excreted to carry out the high concentration of glucose). As urine output increases, most patients develop excessive thirst (polydipsia), which results from the body's efforts to maintain normal hydration despite excessive fluid losses through the kidney. Some patients develop perineal infections, made likely by the presence of glucose in urine.

The alterations in metabolism caused by insulin deficiency and the relative excess of catabolic hormones (catecholamines and steroids) ultimately result in excessive protein and fat breakdown. Protein is metabolized to amino acids and then to glucose, whereas fats are converted to free fatty acids and then to ketone bodies that are released into the circulation. These excess breakdown products may cause a patient to become ketotic or acidotic.

Ketoacidosis is a serious acute complication of diabetes mellitus seen primarily in patients with type 1 diabetes who have little or no endogenous insulin production. These patients are sometimes called ketosis-prone diabetic patients.

Patients with type 2 diabetes who produce enough insulin to suppress lipid breakdown are resistant to ketosis, but patients with type 2 diabetes may still experience ketoacidosis, especially if the system is stressed by an infection or a stroke. The symptoms of ketoacidosis include hyperglycemia, osmotic diuresis with fluid depletion, and acidosis. Ketones are detected in blood. Ketoacidotic coma is associated with mortality rates of 3% to 30%. The mortality rate is highest when treatment is delayed, so the key to survival is early recognition of the signs. Treatment involves controlling hyperglycemia with insulin and treating the fluid and electrolyte imbalances appropriately, often with fluids containing potassium. If the ketoacidosis has been precipitated by an infection, stroke, or heart attack, these underlying conditions must also be controlled to regain control of the diabetes.

Any diabetic person may become comatose as a result of dehydration. As the plasma becomes hyperosmolar (higher solute concentration than normal for blood), water is pulled from body tissues and severe water and electrolyte imbalances occur. Patients in this type of hyperosmolar coma tend to be older than 60 years of age and tend to have an even higher mortality rate than patients in ketoacidotic coma.

Long-Term Complications

Pathologic changes in blood vessels, nerves, and kidneys occur in diabetic patients. Retinal hemorrhages may destroy sight. Other vessels may also be affected, although those changes are not so easily observed early in the disease. At later stages, circulation to the limbs may be impaired. Pathologic changes also occur in kidneys, at first affecting glomerular filtration rate, then progressing to glomerulosclerosis with thickening of capillary basement membranes. Nephrotic syndrome with protein loss in urine and frank kidney failure are late complications of diabetes. Nerve function is impaired, so late in the disease, the patient may lose feeling in the limbs or other parts of the body. Sexual impotence is common among diabetic men.

Some studies suggest that many of the late pathologic changes may be delayed or reduced in severity by strict control of the blood glucose level in diabetes. This strict control is usually not attempted in children because hypoglycemia has the potential to damage developing brains. Hypoglycemia is a more likely side effect of insulin when strict control is attempted. Strict control is also contraindicated for the elderly and patients with severe renal disease because hypoglycemia also places these patients at greater risk.

Clinical trials to assess the value of good control of hyperglycemia take years to plan, complete, and assess. One such trial among nearly 4000 mild type 2 diabetic patients began in 1977 and ended in late 1998. Until this trial and others are fully assessed, the benefits of strict insulin control to produce normal glucose levels in type 2 diabetics cannot be proven to offset the risks, which may include cardiovascular complications. The situation is different for type 1 diabetes. A long-term clinical trial called the Diabetes Control and Complications Trial showed that maintaining blood glucose levels near normal reduced the risk of diabetic retinal damage, kidney damage, and nerve damage by about 60%.

Diagnosis

Diabetes mellitus is diagnosed by applying one or more of the following procedures:

- Fasting blood sugar is determined by obtaining 1 to 3 ml of blood after a 12-hour fast and measuring the glucose content by any of several methods approved for use in clinical laboratories. Most conveniently, the blood is taken in the early morning. The range of normal fasting plasma sugar values is 65 to 110 mg/dl for venous blood. A value of greater than 140 mg/dl in a truly fasting individual suggests the diagnosis of diabetes mellitus. Values between 110 and 140 mg/dl may require further patient evaluation.
- Glucose in urine (**glucosuria**) is conveniently tested in screening programs with commercially available pretreated test strips (Dextrostix), which develop a particular color when exposed to urine containing glucose. Glucose does not routinely appear in urine of nondiabetic persons because a blood glucose level of about 160 mg/dl is required before healthy kidneys pass glucose into urine. Some diabetic patients spill glucose into urine at lower blood glucose concentrations, possibly as a result of impaired renal function.
- An oral glucose tolerance test is used to detect diabetes mellitus. After a 12-hour fast, 50 to 100 g of glucose are taken and blood is sampled at 30- or 60-minute intervals. Glucose levels in plasma are compared with the value ob-

tained just before the glucose was administered. In nondiabetic individuals, plasma glucose levels rise in response to this acute glucose load and immediately trigger the release of insulin from beta cells of the pancreas. As a result of the circulating insulin, glucose levels begin to fall within about 1 hour after the glucose load is ingested and return to normal within 2 hours (Figure 69-1). In contrast, plasma glucose levels of a diabetic person fall more slowly than those of nondiabetic individuals because insulin is not released to aid in disposition of the glucose load. Plasma glucose levels in diabetic persons remain greater than 200 mg/dl of plasma 2 hours after the glucose load.

Long-term hyperglycemia causes a significant fraction of the hemoglobin in blood to be glycosylated. Glycosylated hemoglobin can be assayed to assess how well diabetic persons are controlling their glucose levels with the medications discussed in the next section.

THERAPEUTIC AGENTS: DRUGS TO TREAT DIABETES MELLITUS

Parenteral Agents

▼ insulin

Mechanism of Action

Insulin used in the treatment of diabetes mellitus constitutes replacement therapy. The administered insulin restores the ability of cells to use glucose as an energy source and corrects many associated metabolic derangements.

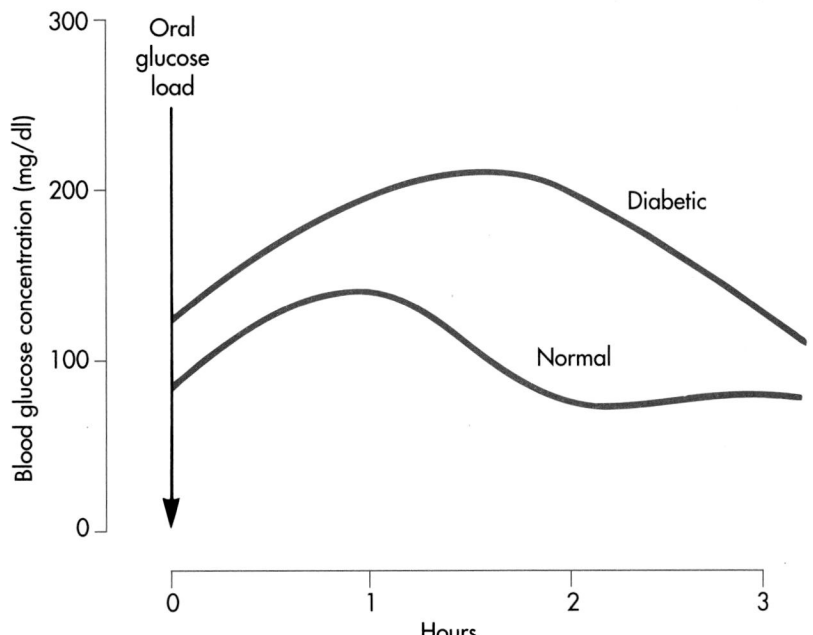

Figure 69-1 Typical oral glucose tolerance tests for normal and diabetic patients. Test is performed preferably in ambulatory patients in morning before eating. Oral glucose load is about 75 g given in solution. Blood is drawn at appropriate intervals (before glucose and 60, 90, 120, and 180 minutes after glucose) and is analyzed for glucose concentration.

Table 69-2   Insulin Preparations and Their Pharmacokinetics

Generic Name/ Class	Trade Name	Source	Dosage	Pharmacokinetics		
				Onset	Peak	Duration
Rapid-Acting: Clear Solutions with No Precipitate						
insulin injection	Humulin-R*	Human	INTRAVENOUS: *Adults and children*—Insulin injection preparations are 100 units/ml; dosage is individualized.	10-30 min	15-30 min	30-60 min
	Insulin-Toronto†	Beef/pork				
	Novolin R	Human				
	Novolin ge Toronto†	Human	SUBCUTANEOUS: *Adults and children*—Insulin injection preparations are 100 units/ml; dosage is individualized, but is usually given 15 to 30 min before meals or bedtime snack.	0.5-1 hr	2-4 hr	5-7 hr
	Regular Iletin†	Beef/pork				
	Regular Iletin I	Beef/pork				
	Regular Iletin II	Purified pork				
	Regular Iletin II†	Pork				
	Regular Insulin	Pork				
	Regular Insulin	Purified pork				
insulin injection	Regular (Concentrated) Iletin II	Purified pork	SUBCUTANEOUS: *Adults and children*—500 units/ml preparation is for insulin-resistant patients only.			24 hr
insulin lispro	Humalog	Human analog	SUBCUTANEOUS: *Adults*—100 units/ml preparation is used primarily for pre-meal injections. This insulin preparation is the only one requiring a prescription.	15-30 min	1 hr	3.5-4 hr
Intermediate-Acting: Uniform Suspensions Intended Only for Subcutaneous Use						
isophane insulin	Humulin N*	Human	SUBCUTANEOUS: *Adults and children*—Isophane insulin preparations are 100 units/ml; dosage is individualized and usually given 30-60 min before meals or bedtime snack.	3-4 hr	6-12 hr	18-28 hr
	Novolin ge NPH†	Human				
	Novolin N	Human				
	NPH Iletin†	Beef/pork				
	NPH Iletin I	Beef/pork				
	NPH Iletin II	Purified pork				
	NPH Iletin II†	Pork				
	NPH-Insulin†	Beef/pork				
	NPH-N	Purified pork				
insulin zinc	Humulin L*	Human	SUBCUTANEOUS: *Adults and children*—Insulin zinc suspensions are 100 units/ml; dosage is individualized, with the dose usually given 30 min before a meal or a bedtime snack.	1-3 hr	8-12 hr	18-28 hr
	Lente Iletin†	Beef/pork				
	Lente Iletin I	Beef/pork				
	Lente Iletin II	Purified pork				
	Lente Iletin II†	Pork				
	Lente Insulin†	Beef/pork				
	Novolin L	Human				
	Novolin ge Lente†	Human				
isophane insulin§/ human insulin‡	Humulin 10/90†	Human 10‡/90§	SUBCUTANEOUS: *Adults and children*—These mixtures are 100 units/ml total insulin; dosage is individualized, with the dose usually given 15-30 min before meals or bedtime snack.	0.5 hr (for 50/50 preparation)	4-8 hr	18-28 hr
	Humulin 20/80†	Human 20‡/80§				
	Humulin 30/70†	Human 30‡/70§				
	Humulin 40/60†	Human 40‡/60§				
	Humulin 50/50*	Human 50‡/50§				
	Humulin 70/30	Human 30‡/70§				
	Novolin 70/30	Human 30‡/70§				
	Novolin ge 10/90†	Human 10‡/90§				
	Novolin ge 20/80†	Human 20‡/80§				
	Novolin ge 30/70†	Human				
	Novolin ge 40/60†	30‡/70§				

*Available in Canada and the United States.
†Available in Canada only.
‡Percentage of insulin content in the form of regular ainsulin (rapid-acting).
§Percentage of insulin content in the form of isophane insulin (intermediate-acting).

Table 69-2   Insulin Preparations and Their Pharmacokinetics—cont'd

Generic Name/ Class	Trade Name	Source	Dosage	Pharmacokinetics		
				Onset	Peak	Duration
Intermediate-Acting: Uniform Suspensions Intended Only for Subcutaneous Use—cont'd						
	Novolin ge 50/50†	Human 40‡/60§ Human 50‡/50§				
Long-Acting: Uniform Suspensions Intended Only for Subcutaneous Use						
extended insulin zinc	Humulin U† Humulin U Ultralente Novolin ge Ultralente†	Human Human Human	SUBCUTANEOUS: *Adults and children—* Extended insulin zinc suspensions are 100 units/ml; dosage is individualized, with the dose usually given 30-60 min before a meal or bedtime snack.	4-6 hr	18-24 hr	36 hr

*Available in Canada and the United States.
†Available in Canada only.
‡Percentage of insulin content in the form of regular insulin (rapid-acting).
§Percentage of insulin content in the form of isophane insulin (intermediate-acting).

Pharmacokinetics

Insulin must be used by injection because it is a protein and therefore would be destroyed in the gastrointestinal (GI) tract. In its natural form, insulin is relatively soluble in water and is quickly absorbed from subcutaneous injection sites. This property is reflected in the pharmacologic behavior of regular insulin for injection (Table 69-2), which is rapidly absorbed, has its peak effect within 2 to 4 hours, and is no longer active after 8 hours. The longer-acting insulin preparations are prepared by crystallizing insulin in the presence of zinc or other agents to form slowly dissolving complexes. These preparations differ from regular insulin and from each other in onset and duration of action because of differences in absorption from the injection site.

Health care professionals must be familiar with the onset and duration of insulin products. With different insulin forms, control can be adjusted to fit the lifestyle and metabolic demands of individual patients. Not only must diabetic patients become proficient in techniques of storing, preparing, and injecting their insulin, but they also must be taught proper testing procedures. To avoid complications, patients must also understand the onset and duration of action of the insulin preparations they are receiving.

As an example of the many patterns of dosage that may be used successfully, consider the following hypothetical case:

A person with type 1 diabetes who has been maintained on a single dose of insulin zinc suspension (lente insulin) before breakfast each morning has started to show hypoglycemia before supper in the evening. To overcome this problem, the physician splits the insulin dose, giving 80% of the daily dose in the morning and the remainder before supper. The rationale for this therapy is simple. Lente insulin injected at around 7 AM reaches its peak effect around dinnertime (see Table 69-2). By decreasing the dose in the morning, the intensity of the hypoglycemic effect before supper is reduced. The small dose of lente insulin administered before supper helps protect the patient

from developing hyperglycemia overnight. After a few days on the new regimen, the patient reports that the hypoglycemia before supper has disappeared but that hyperglycemia is now a problem after the evening meal. This situation is corrected by adding a small amount of a short-acting insulin (e.g., regular insulin injection) to the dose of insulin taken before supper. The short-acting insulin will control the hyperglycemia after eating, and the longer-acting insulin continues to protect from hyperglycemia overnight.

Many individualized schemes for insulin dosage may be devised. In all cases the principle is the same: doses of insulin must be timed so that the patient is protected from hyperglycemia at any time and from hypoglycemia during peak periods of insulin action.

Uses

Insulin is used primarily for type 1 diabetes mellitus, the condition in which beta-cell function is lost and insulin production is very low or absent. Insulin may also be used in type 2 diabetes mellitus that cannot be controlled by diet and/or oral hypoglycemic agents.

Adverse Reactions and Contraindications

Insulin therapy is associated with two important acute side effects. If therapy is inadequate, the person may go into a coma as a result of uncontrolled metabolic derangements; blood glucose concentrations will be high, and ketoacidosis or hyperosmolar coma may result. If insulin overdosage occurs or if a patient does not eat or overexercises, the patient may lapse into coma resulting from hypoglycemia. It is critical for health care professionals to be able to differentiate between these conditions. The distinguishing symptoms are outlined in Table 69-3. Treatment of hypoglycemia consists of elevating blood glucose levels by oral administration of sugar in conscious patients or by glucagon injection or glucose intravenous (IV) infusion in unconscious patients.

Table 69-3   Differential Diagnosis of Diabetic Coma and Hypoglycemic Reactions

Clinical Data	Diabetic Coma	Hypoglycemic Reactions
Symptoms	Thirst	Nervousness
	Abdominal pain	Hunger
	Nausea and vomiting	Sweating
	Headache	Weakness
	Constipation	Stupor
	Shortness of breath (Kussmaul's respiration)	Convulsions
Signs	Facial flushing	Pallor
	Air hunger	Shallow respiration
	Soft eyeballs	Normal eyeballs
	Normal or absent reflexes	Babinski's reflex may be seen
	Acetone breath	
Urine glucose	Positive	Negative or low
Urine acetone	Positive	Negative
Blood glucose	High (greater than 250 mg/dl)	Low (less than 60 mg/dl)
Blood CO$_2$	Low	Normal
Precipitating factors	Untreated diabetes	Insulin overdosage
	Infection or disease appearing in previously controlled diabetic patient	Skipping meals
	High degree of emotional or psychological stress	Excessive exercise before meals
History	Onset of symptoms usually occurs over days	Onset of symptoms is related to type of medication used; regular insulin overdose produces symptoms more rapidly than longer-acting insulins or oral agents

Treatment of diabetic coma requires insulin administration to lower blood glucose concentration.

Many patients receiving insulin therapy have insulin antibodies in their blood. These antibodies may contribute to insulin resistance in some patients.

Insulin may also provoke subcutaneous fat near injection sites to atrophy. This lipoatrophy leads to the formation of hollows or depressions in the skin. Careful rotation of injection sites minimizes this effect. Lipoatrophy is less common with the highly purified insulin preparations.

Three types of insulin are available in the United States: beef, pork, and human. Beef and pork insulin are obtained from the pancreas of animals slaughtered for food. Many commonly used preparations are mixtures of beef and pork insulin that also may contain proinsulin as a contaminant (Table 69-4). Highly purified insulins contain much less proinsulin.

Human insulin comes from two sources. Semisynthetic human insulin is prepared by converting pork insulin to the human form by chemically changing the one differing amino acid. Human insulin is also made by recombinant DNA techniques; human genes for insulin are inserted into bacteria, which then produce large amounts of the protein to be processed and purified.

The hypoglycemic actions of the various forms of insulin are similar; however, the preparations differ slightly in pharmacokinetics and side effects. For example, human insulin preparations have a slightly shorter duration of action than corresponding pork insulin preparations. Dosages may require slight adjustment when switching from one prepara-

tion to another. Human insulin and purified pork insulin are less antigenic than the other types available. Patients may be switched to one of these forms to help control allergic side effects associated with insulin therapy.

Toxicity

Insulin overdose produces hypoglycemia. In severe cases, convulsions or coma may result. The very young and the elderly are especially at risk of developing this condition.

Interactions

Alcohol tends to enhance the hypoglycemic action of insulin. The result can be a greater risk of hypoglycemic reactions, but the risk is usually minimal unless alcohol consumption is moderate to high and the alcohol is taken without food.

Beta-adrenergic agents or corticosteroids may antagonize the actions of insulin (see Table 69-1). Insulin dosages may require adjustment.

Oral Hypoglycemic Agents

▼ Sulfonylureas

Mechanism of Action

Sulfonylureas and related agents (see Table 69-4) block the potassium channel in the membrane of beta cells of the pancreas (see p. 803). This action depolarizes the cell and stimulates release of insulin. Thus these drugs are useful only for patients who produce some insulin on their own (i.e., patients with type 2 diabetes mellitus).

Table 69-4 **Oral Antidiabetic Agents: Sulfonylureas and Related Agents**

Generic Name	Trade Name	Dosage/Range	Time to Peak Effect	Duration of Action
acetohexamide	Dimelor† Dymelor	0.25-1 g/day as a single dose or up to 1.5 g as a divided dose. FDA pregnancy category C.	2-6 hr	8-24 hr
chlorpropamide	Diabinese*	0.1-0.5 g/day, single dose. FDA pregnancy category C.	2-4 hr	24-72 hr
gliclazide	Diamicron†	40-160 mg twice daily.	4-6 hr	24 hr
glimepiride	Amaryl	1-4 mg once a day with the first main meal. FDA pregnancy category C. Maximum daily dose: 8 mg.	2-3 hr	ca. 24 hr
glipizide	Glucotrol	Tablets: 2.5-40 mg/day. Doses >15 mg should be divided. Extended-release tablets: 5-20 mg once daily. FDA pregnancy category C.	Tablets: 1-3 hr; extended-release tablets: 6-12 hr	12-24 hr
glyburide	DiaBeta* Euglucon† Micronase	Nonmicronized tablets: 1.25-20 mg/day. Micronized tablets: 0.75-12 mg once daily. FDA pregnancy category C (Diabeta), B (Micronase).	Nonmicronized: 3.5-4.5 hr; micronized: 2.5-3.5 hr	16-24 hr
repaglinide	Prandin	0.5 mg-4 mg given 15-30 min before each meal. FDA pregnancy category C.	1 hr	<4 hr
tolazamide	Tolinase	0.1-1 g/day; single dose for lower range, divided dose for higher range. FDA pregnancy category C.	3-4 hr	12-24 hr
tolbutamide	Orinase* Mobenol†	0.25-3 g/day, divided doses. FDA pregnancy category C.	3-4 hr	6-12 hr

*Available in Canada and the United States.
†Available in Canada only.

Clinical studies of patients with type 2 diabetes mellitus have shown that many have normal or even above-normal insulin levels in their blood. However, the cells of these patients are resistant to the action of insulin. Therefore insulin action is lost not because insulin is missing but because target cells fail to respond normally. Sulfonylureas also may diminish hepatic glucose production and may directly increase tissue responsiveness to insulin. These actions tend to diminish fasting plasma glucose concentrations and improve glucose use by fat and muscle cells. The effectiveness of sulfonylureas in obese patients with type 2 diabetes mellitus is enhanced by caloric restriction and weight loss. This dietary manipulation also tends to increase the responsiveness of target cells to insulin.

Pharmacokinetics

Sulfonylureas are well absorbed orally, although food may delay absorption of some of the agents. These drugs bind extensively to serum proteins. The sulfonylureas differ from one another primarily in onset and duration of action (see Table 69-4), which is strongly influenced by their hepatic metabolism. For example, tolbutamide is relatively short acting because it is quickly converted to an inactive product. In contrast, acetohexamide and tolazamide must be converted in the body to active products before they become effective. Hence they are intermediate in action. Chlorpropamide, the longest-acting member of the class, is tightly bound to plasma protein, slowly metabolized, and excreted in urine.

Glyburide, glipizide, glimepiride, and repaglinide are many times more potent than other sulfonylureas. For example, 5 mg of glyburide or glipizide has an effect equivalent to that of 250 mg of chlorpropamide or tolazamide. At the dosages used in patients, clinical effects are similar. Glyburide, glipizide, and glimepiride are extensively metabolized and are excreted primarily in urine, with a small amount in bile. Repaglinide is also extensively metabolized in liver, but most of the drug is eliminated in bile with only minor amounts in urine.

Uses

Sulfonylureas are used for the treatment of type 2 diabetes mellitus, along with diet and exercise. They are occasionally combined with insulin.

Adverse Reactions and Contraindications

Side effects of sulfonylurea therapy include GI tract distress and neurologic symptoms such as dizziness, drowsiness, or headache. Allergy to the drugs occurs in some patients, with skin reactions being the most common sign. The incidence of these types of reactions is reported to be less than 5% of patients treated.

Hypoglycemia is a common side effect with sulfonylureas and related agents. It is estimated that about 20% of treated patients will experience hypoglycemia within 6 months. For some of these patients, the hypoglycemia may occur at night and cause no noticeable symptoms; but for others, the symptoms may be obvious. Hypoglycemia is cause for dosage adjustment or change of medication. Glimepiride was reported to cause less than 2% incidence of hypoglycemia in clinical trials, but the drug is new and the incidence in patients treated long term has yet to be fully analyzed.

Weight gain is another common side effect with sulfonylureas, especially if these drugs must be combined with insulin. Gliclazide, glimepiride, and repaglinide may cause less weight gain than other drugs of this class.

Repaglinide causes symptoms of upper respiratory infections such as cough, runny nose, sneezing, and sore throat. Bronchitis and shortness of breath may also be noted.

Sulfonylureas and related drugs are never to be used in type 1 diabetes mellitus or in patients with type 2 diabetes mellitus who are prone to diabetic ketoacidosis. These drugs are also not intended for use during metabolic stress, such as that attending serious acute infections, major surgery or trauma, or severe burns. Insulin therapy is indicated for these conditions.

Toxicity

Hypoglycemia is a danger with sulfonylureas and may be caused by drug overdose, drug interactions, altered drug metabolism, or the patient failing to eat. Sulfonylureas should not be used when renal or liver function is inadequate; normal function of those organs is required for metabolism and elimination of sulfonylureas (see Table 69-4). Older adult patients also occasionally show excessive hypoglycemic reactions to these drugs.

Interactions

Sulfonylureas are implicated in drug interactions that can have serious consequences to the patient. The major interactions occur with ethyl alcohol, phenylbutazone, sulfonamides, salicylates, phenothiazines, and thiazides.

Patients receiving sulfonylureas should avoid alcohol. Several interactions between alcohol and sulfonylureas are possible. Some patients receiving sulfonylureas develop a disulfiram-like reaction when they ingest alcohol. The most striking symptoms of this reaction are unpleasant flushing and severe headache. Other patients taking sulfonylureas become hypoglycemic when they ingest alcohol, probably because ethanol is a hypoglycemic agent in some people.

Hypoglycemia can result when one of several drugs is given to a patient taking sulfonylureas, most importantly the antiinflammatory agents, phenylbutazone and salicylates, and sulfonamide antibiotics. These three types of drugs are all tightly bound to plasma protein and may displace sulfonylureas, which tend to be highly bound to serum protein. Thus blood concentrations of free sulfonylurea are elevated. Because the free drug is the active form, the result is an enhancement of the hypoglycemic effect of the sulfonylurea. In addition to this mechanism, phenylbutazone may block excretion of the active metabolite of acetohexamide, an action that also tends to increase hypoglycemia. Sulfonamides may inhibit the metabolic breakdown of tolbutamide and thereby may enhance its hypoglycemic action. The hypoglycemic effect of glipizide, glyburide, and tolbutamide is also increased by the antifungal agents fluconazole and miconazole.

Phenothiazines such as chlorpromazine may impair the effectiveness of sulfonylureas. Chlorpromazine inhibits the release of insulin from beta cells in the pancreas and elevates adrenal production of epinephrine, a hormone that can raise blood glucose levels (see Table 69-1). These actions of chlorpromazine directly antagonize the hypoglycemic action of sulfonylureas.

Thiazide diuretics possess hyperglycemic activity in addition to their diuretic actions; thus they may impair diabetes control with sulfonylureas.

Beta-adrenergic blocking agents have complex interactions with the sulfonylureas. One of the most dangerous is the tendency of the beta-adrenergic blockers to diminish the intensity of the symptoms of hypoglycemia. Thus patients may become profoundly hypoglycemic before they realize it.

metformin

Mechanism of Action

Metformin is a biguanide that is thought to increase the ability of insulin to bind to peripheral tissues, thus increasing glucose uptake by muscle and other tissues. Metformin is effective only in patients who produce insulin. One advantage of metformin is that it almost never causes hypoglycemia when used alone.

Pharmacokinetics

Metformin is slowly absorbed after oral doses (see Table 69-5). Food delays absorption and lowers the total amount of drug absorbed. Bioavailability is generally low. Absorbed drug is not significantly bound to plasma protein. Metformin is excreted unchanged primarily in urine, with a half-life of 6.2 hours.

Uses

Metformin is used only for the treatment of type 2 diabetes mellitus, alone or with a sulfonylurea.

Adverse Reactions and Contraindications

The most common side effects with metformin are GI effects, including anorexia, flatulence, metallic taste, nausea, stomach pain, vomiting, or weight loss. Some of these effects are transient and may be minimized by using small doses initially and increasing the dosage gradually.

Metformin is not sufficient during traumatic disease or injury in a diabetic patient; insulin is usually required. Metformin is also avoided in patients with significant cardiorespiratory insufficiency, congestive heart failure, heart attack, or severe liver or renal disease or in patients prone to lactic acidosis. In all of these conditions, the risk of potentially fatal lactic acidosis is increased. For the same reason, metformin is avoided in patients undergoing angiography or pyelography because the contrast medium used in these procedures may increase risk of lactic acidosis.

Table 69-5	Oral Antidiabetic Agents: Biguanides, Alpha-Glucosidase Inhibitors, Thiazolidinediones				
Generic Name	Trade Name	Dosage Range		Time to Peak Effect	Duration of Action
Biguanide					
metformin	Glucophage	500 mg twice daily with meals, up to 850 mg 3 times/day with meals. FDA pregnancy category B.		1.8-2.7 hr	6-12 hr
Alpha-Glucosidase Inhibitors					
acarbose	Precose	25-50 mg 3 times/day, at the start of each main meal. FDA pregnancy category B.		1 hr	Hours
miglitol	Glyset	25-100 mg 3 times/day, at the start of each main meal. FDA pregnancy category B.		2-3 hr	4-6 hr
Thiazolidinediones					
troglitazone	Rezulin	400-600 mg once daily with a meal; 200 mg once daily if used with insulin. FDA pregnancy category B.		2-3 hr	Up to 24 hr

Toxicity

Overdoses of metformin may cause hypoglycemia and lactic acidosis.

Interactions

Patients taking metformin should avoid alcohol to prevent excessive risk of hypoglycemia or lactic acidosis. Amiloride, cimetidine, digoxin, morphine, procainamide, quinidine, quinine, ranitidine, triamterene, trimethoprim, and vancomycin may block renal secretion of metformin. Furosemide may increase oral absorption of metformin. The result of both types of interaction is to increase blood concentration of metformin; dosages of metformin may require reduction.

acarbose and miglitol

Mechanism of Action

Acarbose and miglitol are inhibitors of intestinal enzymes that break complex carbohydrates into smaller molecules, including glucose. Alpha-glucosidases are the primary enzymes inhibited. The result of the reversible inhibition of these enzymes is that digestion of complex carbohydrates is slowed and hyperglycemia after eating is decreased.

Pharmacokinetics

Acarbose is only minimally absorbed from the GI tract, so it tends to stay at its site of action, which is the intestinal lumen. Some drug is eventually metabolized and absorbed, but most of the drug is eliminated unchanged in the feces.

Miglitol is absorbed after oral dosage and is almost exclusively eliminated by the kidneys. There is no significant metabolism of this drug.

Uses

Use of acarbose or miglitol is indicated for type 2 diabetes mellitus, when adequate control cannot be maintained by diet alone. If needed, these drugs may also be combined with a sulfonylurea.

Adverse Reactions and Contraindications

GI side effects are the most common reactions to acarbose and miglitol. Symptoms include pain, diarrhea, and flatulence. Nearly all treated patients report one or more of these symptoms, but for many patients, these side effects diminish with time.

Toxicity

Overdose with acarbose or miglitol should not cause hypoglycemia but should be expected to cause more profound interference with digestive processes, leading to worsened diarrhea and other GI symptoms.

Interactions

Corticosteroids and thiazide diuretics may interfere with control of hyperglycemia with acarbose. Intestinal adsorbents such as activated charcoal may interfere with the actions of acarbose or miglitol. Digestive enzyme preparations often contain carbohydrate-splitting enzymes and would thus directly antagonize the effects of both acarbose and miglitol.

Miglitol has a dramatic effect on the pharmacokinetics of propranolol and ranitidine, lowering the bioavailability by 40% to 60%.

troglitazone

Mechanism of Action

Troglitazone acts primarily on target tissues of insulin to decrease insulin resistance. The drug does not stimulate insulin release but depends on the presence of insulin to achieve its desired clinical effect. Troglitazone may decrease glucose output by the liver, in addition to increasing glucose use in target tissues.

Pharmacokinetics

Troglitazone is well absorbed orally, especially when taken with food. The drug is metabolized by liver enzymes and is an inducer of the CYP3A4 system (see Chapter 1). Elimination of troglitazone is primarily in the feces.

Uses

Troglitazone is indicated only for the treatment of type 2 diabetes mellitus. The drug may be added to a regimen of diet and exercise to achieve adequate control. If needed, troglitazone may be used with a sulfonylurea or with insulin.

Adverse Reactions and Contraindications

Pain, including back pain, and infections were common side effects with troglitazone. Dizziness, headache, nausea, and generalized weakness were also noted in up to 11% of treated patients. Edema and jaundice were rare but may signal a dangerous reaction. Edema may follow from the increase in plasma volume caused by troglitazone; this side effect may put predisposed patients at risk of developing impaired cardiovascular function. Jaundice may signal the onset of liver damage, which in rare cases has led to fatalities.

Toxicity

Overdoses of this drug have not been reported, but in cases of overdose, liver and cardiac function should be closely monitored.

Interactions

Cholestyramine may interfere with the absorption of troglitazone; the drugs should not be used together.

Troglitazone is an inducer of CYP3A4 drug-metabolizing enzymes in the liver. Thus drugs that are metabolized by that enzyme system will be eliminated more quickly when given with troglitazone. Drugs affected in this way include calcium channel blocking agents, corticosteroids, HMG-CoA reductase inhibitors (see Chapter 21), and oral contraceptives containing either ethinyl estradiol or norethindrone.

Adjuncts to Drug Therapy

Diet Therapy

Mechanism of Action

Obesity, or more specifically excessive caloric intake, tends to reduce the number of insulin receptors on target tissues. An understanding of this disease mechanism helps in appreciating the rationale for dietary control of diabetes. Reduced caloric intake allows the insulin receptors to increase and makes the available insulin more effective. Dietary restriction may lower insulin requirements in obese diabetic patients and, in many cases, when combined with moderate exercise, may be the only form of therapy required. The effectiveness of sulfonylureas in obese patients with type 2 diabetes mellitus is enhanced by caloric restriction and weight loss.

Careful dietary control is important for all diabetic patients. Successful long-term treatment of the condition often involves counseling by a dietitian and supportive follow-up for the rest of the patient's life.

Nursing Process Overview

Diabetes Mellitus

Assessment

Diabetes occurs in all age groups. Assess vital signs, weight, serum and urine glucose levels, and any signs associated with possible long-term effects, such as decreased circulation to the lower extremities. Assess the condition of skin and nails.

Nursing Diagnoses

- Possible complication: hypoglycemia
- Knowledge deficit related to diabetes mellitus

Patient Outcomes

The nurse will minimize and manage complications of hypoglycemia. The patient will explain how or demonstrate how to measure blood or urine glucose, administer insulin, treat hypoglycemia, manage diet, or perform other aspects of management as needed.

Planning/Implementation

In relation to drug therapy, monitor serum blood glucose and examine other appropriate laboratory work such as glycosylated hemoglobin A_{1c}, serum potassium, or pH. Begin planning for discharge as soon as the patient is diagnosed. Instruct the patient about the medications that have been prescribed, their method of administration, and how to test blood glucose. Refer the patient as appropriate to the hospital or community dietitian, the local visiting nurse association, and the local diabetes association.

Evaluation

Before discharge, verify that the patient understands why the drugs are prescribed and can demonstrate how to administer insulin or other medications correctly. Be certain that the patient understands the symptoms of hyperglycemia and hypoglycemia and how to treat them and other prescribed aspects of care such as foot care, dietary restrictions, and any limitations in activity that have been prescribed. Ensure that the patient can demonstrate how to test for blood glucose levels and can state what to do based on the information obtained from this test.

Nursing Implications Summary

General Guidelines: Treatment of Diabetes Mellitus

Nursing in the Community

➤ Teach the patient and family the signs and symptoms of hyperglycemia and hypoglycemia (see Table 69-3).

➤ The development of hypoglycemia may relate to the time the insulin or the oral agent was taken (see Tables 69-2, 69-4, and 69-5). If possible, obtain a blood glucose level. Whether or not a blood glucose level is obtained, treat by administering a fast-acting carbohydrate such as ½ cup fruit juice, ½ cup cola drink (not diet forms), ½ cup regular gelatin dessert, 4 cubes or 2 packets of sugar, 2 squares of graham crackers, or 2 to 3 pieces of hard candy. A common treatment is a glassful of orange juice containing 2 or 3 teaspoonfuls of sugar. Instruct the patient to wait about 15 minutes after ingesting carbohydrate, then measure blood glucose again. Instruct the patient to have available hard candy or other sources of carbohydrate at all times. Glucagon may be used if the patient is unconscious. Teach family members how to use this, and instruct the patient to have glucagon always available.

➤ If hypoglycemia is severe, is repeated, or occurs without explanation, instruct the patient to consult the physician.

➤ Teach the patient about appropriate dietary restrictions or refer the patient as needed to a dietitian. Losing weight to desirable body weight is helpful in controlling diabetes.

➤ Encourage the patient to participate in a regular exercise program.

➤ Review foot care and other aspects of personal hygiene to prevent infection.

➤ Teach the patient how to test blood glucose level. Review methods of testing and frequency, and supervise the patient performing the test activity for accuracy. If a urine test method is being used, point out to the patient that some drugs may cause urine test results to be inaccurate. Instruct the patient to ask the physician and pharmacist if there is a possibility of drug-urine test interaction when new drugs are prescribed.

➤ Refer the patient as appropriate to the health department or other community-based nursing care agencies for follow-up.

➤ Refer the patient to the American Diabetes Association or local support groups for additional information and resources; examples of such resources include syringes adapted for the visually impaired, information booklets, automatic insulin injectors, and cookbooks.

➤ Encourage diabetic patients to wear a medical identification tag or bracelet.

➤ Instruct the patient to avoid drinking alcoholic beverages.

➤ Instruct the patient to avoid smoking. Patients who begin or stop smoking may require an adjustment in diet or drug dosage.

➤ Warn the patient to inform all health care providers about the diabetes and the type of drug used to control it.

➤ Caution the patient to avoid taking any drug unless first approved by the physician. Many drugs cause changes in blood glucose level. Instruct the patient to monitor blood and/or urine glucose level carefully when starting or stopping a new medication.

➤ The specific regimen prescribed for any patient is based on many factors, including age, type of diabetes, severity of diabetes, weight, resources available, philosophy of the health care team, and other medical problems the patient may have. Although general guidelines are noted in this text, consult other nursing texts and printed resources as needed.

➤ Caution female patients to consult the physician before attempting to conceive because management of diabetes may be modified during pregnancy. A diabetic female who becomes pregnant should notify the physician immediately.

insulin

Drug Administration

➤ Local allergic reactions involving itching, redness, swelling, or stinging at the injection site are usually transient and are common. Anaphylaxis is rare. Insulin resistance occasionally involves antibodies to insulin. It may not be possible to eliminate local allergic reactions. Supervise insulin administration technique because scrupulous attention to technique may lessen local irritation. Record and rotate sites on a systematic basis so that accessible sites are not overused (see Chapter 5). Prepare the dose of insulin as ordered and let it warm to room temperature. Cleanse the injection site carefully and allow skin surface to dry completely. Pinch skin between thumb and fingers of one hand and insert needle into the "pocket" between the subcutaneous fat and muscle; a 45- to 90-degree angle can be used, depending on the amount of subcutaneous fat and the length of the needle. Inject the insulin and withdraw the needle. Apply moderate pressure to the site but do not rub.

➤ If local irritation is severe or persistent, consult the physician about a change in type of insulin.

➤ Systemic reactions are rare and may be caused by the animal source of the insulin (bovine, porcine, or mixed bovine-porcine). Treat symptomatically and notify the physician.

➤ Use regular insulin for patients on "sliding scale" management.

➤ Consult with the physician about diabetes management when patients are permitted nothing by mouth in preparation for surgery or are otherwise unable to maintain usual dietary intake.

➤ For IV use, only regular insulin can be used. Insulin adsorbs to bags, tubing, and other items made of polyvinyl chloride (PVC). To decrease the amount of insulin lost to adsorption to the PVC during continuous infusion (e.g., 100 units regular insulin in 500 ml normal saline), flush the system with 50 ml of the diluted insulin mixture, then store the IV bag or bottle, and tubing for 30 minutes before connecting it to the patient. Titrate the rate of infusion to the patient response, blood glucose levels, and ordered rate of drop of blood glucose level. Also monitor serum electrolyte level, especially potassium.

Continued

Nursing Implications Summary—cont'd

➤ Only buffered regular insulin is used in insulin pumps. Review the manufacturer's instruction sheet with the patient. Some patients follow a regimen that includes continuous infusion of insulin via pump, with periodic subcutaneous injections of additional insulin.

➤ Observe agency policies regarding insulin administration. For example, many hospitals require that insulin doses be checked by two licensed nurses before administration.

➤ Monitor serum and urinary glucose, serum potassium, pH, urinary ketones, and glycosylated hemoglobin A_{1c}.

Nursing in the Community

➤ Review the general guidelines and the information about injection with the patient.

➤ Teach the patient that only syringes marked for units of insulin should be used with insulin. Special syringes are available for doses less than 50 units. Review carefully with the patient the need to obtain the correct concentration and type of insulin and correct syringe.

➤ To mix insulins, instruct the patient to always draw up the regular (unmodified) insulin first, then the other insulin that is ordered. If two modified insulins are to be drawn up together, either can be drawn up first, but the patient should establish a pattern and always draw up the same one first.

➤ Some mixtures of insulin in a syringe must be administered within a few minutes of drawing them up, although others are stable for longer periods. The patient should consult the physician or pharmacist.

➤ Regular insulin is clear, and modified insulins are cloudy. Instruct the patient to not use discolored insulins or ones that appear grainy. Instruct the patient to warm and resuspend insulins by rotating the vials between the hands and to avoid vigorous shaking.

➤ Generally, insulin injected into the abdomen is absorbed the fastest, insulin in the arm is absorbed more slowly, and insulin is absorbed slowest when injected in the thigh. However, several things may influence this. For example, a diabetic patient who jogs has faster absorption from the thigh when jogging and using the thigh muscles. Consider the daily habits of the patient in working out an appropriate plan for diabetes management.

➤ Insulin can be safely kept at room temperature for up to 1 month. Insulin kept at room temperature for longer than 1 month should be discarded. Insulin may be stored in the refrigerator for longer than 1 month. Instruct the patient to not freeze insulin and to check the expiration date.

➤ Teach the patient that when illness occurs, it is important to maintain fluid intake. Consult the physician about specific guidelines for insulin dosage and diet when the patient is sick. Remind the patient to contact the physician with questions about management.

➤ Develop an individualized teaching plan about insulin for patients. Decisions to be made include whether patients will use disposable syringes or will sterilize and reuse glass syringes, whether the patient has the ability (vision, dexterity,

and so on) to draw up and administer the insulin, and what type of glucose test method will be used.

➤ Instruct the patient to use the same brand of syringe at all times. Switching syringes may cause variations in level of blood glucose control as a result of the different volumes between the needle and the end of the calibrated syringe (dead space).

➤ Disposable syringes and needles were designed for one-time use. However, some patients reuse these syringes and needles, usually for economic reasons. If the patient must reuse syringes and needles, review the importance of cleaning the needle and capping the needle between uses. A syringe and needle should be used, even repeatedly, on only one patient, never shared. Finally, the syringe and needle should be reused for a few injections only, not on a continuing basis. If skin irritation is a problem, the patient may want to use a new needle or syringe more often.

➤ Many kinds of specialized insulin injectors are in use, including automatic injectors, insulin "pen" devices, and spray injectors. Review the manufacturer's instructions in teaching the patient how to prepare and use these injectors.

➤ Instruct the patient not to switch type or source of insulin without consulting the physician because a change in dosage is often necessary. Also, tell the patient not to switch the brand of syringe because small variations may be sufficient to cause improper dosage.

➤ Remind the patient to monitor the supply of insulin and syringes on hand to avoid running out unexpectedly.

➤ Instruct the patient with IDDM to carry insulin and syringes with hand luggage to avoid losing them whenever traveling. For large quantities of insulin and syringes, divide them among pieces of luggage so that all are not lost if a piece of luggage is lost. Some states require prescriptions for syringes, so suggest that the patient carry an adequate supply for the entire trip. This is especially important in international travel. Suggest that the patient carry a letter from the physician listing the need for insulin and syringes because this may help if insulin is lost in delayed baggage or in delays at Customs. Discuss in advance with the pharmacist any special considerations for insulin storage.

Oral Hypoglycemic Agents: Sulfonylureas and Related Agents, and metformin

Drug Administration

➤ Review the symptoms of hypoglycemia and hyperglycemia listed in Table 69-3 and teach them to the patient.

➤ Monitor weight.

➤ Monitor complete blood count and white blood cell differential, platelet count, liver function tests, blood glucose, and glycosylated hemoglobin A_{1c}. With patients taking metformin, monitor serum folic acid and vitamin B_{12} concentrations.

Nursing in the Community

➤ See the general guidelines for treating diabetes mellitus.

Nursing Implications Summary—cont'd

➤ Instruct the patient to report any new side effects.

➤ Note the many drug interactions described in this text. Instruct patients to avoid taking any medications unless first discussed with the physician.

➤ See the Patient Problems boxes on constipation (Chapter 24) and photosensitivity (Chapter 58).

➤ See the Patient Problem box in Chapter 57 on disulfiram-like reactions. Some patients develop disulfiram-like reactions when they ingest alcohol and are taking a sulfonylurea.

➤ Remind the patient to take the medication as ordered, even if not feeling well.

➤ Usually, the patient should take ordered doses with the first meal of the day. If a dose is missed, instruct the patient to take it as soon as remembered, unless it is almost time for the next dose, in which case omit the missed dose and resume the regular dosing schedule. The patient should not double up for missed doses.

Alpha-Glucosidase Inhibitors
Drug Administration/Nursing in the Community
➤ See the general guidelines for treating diabetes mellitus.

➤ Review the symptoms of hypoglycemia and hyperglycemia listed in Table 69-3 and teach them to the patient.

➤ Monitor serum and/or urine glucose levels, glycosylated hemoglobin, and with acarbose, serum transaminase levels.

➤ Monitor weight.

➤ Instruct the patient to report any new side effects.

➤ GI symptoms are common but often lessen with time. Instruct the patient to notify the physician of severe or persistent abdominal pain, diarrhea, or flatulence.

➤ Instruct the patient to take doses of acarbose or miglitol three times each day, with the first bite of each meal.

troglitazone
Drug Administration/Nursing in the Community
➤ See the general guidelines for treating diabetes mellitus.

➤ Monitor serum urine glucose levels, glycosylated hemoglobin, liver function tests, and serum transaminase levels.

➤ Monitor weight. Assess for the development of peripheral edema, jaundice, or diarrhea.

➤ Instruct the patient to avoid driving or operating hazardous equipment if dizziness or excessive fatigue develops.

➤ Instruct the patient to report any new side effects.

➤ Instruct the patient to take doses with meals.

➤ When administered alone, this drug should not cause hypoglycemia. However, when administered with insulin or a sulfonylurea, hypoglycemia may develop. Review the symptoms of hypoglycemia and hyperglycemia listed in Table 69-3 and teach them to the patient and family.

CHAPTER REVIEW

Application

1. What three peptide hormones from pancreatic islets affect glucose metabolism?

2. What effect does insulin have on glucose metabolism?

3. What effect does glucagon have on glucose metabolism?

4. What effects do cortisol, epinephrine, and growth hormone have on glucose metabolism?

5. What effect does insulin have on fat and protein metabolism?

6. What is diabetes mellitus? How should you assess for this?

7. What are the characteristics of type 1 diabetes mellitus?

8. What are the characteristics of type 2 diabetes mellitus?

9. What effect does diabetes mellitus have on protein and fat metabolism?

10. What are the long-term complications of diabetes mellitus?

11. How is diabetes mellitus diagnosed?

12. How does insulin therapy relieve the symptoms of diabetes mellitus?

13. Why must insulin be injected?

14. What is the onset and duration of action of regular insulin?

15. What advantages do the insulin preparations containing relatively insoluble insulin complexes have over regular insulin?

16. When does peak hypoglycemic action occur after a dose of insulin injection? NPH insulin? Ultralente insulin?

17. What reaction would be expected from an overdose of insulin? What are signs and symptoms of this reaction?

18. What type of reactions may insulin produce at the site of injection?

19. What is the mechanism of action for the sulfonylureas as hypoglycemic agents?

20. What type of diabetic patient benefits from sulfonylurea therapy?

21. How are sulfonylureas administered?

22. Which sulfonylureas are converted to active forms by the body?

23. Which is the longest-acting sulfonylurea?

24. What side effects occur with sulfonylureas?

25. Why does caloric restriction enhance effectiveness of sulfonylureas?

26. What other drugs may enhance the hypoglycemic effect of sulfonylureas?

27. What reaction may be seen in patients receiving sulfonylureas who ingest ethyl alcohol?

28. How does metformin aid in controlling diabetes mellitus?

Continued

29. What are the most common side effects with metformin?
30. Which patients should not receive metformin?
31. What are the expected signs of overdosage with metformin?
32. What risk is associated with alcohol use by a patient receiving metformin?
33. How do inhibitors of alpha-glucosidase enzymes aid in control of type 2 diabetes mellitus?
34. What are the most common side effects of acarbose and miglitol?
35. What is the mechanism of action of troglitazone?
36. What side effects are common with troglitazone?
37. What organ may be a special target for toxicity with troglitazone?

Critical Thinking

1. What is the duration of action of each of the insulin preparations? What are implications of this information in teaching patients?
2. Which of the drugs used for diabetes are least likely to cause hypoglycemia? Why?

References

Bak LB, Heard KA, Kearney GP: Tube feeding your diabetic patient safely, *Am J Nurs* 96(12):47-49, 1996.

Cirone N: Unmasking a hidden disorder. Diabetes in the elderly. Part I, *Nursing* 26(3):34-39, 1996.

Cirone N, Schwartz N: Finding the balance for drug therapy, Diabetes in the elderly. Part II, *Nursing* 26(3):40-45, 1996.

Depree PA: Lispro insulin, *Nursing* 28(11):54-55, 1998.

Drass JA: Caring for patients with insulin-dependent diabetes mellitus, *Nursing* 26(8):46-47, 1996.

Drass JA: Caring for patients with non-insulin-dependent diabetes mellitus, *Nursing* 26(9):48-49, 1996.

Maffeo R: Helping families cope with type I diabetes, *Am J Nurs* 97(6):36-39, 1998.

Saulie BA, Campbell RK: Pharmacy update: treating erectile dysfunction in diabetes patients, *Diabetes Educ* 23(1):29-33, 35-36, 38, 1997.

Savinetti-Rose B, Bolmer L: Understanding continuous subcutaneous infusion therapy, *Am J Nurs* 97(3):42-49, 1997.

Tomky D: Taking a new look at an old adversary: diabetes, *Nursing* 27(11):41-45, 1997.

Chapter 70

Estrogens, Progestins, and Contraception

OBJECTIVES

After studying this chapter, you should be able to do the following:

- *Describe the use of estrogens in replacement therapy.*

- *Discuss the use of progestins alone or progestins in combination with estrogens as contraceptive agents.*

- *Discuss the drugs that can increase female fertility.*

- *Develop a nursing care plan for a patient receiving a drug discussed in this chapter.*

CHAPTER OVERVIEW

Female reproduction depends on a finely regulated interaction of endocrine tissues. The negative feedback loop that regulates the menstrual cycle involves the hypothalamus, the anterior pituitary, and the ovaries (see Chapter 65). Actions of natural female hormones, as well as clinical uses of synthetic drugs that affect the female reproductive system, are considered in this chapter.

THERAPEUTIC RATIONALE: HORMONES INVOLVED IN FEMALE REPRODUCTION

Classes of Female Hormones

Hormones from many organs are involved in developing and maintaining female reproductive capacity. The hypothalamus supplies gonadotropin-releasing hormone (GnRH), a peptide that acts directly on the anterior pituitary, stimulating synthesis and release of follicle-stimulating hormone (FSH) and luteinizing hormone (LH). In addition, the central nervous system (CNS) neurotransmitter dopamine is the inhibitory factor that regulates the release of prolactin from the anterior pituitary. FSH, LH, and prolactin are the major gonadotropins. These hormones each have a different primary target tissue. FSH stimulates the ovarian cells that form follicles and nurture the maturing ovum. Under the influence of FSH, these cells synthesize the potent steroid estradiol. LH acts primarily on a mature follicle to cause release of the ovum. Prolactin stimulates breast tissue to promote milk production but may affect other reproductive tissues as well.

The most important hormones regulating female reproduction are estrogens and progestins. **Estrogens** are steroids that stimulate female reproductive tissues; **progestins** are steroids that specifically stimulate the uterine lining. Estrogens are produced most abundantly by FSH-stimulated cells of the ovarian follicle. Progesterone, the most important progestin, is synthesized in cells remaining in the follicle after expulsion of an ovum. This tissue is called the corpus luteum.

All of the steroids produced in the ovary are derived from cholesterol. Progestins are formed first and are the precursors of androgens. Androgens, the steroid hormones capable of producing masculinization, are primarily precursors of estrogen synthesis in females. Androstenedione is

817

the androgen precursor of estrone, a circulating estrogen formed mostly in peripheral tissues and not in the ovary. Estradiol, the most abundant circulating estrogen, is formed in the ovary.

Hormones Affecting Female Reproductive Development

At birth the ovary is already in an advanced stage of development and contains between 2 and 4 million oocytes, cells that will form ova. The primordial follicles containing oocytes are not quiescent before puberty but undergo a process called atresia in which oocytes are destroyed and follicles are resorbed. At **menarche,** when menstrual cycles begin during puberty, an estimated 400,000 oocytes remain. Even after ovulation starts, atresia continues and is responsible for the destruction of more than 99% of the follicles present in the ovary.

As puberty begins the immature ovaries are stimulated by increasing amounts of pituitary gonadotropins. As a result, estrogen synthesis is promoted, and estrogen levels in the blood rise. The primary function of estrogens during early puberty is to promote development of the reproductive system. The uterus and fallopian tubes enlarge to adult proportions. The vagina enlarges, and the vaginal epithelium thickens and strengthens. In the breasts, estrogen promotes proliferation of tissues responsible for the production of milk.

The secondary sexual characteristics also depend on estrogens. These hormones promote increased deposition of fat, especially in the breasts and hips. Without estrogens, the typical contours of the female body do not develop.

Estrogens are also involved in regulating the start and the stop of the growth spurt that is characteristic of puberty. Along with other hormones, estrogen causes retention of calcium and phosphorus and thereby promotes bone growth. Estrogens also induce closure of the epiphyses. When this closure occurs, no further increase in height occurs.

Hormones Affecting Ovulation

Ovulation requires proper functioning of the hypothalamus, anterior pituitary, and ovaries in the negative feedback loop described in Chapter 65. FSH and LH are required to act on the developing follicle before a mature ovum may be released to begin its journey down the fallopian tube to the uterus. Estrogen synthesis is required for its action on the follicle and for its ability to trigger the midcycle surge of LH from the anterior pituitary.

Hormones Affecting Endometrial Function

The uterus is composed of smooth muscle (myometrium) and glandular epithelium, or endometrium. The endometrium, which nourishes and supports the ovum during development, is controlled primarily by estrogens and progestins. Estrogens promote proliferation of the endometrium during the first half of the menstrual cycle before ovulation occurs. Progesterone, which is formed in the corpus luteum of the ovary during the second half of the menstrual cycle,

acts on the endometrium and the myometrium. Progesterone reduces myometrial activity, preventing muscular contractions, and promotes development of the secretory capacity of endometrium. Actions on these two tissues aid in establishing the environment in which the fertilized ovum may implant successfully and begin development. Once implantation of the ovum has occurred, progesterone continues to alter the endometrium, ultimately changing the tissue so that a second implantation becomes impossible.

Hormones in Pregnancy

Pregnancy requires that a mature ovum be released from the ovary at the appropriate time, that the ovum be fertilized successfully within about 2 days of its release, and that the ovum be able to implant within the endometrium and to draw nourishment to support the early stages of development. The most important hormone during these first days and weeks of pregnancy is **progesterone.** Without adequate progesterone, the endometrium is sloughed and the fertilized ovum is lost. Luteal progesterone is produced for about the first 10 weeks of pregnancy. Control of progesterone synthesis is exercised by cells of the fetus, which develop into the placenta. A few days after implantation of the ovum in the endometrium, these fetal cells begin to produce a hormone called **human chorionic gonadotropin (HCG);** HCG takes

ALTERNATIVE THERAPIES

Estrogenic Activity

PHYTOESTROGENS

The decision to take or not to take estrogen replacement therapy is a difficult one for many women because it involves weighing relative risks of several possible effects. For many women, the fear of increased risk of uterine or breast cancer persuades them to avoid the powerful synthetic- or animal-derived estrogens used in replacement therapy. Some of these women seek to lessen symptoms of menopause with phytoestrogens, which are plant-derived chemicals that have mild estrogenic effects. Soy products are the best studied for this effect. At least three servings daily of soy-derived foods are needed for an effect, but more concentrated powders are available. A concentrate of red clover that contains the same type of phytoestrogens, which may reduce the hot flashes associated with menopause, is also available. If these weaker phytoestrogens are used with the stronger medically used estrogens, the phytoestrogens will block some of the effects of the stronger agents.

Several other plant-derived products are promoted for their estrogenic effects, but these products are less well studied and may produce other unwanted actions. For example, a product containing black cohosh has sedative and antihypertensive effects that may interfere with drug therapy for hypertension. Some products combine black cohosh, kava, and soy, but these products can produce sedation. A Chinese herbal, dong quai, sold for menopause, has not been documented to relieve menopausal symptoms but does induce photosensitivity and may be carcinogenic.

over control of the corpus luteum and maintains its production of progesterone. By the fifth week of pregnancy the placenta has developed to where it begins to synthesize progesterone directly. Placental progesterone production increases during the remainder of the pregnancy, whereas progesterone production in the corpus luteum virtually disappears.

THERAPEUTIC AGENTS: DRUGS AFFECTING FEMALE SEXUAL FUNCTION

Agents for Replacement Therapy

Estrogens

Mechanism of Action

Many conditions of the female reproductive tract for which women seek medical aid may be treated successfully by replacement therapy. The most common conditions are those that arise as a result of estrogen deficiency. A lack of estrogen during puberty prevents normal growth and sexual development; menarche may not occur. This endocrine malfunction is one of several abnormalities that may be responsible for amenorrhea (no menstrual cycles). **Menopause,** which usually occurs in women in their late forties or early fifties, is the state in which estrogen levels begin to decline. Lower estrogen levels may cause vasomotor symptoms (hot flashes and sweating), osteoporosis (bone loss), and atrophy of vaginal and urethral tissue. Exogenously supplied natural or synthetic estrogens have the same actions described earlier for endogenously formed estrogens and thus can effectively replace the missing natural estrogen.

Other medical problems of the female reproductive system cannot be ascribed to a specific hormone deficiency. Nevertheless, many of these conditions respond to hormones used for some pharmacologic action rather than as replacement therapy. The rationale for therapy for these conditions is listed in Table 70-1.

Pharmacokinetics

Many estrogens are available (Table 70-2). The two naturally occurring steroid estrogens used clinically are **estradiol** and **estrone.** As steroids, these compounds are not water soluble, but they are soluble in oil. With estradiol, slower absorption and longer duration of action may be achieved by using the cypionate or the valerate ester of the natural steroid. Estradiol is absorbed orally if the drug crystals are reduced to particles 1 to 3 mm in diameter. Estradiol is also effectively absorbed transdermally.

Estrone is not well absorbed orally in its natural form but may be used orally if it is converted to the piperazine sulfate (estropipate). Estrone is also the major component of

Table 70-1 Pharmacologic Therapy of Dysfunctions of Female Reproductive System

Clinical Condition	Treatment	Rationale
Hypogonadism	Estrogens	Estrogens are required to promote secondary sex characteristics. Other hormonal support may be required for full fertility.
Amenorrhea	bromocriptine, gonadorelin, or a progestin	Drugs are effective only for specific types of conditions producing amenorrhea.
Menopause		
Vasomotor symptoms	Estrogens	Hot flashes and sweating are relieved by estrogens.
Osteoporosis	Estrogens	Loss of calcium may be slowed while estrogens are taken.
Atrophy of vaginal and urethral tissue	Estrogens	Estrogen support is needed to maintain tissue tone.
Dysfunctional uterine bleeding	Estrogen and progestin	Combination stops bleeding; drug withdrawal induces endometrial sloughing.
Luteal phase defect (infertility)	Progestins	Infertility resulting from inadequate synthesis of progesterone from corpus luteum may be treated by progestin early in pregnancy.
Metastatic breast carcinoma	Estrogens, androgens, or progestins	Tumors show differing sensitivities to these hormones.
Metastatic endometrial carcinoma	Progestins	Natural suppressive effect of progestins on endometrium is retained in some of these tumors.
Galactorrhea	bromocriptine	Drug suppresses prolactin release, thereby preventing excessive stimulation of breast secretory tissue.
Dysmenorrhea	Oral contraceptives or prostaglandin inhibitors	Suppression of ovulation gives relief to some patients. Drugs such as ibuprofen, indomethacin, mefenamic acid, naproxen, and ketoprofen relieve symptoms by preventing excessive production of prostaglandins.
Pelvic endometriosis	Progestins, danazol, goserelin, leuprolide, naferelin	Suppresses proliferation of endometrial tissue. Inhibits gonadotropins, thus preventing proliferation of endometrial tissue.
Anovulation (infertility)	Recombinant human luteinizing hormone, clomiphene, human chorionic gonadotropin, menotropins	Ovulation may be stimulated directly by luteinizing hormone. Clomiphene may promote gonadotropin release, and menotropins supply them directly.
Premenstrual tension	ergotamine, diuretics, or antianxiety agents	Therapy is empiric and often ineffective.

Table 70-2 **Estrogens Used Primarily for Replacement Therapy**

Generic Name	Trade Name	Administration/Dosage‡	Comments
dienestrol	Dienestrol*	VAGINAL: *Adults*—1 application twice daily for 2 wk, tapering to 1 dose 1-3 times/wk for 3 wk, then no drug for 1 wk.	For vaginal and vulval atrophy.
estradiol	Estrace*	ORAL: *Adults*—0.5-2 mg daily or cyclically.	For estrogen replacement or menopausal symptoms. Cyclical regimens may be 3 wk on and 1 wk off drug, or 5 days on and 2 days off.
		VAGINAL: *Adults*—0.2-0.4 mg/day for 2 wk, tapering to 0.1 mg 1-3 times/wk for 3 wk, then no drug for 1 wk. Vaginal insert (Estring): device delivers 7.5 μg/day; replaced every 90 days.	
	Climara Estraderm* FemPatch Vivelle*	TRANSDERMAL: *Adults*—1 patch delivers 0.025-0.1 mg/day; change once or twice weekly, depending on the patch.	
estradiol cypionate	Depo-Estradiol Dura-Estrin	INTRAMUSCULAR: *Adults*—1-5 mg every 3 or 4 wk.	For estrogen replacement.
estradiol valerate	Delestrogen* Femogex†	INTRAMUSCULAR: *Adults*—10-20 mg every 4 wk.	For estrogen replacement.
estrogens, conjugated	Congest† Premarin*	ORAL: *Adults*—0.3-7.5 mg daily or cyclically. INTRAMUSCULAR, INTRAVENOUS: 25 mg every 6-12 hr. VAGINAL: *Adults*—0.3-1.25 mg/day for 3 wk; may repeat after 1 wk with no drug.	For estrogen replacement; intramuscular doses for abnormal uterine bleeding.
estrogens, esterified	Estratab Neo-estrone†	ORAL: *Adults*—0.3-7.5 mg daily or cyclically.	For estrogen replacement.
estrone	Aquest Estragyn 5	INTRAMUSCULAR: *Adults*—0.1 mg-2 mg/wk.	For estrogen replacement; higher dosages for abnormal uterine bleeding.
estropipate	Ogen*	ORAL: *Adults*—0.75-9 mg/day. VAGINAL: *Adults*—3-6 mg/day for 3 wk, then no drug for 1 wk.	For estrogen replacement; vaginal dosing for vaginal or vulval atrophy.
ethinyl estradiol	Estinyl*	ORAL: *Adults*—0.02-0.05 mg 1-3 times/day.	For estrogen replacement.

*Available in Canada and the United States.
†Available in Canada only.
‡All estrogens are FDA pregnancy category X.

various estrogen mixtures described as esterified or conjugated estrogens. These mixtures, which are isolated from the urine of pregnant mares, are relatively cheap and are effective for many purposes. These mixtures can also be taken orally, which makes them a convenient drug form for many patients.

Synthetic estrogens such as **ethinyl estradiol** are also available. Ethinyl estradiol is more potent than naturally occurring estrogens. This drug used orally has a relatively short duration of action but persists in the body longer than any of the natural estrogens.

Nonsteroidal estrogens such as diethylstilbestrol (DES) are oral agents. DES was once widely used to prevent spontaneous abortions, but the children who were in utero at the time of DES treatment may have experienced drug effects. As adults, female offspring have an increased incidence of vaginal adenosis and adenocarcinoma; male offspring are more prone to develop epididymal cysts. DES is currently used only as an antineoplastic agent (see Chapter 56).

Natural estrogens do not persist long in the body because they are rapidly metabolized by the liver and renally excreted. Ethinyl estradiol is less rapidly metabolized and is thus longer acting than natural estrogens.

Uses

Estrogen dosages vary depending on the condition being treated. When used in replacement therapy, estrogen dosages tend to be low. Higher dosages are used to treat conditions such as advanced breast cancer. Table 70-2 gives ranges for dosages of the various preparations, but a drug handbook or the pharmacist should be consulted for the dose of a specific preparation in a specific condition.

Estrogens are also used in combinations with progestins. These combinations are discussed in the section on oral contraceptive drugs.

Adverse Reactions and Contraindications

Side effects of estrogens include overreactions of certain reproductive tissues to the hormones. Breast tenderness is reported by many women who take estrogen. Estrogens stimulate endometrial proliferation, and some evidence suggests that estrogens alone may increase the risk of endometrial cancer; estrogens given cyclically with progestins do not support endometrial hyperplasia and the risk of endometrial cancer is reduced. Estrogens have not been shown to increase the risk of breast cancer in women but may do so in men.

Estrogens are often associated with acute adverse reactions such as nausea and vomiting, anorexia, and mild diarrhea. Malaise, depression, and excessive irritability are also related to estrogen therapy in some women. Estrogens promote salt and water retention and may therefore produce edema in some patients. Atherosclerosis is a definite risk for patients who take estrogens, especially if they have other

Table 70-3 Clinical Summary of Progestins‡

Generic Name	Trade Name	Administration/Dosage	Comments
hydroxyprogesterone	Hylutin	INTRAMUSCULAR: *Adults*—125-375 mg; repeat in 1 wk if needed. FDA pregnancy category D.	For amenorrhea or dysfunctional bleeding.
levonorgestrel*	Norplant	SUBDERMAL IMPLANT: *Adults*—6 capsules implanted; duration 5 yr. FDA pregnancy category X.	For contraception.
medroxyprogesterone	Cycrin Provera*	ORAL: *Adults*—5-10 mg/day for 5-10 days. FDA pregnancy category X.	For amenorrhea, induction of menses, or dysfunctional uterine bleeding.
medroxyprogesterone	Depo-Provera*	INTRAMUSCULAR: *Adults*—150 mg every 3 mo. FDA pregnancy category X.	For contraception; higher dosages for carcinoma.
medroxyprogesterone & conjugated estrogens	Premphase Prempro	ORAL: *Adults*—Dosage of estrogen is 0.625 mg/day. Dosage of progestin is cyclical in Premphase (5 mg on days 14-28) but continuous in Prempro (2.5 or 5 mg/day). FDA pregnancy category X.	For osteoporosis or symptoms of menopause.
megestrol	Megace*	ORAL: *Adults*—800 mg/day for 1 mo, then 400-800 mg for 3 mo. FDA pregnancy category X.	For acquired immunodeficiency syndrome (AIDS)-associated anorexia, cachexia, and weight loss.
norethindrone acetate	Aygestin Norlutate†	ORAL: *Adults*—2.5-10 mg/day on days 5 through 25 of cycle. *For endometriosis:* 5-15 mg/day. FDA pregnancy category X.	For amenorrhea, dysfunctional uterine bleeding, or endometriosis.
progesterone	Prometrium*	ORAL: *Adults*—100-400 mg/day for 10-14 days, adjusted to patient's cycle. Avoid in pregnancy.	For amenorrhea or endometrial hyperplasia.
progesterone	Gesterol Crinone	INTRAMUSCULAR: *Adults*—5-10 mg/day for 6 consecutive days. VAGINAL: *Adults*—45 mg once every other day for 6 doses. FDA pregnancy category D.	For amenorrhea or dysfunctional uterine bleeding; vaginal gel for amenorrhea.
	Progestasert	INTRAUTERINE: *Adults*—1 intrauterine device replaced yearly; contains 38 mg progesterone.	For contraception.

*Available in Canada and the United States.
†Available in Canada only.
‡For oral contraceptive use of progestins, see Table 70-5.

high-risk factors such as smoking. Hypertension has been associated with estrogen use.

Estrogens are routinely avoided in patients with breast cancer because estrogens may promote growth of these tumors. Rarely, metastatic tumors may be treated with estrogens. Vaginal bleeding also precludes the use of estrogens because the bleeding may signal conditions such as endometrial hyperplasia or carcinoma, which would be worsened by estrogens.

Toxicity

High dosages of estrogens in women may produce any of the signs noted previously. Migraine headaches and vomiting may also occur. The vomiting is triggered by effects in the CNS.

Interactions

Estrogens increase the risk of toxicity with hepatotoxic drugs. Both hepatotoxicity and nephrotoxicity of cyclosporine may be enhanced because estrogens inhibit metabolism of cyclosporine. Ritonavir and other human immunodeficiency virus (HIV) protease inhibitors promote metabolism of estrogens, so estrogens are cleared more rapidly from the body.

Progestins

Mechanism of Action

Progestins used as drugs promote all of the actions of the naturally occurring progestins. Some preparations are most effective as progestational agents, whereas others have signif-

icant activities in other areas. For example, some progestins have detectable androgenic effects. Megestrol has a medically useful antianoretic and anticachetic action. These actions and others all arise as the progestin interacts with the steroid receptors inside target cells and alter gene expression.

Pharmacokinetics

Progestins available for medical use include the natural steroid hormone progesterone and synthetic derivatives of that compound (Table 70-3), many of which may be used orally. Injections of progesterone are painful and may produce local inflammation. Progesterone is rapidly metabolized by the liver and eliminated in urine.

Uses

Progestins are used clinically for their effects on the endometrium. High dosages suppress bleeding of the endometrium, and withdrawal induces sloughing of the tissue; thus they may be useful to treat secondary amenorrhea, to treat dysfunctional uterine bleeding, and to induce menses (see Table 70-3). Lower dosages of progestins induce changes in the endometrium and cervical mucus that prevent pregnancy. This use of progestins is discussed in the section on contraceptive agents.

Adverse Reactions and Contraindications

Adverse reactions to progestins may involve several organ systems other than reproductive organs. Some of these reactions are similar to those seen with estrogens, including edema, breast tenderness and swelling, gastrointestinal (GI) disturbances, depression, and weight change. Other reactions include changes in menstrual blood flow, midcycle spotting or breakthrough bleeding, cholestatic jaundice, and rashes. Medroxyprogesterone has been associated with delays in returning to fertility after the drug is withdrawn. Megestrol is associated with hyperglycemia in as many as 16% of treated patients.

Progestins should be avoided during pregnancy because many progestins have some androgenic activity and may cause masculinization of female fetuses. Norgestrel and levonorgestrel have the most androgenic activity, whereas norgestimate and desogestrel (see Table 70-5) have the least.

Patients with a history of thromboembolic disorders or thrombophlebitis should not be treated with progestins. These drugs are also normally avoided in patients with breast tumors or hepatic disease because these conditions may be worsened by progestins.

Toxicity

High dosages of progestins are associated with greater risks of thromboembolitic disease. If blood clots form, patients may note sudden, sharp pains; sudden, severe headaches; or sudden changes in speech, vision, or coordination. Any of these signs are reason to seek medical attention immediately. Fatalities have occurred.

Interactions

Aminoglutethimide lowers serum concentrations of medroxyprogesterone. Drugs such as carbamazepine, phenobarbital, phenytoin, rifabutin, and rifampin may induce enzymes in the liver that metabolize progestins; this action lowers the effect of progestins.

Agents for Infertility or Endometriosis

Loss of fertility in women may occur for many reasons. Therapy depends on evaluating the cause of infertility. In some women the pituitary and ovaries are normal, but

---

Table 70-4 Fertility Agents and Agents for Endometriosis

Generic Name	Trade Name	Administration/Dosage	Comments
bromocriptine	Parlodel*	ORAL: *Adults*—1.25-2.5 mg once at bedtime with food; gradually increase to 2.5 mg 2 or 3 times/day. FDA pregnancy category B.	Inhibitor of prolactin and growth hormone release; used for infertility caused by excessive prolactin.
cabergoline	Dostinex	ORAL: *Adults*—0.25 mg twice weekly; maximum dose is 2 mg/wk. FDA pregnancy category B.	Specific inhibitor of prolactin release.
chorionic gonadotropin	A. P. L.* Profasi*	INTRAMUSCULAR: *Adults*—5000-10,000 units once in an appropriately primed patient. FDA pregnancy category C.	Placental hormone related to LH is used for stimulation of ovulation.
clomiphene	Clomid*	ORAL: *Adults*—50 mg/day on days 5-10 of menstrual cycle. FDA pregnancy category X.	For infertility caused by anovulation; mechanism is probably hypothalamic.
danazol	Cyclomen† Danocrine	ORAL: *Adults*—50-400 mg twice daily. Contraindicated in pregnancy.	Inhibitor of pituitary gonadotropin release; used for endometriosis or fibrocystic breast disease.
follitropin alfa	Gonal-F	SUBCUTANEOUS: *Adults*—75 units once daily for 14 days; increase if needed, but maximum daily dose is 300 units. Length of treatment is normally ≤35 days total. FDA pregnancy category X.	Recombinant follitropin for use in female infertility; indistinguishable from follitropin beta.
follitropin beta	Follistim	SUBCUTANEOUS, INTRAMUSCULAR: *Adults*—75 units once daily for 14 days; increase if needed, but maximum daily dose is 300 units. FDA pregnancy category X.	Recombinant follitropin for use in female infertility; indistinguishable from follitropin alfa.
gonadorelin	Factrel*	SUBCUTANEOUS, INTRAVENOUS: *Adults or children*—0.1 mg once for diagnosis. FDA pregnancy category B.	Stimulates release of FSH and LH from healthy ovary; diagnostic for infertility.
leuprolide	Lupron*	INTRAMUSCULAR: *Adults*—3.75 mg once a month for up to 6 mo. FDA pregnancy category X.	Analog of GnRH used continuously suppresses estradiol and progestins; used for endometriosis.
menotropins	Humegon* Pergonal*	INTRAMUSCULAR: *Adults*—75 units each of FSH and LH daily for 9-12 days. FDA pregnancy category X.	Human urinary menopausal gonadotropins; FSH and LH in preparation induce ovulation.
nafarelin	Synarel*	INTRANASAL: *Adults*—0.2 mg in one nostril in morning; repeat in other nostril in evening. FDA pregnancy category X.	Peptide analog of GnRH, used continuously suppresses estradiol and progestins; used for endometriosis.
urofollitropin	Metrodin*	INTRAMUSCULAR: *Adults*—75-150 units/day. FDA pregnancy category X.	Human urinary menopausal FSH used to induce ovulation.
	Fertinex Fertinorm HP†	SUBCUTANEOUS: *Adults*—75-150 units/day. FDA pregnancy category X.	Subcutaneous route less painful.

LH, Luteinizing hormone; *FSH*, follicle-stimulating hormone; *GnRH*, gonadotropin-releasing hormone.
*Available in Canada and the United States.
†Available in Canada only.

the proper stimulus for follicular development is not transmitted. For these women, **clomiphene** may be effective (Table 70-4). This drug seems to activate the pituitary by hypothalamic mechanisms, and ovarian stimulation is thus achieved. Stimulation of several follicles may be induced by clomiphene, and multiple births have occurred.

In women with pituitary glands that cannot supply sufficient gonadotropins to properly stimulate the ovaries, infertility may also occur. The gonadotropins needed are primarily FSH and LH. Several strategies are possible in this situation. Menotropins are a mixture of compounds extracted from the urine of postmenopausal women; the preparation contains FSH and LH in approximately equal amounts. When LH action alone is required, chorionic gonadotropin may be prescribed. Chorionic gonadotropin is chemically related to LH and possesses many of the same physiologic actions, including the ability to stimulate ovulation. FSH activity can be supplied by hormone isolated from urine of menopausal women (urofollitropin) or by preparations of recombinant protein (follitropin alfa and follitropin beta).

Bromocriptine is a chemical relative of the ergot alkaloids, which are used as oxytocic agents. Bromocriptine is clinically useful because it can inhibit prolactin secretion. Bromocriptine is approved in the United States to control galactorrhea (spontaneous milk production) caused by excessive prolactin secretion usually from functional tumors. Amenorrhea (no menstrual cycles) and infertility also are produced when prolactin secretion is excessive. Bromocriptine suppression of prolactin secretion reverses these symptoms, and fertility becomes possible. Cabergoline is a more specific inhibitor of prolactin release; this newer agent seems to cause less inhibition of growth hormone production than does bromocriptine.

Several analogs of GnRH are available (see Table 70-4). These agents can be used short term to stimulate release of LH and FSH. For example, gonadorelin is used in this way for diagnostic purposes. If the agents are used continuously, they ultimately suppress production of LH and FSH, with the result that estrogen levels fall to postmenopausal levels. This action is useful for endometriosis, a painful condition in which endometrial tissue becomes implanted in the abdominal cavity outside of the uterus. Withdrawing hormonal support causes these tissues to atrophy.

CONTRACEPTIVE AGENTS

Oral Contraceptives

Mechanism of Action

Reversible sterility induced by pharmacologic agents has been possible since the late 1950s, when the oral contraceptive agents became available. These agents contain a combination of estrogen and a progestin or a progestin alone (Table 70-5). The effectiveness of oral contraceptives is very high. Most reports give estimates of 0% to 6% failure rates in

---

RESEARCH HIGHLIGHTS

Women's Responses to Depo-Provera

—Freda MC, Abruzzo-Fogarassy M, Adams NV, et al: *MCN 21(4):183-186, 1996.*

PURPOSE

Depot medroxyprogesterone acetate (Depo-Provera, DMPA) is one of the newest forms of birth control available in the United States. DMPA is administered as an intramuscular injection every 3 months and has a contraceptive efficacy of 99.7%. The purpose of the exploratory study was to ask women who had received this drug to answer questions about their experience with the drug to better understand typical problems and to develop appropriate teaching materials.

METHODS

All women had received DMPA at an inner-city health care facility. There were 72 subjects, 63% Hispanic, 29% African-American, and 8% white. The mean age was 27.7 years, and the mean educational level was 11.4 years of completed schooling. Each subject was asked 14 questions in a semistructured interview format.

RESULTS

Subjects chose DMPA because they forgot to take their [birth control] pills (25%), they disliked the pills (20%), a doctor or midwife advised them to (18%), the method was perceived as easy and safe (18%), and they liked that it is used every 3 months versus daily (12%). A total of 78% expressed satisfaction with the method. The 22% who were dissatisfied disliked the following: too much bleeding, bad headaches, pimples, losing hair, and gaining weight. Despite dissatisfaction by some, 65% planned to have another injection. When asked what they would tell a friend about the drug, common answers included "easy," "safe," "don't have to think about it for 3 months," and "don't get periods all the time." However, 6% stated "you don't have to use condoms," and 18% responded some variation of "it prevents sex diseases," which are incorrect responses. Side effects were reported by 65% of the respondents, including no menstrual periods (31%), headaches (27%), hair loss (27%), irregular periods (22%), and heavy bleeding (19%). Most women were satisfied (93%) with the information they received before beginning the medication.

IMPLICATIONS

Most of the subjects in this study considered this a safe drug to use, with minimal or tolerable side effects. An area of concern was the misunderstanding about the need to use condoms to prevent sexually transmitted diseases. This study emphasizes the need to verify patients' understanding about drug actions and implications so that additional areas of teaching can be identified.

Table 70-5 Oral Contraceptives

Progestin : Estrogen	Progestin : Estrogen	Trade Name	Dose‡
desogestrel: ethinyl estradiol	0.15 mg : 30 μg	Desogen, Marvelon,† Ortho-Cept*	Monophasic: 21 days of active agent, then 7 days with placebo or no drug.
	0.15 mg : 20 μg (21 tablets) and no progestin : 10 μg	Mircette	Biphasic: 21 days of 0.15 mg : 20 μg tablets, then 2 days placebo, followed by 5 days of 10 μg ethinyl estradiol tablets.
ethynodiol diacetate: ethinyl estradiol	1.0 mg : 50 μg	Demulen 1/50, Zovia 1/50 E Demulen 50†	Monophasic: 21 days of active agent, then 7 days with placebo or no drug.
	1.0 mg : 35 μg	Demulen 1/35, Zovia 1/35E	
	2.0 mg : 30 μg	Demulen 30†	
levonorgestrel: ethinyl estradiol	0.1 mg : 20 μg	Alesse, Levlite	Monophasic: 21 days of active agent, then 7 days with placebo or no drug.
	0.15 mg : 30 μg	Levlen, Levora 0.15/30, Min-Ovral†, Nordette	
	0.05 mg : 30 μg (6 tablets), and 0.075 mg : 40 μg (5 tablets), and 0.125 mg : 30 μg (10 tablets)	Tri-Levlen, Triphasil*, Triquilar†, Trivora	Triphasic: 0.05 μg : 30 μg tablets are taken on the first 6 days of the cycle, 0.075 mg : 40 μg tablets the next 5 days and the 0.125 mg : 30 μg tablets the next 10 days, followed by 7 days of placebo or no drug.
norethindrone	0.35 mg	Micronor*, Nor-QD	Continuous.
norethindrone acetate: ethinyl estradiol	1 mg : 20 μg	Loestrin 1/20, Loestrin Fe 1/20, Minestrin 1/20†	Monophasic: 21 days of active agent, then 7 days with placebo, 75 mg ferrous fumarate (Loestrin Fe), or no drug.
	1.5 mg : 30 μg	Loestrin 1.5/30,* Loestrin Fe 1.5/30	
	1 mg : 20 μg (5 tablets), and 1 mg : 30 μg (7 tablets), and 1 mg : 35 μg (9 tablets)	Estrostep	Triphasic: 1 mg : 20 μg tablets are taken on the first 5 days of the cycle, 1 mg : 30 μg tablets the next 7 days, and 1 mg : 35 μg tablets the next 9 days, followed by 7 days of placebo or no drug.
norethindrone: ethinyl estradiol	0.4 mg : 35 μg	Ovcon-35	Monophasic: 21 days of active agent, then 7 days with placebo or no drug.
	0.5 mg : 35 μg	Brevicon,* Genora 0.5/35, Intercon 0.5/35, ModiCon, Necon 0.5/35, Nelova 0.5/35	
	1 mg : 35 μg	Brevicon 1/35,† Genora 1/35, Intercon 1/35, Necon 1/35, N.E.E. 1/35, Nelova 1/35, Norethin 1/35, Norinyl 1+35, Ortho-Novum 1/35	
	0.5 mg : 35 μg (10 tablets), and 1 mg : 35 μg (11 tablets)	Necon 10/11, Nelova 10/11, Ortho-Novum 10-11 Symphasic†	Biphasic: 0.5 mg : 35 μg tablets are taken on the first 10 days of the cycle, the 1 mg : 35 μg tablets the next 11 days, then 7 days with placebo or no drug.
	0.5 mg : 35 μg (7 tablets), and 1 mg : 35 μg (14 tablets)	Jenest	Biphasic: 0.5 mg : 35 μg tablets are taken on the first 7 days of the cycle, the 1 mg : 35 μg tablets the next 14 days, then 7 days with placebo or no drug.
	0.5 mg : 35 μg (7 tablets), and 1 mg : 35 μg (9 tablets), and 0.5 mg : 35 μg (5 tablets)	Tri-Norinyl	Triphasic: 0.5 mg : 35 μg tablets are taken on the first 7 days of the cycle, the 1 mg : 35 μg tablets the next 9 days, the 0.5 mg : 35 μg tablets the next 5 days, then 7 days with placebo or no drug.
	0.5 mg : 35 μg (7 tablets), and 0.75 mg : 35 μg (7 tablets), and 1 mg : 35 μg 7 (tablets)	Ortho-Novum 7/7/7, Ortho 7/7/7†	Triphasic: 0.5 mg : 35 μg tablets are taken on the first 7 days of the cycle, the 0.75 mg : 35 μg tablets the next 7 days, the 1 mg : 35 μg tablets the next 7 days, then 7 days with placebo or no drug.
norethindrone: mestranol	1 mg : 50 μg	Genora 1/50, Intercon 1/50 Necon 1/50, Nelova 1/50M Norethin 1/50 M, Norinyl 1/50,† Ortho-Novum 1/50*	Monophasic: 21 days of active agent, then 7 days with placebo or no drug.

*Available in Canada and the United States.
†Available in Canada only.
‡All oral contraceptives are FDA pregnancy category X.

Table 70-5 Oral Contraceptives—cont'd

Progestin : Estrogen	Progestin : Estrogen	Trade Name	Dose‡
norgestimate: ethinyl estradiol	0.25 mg : 35 μg	Cyclen†, Ortho-Cyclen	Monophasic: 21 days of active agent, then 7 days with placebo or no drug.
	0.18 mg : 35 μg (7 tablets), and 0.215 mg : 35 μg (7 tablets), and 0.25 mg : 35 μg (7 tablets)	Ortho Tri-Cyclen, Tri-Cyclen†	Triphasic: 0.18 mg : 35 μg tablets are taken on the first 7 days of the cycle, the 0.215 mg : 35 μg tablets the next 7 days, the 0.25 mg : 35 μg tablets the next 7 days, then 7 days with placebo or no drug.
norgestrel: ethinyl estradiol	0.3 mg : 30 μg	Lo/Ovral	Monophasic: 21 days of active agent, then 7 days with placebo or no drug.
	0.5 mg : 50 μg	Ovral*	
norgestrel	75 μg	Ovrette	Continuous.

*Available in Canada and the United States.
†Available in Canada only.
‡All oral contraceptives are FDA pregnancy category X.

a year of use for the combined estrogen-progestin agents. This pregnancy rate is in contrast to rates of 2% to 27% failures per year for mechanical devices such as diaphragms, sponges, and condoms.

Estrogen-progestin combinations suppress ovulation. In addition, these drugs change the cervical mucus, making it difficult for sperm to enter the uterus. Changes also occur in the endometrium, making implantation difficult even if fertilization occurs. The preparations that contain progestins alone alter the cervical mucus and the endometrium as the combination products do, but they do not always suppress ovulation. Agents that contain only progestins are less effective than the combined preparations.

To achieve contraception and to simulate normal menstrual cycles, oral contraceptives usually are taken for 21 consecutive days. The increased estrogen and progestin levels suppress the hypothalamus and the anterior pituitary so that no LH is released at the time when ovulation would normally occur. This is the mechanism by which ovulation is suppressed. During the 7 days when hormones are not administered, the endometrium involutes and sloughs off, primarily as a result of loss of progestin activity. This withdrawal period prevents excessive endometrial proliferation.

Pharmacokinetics

The pharmacokinetics of oral contraceptives is the same as previously noted for the individual estrogen or progestin components. Synthetic progestins such as **norethindrone** or **norgestrel** are used in oral contraceptives because oral absorption of these synthetic forms is better than for the natural hormone.

Uses

The oral contraceptive preparations are intended to provide reversible prevention of pregnancy in otherwise healthy women. These preparations are also useful to control irregular or excessive menstrual cycles.

Adverse Reactions and Contraindications

Side effects produced by oral contraceptives may come from the estrogen or the progestin component. Side effects caused by estrogens may include nausea, bloating, breast fullness, edema, hypertension, and cervical discharge. Patients who report these symptoms may be given a preparation with low estrogen such as Loestrin 1/20, Lo/Ovral, or Mircette. Side effects associated with progestins include hair loss, hirsutism, oily scalp, acne, increased appetite and weight gain, tiredness and depression, breast regression, and reduced menstrual blood flow. Oral contraceptives fall into the Food and Drug Administration (FDA) pregnancy category X.

Oral contraceptives are used by millions of women to prevent pregnancy. Oral contraceptives are highly effective, but questions about the safety of these agents have been raised. In particular, the incidence of unexpected serious or fatal medical conditions has been studied in the relatively healthy women who take oral contraceptives. Risk of certain serious medical conditions is now shown to be increased in those who use oral contraceptive compared with similar women who do not take these drugs (Table 70-6).

As with any medication, oral contraceptives must be considered in terms of the risk-to-benefit ratio. Of primary importance may be how much value the patient places on almost complete protection against unwanted pregnancy. Women who desire this high level of control should then consider the safety factors of the medication. Many of the dangerous complications (e.g., stroke, thromboembolic diseases) are rare even among those who use oral contraceptives. The risk of these complications is greater than the risk among women not taking oral contraceptives but much lower than the risk of these complications during pregnancy. Women should also consider other predisposing risk factors such as smoking, obesity, and hypertension. The combination of oral contraceptives with these conditions leads to unacceptable risk for many patients. All women who take oral contraceptives should be urged to stop smoking.

Table 70-6   Oral Contraceptives: Adverse Reactions

Adverse Reaction	Relation to Oral Contraceptives	Comments
Thromboembolytic diseases	Risk increased 2- to 7-fold in users over nonusers. Incidence about 100:100,000 woman years; fatalities 2:100,000 woman years.*	Obesity, family history of thromboembolytic disorders, immobility, or group A blood type may increase risk. Females with group O blood type have lower risk. Directly related to estrogen dosage.
Thrombotic stroke	Risk increased 3.1- to 6-fold. Incidence about 25:100,000 woman years; fatalities 0.5:100,000 woman years.*	Hypertension increases risk.
Hemorrhagic stroke	Risk increased at least 2-fold. Incidence about 10:100,000 woman years.*	Hypertension and heavy smoking are strong risk factors.
Myocardial infarction	Risk increased about 2-fold over nonusers when estrogen doses exceed 50 mg/day.	Synergistic increase in risk if oral contraceptives are used by smokers.
Hypertension	About 15% of patients show increase in blood pressure. Clinical hypertension is less common.	Risk is increased by age, obesity, and parity.
Gallbladder disease	Risk increased an estimated 2-fold.*	Risk may be related to duration of use.
Liver disease	Up to 50% of patients show altered liver function. Incidence 10:100,000 woman years for jaundice. Tumors are rare.	Reversible. Dangerous for patients with preexisting liver disease (hepatitis or cholestasis). Liver tumors may be related specifically to mestranol.
Hepatocellular carcinoma	Risk of this rare tumor increases after 8 yr of oral contraceptive use.	This tumor occurs in less than 1 woman per 1 million long-term users of oral contraceptives.
Carbohydrate metabolism	Many patients show reduced glucose tolerance.	Important only in prediabetic women who may become insulin dependent. Related to dose and potency of progestin.
Lipid metabolism	Many patients have increased serum triglyceride levels.	Reversible effect; relationship to coronary artery disease in these patients is unknown.
Melasma	3%-4% of patients treated.	Increased sensitivity to sunlight also occurs. Reversible.
Headaches	Increased or worsened in about one fifth of patients.	Chronic headache may presage stroke.
Visual disturbances	Have been associated with use of oral contraceptives.	Temporary blindness, blind spots, and changes in field of vision have been reported.
Endometrial cancer	1 yr of treatment confers 15 yr of protective effect against endometrial cancer.	Risk is increased by estrogens alone but is reduced by progestins.
Ovarian cancer	3 yr of use confers up to 10 yr protective effect.	Short-term use confers no protection that can be documented.
Cervical cancer	Risk is increased 2-fold after 5 yr use and continues to increase with longer use.	Frequency of coitus and number of sexual partners are also important risk factors.
Breast cancer	No relationship established.	Risk may depend on age or duration of use.
Benign fibrocystic breast disease	40% reduction in incidence for 2 yr after use.	Data based on estrogen doses of 50 mg or more; effect of low dosage unknown.
Permanent infertility	No relationship established.	Most patients quickly return to fertility when oral contraceptives are discontinued.
Outcome of later pregnancies	No increased risk to mother or fetus has been demonstrated.	Data are for pregnancies begun after oral contraceptives have been discontinued.

*Risk may be less with the lower dose estrogen products currently in use.

Some medical conditions are improved or the symptoms are lessened by oral contraceptives. Many patients report a reduction in menstrual disorders and especially in dysmenorrhea. Menstrual blood flow usually is reduced, and anemia is prevented or lessened in many women. Benign breast tumors may be improved over time by oral contraceptive therapy, but patients with carcinoma of the breast, cervix, liver, uterus, or vagina should not take these drugs because these cancers may be stimulated by estrogens.

Current medical data suggest that oral contraceptives are safe in young women in whom other risk factors are minimized. Women with a history of hypertension or thromboembolytic disease probably should not receive the drugs.

Women who choose to take oral contraceptives should undergo thorough physical examinations yearly. The dosage of estrogen and progestin should be the lowest dosage that achieves contraception and prevents unwanted side effects such as breakthrough bleeding.

Careful history taking may reveal symptoms that the patient has not linked to oral contraceptive use. Migraine headaches, dizziness, and visual disturbances often are not related by the patient to oral contraceptive use and may not be mentioned spontaneously. Breakthrough bleeding, excessive cervical mucus formation, breast tenderness, and other changes in the reproductive tract usually are quickly connected to oral contraceptive use by patients. These symptoms may be more annoying than serious. Severe headaches or visual disturbances are often early signs of impending stroke and may be sufficient cause to discontinue the medications.

The first oral contraceptives contained more estrogens than the agents available today. These lower estrogen combinations are usually as effective as the older agents and may be associated with a lower incidence of side effects (see Table 70-6).

Toxicity

Acute overdoses with oral contraceptives often cause nausea and vomiting. Withdrawal vaginal bleeding may also occur. Higher dosages over longer periods are associated with greater risk of thromboembolitic complications.

Interactions

Oral contraceptive agents are subject to the same interactions as the estrogen and progestin components. Hepatotoxic medications should be avoided. Hepatic enzyme inducers may impair effectiveness of the oral contraceptives and lead to unexpected pregnancy. Oral contraceptives interfere with the activity of bromocriptine and anticoagulants and increase the toxicity of tricyclic antidepressants.

Contraceptive Implants and Intrauterine Devices

When long-term pharmacologic contraception is desired, systemic absorption can be achieved without the need for daily oral dosing. Because most forms of the steroid hormones such as estrogens and progestins are relatively insoluble in water, they are slowly absorbed from tissue sites when injected. This property can be used to advantage by confining the drugs to insoluble polymers that can then be implanted under the skin. Small amounts of drug are continuously released over very long periods. One example of such an application is the contraceptive Norplant. Six slender capsules, each containing 36 mg of the synthetic progestin levonorgestrel, are implanted subdermally. This application affords contraceptive protection for up to 5 years.

Long-term contraception can also be achieved with intrauterine devices (IUDs) that release active agents directly to the target tissues. For example, the natural progestin progesterone is used in an IUD (Progestasert) in this way. The very small amounts of progesterone released are retained within the reproductive tract rather than being systemically absorbed. The effectiveness of this device depends on the mechanical effects of the IUD and on the pharmacologic effects of progesterone. This device provides contraception for up to 12 months. IUDs that release copper are also available. These devices tend to cause local inflammatory responses that affect the ability of an ovum to implant. The copper released by the devices may also affect viability of the sperm and mobility of the ovum. These copper-releasing IUDs provide contraception for 24 months (Copper-T 200), 30 months (Copper-T 200 Ag, Copper-T 380S), or 10 years (Copper-T 380A).

Nursing Process Overview

Drugs Acting on the Female Reproductive System

Assessment

Drugs acting on the female reproductive system provide replacement therapy, stimulate or inhibit ovulation and conception, and treat hormonally sensitive tumors. Obtain a complete patient assessment, focusing on the problem being addressed by the drug. Monitor the vital signs, blood pressure (BP), weight, and description of the menstrual cycle; assess the patient's breasts and condition of skin.

Nursing Diagnoses

- Potential complication: vascular disorders
- Self-concept disturbance: acne and weight gain related to drug therapy

Patient Outcomes

The nurse will minimize and manage vascular complications. The patient will discuss concerns related to self-concept and will state two positive features about himself or herself.

Planning/Implementation

Continue to monitor the pulse, BP, and weight. Explain patient activities needed in detail to help ensure success. For example, activities such as using alternative birth control measures during the first month of birth control pill therapy, keeping basal temperature charts to monitor possible ovulation, and saving urine specimens to measure hormone or drug excretion need thorough explanations. Monitor calcium levels in patients being treated for cancer.

Evaluation

Before discharge, verify that the patient understands why and how to take the drug, what possible side effects might occur, which side effects require immediate medical attention, and what risks are associated with therapy.

Nursing Implications Summary

Estrogens

Drug Administration

➤ Assess vital signs, BP, weight, history of weight gain or loss, nausea and vomiting, breasts for enlargement, complaints of breast pain, and mammogram if available. Assess dependent areas for edema.

➤ Monitor liver function tests and serum lipid profile. Monitor x-ray films of the hand and wrist in children to monitor bone age.

➤ Patients with metastatic bone cancer who are started on hormonal therapy may develop severe hypercalcemia. Monitor serum electrolyte levels (see Table 17-1).

Nursing in the Community

➤ Teach the patient to take drug as ordered even if not feeling well. Nausea may develop during the first few weeks of therapy but should diminish with regular use. Instruct the patient to take doses with meals or food, or just after eating, to lessen GI symptoms.

➤ Emphasize the importance of regular follow-up visits to monitor for side effects and effectiveness.

➤ Instruct the patient to notify the physician if any of the following develop: breast pain, discharge from breasts, lumps in breast, changes in vaginal bleeding such as breakthrough bleeding or amenorrhea, stomach cramps, nausea, vomiting, diarrhea, loss of appetite, headache, or jaundice.

➤ For men taking estrogens for breast or prostate cancer, review symptoms of possible thromboembolism: severe or sudden headache, shortness of breath, sudden slurred speech, changes in vision, or weakness or numbness in the arm or leg.

➤ Teach the patient to perform monthly breast self-examination. Encourage regular mammograms if recommended by the physician. This is true for men or women taking estrogens.

➤ Encourage female patients to have regular Pap smears.

➤ Drug may cause tenderness, swelling, or bleeding of gums. Encourage the patient to brush and floss teeth carefully and regularly, to see a dentist regularly, and to have teeth professionally cleaned periodically.

➤ Instruct the patient to notify the physician immediately if pregnancy is suspected.

➤ Encourage the patient to avoid or limit smoking while taking this drug.

➤ Teach proper injection technique if the patient is to administer intramuscular (IM) forms at home.

➤ To use transdermal patch: See the manufacturer's instruction leaflet. Wash and dry hands before and after handling patches. Apply patch to a clean, dry, nonoily area of abdomen or buttocks. Avoid areas with excess hair, cuts, or irritation. Avoid the waist, other areas that may be rubbed with clothing. Do not apply to breasts. Apply patch firmly for about 10 seconds. If patch falls off or comes loose, reapply or apply a new patch. Apply each new patch to a different area, allowing at least a week to pass before an area is used again.

➤ To administer vaginal cream: See the manufacturer's instructions. For daily application, instruct the patient to use at bedtime. Tampons should be avoided, but a sanitary napkin may be worn to protect clothing. Instruct the patient not to use this medication as a lubricant during sexual intercourse; regular absorption by the male partner through the skin of the penis may cause side effects. This drug may also weaken diaphragms, cervical caps, or condoms; check with the physician or pharmacist.

➤ Remind the patient to notify all health care providers of all drugs being used before having laboratory work done. Regular use of estrogens may influence some test results.

Progestins

Drug Administration

➤ If drug is used in an estrogen-progestin combination product for birth control, see the section on birth control following.

➤ Assess vital signs, BP, menstrual history, weight, and history of weight gain or loss. Assess dependent areas for edema. Assess skin for hair loss, acne, and changes in hair growth. Perform mental status examination. Assess vision.

➤ Monitor liver function tests.

Nursing in the Community

➤ If the patient is using a combination estrogen-progestin product for birth control, see the section on birth control (following).

➤ Emphasize the importance of returning for regular follow-up visits to monitor for drug effectiveness and side effects.

➤ Spotting or breakthrough bleeding during the first 3 months of therapy is not unusual. Instruct the patient to notify the physician of heavy or prolonged bleeding or amenorrhea. When a progestin is used continuously as a contraceptive (not a combination estrogen-progestin), breakthrough bleeding or spotting is common.

➤ Instruct the patient to notify the physician of sudden or severe headache; changes in vision; pain in the chest, leg, or groin; shortness of breath; slurred speech; an increase or decrease in weight of more than 2 pounds per day or 5 pounds in 1 week; discharge from breasts; depression; GI pain; swelling of feet or legs; acne; or thinning of hair.

➤ This drug may cause tenderness, swelling, or bleeding of the gums. Encourage the patient to brush and floss teeth carefully and regularly, to see a dentist regularly, and to have teeth professionally cleaned periodically.

➤ Women who are fertile and sexually active should use a birth control method while taking this drug, unless the drug is being used daily as a contraceptive. Notify the physician immediately if pregnancy is suspected or if 45 days have elapsed since the last menstrual period.

➤ Encourage female patients to have regular Pap smears.

➤ For IM administration, review proper injection technique with the patient.

➤ For vaginal suppository, review proper insertions technique with the patient.

Nursing Implications Summary—cont'd

➤ This drug may alter laboratory results. Remind the patient to tell the physician before having laboratory work performed that progestins are being used.

➤ Instruct the patient to talk with the pharmacist or physician each time another drug is prescribed or discontinued because other drugs may interfere with the effectiveness of a progestin being used as a contraceptive. Another form or birth control may be needed temporarily.

➤ Levonorgestrel implant capsules (Norplant), used as a contraceptive: The implants are inserted under the skin of the upper arm by a physician or trained professional. Instruct the patient to keep gauze in place on the insertion site for 24 hours, then remove it. Leave strips of tape in place for 3 days. Full contraceptive protection begins within 24 hours if the insertion is performed within 7 days of the beginning of a menstrual period. Contraceptive protection should last for 5 years. The implants should be removed and replaced if desired after 5 years.

➤ For medroxyprogesterone injection form, used as a contraceptive: Instruct the patient to return at 3-month intervals for injection of this contraceptive. Full contraceptive protection begins immediately if the patient receives the injection within the first 5 days of a menstrual period or within 5 days of delivering a baby if the mother is not breast-feeding. Emphasize the importance of returning on schedule for later injections.

➤ For medroxyprogesterone and conjugated estrogens (Premphase, Prempro): Instruct the patient to take doses with meals to prevent nausea. Tolerance to nausea should develop in a few weeks. Menstrual bleeding may begin again but should stop by 10 months with continued therapy. Breakthrough bleeding may occur for up to 3 months. Instruct the patient to notify the physician if excessive or persistent bleeding occurs. Encourage the patient to have regular mammograms, as directed by the physician.

General Guidelines: Fertility Agents
Nursing in the Community

➤ Teach the patient to keep a record of basal body temperature, consistency of vaginal mucus, and 24-hour urine specimen as prescribed by the physician.

➤ Ensure the patient understands the best time of the month to have intercourse to attempt to get pregnant on the basis of the drugs being used.

➤ Provide emotional support. Treatment of infertility problems may be prolonged and discouraging.

➤ Encourage the patient to return as directed for blood tests, ultrasounds, examinations, additional medications, and other therapies as prescribed.

➤ Remind the patient to keep all drugs out of the reach of children.

➤ Instruct the patient to notify the physician immediately if pregnancy is suspected because these drugs should usually not be continued during pregnancy.

bromocriptine
Drug Administration

➤ Assess mental status. Assess for signs of depression, including lack of interest in personal appearance, withdrawal, anorexia, and insomnia.

➤ Monitor pulse and BP. Check stools and emesis for occult blood.

➤ If drug is used for female fertility problems, assess date of last menstrual period and other measures used to treat infertility. If used to treat male hypogonadism or male fertility problems, see Chapter 72.

➤ If drug is used for acromegaly, assess ring and shoe size, height, and weight.

➤ If drug is used for Parkinson's disease, assess other current treatments, ability to perform activities of daily living, and signs of disease (e.g., masklike facial expression, tremor, rigidity, salivation, shuffling gait). See Chapter 62.

Nursing in the Community

➤ Review the anticipated benefits and possible side effects of drug therapy with the patient. Tell the patient to report any new side effects.

➤ Suggest that the patient take the first dose while lying down or at bedtime because dizziness is more likely to occur with first dose. Warn the patient to avoid driving or operating hazardous equipment if drowsiness develops.

➤ See the Patient Problems boxes on constipation (Chapter 24), dry mouth (Chapter 23), and orthostatic hypotension (Chapter 13).

➤ When used to treat Parkinson's disease, full benefit of this drug may not be seen for several weeks. Provide emotional support. See Chapter 62.

➤ See the general guidelines for infertility.

➤ Instruct the patient to take doses with meals or a snack to lessen gastric irritation.

➤ Encourage the patient to avoid drinking alcoholic beverages; see the Patient Problems box in Chapter 57 on alcohol use and disulfiram.

➤ Depending on the patient's age and reason for taking bromocriptine, counsel about methods of birth control as appropriate. Oral contraceptives should not be used.

cabergoline
Drug Administration/Nursing in the Community

➤ Monitor BP and serum prolactin.

➤ Assess the patient for abdominal pain, anorexia, edema, hot flashes, diarrhea, acne, and GI discomfort. See the Patient Problems boxes on orthostatic hypotension (Chapter 13) and dry mouth (Chapter 23).

➤ Warn the patient to avoid driving or operating hazardous equipment if vertigo or dizziness develops.

➤ Instruct the patient to notify the physician immediately if pregnancy is suspected.

➤ This drug may be used for treatment of Parkinson's disease, but dosages are much higher for this disease. Side effects at

Continued

Nursing Implications Summary—cont'd

these dosages include dyskinesia, hallucinations, heart failure, pleural effusion, and GI ulceration.

chorionic gonadotropin
Drug Administration/Nursing in the Community
➤ Review the anticipated benefits and possible side effects of drug therapy with the patient. Remind the patient to notify the physician if any unexpected side effects develop or if any side effects are severe or persistent. Instruct the patient to monitor daily basal body temperature if prescribed.
➤ Remind women of common side effects, including breast enlargement, headache, irritability, edema, fatigue, depression, or stomach or pelvic pain.
➤ This drug may be used to treat cryptorchidism if no anatomic obstruction is present. See Chapter 72.
➤ Warn the patient to avoid driving or operating hazardous equipment if excessive fatigue or visual changes occur and to notify the physician.
➤ See the general guidelines for fertility agents.

clomiphene citrate
Drug Administration/Nursing in the Community
➤ Review the anticipated benefits and possible side effects of drug therapy with the patient. Common side effects include breast discomfort, headache, heavy menstrual periods, and nausea or vomiting. Instruct the patient to notify the physician if abdominal pain, blurred or double vision, or jaundice develops. Encourage the patient to notify the physician if any unexplained side effects develop.
➤ Typical instructions for taking this drug are to count the first day of the menstrual cycle as day 1. Begin clomiphene in the dose ordered on day 5, and continue daily until the prescribed number of doses is completed. Review instructions with the patient, and ensure that she understands the dosing schedule. In addition, the physician may want the patient to use an ovulation prediction kit; review the manufacturer's instructions with the patient. Advise the couple to have frequent intercourse at or around the time ovulation is anticipated.
➤ The drug may also be prescribed for men; review the physician's prescription with the patient.
➤ Warn the patient to avoid driving or operating hazardous equipment if changes in vision, dizziness, or light-headedness occurs and to notify the physician.
➤ See the general guidelines for infertility.
➤ Monitor liver function tests, HCG levels, and urinary LH levels.

danazol
Drug Administration
➤ This drug may be used to treat endometriosis, fibrocystic breast disease, hereditary angioedema, and hematologic disorders, including idiopathic thrombocytopenic purpura. It has weak androgenic and anabolic properties (see Chapter 72).

➤ Assess for weight gain. Inspect for acne, edema of dependent areas, and hirsutism. Monitor BP and liver function tests.

Nursing in the Community
➤ Review the anticipated benefits and possible side effects of drug therapy. Encourage the patient to notify the physician if any unexpected side effects develop. Common side effects in women include reduction in breast size, hirsutism, weight gain, deepening of voice, and emotional lability. Side effects caused by the androgenic properties of the drug may be less noticeable in male patients.
➤ Tell the female patient that menstrual periods may diminish or cease while taking this drug (depending on the dosage). She should keep a record of menstrual periods. Instruct her to use birth control measures while taking danazol and for 2 months after stopping therapy but not to use birth control pills. Tell the patient to notify the physician if pregnancy is suspected.
➤ Side effects are dose related but may be intolerable to some patients. Remind the patient to take drugs as ordered for best effects and not to discontinue therapy without consulting the physician.
➤ Warn diabetic patients to monitor blood glucose levels carefully while taking this drug; a change in diet or insulin dosage may be needed.
➤ See the Patient Problems box in Chapter 58 on photosensitivity.

follitropin
Drug Administration/Nursing in the Community
➤ Monitor daily basal body temperature. Monitor serum progesterone, serum estradiol, and/or ultrasound of ovaries and uterus. In male partners, monitor sperm count and determinations of sperm motility, and serum testosterone.
➤ Monitor patients for abdominal or pelvic pain, nausea, rapid weight gain, vomiting, diarrhea, breast tenderness, skin changes, acne, mood swings, and headache.
➤ Teach patients appropriate administration technique (subcutaneous or IM injection; depends on preparation). Review the manufacturer's patient instruction leaflet.
➤ Instruct patients not to double up for missed doses. Instruct patients to call the physician if a dose is missed.
➤ Emphasize the importance of regular monitoring by the physician, during treatment and for up to 2 weeks after the last dose of drug.

gonadorelin
Drug Administration/Nursing in the Community
➤ Except for allergic reaction, usually after multiple doses, no serious side effects have been reported with this drug. Warn the patient that itching may occur at the injection site. Consult the manufacturer's literature. See the general guidelines for infertility.
➤ Monitor serum LH levels.

Nursing Implications Summary—cont'd

leuprolide

Drug Administration/Nursing in the Community

➤ This drug is used to treat cancer of the prostate (see Chapter 56) and endometriosis.

➤ For endometriosis, assess menstrual history and previous treatment for infertility.

➤ Review the side effects with the patient: hot flashes, nausea or vomiting, weight gain, or trouble sleeping. Men may experience constipation, decreased size of testicles, transient bone pain, impotence or decreased libido, and loss of appetite. Women may experience decreased libido, breast tenderness, mood changes, vaginitis, and amenorrhea or spotting. Instruct the patient to notify the physician of any unexpected sign or symptom.

➤ Read the physician's orders carefully; there is an injectable subcutaneous form and an IM depot form. The depot form should be administered by the physician. If the patient is to self-administer at home, review the patient instruction leaflet supplied with the subcutaneous form.

➤ Perform a pregnancy test before treating for endometriosis, unless starting drug during menstrual period. For prostate cancer, monitor serum acid phosphatase and/or prostate-specific antigen.

menotropins

Drug Administration/Nursing in the Community

➤ Review the anticipated benefits and possible side effects of drug therapy with the patient. Tell the patient to report any new, severe, or persistent side effects.

➤ Teach the female patient to record basal body temperature if prescribed.

➤ This drug is often administered with chorionic gonadotropin. Side effects are often related to excessive ovarian stimulation and include abdominal discomfort, nausea and vomiting, diarrhea, increased weight, and hypertension.

➤ The drug may also be administered to men. See Chapter 72.

➤ If the patient is to self-administer, teach IM injection technique.

➤ See the general guidelines for infertility.

nafarelin

Drug Administration/Nursing in the Community

➤ Assess menstrual history and history of infertility.

➤ Review the possible side effects with the patient, including breakthrough bleeding, heavy menstrual periods, amenorrhea or spotting, pelvic pain or bloating, joint pain, headache, rash, breast pain, depression, and weight changes. Instruct the patient to report new, severe, or persistent side effects to the physician.

➤ Administer doses as a nasal spray. Review the manufacturer's patient instruction leaflet.

➤ The drug may cause vaginal drying. Encourage the use of a water-soluble lubricant during sexual intercourse.

urofollitropin

Drug Administration/Nursing in the Community

➤ Review the anticipated benefits and possible side effects of drug therapy with the patient. Tell the patient to report any new, severe, or persistent side effects.

➤ Common side effects include bloating, pelvic pain, nausea and vomiting, and breast tenderness.

➤ See the general guidelines for drugs for infertility.

➤ Instruct the patient to record daily basal body temperature if prescribed.

➤ If the patient is to self-administer this drug, teach injection technique.

Oral Contraceptives

Drug Administration

➤ Monitor BP, pulse, and weight. Assess for skin changes.

➤ Instruct the patient to report leg pain, sudden onset of chest pain, shortness of breath, coughing up blood, dizziness, changes in vision or speech, or weakness or numbness of an arm or leg because these may indicate pulmonary embolism or other thromboembolic problems.

➤ Assess for signs of depression, including withdrawal, insomnia, anorexia, and lack of interest in personal appearance.

➤ Assess tactfully for changes in libido. The patient may be reluctant to discuss this problem.

➤ Monitor complete blood count and liver function tests.

➤ For discussion of IM administration of oil-based suspension, see Chapter 5.

Nursing in the Community

➤ Review the anticipated benefits and possible side effects of drug therapy with the patient. Review Table 70-6. Tell the patient to notify the physician if any new side effects develop.

➤ Teach the patient when to begin first dose of oral contraceptive and to take doses in order. It may take up to 1 week for full contraceptive effect to develop. During this period, instruct patient to use an additional/different form of birth control to prevent pregnancy. Some physicians recommend that an alternate form of birth control be used for the first cycle of birth control pills.

➤ Counsel or refer the patient as needed about stopping smoking, losing weight to achieve desirable weight, and modifying diet to decrease cholesterol and triglycerides.

➤ Warn diabetic patients to monitor blood glucose levels carefully because these drugs may alter glucose levels.

➤ Tell the patient to take doses with meals or a snack to lessen nausea. This side effect usually lessens with continued use. The patient should try taking the dose at bedtime rather than in the morning.

➤ Warn the patient to avoid driving or operating hazardous equipment if changes in vision occur and to notify the physician.

➤ Instruct the female patient to report any vaginal bleeding or menstrual irregularities and to notify the physician immediately if pregnancy is suspected.

Continued

Nursing Implications Summary—cont'd

➤ Remind the patient to inform all health care providers of all medications being used. It may take several months for these drugs to be completely eliminated even when the patient has stopped taking them, so the patient should be reminded to inform health care providers for up to several months after therapy has stopped. This is also important when diagnostic blood work is performed; recent or current use of oral contraceptives may influence test results.

➤ See the instruction leaflet supplied with oral contraceptive for instruction about missed doses. The guidelines vary somewhat depending on the product being used.

➤ Many drugs interfere with effectiveness of birth control pills. Teach the patients to ask the physician or pharmacist about this possibility when a new medication is taken.

➤ If a patient discontinues oral contraceptives to become pregnant, recommend that she use an alternative form of birth control for 2 months after stopping the pills to ensure more

complete excretion of the hormonal agents before conceiving and thus reducing the potential effects of the medications on the fetus.

➤ Teach the patient how to do a breast self-examination and encourage her to perform this monthly.

➤ A patient taking estrogens may develop brown areas on the skin. See the Patient Problems box in Chapter 58 on photosensitivity.

➤ Tell the patient taking birth control pills that the drugs work best when used regularly. Advise the patient to keep an additional month's supply on hand to avoid running out of pills.

➤ Remind the patient to keep all medications out of the reach of children.

➤ For implant dosage form: Levonorgestrel (Norplant) is described under the previous section on progestins.

➤ IM medroxyprogesterone used as a contraceptive is discussed previously under progestins.

 CHAPTER REVIEW

Application

1. What are gonadotropins?
2. How are the synthesis and release of FSH, LH, and prolactin regulated?
3. What are the major steroid hormones that affect the female reproductive tract?
4. What are the functions of estrogens during puberty?
5. What hormones regulate ovulation?
6. What effect do estrogens have on the endometrium in an adult woman?
7. What effects does progesterone have on the endometrium and myometrium?
8. What is the function of progesterone in pregnancy?
9. What is the role of HCG in pregnancy?
10. What side effects are characteristic of pharmacologic use of progestins?
11. What is the mechanism of action of clomiphene, and what is its medical use?
12. What hormones are contained within menotropins?
13. What is the mechanism of action of bromocriptine, and how is it currently used?

14. What is the mechanism of action of gonadorelin, and what is its medical use?
15. What is the mechanism of action of urofollitropin, and what is its medical use?
16. What types of agents are used to produce pharmacologic contraception?
17. What is the mechanism of action of the oral contraceptive agents?
18. By what mechanisms do progesterone-releasing IUDs prevent pregnancy?

Critical Thinking

1. What side effects and toxic reactions are seen with long-term use of estrogens? How should you assess for these?
2. What side effects occur with use of the oral contraceptives? What should you teach about these side effects?
3. Your patient has just been switched from a monophasic 21-day preparation (21 days of drug, 7 days of no drug) to a monophasic 28-day preparation (21 days of drug, 7 days of placebo). What advantages might this switch confer to the patient? What should you say if the patient asks what is in the extra 7 tablets?

References

Lichtman R: Perimenopausal and postmenopausal hormone replacement therapy. Part 1: an update of the literature on benefits and risk, *J Nurse Midwife* 41(1):3-28, 1996.

Lichtman R: Perimenopausal and postmenopausal hormone replacement therapy. Part 2: hormonal regimens and complemen-

tary and alternative therapies, *J Nurse Midwife* 41(3):195-210, 1996.

Scharbo-Dehaan M: Hormone replacement therapy, *Nurse Pract* 21(12)part 2:1-15, 1996.

Smith A, Hughes P: The estrogen dilemma, *Am J Nurs* 98(4):17-20, 1998.

Drugs for Labor and Delivery

OBJECTIVES

After studying this chapter, you should be able to do the following:

- *Compare the actions and uses of the three classes of oxytocic drugs.*
- *Explain how ritodrine may control premature labor.*
- *Develop a nursing care plan for a patient receiving a drug discussed in this chapter.*

CHAPTER OVERVIEW

A successful pregnancy and postpartum period depends on the proper functioning of several systems of the body. This chapter reviews the endocrine control of pregnancy and discusses drugs used to facilitate delivery of the fetus. It also discusses drugs used to protect the fetus from premature delivery and drugs used in the postpartum period to control uterine bleeding.

THERAPEUTIC RATIONALE: CHILDBIRTH AND POSTPARTUM CARE

Physiology of Childbirth

The pharmacologic management of labor and delivery is easily understood when put into the context of the physiologic processes involved. During pregnancy, high progesterone levels aid in maintaining the pregnancy by suppressing contractions of the **myometrium,** the powerful muscle layer in the uterine wall. As the pregnancy comes to term, progesterone levels begin to decrease, allowing the uterus to begin to produce prostaglandins. **Prostaglandins** are involved in regulating myometrial activity. These derivatives of fatty acids are readily formed in their target tissues and are rapidly degraded without persisting in blood for any appreciable time. In the uterus, these hormones induce very powerful myometrial contractions. Prostaglandins, especially PGE_2 and $PGF_{2\alpha}$, may play a role in natural induction of labor. Prostaglandin levels rise in the amniotic fluid and other pelvic reproductive tissues as term approaches. This increasing concentration of prostaglandins has been suggested to be the stimulus causing Braxton Hicks contractions, the mild myometrial contractions occurring during the final few

weeks of pregnancy. Oxytocin, a hormone produced by the posterior pituitary, is also capable of inducing uterine contractions. The uterus increases its sensitivity to oxytocin at term and during the puerperium (period immediately after birth).

Parturition, the process of giving birth, is divided into three phases. During stage I, uterine contractions begin to increase in frequency and intensity and the cervix begins to dilate. In stage II, uterine contractions occur at the rate of about one every 2 minutes. The cervix is fully dilated, and uterine contractions bring about the delivery of the infant. During stage III of labor, the frequency of contractions decreases and the placenta separates from the uterus and is expelled. Uterine contractions continue for hours to days, with the frequency and intensity of the contractions diminishing with time.

When contractions occur during labor and delivery, the myometrium compresses major blood vessels supplying oxygen to the fetus. The result is that during a contraction, the fetus is relatively anoxic (starved for oxygen). When the uterus relaxes between contractions, oxygenated blood quickly returns to the fetus. If the uterus is overstimulated and fails to relax sufficiently between contractions, the prolonged anoxia can harm the fetus. Induction of labor with one of the oxytocic drugs carries with it the risk of producing this condition. Therefore all patients in whom labor is being induced should receive continuous care, and fetal monitoring should be done when possible. Oxytocin is the drug of choice to induce or stimulate labor because it seems to allow the uterus to relax between contractions. The ergot alkaloids and other oxytocic drugs tend to increase the overall tone of the myometrium and the strength of contractions; therefore they carry a greater risk of producing fetal anoxia.

Uterine contractions that occur after delivery have two beneficial effects on the mother. First, they are responsible for expulsion of the afterbirth and produce a general cleansing of the uterus. Second, these contractions aid in controlling postpartum bleeding by clamping the vessels that were ruptured by the birth process. If bleeding is a problem at this stage, the physician may use an agent with a longer and more continuous action such as one of the ergot alkaloids.

THERAPEUTIC AGENTS: DRUGS FOR LABOR AND DELIVERY

Oxytocic Drugs

▼ oxytocin

Mechanism of Action

Oxytocin interacts with specific receptors in the myometrium and raises the level of calcium inside these smooth muscle cells; this action induces contraction of the myometrium (Table 71-1). The uterus is relatively insensitive to the action of oxytocin until labor has started. Oxytocin also acts on breast tissue; it stimulates the myoepithelium of the breast and promotes milk letdown. Suckling by the infant sets off a reflex action in which oxytocin release is stimulated. The central nervous system (CNS) controls this process; the sight of the infant is sufficient in some women to induce oxytocin release and milk letdown. Oxytocin action is responsible for the improved uterine muscle tone in nursing mothers and for the more rapid return of the uterus to the pregravid (before birth) size in these women.

Pharmacokinetics

Oxytocin is a peptide and is therefore quickly broken down by enzymes in target tissues and in plasma. Oxytocin has a quick onset of action by intranasal, intramuscular (IM), or intravenous (IV) routes, but the effect disappears within 3 hours. Effects of intranasal doses on milk letdown are lost within 20 minutes.

Uses

Oxytocin is used to induce or augment labor. In addition, it may be used to control postpartum bleeding by inducing contraction of the myometrium. The intranasal route is used to promote milk letdown and facilitate breast-feeding. Oxytocin may be used to induce or complete an abortion.

Adverse Reactions and Contraindications

Adverse reactions to oxytocin are rare. Possible reactions include allergies, arrhythmias, changes in blood pressure (BP), uterine rupture, and water intoxication.

Oxytocin should be avoided in patients with a history of allergy to the drug. It should not be used to augment or induce labor in a patient who cannot support a vaginal delivery or in a patient with hypertonic uterine contractions.

Toxicity

High dosages of oxytocin may cause hypotension with a rebound of hypertension. Reflexive tachycardia and other cardiac arrhythmias have also been noted. In rare cases, the intensity of the uterine contractions can rupture the uterus and may cause the death of the mother.

Interactions

Oxytocin may cause excessively strong uterine contractions if combined with other oxytocic agents or with intraamniotic urea or sodium chloride.

Ergot Alkaloids: ergonovine and methylergonovine

Mechanism of Action

Ergot alkaloids have been known as poisons since the Middle Ages, when it was noted that people who ate grain contaminated with the fungus that produces these alkaloids developed dry gangrene. This extreme reaction is caused by the potent vasoconstrictive effect of ergot alkaloids. Blood flow to the limbs may be reduced so severely that the tissues die, and the limbs eventually fall away with little bleeding. In addition, pregnant women who ate the affected grain entered an abrupt and devastating labor that expelled fetuses at any stage of development. The preparations used today have less vasoconstrictive activity but retain the ability to directly increase the force and frequency of myometrial contractions.

Pharmacokinetics

Oral doses of ergonovine or methylergonovine produce effects on uterine contractions within 15 minutes. IM doses take effect within 5 minutes. Effects are maintained for about 3 hours. Hepatic metabolism inactivates these drugs, and the metabolites are excreted in urine.

Uses

Ergot alkaloids are indicated for postpartum hemorrhage after delivery of the placenta.

Adverse Reactions and Contraindications

Reactions to ergot alkaloids include angina and bradycardia. Other cardiac arrhythmias, myocardial infarction, and severe hypertension are rare but can occur. More common effects include nausea and uterine cramping.

Ergot alkaloids are usually avoided in patients with significant cardiovascular disease, peripheral vascular disease,

Table 71-1 **Oxytocic Drugs**

Generic Name	Trade Name	Administration/Dosage	Comments
oxytocin	Pitocin Syntocinon*	INTRAVENOUS: *Adults—For induction or augmentation of labor:* 0.5-2 mU/min gradually increased to 20 mU/min. *For postpartum hemorrhage or abortion:* 10 U at 20-100 mU/min. INTRANASAL: *Adults—Lactation stimulant:* 1 spray of 40 U/ml solution before nursing. FDA pregnancy category X.	May produce uterine hypertonicity with fetal or maternal injury; monitor uterine contractions and status. Onset of action within 2-3 min, also causes nasal vasoconstriction.
Ergot Alkaloids			
ergonovine	Ergotrate*	ORAL, SUBLINGUAL: *Adults—To control postpartum bleeding:* 0.2-0.4 mg every 6-12 hr for 48 hr. INTRAVENOUS: *Adults—To control postpartum bleeding:* 0.2 mg given over 1 min; repeat every 2-4 hr up to 5 doses.	Produces strong tetanic contractions; avoid use until placenta is delivered.
methylergonovine	Methergine	ORAL: *Adults—To control postpartum bleeding:* 0.2-0.4 mg every 6-12 hr for 48 hr. INTRAVENOUS, INTRAMUSCULAR: *Adults—To control postpartum bleeding:* 0.2 mg; repeat every 2-4 hr up to 5 doses. Give intravenous doses over 1 min.	Produces strong tetanic contractions; avoid use until placenta is delivered.
Prostaglandins			
carboprost	Hemabate Prostin/15M†	INTRAMUSCULAR: *Adults—To control postpartum bleeding:* 0.25 mg by deep intramuscular injection; repeat every 90 min up to total dose of 2 mg. FDA pregnancy category C. INTRAAMNIOTIC: *Adults—To induce abortion:* 2.5 mg over 5 min.	Two thirds of patients experience vomiting and diarrhea.
dinoprost†	Prostin F₂ Alpha†	INTRAAMNIOTIC: *Adults—To induce abortion:* 5 mg at 1 mg/min; then 35 mg over 5 min. Repeat in 24 hr.	Up to 57% of patients experience vomiting or other gastrointestinal symptoms.
dinoprostone	Cervidil Prepidil* Prostin E₂*	INTRACERVICAL: *To induce cervical ripening:* 0.5 mg in cervical canal. Maximum dose: 1.5 mg in 24 hr. FDA pregnancy category C. INTRAVAGINAL: *Adults—For induction of labor:* 1 mg repeated in 6 hr. *To induce abortion:* 20 mg repeated every 3-5 hr up to maximum of 240 mg in 48 hr.	Patients should remain supine for 10-30 min after dosing.

*Available in Canada and the United States.
†Available in Canada only.

hypertension, eclampsia, or preeclampsia. These conditions are worsened by the vasoconstrictive effects of the drugs.

Toxicity

High dosages of these drugs are associated with peripheral vasospasm or vasoconstriction, angina, miosis, confusion, respiratory depression, seizures, or unconsciousness. Uterine tetany may occur.

Interactions

Vasoconstrictors may be more potent in the presence of the ergot alkaloids, which are themselves vasoconstrictors.

Prostaglandins: carboprost, dinoprost, and dinoprostone

Mechanism of Action

Prostaglandins are potent stimulators of the myometrium and have been successfully used to induce abortion during the second trimester, when the uterus is resistant to oxytocin. Dinoprostone also facilitates dilation of the cervix.

Pharmacokinetics

Prostaglandins are rapidly degraded in the blood and are unstable to gastric acid.

Dinoprost is administered by transabdominal instillation into the amniotic fluid. Given this way, the drug stays primarily within the uterus and persists in action for hours. Dinoprostone is administered as a gel or suppository directly into the vagina. Intravaginal delivery keeps the drug at the site of action and avoids rapid degradation carried out in maternal lung and liver. Carboprost can be given by deep IM injection.

Uses

Prostaglandins are used primarily as abortifacients. Dinoprost given by IV infusion or dinoprostone administered as an intravaginal gel may be used to induce labor, although oxytocin is usually preferred. Dinoprostone is also used to soften the cervix to facilitate vaginal delivery.

Adverse Reactions and Contraindications

These drugs very often cause significant gastrointestinal (GI) side effects, including diarrhea, nausea, vomiting, and stomach cramps. Fever, chills, and flushing are also noted.

Less common but more serious reactions include anaphylaxis, arrhythmias, bronchoconstriction, chest pain, hypertension, and peripheral vasoconstriction. Because of these potential problems, these drugs are usually avoided in patients with significant cardiovascular disease or those with a history of asthma or pulmonary disease.

Toxicity

Overdoses may cause the exaggerated responses already noted as well as uterine cramping or tetany.

Interactions

Prostaglandins are usually not combined with oxytocin because the risk of uterine tetany or uterine laceration is increased.

Uterine Relaxants

▼ ritodrine

Mechanism of Action

Specific uterine relaxation in cases of hypertonicity or premature labor is not yet possible, but several types of compounds produce uterine relaxation along with other reactions. For example, premature labor is sometimes treated with agents that stimulate beta$_2$-adrenergic receptors because stimulation of these receptors in the uterus causes relaxation of the myometrium. Agonists of beta$_2$-adrenergic receptors cause side effects throughout the body, however, as a result of beta-adrenergic receptor stimulation in other tissues. The best beta$_2$-adrenergic agonist for use in halting premature labor is **ritodrine.** This agent effectively relaxes the myometrium but also affects the peripheral vasculature and other tissues (Table 71-2).

Pharmacokinetics

Ritodrine may be used orally or intravenously. Ritodrine usually is administered intravenously when premature labor begins. When contractions have been controlled for 12 to 24 hours, the patient may be started on oral ritodrine, and the IV infusion may be discontinued. The onset of action after oral doses is within 30 minutes, but IV administration produces effects within 5 minutes. The drug is inactivated in the liver and eliminated by the kidneys.

Uses

Ritodrine is used to halt spontaneous labor when it appears after the twentieth week of pregnancy and before the thirty-sixth week. Spontaneous labor beginning before the twentieth week often is associated with irreversible problems in fetal development and may not be interrupted.

Adverse Reactions and Contraindications

The heart is sensitive to stimulation by ritodrine, suggesting that the drug is also an agonist with some activity on beta$_1$-adrenergic receptors. The major side effects noted with this drug have been heart palpitations, nausea and vomiting, trembling, flushing, and headache. These effects appear transient and rarely warrant termination of therapy. Patients should be observed for undue tachycardia or signs of cardiac distress. The fetal heart may also be stimulated by ritodrine. Ritodrine increases the workload of the mother's heart and is contraindicated in patients with preexisting cardiac disease. Pulmonary edema may occur in up to 15% of patients receiving intravenous ritodrine.

Toxicity

Overdoses of ritodrine may produce excessive beta-adrenergic stimulation, especially noticed as cardiovascular symptoms.

Interactions

Beta-adrenergic blockers inhibit the effects of ritodrine, whereas beta-adrenergic agonists may increase the risk of

Table 71-2 Drugs Used to Control Premature Labor

Generic Name	Trade Name	Administration/Dosage	Comments
isoxsuprine	Vasodilan†	INTRAMUSCULAR: *Adults*—5-10 mg 2 or 3 times/day. FDA pregnancy category C.	Canadian preparation, not approved for this use in the United States.
ritodrine	Yutopar*	INTRAVENOUS: *Adults*—0.05-0.1 mg/min increased by 0.05 mg every 10 min up to maximum of 0.35 mg/min. FDA pregnancy category B. ORAL: *Adults*—10 mg 30 min before intravenous infusion is terminated; then 10 mg every 2 hr for 24 hr; maintain with 10-20 mg every 4-6 hr. Extended-release capsules: 40 mg 30 min before intravenous infusion is terminated; then 40 mg every 8 hr for 24 hr; maintain with 40 mg every 8-12 hr. FDA pregnancy category B.	Ritadrine is the preferred drug to control premature labor.
terbutaline	Bricanyl*	INTRAVENOUS: *Adults*—0.01 mg/min increasing up to 0.08 mg/min. FDA pregnancy category B. SUBCUTANEOUS: *Adults*—0.25 mg every hr until contractions cease. FDA pregnancy category B. ORAL: *Adults*—2.5 mg every 4-6 hr until term. FDA pregnancy category B.	Primary use is to control bronchospasms; alternate for control of premature labor.

*Available in Canada and the United States.
†Available in Canada only.

cardiovascular side effects. Corticosteroids may increase the risk of pulmonary edema because of their effects on fluid balance.

Other Drugs to Halt Premature Labor

CNS depressants may halt premature labor. For example, ethanol, which is an inhibitor of oxytocin release and a CNS depressant, has been used to halt premature labor. The levels required to relax the uterus are sufficient to produce acute alcohol intoxication. Controlled clinical trials have suggested ritodrine is more effective and less toxic.

General anesthetics may also relax the uterus. Enflurane and halothane are the preferred agents. In addition to CNS effects, these agents may act directly on the myometrium and may also slow catecholamine release from the adrenal gland, thus reducing endogenous stimulators of myometrial activity.

Progesterone is the natural steroid that normally functions as a uterine relaxant. The use of this or other progestins is not recommended in cases of uterine hypertonicity during delivery because the hormone may not reach the uterus in sufficient quantities to relax the uterus quickly and effectively. Use of progesterone during earlier stages of pregnancy may cause undesirable effects on the developing fetus.

Nursing Process Overview

Drugs for Labor and Delivery

Assessment
Assess the vital signs, blood pressure, history of previous pregnancies and deliveries, fetal heart tones, and fetal position.

Nursing Diagnoses
- Potential complication: preterm labor
- Potential complication: fetal distress

Patient Outcomes
The nurse will minimize and manage complications of preterm labor. The nurse will manage and minimize episodes of fetal distress.

Planning/Implementation
Continue to monitor vital signs and BP. Assess frequency, duration, and force of contractions. With oxytocics, monitor the mother and infant closely, and use an IV monitoring device. Provide emotional support. Monitor intake, output, and specific gravity. Initiate and maintain fetal monitoring, as appropriate.

Evaluation
Ideally, all pregnancies would continue to term, with successful delivery of a healthy child or children. Emphasize the importance of follow-up visits.

Nursing Implications Summary

oxytocin

Drug Administration
- See Table 71-1. Monitor level of consciousness, weight, and intake and output. Monitor BP and pulse. Auscultate lung and heart sounds. Monitor frequency, duration, and force of contractions. Monitor resting uterine tone.
- Monitor fetal heart sounds; notify the physician of significant changes in rate or rhythm; follow agency protocol.
- Monitor serum electrolyte levels and complete blood cell (CBC) and platelet counts.
- Do not leave patient unattended when IV oxytocin is being used.
- Monitor vaginal bleeding.
- Have drugs, equipment, and personnel available to treat acute allergic reactions in settings where oxytocin is administered.
- For IV use, dilute as ordered or according to agency protocol. Use a microdrip infusion set or an infusion monitoring device. Measure dose according to the physician's order and patient response.
- Administer using a Y-setup or via stopcock, with normal saline in primary line. In the event of an adverse reaction, oxytocin can be stopped but IV access can be maintained.
- Oxytocin challenge test may be done in antepartum period to assess uteroplacental insufficiency. The test should be done by a physician.

Nursing in the Community
- Review the anticipated benefits and possible side effects of drug therapy. Instruct the patient to call for assistance if any new side effects develop.
- For intranasal spray, instruct the patient to sit upright to use spray; for nose drops, tell the patient to tilt head back to administer drops. Administer dose 2 to 3 minutes before nursing or pumping breasts. When intranasal use is prescribed to promote milk ejection, review with the mother other actions that may also aid in milk ejection, such as relaxing, massaging breasts, staying well hydrated, getting enough sleep, and cuddling the infant before trying to nurse.

Continued

Nursing Implications Summary—cont'd

Ergot Alkaloids

Drug Administration

➤ See Table 71-1. Monitor level of consciousness, weight, and intake and output. Monitor BP and pulse. Auscultate lung and heart sounds. Monitor uterine response, and assess vaginal bleeding.

➤ Assess the patient for chest pain, headache, shortness of breath, itching, pale or cold hands or feet, diarrhea, and dizziness.

➤ Monitor serum electrolyte level and CBC and platelet counts.

➤ Have drugs, equipment, and personnel available to treat acute allergic reactions in settings where ergot alkaloids are administered.

➤ For IV use in an emergency, either drug may be administered undiluted. Administer at a rate of 0.2 mg or less over 1 minute. Administer via Y-setup or stopcock. IM or oral route is preferred.

➤ Read drug labels carefully; do not confuse ergotamine with ergonovine.

Nursing in the Community

➤ Review the anticipated benefits and possible side effects of drug therapy with the patient. Instruct the patient to call for assistance if any new side effects develop.

➤ Remind the patient to keep all health care providers informed of all medications and herbal remedies that are currently being used.

➤ Warn the patient to avoid smoking while using ergot alkaloids.

Prostaglandins

Drug Administration

➤ See Table 71-1. Monitor level of consciousness, weight, and intake and output. Monitor BP, pulse, and temperature. Auscultate lung and heart sounds. Monitor force, duration, and frequency of uterine contractions. Assess resting uterine tone frequently.

➤ Keep siderails up. Have a suction machine available.

➤ Monitor serum electrolyte level and CBC and platelet counts.

➤ Monitor vaginal bleeding. Palpate the fundus regularly.

➤ GI symptoms are common; antidiarrheal and antiemetic medications may be ordered concomitantly or prophylactically.

➤ Remain with the patient at least 30 minutes after the dose is administered to monitor for anaphylaxis: shortness of breath or difficulty breathing, tachycardia, hives, tightness in chest, or swelling of face.

Nursing in the Community

➤ Review with the patient the anticipated benefits and possible side effects of drug therapy. Instruct the patient to report the development of severe or persistent headache, shortness of breath, chest pain, tightness in chest, fever, foul-smelling vaginal discharge, or increased uterine bleeding. Instruct the patient to call if any unexpected side effects develop.

➤ Provide emotional support. Refer for counseling if appropriate.

➤ Emphasize the importance of follow-up visits.

isoxsuprine

Drug Administration

➤ This drug is also discussed in Chapter 15.

➤ Monitor BP, pulse, uterine contractions, and fetal heart tone. Assess the patient and fetus frequently. Fetal monitoring may be indicated.

➤ Stay calm. Provide reassurance to the mother as much as possible. This drug may increase the subjective sense of anxiety and may cause tachycardia, tightness in the chest, tremor, and other symptoms.

Nursing in the Community

➤ Review the anticipated benefits and possible side effects of drug therapy with the patient.

➤ Review with the patient the limits of activity.

➤ Tell the patient to notify the physician if labor begins again, membranes rupture, or contractions increase in frequency or duration.

➤ Instruct patient to avoid smoking while taking isoxsuprine. See the Patient Problems box in Chapter 13 on orthostatic hypotension.

➤ Instruct the patient to take oral doses with meals, milk, or a snack to lessen gastric irritation.

ritodrine

Drug Administration

➤ Review the information about beta$_2$-adrenergic receptors in Chapter 12.

➤ Monitor BP, pulse, uterine contractions, and fetal heart tones. Assess the patient and fetus every 5 minutes when initiating IV therapy, every 15 to 30 minutes when the patient is stable, and every 4 hours when the patient is taking oral maintenance doses (or according to agency protocol). Fetal monitoring may be indicated.

➤ Monitor CBC and maternal and neonatal fluid and electrolyte status.

➤ For IV administration, dilute 150 mg in 500 mg D5W to make a dilution of 0.33 mg/ml, or dilute as agency protocol directs. Use a minidrip infusion set or an infusion control device. The dosage may be titrated to patient response.

➤ Stay calm. Provide reassurance to the mother as possible. The drug may increase the subjective sense of anxiety and may cause tachycardia, tightness in the chest, tremor, and other symptoms.

Nursing in the Community

➤ Review the anticipated benefits and possible side effects of drug therapy with the patient.

➤ Review with the patient the limits of activity.

Nursing Implications Summary—cont'd

➤ Remind the patient to keep all health care providers informed of all drugs and herbal remedies being used.

➤ Tell the patient to notify the physician if labor begins again, membranes rupture, or contractions increase in frequency or duration.

terbutaline
Drug Administration
➤ See Table 71-2. This drug is also used as a bronchodilator; see Chapter 28.

➤ Read order carefully. IV and subcutaneous doses are significantly different.

➤ Monitor BP, pulse, uterine contractions, and fetal heart tones. Assess the patient and fetus every 5 minutes when initiating IV therapy, every 15 to 30 minutes when the patient is stable, and every 4 hours when the patient is taking oral maintenance doses (or according to agency protocol). Fetal monitoring may be indicated.

➤ For IV administration, dilute 5 mg in 1000 ml D5W to make a concentration of 5 μg/ml, or dilute as agency protocol directs. Use a minidrip infusion set or an infusion control device. The dosage may be titrated to patient response.

➤ Stay calm. Provide reassurance to the mother as possible. This drug may increase the subjective sense of anxiety and may cause tachycardia, tightness in the chest, tremor, and other symptoms.

Nursing in the Community
➤ Review the anticipated benefits and possible side effects of drug therapy with the patient.

➤ Review with the patient the limits of activity.

➤ Remind the patient to keep all health care providers informed of all drugs and herbal remedies being used.

➤ Tell the patient to notify the physician if labor begins again, membranes rupture, or contractions increase in frequency or duration.

CHAPTER REVIEW

Application

1. How does oxytocin stimulate uterine contractions?
2. How do the uterine contractions produced by prostaglandins differ from those produced by oxytocin?
3. What is the desired effect of intranasal administration of oxytocin?
4. What are the ergot alkaloids?
5. What is the only clinical indication for ergonovine and methylergonovine?
6. What is the other significant action of ergot alkaloids? How does this action lead to potentially serious side effects?
7. What is the source of natural prostaglandins?
8. Why are prostaglandins best administered intraamniotically or intravaginally?
9. What is the most common side effect with prostaglandins?
10. What is the mechanism of action of ritodrine?
11. What is the clinical use of ritodrine?
12. Why are cardiovascular effects seen with ritodrine?

Critical Thinking

1. Your patient is experiencing her first pregnancy. She is worried about premature labor. What symptoms would you teach her to watch for? How can a patient differentiate between Braxton Hicks contractions and the contractions of labor?

REFERENCES

Burton J: When your patient is pregnant: a guide for the medical-surgical nurse, *Am J Nurs* 97(3):16F, 16H, 16J, 1997.

Viamontes CM: Pharmacologic intervention in the management of preterm labor: an update, *J Perinat Neonat Nurs* 9(4):13-30, 1996.

Drugs Acting on the Male Reproductive System

OBJECTIVES

After studying this chapter, you should be able to do the following:

- *Describe the uses of androgens.*
- *Describe the uses and abuses of anabolic steroids.*
- *Develop a nursing care plan for the patient receiving androgens.*

CHAPTER OVERVIEW

The major reproductive hormones in men are androgens. These steroids are synthesized primarily in the testes and to a lesser extent in the adrenal glands. Within the testes the status of interstitial or Leydig's cells and the seminiferous tubular cells is most important for determining male sexual potential. Leydig's cells synthesize testosterone, the primary masculinizing steroid hormone. The seminiferous tubules contain the germ cells that in the adult male produce functional sperm. The endocrine control of male sexual development and function, the actions of natural male hormones, and the clinical uses of synthetic and natural drugs acting on the male reproductive system are discussed in this chapter.

THERAPEUTIC RATIONALE: DEVELOPMENT AND REGULATION OF MALE SEXUAL FUNCTION

In adult males, sexual function depends on the proper interaction of the hypothalamus, anterior pituitary, and the testes. Regulation of testicular function is by a negative feedback loop (see Chapter 65). The primary hormones in this cycle are testosterone from the testes, luteinizing hormone (LH) and follicle-stimulating hormone (FSH) from the anterior pituitary, and gonadotropin-releasing hormone (GnRH) from the hypothalamus. When testosterone levels in blood are low, GnRH is released from the hypothalamus to enter the anterior pituitary through a portal venous system. Under the influence of GnRH, both LH and FSH are released from the pituitary into general circulation, where they act in males on testicular tissues to stimulate production of androgens.

The action of these regulatory hormones is slightly different during the three stages of life in which they act. During fetal development, Leydig's cells develop in the embryonic testes as a result of stimulation with the maternal hormone human chorionic gonadotropin (HCG). These embryonic cells produce the small amounts of testosterone necessary for the development of the male external genitalia; without testosterone, genetically male infants are born with female genitalia. After birth, Leydig's cells regress because the stimulus of HCG is no longer available.

The second period of life when these regulatory processes are most important is puberty. In childhood, very low concentrations of gonadotropins are found in blood. With the onset of puberty the anterior pituitary begins to synthesize and release greater quantities of LH and FSH. The targets for LH in males are Leydig's cells, where LH stimulates testosterone production. FSH acts directly on cells in seminiferous tubules to prepare that tissue for spermatogenesis. This process cannot be completed unless testosterone from Leydig's cells is also present. With FSH and testosterone acting on the seminiferous tubules, mature sperm can be produced. Testosterone acts not only within the testes but also throughout the body at this stage of life. These actions are discussed in the next section.

The third period of life to be considered is sexual maturity. During this time, LH is important in the maintenance of sexual function because it is still required for the synthesis of testosterone, which maintains spermatogenesis.

The major steroid affecting male sexual function is testosterone. This hormone is synthesized in the Leydig's cells and in the adrenal cortex. Testosterone is a potent **androgen,** a substance that stimulates growth of the organs of the male reproductive tract. Testosterone is responsible for the enlargement and maturation of the penis, scrotum, seminal vesicles, prostate gland, and other accessory tissues of the male reproductive tract. These actions constitute the primary sexual effects on the male.

Testosterone is also responsible for the development of secondary sexual characteristics. The increased testosterone level during puberty stimulates growth of facial and pubic hair and hair on chest and armpits. Sustained levels of testosterone trigger the onset of baldness in genetically predisposed males. The other dramatic changes that occur in the pubertal male are also related to the increased testosterone levels and include lowering of the voice caused by thickening of the vocal cords, stimulation of sebaceous glands, and stimulation of the libido. Psychologists who work with primates other than humans have related aggression to high testosterone levels.

In addition to these primary and secondary sexual effects, testosterone also has profound effects on metabolism. Androgens are anabolic (i.e., they stimulate synthetic rather than degradative processes). Testosterone increases nitrogen retention, protein formation, and overall metabolic rate. This anabolic action is responsible for the increase in muscle mass associated with puberty and the distribution of this mass in the male pattern. In addition, calcium is retained, and the size and strength of bone are enhanced. Blood-forming cells are also affected so that more red blood cells may be formed.

Although testosterone is the major circulating androgen in human males, it is not the only metabolically important androgen. Testosterone is transformed within many target cells to dihydrotestosterone, which is a more potent androgen than testosterone. Small amounts of another androgen, androstenedione, may also affect various tissues of the body.

Testosterone and androstenedione are close chemical relatives of the estrogens, steroid hormones that have feminizing effects. Some tissues in the brain, breasts, and testes can convert androgens to estrogens. Therefore low estrogen concentrations are found in the blood of healthy adult men. These estrogens have no obvious influence on healthy men, but under certain circumstances, estrogen concentrations may increase and produce pathologic signs such as breast development.

THERAPEUTIC AGENTS: DRUGS AFFECTING DEVELOPMENT AND REGULATION OF MALE SEXUAL FUNCTION

Androgens

▼ fluoxymesterone, methyltestosterone, and testosterone

Mechanism of Action

The androgens are steroids that diffuse into cells and bind to receptors that move to the nucleus of the cell and affect gene expression. These changes bring about a change in the proteins that are produced, and cell function is altered. The effect on the body is as described previously for naturally produced androgens.

Pharmacokinetics

Testosterone in its natural form is not water soluble and therefore is used as an aqueous suspension suitable only for intramuscular (IM) injection (Table 72-1). In this form the drug has a short duration of action and produces somewhat erratic clinical responses. Testosterone can be absorbed from the gastrointestinal (GI) tract; however, this route of administration does not produce clinically useful testosterone concentrations in blood because the steroid absorbed from the intestine passes directly into portal circulation to the liver before it circulates to the rest of the body. The liver can inactivate testosterone rapidly by forming less active metabolites or by converting the steroid to a glucuronide or to sulfated derivatives.

Testosterone esters are much more useful than testosterone for producing sustained androgenic effects. Two preparations commonly used clinically are testosterone enanthate and testosterone cypionate (see Table 72-1). Both are supplied in forms that are slowly absorbed from IM sites and therefore are effective for 3 to 4 weeks. This increased convenience for the patient is at the cost of less flexibility in control. Another testosterone ester, testosterone propionate, has a short duration of action more similar to that of testosterone.

Orally absorbed androgens have been developed. Methyltestosterone and fluoxymesterone are examples. These compounds are effective orally because they are resistant to the action of liver enzymes that degrade testosterone. Unfortunately, these compounds are also associated with liver toxicity of various types, including cholestatic jaundice.

Uses

Androgenic drugs are primarily used in replacement therapy for patients who have reduced endogenous androgen production. For some patients the loss of androgens occurs early and prevents the normal changes of puberty. Androgen loss after puberty may cause a loss in libido or sexual desire or may cause mild feminizing tendencies. Aging males produce less testosterone than younger men and may experience a loss of sexual drive. Some older men have more severe symptoms suggestive of a male climacteric or male

Table 72-1 Androgens

Generic Name	Trade Name	Administration/Dosage	Comments
fluoxymesterone	Android-F Halotestin*	ORAL: *Adults—Replacement therapy in males:* 5-20 mg/day. *For breast cancer in females:* 10-40 mg/day. FDA pregnancy category X. *Children—For delayed puberty in boys:* 2.5-10 mg/day for 4-6 mo.	Relatively short-acting agent; risk of liver toxicity.
methyltestosterone	Android Metandren† Testred Virilon	ORAL: *Adults—Replacement therapy in males:* 10-50 mg/day. *For breast cancer in females:* 50-200 mg/day. FDA pregnancy category X. *Children—For delayed puberty in boys:* 5-25 mg/day for 4-6 mo.	Relatively short-acting agent; risk of liver toxicity.
testosterone	Andro Histerone Malogen† Testaqua	INTRAMUSCULAR: *Adults—Replacement therapy in males:* 25-50 mg 2 or 3 times/wk. *For breast cancer in females:* 50-100 mg 3 times/wk. FDA pregnancy category X. *Children—For delayed puberty in boys:* 100 mg/mo for 4-6 mo.	Aqueous suspension for intramuscular use only.
testosterone	Androderm Testoderm	TRANSDERMAL PATCH: *Adults—*4- or 6-mg patch placed on scrotal area daily (Testoderm); 5-mg patch applied to back, abdomen, upper arms, or thighs every 22-24 hr.	For replacement therapy only.
testosterone	Testopel pellets	SUBCUTANEOUS: *Adults—Replacement therapy in males:* 150-450 mg replaced every 3-4 mo. Each pellet contains 75 mg testosterone.	For replacement therapy in adult males only.
testosterone cypionate	Andronate Depotest Virilon-IM	INTRAMUSCULAR: *Adults—Replacement therapy in males:* 50-400 mg every 2-4 wk. *For breast cancer in females:* 200-400 mg every 2-4 wk. FDA pregnancy category X. *Children—For delayed puberty in boys:* 100 mg/mo for 4-6 mo.	Very long-acting preparation for intramuscular use only.
testosterone enanthate	Delatest Delatestryl* Everone	INTRAMUSCULAR: *Adults—Replacement therapy in males:* 200-400 mg every 2-4 wk. *For breast cancer in females:* 200-400 mg every 2-4 wk. FDA pregnancy category X. *Children—For delayed puberty in males:* 100 mg/mo for 4-6 mo.	Very long-acting preparation for intramuscular use only.
testosterone propionate	Malogen† Testex	INTRAMUSCULAR: *Adults—Replacement therapy in males:* 25-50 mg 2 or 3 times/wk. *For breast cancer in females:* 50-100 mg 3 times/wk. FDA pregnancy category X. *Children—For delayed puberty in boys:* 100 mg/mo for 4-6 mo.	For intramuscular use only.

*Available in Canada and the United States.
†Available in Canada only.

menopause. These conditions and others related to specific malfunctions of the male sexual organs may be treated with testosterone or one of the other androgenic compounds (see Table 72-1). For patients with reduced natural testosterone production, this treatment constitutes replacement therapy.

Androgens have been used for various conditions in females, such as relief of dysmenorrhea, menopausal symptoms, and postpartum breast engorgement, but other agents now are preferred (see Chapter 70). Androgens are still indicated for treatment of certain advanced breast carcinomas (see Chapter 56). The high dosages used for this purpose exceed those required for replacement therapy and may be expected to cause masculinization (see Table 72-1).

Adverse Reactions and Contraindications

The reactions experienced with androgens differ in men and women. Men often report urinary tract infections, bladder irritation, tender breasts, gynecomastia, or priapism. Women, who generally receive higher dosages than men, ex-

perience menstrual irregularities or virilism. Virilism may also be noted in boys who receive androgens.

Less common symptoms in men and women include edema, erythrocytosis, hypercalcemia, liver dysfunction, nausea, or vomiting. Acne, diarrhea, and changes in libido are also possible. Men may also experience pain in the scrotum or groin; difficulty in urination may signal changes in the prostate gland. Androgens are usually avoided in men with known prostatic or breast carcinoma because androgens often stimulate growth of these tumors.

Toxicity

The most important toxicity of androgens is directed to the liver.

Interactions

Androgens increase effects of anticoagulants; dosages must be adjusted. Hepatotoxic drugs are avoided with androgens because of the risk of additive damage to the liver.

Table 72-2 **Nonandrogenic Agents Used for Male Hypogonadism**

Generic Name	Trade Name	Administration/Dosage	Comments
bromocriptine	Parlodel*	ORAL: *Adults*—1.25-2.5 mg at bedtime with snack. Increase gradually as needed to maximum of 7.5 mg/day.	Effective for male gonadism when symptoms are related to hyperprolactinemia.
chorionic gonadotropin	A.P.L.*	INTRAMUSCULAR: *Adults—For male infertility:* 1000-4000 units 2 or 3 times/wk for 6 mo or longer. *Children—For prepubertal cryptorchidism:* 1000-5000 units 2 or 3 times/wk until testes descend or until 10 doses have been given.	Substitutes for luteinizing hormone action.
gonadorelin	Factrel*	SUBCUTANEOUS, INTRAVENOUS: *Adults and children >12 yr*-0.1 mg once.	For diagnosis of hypogonadism.
menotropins	Humegon* Pergonal*	INTRAMUSCULAR: *Adults*—75 units of follicle-stimulating hormone and 75 units of luteinizing hormone 3 times/wk after pretreatment with chorionic gonadotropin and with continuing administration of chorionic gonadotropin. Dosages may be increased after 4 mo if spermatogenesis has not occurred.	Used with chorionic gonadotropin to stimulate sperm production in men with failure of hypothalamus or pituitary.

*Available in Canada and the United States.

ALTERNATIVE THERAPIES

Prostate Disorders

SAW PALMETTO

The drug consists of the dried fruits of *Serenoa repens* (Bartr.) Small. It is a member of the palm family and grows wild in Georgia and Florida.

Saw palmetto fruits and their preparations are used widely in Germany, France, and Italy for the treatment of symptoms associated with benign prostatic hyperplasia (BPH). Liposterolic extracts of the fruit have been shown to exert antiandrogenic and antiinflammatory actions. Its effectiveness against BPH is supported by results of placebo-controlled, double-blind studies in more than 2000 BPH patients in Germany. Stomach upset has been reported as a side effect of saw palmetto extract.

Preparations of saw palmetto are freely available without prescription in the United States, but nurses should caution against its unsupervised use and urge anyone who thinks they may have BPH to consult their physician first.

Saw palmetto has also been claimed to promote female breast enlargement. There is no evidence to support this claim.

Nonandrogens Used for Male Hypogonadism

In males, the hormones LH and FSH promote production of testosterone from the testes. A failure of the pituitary to produce these hormones will lead to male hypogonadism and infertility. Thus administering LH and/or FSH may correct the situation for men whose infertility is not caused by primary inability of the testes to produce androgens. A third hormone of the anterior pituitary involved in male sexual function is prolactin. The role of prolactin in men is unclear, but men with pituitary tumors that secrete large quantities of prolactin often have decreased libidos and low concentrations of LH, FSH, and testosterone in their blood. Prolactin seems to suppress synthesis and release of LH and FSH from the pituitary gland and may directly interfere with the actions of these hormones on testes.

Agents that are used directly to treat hypogonadism in males include many agents that also have use in dealing with female fertility. For example, chorionic gonadotropin is used for male hypogonadism because it acts as LH on the testes (Table 72-2). Likewise, menotropins contain both LH and FSH and thus have effects on testicular function. Bromocriptine is useful only in men whose infertility is related to overproduction of prolactin.

Gonadorelin is useful for diagnosis of male hypogonadism because this hormone normally stimulates a rise in serum LH in males with intact pituitary function. Failure of the agent to increase LH implies that pituitary function is lacking and that LH, or an androgen, may need to be supplied.

Anabolic Steroids

In addition to androgenic properties, the natural male steroids also possess anabolic properties that may be useful in certain clinical situations. Relatives of the natural hormones have been developed, which maximize the anabolic properties and minimize androgenic effects (Table 72-3). These **anabolic steroids** may be used to treat conditions for which increased nitrogen retention and protein formation are desirable. Accordingly, these drugs may alleviate the catabolic state produced by severe trauma. Patients who have extensive burns or have had surgery may benefit from the action of the anabolic steroids. The effects of anabolic hormone on red blood cell formation make these drugs valuable in the treatment of certain forms of anemia.

Although a few anabolic compounds are relatively weak androgens, all anabolic steroids possess some androgenic properties. These androgenic effects may be unseen in healthy men, but they may become obvious when the compounds are used to treat women or children. Patients receiving these compounds may develop increased libido. Men may develop priapism (continuous erection). Women may show androgen-induced changes, such as inappropriate hair development, voice changes, or personality alterations. Children should be watched closely for precocious sexual development. These compounds, while promoting bone growth in children, also promote fusion of the epiphyses, which permanently halts skeletal growth. Therefore full adult height may be reduced in spite of a growth spurt when the drugs are first given. For this reason and because of the effects on sexual development, these drugs are less than ideal for therapy in children.

Anabolic steroids are inappropriate for use in athletes who seek to increase bone or muscle mass. In healthy young men the anabolic effects are minimal, but the side effects can be serious (altered liver function, reduced gonadotropin lev-els, lowered testosterone synthesis, and depressed spermatogenesis). In healthy young women, bone and muscle mass may be increased more dramatically but at the cost of virilization and menstrual disturbances.

Drugs for Erectile Dysfunction

Sildenafil (Viagra) is widely used to treat erectile dysfunction in males, but the drug does not change levels of androgens. Instead, sildenafil acts as a local vasodilator, inhibiting phosphodiester type 5 in the corpus cavernosum and thus allowing adequate blood flow to produce an erection. General vasodilators are discussed in Chapter 15. Sildenafil is metabolized in the liver and should be avoided in patients with severe liver or renal impairment. Visual disturbances or cardiac symptoms may signal dangerous reactions to the drug.

Table 72-3 Anabolic Steroids

Generic Name	Trade Name	Administration/Dosage	Comments
nandrolone decanoate	Deca-Durabolin* Hybolin	INTRAMUSCULAR: *Adults—For deep intramuscular injection:* 50-200 mg. Repeat doses every 1-4 wk. FDA pregnancy category X. *Children—*25-50 mg; repeat every 3-4 wk.	Refractory anemias.
oxandrolone	Oxandrin	ORAL: *Adults—Tablets:* 2.5 mg 2-4 times/day. FDA pregnancy category X. *Children—*0.25 mg/kg intermittently.	To produce weight gain after severe trauma.
oxymetholone	Anapolon†	ORAL: *Adults and Children—Tablets:* 1-5 mg/kg body weight/day up to 100 mg total daily dose. FDA pregnancy category X. *Neonates—*0.175 mg/kg or 5 mg/m².	Anemias or hereditary angioedema.
stanozolol	Winstrol	ORAL: *Adults—Tablets:* 2 mg 3 times/day initially. Reduce dose when response allows. FDA pregnancy category X. *Children—*1 mg twice daily with meals, only during attack.	Hereditary angioedema.

*Available in Canada and the United States.
†Available in Canada only.

Nursing Process Overview

Drugs Acting on the Male Reproductive System

Assessment

Perform a complete patient assessment before initiating drug therapy. Assess the vital signs, blood pressure (BP), weight, serum calcium level, height, and serum and urine glucose. Focus part of the assessment on the presenting problem. For example, in treatment of reduced androgen production, assess development of secondary sexual characteristics. In the patient receiving androgen therapy for its anabolic effects, assess nutritional needs, level of mobility, and intake and output.

Nursing Diagnoses

- Body image disturbance: acne related to androgen therapy
- Body image disturbance: masculinization of women related to androgen therapy

Patient Outcomes

The patient will discuss feelings related to body image changes.

Planning/Implementation

Monitor the vital signs and other data mentioned in the assessment. Review possible and probable side effects. Refer the patient receiving steroids for their anabolic effects to the hospital or community dietitian.

Evaluation

Before discharge, verify that the patient understands how and why to take the drugs, what side effects are expected, which side effects require immediate notification of the physician, how to treat side effects that may be troublesome but are not serious, and what parameters should be measured regularly at home to monitor drug effectiveness.

Nursing Implications Summary

Androgens

Drug Administration

➤ Assess mental status and neurologic function.

➤ Assess for signs of depression, including insomnia, lack of appetite, loss of interest in personal appearance, and withdrawal.

➤ Monitor weight, pulse, and BP. Assess for edema and skin changes. Auscultate lung and heart sounds.

➤ Assess for signs of liver dysfunction, including right upper quadrant abdominal pain, malaise, fever, jaundice, and pruritus.

➤ When the drug is used for treatment of hypogonadism, assess for development of secondary sexual characteristics: deepening of voice, growth of pubic hair, or growth of the penis. Assess for acne.

➤ When the drug is used to treat breast cancer, assess for signs of hypercalcemia: confusion, depression, nausea, increased thirst, increased urination, constipation, or vomiting.

➤ When the drug is used in women, assess for virilization: deeper voice, hoarseness, enlargement of clitoris, decreased breast size, vaginal drying, acne, changes in hair growth patterns, abnormal menstrual periods, or amenorrhea.

➤ When the drug is prescribed for children, review the proposed long-term treatment plan. Therapy for children is often intermittent to allow drug-free periods to permit normal bone growth. The child's progress may be monitored with regular x-ray studies of wrists and hands to monitor bone maturation. Monitor weight and height.

➤ Do not substitute testosterone cypionate or testosterone enanthate for testosterone propionate or testosterone base because there are different durations of action.

➤ Chapter 5 discusses IM administration of oil-based suspensions.

➤ For buccal tablets, instruct the patient to place tablets in the mouth between the upper or lower gum and the cheek and to allow the tablet to dissolve. While the tablet is in place, the patient should refrain from eating, drinking, chewing, or smoking. Instruct the patient to rotate sites with each dose. Remind the patient to maintain a program of good regular oral hygiene and to report any oral irritation to the physician.

➤ For transdermal form applied to the scrotum, instruct the patient to dry-shave a small area on scrotum and apply the patch to the scrotum once daily. Chemical hair removers should not be used. Review the patient instruction leaflet dispensed with drug.

➤ For transdermal form not applied to scrotum, apply to dry skin of back, abdomen, upper arms, or thigh. Men older than age 65 should not use the back because absorption is poor via this route. Review the patient instruction leaflet dispensed with drug.

➤ For implant form: Implantation requires a brief procedure that can be done on an outpatient basis. The area for implantation is anesthetized with a local anesthetic. A small incision is made, and the physician inserts and releases each implant into a fanlike track using a special trocar. The usual site of application is the lower abdomen. After the procedure, the patient may experience minor discomfort until the small incision heals. Sutures are not required. Steri-Strips, covered by a water-resistant dressing, are use to for approximately 1 week, until the insertion site heals.

➤ Monitor complete blood cell count (CBC) and differential, serum electrolyte level, and liver function tests.

Nursing in the Community

➤ Review the anticipated benefits and possible side effects of drug therapy with the patient. Tell the patient to report any new side effects.

➤ Remind the patient to take these drugs as ordered and not to increase doses unless directed to do so by the physician.

➤ Assess the patient tactfully for side effects such as decreased ejaculatory volume, and in females, amenorrhea, menstrual irregularities, virilization, and clitoral enlargement. Children may experience premature virilization. Patients may be reluctant to discuss these problems, or children may not know how to do so. Provide emotional support. Remind the patient to take drugs as ordered for best effects and not to stop taking the drug without notifying the physician.

➤ Instruct men to notify the physician if priapism develops.

➤ Tell the patient to take oral doses with meals or a snack to lessen gastric irritation.

➤ Warn diabetic patients to monitor blood glucose levels frequently for the first 2 weeks of therapy and after androgen therapy is completed because a change in insulin dosage or diet may be needed.

➤ Warn the patient using a scrotal patch that testosterone from the patch may be transferred to female sexual partners. Assess female sexual partners for increases in acne or changes in body hair distribution.

NONANDROGENIC AGENTS USED FOR MALE HYPOGONADISM

bromocriptine

Drug Administration/Nursing in the Community

➤ This drug is discussed in Chapters 62, 65, and 70.

➤ When used to treat male infertility, monitor serum FSH and LH, serum prolactin, serum testosterone, and sperm counts. See other nursing care guidelines in Chapter 70.

chorionic gonadotropin

Drug Administration/Nursing in the Community

➤ See Chapter 70 for general nursing care guidelines.

➤ For prepubertal cryptorchidism, assess the patient for enlargement of the penis or testes, growth of pubic hair, or rapid increases in height.

➤ Monitor serum testosterone and sperm count.

Continued

Nursing Implications Summary—cont'd

gonadorelin
➤ This drug is also discussed in Chapter 70.

menotropins
Drug Administration/Nursing in the Community
➤ The drug is also discussed in Chapter 70.
➤ Monitor serum testosterone and sperm count.
➤ Assess for breast enlargement, shortness of breath, irregular heartbeat, dizziness, anorexia, headache, and nosebleeds.

Anabolic Steroids
Drug Administration
➤ Assess mental status. Assess for signs of depression, including lack of interest in personal appearance, insomnia, loss of appetite, and withdrawal.
➤ Monitor weight, BP, and pulse. Assess for edema and skin changes.
➤ When drug is used for anemia, take diet history if needed. Assess for shortness of breath, activity tolerance level, ability to perform activities of daily living, malaise, fatigability, and paleness.
➤ Assess prepubertal boys for darkening of the skin and development of secondary sexual characteristics.
➤ When drug is used for treatment of breast cancer, assess for signs of hypercalcemia: confusion, depression, nausea, increased thirst, increased urination, constipation, or vomiting.
➤ Assess women for virilization: deepening of the voice, hoarseness, enlargement of clitoris, decreased breast size, vaginal drying, acne, changes in hair growth patterns, abnormal menstrual periods, or amenorrhea.

➤ Monitor CBC, white blood cell differential, iron and total iron-binding capacity, serum calcium, serum cholesterol, and liver function tests.

Nursing in the Community
➤ Review the anticipated benefits and possible side effects of the drug therapy with the patient. Tell the patient to take drugs only as ordered and not to share drugs with others. Anabolic steroids should not be used to change body size or function or for athletic purposes.
➤ Teach the patient to take oral doses with meals or a snack to lessen gastric irritation. If GI symptoms are severe or persistent, instruct the patient to notify the physician.
➤ Assess tactfully for changes such as hirsutism and virilization in females or gynecomastia and decreased libido in males. Provide emotional support as needed. Remind the patient to take medications as ordered and not to stop medications without notifying the physician.
➤ Instruct men to notify the physician if priapism develops.
➤ Warn diabetic patients to monitor blood glucose levels carefully when starting or ending therapy with steroids because an adjustment in insulin dosage or diet may be necessary.
➤ A patient who has been burned, traumatized, or immobilized should be informed that the effectiveness of anabolic steroids may be enhanced by concomitant use of a diet high in calories and protein. Continue regular physical therapy to help reduce bone demineralization.

DRUGS FOR ERECTILE DYSFUNCTION
sildenafil
Drug Administration/Nursing in the Community
➤ See manufacturer's literature for current information.

 # CHAPTER REVIEW

Application
1. Which three organs produce hormones that affect male sexual development and function?
2. What is the function of GnRH in the adult male?
3. What is the function of LH in the adult male?
4. What is the function of FSH in the adult male?
5. What is the function of testosterone during fetal development in males?
6. What is the primary natural androgenic steroid?
7. What is the most common clinical use of androgen steroids?
8. Why is testosterone not administered by the oral route?

9. What two androgenic steroids are well absorbed orally?
10. What is the major effect of the anabolic steroids?
11. What side effect is commonly associated with anabolic steroids?

Critical Thinking
1. What effect does testosterone have on metabolism? How should you assess for this?
2. What advantages do testosterone esters such as testosterone enanthate have over testosterone for long-term replacement therapy of androgen deficiency?
3. What disadvantages do the orally administered androgenic steroids possess compared with other androgenic agents?

Chapter 73

Drugs to Treat Glaucoma

KEY TERMS

acute (closed-angle) glaucoma, p. 847
chronic (open-angle) glaucoma, p. 847

KEY DRUGS ▼

dipivefrin, p. 851
pilocarpine, p. 852
timolol, p. 851

OBJECTIVES

After studying this chapter, you should be able to do the following:

- *Differentiate between chronic and acute glaucoma.*

- *Discuss the categories of drugs to treat glaucoma, including cholinomimetic drugs, adrenergic drugs, beta-blockers, carbonic anhydrase inhibitors, and osmotic agents.*

- *From a list of drugs used in the treatment of glaucoma, develop a teaching plan to prepare patients for discharge.*

CHAPTER OVERVIEW

The key functions of the eye are controlled by the autonomic nervous system. Selected drugs with autonomic actions are used to treat glaucoma. These drugs are presented in this chapter.

THERAPEUTIC RATIONALE: GLAUCOMA

Glaucoma is the third leading cause of visual impairment and blindness in the United States. Blindness results from damage to the optic nerve caused by an increased intraocular pressure. The detection and treatment of glaucoma is important. About 3 million people in the United States are estimated to have glaucoma, half being unaware of their condition. The risk factors for glaucoma are indicated in Box 73-1. An estimated 150,000 people in the United States are estimated to be blind as a consequence of glaucoma.

The increase in intraocular pressure is caused by the accumulation of aqueous humor in the space between the lens and cornea. Aqueous humor is a protein-poor fluid formed by the ciliary body. As illustrated in Figure 73-1, this fluid is normally reabsorbed through the trabecular spaces into Schlemm's canal in a region of the cornea called the anterior chamber. If the aqueous humor cannot be reabsorbed through the anterior chamber, the fluid accumulates and intraocular pressure increases. If the intraocular pressure is not relieved, the optic nerve becomes damaged, resulting in blindness.

Chronic (open-angle) glaucoma is the more common form of glaucoma and is very gradual in its onset. The defect is a slow degeneration of the anterior chamber that impairs the uptake of aqueous humor (see Figure 73-1). Traditionally, drug therapy, applied as eyedrops, has been used to improve the uptake of aqueous humor and thereby lower intraocular pressure. The most commonly prescribed drugs are beta-blockers, epinephrine, and miotics.

Laser surgery is an effective method for treating the drainage area to improve fluid outflow. In the United States, laser surgery is used when drug therapy fails. Laser treatment properly performed has minimal side effects. The need for medication is usually greatly reduced. Current studies are examining whether laser treatment may be the preferred first treatment for glaucoma. There is also filtration surgery for treating glaucoma in which conventional surgical instruments are used to open a passage for draining of excess aqueous humor.

Acute (closed-angle) glaucoma is characterized by the iris bulging up to shut off access of the aqueous humor to the anterior chamber (see Figure 73-1). This creates an emergency because the buildup of intraocular pressure may

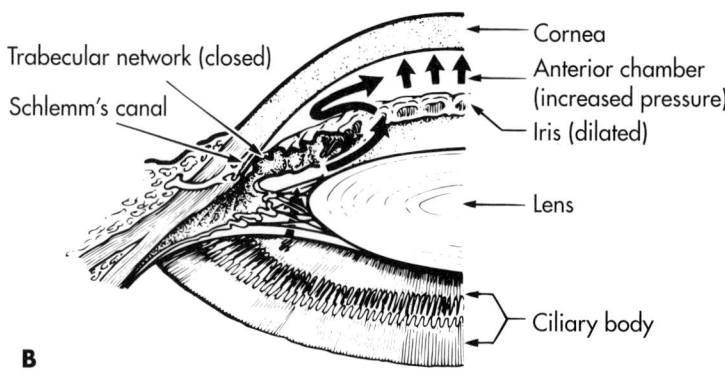

Figure 73-1 **A,** Normal eye or eye with chronic glaucoma. Flow of aqueous humor is shown from ciliary body and around iris. Aqueous humor is normally absorbed into body through trabecular network into Schlemm's canal. In chronic glaucoma, aqueous humor accumulates because trabecular network degenerates. **B,** Eye in acute glaucoma. Flow of aqueous humor is stopped because iris has blocked trabecular network and Schlemm's canal. Aqueous humor can accumulate quickly to cause a significant rise in ocular pressure that may damage optic nerve.

Box 73-1   Risk Factors for Glaucoma

- Advancing age (>40 years old)
- Intraocular pressure >20 mm Hg
- Family history of glaucoma
- African-American background
- Diabetes mellitus
- High myopia
- Systemic vascular disease

---

rapidly become severe, damaging the optic nerve and causing blindness. Emergency treatment consists of a cholinomimetic drug, a carbonic anhydrase inhibitor, epinephrine, and an osmotic diuretic. This drug regimen provides transient treatment while the patient is being prepared for eye surgery in which the iris is cut to allow fluid access to the anterior chamber once again.

THERAPEUTIC AGENTS: DRUGS TO TREAT GLAUCOMA

For a summary of the drugs commonly used to treat glaucoma, see Table 73-1.

Four major types of drugs are used to treat glaucoma: beta-blockers, adrenergic agonists, miotics (cholinomimetics), and carbonic anhydrase inhibitors. These drug classes act either by decreasing production of aqueous humor or by increasing the drainage of aqueous humor.

A beta-blocker formulated for ophthalmic administrations is commonly the first drug prescribed to treat chronic glaucoma. Beta-blockers decrease production of aqueous humor. They are effective, have a low rate of local or systemic side effects, and are applied twice a day.

The adrenergic agonist epinephrine is the alternative drug to initiate therapy. However, it can cause local allergy and ocular redness. Adrenergic drugs increase drainage of aqueous humor.

Pilocarpine is a cholinomimetic with few systemic effects when applied to the eye, but it has a short duration of action and causes blurred vision. Pilocarpine is third choice to initiate treatment. Cholinomimetics increase drainage of aqueous humor.

Several new drugs have been released to treat glaucoma. Brinzolamide and dorzolamide are carbonic anhydrase inhibitors that can be applied directly to the eye, unlike previous drugs of this class that had to be taken systemically.

Table 73-1   Drugs to Treat Glaucoma

Generic Name	Trade Name	Administration/Dosage	Comments
Beta-Blockers			
betaxolol	Betoptic*	TOPICAL: 1 drop of 0.5% solution twice daily. FDA pregnancy category C.	Cardioselective (beta-$_1$) beta-adrenergic antagonist.
carteolol hydrochloride	Ocupress	TOPICAL: 1 drop of 1% solution twice daily. FDA pregnancy category C.	Nonselective beta-adrenergic antagonist.
levobunolol	Betagan*	TOPICAL: 1 drop of 0.25% solution once or twice daily or 1 drop 0.5% solution once daily. FDA pregnancy category C.	Nonselective beta-adrenergic antagonist.
metipranolol	Optipranolol	TOPICAL: 1 drop 0.3% solution twice daily. FDA pregnancy category C.	Nonselective beta-adrenergic antagonist.
timolol maleate	Timoptic* Apo-Timop†	TOPICAL: 1 drop of 0.25% solution twice daily; if not sufficient, 0.5% solution is used. FDA pregnancy category C.	Nonselective beta-adrenergic antagonist.
Adrenergic Drugs			
apraclonidine hydrochloride	Iopidine	TOPICAL: 1 drop 0.5% solution 2 or 3 times/day.	Also used to prevent acute transient spikes in intraocular pressure after laser surgery for glaucoma.
brimonidine tartrate	Alphagan	TOPICAL: 1 drop 0.2% solution 3 times/day. FDA pregnancy category B.	New alpha$_2$-adrenergic agonist like apraclonidine.
dipivefrin hydrochloride	Propine*	TOPICAL: 1 drop 0.1% solution twice daily.	Dipivefrin is converted to epinephrine by esterases in cornea and anterior chamber.
epinephrine borate	Epinal* Eppy	TOPICAL: 1 drop of 0.25%-2.0% solution once or twice daily. FDA pregnancy category C.	Persons with darkly pigmented irises may require higher concentration of solution.
epinephrine hydrochloride	Epifrin* Glaucon*	Same as epinephrine borate.	See above.
Cholinomimetic Drugs (Weak Miotics)			
carbachol	Isopto Carbachol* Miostat*	TOPICAL: 1 drop 0.75%-3% solution 3 times/day. Onset: 15-30 min.	Carbachol is direct-acting cholinomimetic and miotic for treating chronic glaucoma.
pilocarpine hydrochloride	Isopto Carpine* Pilocar Various others	TOPICAL: 1 drop, 0.5%-4% up to 4 times/day. Onset: 15-30 min. Ocular insert: 1 system inserted every 7 days. FDA pregnancy category C.	Pilocarpine hydrochloride is direct-acting cholinomimetic and miotic; it is drug of choice for acute and chronic glaucoma.
pilocarpine nitrate	PV Carpine† Pilofrin Liquifilm Pilagan	TOPICAL: 1 drop, 1%-4% 2-4 times/day. Onset: 15-30 min. FDA pregnancy category C.	Pilocarpine nitrate is direct-acting cholinomimetic and miotic; it is drug of choice for acute and chronic glaucoma.
Cholinomimetic Drugs (Strong Miotics)			
demecarium bromide	Humorsol	TOPICAL: 1 drop 0.125%-0.25% solution every 12-48 hr. Onset: 12 hr. FDA pregnancy category X.	Demecarium bromide is irreversible acetylcholinesterase inhibitor; it is potent miotic for resistant chronic glaucoma. Cataracts can develop with long-term administration.
echothiophate iodide	Phospholine Iodide*	TOPICAL: 1 drop 0.03%-0.06% every 12-48 hr. Onset: 12 hr. FDA pregnancy category X.	Same as for demecarium.
isoflurophate	Floropryl	TOPICAL: $\frac{1}{4}$ in strip of 0.025% ointment every 12-72 hr. Onset: 12 hr. FDA pregnancy category C.	Same as for demecarium.
Carbonic Anhydrase Inhibitors			
acetazolamide	Acetazolam† AK-Zol Apo-Acetazolamide† Diamox* Others	ORAL: *Adults*—250 mg every 6 hr. *Children*—10-15 mg/kg body weight/day in divided doses; timed-release capsules taken every 12-24 hr but may not be as effective.	Acetazolamide is a weak diuretic.
acetazolamide sodium	Diamox, Parenteral*	INTRAVENOUS, INTRAMUSCULAR: *Adults*—500 mg repeated in 2-4 hr if necessary. *Children*—5-10 mg/kg body weight every 6 hr.	Intravenous or intramuscular route is used for rapid initial lowering of intraocular pressure.
brinzolamide	Azopt	TOPICAL: 1 drop 1% suspension 3 times/day.	New drug. Topical application minimizes side effects.

*Available in Canada and the United States.
†Available in Canada only.

Continued

Table 73-1	**Drugs to Treat Glaucoma—cont'd**		
Generic Name	**Trade Name**	**Administration/Dosage**	**Comments**
Carbonic Anhydrase Inhibitors—cont'd			
dichlorphenamide	Daranide	ORAL: *Adults*—100 mg twice daily initially; maintenance dose is 25-50 mg 1-3 times/day.	Carbonic anhydrase inhibitor taken systemically to treat glaucoma.
dorzolamide hydrochloride	Trusopt	TOPICAL: 1 drop 2% solution 3 times/day. FDA pregnancy category C.	Topical application minimizes side effects.
methazolamide	Neptazane*	ORAL: *Adults*—50-100 mg 2 or 3 times/day.	Carbonic anhydrase inhibitor taken systemically to treat glaucoma.
Prostaglandin Analog			
latanoprost	Xalatan	TOPICAL: 1 drop 0.005% solution once a day in the evening.	New drug class for the treatment of glaucoma.
Osmotic Agents			
glycerin	Glyrol Osmoglyn	ORAL: *Adults and children*—1-1.5 g/kg body weight as 50% or 75% solution once or twice daily.	Nurse may flavor glycerin with instant coffee or lemon juice to increase palatability. Nurse may chill it with chipped ice. Glycerin may cause hyperglycemia in diabetic patients.
mannitol	Osmitrol*	INTRAVENOUS: *Adults and children*—0.25-2 g/kg body weight as 15% or 25% solution infused over 30-60 min.	Nurse may discontinue it when intraocular pressure is decreased, even though full dose has not been given.
urea	Ureaphil	INTRAVENOUS: *Adults*—0.5-2 g/kg body weight as 30% solution infused at 60 drops/min. *Children*—0.5-1.5 g/kg body weight of 30% solution infused over 30 min.	Urea should be infused carefully. Patients with hereditary fructose intolerance should not be given urea made up in invert sugar.

*Available in Canada and the United States.
†Available in Canada only.

Brimonidine is a selective alpha$_2$-adrenergic agonist. Latanoprost is a prostaglandin F$_{2alpha}$ analog. These new drugs may alter the pharmacologic management of glaucoma.

The drugs discussed previously are all applied directly to the eye. In resistant cases of glaucoma, systemic drugs are added. A carbonic anhydrase inhibitor is the next drug added because, aside from being weak diuretics, carbonic anhydrase inhibitors are also effective in decreasing the production of aqueous humor.

Osmotic agents such as glycerin, isosorbide, urea, and mannitol provide an immediate but short-term reduction in intraocular pressure by drawing fluid from the eyeball to the hyperosmotic blood.

Beta-Blockers: General Characteristics

Mechanism of Action

Beta-adrenergic blockers act in the eye to decrease the production of aqueous humor. This action lowers intraocular pressure.

Pharmacokinetics

The beta-blockers are applied as ophthalmic solutions directly to the eye. The onset of action is 30 to 60 minutes, and the duration of action varies with the beta-blocker used. The drug is removed by gradual systemic uptake and excretion.

Uses

An ophthalmic preparation of one of the beta-blockers is the drug of choice for the initial treatment of chronic glaucoma. The major advantage of beta-blockers is that neither pupil size nor reactivity to light is altered. This is of particular benefit for young patients with active accommodation and for older adult patients with opaque lenses who cannot tolerate miotics. Some irritation and blurred vision may occur at the start of therapy, but these effects usually disappear with continued administration.

Adverse Reactions and Contraindications

Beta-blockers applied to the eye may cause ocular pain, dizziness, or headaches. The eyes may be red, and occasionally, the irritation can be severe. Other occasional side effects include blurred vision, different size of pupils, discoloration of pupil, and double vision.

Systemic concentrations of beta-blockers administered to the eye are seldom significant. Nevertheless, patients with severe cardiovascular disease or severe asthma should not take these drugs. The systemic absorption of beta-blockers may worsen asthma or may mask signs of hyperthyroidism or hypoglycemia in diabetic patients taking insulin.

Interactions

Beta-blockers provide an additive reduction in intraocular pressure when administered with topical miotics or systemically administered carbonic anhydrase inhibitors.

Specific Beta-Blockers for Ophthalmic Use

betaxolol

Betaxolol (Betoptic) is a selective beta$_1$-blocker and is preferred for patients with pulmonary problems (especially asthma) being treated for glaucoma. Betaxolol is effective for about 12 hours. The ophthalmic suspension form appears to be less irritating than the ophthalmic solution form. In general, betaxolol produces more eye irritation than the other beta-blockers.

carteolol

Carteolol (Ocupress) is effective for 6 to 8 hours after administration. Decreased night vision has been reported for carteolol.

levobunolol

Levobunolol (Betagan) has a longer onset of action (60 minutes) than the other beta-blockers. It is effective for up to 24 hours after a single dose.

metipranolol

Metipranolol (Optipranolol) is effective for up to 24 hours after administration.

▼ timolol

Timolol (Timoptic) is used not only for treating chronic glaucoma but also for treating glaucoma related to specific causes. It is as effective as pilocarpine or epinephrine in lowering intraocular pressure and is generally better tolerated.

Adrenergic Drugs

epinephrine

Mechanism of Action

Epinephrine (Epifrin, Epinal, Eppy, Glaucon) is an adrenergic agonist that stimulates alpha- and beta-adrenergic receptors (see Chapter 12). The vasoconstrictive effect resulting from stimulation of alpha-receptors decreases the production of aqueous humor and leads to a decrease in intraoptic pressure. Epinephrine dilates the pupil (mydriasis) by stimulating the dilator muscles.

Pharmacokinetics

Ophthalmic solutions of epinephrine are available as bitartrate, hydrochloride, or borate salts. The onset of action is in 1 hour and persists for 12 to 24 hours. Epinephrine is taken up by nerve endings.

Uses

Epinephrine is used to treat chronic glaucoma, commonly given with pilocarpine or a carbonic anhydrase inhibitors. It may also be combined with a beta-blocker or hyperosmotic agent. Epinephrine is also applied to the eye during eye surgery to reduce hemorrhaging and conjunctival congestion.

Adverse Reactions and Contraindications

When applied to the eye, epinephrine can produce a burning or stinging sensation and watering of the eyes. Epinephrine can also cause a headache or browache. With repeated use, a reactive redness of the eye, allergic conjunctivitis, or contact dermatitis may develop, requiring discontinuance in about 20% of patients taking epinephrine.

CASE STUDY
Glaucoma and the Elderly

Mrs. Steele, a 72-year-old grandmother, was taken to an urgent care center by her daughter after a fall at home. She has been treated for hypertension for 8 years, and was diagnosed 2 days ago with glaucoma. Further assessment reveals that her blood pressure is 118/68 lying, and 90/48 standing, her pulse is 46 beats/min, and the electrocardiograph shows sinus bradycardia. Her medications include timolol maleate (Blocadren), 40 mg/day, and betaxolol HCl (Betoptic), 0.5% solution 1 drop in each eye twice daily.

1. What could be an explanation for her fall?
2. What patient teaching would have monitored for this potential problem?
3. How can systemic absorption of ophthalmic medications be reduced or prevented?
4. What alternative medication, if any, may be suggested for the glaucoma?

Although systemic effects are uncommon, care should be used when a patient has a history of hypertension, arrhythmias, hyperthyroidism, or a recent heart attack.

Interactions

Additive reduction in intraocular pressure is seen when epinephrine is administered with topical miotics, topical beta-blockers, or systemically administered carbonic anhydrase inhibitors. Epinephrine may sensitize the heart to arrhythmias when used with halogenated hydrocarbon anesthetics or digitalis glycosides.

Other Adrenergic Drugs
apraclonidine

Apraclonidine (Iopidine) is an alpha-adrenergic agonist that acts by reducing aqueous humor formation. It can be added to glaucoma therapy short term to reduce elevated intraocular pressure. However, apraclonidine will not add any benefit to a combination of a beta-blocker and a carbonic anhydrase inhibitor. Apraclonidine is also used to prevent acute, transient spikes in intraocular pressure after laser surgery for glaucoma. The drug is administered 1 hour before surgery and again just before surgery. Side effects include upper lid elevation, conjunctival blanching, and mydriasis.

brimonidine

Brimonidine (Alphagan) is a new alpha-adrenergic agonist for ophthalmic use. It decreases aqueous humor production to lower intraocular pressure in glaucoma. It has minimal cardiovascular or pulmonary effects after application.

▼ dipivefrin

Dipivefrin (dipivalyl epinephrine) is another form of epinephrine used for the treatment of chronic glaucoma. Dipivefrin (Propine) is a prodrug that is inactive but is converted to epinephrine by esterases in the cornea and anterior chamber of the eye. Dipivefrin is more lipid soluble than epinephrine and therefore concentrates in the eye more readily than epinephrine. It produces less burning and irritation than epinephrine and causes fewer allergic reactions.

Cholinomimetics
▼ pilocarpine and carbachol
Mechanism of Action
Pilocarpine (PV Carpine, Ocusert Pilo-20/Pilo-40 Systems, Pilopine HS Gel) and **carbachol** (Miostat) are direct-acting cholinomimetic drugs formulated for ophthalmic application in treating glaucoma.

Pilocarpine and carbachol mimic the action of the neurotransmitter acetylcholine (see Chapter 11). In the eye, cholinomimetic drugs produce contraction of the sphincter (circular) muscles, which constricts the pupil, a process called miosis. Therapeutic effectiveness results from the spread of the trabecular spaces of the anterior chamber when the sphincter muscles contract. The larger area allows improved uptake of the aqueous humor, which relieves intraocular pressure.

Pharmacokinetics
Pilocarpine administered as drops of a 1% or 2% solution produces miosis in 15 to 30 minutes and lasts for 2 to 4 hours.

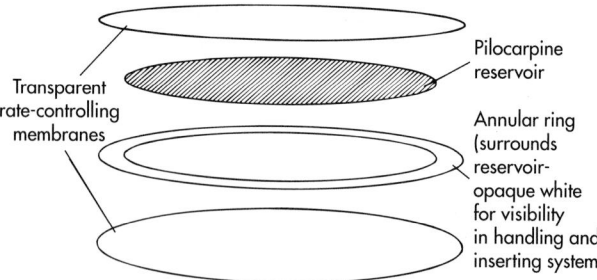

Transparent rate-controlling membranes

Pilocarpine reservoir

Annular ring (surrounds reservoir-opaque white for visibility in handling and inserting system)

Figure 73-2 Ocusert ocular therapeutic system for delivery of pilocarpine for treatment of glaucoma. Flexible wafer is placed under eyelid and provides drug for 1 week. Eyelid is shown displaced to expose device. Expanded view denotes purpose of each component. *(Courtesy ALZA Corp.)*

To increase the duration of action, pilocarpine may also be administered as a gel, which lasts 18 to 24 hours. A more sophisticated delivery system is the Ocusert system (Figure 73-2). This drug delivery system is placed in the upper or lower cul-de-sac of the eye and allows pilocarpine to slowly diffuse out. The system is designed to deliver pilocarpine over 7 days, but the duration varies with the individual.

Carbachol is more potent and slightly longer acting than pilocarpine.

Uses
Beta-blockers are now more commonly prescribed for the initial therapy for glaucoma, but pilocarpine is still widely used alone or in combination with beta-blockers and other agents to control glaucoma. Pilocarpine is also used in the emergency treatment of acute-angle glaucoma, both before and after surgery. Pilocarpine is also used to counteract the effects of cycloplegics and mydriatics after ophthalmoscopic examinations.

Carbachol is used as a replacement drug when the eyes have become resistant or intolerant to pilocarpine. Carbachol is also used to induce miosis during ocular surgery.

Adverse Reactions, Contraindications, and Toxicity
Pilocarpine is well tolerated. Because it is applied in small amounts directly to the eye, systemic effects are uncommon. The most common reaction is some stinging and local irritation. Ciliary spasm and miosis may be troublesome when starting therapy. Miosis makes vision in dim light poor, so patients should be cautioned against driving at night.

The Ocusert system may migrate and produce pain, but this is uncommon. Patients with loose lids may be unable to retain the system and may need to check for its presence each morning.

Patients with acute iritis or other conditions in which pupillary constriction is undesirable should not take pilocarpine or carbachol.

Interactions
Pilocarpine can be administered with carbonic anhydrase inhibitors, epinephrine, or beta-blockers to control glaucoma because the mechanisms of actions vary and are therefore synergistic when combined. Pilocarpine and carbachol counteract the anticholinergic effects of atropine and other anticholinergics.

Anticholinesterase Miotics
Mechanism of Action
Demecarium (Humorsol), **echothiophate** (Phospholine), and **isoflurophate** (Floropryl), the anticholinesterase miotics, inhibit the degradation of acetylcholine. The increased amount of acetylcholine then causes miosis. As with the direct-acting miotic pilocarpine therapeutic effectiveness results from the spread of the trabecular spaces of the anterior chamber when the sphincter muscles contract. The larger area allows improved uptake of the aqueous humor, which relieves intraocular pressure.

Pharmacokinetics

The anticholinesterase miotics are applied directly to the eye and are very long acting. Miosis begins in about 1 hour and lasts for up to 1 month after the drug is discontinued. Reduction in intraocular pressure begins in 4 hours and lasts about 1 to 2 days after the drug is discontinued.

Uses

Demecarium, echothiophate, and isoflurophate are potent miotics. They are generally used only for patients with chronic glaucoma that is not well controlled by other agents.

Adverse Reactions and Contraindications

Miotics inhibit accommodation, so patients taking these drugs have poor vision in dim light. Other common local effects can include browache, ocular pain, ciliary and conjunctival congestions, tearing, and twitching of the eyebrows. In patients older than 60 years of age, the development of cataracts can be accelerated.

The anticholinesterase inhibitors, especially echothiophate and demecarium, occasionally cause systemic cholinergic effects, including muscle weakness, hypersalivation, sweating, nausea, vomiting, abdominal pain, urinary incontinence, diarrhea, bradycardia, severe hypotension, and bronchospasm.

The anticholinesterase inhibitors are contraindicated during pregnancy. They are contraindicated for patients with retinal detachment or uveitis and for patients with glaucoma associated with iridocyclitis. Patients with myasthenia gravis are not good candidates for treatment with anticholinesterase miotics.

Toxicity

Symptoms of systemic toxicity include ataxia, confusion, seizures, coma, and muscle paralysis. The most common symptoms in children are abdominal cramps and diarrhea, with a runny nose and tearing.

Interactions

Other agents with anticholinesterase activity should be avoided when an anticholinesterase miotic is taken because of the additive toxicity. Drugs to avoid include atropine, anticholinesterases for treatment of myasthenia gravis, and pesticides with anticholinesterase activity.

Demecarium, echothiophate, and isoflurophate can decrease plasma concentrations of plasma cholinesterases, thereby enhancing the neuromuscular blockade of succinylcholine. This effect can be present for several weeks or months after the anticholinesterase has been discontinued.

Carbonic Anhydrase Inhibitors

acetazolamide

Mechanism of Action

Carbonic anhydrase inhibitors decrease the formation of aqueous humor by 50% to 60% by blocking ocular carbonic anhydrase. A fall in intraocular pressure is seen only in individuals with glaucoma. The fall in intraocular pressure is negligible in individuals with normal ocular pressure.

Pharmacokinetics

Carbonic anhydrase inhibitors are given orally and distributed throughout the body. Acetazolamide (Diamox) formulated in tablets has an onset of action in about 1 hour, with a duration of action of 8 to 12 hours. The bioavailability of acetazolamide varies significantly with some brands. Formulated in extended-release capsules, acetazolamide has an onset of action of 2 hours and a duration of action of 18 to 24 hours. The drug is excreted unchanged in the urine.

Uses

Acetazolamide is used principally as an adjunct in the treatment of chronic glaucoma when other drugs alone do not control intraocular pressure. Acetazolamide is also used with osmotic agents, miotics, and beta-blockers for the emergency treatment of acute (closed-angle) glaucoma on a short-term basis only. Acetazolamide is also used as an anticonvulsant and in the treatment of altitude sickness. Carbonic anhydrase inhibitors are weak diuretics but are no longer used for this purpose.

Adverse Reactions and Contraindications

Acetazolamide is generally not well tolerated for prolonged therapy. Malaise, weight loss, fatigue, headache, nervousness, loss of libido, impotence, and tingling sensations are all common side effects. Infants show a failure to thrive. Occasionally, acetazolamide causes confusion, ataxia, tremor, and tinnitus. Diuresis is common initially but usually subsides. Hypokalemia is a problem if other drugs are taken that lower body potassium.

Acetazolamide may precipitate acute pulmonary failure in patients with chronic obstructive lung disease. Gout may also be precipitated in patients with a history of this disease. Acetazolamide is also teratogenic and should be avoided in pregnancy. Patients with renal failure develop excessively high concentrations of the drug.

Interactions

Acetazolamide is highly bound to plasma protein. Diflunisal, a nonsteroidal antiinflammatory drug, has been reported to displace bound acetazolamide, thereby increasing side effects.

Acetazolamide increases the pH of the urine to the alkaline range, which decreases the excretion of several drugs, including amphetamines, anticholinergics, mecamylamine, and quinidine. These drugs may reach toxic levels if their dosage is not lowered. The bacteriostatic activity of methenamine is decreased in an alkaline urine.

Other Carbonic Anhydrase Inhibitors

brinzolamide

Brinzolamide (Azopt) is a new topical carbonic anhydrase inhibitor used for the treatment of glaucoma.

dichlorphenamide

Dichlorphenamide (Daranide) has an onset of action of 30 to 60 minutes and a duration of action of 6 to 12 hours.

dorzolamide

Dorzolamide (Trusopt) is the first carbonic anhydrase inhibitor formulated for direct application into the eye. The most common side effect is a bitter taste. The drug is systemically absorbed and accumulates in red blood cells bound to carbonic anhydrase. The systemic concentration is considered too low to have an effect on renal or pulmonary function. However, patients with a history of kidney stones should not be given dorzolamide.

Cosopt is a combination drug for ophthalmic application containing dorzolamide and timolol. It is administered once a day.

methazolamide

Methazolamide (Neptazane) has an onset of action of 2 to 4 hours and a duration of action of 10 to 18 hours. It is not as highly protein bound as acetazolamide. Only 25% of the drug is excreted unchanged in the urine.

Prostaglandin Analog

latanoprost

Latanoprost (Xalatan) is an analog of prostaglandin $F_{2-alpha}$. It acts to increase the outflow of aqueous humor. Thus it the first prostaglandin analog used for the treatment of glaucoma. It is applied once a day in the evening. A few patients have gradual changes in eye color as a result of an increased amount of brown pigment in the iris. Other local effects can include stinging, blurred vision, redness, and the feeling of having a foreign body in the eye.

Specific Osmotic Agents

The osmotic agents are used as short-term treatment only to lower the intraocular pressure of glaucoma before surgery or as an emergency treatment of acute (closed-angle) glaucoma. Glycerin and isosorbide are administered orally, whereas mannitol and urea are administered intravenously.

glycerin

Glycerin (Glyrol, Osmoglyn) lowers intraocular pressure 1 hour after ingestion, and the effect lasts 5 hours. Because glycerin is metabolized, it does not cause diuresis; however, glycerin can cause hyperglycemia in diabetic patients. Headache, nausea, and vomiting are additional side effects of glycerin.

mannitol

Mannitol (Osmitrol) is effective in lowering intraocular pressure in 30 to 60 minutes, with the effect lasting 6 to 8 hours. Mannitol produces a pronounced diuresis and often causes headache, nausea and vomiting, and dehydration.

urea

Urea (Ureaphil) is less satisfactory than mannitol because it can penetrate the eye and cause a rebound increase in intraocular pressure when the systemic osmotic effect is over, 8 to 12 hours after administration. Urea is also highly irritating on injection.

Nursing Process Overview

Drugs to Treat Glaucoma

Assessment

Patients requiring treatment of glaucoma may have no visible signs of their condition. Assess the patient, focusing on symptoms related to the eye. Check peripheral vision, and test visual acuity using a Snellen chart. Question patients about recent difficulties driving or ambulating. Examine the eyes for signs of infection, exudate, excessive tearing or dryness, or other deviations.

Nursing Diagnoses

- Risk for injury related to impaired vision related to specific eye problem

Patient Outcomes

The patient will sustain no injury related to impaired vision.

Planning/Implementation

The drugs discussed in this chapter are used to treat glaucoma. Other eye medications include antibiotics, glucocorticoids, and lubricants. Caution the patient about side effects, particularly those related to vision. Inform the patient about possible systemic side effects (see Table 73-1).

Evaluation

Drugs used to treat glaucoma are successful if the intraocular pressure is lowered to within safe limits. Before discharge, ensure that the patient understands why the drug is being used, how to administer the drug correctly, what potential local and systemic side effects may occur, which signs and symptoms require medical evaluation, and why continuing therapy is needed (if ordered).

Nursing Implications Summary

General Guidelines: Drugs to Treat Glaucoma
Drug Administration

➤ Wash hands carefully before administering eye medications to avoid contaminating the eye or applicator. Wash hands after administering eye medications to rinse off any residue that might accidentally be rubbed into your eye. Use a separate bottle or tube of medication for each patient to avoid accidental cross-contamination; wash hands between seeing patients.

➤ Place the ordered dose of eye medication in the lower conjunctival sac, never directly onto the cornea. Avoid touching any part of the eye with the dropper or applicator. For additional information about administration, see Chapter 5.

➤ To prevent overflow of medication into nasal and pharyngeal passages, thus reducing systemic absorption, occlude (or teach the patient to occlude) the nasolacrimal duct with one finger for 1 to 2 minutes after instilling the medication. This is especially important when these medications are used in infants or children.

➤ When two or more eye medications are administered, wait at least 3 minutes between administering drugs. Administer drops or liquid preparations before ointments. Administer glucocorticoid preparations before other drugs. If in doubt, consult the physician.

➤ Monitor the pulse of a patient receiving beta-blockers, and instruct the patient to do the same. If the pulse is less than 50 to 60 beats/min in an adult, withhold the next dose of medication and notify the physician. Reassess whether the patient is occluding the nasolacrimal duct correctly after administration of each dose.

➤ Use 1 drop of a 1% or 2% epinephrine solution to reverse the redness caused by potent acetylcholinesterase inhibitors; consult the physician.

➤ Use pralidoxime (PAM), 0.1 to 0.2 ml of a 5% solution, to reverse the action of the irreversible acetylcholinesterase inhibitors. PAM must be injected subconjunctivally to be effective in the eye (see Chapter 11).

➤ Glycerin may cause hyperglycemia. Monitor blood glucose levels, especially in diabetic patients.

➤ See Chapter 14 for additional information about carbonic anhydrase inhibitors, mannitol, and urea.

Nursing in the Community

➤ Teach the patient how to instill medication correctly, and supervise instillation until the patient can do it safely (see section on drug administration and Chapter 5). Instruct the patient to read labels carefully to ensure administration of correct drug and correct strength. Remind the patient to keep these and all drugs out of the reach of children.

➤ Some of these drugs are dispensed with a special cap (Compliance cap or "C" cap) to help patients keep track of their doses. See manufacturer's leaflet or demonstrate how to turn cap after each use to keep track of doses.

➤ Warn the patient to avoid driving or operating hazardous equipment if vision is blurred. If the patient is using eye medications that cause pupillary constriction, caution the patient to be careful driving at night or doing any potentially dangerous activities in dim light because vision may be impaired.

➤ If photophobia occurs, instruct the patient to wear sunglasses and to avoid bright lights. Instruct the patient not to wear sunglasses after dusk.

➤ Instruct the patient to administer missed doses as soon as they are remembered, unless within 1 to 2 hours of the next dose, in which case omit the missed dose and resume regular dosing schedule. Instruct the patient not to double up for missed doses.

➤ Instruct the patient to lie down if headache occurs after doses of glycerin. To make doses of glycerin or isosorbide more palatable, encourage the patient to chill them over crushed ice and to flavor glycerin with instant coffee or lemon juice.

➤ Inform diabetic patients that beta-blockers may affect blood glucose levels. Instruct these patients to monitor blood glucose levels. Observe patients' drug administration technique. Occluding the nasolacrimal duct may decrease systemic drug absorption.

➤ Inform a patient with glaucoma that it cannot be cured, only controlled. Reinforce the importance of using medications to treat glaucoma as prescribed and not to discontinue these medications without consulting the physician. Drugs used to treat glaucoma may cause pain and blurred vision, especially when therapy is begun. Inform the patient that this may diminish with time. Encourage the patient to try cold compresses to relieve painful eye spasm.

➤ Instruct the patient to report the development of any eye irritation.

➤ Instruct a patient using eye gel to store the gel at room temperature or in the refrigerator but not to freeze it. Unused gel kept at room temperature should be discarded after 8 weeks. After each use, instruct the patient to wipe the tip of the tube with tissue and replace the cap tightly.

➤ Soft contact lenses may absorb certain eye medications, and preservatives in eye medications may discolor the contact lenses. Encourage a patient wearing contact lenses to question the physician or pharmacist carefully about special precautions to observe.

➤ For sustained-release forms: Instruct the patient to review carefully the manufacturer's instruction sheet. The eye system is inserted into the upper or lower cul-de-sac of the eye, and the drug is released slowly; the system should be replaced weekly. Instruct the patient to check each morning and evening to make sure the system is still in place. If the unit does not seem to be working, is damaged, or is releasing too much medication, instruct the patient to remove it and

Continued

Nursing Implications Summary—cont'd

insert a new one. Because vision may change in the first few hours after the eye system is inserted, advise the patient to replace it at bedtime. Instruct the patient to store the eye system in the refrigerator but to avoid freezing it.

➤ For patients using isoflurophate eye ointment: This drug loses its effectiveness when exposed to moisture, so caution the patient not to wash the tip of the ointment tube or allow it to touch moist surfaces, including the eye itself. To clean off tip of tube, instruct the patient to wipe with a dry tissue.

➤ For patients using anticholinesterase miotics (cholinomimetics) (e.g., demecarium, isoflurophate, echothiophate): See

Interactions. Caution patients who are farmers, gardeners, workers in plants that produce these pesticides, or residents of areas where pesticides or insecticides are sprayed to avoid contact with these sprays and to wear a mask over the nose and mouth if they must be in the area when spraying occurs. Examples of these pesticides and insecticides include Sevin, diazinon, malathion, and parathion.

➤ Many of these medications are contraindicated during pregnancy. Instruct women to notify the physician if they become pregnant or are planning to become pregnant.

CHAPTER REVIEW

Application

1. Describe glaucoma and the role of aqueous humor.
2. Differentiate between chronic and acute glaucoma.
3. How are carbonic anhydrase inhibitors and osmotic agents used to treat glaucoma?
4. When two or more eye medications are ordered to be given at the same time, what are the guidelines for the sequence of administrations?
5. What are the abbreviations for left eye, right eye, and both eyes that may be used when eye medications are ordered? (See Chapter 5.)

Critical Thinking

1. How are cholinomimetic drugs used to treat glaucoma? Which drugs might a nurse administer in the treatment of glaucoma?
2. What role do drugs acting as adrenergic receptors play in the treatment of glaucoma? Describe the actions of epinephrine and timolol.
3. How would you determine whether a patient is administering ordered eye medications correctly?

REFERENCES

Miller CA: Drug consult. Keeping an eye on the hidden effects of eye drops. *Geriatr Nurs* 19(5):293-294, 1998.

Whitaker R Jr, Whitaker VB, Dill C: Glaucoma: what the nurse practitioner should know, *Nurse Pract Forum* 9(1):7-12, 1998.

Other Ophthalmic Agents

OBJECTIVES

After studying this chapter, you should be able to do the following:

- *Define miosis, mydriasis, and cycloplegia, and give examples of when they are therapeutically produced.*
- *Discuss the use of anticholinergic drugs for the eye.*
- *Discuss the use of nonsteroidal antiinflammatory drugs for the eye.*

CHAPTER OVERVIEW

The key functions of the eye are controlled by the autonomic nervous system. Selected drugs with autonomic actions are used in eye examinations, eye surgery, and glaucoma treatment. These ophthalmic drugs are presented in this chapter.

THERAPEUTIC RATIONALE: EXAMINING THE EYE

An internal examination of the eye requires dilation of the pupil (**mydriasis**) and paralysis of accommodation (**cycloplegia**). These actions require the use of parasympathetic and sympathetic drugs.

The autonomic nervous system controls the amount of light entering the eye and in focusing images. The amount of light penetrating the eye is controlled by the size of the pigmented iris, which contains two sets of muscles—the sphincter and dilator muscles. The sphincter muscles are circular muscles with muscarinic receptors innervated by the parasympathetic nervous system. As shown in Figure 74-1, the pupil is constricted when the sphincter muscles contract so that only a small surface on the eye transmits light. The dilator muscles contain alpha-receptors innervated by the sympathetic nervous system. **Miosis** refers to a constricted pupil and is achieved primarily by stimulating the muscarinic receptors of the sphincter muscles. *Mydriasis* refers to a dilated pupil and is achieved by blocking the muscarinic receptors of the sphincter muscles or by stimulating the alpha-receptors of the dilator muscles.

The cornea and the lens determine the focus of images onto the retina. The cornea accomplishes the coarse focusing, but the fine focusing for sharp images and near vision is accomplished by the lens. The shape of the lens is controlled by muscarinic receptors of the parasympathetic nervous system. As diagrammed in Figure 74-1, the accommodation for near vision requires the contraction of ciliary muscles to change the shape of the lens. Ligaments normally pull the lens to keep it relatively flat. Contraction of the ciliary muscles relaxes the ligaments so that the lens becomes more round as required for near vision. *Cycloplegia* refers to the paralysis of the ciliary muscles by drugs that block muscarinic receptors. Cycloplegia causes blurred vision because the shape of the lens can no longer be adjusted to near vision.

THERAPEUTIC AGENTS: DRUGS TO ACHIEVE MYDRIASIS

Mydriasis is achieved with anticholinergic drugs or with adrenergic drugs. Anticholinergic drugs also cause cycloplegia. Prostaglandin inhibitors prevent miosis related to prostaglandin synthesis. Drugs from all these classes are listed in Table 74-1.

Anticholinergics: General Characteristics

Mechanism of Action

Classic anticholinergic actions include dilated pupils (mydriasis) and blurred vision (cycloplegia). Anticholinergic drugs block the muscarinic receptors of the sphincter

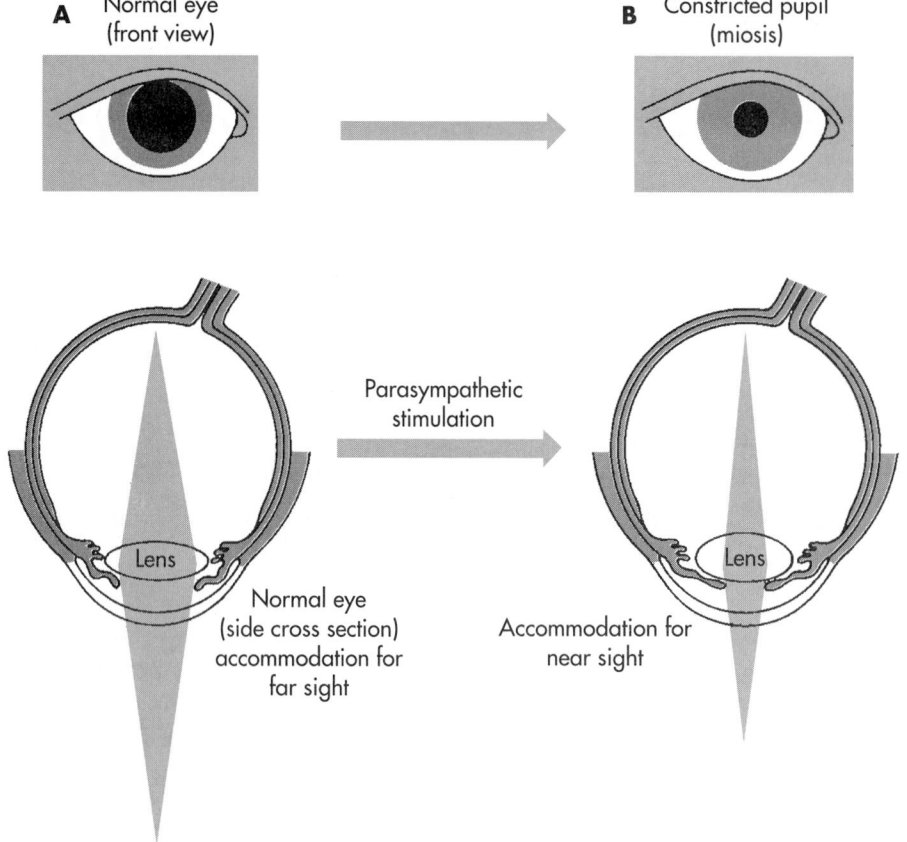

A, Normal eye
(front view)

B, Constricted pupil
(miosis)

Parasympathetic
stimulation

Lens

Lens

Normal eye
(side cross section)
accommodation for
far sight

Accommodation for
near sight

Figure 74-1 **A,** Normal eye. Effects of parasympathetic nervous system on eye are mediated through muscarinic receptors. **B,** Pupil is made smaller because circular muscles contract. Accommodation is made by contracting muscles to thicken lens.

muscles, so the pupil cannot contract (see Figure 74-1). The ciliary muscles controlling the shape of the lens are also paralyzed, so the eye can no longer accommodate and produce focused images.

Pharmacokinetics

These agents are solutions or ointments instilled in the eye. The onset and duration of action depend on the agent and the strength of the solution. The drug is gradually removed through systemic circulation.

Uses

The major use of the anticholinergic drugs is to induce mydriasis and cycloplegia for examination of the eye. Accurate measurement of lens refraction requires both actions. Some anticholinergics are used in the treatment of inflammation of the eye (uveitis). The relaxation of sphincter and ciliary muscles hastens healing of inflammatory conditions, especially after eye surgery.

Adverse Reactions and Contraindications

Systemic reactions may occur when the anticholinergic drug is absorbed into the body, particularly with atropine. Systemic reactions are associated with anticholinergic effects such as dry mouth and dry skin, fever, thirst, confusion, and

hyperactivity. Children are the most prone to systemic toxicity from ophthalmic drugs.

Acute (closed-angle) glaucoma may occur in certain patients when the iris crowds the anterior chamber. Patients with keratoconus (protrusion of the central cornea) or Down's syndrome are especially sensitive to the mydriatic effect of anticholinergic drugs.

Interactions

Physostigmine salicylate, an indirect-acting cholinergic drug, is an effective antidote to reverse systemic anticholinergic toxicity but not for hypotensive reactions.

Specific Anticholinergic Drugs
▼ atropine

Atropine (Atropair, Ocu-Tropine, others) is the drug of choice for use in children because it is potent and long acting and children have an active accommodation. Mydriasis may last 12 days, although accommodation usually returns in 6 days. Because atropine is applied for 3 days, the child should be watched for systemic reactions and application discontinued if any reactions appear. The child will also require protection from bright light.

Atropine is also used before surgery (often with phenylephrine) to produce mydriasis and for other conditions re-

Table 74-1 Drugs for Mydriasis and Cycloplegia

Generic Name	Trade Name	Administration/Dosage	Comments
Anticholinergic Drugs for Mydriasis and Cycloplegia			
atropine sulfate	Atropair Atropisol* Isopto-Atropine* Minims Atropine† Ocu-Tropine Others	TOPICAL SOLUTIONS: 0.5%-3%. *Adults*—1 drop of 1%-3% solution to each eye. Frequency of administration depends on condition being treated. *Children <8 yr*—1 drop of 0.125%-0.5 solution. *Children >8 yr*—0.25%-1% solution 3 times/day for 3 days before and once on morning of day refraction is measured. Duration: 6 days.	For children, for refraction measurements. For adults, to relax eye muscles during surgery or treatment of eye inflammation.
cyclopentolate hydrochloride	AK-Pentolate* Cyclogyl* I-Pentolate Minims Cyclopentolate† Pentolair Others	TOPICAL SOLUTIONS: 0.5%, 1%, and 2%. *Adults*—1 drop of solution in each eye, repeated after 5 min. Patients with darker irises and children require stronger solutions. *Children*—1 drop of solution in eye, repeated after 10 min. Onset: 25-75 min. Duration: 6-24 hr.	To aid in measuring refraction.
homatropine hydrobromide	AK-Homatropine Isopto Homatrine* I-Homatrine† Spectro-Homatrine	TOPICAL SOLUTIONS: 2% and 5%. *Adults—For refraction:* 1 drop of 5% solution is applied 2 or 3 times at 10-min intervals. Duration: 2 days.	To aid in refraction measurements in adults; to aid in treating mild eye inflammation.
scopolamine hydrobromide	Isopto Hyoscine	TOPICAL SOLUTION: 0.25%. *Adults*—1 drop of solution or ointment to each eye. 1 or more times daily, depending on condition being treated. *Children*—1 drop of solution or ointment twice daily for 2 days before refraction measurement. Duration: 3 days.	For children, to measure refraction. For adults, to treat eye inflammation.
tropicamide	I-Picamide Mydriacyl* Minims Tropicamide† Tropicacyl Various others	TOPICAL SOLUTIONS: 0.5% and 1%. *Adults and children*—1 drop in each eye; repeated in 5 min. Onset: 20-35 min. Duration: 2-6 hr.	To aid in measuring refraction.
Adrenergic Drugs for Mydriasis Only			
phenylephrine hydrochloride	AK-Dilate* Dilatair Mydfrin* Ocu-Phrin* Others	TOPICAL: 1 drop of 2.5% solution.	To obtain maximum mydriasis in 60-90 min. To obtain recovery in 6 hr.
Alpha-Adrenergic Blocker			
dapiprazole hydrochloride	Rev-Eyes*	TOPICAL: 1 drop 0.5% solution after completion of the retinal examination, followed by another drop in 5 min.	To counteract mydriasis induced by phenylephrine and, to a lesser degree, by tropicamide.
Prostaglandin Inhibitors			
diclofenac	Voltaren Ophthalmic Voltaren Ophtha†	TOPICAL: 1 drop 0.1% solution 4 times/day.	To treat inflammation after cataract surgery.
flurbiprofen sodium	Ocufen*	TOPICAL: 1 drop 0.03% solution instilled every 30 min beginning 2 hr before surgery; total dose: 4 drops.	To prevent miosis during surgery. (Nonsteroidal antiinflammatory drug is applied topically.)
suprofen	Profenal	TOPICAL: 2 drops 1% solution are applied 3, 2, and 1 hr before surgery; 2 drops may be applied every 4 hr during waking hours day before surgery.	To prevent miosis during surgery. (Nonsteroidal antiinflammatory drug is applied topically.)

*Available in Canada and the United States.
†Available in Canada only.

quiring prolonged mydriasis. Atropine may cause contact dermatitis of the eyelids.

cyclopentolate

Cyclopentolate (Cyclogyl) is a rapidly acting mydriatic and cycloplegic drug. It is effective in 25 to 75 minutes, and ac-commodation returns in 6 to 24 hours. Cyclopentolate is used as for aiding refraction, for ophthalmoscopy, and for preoperative mydriasis. Systemic reactions have been reported. A combination of cyclopentolate and phenylephrine (Cyclomydril) is used and is the combination of choice for use with premature infants.

homatropine

Homatropine (AK-Homatropine) is applied two or three times at 10-minute intervals to produce mydriasis and cycloplegia, which are achieved in 60 minutes. Recovery may take 2 days.

scopolamine

Scopolamine (Isopto Hyoscine) is a potent mydriatic and is used like atropine, but cycloplegia lasts for only 3 days instead of 6 days. Scopolamine can be used in patients who are allergic to atropine.

tropicamide

Tropicamide (Mydriacyl) acts rapidly, taking effect in 20 to 35 minutes. Accommodation returns in 2 to 6 hours. Systemic side effects are rare. This agent is most commonly used for routine eye examinations.

Adrenergic Drugs

The adrenergic drug phenylephrine is used as a mydriatic when only the interior structures of the eye are examined and cycloplegia is not required. The alpha-adrenergic blocker dapiprazole is used to reverse the mydriasis produced by phenylephrine.

▼ phenylephrine

Phenylephrine (AK-Dilate, Dilatair, Mydfrin, Ocu-Phrin) acts on the alpha-receptors of the dilator muscles to produce mydriasis without cycloplegia. Dilation is maximal in 60 to 90 minutes, and recovery occurs in 6 hours. Cyclomydril is a combination of cyclopentolate and phenylephrine used when maximal dilation is required.

Phenylephrine is also used in the treatment of uveitis and postoperative inflammation. Dilute solutions of phenylephrine are used to bring temporary relief of the redness of the eyes caused by minor eye irritations.

dapiprazole

Dapiprazole (Rev-Eyes) is an alpha-adrenergic blocking agent used to reverse the mydriasis produced by phenylephrine and to a lesser degree tropicamide. Dapiprazole acts rapidly but is slower acting in more heavily pigmented brown eyes than in blue or green eyes. About 50% of patients experience a burning sensation when the drops are applied. About 80% have a redness of the eye (conjunctival injection) lasting about 20 minutes.

Prostaglandin Inhibitors

Flurbiprofen (Ocufen) and suprofen (Profenal) are nonsteroidal antiinflammatory drugs (NSAIDs) specifically for ophthalmic use (see Table 74-1). Ophthalmic surgery may stimulate the synthesis of prostaglandins in the eye. Prostaglandins are chemical transmitters synthesized in response to stimulation, locally in tissues. In the eye, newly synthesized prostaglandins cause a miosis that resists the mydriatic action of atropine. The locally applied NSAIDs prevent miosis during surgery.

Diclofenac (Voltaren Ophthalmic) is an NSAID used ophthalmically to treat inflammation after cataract surgery.

Nursing Process Overview

Drugs to Treat Eye Conditions

Assessment

Patients requiring treatment of eye conditions may have no visible signs of their condition. Assess the patient, focusing on symptoms related to the eye. Check peripheral vision, and test visual acuity using a Snellen chart. Question the patient about recent difficulties driving or ambulating at home; such difficulties might include tripping or bumping into objects. Examine the eyes for signs of infection, exudate, excessive tearing or dryness, or other deviations.

Nursing Diagnoses

- Risk for injury related to impaired vision related to specific eye problem
- Altered home maintenance management related to insufficient knowledge about eye medications, their use, or their instillation

Patient Outcomes

The patient will sustain no injury related to impaired vision. The patient will demonstrate correct use of eye medications

Planning/Implementation

The drugs discussed in this chapter are used to assist evaluation of eye problems or to treat specific problems. Other eye medications include antibiotics, glucocorticoids, and lubricants. Caution the patient about side effects, particularly those related to vision. Blurred vision, photophobia, and other symptoms can be frightening when they occur without warning. Teach the patient about possible systemic side effects.

Evaluation

Drugs used to assist in diagnostic evaluation of the eye are successful if they aid in the examination without producing serious side effects. Before discharge, ensure that the patient understands why the drug is being used, how to administer the drug correctly, what potential local and systemic side effects can occur, which signs and symptoms require medical evaluation, and why continuing therapy is needed (if ordered).

Nursing Implications Summary

Drugs Affecting the Eye
Drug Administration

➤ Wash hands carefully before administering eye medications to avoid contaminating the eye or applicator. Wash hands after administering eye medications to rinse off any residue that might accidentally be rubbed into your eye. Use a separate bottle or tube of medication for each patient to avoid accidental cross-contamination; wash hands between seeing patients.

➤ Place the ordered dose of eye medication in the lower conjunctival sac, never directly onto the cornea. Avoid touching any part of the eye with the dropper or applicator. For additional information on administration, see Chapter 5.

➤ To prevent overflow of medication into nasal and pharyngeal passages, thus reducing systemic absorption, occlude (or teach the patient to occlude) the nasolacrimal duct with one finger for 1 to 2 minutes after instilling the medication.

➤ When two or more eye medications are administered, wait at least 3 minutes between administering drugs. Administer drops or liquid preparations before ointments. Administer glucocorticoid preparations before other drugs. If in doubt, consult the physician.

➤ Use atropine and the belladonna alkaloids cautiously in older adult patients because these drugs may precipitate an acute attack of glaucoma.

Nursing in the Community

➤ Teach the patient how to instill medication correctly, and supervise instillation until the patient can do it safely (see Drug Administration and Chapter 5). Instruct the patient to read labels carefully to ensure administration of correct drug and correct strength. Remind the patient to keep all drugs out of the reach of children.

➤ Warn the patient to avoid driving or operating hazardous equipment if vision is blurred. Caution adults that they may be unable to drive home after eye examinations in which medications to dilate the pupil (mydriatics) or drugs to paralyze the ciliary muscle (cycloplegics) were used; a friend or family member should drive until the effects of the medication wear off.

➤ If photophobia occurs, instruct the patient to wear sunglasses and to avoid bright lights. Instruct the patient not to wear sunglasses after dusk.

➤ Instruct the patient to administer missed doses as soon as they are remembered, unless within 1 to 2 hours of the next dose, in which case omit the missed dose and resume regular dosing schedule. Instruct the patient not to double up for missed doses.

➤ In infants, atropine eyedrops may contribute to abdominal distension. Instruct caregivers to keep a record of bowel movements of infants. In the health care setting, auscultate bowel sounds of infants and children receiving atropine eyedrops.

➤ Instruct the patient to report the development of any eye irritation.

➤ Soft contact lenses may absorb certain eye medications, and preservatives in eye medications may discolor the contact lenses. Encourage a patient wearing contact lenses to question the physician carefully about special precautions to observe.

➤ See Chapter 73 for information about eye gel and sustained-release forms.

 ## CHAPTER REVIEW

Application

1. Which anticholinergic drugs might you administer in the eye?

2. When two or more eye medications are ordered to be given at the same time, what are the guidelines for the sequence of administrations?

3. What are the abbreviations for left eye, right eye, and both eyes that may be used when eye medications are ordered? (See Chapter 5.)

Critical Thinking

1. Explain what you would observe in a patient given a drug to produce miosis, mydriasis, or cycloplegia.

2. What would you observe when anticholinergic drugs are applied to the eye? How are these actions medically useful?

3. What action is mediated by the alpha-adrenergic receptor in the eye? Which drugs might you administer for this effect?

4. How would you determine whether a patient is administering ordered eye medications correctly?

P-450 Drug-Metabolizing Enzymes

CYP3A4: Responsible for metabolism of about 60% of drugs metabolized by P-450 enzymes.

Inducers:	anticonvulsants	Examples of drugs metabolized:	benzodiazepines
	glucocorticoids		codeine
	rifampin		cyclosporine
Inhibitors:	cimetidine		dextromethorphan
	ciprofloxacin		diltiazem
	econazole		estrogens
	erythromycin		fentanyl
	grapefruit juice		halothane
	itraconazole		lidocaine
	ketoconazole		methadone
	norfloxacin		midazolam
			nifedipine
			omeprazole
			paclitaxel
			progesterone
			ritonavir
			saquinavir
			tacrolimus
			testosterone

CYP2D6: Responsible for metabolism of about 25% of drugs metabolized by P-450 enzymes.

Inducers:	unknown	Examples of drugs metabolized:	clomipramine
			codeine
			dextromethorphan
Inhibitors:	amitriptyline		lovastatin
	quinidine		methamphetamine
			metoprolol
			propranolol

CYP2C: Responsible for metabolism of about 20% of drugs metabolized by P-450 enzymes.

Inducers:	phenobarbital	Examples of drugs metabolized:	diazepam
			imipramine
Inhibitors:	azole antifungals		phenytoin
	fluoxetine		mephenytoin
	phenylbutazone		tolbutamide
			warfarin

CYP1A2: Usually minor contributor to drug metabolism.

Inducers:	cigarette smoke	Examples of drugs metabolized:	acetaminophen
			aflatoxin B1
Inhibitors:	fluvoxamine		caffeine
	grapefruit juice		phenacetin
			methadone
			theophylline
			verapamil

CYP2E1: Usually minor contributor to drug metabolism.

Inducers:	ethanol (chronic)	Examples of drugs metabolized:	acetaminophen
	isoniazid		dextromethorphan
			ethanol
Inhibitors:	4-methylpyrazole		halothane
			enflurane

*Summary of Drugs with Common Side Effects**

Drugs That Cause Central Nervous System Depression

alcohol
anesthetics
anticonvulsants
antidepressants
antihistamines, H-1
barbiturates
benzodiazepines
beta-adrenergic blocking agents
chloral hydrate
fluoxetine
haloperidol
meclizine
meprobamate
opioid analgesics
paregoric
paroxetine
phenothiazines
rauwolfia alkaloids
scopolamine

Drugs That Cause Hearing Loss

aminoglycoside antibiotics
bumetanide
carboplatin
chloroquine
cisplatin
ethacrynic acid
furosemide
quinidine
salicylates
vancomycin

Drugs That Induce Hepatic Drug-Metabolizing Enzymes

alcohol, chronic
barbiturates
carbamazepine
glutethimide
griseofulvin
nevirapine
phenytoin
primidone
rifampin
saquinavir
troglitazone

Drugs That Inhibit Hepatic Drug-Metabolizing Enzymes

alcohol, acute
allopurinol
antidepressants
azole antifungals
cimetidine
clarithromycin
contraceptives containing estrogen
diltiazem
erythromycin
fluoroquinolones
isoniazid
metoprolol
omeprazole
paroxetine
phenylbutazone
propranolol
quinidine
valproic acid
verapamil

Drugs That Are Hepatotoxic

acetaminophen
alcohol
anabolic steroids
androgens
ACE inhibitors
anti-inflammatory drugs
azole antifungals
carbamazepine
carmustine
erythromycin
estrogens
ethionamide
halothane
HMG-CoA reductase inhibitors
isoniazid
labetalol
niacin
pemoline
phenothiazines
phenytoin
propylthiouracil
rifampin
sulfonamides
valproic acid
vitamin A
zidovudine

Drugs That Are Nephrotoxic

acyclovir
aminoglycosides
amphotericin B
analgesics
ciprofloxacin
cisplatin
cyclosporine
edetate
lithium
methoxyflurane
rifampin
sulfonamides
tetracyclines
vancomycin

Drugs That Cause Pancreatitis

alcohol
asparaginase
azathioprine
estrogens
furosemide
methyldopa
pentamidine
sulfonamides
sulindac
tetracyclines
thiazides
valproic acid

Drugs That Cause Peripheral Neuropathy

chloramphenicol
cisplatin
dapsone
ethambutol
ethionamide
hydralazine
isoniazid
lithium
metronidazole
nitrofurantoin
nitrous oxide
phenytoin
stavudine
vincristine
zalcitabine

*These lists are not exhaustive but are intended to list more common agents with the activity noted.

Appendix C

Suggested Answers to Case Studies

CHAPTER 1

Pharmacokinetics

1. For any drug given on a regular schedule, it takes about four half-lives to achieve a plateau concentration in blood. The half-life of clemastine is about 12 hours; therefore the plateau would be achieved in about 48 hours (4 × 12 hours).

2. After 4 days of taking the original dosage, the patient complained of dry mouth and other symptoms that suggested drug side effects. The symptoms were like those produced by anticholinergic drugs (see Chapter 11). Clemastine is known to cause anticholinergic effects (see Chapter 29). Because 4 days was long enough for the plateau concentration to have been achieved and because the symptoms that developed were consistent with anticholinergic side effects, the dosage of clemastine was lowered.

3. Because the dosage interval has been lengthened but the amount of drug is given in a single dose is the same, the effect is to give a longer period for drug elimination during each dosing interval; therefore the plateau concentration of drug falls to a new, lower level. This new plateau is below the threshold for toxicity and should thus minimize dose-related side effects of the drug. These changes are shown in Figure A-1.

4. On the once-daily dosage schedule James seems to be losing control of his allergic symptoms at the end of each dosing interval. One possible explanation is that the wide swings in concentrations of drug in the blood produced by this regimen cause the trough (lowest) levels to fall below the minimum effective concentration for this patient (see Figure A-1).

5. Figure A-1 shows that after an initial slight fall in average blood concentration, the final dosage regimen causes blood levels to return to the previous plateau within four half-lives. The advantage with the dosing regimen of 1.34 mg every 12 hours is that the fluctuations in blood levels are smaller than with 2.68 mg given every 24 hours. Therefore the trough values do not fall into the ineffective range.

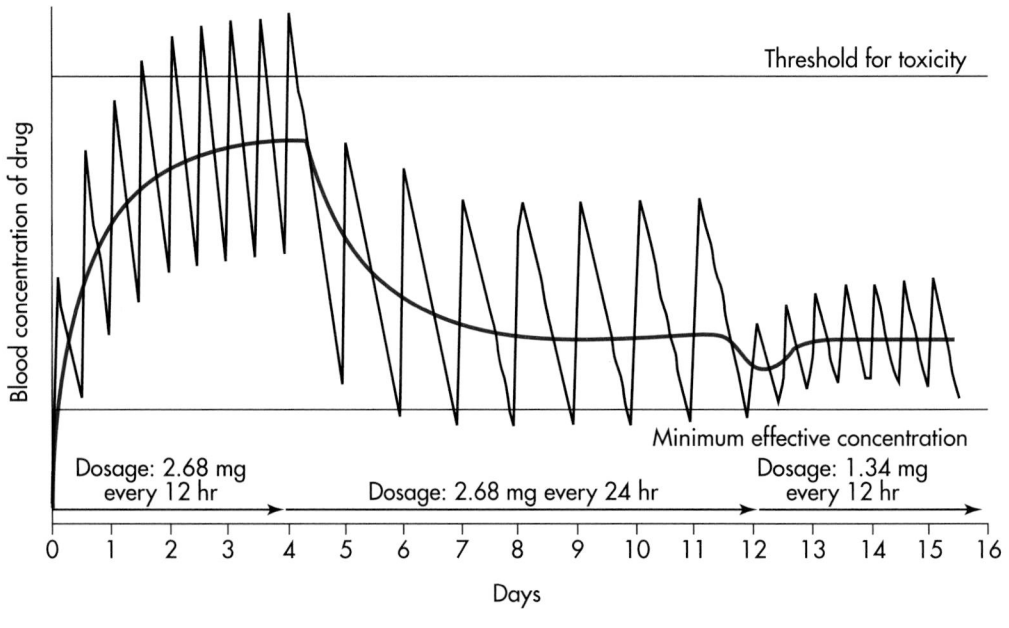

Figure A-1

CHAPTER 7

Over-the-Counter Medications

1. Tylenol would *not* be the antipyretic of choice because of the acetaminophen content! Jane needs to be seen by her physician as soon as possible to rule out wound infection or sepsis. If the physician orders an antipyretic, it would be aspirin, not acetaminophen.

2. The labels on the over-the-counter drugs state that the maximum dosage of acetaminophen should not exceed 4 g/day; adults who take more than 2.6 g in 24 hours may show mild symptoms of liver damage. According to Jane's report, the medications she took contained acetaminophen as follows:
   - Sinutabs Without Drowsiness, 2 tablets twice a day: acetaminophen 500 mg $\times$ 2 = 1000 mg
   - Excedrin, 1 tablet, twice a day for headache: acetaminophen 250 mg $\times$ 2 = 500 mg
   - Excedrin PM, 1 tablet at bedtime for sleep: acetaminophen 500 mg = 500 mg
   - Vicodin, 1 tablet, every 4 hours while awake for pain: acetaminophen 500 mg $\times$ 4 = 2000 mg
   - Total acetaminophen dosage = 4000 mg (4 g).
   Taking Tylenol for her fever would have added 650 mg to this total, resulting in 4650 mg of acetaminophen that day! There is a very real possibility of liver damage at this dosage.

3. Adults who take more than 2.6 g in a 24-hour period may show mild symptoms of liver damage, such as loss of appetite, nausea, vomiting, and slight jaundice. When an excessive amount of acetaminophen is ingested, unconjugated metabolites of the drug bind to and destroy liver cells.

4. Discuss Jane's use of over-the-counter medications for her symptoms; encourage her to read the labels of the medications and to discuss with her pharmacist or the physician whether the medication is safe to use with other medications she is taking. The pharmacist can help her choose the product that contains only the drug needed. Suggestions for alternatives to the acetaminophen-containing drugs need to be made. Last, explore non-pharmacologic measures for some of her problems (e.g., other measures to promote sleep).

CHAPTER 9

Lead Poisoning: Detection and Treatment in Children

1. Examples of resources found from an Internet search:
   - What Every Parent Should Know about Lead Poisoning in Children http://www.cdc.gov/nceh/programs/lead/faq/cdc97a.htm
   - Facts on . . . Lead (Centers for Disease Control and Prevention) http://www.cdc.gov/nceh/programs/lead/guide/1997/docs/factlead.htm

2. Potential sources of lead exposure for children include deteriorated paint in older housing and dust and soil that are contaminated with lead from old paint and from past emissions of leaded gasoline. Young children may ingest lead by eating paint chips or chewing on a surface painted with lead-based paint, such as a windowsill.

3. Very high blood levels of lead may cause seizures, coma, and death. The longer the elevated blood lead level persists and the higher it goes, the greater the chance that learning disabilities, behavioral problems, and mental retardation may result.

4. Intramuscular is the preferred route for edetate calcium disodium, and the dosage for children is 35 mg/kg twice daily. For a child weighing 12 kg, the dosage would be 420 mg/dose. The drug will be discontinued for 4 days or more after 3 to 5 days of therapy.

5. The lead chelate produced by this medication is excreted in the urine, and the chelation can cause toxic effects such as renal damage and irregularities in cardiac rhythm. Dosages must be monitored closely.

CHAPTER 13

Hypertension: Compliance Issues and Lifestyle Modifications

1. Beta-blockers in combination with diuretics are effective in African-Americans, whereas beta-blockers alone are generally less effective as single agents.

2. He is most likely referring to sexual dysfunction, or impotence. Other common side effects of beta-blockers include sleep disturbances, fatigue, reduced exercise tolerance, and depressed mood. The nurse needs to further explore Mr. Todd's complaints to pinpoint the specific problems.

3. Obesity and high salt intake are factors that worsen hypertension. African-Americans often have a higher prevalence of salt sensitivity, which can be modified with dietary changes. He should learn which foods have a high sodium content and should be taught to avoid adding salt to food. A supervised exercise program may also be helpful for losing the weight and improving cardiovascular tone. In addition, reducing alcohol and caffeine consumption is helpful in the management of hypertension.

4. If the patient reduces his weight and salt intake, the dosage of the drug may also be reduced over time. This reduction of dosage may result in fewer of the undesirable side effects of the antihypertensive medications. Drug therapy can rarely be discontinued after the blood pressure is brought into a normal range.

CHAPTER 14

Diuretics and Electrolyte Imbalance

1. Because of the therapy with Aldactone, a potassium-sparing diuretic, the possibility of hyperkalemia must be considered. A stat serum potassium should be ordered and an electrocardiogram (ECG) must also be done to check for changes in the ECG.

2. Subacute hyperkalemia is treated with cation exchange resins, such as Kayexalate, which exchange sodium for potassium in the intestine. The effect is not usually evident for several hours to 1 day after administration. Therefore careful observation to prevent injury from falls resulting from weakness and cardiac monitoring for arrhythmias is important.

3. While taking the chlorothiazide diuretic, Mr. Greene was probably also taking a potassium supplement and was taught to eat foods high in potassium. Now the opposite is in effect. He should no longer be taking the potassium supplement, and he should avoid foods high in potassium, such as citrus fruits and juices; bananas; grape, cranberry, apple, pear, and apricot juices; cereals; and leafy vegetables.

4. Certain salt substitutes are made of potassium salts. He should read the label very carefully and not use potassium-based salt substitutes.

CHAPTER 18

Polypharmacy and the Elderly

1. Older adults often have many medical problems that require multiple medications. Because of this, excessive drug use—or polypharmacy—may occur. This pattern results from attempts to treat several medical problem simultaneously and leads to a high risk of interactions and adverse drug reactions. Sometimes the patient may become confused by the number of medications being taken and may take the drugs in incorrect amounts and at wrong times. Last, seeing more than one primary care physician may result in multiple prescriptions.

2. The elderly are more prone to electrolyte imbalances, including hypokalemia, which can increase drug toxicity. Complaints of fatigue, weakness, and mood alteration may indicate digoxin toxicity and yet be mistaken for a normal part of aging or of heart disease. In addition, use of opioids such as Darvon may cause orthostatic hypotension, dizziness, or drowsiness.

3. Ask Mrs. Craine and her son to bring in *all* of her current medications to the physician/nurse with each visit on a regular basis to confirm whether the medications are still needed. In addition, any nonprescription drugs should also be brought in. They should be told that she should check with her physician before taking any over-the-counter medications to prevent interactions. Emphasize that over-the-counter medications are not to be treated less seriously just because they have not been prescribed by her physician. By establishing care with one physician, the chances of receiving multiple medications may be reduced. Using one pharmacy consistently will also aid in tracking the medications she is currently taking. In addition, Mrs. Craine should be taught that she should *not* borrow her son's sleeping pills (or any other medications), and the nurse should explore alternative methods to help her get to sleep.

4. The digoxin level is within normal limits (0.8 to 1.6 ng/L), and the potassium level is also normal (3.5 to 5 mEq/L). To help Mrs. Craine remember to take her medications, first ask her how she manages her medications daily. Does she set them out in the morning for the day or does she get them as needed from the bottles? Explore with Mrs. Craine some methods for remembering to take her medications until an acceptable solution is found. One possibility is making a calendar that includes an area to check off as medications are taken. Preparing her daily dosages in special containers or cups might also be helpful. The nurse should assist Mrs. Craine in finding a method that works for her and that still allows a degree of independence in her self-care.

CHAPTER 20

Oral Anticoagulants

1. The vitamin K content of the dark leafy green vegetables, Ensure supplement, and possibly in the multivitamins will reduce the effectiveness of the warfarin.

2. Bufferin contains aspirin, which is contraindicated in the use of anticoagulants. He needs to check with his physician before taking any over-the-counter medications. Alcohol intake has an effect on the liver, and 2 to 3 drinks may increase the tendency to bleed.

3. Instruct the patient to notify the physician for any signs of bleeding such as nosebleeds, bleeding gums, blood in the urine or stool, severe headache, unexplained bruising, or stiff neck. Suggest that the patient wear a medical identification bracelet or necklace to indicate the use of anticoagulants. Instruct him to use an electric razor, to brush teeth with a soft-bristle toothbrush, and to avoid flossing. Rough contact activities should also be avoided while on anticoagulants.

4. If the amount of unbound warfarin increases in the blood, the anticoagulant effect of the drug will also increase. This could result in untoward bleeding if not detected.

CHAPTER 22

Anemia and Pregnancy

1. Iron deficiency anemia develops when the intake of iron is inadequate to meet the demand. As a result, the newly made red blood cells are small and lighter in color because there is insufficient hemoglobin to fill the cells. In pregnancy, the placenta and fetus place an additional demand on the iron stores of the woman. Iron deficiency anemia is easily treated with iron supplementation.

2. The ferrous fumarate iron salts contain the largest amount of iron per gram of salt: 33% elemental iron.

3. Dietary sources of iron include red meats, dark green leafy vegetables, dried fruits, molasses, whole grains, enriched breads and cereals, and organ meats. Dietary iron must be converted by gastric juices before it can actually

be absorbed. Foods such as orange juice, fish, and ascorbic acid (vitamin C) may enhance iron absorption. However, eggs, beans, corn, and cereal products that contain phytates may actually impair iron absorption.

4. The tablets should be swallowed whole and never crushed. Antacids and milk interfere with its absorption and should be taken at least 1 hour before or after the dose. The patient should be told to expect her stools to turn black or dark green. To avoid esophageal irritation, she should not lie down for 15 to 30 minutes after taking the tablet. She should notice an increase in her energy and appetite soon after beginning therapy, and subsequent blood tests should show an increase in normal red blood cells and normal levels of hemoglobin.

CHAPTER 24
Laxative Use and Abuse

1. The decreased physical activity during this postoperative period as well as a low-fiber diet and the constipating side effects of the opioid analgesic all may contribute to constipation. It is Mrs. Lankford's health belief that one should have a large bowel movement every day or else one is constipated.

2. Surfak is a stool softener (wetting agent) that is commonly prescribed after surgery and inhibits the absorption of water so that the fecal mass remains large and soft. Citrucel is a bulk-forming laxative that acts by retaining water so that the stool remains large and soft. Dulcolax is a stimulant (irritant) cathartic that usually forms a stool within 6 to 12 hours. There is a duplication of the actions of the stool softener and the bulk-forming laxative.

3. Mrs. Lankford should be taught to recognize "true" constipation and how to prevent it and treat it properly should it occur. Signs and symptoms that indicate constipation include abdominal discomfort; feeling a need to defecate but inability to do so; dry, firm, hard stools when bowel movements do occur; and infrequent defecation. Stimulant laxatives are the most commonly abused laxatives. If a stimulant laxative is used for more than 1 week, the large intestine loses its tone and becomes less responsive to any stimulation. Continued use may lead to diarrhea that may result in dehydration and electrolyte losses. These agents should be used only if other means do not promote proper bowel elimination.

4. Nonpharmacologic means to promote bowel elimination include adequate water intake (2500 to 3000 ml of water a day if not contraindicated), adequate exercise (as her knee permits increased activity), and adequate amounts of dietary fiber. Good sources of dietary fiber include fruits and vegetables, especially those that are raw and unpeeled or with edible seeds, whole grains, and whole grain products such as bread, cereals, pastas, bran, oats, beans, and beans. She may also try drinking prune juice daily. Switching to a nonnarcotic analgesic will remove one of the possible contributing factors.

CHAPTER 26
Gastrointestinal Tract Ulceration

1. Maalox is an antacid, which neutralizes the stomach acid. Famotidine, a H_2-receptor antagonist, inhibits the binding of histamine to the H_2 receptors located on the parietal cells in the stomach, resulting in a reduction in gastric acid secretion. In the absence of normal mucosal defenses, gastric acid injures the gastrointestinal (GI) tract mucosa. Therefore neutralizing it or reducing its secretion will promote healing of GI tract ulceration.

2. Antacids were once the drugs of choice for the treatment of GI tract ulceration. However, with the introduction of the H_2 antagonists and proton pump inhibitors, antacids now play a secondary role in treatment. To be effective, antacids need to be taken 1 and 3 hours after meals, or approximately 7 times a day. In addition, most individuals find them unpleasant to take, which creates compliance a problem. The newer agents are as effective in healing ulcerations and are better tolerated by most individuals.

3. Omeprazole is the prototype of a new class of antiulcer agents, the proton pump inhibitors. Omeprazole inhibits function of an enzyme in the parietal cells of the stomach, H^+-K^+-ATPase, that generates gastric acid. This is the final common pathway for acid secretion regardless of the type of stimulus (e.g., gastrin, acetylcholine, histamine). The H_2-receptor antagonists block only the effects of histamine as a stimulant of gastric acid secretion. This is why the proton pump inhibitors are even more effective than the H_2 antagonists for suppressing gastric acid secretion.

4. Smoking has been associated with an increased incidence of ulcer disease and may slow healing. Alcohol ingestion may also be an aggravating factor for some individuals. Mr. Hanson's biopsies are positive for *Helicobacter pylori*.

5. *H. pylori* is a gram-negative bacillus that resides in the GI tract of many individuals. Although only a minority of these individuals will develop peptic ulcer disease, this organism is now recognized as the cause of more than 90% of duodenal ulcers and approximately 80% of gastric ulcers. Eradication of this organism has been shown to promote ulcer healing and prevent recurrences. Drug regimens include two or three antibiotics combined with a proton pump inhibitor taken for 7 to 14 days.

   Discharge orders are written and Mr. Hanson's prescriptions include metronidazole 400 mg orally three times daily for 14 days, amoxicillin 500 mg orally three times daily for 14 days, and omeprazole 40 mg orally once daily for 14 days.

6. Compliance should be emphasized. The antibiotic therapy often leads to noncompliance because of the number of pills the patient must take each day, the length of therapy, and unpleasant side effects. It is imperative for Mr. Hanson to finish his full course of medications because the *H. pylori* organism is difficult to eradicate and is likely to develop resistance if the full course of

antibiotics is not completed. Nausea, diarrhea, abdominal pain, rash, headache, and dizziness are common side effects of these antibiotics. In addition, Mr. Hanson should avoid drinking alcohol while taking the metronidazole because a disulfiram-like reaction (severe flulike symptoms) may occur when combining these two drugs. The incidence of side effects with omeprazole is low.

CHAPTER 34
Chronic Pain

1. The World Health Organization (WHO) recommends a "step approach" to cancer pain relief. This analgesic ladder begins with drug regimens using nonopioid analgesics such as acetaminophen and ibuprofen in maximum recommended doses. If pain is not relieved, the patient should progress to second-level therapy that includes weaker opioids (e.g., oxycodone) in combination with nonopioids (e.g., acetaminophen, ibuprofen). The weaker opioids and nonopioids are used in combination because they have different mechanisms of action. Third-level therapy for more resistant pain includes using the strong opioids (e.g., morphine). The goal of this approach is to adequately manage pain and promote a better quality of life while at the same time delaying the development of drug tolerance and dependence.

2. The WHO ladder also recommends use of adjuvant agents in chronic pain management. These are drugs that are usually used for conditions other than pain relief but that augment pain relief when used in combination with analgesics. Antianxiety agents, antidepressants, and neuroleptics are examples of classes of adjuvant drugs. It is important to remember that the adjuvants do not have analgesic properties in and of themselves and, in general, should not replace the nonopioid or opioid analgesics.

3. Concern that addiction to opioids will occur is a common but erroneous belief among both health care providers and patients receiving these medications. Studies have shown that the incidence of addiction in patients receiving narcotics is actually quite small. The goal for treatment of chronic cancer pain should be to maximize comfort, and this usually requires opioids. During the course of treatment, use of opioids in increasing doses and potencies usually reflects development of tolerance and/or progression of the disease process. Tolerance is a physiologic response of the body that occurs with repeated use of opioids, resulting in a need for larger doses or use of more potent agents to achieve analgesia. Addiction, on the other hand, is a behavioral compulsion to take drugs for their psychological effects. The nurse should explain the concept of tolerance to Warren and reinforce the primary goal of comfort.

4. The nurse should first assess the sensory components of Warren's pain. These components include location, intensity (preferably using a numerical pain scale), quality, and pattern. Remember that the patient, not the health care professional, is the expert on his or her pain. Additional data would also include Warren's expectations for pain relief and what pain control behaviors (e.g., watching television, visiting with family) are effective in helping him control his pain. These assessments will assist the nursing in planning Warren's care. The nurse should also assess Warren's baseline level of consciousness, blood pressure, heart rate, and respiratory rate before initiating the morphine patient-controlled analgesia (PCA). These data will assist the nurse in identifying common adverse effects of the morphine when reassessing Warren for the effects of the morphine after initiating the PCA therapy.

5. The PCA method of pain management allows Warren, who is the best judge of his pain level, to have control over his pain management instead of being dependent on the nursing staff for pain management. Studies have shown that standard doses of opioid analgesics provide adequate pain relief for only 70% of recipients. The PCA approach will allow Warren to titrate the medication for his needs and also precludes him having to wait for pain medication when he experiences breakthrough pain. The continuous infusion establishes a relatively constant plasma morphine concentration within a therapeutic range, thus minimizing the "peaks and valleys" that occur with intermittent dosing. A continuous infusion also has the advantage of providing analgesia while Warren is sleeping.

6. Opioid analgesics such as morphine can cause sedation, respiratory depression, and nausea and vomiting. In general, tolerance to these side effects develops after an individual has been taking opioids for a while. Because Warren has been taking opioids for months, he is at a lower risk of experiencing these adverse effects (compared with a postoperative patient who has not been receiving opioids and has just been started on a morphine PCA). One additional consideration, however, is that patients with preexisting pulmonary disease such as lung cancer and emphysema may be at a higher risk for developing the respiratory depressant effects of opioids. Constipation and urinary retention are two other adverse effects of morphine. Despite having developed tolerance to opioids, Warren still has some risk for developing any of the adverse effects of morphine, especially because he will now be receiving the drug via the intravenous route. His nurses should be monitoring him for these adverse effects.

7. Although nonpharmacologic pain relief strategies are not substitutes for drug therapy, many patients benefit from a treatment plan using both approaches. Warren may benefit from relaxation therapy, guided imagery, massage, or hypnosis. Heat and cold therapy should be avoided over irradiated areas. Heat should also be avoided over malignancy sites in nonterminal patients because it has been shown to increase malignancy growth rates.

8. Opioids should be given around-the-clock for control of the persistent or continuous chronic pain from cancer. Fentanyl is an opioid that has a greater potency than morphine and is useful in treating chronic pain. The drug is released from the patch into the skin slowly over 3 days, after which it should be removed and a new one applied. The hydromorphone is another potent opioid which Warren can take on a prn basis to manage his breakthrough pain.

CHAPTER 39
Children and Immunizations

1. To improve communication with this patient, either locate an interpreter from the hospital's resource bank or call the local chapter of the American Red Cross to locate one. Another strategy would be to find a family member or friend who speaks English. The hospital should also have "interpreter cards" that have pictures or words from Spanish-to-English or English-to-Spanish to facilitate communication.

2. First, find out if the husband has medical coverage through his factory position. If not, refer the patient to the public health department for assistance in obtaining medical care for the toddler, including immunizations.

3. Following is the schedule for immunizations recommended in the United States:
   - Age 2 months: DTaP (or DTP)-1, HepB-1, PV-1, Hib-1
   - Age 4 months: DTaP (or DTP)-2, HepB-2, PV-2, Hib-2
   - Age 6 months: DTaP (or DTP)-3, PV-3, Hib-3
   - Age 12-15 months: DTaP (or DTP)-4, MMR-1, Hib-4, Var

4. Some Hispanics view good health as being the result of good luck and good living. Likewise, they view illness as being a result of bad luck or bad actions. These individuals may seek to restore health by seeking "cold" remedies or foods and "hot" remedies or foods to counteract "hot" illnesses and "cold" illnesses, respectively. In addition, certain rituals such as lighting of candles may be used. However, beliefs will vary from patient to patient; therefore always perform a cultural assessment first to explore these beliefs. For more information, refer to a text on cultural considerations.

CHAPTER 44
Child with Otitis Media

1. Gather more data concerning each use of antibiotics:
   - Did the child get all of the medication?
   - Did the ears clear? Was this validated by the doctor with an ear recheck?
   - Does the child's fever respond to an antipyretic? Which one does the mother use?
   - What do the parents know about second-hand smoke?

2. Most common bacteria causing otitis media are *Streptococcus pneumoniae*, *Haemophilus influenzae*, and *Moraxella catarrhalis*. Any virus can settle in the inner ear.

3. Elements in Jay's history include the smoking by the parents, other relatives, and friends; amount of time spent in day care; and possibly the large tonsils.

4. Potential lack of knowledge concerning second-hand smoke and eustachian tube dysfunction; potential for allergies (animal dander)

5. Azithromycin (Zithromax): macrolide that is indicated for community infections; the child has had a number of penicillins, cephalosporins, and sulfa drugs for previous infections. A danger in prescribing multiple antibiotics is that the child will become resistant to them all. The dosage is 10 mg/kg once on day 1 and 5 mg/kg once daily on days 2, 3, 4, and 5. Jay would receive 150 mg on day 1 and 75 mg on days 2 through 5. If using the 200 mg/5 ml strength, the child will receive 3.8 ml on day 1 and 1.9 ml on days 2 through 5. Other considerations with azithromycin include the following:
   - Give on empty stomach (1 hour before meals or 2 hours after meals).
   - The child is not taking any drugs that would interact with azithromycin.
   - Adverse effects would be gastrointestinal upset.
   - Other antibiotics that could be considered are loracarbef (Lorabid), a carbacephem that can be used for otitis media (suspension form only), and erythromycin ethylsuccinate (Pediazole), a good second-line combination antibiotic of a macrolide plus a sulfonamide.

6. Another pharmacologic preparation to use would be a nonsteroidal antiinflammatory drug (NSAID) such as ibuprofen for fever and discomfort. NSAIDs have an advantage over acetaminophen because acetaminophen reduces fever but has no antiinflammatory properties. An antihistamine or a decongestant or a combination of the two may also be ordered. Preferred use is a one-ingredient drug rather than a combination, so a sympathomimetic such as pseudoephedrine HCl (Sudafed) is suggested. However, parents could try different decongestants and/or antihistamine preparations until they find one that works for the child. Nonpharmacologic interventions include fluids and rest for the child and smoking cessation for the parents. Good nutrition and hygiene can be taught as best as possible to a 3-year-old child to enhance the immune system (because stopping day care is not an option).

7. Educational points to cover with the parents include the following:
   - Research-supported link between second hand smoke and recurrent otitis media (see *http://www.kidshealth.org/parent/common/otitis_media.html* and References)
   - Way to give antibiotic and other pharmacologic preparations if needed
   - Signs and symptoms to watch for; when to call back

- Office visit for ear recheck with otoscope; repeat tympanogram for comparison
- Parents recall of patient behavior, administration of all medication

CHAPTER 49
Urinary Tract Infection

1. Because these two drugs have a wide spectrum of antimicrobial activity, most pathogens causing urinary tract infections (UTIs) are susceptible to them. In addition, these urinary antiseptics are concentrated in the urine, at the site of the infection.

2. The different mechanisms of action of these two drugs explains why they are commonly prescribed together. Susceptible bacteria must synthesize tetrahydrofolic acid (THFA), the active form of folic acid, from precursors to produce bacterial DNA, RNA, and proteins. Sulfamethoxazole inhibits an enzyme that converts the precursor PABA into another THFA precursor, dihydropteroic acid. Trimethoprim, on the other hand, inhibits the action of another enzyme, dihydrofolate reductase, also essential in the synthesis of THFA. Because these two drugs inhibit different enzymes required for the process of converting precursors into THFA, their effects are synergistic. This means that the combined effects of these two drugs when administered together are greater than the sum of the effects of the drugs if they were administered individually.

3. Although these drugs are usually well tolerated, side effects can develop. The most common side effects include nausea, vomiting, and development of skin rashes. Carla should contact the clinic if any of these effects, other than mild nausea, occur.

4. The sulfonamides can cause hemolytic anemia in persons who have a genetic deficiency of glucose-6-phosphate dehydrogenate (G6PD), an enzyme within red blood cells. This trait is more common among African-Americans and persons of Mediterranean descent. Rarely, sulfamethoxazole can also cause hemolytic anemia, agranulocytosis, leukopenia, and thrombocytopenia. Carla should contact a health care provider if she experiences a fever, sore throat, mouth sores, bleeding, or excessive bruising.

5. The sulfonamides can cause crystalline aggregates to form in the urine, which in turn can cause irritation or stone formation within the kidneys or urinary tract. The risk of crystalluria is reduced if the patient increases her daily fluid intake, which will increase urine flow through the urinary system. The sulfonamides also cause photosensitivity. Photosensitive skin rashes or sunburn can be avoided by using sunscreens or avoiding excessive sun exposure. This teaching is especially important given Carla's plans to vacation in Mexico.

6. Phenazopyridine is a nonopioid urinary analgesic. It acts locally on the mucosa of the urinary tract, producing analgesia. It has been prescribed to decrease the pain and burning Carla has with urination. The nurse should tell Carla that this drug causes the urine to become bright orange, which can stain undergarments.

7. Given Carla's history, the following points should be emphasized:
   - Maintaining a fluid intake of 2 to 3 L/day ensures an adequate urine flow to flush bacteria from the urinary tract.
   - In women, the urinary meatus is closer to the anus than in men. This is why women have a higher incidence of UTIs than men. Wiping the perineal area from front to back after voiding will decrease the risk of gram-negative gastrointestinal tract bacteria infecting the urinary tract.
   - Women who are sexually active have an increased incidence of UTIs. Voiding within 15 minutes after sexual intercourse aids in flushing bacteria out of the lower urinary tract.
   - Using bubble baths, perfumed soaps or sanitary pads, feminine hygiene sprays, or bath powders in the perineal area should be avoided because they are irritants and can predispose the patient to UTIs.
   - Showering rather than taking baths will decrease the perineal exposure to bacteria that can cause UTIs.
   - Use of the diaphragm with contraceptive jelly increases the incidence of UTIs. Carla may want to consider another form of birth control.
   - Wearing nylon underwear or tight clothing such as jeans can contribute to a moist, warm environment in the perineal area, which encourages growth of bacteria.
   - Retention of urine in the bladder promotes infection. Therefore the patient should void when the urge is first felt.
   - Patients who have received a prescription for antibiotics should take the full course of therapy even after symptoms have subsided. This prevents recurrence of the infection and aids in preventing the development of bacterial resistance.

CHAPTER 52
Acquired Immunodeficiency Syndrome

1. Contact the local community service board/social services department for a referral to the appropriate substance abuse counseling program. In addition, inquire about local acquired immunodeficiency syndrome (AIDS) support groups that may offer assistance with the medications.

2. *HAART* stands for "high-activity antiretroviral therapy" and consists of the use of three or four anti–human immunodeficiency virus (HIV) drugs in combination. By choosing drugs with different mechanisms of action, a potent antiviral effect may be achieved by attacking the virus through two independent mechanisms. In addition, the chance for resistance to the drugs is lowered.

3. She should be taught to take the medication on an empty stomach and exactly as prescribed. She should be advised

to report signs of infection (e.g., increased temperature, sore throat, flu symptoms) and to avoid crowds and persons with known infections. She should be advised to report signs of anemia, such as fatigue, headache, faintness, irritability, and shortness of breath. She should also be advised to report bleeding. One rare effect is that hair may be lost during therapy. She should not use any other over-the-counter medications without consulting the physician. Last, she should not have sexual contact without use of a condom, needles should not be shared, and blood should not come into contact with another's mucous membranes. She and her mother should be taught about the ways that HIV is contracted so that she can protect her children and others and so that she can reduce the fears of those who live in the same household.

4. Antiviral drugs have dose-limiting side effects such as bone marrow suppression, meaning that the patient with an HIV infection has to be switched to a different agent. She will probably continue receiving antiviral drug therapy as long as the side effects and adverse effects of the medications can be managed.

CHAPTER 59

Depression

1. Tricyclic antidepressants (TCAs) have a complex and dosage-related effect on the heart. The anticholinergic action increases the heart rate, which is not appropriate for a person with coronary artery disease. The diseased heart may not respond well to an increase in the cardiac workload. At high concentrations of the TCAs, quinidine-like side effects of decreased heart rate, myocardial contractility, and coronary blood flow also present a special concern for those with cardiac disease. In addition, intentional overdosage with TCAs often results in death.

2. Sertraline HCl is safer for Mr. Brown because of the lack of anticholinergic effects and cardiac conduction distur-

bances. In addition, overdoses of selective serotonin reuptake inhibitors (SSRIs) such as sertraline are not as likely to be fatal; therefore they are safer than the TCAs.

3. SSRIs are bound to protein plasma and therefore may displace other drugs that are bound to protein, such as oral anticoagulants and phenytoin. In addition, the central nervous system depression of other drugs may be potentiated by the SSRIs.

4. Several weeks of therapy may be necessary before the full effects of a drug regimen can be evaluated. In addition, the side effects that may be present may lessen with continued use. The family should be informed of this.

CHAPTER 73

Glaucoma and the Elderly

1. The sinus bradycardia may be caused by the concurrent administration of two beta-blocker medications. The timolol maleate is taken orally, and the eye medication, betaxolol HCl (Betoptic) 0.5% solution, may have been absorbed systemically. Beta-blockers prevent sympathetic stimulation of the heart and thus may cause excessive slowing of the heart rate and even syncope.

2. Instructing the patient, and a family member, to check her pulse before taking the beta-blocker medication may have detected an impending problem. If the pulse is slower than 50 to 60 beats/min, withhold the next dose and notify the physician.

3. To prevent overflow of the medication into nasal and pharyngeal passage, thus reducing systemic absorption, teach the patient how to occlude the nasolacrimal duct with one finger for 1 to 2 minutes after instilling the medication.

4. Pilocarpine, a cholinomimetic agent, is a direct-acting miotic that is the drug of choice for acute and chronic glaucoma. The dosage is 1 drop of 1% to 2% solution every 6 to 8 hours.

Disorders Index

Page numbers in *italics* indicate illustrations;
t indicates table.

Comprehensive Index

Page numbers in *italics* indicate illustrations; *t* indicates table; generic drug names are set in *lower case italics;* trade names are set in SMALL CAPS

883

Children—cont'd
pain assessment in, 404-407
pain management for, 413
poisoning of, 100, 101, 310
CHILDREN'S ASPIRIN *(aspirin)*, 367*t*
Chlamydial infection, 498*t*, 532, 534, 545
chlophedianol, 360, 360*t*
chloral hydrate, 30*t*, 672, 672*t*
chlorambucil, 617*t*, 628*t*, 629-630, 642
chloramphenicol, 10, 16, 16*t*, 531*t*, 533-536
chlordiazepoxide, 30*t*, 665, 666, 667*t*, 678
for alcohol withdrawal, 95, 97
Chloride ion sites, renal, 162
CHLOROMYCETIN *(chlorophenicol)*, 531*t*
chloroprocaine, 419*t*, 420
CHLOROPTIC *(chlorophenicol)*, 531*t*
chloroquine
for amebic disease, 595*t*, 597
for malaria, 596*t*, 597-598, 608
chlorothiazide, 167*t*, 170, 174
chlorothiazide + methyldopa, 168*t*
chlorothiazide + reserpine, 168*t*
chlorphenesin, 751*t*, 752, 753
chlorpheniramine, 353*t*, 354, 356
CHLORPROMANYL *(chlorpromazine)*, 683*t*
chlorpromazine
as antiemetic, 307*t*, 311, 687
as antipsychotic, 682, 683*t*, 695
chlorpropamide, 16*t*
for diabetes insipidus, 762
for diabetes mellitus, 808-810, 809*t*
chlorprothixene, 685*t*
chlortetracycline, 88
chlorthalidone, 136, 167*t*
chlorthalidone + atenolol, 168*t*
chlorthalidone + clonidine, 168*t*
chlorthalidone + reserpine, 168*t*
CHLOR-TRIMETRON *(chlorpheniramine)*, 353*t*
chlorzoxazone, 751*t*, 752, 753
Cholecalciferol, 791, 794
CHOLEDYL *(oxtriphylline)*, 340*t*
Cholelithiasis, 326
Cholera, 532
vaccine for, 450, 451*t*
Cholestatic hepatitis, 524
antipsychotic-induced, 690
Cholesterol, 266-269
atherosclerosis and, 135, *268*, 268-269
degradation of, 268
drugs to lower blood levels of, 270-274, 271*t*
lifestyle modifications to lower blood levels
of, 270
diet, 269, 270
cholestyramine, 271*t*, 272, 275
Choline acetylase, 115
Cholinergic antagonists; *see* Anticholinergic
drugs
Cholinergic nervous system, 116, 117*t*
mechanisms controlling bronchioles, 334
mechanisms of cholinergic control, 120-124
Cholinergic poisoning, 106*t*
Cholinergic receptors, 3, 120-121
choline salicylate, 367*t*, 371
Cholinomimetic drugs, 121-122; *see also*
Acetylcholinesterase inhibitors
administration of, 291
bronchospasm induced by, 334

Cholinomimetic drugs—cont'd
for glaucoma, 848, 849*t*, 852-853
to increase gastrointestinal motility, 121, 285-287, 287*t*
for myasthenia gravis, 478-481, 480*t*
receptors for, 122*t*
uses of, 121-122, 122*t*
chondroitin sulfate, 374
CHOP, 620*t*
Choriocarcinoma, 613, 614*t*
chorionic gonadotropin
for females, 819*t*, 822*t*, 823, 830
for male hypogonadism, 843*t*, 845
Chorioretinitis, glucocorticoids for, 471
Christmas disease, 257
Chromosomes, 614-615
Chronic obstructive pulmonary disease, 334-335; *see also* Asthma
alpha₁-proteinase inhibitor for, 344, 349
antihypertensive drugs for patients with, 137
CHRONULAC *(lactulose)*, 296*t*
Chvostek's sign, 214
Chylomicrons, 266-267
CIBACALCIN *(calcitonin human)*, 795*t*
CIBALITH-SI *(lithium)*, 707*t*
ciclopirox olamine, 570*t*
cidofovir, 584*t*, 586, 590-591
CIDOMYCIN *(gentamicin)*, 540*t*
cimetidine, 21, 318, 319*t*, 323, 352
CINOBAC *(cinoxacin)*, 519*t*
cinoxacin, 519*t*, 520
cinoxate, 87
CIN-QUIN *(quinidine sulfate)*, 233*t*
CIPRO *(ciprofloxacin)*, 518*t*
ciprofloxacin, 498, 518, 518*t*, 519
Circulation
enterohepatic, 10
to heart, 177, *178*
portal, 757
cisapride, 286, 287, 287*t*, 291-292
cisatracurium, 436*t*, 437, 439
cisplatin, 309, 620*t*, 621, 628*t*, 629, 642
citalopram, 699*t*, 702
CITANEST *(prilocaine)*, 419*t*
CITRACAL *(calcium citrate)*, 794*t*
citric acid, 359
CITROMA *(magnesium citrate)*, 296*t*
CITRUCEL *(methylcellulose)*, 296*t*
cladribine, 633-634, 633*t*, 644
CLAFORAN *(cefotaxime)*, 512*t*
CLARIPEX *(clofibrate)*, 271*t*, 272
clarithromycin, 523*t*, 560
for *Helicobacter pylori*, 320*t*, 322
CLARITIN *(loratadine)*, 353*t*, 354
Clark's rule, 76
Claviceps purpurea, 399
CLAVULIN *(amoxicillin + potassium clavulanate)*, 507*t*
clemastine, 353*t*
CLEOCIN *(clindamycin)*, 26, 526*t*
clidinium, 290, 290*t*
clindamycin, 26, 525-526, 526*t*, 528-529
Clinical toxicology, 100-112; *see also* Poisoning;
Toxicity
CLINORIL *(sulindac)*, 369*t*, 373
clioquinol, 570*t*
clobetasol propionate, 470*t*

clocortolone pivalate, 470*t*
CLODERM *(clocortolone pivalate)*, 470*t*
clofazimine, 559*t*, 560, 563-564
clofibrate
for diabetes insipidus, 762
to lower serum cholesterol level, 271*t*, 272-273, 275
CLOMID *(clomiphene)*, 822*t*
clomiphene, 819*t*, 822*t*, 823, 830
clomipramine, 699*t*, 704
clonazepam
for anxiety, 665, 666, 667*t*
for seizures, 727*t*, 730-731
clonidine, 128, 129*t*, 130
for hypertension, 134*t*, 142*t*, 151-152
for opioid withdrawal syndrome, 390
clopidolgrel, 251*t*, 252
CLOPRA *(metoclopramide)*, 287*t*, 308*t*
clorazepate
for anxiety, 665, 666, 667*t*
for seizures, 727*t*, 731
Closed-angle glaucoma, 847-848, *848*
Clostridium botulinum infection, 102*t*
antitoxin for, 453, 454*t*
Clostridium difficile infection, 504, 525
clotrimazole, 570*t*
Clotting factors, 244
cloxacillin, 507*t*, 509
clozapine, 692, 692*t*, 695
CLOZARIL *(clozapine)*, 692, 692*t*
Cluster headaches, 396
CMF, 620*t*
Coagulation of blood, 244-246
anticoagulant drugs and, 246-250, 247*t*, 258-261
antiplatelet drugs and, 250-252, 251*t*, 261-262, 369
hemostatic drugs and, 254-258, 255*t*-256*t*, 263-265
role of calcium in, 245-246
steps in, 244-245, *245*
thrombolytic drugs and, 252-254, 253*t*, 262-263
COBEX *(cyanocobalamin)*, 279*t*
cocaine
abuse of, 93*t*, 94*t*, 95-96
for local anesthesia, 418*t*, 420
poisoning with, 102*t*
during pregnancy, 16*t*
withdrawal from, 93
Coccidioidomycosis, 566, 567
Cocoa butter, 87, 88
codeine, 382, 383*t*, 384, 387*t*, 388-389
adverse effects of, 83
classification as controlled substance, 30-31, 30*t*
combined with aspirin, 369
for cough, 83-84, 360, 360*t*, 385
for diarrhea, 298, 299*t*, 300
dosage of, 411*t*
in headache remedies, 397*t*
metabolism of, 6, 9, 9*t*
poisoning with, 102*t*
Cod liver oil, 88
COE-TWO *(potassium bitartrate and sodium bicarbonate)*, 296*t*
COGENTIN *(benztropine)*, 740, 741*t*, 742

extended insulin zinc, 807t
Extracorporeal shock-wave lithotripsy, 328
Extrapyramidal reactions, 688-689, 688t
EXTRA STRENGTH EXCEDRIN *(acetaminophen),* 397t
Extravasation of drug, 211t
Eye medications
  administration of, 65-66, 66, 861
  antiviral agents, 586-587, 587t, 592
  cholinomimetic, 121
  for eye examination, 857
  for glaucoma, 847-856
  glucocorticoids, 470t, 471, 475
  muscarinic receptor antagonists, 124
  mydriatic drugs, 857-860, 859t
  nursing implications for, 861
  nursing process overview for, 860
  over-the-counter, 84-86

F
Factor IX complex, 256t, 257, 265
Factor VIII, 257
FACTREL *(gonadorelin),* 822t, 843t
famciclovir, 584t, 585, 591
Family history of drug abuse, 92
famotidine, 318, 319t, 323-324, 352
FAMVIR *(famciclovir),* 584t
Fanconi syndrome, 532-533
FANSIDAR *(sulfadoxine + pyrimethamine),* 546t
FARESTON *(toremifene),* 651t
FASTIN *(phentermine),* 716t
Fat emulsions, 208, 209t, 215
Fat metabolism
  insulin and, 803
  oral contraceptives and, 826t
Fecal drug elimination, 10
Federal drug laws, 25-27, 26t
Feedback loop for hormones, 766, 766-767
Feeding tube, drug administration via, 52-53
felbamate, 727t, 731, 736
FELBATOL *(felbamate),* 727t, 731
FELDENE *(piroxicam),* 369t, 373, 411t
felodipine
  for angina, 182t, 184-185
  for hypertension, 134t, 141t, 150
felodopam, 153t
FEMARA *(letrozole),* 651t
FEMIRON *(ferrous fumarate),* 279t
fenofibrate, 271t, 272-273
fenoprofen, 367t, 372
fenoterol, 339t, 341-342
fentanyl, 384, 386, 412
  for anesthesia, 427, 428t, 430, 432
FEOSOL *(ferrous sulfate),* 279t
FERGON *(ferrous gluconate),* 279t
FER-IN-SOL *(ferrous sulfate),* 279t
FERO-GRADUMET *(ferrous sulfate),* 279t
ferrous fumarate, 279t, 280
ferrous gluconate, 279t, 280
ferrous sulfate, 279-280, 279t
Fertility agents, 819t, 822-823, 822t, 829-831
FERTINEX *(urofollitropin),* 822t
FERTINIC *(ferrous gluconate),* 279t
FERTINORM HP *(urofollitropin),* 822t
Fetal alcohol syndrome, 675
Fetal antiepileptic drug syndrome, 725
Fetal drug effects, 15-16, 16t, 17t, 27-28;
  see also Pregnancy

Fetal immunity, 448
Fever
  acetaminophen for, 366
  aspirin for, 369
  nonsteroidal antiinflammatory drugs for, 372
  role of prostaglandins in, 365
fexofenadine, 353t, 354
Fiber, dietary, 295
  effect in tube-fed elderly patients, 300
FIBERALL *(psyllium hydrophilic muciloid),* 296t
FIBERCON *(polycarbophil),* 296t
Fibric acid derivatives, 271t, 272-273
Fibrin, 244, 246, 252
FIBRINDEX *(thrombin),* 255t
Fibrinogen, 244
Fibrocystic breast disease, oral contraceptives
  and, 826t
"Fight or flight" response, 117-118, 129
filgrastim, 458-459, 458t, 464
FIORICET *(butalbital),* 397t
First-pass effect, 6
FLAGYL *(metronidazole),* 320t, 322, 595t
FLAMAZINE *(silver sulfadiazine),* 547t
FLAREX *(fluorometholone acetate),* 470t
FLAXEDIL *(gallamine triethiodide),* 436t, 437
flecainide
  for arrhythmias, 230t-232t, 235, 241
  for older adults, 233
FLEET PHOSPHO-SODA *(sodium phosphates),* 296t
FLEET RELIEF *(pramoxine),* 418t
FLEXERIL *(cyclobenzaprine),* 751t, 752, 753
FLEXOJECT *(orphenadrine),* 751t
floctafenine, 368t, 372
FLONASE *(fluticasone),* 470t
FLORINEF *(fludrocortisone),* 774t
FLORONE *(diflorasone diacetate),* 470t
FLOROPRYL *(isoflurophate),* 121, 849t, 852
FLOVENT *(fluticasone),* 337t, 470t
FLOXIN *(ofloxacin),* 518t
floxuridine, 633t, 634, 645
FLUANXOL *(flupenthixol),* 685t
flucinolone, 470t
fluconazole, 566t, 568-571, 573
flucytosine, 566t, 568, 573
fludarabine, 617t, 633t, 634-635, 645
FLUDARA *(fludarabine),* 633t
fludrocortisone, 774-775, 774t, 777
Fluids and electrolytes, 202-216; *see also* Water
  in diabetes insipidus, 761
  diuretic-induced imbalances of, 170
  drinks for replacement of, 298
  hydrating solutions, 206
  indications for fluid therapy, 204-206
    common electrolyte imbalances,
      205-206, 205t
    diarrhea, 298
    fluid excess, 205
    loss of extracellular fluid volume, 204-205
  intravenous hyperalimentation, 208, 209t
  nursing implications for patient receiving in-
    travenous fluids, 210-216
  nursing process overview for, 210
  plasma expanders, 207-208, 208t
  problems related to intravenous infusion,
    211t
  regulation of salt and water balance,
    202-204, 203

solutions to correct specific electrolyte imbal-
    ances, 206-207, 207t
  pediatric sensitivity to benzyl alcohol
    in, 207
  therapy for shock, 193
FLUMADINE *(rimantadine),* 584t
flumazenil, 105, 106t, 110, 665, 668-669,
  668t, 679
flumethasone pivalate, 470t
flunarizine, 400
flunisolide, 336, 337t, 470t
flunitrazepam, 96-97
FLUOCET *(fluocinolone acetonide),* 470t
FLUOCIN *(fluocinonide),* 470t
FLUODERM *(fluocinolone acetonide),* 470t
fluorometholone, 470t
FLUOR-OP *(fluorometholone),* 470t
FLUOROPLEX *(fluorouracil),* 633t
Fluoroquinolone antibiotics, 517-521, 518t
  adverse reactions and contraindications to,
    518-519
  interactions with, 519
  mechanism of action of, 517
  nursing implications for, 520-521
  nursing process overview for, 520
  pharmacokinetics of, 517-518
  resistance to, 517
  toxicity of, 519
  for urinary tract infections, 520
  use in children, 17, 519
  uses of, 518
fluorouracil, 617t, 620t, 633t, 634, 645
FLUOTHANE *(halothane),* 426, 426t
fluoxetine
  for depression, 699t, 702
  for migraine prophylaxis, 400
fluoxymesterone, 841-843, 842t
flupenthixol, 685t, 695
fluphenazine, 683t, 695
flurandrenolide, 470t
flurazepam, 665, 666, 667t
flurbiprofen, 368t, 372
  to achieve mydriasis, 859t, 860
FLUROSYN *(fluocinolone acetonide),* 470t
FLUSHIELD *(influenza vaccine),* 451t
flutamide, 649, 650-651, 651t, 657
fluticasone, 336, 337t, 470t
fluvastatin, 271, 271t
FLUVIRAL *(influenza vaccine),* 451t
FLUVIRIN *(influenza vaccine),* 451t
fluvoxamine, 699t, 702
FLUZONE *(influenza vaccine),* 451t
FML *(fluorometholone),* 470t
FOLEX *(methotrexate),* 633t
folic acid, 209, 279t, 281, 283
Follicle-stimulating hormone
  female reproduction and, 817-818
  infertility and, 823
  male sexual function and, 840, 843
  sexual development and, 763t, 764-766, *765*
FOLLISTIM *(follitropin alfa),* 822t
follitropin alfa, 822t, 823, 830
follitropin beta, 822t, 823, 830
FOLVITE *(folic acid),* 279t
fomepizole, 106t
Food, Drug, and Cosmetics Act, 25, 26t
Food and Drug Administration, 28-29

Chapter 1
Drugs in the Body: Pharmacodynamics and Pharmacokinetics

Define the following:

1. Pharmacokinetics

2. Pharmacodynamics

3. Plateau Principle

4. Affinity

5. Antagonist

6. First-pass effect

7. Half-life

8. Therapeutic index

Match the terms below to the phases of pharmacokinetics they affect.

9. __a__ Bioavailability   a. Absorption

10. __d__ Half-life   b. Distribution

11. __c__ Biotransformation   c. Metabolism

12. __b__ Enterohepatic circulation   d. Elimination

13. __a__ Drug pH

14. Describe the role of receptors and the action of agonists and antagonists.

List an advantage and a disadvantage of the following drug administration routes.

Route	Advantage	Disadvantage
15. Oral		
16. Sublingual		
17. Subcutaneous		
18. Intramuscular		
19. Intravenous		
20. Aerosol		

Match the defintions below to the terms.

1. _____ The result of one drug increasing the concentration of another drug

2. _____ Common measure of renal function

3. _____ Drug interaction in which the effects of both are increased

4. _____ Increased efficiency of the liver metabolism of drugs

5. _____ Usual adverse effect caused by a drug

6. _____ A condition that may result in the destruction of red blood cells

a. Synergism

b. Iatrogenic

c. Potentiation

d. Creatinine clearance

e. G6PD deficiency

f. Induction

7. Explain why neonates may respond to medications quite differently than adults or older children.

8. List factors that increase risk when older adults take medications.

9. How does renal function affect drug therapy?

10. How does a full stomach affect drug absorption?

Match the drugs below to their FDA pregnancy categories.

11. _____ tobramycin

12. _____ morphine

13. _____ Thyroid hormones

14. _____ hydrochlorothiazide

15. _____ methotrexate

16. _____ captopril

17. _____ cimetidine

a. A

b. B

c. C

d. D

e. X

Chapter 3
Legal Implications of Drug Therapy

Define the following:

1. Orphan drug

2. Generic name

3. Trade name

4. Food, Drug, and Cosmetic Act

5. Carcinogenic

6. Double-blind design

7. Placebo effect

8. Addiction

9. Durham-Humphrey Amendment

10. Scheduled drugs

11. Teratogens

12. List four organizations involved in drug regulation and their functions.

Match each schedule classification to its definition.

13. _____ Schedule III

14. _____ Schedule V

15. _____ Schedule II

16. _____ Schedule I

17. _____ Schedule IV

a. Drugs with a high potential for abuse; not used in medicine

b. Drugs that may cause mild dependence

c. Drugs that cause a moderate amount of dependence

d. Drugs with a high potential for abuse/dependence but that have medical use

e. Drugs that have limited potential for causing mild dependence

18. List nursing interventions for a patient receiving a controlled substance.

Chapter 4
Application of the Nursing Process to Drug Therapy

1. List the five phases of the nursing process.

Match each of the "five rights" to its appropriate example.

2. _____ Right drug

3. _____ Right route

4. _____ Right dose

5. _____ Right time

6. _____ Right patient

a. Checking name band against medication administration form.

b. Giving a sleeping pill at 9:00 PM when order reads "HS."

c. Checking the drug handbook for use of ordered medication.

d. Using appropriate math when calculating medication.

e. Determining the appropriate way to administer a medication.

7. Identify five safety points to teach patients receiving medications.

8. Develop an assessment tool for a parent of a 3-year-old child receiving medication.

9. Describe two methods for helping patients remember to take their pills.

10 List three causes of medication errors.

Chapter 5
Drug Administration

Define the following:

1. Unit dose

2. Sustained-release drug

3. Sublingual

4. Troche

5. Intradermal

6. Z-track technique

7. Peripherally inserted central catheter

8. Suppositories

9. Transdermal

10. Intraosseous

11. List important data that the nurse should document when administering medications.

12. Describe the following parenteral routes used in medication administration.

    Intravenous:

    Intramuscular:

    Subcutaneous:

13. List nursing concerns related to the administration of eye medications.

Continued

14. Compare the proper techniques for administrating ear medications for adults and children age 3 and younger.

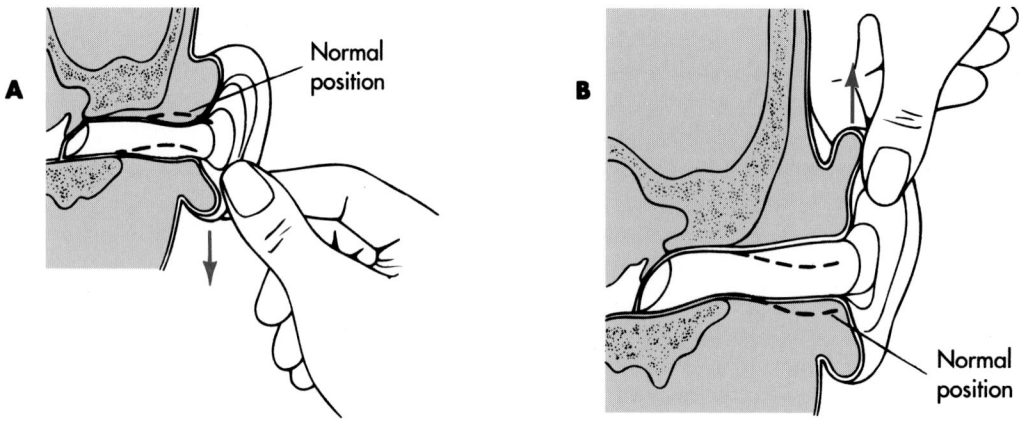

15. Which oral drug forms should *not* be crushed and chewed?

16. Identify the unique difficulties experienced by older adults receiving multiple drugs.

Chapter 6
Calculating Drug Dosages

Define the following:

1. Body surface area

2. Clark's rule

3. Young's rule

4. Solution

5. prn

6. Explain the following drug orders. Classify the order as a routine order (RO), stat order (STAT), prn order (PRN), or single order (S).

Classification   **Explanation of Drug Order**

a. _____ Demerol 100 mg IM stat

b. _____ MOM 30 ml PO HS

c. _____ Seconal 100 mg PO HS prn

d. _____ Lanoxin 0.25 mg PO QD

e. _____ Dilantin 100 mg PO

The following abbreviations are commonly used in relation to medication administration. Match each definition with the term(s) that best describe it.

7. ac

8. bid

9. $\bar{c}$

10. OD

11. qid

12. tid

13. QD

14. OU

a. Before meals

b. After meals

c. With

d. Without

e. Right eye

f. Left eye

g. Both eyes

h. Twice daily

i. Three times daily

j. Four times daily

k. Every other day

l. Every day

m. Every hour

Continued

15. Convert:

    a. 1 T = _____ oz = _____ cc

    b. 1 oz = _____ ml

    c. 0.5 g = _____ mg

    d. 2000 cc = _____ L

    e. 100 mg = _____ g

    f. 1 mg = _____ μg

    g. 1 lb = _____ oz

    h. 164 kg = _____ lb

    i. 64 gal = _____ L

    j. 1 g = _____ gr

Calculate the following:

16. How many cc of 25% Lysol stock solution are needed to prepare 1 L of 2.5% solution?

17. How many cc of 75% stock solution are necessary to prepare 300 ml of 5% dilute solution?

18. The doctor orders morphine sulfate 10 mg IV q3h prn for pain. Available in stock is morphine sulfate 16 mg/cc. How many cc will the nurse need to give?

19. The nurse is to infuse 500 cc of packed red blood cells over 4 hours. The administration set has a drop factor of 10. How many drops/min should be infused?

20. The order is 1500 ml 5% dextrose with normal saline to infuse in 16 hours. How many milliliters will infuse in 1 hour?

21. The order is 100 ml 5% dextrose and 0.45% saline that contains 100 U regular insulin. It is to infuse at 12 U/hr. The drop factor is 60. What is the gtt/min flow rate?

22. If 200 ml of DW IV is left in a bottle at 7 PM, at what time will the infusion be completed if the drop factor is 15 and the drop rate is set at 40 gtt/min?

23. You are to give carbamazepine to a child who weighs 70 lb and is 45 inches in height. Using the nomogram in the text in Figure 6-1, state this child's BSA and calculate the proper dosage range for this child. The adult dosage range is 200 to 1200 mg/day.

Chapter 7
Over-the-Counter Drugs and Self-Medication

1. State common properties of over-the-counter (OTC) drugs.

2. Summarize the following legislative acts:

   a. Pure Food and Drug Act of 1906

   b. The Sherley Amendment (1912)

   c. The 1938 Food and Drug Act

   d. The Durham-Humphrey Amendment of 1952

   e. The Kefauver-Harris Amendment of 1962

3. Describe each of the three categories of OTC drugs:

   a. Category I

   b. Category II

   c. Category III

4. List at least five classifications of OTC drugs and state a therapeutic use for each.

5. Describe the intent of the Dietary Supplement Health and Education Act of 1994.

6. Discuss some of the cautions necessary when considering herbal remedies for sale in the United States.

7. Develop a teaching plan for a patient taking OTC drugs.

Chapter 8
Issues of Drug Abuse

Define the following:

1. Drug abuse

2. Drug dependence

3. Tolerance

4. Withdrawal

5. Physical dependence

Match the drug in Column A to its desired effect in Column B and withdrawal effect in Column C.

Column A	Column B	Column C
6. alcohol ____	1. Relaxation	a. Seizures
____	2. Distorted perception	b. Headaches
7. PCP ____	3. Mild stimulation	c. Irritability
____	4. Euphoria	d. Depression
8. marijuana ____		e. Tremors
____		f. None
9. cocaine ____		
____		
10. benzodiazepines ____		
____		
11. LSD ____		
____		
12. caffeine ____		
____		
13. nicotine ____		
____		

14. Identify important data necessary to obtain during the assessment phase of the nursing process.

Chapter 9
Care of the Poisoned Patient

Define the following:

1. Toxicokinetics

2. Toxicodynamics

3. Competitive antidote

4. Chelate

Match each poison to its antidote.

5. _____ lead   a. naloxone (Narcan)

6. _____ cyanide   b. deferoxamine mesylate (Desferal)

7. _____ morphine   c. acetylcysteine (Mucomyst)

8. _____ acetaminophen   d. edetate calcium disodium

9. _____ iron   e. amyl nitrate

10. List the three major points that determine whether vomiting or gastric lavage should be used to empty the stomach in cases of poisoning.
    a.

    b.

    c.

Discuss the action of the following nonspecific antidotes for poison removal.

11. gastric lavage

12. ipecac syrup

13. activated charcoal

14. List two nursing diagnoses and three nursing interventions appropriate in the care of a poisoned patient.

Chapter 10
Introduction to Autonomic Pharmacology

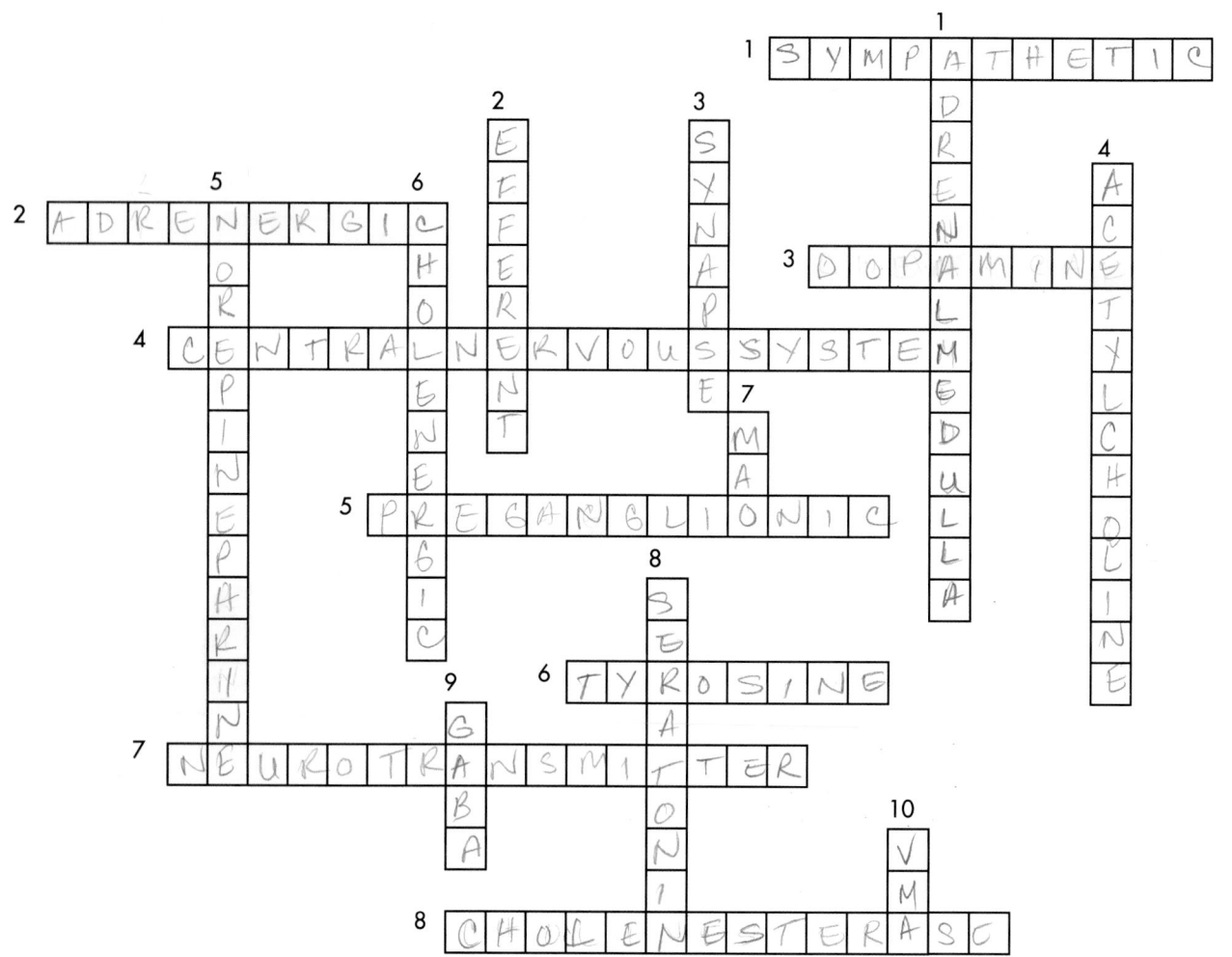

Across

1. Nervous system initiating the "fight or flight" response
2. Synonym for 1 across
3. A neurotransmitter
4. Includes the brain and spinal cord
5. Neuron with cell body in spinal cord
6. Amino acid necessary for synthesis of norepinephrine
7. Chemical synthesized in nerve cells
8. Enzyme that degrades acetylcholine

Down

1. Gland that converts norepinephrine to epinephrine
2. Relays information from the central nervous system to the peripheral nervous system
3. Space between a neuron and a cell
4. Major neurotransmitter affecting both the parasympathetic and sympathetic nervous system
5. Major neurotransmitter affecting the sympathetic nervous system
6. Synonym for parasympathetic nervous system
7. Monoamine oxidase
8. A neurotransmitter
9. An inhibitory neurotransmitter
10. Metabolite of norepinephrine and epinephrine

Chapter 11
Mechanics of Cholinergic Control

Define the following:

1. Cholinergic — parasympathetic nervous system

2. Muscarine — mimics acetylcholine at postganglionic receptors

3. nicotine — " " skeletal muscle/ganglionic receptors

4. Direct-acting cholinomimetic drug — mimic acetylcholine

5. Indirect-acting cholinomimetic drug — inhibit acetylcholinesterase

Match the physiologic response to the specific receptor.

6. _a_ Salivation   a. Muscarinic

7. _a_ Miosis   b. Nicotinic

8. _b_ Smooth muscle contraction

9. _a_ Diarrhea

10. _b_ Increased muscle strength

11. Describe the action of atropine. Blocks acetylcholine at the muscarinic receptors. Affects smooth muscle, the heart & exocrine glands

12. List important concepts to teach a patient receiving atropine systemically.
Dry mouth, ↑ HR, photophobia, constipation, N+V, urinary hesitancy/retention, skin dry/flushed → may develop temp 2° inability to sweat.

For the following agents, list its classification and therapeutic use.

	Classification	Therapeutic Use
13. edrophonium (Tensilon)	nicotinic	dx myasthenia gravis, myasthenic vs. cholinergic crisis
14. demacarium (Humorsol)	muscarinic	constriction of pupil
15. bethanchol (Urecholine)	muscarinic	stimulates atonic bladder/intestine
16. pralidoxime (Protopam)	musc/nico.	reactivates acetylcholinesterase
17. pilocarpine (Pilocar)	musc.	constriction of pupil

Chapter 12
Mechanisms of Adrenergic Control

Match the physiologic effect to the receptor stimulated.

1. __c__ Increased heart rate

2. __b__ Central nervous system control of sympathetic tone

3. __a__ Constriction of arterioles and veins, causing increased blood pressure

4. __d__ Dilation of bronchioles

5. __c__ Increased impulse conduction speed in cardiac tissue

6. __a__ Dilation of the pupil

7. __d__ Relaxation of uterine smooth muscle

8. __a__ Nasal decongestion

9. __c__ Increased force of ventricular contraction

a. Alpha$_1$ adrenergic

b. Alpha$_2$ adrenergic

c. Beta$_1$ adrenergic

d. Beta$_2$ adrenergic

10. List the side effects of epinephrine.

restless, nervous, insomnia, ↑ B/p & HR

11. Identify three naturally occurring catecholamines.

epinephrine, norepinephrine, dopamine

12. Name two alpha-adrenergic receptor antagonists and two beta-adrenergic receptor antagonists and their main therapeutic uses.

alpha: Dibenzyline - Raynaud's / HTN 2° pheochromocytoma
Minipress - chronic HTN / BPH
beta: atenolol - HTN / angina
betaxolol - glaucoma

13. Identify safety needs of a patient receiving an alpha-adrenergic antagonist.

May faint 2° orthostatic hypotension

Chapter 13
Antihypertensive Drugs

Define the following:

1. Hypertension

2. Adrenergic blockers

3. ACE inhibitors

4. Calcium channel blockers

5. Diuretics

6. Describe the renin-angiotensin-aldosterone mechanism

7. List the special needs of the older adult receiving antihypertensives.

8. List the lifestyle changes necessary for patients with hypertension.

9. State the reason(s) that beta blockers should not be discontinued abruptly.

10. What issues may influence patient compliance with antihypertensive drug therapy?

11. Discuss the assessment needed when planning the care of the hypertensive patient.

Chapter 14
Diuretics

Match the diuretic to the site of the nephron it influences.

1. _____ furosemide

2. _____ acetazolamide

3. _____ hydrochlorothiazide

4. _____ spironolactone

5. _____ dichlorphenamide

6. _____ bumetanide

a. Proximal tubule

b. Distal tubule

c. Loop of Henle

Match the diuretic to its classification.

7. _____ methazolamide

8. _____ spironolactone

9. _____ bumetanide

10. _____ chlorthalidone

11. _____ ethacrynic acid

12. _____ quinethazone

13. _____ triamterene

14. _____ furosemide

15. _____ mannitol

16. _____ acetazolamide

17. _____ hydrochlorothiazide

a. Thiazides and related drugs

b. Loop diuretics

c. Osmotic diuretics

d. Carbonic anhydrase inhibitors

e. Potassium-sparing diuretics

18. List special nursing considerations for administering diuretics to an older adult patient.

19. List five foods high in potassium.

20. What important dietary concern is necessary for the patient who is now taking spironolactone?

Chapter 15
Antianginals and Other Vasodilators

Define the following:

1. Raynaud's disease

2. Angina pectoris

3. Nitrates

4. Vasodilators

5. Differentiate classic angina, variant angina, and unstable angina.

6. List the various dosage forms of nitroglycerin.

7. List the three therapeutic objectives for the use of antianginal agents.
    a.

    b.

    c.

8. Identify patient education strategies when administering via transdermal delivery system.

9. Describe how beta-blockers are used for prophylactic therapy.

Chapter 16
Drugs to Treat Hypotension and Shock

Define the following:

1. Shock

2. Anaphylactic shock

3. Reflex bradycardia

4. Sympathomimetic drug

5. Develop a table comparing and contrasting the following drugs:

Drug	Action	Side Effect	Advantages/ Disadavantages
a. dobutamine HCl			
b. dopamine HCl			
c. epinephrine HCl			
d. isoproterenol HCl			
e. levarterenol bitartrate			
f. memphentermine sulfate			

6. Describe the complications that occur if extravasation of sympathomimetic drugs occurs, and explain the appropriate actions to take.

7. Name an alternative route for epinephrine if the intravenous route is unavailable.

8. Differentiate the three levels of dosages for dopamine.
   a.

   b.

   c.

Chapter 17
Fluids and Electrolytes

1. Differentiate the following:

   a. Osmosis and diffusion

   b. Acidosis and alkalosis

   c. Intracellular fluid and extracellular fluid (be sure to name the two main fluid compartments of extracellular fluid)

2. Describe the signs and symptoms of the following:

   a. Fluid volume deficit

   b. Fluid volume excess

3. Complete the following table:

Solute	Signs of Deficiency (state terminology)	Signs of Excess (state terminology)
a. sodium		
b. potassium		

4. Describe the main therapeutic uses for the following:

   a. sodium chloride in water

   b. Ringer's solution and lactated Ringer's solution

   c. dextrose in water

   d. potassium chloride

   e. human albumin

5. List three potential problems and a corresponding nursing action associated with intravenous infusions.

Problem	Nursing Action
a.	
b.	
c.	

6. List nursing care strategies for a patient receiving parenteral nutrition.

Chapter 18
Drugs to Control Congestive Heart Failure

Define the following:

1. Inotropic

2. Congestive heart failure

3. Loading dose

4. Contractility

5. Afterload

6. Create a table that describes the following:

	Desired Effect When Treating Congestive Heart Failure	Potential Adverse Effects
a. Angiotensin-converting enzyme		
b. Diuretics		
c. amrinone		

7. List adverse reactions associated with digoxin.

8. List at least three factors that may predispose a patient to digitalis toxicity.

9. Describe the patient education strategies required for a patient receiving cardiac glycoside therapy.

Chapter 19
Drugs to Control Cardiac Arrhythmias

Define the following:

1. Arrhythmia

2. Bradycardia

3. Tachycardia

4. Reentry phenomenon

5. PVCs

6. Refractory period

Match the antiarrhythmic drug to its classification. Summarize the effects of each classification.

7. _____ procainamide

8. _____ mexiletine

9. _____ verapamil

10. _____ quinidine

11. _____ esmolol

12. _____ propafenone

13. _____ bretylium

14. _____ lidocaine

a. Group IA _____

a. Group IB _____

a. Group IC _____

a. Group II _____

a. Group III _____

a. Group IV _____

15. Identify nursing considerations for patients receiving antiarrhythmic agents.

16. Identify the components of the normal electrocardiogram.

Chapter 20
Agents Affecting Blood Coagulation

Define the following:

1. Thrombus

2. Embolus

3. Thrombolytic

4. Anticoagulant

5. Define aPTT and state the drug it monitors for appropriate levels.

6. Define PT and state the drug it monitors for appropriate levels.

Match the drug with the reaction it causes when given with anticoagulants.

7. _____ rifampin

8. _____ quinidine

9. _____ vitamin K

10. _____ aspirin

11. _____ cimetidine

12. _____ cholestyramine

13. _____ ibuprofen

14. _____ barbituates

a. Increases effect of an anticoagulant

b. Decreases effect of an anticoagulant

15. Identify risks associated with coadministration of thrombolytics and anticoagulants.

16. Identify nursing implications for the patient receiving thrombolytics.

17. Name the antidote for an overdose of oral anticoagulants.

18. Name the antidote for an overdose of heparin.

Chapter 21
Drugs to Lower Blood Lipid Levels

Define the following:

1. Hyperlipidemia

2. Atherosclerosis

3. High-density lipoproteins

4. Lipoproteins

5. Low-density lipoproteins

6. Chylomicrons

7. List two drugs that interact with bile acid sequestering agents and the effects they produce.

Drug	Effects
a.	
b.	

8. List education strategies appropriate for a patient receiving clofibrate.

9. List adverse reactions of bile acid sequestrants.

10. What does the patient need to know regarding the timing of doses of HMG-CoA reductase inhibitors (Statins)?

Chapter 22
Drugs to Treat Anemia

Define the following:

1. Hematopoieses

2. Erythropoietin

3. Anemia

4. Iron

5. RBC

6. List and describe types of anemias.

Anemia Type	Characteristics	Drug(s) of Choice for Treatment
a.		
b.		
c.		
d.		

7. List foods high in iron.

8. Describe the nursing considerations for a patient receiving iron therapy.

9. Describe the mechanism of action of epoetin alfa, and state when effects are seen.

Chapter 23
Drugs Affecting Motility: Cholinergic Stimulants and Anticholinergics/Antispasmodics

1. Describe how the autonomic nervous system affects the gastrointestinal system.

2. List two gastrointestinal stimulants and their adverse reactions.

   Stimulant   **Adverse Reactions**

   a.

   b.

3. Develop a table describing three gastrointestinal antispasmodics.

   Drug   **Action**   **Contraindications**

   a.

   b.

   c.

4. Describe xerostomia and nursing measures to diminish discomfort.

Chapter 24
Laxatives and Antidiarrheals

Define the following:

1. Constipation

2. Laxatives

3. Diarrhea

4. Absorbents

5. Suggest nursing diagnoses for the use of antidiarrheals and appropriate nursing interventions.

6. List measures, including recommended foods, the nurse can suggest to prevent or treat constipation.

Match each drug with its laxative classification.

Drug

7. _____ magnesium sulfate

8. _____ lactulose

9. _____ methylcellulose

10. _____ docusate sodium

11. _____ mineral oil

12. _____ bisacodyl

13. _____ sodium phosphate

Classification

a. Bulk-forming

b. Stimulants

c. Osmotics

d. Stool softeners

e. Lubricants

f. Miscellaneous

For each medication classification, describe the mechanism of action.

14. Bulk-forming laxative

15. Wetting agent

16. Stimulant cathartic

17. Saline cathartic

18. Opioid-related drugs

1. Describe the body systems involved when vomiting occurs.

2. Name conditions commonly associated with nausea and vomiting.

Match the drug with its mode of action.

Drug	**Action**
3. _____ hyroxyzine HCl	a. Anticholinergic
4. _____ granisetron HCl	b. Antihistamine
5. _____ nabilone	c. Antidopaminergic
6. _____ scopolamine	d. Antiserotinergic
7. _____ chlorpromazine HCl	e. Cannabinoid
8. _____ ondansetron	
9. _____ dimenhydrinate	
10. _____ metoclopramide	
11. _____ prochlorperazine	

12. Describe the recommended treatment for nausea and vomiting in pregnancy.

13. Develop a nursing care plan for a patient receiving an antiemetic.

Chapter 26
Drugs to Treat Acid Reflux and Ulcers

Indicate the actions of antacids and histamine H_2-receptor antagonists by putting an A (antacids); H (histamine H_2-receptor antagonists); B (both); or N (neither) in front of the following possible actions.

1. _____ Neutralize hydrochloric acid

2. _____ Increase gastric pH

3. _____ Buffer gastric acid

4. _____ Inhibit secretion of gastric acid

5. _____ Decrease gastric pH

6. _____ Promote healing of gastric and duodenal ulcers

7. Describe the action of sucralfate and its use in the treatment of patients with ulcers.

8. What information should be given to parents of a child receiving an antacid and an H_2-receptor blocker for a gastric ulcer?

9. Describe the differences between H_1-and H_2-receptor antagonists.

10. Describe the role of *Helicobacter pylori* as a cause of ulcers and the treatment for this condition.

11. State the nursing implications for the acid (proton) pump inhibitors lansoprazole and omeprazole.

Chapter 27
Drugs to Treat Gallbladder and Pancreatic Diseases

Define the following:

1. Gallstone

2. Cholelithiasis

3. Cholecystitis

4. Pancreatic enzymes

5. Describe the main adverse reactions to therapy with chenodiol.

6. If a pregnant patient has been diagnosed with uncomplicated gallstones, which drug (if any) could she safely receive for pharmacologic therapy?

7. When teaching the patient receiving pharmacologic therapy for gallstones, what should you explain about the duration of treatment?

8. Describe the patient education principles for the patient taking pancreatic enzyme replacements.

Chapter 28
Drugs to Treat Asthma and Other Pulmonary Diseases

Define the following:

1. Bronchodilators

2. Asthma

3. Extrinsic asthma

4. COPD

5. Respiratory distress syndrome

6. List the three ways asthma restricts the airways.

7. Describe two ways aerosol drugs can be administered.

   a.

   b.

8. Describe the action of theophylline.

9. List steps to describe in teaching a patient how to use an inhaler.

10. Describe patient education principles for the patient taking leukotriene modifiers.

11. Differentiate "controller medications" and "reliever medications" for the treatment of asthma and provide examples for each category.

Match each of the following terms with its definition.

1. ____ Rhinitis   a. Hives

2. ____ Eczema   b. Swelling caused by plasma leakage

3. ____ Purpura   c. Inflamed areas of skin

4. ____ Urticaria   d. Inflammation of nasal mucosa

5. ____ Angioedema   e. Red spots on the skin caused by leakage of blood

6. What are the side effects of antihistamines?

7. Define *anaphylaxis*.

8. Identify learning needs of patients receiving antihistamines.

9. What is an advantage of the newer antihistamines, such as astemizole and loratadine, over the older ones?

Chapter 30
Drugs to Control Bronchial Secretions

Define the following:

1. Antitussive

2. Expectorant

3. Mucolytic

4. Rebound congestion

5. Cough

6. List nursing interventions for a patient receiving acetylcysteine (Mucomyst).

7. What home teaching should be given to a patient using nasal decongestants?

8. List two antitussives and their adverse reactions.

9. Describe the proper application of nasal decongestant nose drops.

Chapter 31
Aspirin, Acetaminophen, NSAIDs, and Drugs to Treat Gout

Define the following:

1. Analgesia

2. NSAIDs

3. Acetylsalicylic acid

4. Prostaglandins

5. Gout

6. List three drugs that interact with NSAIDs and their adverse, interactive effects.

      Drug   **Effect**

   a.

   b.

   c.

Specify the actions for each drug listed. Some may have more than one action.

Drugs	Primary Actions
7. ____ acetaminophen	a. Antipyretic
8. ____ aspirin	b. Antiinflammatory
9. ____ ibuprofen	c. Analgesic
10. ____ indomethacin	d. Inhibit platelet aggregation

11. What are the potential gastrointestinal side effects of indomethacin and how can they be reduced?

12. List the treatment goals for gout.

13. Develop a nursing care plan for a patient receiving probenecid.

Chapter 32
Opioids (Narcotic Analgesics)

Define the following:

1. Neuropeptides

2. Chemoreceptor trigger zone

3. Drug dependence

4. Acute pain

5. Drug tolerance

6. List three known neuropeptides.

7. State the important assessment parameters for vital signs that should be checked before administration of opiates and relevant nursing actions.

Match opioid receptors with their physiologic characteristics.

Receptor	Characteristic Response
8. ____ Mu	a. Spinal analgesia, miosis, sedation, and appetite regulation
9. ____ Kappa	b. Central analgesia, euphoria, respiratory depression, and physical dependence
10. ____ Delta	c. Analgesia both spinally and in brain structures

11. Describe the symptoms of withdrawal syndrome.

12. Describe briefly the recommended steps for pain management for patients with chronic pain.

13. Explain the action and use of naloxone.

Chapter 33
Drugs to Treat Headaches

State the characteristics of the following:

1. Tension headache

2. Migraine headache

3. Cluster headache

4. How does caffeine influence the effect of ergotamine?

5. Name the drugs used for acute and prophylactic treatment of migraine headaches.

6. What are the safety concerns regarding the drugs used for headaches that the nurse should discuss with the patient during education sessions?

7. Name some of the nonpharmacologic interventions that may assist in the prevention or treatment of headaches.

Chapter 34
Management of the Patient in Pain

1. Compare and contrast pharmaceutical methods of pain relief.

2. List factors that interfere with pain relief.

3. Identify objective and subjective assessment data necessary in planning care of a patient experiencing pain.

4. Name the nursing diagnoses that may be appropriate for the patient in pain.

5. Describe nonpharmacologic approaches to pain control and management.

Chapter 35
Local Anesthetics

1. Compare the following forms of anesthesia:

   a. Infiltration:

   b. Epidural:

   c. Saddle block:

   d. Caudal anesthesia:

   e. Nerve block anesthesia:

   f. Surface anesthesia:

2. Describe adverse reactions of local anesthetics.

3. Develop a teaching plan for a patient receiving local anesthetics.

4. Which drugs can be used both topically and by injection to produce anesthesia?

Chapter 36
General Anesthetics

Define the following:

1. MAC

2. Balanced anesthesia

3. Malignant hyperthermia

4. Dissociative anesthetic

5. Conscious sedation

6. Deep sedation

7. Neuroleptanalgesia

8. Define *emergence* and state the important nursing implications for this period of time.

9. Which inhalation anesthetics are the most widely used agents in the United States? Which agent is used often for pediatric patients but not for adults? Which agent is *not* used in the United States?

10. What differences, if any, are there in the anesthesia requirements for pediatric patients and for older adults?

11. Develop a nursing diagnosis, goal, and interventions for an elderly patient receiving a general anesthetic.

Define the following:

1. Neuromuscular-blocking drugs

2. Nondepolarizing blocking drugs

3. Depolarizing neuromuscular-blocking drugs

4. State the uses for neuromuscular-blocking drugs.

5. Complete the following table comparing tubocurarine and succinylcholine.

Drug	Action	Duration	Adverse Reactions
a. tubocurarine			
b. succinylcholine			

6. List nursing diagnoses and nursing interventions for a patient receiving neuromuscular-blocking drugs.

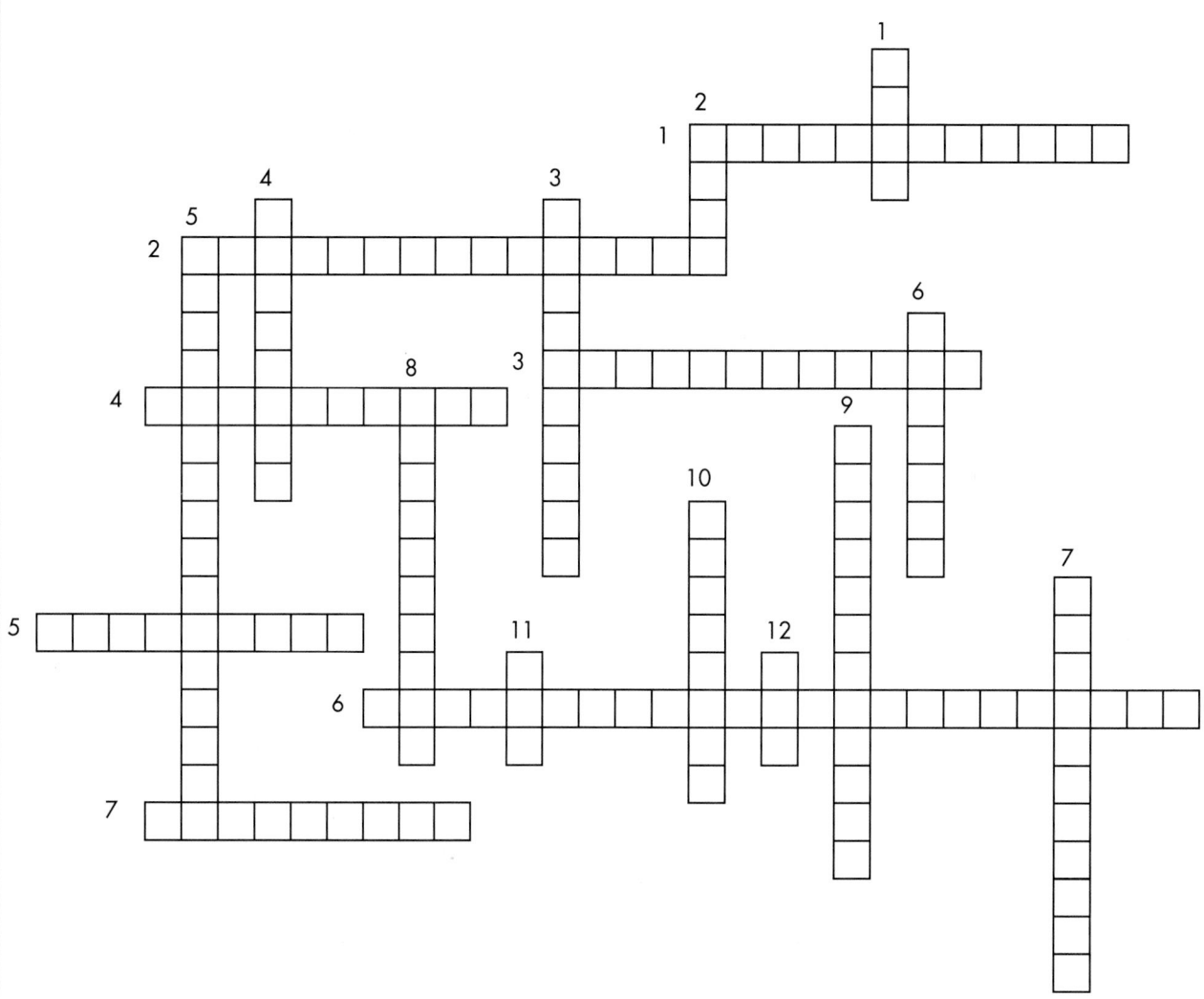

Across

1. The ingestion and destruction of foreign particles by cells of the immune system
2. IgG, IgM, IgA, IgE, and IgD
3. Forms of cytokines which influence leukocytes
4. Soluble proteins of humoral immunity that bind a foreign substance
5. Type of WBC; upon differentiation become macrophages
6. Factor that controls differentiation of hematopoietic stem cells to produce new leukocytes
7. Soluble factors that increase communication within the immune system

Down

1. White blood cells
2. Polymorphonuclear neutrophil leukocytes
3. Immune cells that destroy own body cells
4. Protection against foreign invaders
5. Depletion of ability to fight infections and disease
6. Protein that stimulates antibody production
7. White blood cells that are divided into T cells and B cells
8. Cytokine that is mainly produced by T cells and has antiviral actions
9. Neoplastic diseases that arise from abnormal proliferation of B cells and plasma cells
10. Neoplastic diseases arising from B cells and plasma cells
11. Tumor necrosis factor
12. Human leukocyte antigen

Chapter 39
Immunizations

1. Define immunostimulation and its therapeutic result.

2. Discuss two current developments in immunization therapy.

3. Compare active and passive immunity as indicated by the following headings:

	Definition	Sources	Duration
a. Active immunity			
b. Passive immunity			

Identify each immune agent as causing either (A) active or (B) passive immunity:

4. _____ Varciella-zoster immune globulin

5. _____ Botulism antitoxin

6. _____ Cholera

7. _____ Influenza

8. _____ Hepatitis B immune globulin

9. _____ Rabies

10. _____ Antivenins

11. _____ Diphtheria and tetanus toxoids

12. _____ Diphtheria antitoxin

13. _____ Typhoid

14. _____ Rh_0 (D) immune globulin

15. _____ Polio

16. List the recommended childhood immunizations and the time frame for each.

17. Describe immunity in the fetus and newborn.

Chapter 40
Immunomodulators and Care of Patients with Altered Immune Function

Define the following:

1. Colony-stimulating factors

2. cyclosporine

3. Immunosuppressants

4. Progenitor cells

5. filgrastim

6. sargramostim

7. List the most commonly reported adverse effects of cyclosporine.

8. Differentiate the action of colony-stimulating factors and cell-stimulating agents and name examples of each.

9. Develop a nursing care plan for a patient receiving filgrastim.

Chapter 41
Glucocorticoids to Treat Inflammatory Conditions

1. List four uses for glucocorticoids.

2. State the adverse effects of long-term glucocorticoid use on the following body systems and functions.

   Body System/Function   **Adverse Effects**

   a. Bones

   b. Behavior/mood

   c. Endocrine

   d. Skin

   e. Growth in children

3. Identify two drugs that interact with glucocorticoids and their effects.

   Drug   **Effect**

   a.

   b.

4. Explain the rationale behind the gradual tapering of glucocorticoid doses before discontinuing the drug.

5. Identify two nursing diagnoses and interventions important in the care plan prepared for a patient receiving glucocorticoids.

Chapter 42
Drug Treatment of Selected Autoimmune Diseases

Define the following:

1. Myasthenia gravis

2. Rheumatoid arthritis

3. Systemic lupus erythematosus

4. Multiple sclerosis

5. Autoimmune disease

6. Describe the use of edrophonium with myasthenia gravis. What is the preferred drug for the treatment of this disease?

7. List common DMARDs used for patients with rheumatoid arthritis.

8. Name the goal of drug therapy for patients with systemic lupus erythematosus and list examples of agents used.

9. List the education needs of a patient with multiple sclerosis.

Chapter 43
Introduction to the Use of Antiinfective Agents

Define the following:

1. Procaryotic cells

2. Eucaryotic cells

3. Therapeutic index

4. Bacteriostatic

5. Bactericidal

Match the organism to its microbial classification.

6. _____ *Staphylococcus*

7. _____ Herpes simplex

8. _____ *Proteus*

9. _____ *Streptococcus*

10. _____ *Histoplasma*

11. _____ *Escherichia (E. coli)*

12. _____ Syphilis

13. _____ *Shigella*

14. _____ *Candida*

15. _____ Tuberculosis

a. Gram + bacteria

b. Gram − bacteria

c. Virus

d. *Mycobacteria*

e. *Spirochete*

f. Fungi

16. List the five ways that antibiotics acheive selective toxicity on microorganisms.

17. Develop an education plan for a patient receiving an antimicrobial.

Chapter 44
Penicillins, Cephalosporins, and Related Drugs

Define the following:

1. Beta-lactam antibiotic

2. penicillin

3. cephalosporin

4. MRSA

5. Transpeptidase

6. Broad-spectrum antibiotic

7. List interactions of beta-lactam antibiotics

8. Describe the two most common adverse reactions to beta-lactam antibiotics.

9. Explain the rationale behind the use of repository penicillins.

Match the drug with its corresponding classification

Drug

10. _____ methicillin
11. _____ ticarcillin
12. _____ cefoxitin
13. _____ amoxicillin
14. _____ cefotaxime
15. _____ nafcillin
16. _____ cephalothin
17. _____ procaine Penicillin G
18. _____ ampicillin
19. _____ cefazolin
20. _____ penicillin G

Classification

a. First-generation cephalosporin
b. Second-generation cephalosporin
c. Third-generation cephalosporin
d. Penicillinase-resistant penicillins
e. Extended-spectrum penicillins
f. Repository penicillins
g. Anti-*Pseudomonas* penicillins
h. Narrow-spectrum penicillins

21. Develop a nursing care plan for a patient receiving an antimicrobial.

Chapter 45
Quinolones

1. Describe the action of quinolones.

2. Discuss quinolones' adverse effects.

Fill in the following table with drug interactions occurring with quinolone antibiotics.

Drug	Interaction
3. theophylline	
4. didanosine	
5. warfarin	
6. caffeine	
7. Antacids	
8. sodium bicarbonate	

9. List three fluoroquinolones and their primary uses.

10. List two nursing diagnoses appropriate for a patient receiving quinolones.

Chapter 46
Macrolides, Clindamycin, and Miscellaneous Penicillin Substitutes

Define the following:

1. VRE

2. Macrolide

3. Red man's syndrome

4. Bacteremia

5. Cholestatic hepatitis

6. Describe pseudomembranous colitis and the causative organism.

7. Identify nursing care concerns of an elderly patient receiving vancomycin.

Provide the action, uses, and adverse effects for each drug listed.

Drug	Action	Uses	Adverse Effects
8. erythromycin			
9. clindamycin			
10. vancomycin			
11. spectinomycin			

12. Describe nursing interventions for proper administration of intravenous vancomycin.

Chapter 47
Tetracyclines and Chloramphenicol

1. Describe the mode of action of tetracyclines.

2. List diseases tetracyclines are effective in controlling.

3. What are the special considerations given when administering tetracycline to pediatric patients?

4. Develop a nursing care plan for a patient receiving chloramphenicol.

5. What characteristics make doxycycline and minocycline different from other tetracyclines?

6. Describe education principles regarding food and drug interactions for the patient taking oral tetracyclines.

Chapter 48
Aminoglycosides

1. List four drugs classified as aminoglycosides.

2. Describe the three significant dose-dependent toxicities that may occur with aminoglycosides.
    a.

    b.

    c.

3. Which nursing considerations would be appropriate for an elderly patient taking aminoglycosides?

For each of the following aminoglycosides, write a trade name and state the primary uses.

Generic name	Trade name	Primary uses
4. tobramycin		
5. kanamycin		
6. amikacin		
7. gentamicin		

8. What serum diagnostic tests should be monitored for the patient receiving aminoglycoside therapy?

9. What is the difference between peak and trough drug levels?

10. Develop a teaching plan for a patient receiving gentamicin.

Define the following:

1. UTI

2. Crystalluria

3. G6PD

4. What is the purpose of the addition of phenazopyridine to sulfonomide preparations for the treatment of UTIs?

5. What should the patient be told about his or her urine when either nitrofurantoin or phenazopyridine is prescribed?

6. Compare the adverse effects that can occur in geriatric and pediatric patients receiving sulfonamides.

7. List two drugs that interact with trimethoprim and their effects.

Drug	Effect
a.	
b.	

8. Develop a teaching plan for an adolescent receiving nitrofurantoin.

Define the following:

1. AIDS

2. HIV

3. Tuberculosis

4. Leprosy

5. dapsone

6. Discuss transmission of the tubercle bacilli and interventions to prevent the spread of tuberculosis.

7. List the learning needs of an elderly client receiving isoniazid.

8. Develop a nursing care plan for a client taking dapsone.

9. State the rationale behind multiple drug therapy for *M. tuberculosis.*

10. Why is drug therapy for leprosy long term?

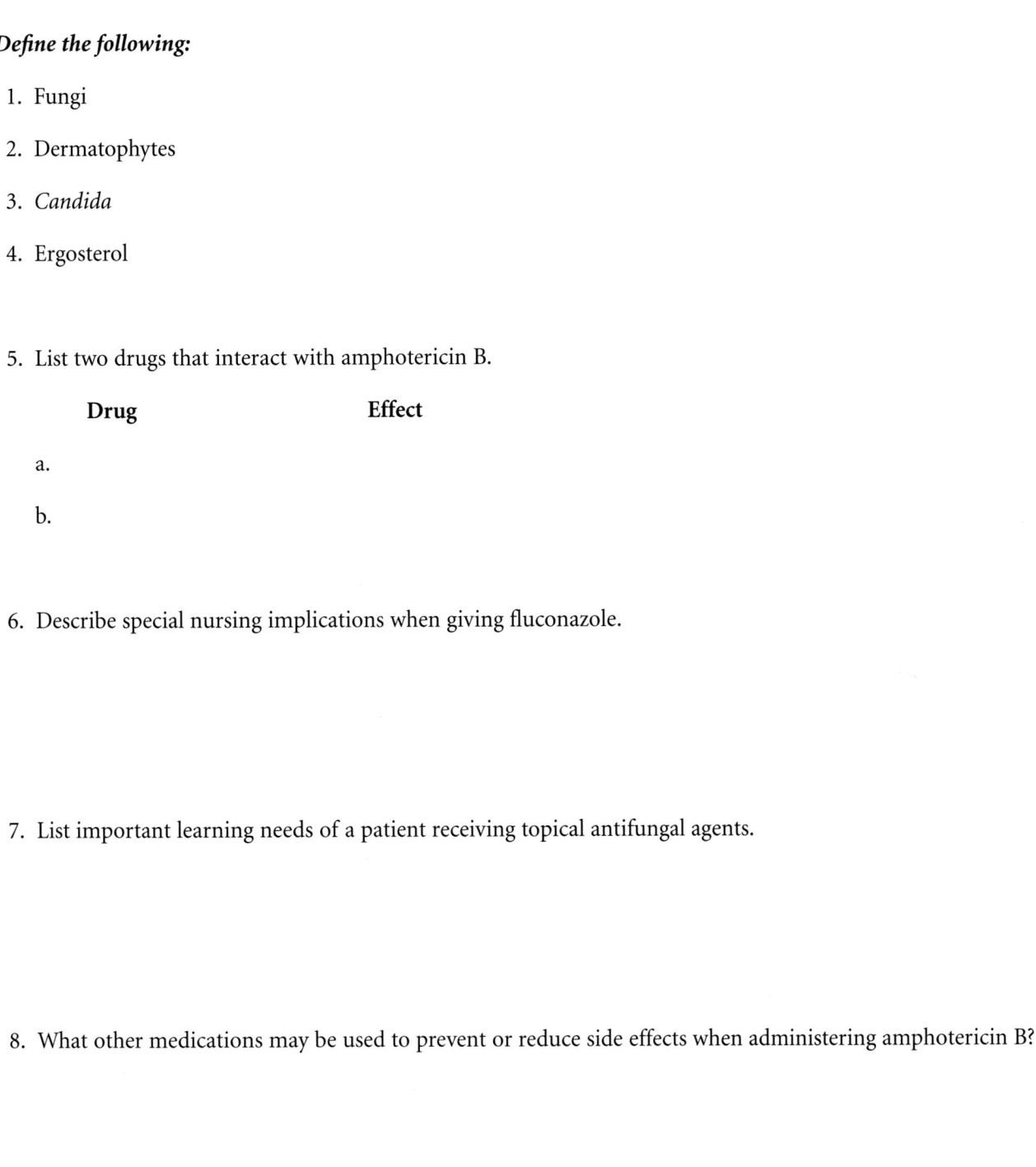

Chapter 51
Antifungal Agents

Define the following:

1. Fungi

2. Dermatophytes

3. *Candida*

4. Ergosterol

5. List two drugs that interact with amphotericin B.

      Drug   **Effect**

  a.

  b.

6. Describe special nursing implications when giving fluconazole.

7. List important learning needs of a patient receiving topical antifungal agents.

8. What other medications may be used to prevent or reduce side effects when administering amphotericin B?

1. Define *HAART.*

2. Describe the action of antiviral drugs.

3. List side effects/adverse reactions of amantadine.

4. Describe patient education for the patient receiving acyclovir for treatment of genital herpes.

5. List administration concerns when giving ribavirin to pediatric patients.

6. Describe the mechanism of action of zidovudine and its effectiveness against HIV.

7. Describe opportunistic infections.

Define the following:

1. Amebic disease

2. Malaria

3. *Cryptosporidia*

4. Enterobiasis

5. *Pneumocystis carinii*

6. Explain the life cycle of a malarial parasite.

7. Describe the dangers of giving chloroquine to infants and children.

Match the following drugs to their therapeutic use classifications.

8. _____ piperazine   a. Ameba

9. _____ chloroquine   b. Malaria

10. _____ niclosamide   c. Parasites

11. _____ mebendazole   d. Helminths

12. _____ diloxanide

13. _____ metronidazole

14. _____ quinine

15. _____ pentamidine

16. Describe food and/or drug interactions that may occur during therapy with metronidazole.

17. State patient teaching points for a patient with a helminthic infestation.

Chapter 54
Introduction to Cancer Chemotherapy

1. State the defining properties of cancer cells.

Define the following:

2. Tumor promoters

3. Oncogenes

4. Carcinogenesis

5. Chemotherapy

6. Explain dose-limiting toxicity.

7. List the phases of the cell cycle and describe what happens in each phase.

In addition to malignant cells, some normal cells in the body are commonly affected by antineoplastic agents. Fill in the following chart with the adverse effect most likely to be produced by the affected cells, and provide interventions for each side effect.

Normal Cells Attacked	Adverse Response Seen	Interventions
8. Gastrointestinal tract		
9. Bone marrow		
10. Hair follicles		
11. Mouth		

Chapter 55
Cytotoxic Drugs to Treat Cancer

Match the drug action to the appropriate antineoplastic agent listed on the left.

Drug Action	Antineoplastic Agent
1. _____ Blocks DNA synthesis (S-phase inhibitor)	a. asparaginase
2. _____ Prevents or arrests mitosis	b. bleomycin
3. _____ Directly attacks DNA	c. vinblastine
4. _____ Blocks RNA or protein synthesis	d. methotrexate

For each drug listed, name the side effects/adverse reactions that may be seen.

5. cisplatin

6. cyclophosphamide

7. asparaginase

8. paclitaxel

9. Develop a teaching plan for the patient receiving procarbazine as chemotherapy. Be sure to specify food-drug interactions.

10. Name some precautions the health care worker should take when preparing or administering chemotherapeutic agents.

Chapter 56
Tissue-Specific Anticancer Agents

Match the cytotoxic agent with the type of cancer it is effective against.

1. _____ Streptozocin

2. _____ interferon alfa-2a

3. _____ tamoxifen

4. _____ goserelin

5. _____ Milotane

6. _____ megestrol

7. _____ estramustine

8. _____ leuprolide

9. _____ interferon alfa-n1

a. Prostate cancer

b. Breast cancer

c. Kaposi's sarcoma

d. Adrenal cancer

e. Pancreatic cancer

f. Melanoma

10. How does prednisone, a glucocorticoid, work against cancer?

11. List three adverse reactions of estrogens.

12. Develop a nursing care plan for a patient receiving interferons.

Chapter 57
Sedative-Hypnotic and Antianxiety Drugs

Define the following:

1. Anxiety disorders

2. Phobia

3. REM sleep

4. Insomnia

5. List data necessary to collect from a patient receiving sedative-hypnotics during the assessment phase of the nursing process.

6. Develop a care plan (nursing diagnoses, goal, and intervention) for a pediatric patient receiving an antianxiety drug.

7. What are nonpharmacologic approaches the patient may take to try to resolve insomnia?

8. Differentiate *sedatives* and *hypnotics.*

9. Describe the important points to include in a teaching plan for the patient who is to receive disulfiram.

Chapter 58
Antipsychotic Drugs

Define the following:

1. Neuroleptic

2. Psychosis

3. Organic psychosis

4. Toxic psychosis

5. Antipsychotic drugs

6. Neuroleptic malignant syndrome

7. Describe photosensitivity and measures that should be taken to prevent problems with this.

8. Describe the mechanism of action of phenothiazines.

9. Define the four extrapyramidal syndromes that may occur with antipsychotic drug therapy and state whether they are reversible or irreversible.

10. Develop a teaching plan for a patient taking antipsychotic drugs.

11. State the advantages of atypical antipsychotics.

Chapter 59
Antidepressant and Antimanic Agents

Define the following:

1. Depression

2. Dysthymia

3. Bipolar disorder

4. Serotonin syndrome

5. Name the four categories of antidepressants and the botanical that is often used for depression.

6. State the advantages of therapy with SSRIs versus tricyclic antidepressants.

7. Describe the patient teaching regarding diet and MAO inhibitors.

8. Explain the rationale behind regular monitoring of lithium drug levels.

9. What should the patient and family be told regarding the onset of therapeutic effects of antidepressant medications?

10. List two nursing interventions for the following adverse reactions of tricyclic antidepressants.

Adverse Reaction	Nursing Interventions
a. Sedation	1.
	2.
b. Anticholinergic effects	1.
	2.
c. Cardiac effects	1.
	2.

Chapter 60
Central Nervous System Stimulants

Define the following:

1. Anorexiants

2. Analeptics

3. Attention-deficit hyperactivity disorder

4. Amphetamines

5. Narcolepsy

6. List important concepts to teach the patient who is receiving amphetamines.

7. List drug interactions that can occur with anorexiants.

8. List adverse reactions of methylphenidate hydrochloride, including pediatric concerns.

9. What agents may be used for respiratory depression?

Chapter 61
Anticonvulsants

1. What is the physiologic mechanism producing the symptoms of epilepsy?

2. Name two adverse reactions of carbamazipine.

3. What disorders are commonly treated with valproic acid?

4. Answer each of the following statements with *T* for true and *F* for false.

   a. _____ IV phenytoin should be mixed with 0.9% sodium chloride to prevent precipitation.

   b. _____ Ethosuximide is a drug of choice for typical absence seizures.

   c. _____ Phenytoin is noted for a lack of drug interactions.

   d. _____ Diazepam is used for status epilepticus.

5. Develop a nursing care plan, including nursing diagnoses, goals, and interventions, for a child receiving an anticonvulsant.

Match the anticonvulsant with the adverse reaction(s) it is associated with.

6. _____ Drowsiness, hangover-type effects   a. phenobarbital

7. _____ Liver failure   b. phenytoin

8. _____ Hiccups, headaches   c. valproic acid

9. _____ Hirsutism   d. ethosuximide

10. Describe the potential oral adverse effects of phenytoin and measures to reduce them.

11. Define the following types of seizures:

    a. Generalized seizures

    b. Partial seizures

    c. Status epilepticus

    d. Tonic-clonic epilepsy

    e. Absence epilepsy

Chapter 62
Drugs to Treat Parkinson's Disease and Alzheimer's Disease

Define the following:

1. Parkinson's disease

2. Akinesia

3. Bradykinesia

4. Rigidity

5. Alzheimer's disease

6. Describe the basic pathophysiology of Parkinson's disease, and list some of the signs and symptoms seen in the patient.

7. Describe the main pharmacologic actions of antiparkinsonian agents.

8. List nursing interventions appropriate for a patient receiving levodopa.

9. Describe drug therapy for a patient with Alzheimer's disease.

Chapter 63
Centrally Acting Skeletal Muscle Relaxants

Define the following:

1. Spasticity

2. Muscle spasms

3. GABA

4. Describe the method of action for centrally acting skeletal muscle relaxants.

5. Compare the action of dantrolene with other agents used to relieve muscle spasms.

6. List the more common adverse effects of the muscle relaxant dantrolene.

7. Develop a nursing care plan, including nursing diagnoses, goals, and interventions, for a patient receiving baclofen.

8. What precautions should be taken regarding drug interactions with centrally acting skeletal muscle relaxants?

Chapter 64
Introduction to Endocrinology

Define the following:

1. Hormone

2. Endocrine glands

3. Target tissues

4. TSH

5. ADH

6. Prohormones

7. Hypothalamus

8. Recombinant proteins

9. Compare the two types of hormones based on their chemical compositions.

10. List and explain the three primary clinical uses of hormones, and provide an example of each.

   a.

   b.

   c.

Chapter 65
Drugs Affecting the Pituitary Gland

Define the following:

1. Neurohypophysis

2. Oxytocin

3. ADH

4. Adenohypophysis

5. Growth hormone

6. Negative feedback

7. Differentiate the effects of growth hormone deficiency and excess.

8. Describe diabetes insipidus and state the cause.

9. Describe SIADH and state the cause.

Match each hormone with the gland from which it is secreted.

10. ____ FSH

11. ____ TSH

12. ____ LH

13. ____ Vasopressin

14. ____ ACTH

15. ____ Oxytocin

a. Anterior pituitary

b. Posterior pituitary

16. Describe intervention, education, and evaluative strategies for a child receiving somatropin.

Define the following:

1. Mineralocorticoids

2. Renin-angiotensin system

3. Glucocorticoid

4. Adrenal insufficiency

5. Addison's disease

6. Aldosterone

7. List the symptoms of acute adrenal insufficiency.

8. Differentiate the function of the adrenal cortex and that of the adrenal medulla.

9. Identify two drugs that interact with mineralocorticoids and their effects.

	Drug	**Effect**
a.		
b.		

10. Name the major glucocorticoid produced, and describe Cushing's syndrome.

For the following, state whether the action is classified as a glucocorticoid action (a) or a mineralocorticoid action (b).

11. _____ Antiinflammatory and immunosuppressive activity

12. _____ Sodium retaining activity with potassium loss

13. _____ Metabolic effects on carbohydrate, protein, and fat metabolism

14. List assessment data important to obtain from a patient receiving fludrocortisone.

Chapter 67
Drugs Affecting the Thyroid Gland

1. Define T_3 and T_4 and state their role in the body. Which one is considered the most important metabolic regulator?

2. Describe the role of TSH.

3. Define *euthyroid.*

4. For each disease listed, state whether there is an excess or deficiency of thyroid hormone, and describe the symptoms:

Disease	Excess or Deficiency?	Symptoms
a. Myxedema		
b. Graves' disease		

5. Describe the thyroid uptake of radioiodine test and factors that may alter results.

6. Describe the education needs for the patient taking levothyroxine.

Chapter 68
Drugs Affecting Calcium Metabolism

1. Describe the effect of calcium on the body and its serum concentration range.

2. Describe the role of vitamin D and state sources.

3. State the effects of vitamin D deficiency and excess.

Define the following:

4. Calcitonin

5. Parathyroid hormone

6. Osteoporosis

7. Paget's disease

8. Define and state the symptoms of the following:

   a. Hypercalcemia

   b. Hypocalcemia

9. List foods high in calcium, and state dietary requirements across the life span.

10. Describe the education needs for the patient taking calcium replacement therapy.

Chapter 69
Drugs to Treat Diabetes Mellitus

Define the following:

1. Glucosuria

2. Ketoacidosis

3. Insulin

4. Oral hypoglycemic agents

5. Differentiate between type 1 and type 2 diabetes.

6. List special nursing interventions related to insulin administration.

7. Match signs and symptoms to blood glucose disorders.

   a. _____ Hunger   HYPER—Hyperglycemia
   b. _____ Thirst   HYPO—Hypoglycemia
   c. _____ Kussmaul's respirations   DC—Diabetic coma
   d. _____ Polyuria
   e. _____ Pallor
   f. _____ Weakness
   g. _____ Acetone breath
   h. _____ Nervousness
   i. _____ Glucosuria
   j. _____ Abdominal pain

8. State the timing of peak effects of the following insulin preparations. Specify which can be administered via the intravenous route:
   a. Humulin N (isophane) insulin
   b. Regular insulin
   c. Humulin U Ultralente

9. Describe the teaching plan for the patient with type 2 diabetes who is taking an oral hypoglycemic agent.

Chapter 70
Estrogens, Progestins, and Contraception

Define the following:

1. Menopause

2. Estrogen

3. Progestin

4. Menarche

5. hCG

Match the drug with the condition in which it is given.

6. _____ Infertility   a. Oral contraceptives

7. _____ Advanced breast cancer   b. estrogens

8. _____ Dysmenorrhea   c. progestins

9. _____ Secondary amenorrhea   d. bromocriptine

10. _____ Menopause

11. _____ Galactorrhea

12. Indicate which of the following are adverse effects (A) or contraindications (C) of oral contraceptives.

   a. _____ Breast cancer

   b. _____ Weight gain

   c. _____ Nausea

   d. _____ Depression

   e. _____ Pregnancy

   f. _____ Hypertension

   g. _____ Acne

   h. _____ Thrombosis

13. List the learning needs of a patient receiving clomiphene.

Chapter 71
Drugs for Labor and Delivery

Define the following:

1. Prostaglandins

2. Myometrium

3. Oxytocin

4. Ergot alkaloids

5. Parturition

6. List adverse reactions to ergonovine.

7. State how ritrodine is used in labor and delivery.

8. Develop a teaching plan for the patient who is taking isoxsuprine at home for preterm labor.

9. State the use(s) for the following drugs for labor and delivery:

   a. terbutaline

   b. dinoprostone

   c. oxytocin

   d. ergonovine

Chapter 72
Drugs Acting on the Male Reproductive System

1. Describe the actions of androgens.

2. List the uses of testosterone.

3. State two drugs that interact with testosterone and their effects.

   Drug   **Effect**

   a.

   b.

4. Discuss the effects of anabolic steroids and learning needs of an adolescent taking these agents.

5. Discuss the use of androgens in females, as well as side effects that may be of concern to females.

Chapter 73
Drugs to Treat Glaucoma

1. Define *glaucoma,* and describe the two types.

2. List four possible nursing diagnoses for a patient receiving ophthalmic drugs.

3. For the following systemic drugs, state the effects on the eye:

   Drug   **Effect**

   a. acetazolamide

   b. glycerin

   c. mannitol

   d. urea

4. State the actions of the following drugs that are used to treat glaucoma, and give an example of each:

   a. Beta-blockers

   b. Adrenergic agonists

   c. Cholinomimetics

5. Describe how to instill eyedrops and eye ointments in children and adults.

6. Identify adverse systemic effects from antiglaucoma agents.

7. State important points to include when teaching the patient about drugs used to treat glaucoma.

Chapter 74
Other Ophthalmic Drugs

Define the following:

1. Accommodation

2. Cataract

3. Uveitis

4. Miosis

5. Mydriasis

6. Cycloplegia

7. When are mydriasis and cycloplegia necessary?

8. Describe the effect of the adrenergic drug phenylephrine on the eye.

9. Describe the action of anticholinergic drugs on the eye.

10. Describe the action of prostaglandin inhibitors on the eye.

11. Describe the nursing considerations for a patient receiving drugs for the eye.

Chapter 1: Drugs in the Body: Pharmacodynamics and Pharmacokinetics

1. The study of how drugs enter the body, reach their site of action, and are removed from the body
2. The study of drug action at the level of the drug target
3. When a drug is given repeatedly at fixed dosage intervals and a concentration in the blood reaches a plateau
4. Ability to bind with a receptor
5. Drug that prevents natural substances from stimulating a receptor
6. When drugs are absorbed from the small intestines and transported by portal circulation directly to the liver before being circulated to the rest of the body
7. The time it takes for a drug to be eliminated from the circulation by $1/2$
8. The ratio of the dose of the drug lethal in 50% of tested population to the dose of the drug therapeutically effective in 50% of the tested population
9. a
10. d
11. c
12. b
13. a
14. An agonist is a substance (or drug) that has high affinity for a receptor and binds with that receptor. An antagonist is a substance that prevents binding of an agonist to a receptor or binds with the receptor but causes no cellular response
15-20. See Table 1-2 in text on page 8.

Chapter 2: Effects of Life Span, Genetics, and Medical Conditions on Drug Therapy

1. c
2. d
3. a
4. f
5. b
6. e
7. Immature liver and kidneys increase the incidence of adverse effects.
8. Altered CNS function may mask signs of drug toxicity; reduced renal function and changes in ratio of body water, body fat, and lean muscle mass may influence distribution and change rates of excretion; altered serum albumin may occur, resulting in altered drug binding; older adults may be taking more than one drug because of the increased incidence of chronic disease.
9. Dosages must be altered to compensate for reduced renal function for drugs that are primarily excreted through renal processes.
10. Food may interact with drugs and alter the effect of therapy by altering the absorption of orally administered drugs. A few drugs are better absorbed on a full stomach, but most drugs are absorbed more slowly or less completely when taken with food.
11. d
12. c
13. a
14. b
15. e

Chapter 2: Effects of Life Span, Genetics, and Medical Conditions on Drug Therapy—cont'd

16. d
17. b

Chapter 3: Legal Implications of Drug Therapy

1. A medicine that has not been profitable to develop or market
2. Name applied to drug no matter who manufactures it (nonproprietary)
3. Proprietary name of a drug belonging to specific company
4. 1938 law that required that a drug be proven safe before it was marketed
5. Cancer-producing effects
6. Highly effective clinical trial method in which patients are randomly assigned to a drug or placebo, and no one knows which patient is getting which drug
7. Clinical improvement in response to an inert element/chemical; however, if patient feels it will help, it often does help
8. Body becomes dependent on a substance and suffers harm if withdrawn
9. Established in 1952, designating certain drugs needing "caution" legends
10. Schedule describing controlled substances (addictive agents); see Table 3-4 in text on page 30
11. Drugs that cause fetal abnormalities
12. See Table 3-2 in text on page 27.
13. c
14. e
15. d
16. a
17. b
18. See Nursing Process Overview in text on page 31.

Chapter 4: Application of the Nursing Process to Drug Therapy

1. Assessment, nursing diagnosis, patient outcomes, planning/implementation, evaluation
2. c
3. e
4. d
5. b
6. a
7. See box in text on page 38.
8. See box in text on page 39.
9. See box in text on page 39.
10. Three of the following: drug ordered for wrong patient, wrong dose, poor writing causing mix-up in drug, error in calculation, wrong route, wrong patient, wrong documentation.

Chapter 5: Drug Administration

1. Medication in which each dose is individually wrapped, labeled, and supplied to patients
2. Form of drug that maintains release of drug over a sustained period
3. Drug given and absorbed under the tongue

4. Tablet form that is held in mouth and slowly dissolved

5. Parenteral route, drug given with a $^5/_8$-inch needle at a 15-degree angle just below the epidermis

6. Method of IM injection that prevents leaking of drug in subcutaneous tissue

7. PICC: central line administered via peripheral arm vein

8. Drug mixed with a substance that allows them to remain solid at room temperature but melt within the body

9. Drug administered through the skin by way of a patch or other adhesive tissue

10. Drugs administered through the bone marrow

11. Name of drug, dose route, time, assessment data, patient response, and effectiveness; information needs to be accurate, complete, and signed by the nurse

12. Intravenous: drug given directly into the vascular route
Intramuscular: drug given at a 90-degree angle into the muscle with a 1- to $1^1/_2$-inch needle
Subcutaneous: drug given at a 45- to 90-degree angle into subcutaneous tissue with a $^5/_8$- to 1-inch needle

13. Administer drugs in lower conjunctiva. When administering drops, gently apply pressure to inner canthus of eye to prevent loss of drug into nose. Do not touch eye with dropper. Warn patient about potential vision difficulty.

14. See Figure 5-24, page 67.

15. See Box 5-2, page 51.

16. See text page 47.

Chapter 6: Calculating Drug Dosages

1. Most accurate measure of calculating pediatric dose (see Figure 6-1 in text on page 76)

2. Method of calculating pediatric dosage based on child's weight to average weight of adult

$$\frac{\text{Weight of child}}{150} \times \text{Adult dose}$$

3. Method of calculating pediatric dosage based on child's age; applies to children 1-12 years of age

$$\frac{\text{Age of child}}{\text{Age of child} + 12} \times \text{Adult dose}$$

4. A given mass of solid substance dissolved in known volume of fluid

5. According to circumstance

6. a. (STAT): Give 100 mg of Demerol into muscle right away.
   b. (S): Give Milk of Magnesia 30 cc (1 oz) per mouth at hour of sleep.
   c. (PRN): Give Seconal 100 mg per mouth at hour of sleep as needed.
   d. (RO): Give Lanoxin 0.25 mg per mouth every day.
   e. (S): Give Dilantin 100 mg per mouth.

7. a

8. h

9. c

10. f

11. j

12. i

13. l

14. g

15. a. $^1/_2$, 15
    b. 30
    c. 500
    d. 2
    e. 0.1
    f. 1000

Chapter 6: Calculating Drug Dosages—cont'd

    g. 16
    h. 360.8
    i. 256
    j. 15

16. 100 cc
17. 20 cc
18. 0.625 cc
19. 21 gtts/min
20. 93.7 ml
21. 12 gtts/min
22. BSA = 1.0 m^2 (approximately)
    118-706 mg/day

Chapter 7: Over-the-Counter Drugs and Self-Medication

1. Low doses and fixed combination of ingredients
2. a. Pure Food and Drug Act of 1906: Required that package labels accurately list the ingredients of medicinal products, and ingredients present but not listed were deemed "adulterants"

   b. The Sherley Amendment (1912): Forbade false and fraudulent labeling claims

   c. The 1938 Food and Drug Act: Required proof of safety for all medicinal products intended for sale

   d. Durham-Humphrey Amendment of 1952: Differentiated drugs safe enough for sale without a prescription and drugs deemed sufficiently dangerous or unsuitable for self-medication that required sale by prescription only

   e. Kefauver-Harris Amendment of 1962: Required proof of efficacy and safety and lack of teratogenicity for all drugs

3. a. Category I: Recognized as safe and effective for the claimed therapeutic indications

   b. Category II: Not recognized as safe and effective

   c. Category III: Additional data needed to decide safety or effectiveness

4. Possible classifications include analgesics, cold remedies, cough remedies, decongestant nose drops and nasal sprays, sleeping aids, ophthalmic products, acne medications, sunscreen products, topical antiinfective drugs, and hemorrhoidal products. See pages 81-89 for discussion under each category for therapeutic uses.

5. The Dietary Supplement Health and Education Act of 1994 permits the sale of herbal remedies as dietary supplements as long as therapeutic claims do not appear on the label. Manufacturers of herbal remedies are not required to provide evidence of product safety and effectiveness.

6. Herbal remedies are not FDA-approved drugs; their labeling cannot be relied on to provide proper instructions for use or cautionary warnings. These products do not have FDA-enforced standards of quality and may contain subtherapeutic amounts of constituents. Many have unproven safety, especially for pregnant and nursing mothers and young children and infants.

7. See Nursing Implications Summary in text on page 89.

Chapter 8: Issues of Drug Abuse

1. Drug use becomes a problem, causing social and personal difficulties
2. Physiologic effects appear as a result of drug use, or when there is loss of control over drug use
3. Decreasing effect of a drug on the body over time

4. Symptoms that occur when drug is withheld, usually the opposite of drug action
5. Physical need for drug; the lack of the drug produces withdrawal symptoms
6. 4, e
7. 4, f
8. 1, f
9. 4, d
10. 1, e and a
11. 2, f
12. 3, b
13. 1, c
14. See Nursing Process Overview in text on page 224.

Chapter 9: Care of the Poisoned Patient

1. Deals with action of a poison over time; encompasses absorption, distribution, metabolism, and excretion
2. Describes the harmful effects a poison produces on the body
3. Antidote that competes with and removes a poison from a receptor
4. Antidote that binds with a heavy metal to promote elimination
5. d
6. e
7. a
8. c
9. b
10. a. Induction of vomiting is not appropriate when the patient might aspirate the vomitus, especially in cases of absent gag reflex, unconsciousness, or seizures.
    b. Vomiting is not indicated when the regurgitated material can be damaging to the esophagus and lungs.
    c. Induction of vomiting can take 20 to 30 minutes and should not be used when time is critical.
11. Gastric lavage is "washing" the stomach with saline to remove contents via a large bore tube until the returned fluid is clear. Large-bore tubing is used so that tablets can be removed.
12. Ipecac syrup is an emetic that induces vomiting within 30 minutes, thus emptying the stomach contents.
13. Activated charcoal absorbs a number of drugs and chemicals and prevents their absorption into the body. The charcoal is eliminated in the feces.
14. See Nursing Process Overview in text on page 108.

Chapter 10: Introduction to Autonomic Pharmacology

Across
1. Sympathetic
2. Adrenergic
3. dopamine
4. Central nervous system
5. Preganglionic
6. Tyrosine
7. Neurotransmitter
8. Cholinesterase

Down
1. Adrenal medulla
2. Efferent

Chapter 10: Introduction to Autonomic Pharmacology—cont'd

3. Synapse
4. acetylcholine
5. norepinephrine
6. Cholinergic
7. MAO
8. Serotonin
9. GABA
10. VMA

Chapter 11: Mechanisms of Cholinergic Control

1. Synonymous with parasympathetic nervous system
2. Chemical found in mushrooms that mimics acetylcholine by slowing the heart rate or stimulating smooth muscle
3. Cholinergic agonist found in tobacco that mimics the effects of acetylcholine at the skeletal muscle and ganglionic receptors
4. Mimics the action of acetylcholine directly; chemically related to acetylcholine
5. Mimics the action of acetylcholine indirectly by inhibiting acetylcholinesterase (inhibits the degradation of acetylcholine)
6. a
7. a
8. b
9. a
10. b
11. Atropine blocks acetylcholine at muscarinic receptors. It affects smooth muscle, cardiac muscle, and exocrine glands.
12. Teach the patient that he or she will have decreased sweating, so hyperthermia can occur; the patient will also have blurred vision, dizziness, or light-headedness, so there is a risk of injury. In addition, both urinary (retention) and bowel (constipation) elimination can be affected.
13-17. See Table 11-1 on page 122.

Chapter 12: Mechanisms of Adrenergic Control

1. c
2. b
3. a
4. d
5. c
6. a
7. d
8. a
9. c
10. More common: nervousness, restlessness, and insomnia.
    Less common: hypertension, tachycardia, tremors, sweating, nausea, vomiting, pallor, and weakness
11. Norepinephrine, epinephrine, dopamine
12. See Table 12-2 in text on page 129.
13. Fainting may occur as a result of orthostatic hypotension (blood pooling in the legs and draining from the head); thus they are at risk for injury from falling.

Chapter 13: Antihypertensive Drugs

1. Pressure measured in blood vessels (SBP >140 and DBP >90)

2. Drugs that block the sympathetic nervous system neurotransmitters

3. Angiotensin-converting enzyme inhibitors: agents that decrease effect of renin-angiotensin system, thus lowering blood pressure

4. Drugs that lower blood pressure by affecting movement of calcium into cells, decreasing contraction of smooth muscle

5. Drugs that cause diuresis, which leads to reduction of body salt and water (extracellular fluid), which results in reduction of arterial blood pressure

6. This mechanism regulates blood pressure by increasing or decreasing blood volume through kidney function. When blood flow through the kidneys is reduced, reduced renal arterial pressure causes release of renin into the circulation. Renin catalyzes cleavage of a plasma protein to form angiotensin I, which is converted by angiotensin-converting enzyme (ACE) to angiotensin II.

   Angiotensin II stimulates secretion of aldosterone, which promotes reabsorption of sodium by kidneys. The increased sodium elevates osmotic pressure in the plasma and a release of antidiuretic hormone from the hypothalamus. Angiotensin II acts on the kidney tubules to promote reabsorption of water.

   Excessive fluid retention is controlled by a negative-feedback mechanism operating within this system so that fluid balance is restored to a normal level. Thus the renin-angiotensin-aldosterone system involves slow adjustments to changes in fluid volume.

7. Patients are at increased risk of cerebrovascular (CV) morbidity and mortality. Nonpharmacologic means of blood pressure reduction are indicated. Antihypertensive drugs should be started with smaller-than-usual doses, increased with smaller dosages, and scheduled at less frequent intervals because the elderly are more sensitive than younger patients to volume depletion and sympathetic inhibition. They commonly have impaired CV reflexes, making them more susceptible to hypotension.

   In patients with isolated systolic hypertension who are treated with antihypertensive drugs, the systolic pressure should be cautiously decreased to 140 to 160 mm Hg. Only if this level is tolerated without side effects should consideration be given to further lowering the value. The elderly patient's response to both nonpharmacologic and pharmacologic therapies should be monitored closely.

8. Lifestyle changes include restriction of dietary sodium, fats, and cholesterol, weight loss if overweight, stopping smoking, reducing caffeine intake, limiting alcohol intake, and increasing aerobic physical activity.

9. Beta-blockers should not be discontinued abruptly because such an action may exacerbate angina, myocardial infarction, or ventricular arrhythmias.

10. Poor compliance may result if the patient feels worse, or not better, while taking the medications. Or, the patient may feel reluctant to discuss side effects such as impotence and may discontinue a drug if this or other side effects occur. In addition, the cost may be prohibitive.

11. See Nursing Process Overview in text on page 154.

Chapter 14: Diuretics

1. c
2. a
3. b
4. b
5. a
6. c
7. d
8. e
9. b

Chapter 14: Diuretics—cont'd

10. a
11. b
12. a
13. e
14. b
15. c
16. d
17. a
18. See box in text on page 166 and Nursing Implications Summary in text on page 172.
19. Foods high in protein include citrus fruits and juices; bananas; grape, cranberry, apple, pear, and apricot juices; cereals; leafy vegetables; meat; fish and fowl; coffee, tea, and cola beverages; nuts; and peanut butter.
20. Emphasize the need to limit intake of potassium-rich foods, including salt-substitutes that contain potassium. In addition, previously prescribed potassium supplements need to be stopped (consult with physician).

Chapter 15: Antianginals and Other Vasodilators

1. Vasospastic disease causing decreased circulation and oxygen to toes and fingers
2. "Choking of the chest"; result of insufficient oxygen to the heart muscle
3. Drugs that dilate peripheral blood vessels
4. Drugs that improve blood flow by increasing the size of the blood vessels
5. Classic angina: Stable angina, or exertional angina; large coronary arteries are obstructed by atherosclerosis to the point that blood flow cannot increase to supply increased oxygen demand of the cardiac muscle

   Variant angina: Prinzmetal's angina; caused by spasms of the large coronary arteries that result in obstruction of blood flow

   Unstable angina: Angina that has a changing intensity; pain comes at decreasing levels of activity and often at rest
6. Sublingual, lingual aerosol, extended-release buccal forms, extended release capsules and tablets, topically (ointment or transdermal delivery system), intravenously
7. a. To decrease duration and intensity of pain during an attack
   b. To prophylactically decrease frequency of attacks and improve work capacity even though angina may occur
   c. To prevent or delay the onset of myocardial infarction
8. See Nursing Implications Summary in text on page 189.
9. Beta-blockers cause a decrease in resting heart rate, thus decreasing cardiac workload; also used to prevent sudden death after a heart attack; also has antiarrhythmic and antiplatelet functions.

Chapter 16: Drugs to Treat Hypotension and Shock

1. Disruption in circulation; often the blood pressure is too low to force blood through vital tissues
2. Result of massive histamine release caused by allergic reaction and causing profound respiratory and cardiovascular failure
3. Slow heart rate that results from stimulation of the vagus nerve
4. Drugs that mimic the sympathetic nervous system
5. See Table 16-1 in text on page 194.

6. If extravasation of sympathomimetic drugs occurs, vasoconstriction leading to tissue necrosis or sloughing can occur. Discontinue the infusion, and infiltrate the site with a solution of 5 to 10 ml of phentolamine diluted in 10 to 15 ml of normal saline solution, using a fine hypodermic needle.

7. Epinephrine can be administered via an endotracheal tube.

8. a. At low dosages, dopamine causes vasodilation.

   b. At moderate dosages, cardiac contractility is stimulated.

   c. At highest dosages, heart rate and blood pressure are increased.

Chapter 17: Fluids and Electrolytes

1. a. Osmosis: Water moving through a semipermeable membrane from an area of lower concentration of solutes to an area of higher concentration

   Diffusion: Movement of solutes from an area of higher concentration to an area of lesser concentration

   b. Acidosis: State of increased serum acidity or increased hydrogen ions or decreased bicarbonate ions in the blood

   Alkalosis: State of decreased serum acidity; increased bicarbonate ions or hydrogen ions in the blood

   c. Intracellular fluid: Fluid compartment inside of the cells

   Extracellular fluid: Fluid compartment outside of the cells; further divided into the intravascular (plasma) and interstitial fluid compartments

2. Fluid volume deficit: Weight loss in excess of 5% of normal body weight, dry lips and eyes, decreased blood pressure, depressed CNS activity, and diminished skin turgor

   Fluid volume excess: Swelling and edema, bounding pulse, distension of the jugular vein, difficult or noisy breathing, and warm, moist skin

3. a. Sodium terminology:
      Deficiency: hyponatremia; excess: hypernatremia

   b. Potassium terminology:
      Deficiency: hypokalemia; excess: hyperkalemia
      Refer to Table 17-1 in text on page 205 for signs of deficiency and excesses.

4. a. Replaces extracellular fluid volume and treats sodium depletion and metabolic alkalosis

   b. Replace fluid, sodium, and other electrolytes

   c. Provides fluid for rehydration and some calories

   d. Potassium replacement

   e. Expands plasma volume

5. a. Pain, slow rate of infusion.

   b. Occlusion, check clamps and tubing, check site.

   c. Phlebitis, DC IV notify doctor and apply warm soaks to site.

   Also see Table 17-5 in text on page 211.

6. Maintain aseptic technique, monitor for blood glucose levels and signs of infection, use pump to administer IV, and gradually decrease rate.

Chapter 18: Drugs to Control Congestive Heart Failure

1. Influencing myocardial contractility

2. Failure of the heart to adequately pump the blood delivered to it, resulting in symptoms of insufficient cardiac output

3. A dose designed to raise the concentration of the drug in the blood rapidly to the therapeutic range

4. The strength of the muscular contraction of the heart

5. The resistance against which the heart works; determined by blood volume and pressure

Chapter 18: Drugs to Control Congestive Heart Failure—cont'd

6. a. Desired effect: Produces vasodilation, which reduces systemic and pulmonary vascular resistance, and improves cardiac output without increasing cardiac workload

   Potential adverse effects: Renal impairment, hypotension, continuing dry cough

   b. Desired effect: Control pulmonary edema that accompanies congestive heart failure and may decrease the pressure forcing blood into the heart, thus improving contractility of the heart

   Potential adverse effects: Volume depletion, excessive dehydration, electrolyte imbalances

   c. Desired effect: Rapid increase in cardiac output

   Potential adverse effects: Increased risk of sudden death from cardiac arrhythmias

7. Irregular heart rate, hypotension, visual disturbance (white and/or yellow "halos" around objects), gastric upset, weight gain, diarrhea, and anorexia

8. Should include three of the following: conditions causing potassium loss, hypercalcemia, and pathologic conditions such as kidney, liver, and severe heart disease.

9. Instruct the patient to take at the same time each day, not to skip or double up doses, to check with the physician if taking other drugs, and to avoid licorice; teach the patient how to take his or her pulse and when to notify physician (if pulse <60 beats/min and/or if patient is experiencing side effects).

Chapter 19: Agents to Control Cardiac Arrhythmias

1. Any deviation from normal rate or pattern of heartbeat

2. Slow heart rate

3. Fast heart rate

4. Action potential from a single impulse to beat passes more than once through the same group of cells

5. Premature ventricular contractions

6. Time span in which ventricular cells cannot be stimulated to beat again

7. a, Group IA: Block sodium channels, thus lowering automaticity

8. b, Group IB: Decrease excitability and automacity

9. f, Group IV: Block calcium channels, depressing depolarization and lengthening repolarization, resulting in slower heart rate

10. a, Group IA: Block sodium channels, thus lowering automaticity

11. d, Group II: Block beta-adrenergic receptors to treat arrhythmias driven by excessive sympathetic stimulation

12. c, Group IC: Profoundly slow conduction, especially in conductive fibers

13. e, Group III: Prolong repolarization phase thereby lengthening the duration of refractoriness

14. b, Group IB: Decrease excitability and automacity

15. Monitor vital signs. Do not give if heart rate is <60 or >130 beats/min. Monitor ECG. Assess for signs and symptoms of congestive heart failure (edema, coarse breath sounds, I&O, and increased weight). Monitor lab values: blood urea nitrogen, liver function tests, and serum drug levels. Use microtubing with IV. Keep patient supine and siderails up.

16. Refer to Figure 19-2 in text on page 229.

Chapter 20: Agents Affecting Blood Coagulation

1. A blood clot

2. A dislodged thrombus

3. Drug that degrades blood clots

4. Drug that interferes with blood coagulation

5. Activated partial thromboplastin time; it monitors heparin levels

6. Prothrombin time; it monitors oral anticoagulants, such as warfarin

7. b

8. a

9. b

10. a

11. a

12. b

13. a

14. b

15. Increased risk of bleeding hemorrhage

16. Monitor side effects, especially nausea, vomiting, fever, muscle aches, and dyspnea, because they can mimic underlying medical conditions. Be alert for hemorrhage, hypotension, mental changes, and neurologic status. Monitor ECG; arrhythmias commonly occur.

17. vitamin K

18. protamine sulfate

Chapter 21: Drugs to Lower Blood Lipid Levels

1. Metabolic disorder characterized by increased concentrations of cholesterol and triglycerides

2. Disorder with a strong correlation to high levels of circulating triglycerides and cholesterol

3. Also known as HDLs ("good cholesterol"); are the smallest and most dense lipoproteins, containing about 20% cholesterol and 5% triglycerides; they carry cholesterol and triglycerides from body cells of membranes to the liver, where they are metabolized and excreted; high levels of HDL lower potential risk for cerebrovascular disease

4. Lipid compounds bound to plasma proteins which act as carriers

5. Also known as LDLs ("bad cholesterol"), or beta lipoproteins; contain the major portion of cholesterol in the blood and may be considered most harmful, associated with high potential risk of atherosclerosis; consist of 50% cholesterol and 5% triglycerides

6. Largest particles and the least dense of the lipoproteins; consist of 90% triglycerides; produced in the small intestine during absorption of a fatty meal and cleared from bloodstream by lipoprotein lipase after 12 to 14 hours

7. Answers should contain two of the following drugs and their effects. *Oral anticoagulants, coumarins, or indanediones:* decrease absorption of oral anticoagulants and vitamin K; *digitalis glycosides, especially digitoxin:* half-life of digitalis glycosides, as well as gastrointestinal absorption, may be reduced; *oral penicillin G, oral tetracyclines, or oral vancomycin:* decreased absorption of antibiotics has been reported; *thyroid hormones:* decreased absorption of thyroid products is reported.

8. Before initiating clofibrate therapy, advise the patient to adhere to the diet prescribed by the physician. Encourage weight reduction and physical exercise. Warn the patient that a paradoxic rise may occur in 2 or 3 months, but afterward, a further decrease is customary. Instruct the patient to keep clinical appointments. If serum cholesterol and triglyceride levels are not lowered within 3 months, discontinue drug therapy. Advise patient to report flulike symptoms. Instruct the patient to check with the physician about alcohol intake because its use may be restricted to prevent hypertriglyceridemia.

9. Adverse reactions include constipation, bloating, epigastric fullness, nausea, and flatulence.

10. Pravastatin and simvastatin need to be taken in the evening or at bedtime. Lovastatin should be taken with the evening meal if ordered once a day; if ordered more than once a day, each dose should be taken with a meal or snack.

Chapter 22: Drugs to Treat Anemia

1. Production of new RBCs
2. Growth factor produced by the kidney that promotes hematopoiesis
3. Condition in which there is a deficiency of RBCs and/or hemoglobin
4. Essential component of key proteins and hemoglobin
5. Cell produced in bone marrow, essential for oxygen

6.

Anemia Type	Characteristics	Drug(s) of Choice for Treatment
a. Iron deficiency	Inadequate intake of iron to produce RBCs; results from blood loss or rapid growth	iron salts
b. Megaloblastic macrocytic	Large immature RBCs caused by a deficiency in B_{12} and folic acid	folic acid
c. Pernicious anemia	Vitamin B_{12} needs a binding protein (intrinsic factor) to be absorbed in the stomach; this condition is caused by a relative or complete lack of characteristic intrinsic factor	vitamin B_{12} (cyanocobalamin)
d. Chronic renal failure	Reduced production of RBCs because of decreased production of erythropoietin	epoetin alfa

7. Foods high in iron include red meats, organ meats, legumes and nuts, green leafy vegetables, whole grains, enriched breads/cereals, molasses, brewers' yeast, dried fruits, and oysters.
8. See Nursing Implications Summary in text on page 282.
9. The human hormone erythropoietin; this drug stimulates the production of red blood cells. The effect is seen in 1 to 2 weeks.

Chapter 23: Drugs Affecting Motility: Cholinergic Stimulants and Anticholinergics/Antispasmodics

1. External innervation of the gastrointestinal system is supplied by the division of the autonomic nervous system, which correlates activities between different regions of the gastrointestinal system and also between this system and other parts of the body. See Figure 23-1 in the text on page 286.

2.

Stimulant	Adverse Effects
a. bethanechol	Salivation, flushing, sweating, nausea, belching, and abdominal cramps
b. cisapride	Diarrhea, abdominal cramps, nausea, headache, fatigue, and rarely, seizures
c. metoclopramide	Restlessness, drowsiness, fatigue, and lassitude

3. See Table 23-2 in text on page 290.
4. See Patient Problem Box in text on page 289.

Chapter 24: Laxatives and Antidiarrheals

1. Abnormally infrequent and difficult fecal evacuation
2. Drugs given to reduce constipation
3. Abnormal passage of stools with increased frequency, fluidity, or weight and increase in stool water excretion
4. Drugs that coat walls of gastrointestinal tract, absorbing bacteria or toxins and causing diarrhea to pass toxins out with the stools
5. Refer to Nursing Process Overview and Patient Problems Box in text on page 302

6. Instruct the patient to increase daily fluid intake to 2500 to 3000 ml, to drink an 8-oz glass of water before each meal and with each meal; to increase daily dietary intake of fiber in food such as bran cereals, fruits, and vegetables (see Dietary Considerations on page 295), and to exercise regularly. Also instruct in proper use of laxatives, especially over-the-counter medications.

7. c

8. f

9. a

10. d

11. e

12. b

13. c

14. Retain water so that the stool remains large and soft

15. Inhibit the absorption of water so that the stool remains large and soft

16. Directly stimulate the motility of the large intestine, and inhibit the reabsorption of water in the large intestine

17. Attract water osmotically into the lumen of the large intestine, and the resulting bulk stimulates peristalsis

18. Decrease the tone of the small and large intestines to slow the transit of material (for treatment of diarrhea)

Chapter 25: Antiemetics

1. See Figure 25-1 in text on page 307.

2. Motion sickness, anesthesia, radiation therapy, and chemotherapy

3. b

4. d

5. e

6. a

7. c

8. d

9. b

10. c

11. c

12. Have the patient sip water or tea and eat small meals.

13. See Nursing Implications Summary in text on page 314.

Chapter 26: Drugs to Treat Acid Reflux and Ulcers

1. A

2. N

3. A

4. H

5. B

6. H

7. Sucralfate binds to proteins in ulcerated tissue and coats them, providing protection from gastric secretions.

8. Inform them not to give these drugs together but at least 1 to 2 hours before or after because antacids interfere with absorption of H_2-receptor antagonists.

9. H_1 receptors are located in the gastrointestinal tract, and H_2 receptors are located in other areas of the body. The histamine antagonists have the same action but completely different effects.

Chapter 26: Drugs to Treat Acid Reflux and Ulcers—cont'd

10. This bacterium attaches to the mucus-secreting gastric epithelial cells that line the stomach and survives by breaking down urea to neutralize the acid in its microenvironment. This leads to the loss of mucus that protects the lining of the stomach and duodenum from acid. Eradication can be achieved with a combination therapy that includes suppression of acid production and antibiotics.

11. See Nursing Implications Summary in text on page 323.

Chapter 27: Drugs to Treat Gallbladder and Pancreatic Diseases

1. Stones composed principally of cholesterol and result when crystals form from bile supersaturated with cholesterol, compounded by poor motility of the gallbladder

2. Presence of gallstones

3. Inflammation of the gallbladder

4. Digestive enzymes secreted by the pancreas, lipase, amylase, trypsin, and chymotrypsin, which are important in the digestion of fat, carbohydrate, and protein

5. The major side effect is diarrhea, which is usually mild and transient. Occasional constipation, gas, or frequent urge for a bowel movement may occur.

6. Animal studies have indicated that chenodiol damages fetal organs; for ursodiol, animal studies have not shown adverse effects on the fetus, and it is not contraindicated in pregnancy.

7. They work slowly and must be taken daily for up to 2 years to dissolve gallstones.

8. See Nursing Implications Summary on page 330.

Chapter 28: Drugs to Treat Asthma and Other Pulmonary Diseases

1. Drugs that dilate the bronchioles

2. Reversible constriction of the bronchioles

3. Bronchial constriction primarily caused by allergic response

4. Chronic obstructive pulmonary disease

5. Hyaline membrane disease caused by deficiency in surfactant leading to collapse of alveoli

6. Hypersecretion of mucus, mucosal edema, and bronchial constriction

7. a. Metered aerosol: One inhalation delivers a given amount of drug.

   b. Nebulizer aerosol: Solution of drug is given via a nebulizer, which disperses the drug in tiny drops to be taken into the lungs by deep inhalation.

8. Theophylline acts by increasing cellular cyclic adenosine monophosphate (cAMP) concentrations by inhibiting the degradation of cAMP by the enzyme phosphodiesterase.

9. See Nursing Implications Summary in text on page 346.

10. See Nursing Implications Summary in text on page 347.

11. *Controller medications* treat the underlying inflammatory condition, with the goal of preventing or decreasing the severity of asthmatic episodes. Such medications include inhaled corticosteroids, inhaled cromolyn or nedocromil, oral long-acting theophylline, leukotriene modifiers, and a long-acting beta$_2$-agonist or oral slow-release beta$_2$-agonist.

    Reliever medications control asthmatic episodes and include short-acting inhaled beta$_2$-agonists, oral short-acting theophylline, and inhaled anticholinergics.

Chapter 29: Antihistamines

1. d
2. c
3. e

4. a

5. b

6. Side effects include drowsiness, dry mouth, dizziness, nervousness, blurred vision, constipation, and tachycardia.

7. Systemic allergic response indicated by generalized itching and tingling sensation and a feeling of apprehension, profound hypotension leading to shock may follow, and bronchiole constriction may cause a choking sensation.

8. Warn the patient to avoid driving or operating hazardous machinery and using alcohol or other CNS depressants. Instruct the patient about adverse reactions, when to notify the physician, how and when to take various forms of antihistamines, and to use over-the-counter drugs carefully.

9. These drugs blunt allergic reactions effectively but without the sedation commonly associated with the older antihistamines.

Chapter 30: Drugs to Control Bronchial Secretions

1. Cough suppressant drug

2. A drug that increases production of mucus

3. A drug that breaks up viscous mucus

4. Increased nasal congestion following use of nasal spray

5. A protective reflex initiated by irritation in the airway

6. Monitor the amount of mucus produced; have tissues, oral care items, and suction available. Teach what to expect, side effects, and purpose of the drug. Do treatment before meals to prevent nausea and vomiting. Administer good oral care immediately after use and expectoration.

7. Inform the patient that the more frequently nasal sprays are used, the less effective they are; thus they should be used for only 3 to 5 days. Overdose can occur with frequent repeated doses, causing systemic symptoms. Nasal decongestants can cause rebound congestion and discomfort.

8. Codeine: Drowsiness, nausea, dizziness, drug dependence

   Dextromethorphan: Drowsiness and dizziness (rare)

   Hydrobromide: Drowsiness and dizziness (rare)

   Diphenhydramine: Drowsiness and dry mouth

9. The patient should be lying on a bed with the head hanging over the edge and turned to one side. The drops are instilled into the upper nostril. After a few seconds, the head is turned to allow administration to the other nostril. Use of this lateral head-low position allows the drops to coat the nasal mucosa without being immediately swallowed.

Chapter 31: Aspirin, Acetaminophen, NSAIDs, and Drugs to Treat Gout

1. Relief of pain

2. Nonsteroidal antiinflammatory drugs

3. Aspirin

4. Local mediators involved in inflammatory pathways; can cause pain, fever, edema, and erythema

5. A metabolic disease in which uric acid is elevated, causing joint damage, inflammation, and pain

6.
Drug	Effects
a. acetaminophen	Increased risk of renal damage
b. Anticoagulants	Increased risk for gastrointestinal upset and bleeding
c. aspirin	Increased gastrointestinal upset and inhibition of platelets

7. a, c

8. a, b, c, d

9. a, b, c

Chapter 31: Aspirin, Acetaminophen, NSAIDs, and Drugs to Treat Gout—cont'd

10. b, c
11. Gastrointestinal disturbances such as nausea, vomiting, loss of appetite, indigestion, and diarrhea are common but can be reduced by taking the drug after meals. Occasionally, ulceration along the gastrointestinal tract may occur and become serious if bleeding or perforation results.
12. The goals are to end the acute attack, prevent a recurrence, prevent uric acid stones, and reduce complications.
13. See Nursing Process Overview in text on page 377.

Chapter 32: Opioids (Narcotic Analgesics)

1. Naturally occurring neurotransmitters that bind with receptors mimicking morphine
2. Located in medulla and stimulated by morphine, causing nausea and vomiting
3. Continued desire or craving for a drug; has both physiologic and psychologic components
4. Pain lasting for short periods
5. Repeated use of a drug resulting in a lesser response
6. Endorphins, enkephalins, and dynorphins
7. If respiratory rate is less than 12 breaths/min in an adult, hold additional doses unless ventilatory support is provided. If bradycardia develops (pulse <60 beats/min in an adult or 110 beats/min in an infant), withhold the dose and notify the physician. Hypotension may occur in older adults, the immobilized, and patients receiving other medications with hypotensive effects. Monitor blood pressure carefully.
8. b
9. a
10. c
11. *Physical reactions:* Rhinorrhea, piloerection, tearing, sweating, yawning, abdominal cramping, muscle twitching, hot and cold flashes, nausea and vomiting, and diarrhea
    Psychologic reactions: Restlessness, anxiety, insomnia, and irritability
12. Give NSAIDs—low-dose narcotics and then stronger narcotics. Also helpful are nonpharmacologic measures. Treatment needs to be individualized and frequently evaluated.
13. Naloxene displaces an opioid from a receptor without an effect of its own. It is useful in opiate overdose.

Chapter 33: Drugs to Treat Headaches

1. Tension headaches are characterized by a throbbing, tight pain felt in the front half of the head, especially around the eyes, and lasting half an hour or more.
2. Migraine headaches last from 4 to 24 hours with pain on one side of the head and can be nondescript and throbbing or a severe stabbing pain. Nausea and vomiting are common, as is sensitivity to light, scalp tenderness, and light-headedness.
3. Cluster headaches begin suddenly, reach a peak in a few minutes, and persist for 30 to 120 minutes. The pain is described as sharp, boring, and excruciatingly severe. Pain is clustered on one side of the head around the eye, with lacrimation, eyelid drop, runny nose, congestion, and facial sweating.
4. Caffeine increases the rate and extent of absorption of ergotamine. Without caffeine, the onset of action is about 2 hours; with caffeine, the onset of headache relief is reduced to about 1 hour.
5. See Table 33-2 in text on page 398 for drugs used for acute treatment. Drugs used for prophylactic treatment include methysergide, amitryptyline, beta-adrenergic blockers, calcium channel blockers, divalproex, and lithium.
6. Many of these drugs cause drowsiness and dizziness. Caution the patient to avoid driving or engaging in potentially dangerous activities until the effects of the medication are known. Remind the patient to avoid alcohol or other drugs that depress the CNS.
7. Nonpharmacologic interventions include avoiding alcohol, which may aggravate headaches; and avoiding smoking and cold temperatures, which may intensify vasoconstriction.

Chapter 34: Management of the Patient in Pain

1. *Oral:* Easily given at home; takes longer for effect, but action is more sustained because blood levels are more constant

   Injectable: Faster acting but painful and frightening, especially for children; harder to administer in the home

   PCA: Patient controlled, quick but short acting; patient or family needs to activate release button, continuous pain relief can occur

   Epidural: Small doses of drug can cause widespread anesthesia without excessive CNS depression; must be inserted by an anesthesiologist or nurse anesthetist, and patient needs to be in a health care facility; patient can control drug delivery similar to PCA pump

   Topical: Used for local anesthesia only; however, large amounts can lead to systemic effects; useful for diagnostic tests

2. The patient has a lack of understanding concerning the drug and its effects. Health care professionals have misconceptions about patient behaviors, pain relief, and drugs. Health professionals often let their own experiences influence views of pain.

3. *Objective data:* Vital signs, signs of pain (grimacing, sweating, dilated pupils, restlessness, immobility, crying, guarding); assess area of pain (e.g., swelling, discoloration, drainage), monitor laboratory values.

   Subjective data: Verbal complaints of pain; ask for description and location of pain, determine previous measures that relieved pain, use subjective tools to measure pain.

4. Possible nursing diagnoses include the following:
   • Pain
   • Anxiety
   • Altered health maintenance
   • Impaired physical mobility
   • Sleep pattern disturbance
   • Fatigue
   • Fear

5. Cognitive-behavioral measures include relaxation, distraction, music therapy, imagery, and prayer. Physical agents/approaches include massage, exercise, and transcutaneous electrical nerve stimulation (TENS).

Chapter 35: Local Anesthetics

1. a. Superficial injection of a small amount of local anesthetic; involves small areas.
   b. Local anesthesia administered outside of the dura mater; can involve large areas (see Figure 67-1 in text on page 800)
   c. Form of spinal anesthesia; a low spinal, affecting nerves innervating the perineum (shape of saddle)
   d. A form of epidural anesthesia injected at the base of the spine; affects only the pelvic region and legs (see Figure 35-1 in text on page 420)
   e. The injection of a local anesthetic along a nerve before it reaches the surgical site
   f. Local anesthetics applied as drops, sprays, lotions, creams, or ointments (see Table 35-2 in text on page 418)

2. Systemic absorption leads to CNS stimulation: anxiety, tingling, and tremors. High plasma levels lead to CNS depression: severe hypotension, respiratory depression, and coma.

3. See Nursing Implications Summary in text on page 421.

4. Lidocaine (Xylocaine), dibucaine (Nupercaine), and tetracaine (Pontocaine) can be used topically and by injection.

Chapter 36: General Anesthetics

1. Minimum alveolar concentration; amount of drug necessary to produce insensitivity to pain in anesthesia

2. The induction of anesthesia by using a combination of drugs, each for its specific effect, rather than by using a single drug with multiple effects

Chapter 36: General Anesthetics—cont'd

3. A rare but very dangerous adverse effect of inhaled, fat-soluble anesthetics in which the patient's temperature suddenly escalates and, if not treated appropriately and promptly, may cause death

4. Anesthetic that produces a cataleptic state in which the patient appears to be awake but detached from his or her environment and unresponsive to pain

5. The use of IV benzodiazepines and opioid analgesics to confer amnesic, sedative, and analgesic effects without complete loss of consciousness

6. A controlled state of anesthesia in which the patient has decreased consciousness and is not easily aroused; produces a loss of protective reflexes, an inability to maintain an open airway, and lack of response to surgical stimuli

7. The combination of fentanyl and droperidol to produce a quiet state with reduced motor activity, reduced anxiety, and indifference to the surroundings

8. Emergence is the time during which the patient regains consciousness after the anesthetic has been discontinued. The patient's vital signs are carefully monitored in a recovery room, and symptoms of pain or nausea and vomiting must be watched for and treated appropriately.

9. Nitrous oxide, desflurane, and isoflurane are the most widely used in the United States. Halothane is used mainly for pediatric anesthesia. Diethyl ether is not used in the United States.

10. In general, pediatric patients require higher concentrations of inhalation anesthetics, and geriatric patients require lower concentrations. Geriatric patients are also more likely to react with hypotension and circulatory depression.

11. The nursing plan should follow the general stages for an anesthetic but should include attention to the geriatric patient's greater potential for drug interactions and side effects, an increased and prolonged drug effect, and mortality rates four to eight times higher. See Nursing Implications Summary in text on page 431.

Chapter 37: Neuromuscular-Blocking Drugs

1. Agents that occupy acetylcholine receptors in muscles and produce muscle relaxation for intubation and surgery (see Figure 37-1 in text on page 435)

2. Drugs that bind with receptors without causing depolarization of muscle membrane

3. Agents that bind with receptors, causing muscle membrane depolarization

4. They provide muscle relaxation during surgery without using deep general anesthesia. They are also used with light anesthesia for endotracheal intubation, to relieve spasm of the larynx, to prevent convulsive muscle spasms during electroconvulsive therapy for depression, and to allow breathing to be controlled totally by a respirator during surgery.

Drug	Action	Duration	Adverse Reactions
a. tubocurarine	Nondepolarizing neuromuscular agent, binds to the receptor without initiating depolarization of the muscle	60 minutes, with range of 25-90 minutes	Hypotension and bronchospasm possible
b. succinylcholine	Depolarizing neuromuscular agent, binds to the receptor for acetylcholine and causes depolarization of the muscle membrane	5 minutes	Causes fasciculations (muscle twitching) before muscles are paralyzed, thereby possibly causing stiffness and soreness 12 to 24 hours after the drug is given

6. See Nursing Process Overview in text on page 438.

Chapter 38: Introduction to the Immune System

Across
1. Phagocytosis
2. Immunoglobulins
3. Interleukins
4. Antibodies
5. Monocytes
6. Colony-stimulating factor
7. Cytokines

Down
1. WBCs
2. PMNS
3. Autoimmune
4. Immunity
5. Immune deficiency
6. Antigen
7. Lymphocyte
8. interferon
9. Gammopathies
10. Myelomas
11. TNF
12. HLA

Chapter 39: Immunizations

1. Immunostimulation is the activation of T cells and B cells by an antigen. Once an antigen activates the immune system, some of the T cells and B cells become memory cells; the next time the antigen is encountered, the immune system can start an active and vigorous response.

2. Two developments are new adult vaccines for Lyme disease and therapeutic vaccines against skin and other cancers.

3.

	Definition	Sources	Duration
a. Active immunity	Administration of substances such as vaccines that stimulate the immune system to respond against a foreign material; once the immune response has occurred, specific cells in the immune system "remember" the response, and an immune response occurs rapidly on a subsequent encounter with the antigen	Vaccines: killed or attenuated bacteria or viruses Toxoids: immunogenic proteins from the pathogen in question	Years
b. Passive immunity	Administration of preformed substances, such as immune serum or antibodies, that can immediately combine with the foreign agent to which they are directed	Antivenins and antitoxins prepared from the serum of horses inoculated with the toxin	Weeks

4. b
5. b

Chapter 39: Immunizations—cont'd

6. a
7. a
8. b
9. a
10. b
11. a
12. b
13. a
14. b
15. a
16. See Table 39-1 in text on page 449.
17. The fetus is protected from bacterial and viral infections and from microbial toxins by maternal immunoglobulin G (IgG) antibodies, which pass through the placenta to confer passive immunity. IgG is the only antibody that can cross the placenta. Newborn infants do not have fully functional immune systems, but human milk contains factors that aid the newborn response against infectious agents. These factors include antibodies, factors that enhance the growth of beneficial intestinal flora, and inhibitory factors such as lysozyme, lactoferrin, interferon, and leukocytes.

Chapter 40: Immunomodulators and Care of Patients with Altered Immune Function

1. Proteins that regulate development of precursor blood cells
2. Blocks release of IL-2, thus inhibiting cytotoxic T-lymphocytes and suppressing cell-mediated immunity
3. Drugs that suppress immune cells, thus impairing immune function
4. Present in bone marrow; produces specific blood cells
5. Granulocyte colony-stimulating factor; binds to receptors on specific progenitor cells in bone marrow and causes them to increase production of neutrophil granulocytes
6. Granulocyte-macrophage colony-stimulating factor; binds to receptors on a less differentiated progenitor cell than filgrastim and therefore promotes the production of more that one type of cell, such as neutrophils and monocyte-macrophages
7. The most common effects are gingival hyperplasia, hirsutism, hypertension, nephrotoxity, increased risk for infection, hypokalemia, hepatotoxicity, and pancreatitis.
8. Colony-stimulating factors bind to receptors on specific progenitor cells in bone marrow and cause them to increase production of leukocytes. Examples are filgrastim and sargramostim.

   Cell-stimulating agents improve immune function by stimulating the activity of cells already formed. Examples are aldesleukin, interferon-gamma, levamisole, and pegademase.
9. See Nursing Process Overview in text on page 463.

Chapter 41: Glucocorticoids to Treat Inflammatory Conditions

1. Should include any four of the following: allergic states, such as acute stages of asthma as well as prophylactic treatment for asthma; dermatologic disorders; gastrointestinal disorders such as inflammatory bowel disease; hematologic disorders; joint inflammation; neoplastic diseases; ophthalmic diseases or rheumatic diseases.
2. Refer to Box 41-1 in text on page 472.

3.
Drug	Effect
Antibiotics cyclosporine estrogen	Slows metabolism and clearance of glucocorticoids

isoniazid
ketoconazole
carbamazepine   Increased metabolism and clearance of glucocorticoids
phenobarbital
phenytoin
rifampin
aminoglutethimide

4. Prolonged therapy suppresses the hypothalamic-pituitary-adrenal axis regulating the natural production of cortisol. Gradual tapering of the dose allows the adrenal gland to resume functioning, thereby avoiding an adrenal crisis.

5. See Nursing Process Overview in text on page 473.

Chapter 42: Drug Treatment of Selected Autoimmune Diseases

1. Disease in which skeletal muscles quickly become fatigued because of deficiency of receptors to acetylcholine

2. An autoimmune disease that involves connective tissue, primarily synovial membrane

3. Chronic, inflammatory multisystem disorder of the immune system

4. A crippling autoimmune disease in which the myelin sheath of nerve fibers of the brain and spinal cord are destroyed

5. Diseases in which the immune system is turned against some component of the host's body

6. Edrophonium is used as a diagnostic agent when determining the presence of myasthenia gravis and, when the diagnosis is known, to test for myasthenic crisis. The preferred drug of treatment is pyridostigmine.

7. See Table 42-2 in text on page 483.

8. Drug therapy is directed at controlling symptoms and to prevent or control serious complications as a result of organ damage by the inflammatory process. See Table 42-3 in text on page 488 for examples of agents used.

9. See Nursing Process Overview in text on page 491.

Chapter 43: Introduction to the Use of Antiinfective Agents

1. Cells that have genetic material that exists free within cell protoplasm (e.g., bacteria)

2. Cells that have membrane-bound nuclei that contain genetic material (e.g., human cells)

3. The ratio of the drug dose that kills 50% of test animals to the dose that is effective in 50% of test animals; a large therapeutic index indicates a wide margin of safety

4. Drug that halts bacteria reproduction but does not kill

5. Drug that kills bacteria directly

6. a

7. c

8. b

9. a

10. f

11. b

12. e

13. b

14. f

15. d

16. Inhibiting cell wall formation, blocking protein synthesis, disrupting cell membranes, interfering with nucleic acid synthesis, or preventing synthesis of folic acid

17. See Nursing Implications Summary in text on page 501.

Chapter 44: Penicillins, Cephalosporins, and Related Drugs

1. Group of antibiotics, including penicillins and cephalosporins
2. First antibiotic developed; has many different types, affecting a wide range of organisms
3. Broad-spectrum beta-lactam antibiotics classified according to generations (first-, second-, and third-generation)
4. Methicillin-resistant *Staphylococcus aureus*
5. A bacterial cell wall enzyme inhibited by beta-lactam antibiotics
6. Antibiotic that affects many different types of bacteria
7. Penicillins are incompatible with common IV solutions; check insert before mixing or adding to solution. Beta-lactams are incompatible with aminoglycoside, methotrexate, and probenecid. Individual drugs may cause further interactions.
8. Allergies, manifested as skin rashes and urticaria to anaphylactic reactions, are the most common adverse reactions. The second most common reaction is gastrointestinal tract distress, such as nausea, vomiting, and diarrhea.
9. Repository penicillins were designed for slow absorption from IM injection sites, creating a long duration of action.
10. d
11. g
12. b
13. e
14. c
15. d
16. a
17. f
18. e
19. a
20. h
21. See Nursing Implications Summary in text on page 515.

Chapter 45: Quinolones

1. Quinolones interfere with DNA replication in bacteria by inhibiting the functioning of DNA gyrase.
2. CNS side effects include headache, dizziness, tinnitus, insomnia, shakiness, changes in vision, and seizures. Damage to cartilage and permanent joint impairment may occur, especially in children.
3. Increases theophylline levels
4. Reduces absorption of quinolones
5. Increases bleeding episodes
6. Decreases excretion of caffeine
7. Reduces absorption of quinolones
8. May cause quinolones to crystallize in urine
9. See Table 45-1 in text on page 518.
10. Knowledge deficit related to the need to increase fluid intake and risk for injury related to potential adverse reactions/toxicity

Chapter 46: Macrolides, Clindamycin, and Miscellaneous Penicillin Substitutes

1. Vancomycin-resistant enterococci, an infection that is difficult to treat
2. Antibiotics (with large molecules) that bind to bacterial ribosomes and thus prevent bacterial protein synthesis; bacteriostatic at low dosages, but bactericidal at higher dosages
3. A side effect of vancomycin administration in which the skin flushes and nausea and itching may occur
4. Bacteria shed into the blood; caused by VRE; has a high mortality rate
5. Damage to the liver by direct drug toxicity or an immune reaction that may appear 10 to 12 days after erythromycin therapy
6. The causative organism of pseudomembranous colitis is *Clostridium difficile*. With use of antibiotics, the normal flora of the gastrointestinal tract is destroyed, allowing an overgrowth of *C. difficile*.
7. See Geriatric Considerations box in text on page 527.

Drug	Action	Uses	Adverse Effects
8. erythromycin	Binds to bacterial ribosomes and thus prevents bacterial protein synthesis	Gram-positive bacteria (especially in patients allergic to penicillins); some atypical pneumonias such as those caused by *Mycoplasma pneumoniae* and *Legionella pneumophila;* diptheria	Gastrointestinal tract problems, such as abdominal discomfort, cramping, nausea, vomiting, and diarrhea
9. clindamycin	Inhibits the action of bacterial ribosomes and halts protein synthesis	Primarily effective against gram-positive organisms and several anaerobic organisms	Colitis, ranging from mild diarrhea to a severe life-threatening condition called pseudomembranous colitis; also, gastrointestinal tract irritation from nausea and vomiting to glossitis and stomatitis
10. vancomycin	Prevents synthesis of bacterial cell walls by blocking peptidoglycan strand formation	Serious or life-threatening staphylococcal or streptococcal infections	Nausea, flushing (red man's syndrome), and itching
11. spectinomycin	Inhibits protein synthesis	Gonorrhea	Nausea, chills, dizziness, pain at the injection site, urticaria, or fever

Chapter 47: Tetracyclines and Chloramphenicol

1. Tetracyclines block bacterial growth by inhibiting protein synthesis through the blocking of messenger RNA.
2. Tetracyclines are effective for gram-negative bacteria, Rocky Mountain spotted fever, typhus, Q fever, tick fever, *Chlamydia,* and *Mycoplasma pneumoniae.*
3. See Pediatric Considerations box in text on page 533.
4. See Nursing Process Overview in text on page 535.

Chapter 47: Tetracyclines and Chloramphenicol—cont'd

5. Both drugs pass freely through gastrointestinal tract membranes and are much more completely and rapidly absorbed than most other tetracyclines. In addition, they both have a longer elimination half-life (12 to 15 hours).

6. Instruct the patient not to take oral tetracyclines within 1 to 2 hours of having milk or milk products, or antacids, calcium supplements, choline and magnesium salicylate combinations, magnesium salicylate, magnesium-containing laxatives, or sodium bicarbonate. Also, instruct the patient not to take iron or vitamins with iron within 2 to 3 hours of tetracycline doses.

Chapter 48: Aminoglycosides

1. Aminoglycosides include gentamicin, streptomycin, tobramycin, netilmicin, kanamycin, and amikacin.

2. a. Ototoxicity: May cause hearing loss, loss of equilibrium, or both
   b. Renal toxicity: Damage to both tubules and glomeruli
   c. Neuromuscular blockade: Manifested by respiratory paralysis

3. See Geriatric Considerations Box in text on page 539.

4-7. See Table 48-1 in text on page 540.

8. Monitor serum creatinine level, blood urea nitrogen (BUN), and urinalysis for renal function; liver function tests; serum electrolyte level; complete blood count; white blood cell differential; platelet count; and peak and trough serum drug levels.

9. Peak levels indicate serum levels after a dose is given and reflect the highest serum level for that patient at that dose. Trough levels are drawn shortly before a dose is given and reflect the lowest serum level for that patient at that dose.

10. See Nursing Implications Summary in text on page 541.

Chapter 49: Sulfonamides, Trimethoprim, and Drugs to Treat Urinary Tract Infections

1. Urinary tract infection

2. Drug crystallization in urine

3. Glucose-6-phosphate dehydrogenase

4. This drug is excreted in urine and exerts an analgesic effect on the mucosa of the urinary tract, therefore relieving the pain, burning, and itching associated with the urinary tract infection.

5. The nitrofurantoin may cause the urine to turn rusty-yellow to brown; the phenazopyridine turns the urine reddish orange and may stain clothing. Both color changes are harmless.

6. See life span considerations boxes in text on pages 546 and 547.

7.

Drug	Effect
a. methotrexate, pyrimethamine, or trimetrexate	Antifolate activity leading to megaloblastic anemia
b. sulfonamides	Increased effect

8. Remember developmental data concerning adolescents. See Nursing Implications Summary in text on page 550.

Chapter 50: Drugs to Treat Tuberculosis and Other Mycobacterial Infections

1. Acquired immunodeficiency syndrome

2. Human immunodeficiency virus; causes AIDS

3. Respiratory and systemic infection caused by *Mycobacterium tuberculosis*

4. Infectious disease that deadens nerves, leading to tissue damage and loss, caused by *Mycobacterium leprae;* also called Hansen's disease

5. An antifolate effective against leprosy

6. Baccili are transmitted by airborne droplets, not by objects. Shared enclosed environment with infected person creates high risk of contamination. Transmission is blocked by good room ventilation, ultraviolet light, and specific drug therapy.

7. Encourage compliance with full course of drug. Regular visits and eye examinations are necessary. Report vision changes promptly. Do not use alcohol or antacids with isoniazid. Patients should use other glucose tests because the drug may produce false-positive results with copper sulfate tests.

8. See Nursing Process Overview in text on page 563.

9. When two drugs with different mechanisms are administered together, the organism must acquire two independent mutations to become resistant to both drugs. Because mutations are rare, the likelihood of simultaneously acquiring two specific mutations is small. Using three or more drugs lowers the probability of developing resistance even further.

10. Therapy is long term, maybe even for life, because the causative agent of leprosy, *Mycobacterium leprae,* is slow-growing and may remain dormant for long periods in humans.

Chapter 51: Antifungal Agents

1. Single-cell eukaryote organism

2. Fungi whose growth is restricted to skin of humans

3. Yeast that normally lives on skin and is thus opportunistic

4. Substance on outer membranes of fungi; is what antifungal agents bind to, causing cell death

5.

Drug	Effect
a. Nephrotoxic drugs	Increased renal damage
b. sodium chloride	Incompatible
c. benzyl alcohol	Incompatible
d. Bone marrow depressants	Increased risk of anemia
e. Digitalis glycosides	Increased risk of digitalis toxicity from hypokalemia
f. Corticosteroids	Hypokalemia

6. Monitor laboratory values: blood urea nitrogen, creatinine, and liver function tests. Monitor adverse reactions: hepatotoxicity, gastrointestinal tract disease, thrombocytopenia, and headache. Administer over 1 hour.

7. See Nursing Implications Summary in text on page 574.

8. Corticosteroids to prevent side effects
   Antiemetics, 30 minutes before starting infusion, to help prevent nausea and vomiting
   Acetaminophen to treat fever or headache
   Codeine or other analgesics to treat headaches
   Heparin to prevent thrombophlebitis
   IV meperidine to treat rigors (shaking chills)
   Mannitol to reduce nephrotoxic effects
   Potassium-sparing diuretic to limit hypokalemia
   Diphenhydramine to prevent chills

Chapter 52: Antiviral Agents and Drugs to Treat AIDS

1. High Activity Antiretroviral Therapy refers to any one of several combinations of anti-HIV drugs that greatly reduce the viral load in patients.

2. Antiviral drugs currently available inhibit reproduction but do not eradicate latent viruses. Antivirals need to be given prophylactically because by the time signs and symptoms appear, viral multiplication has already occurred.

3. Reactions included are CNS stimulation, ataxia, slurred speech, anorexia, nausea, constipation, dry mouth, blurred vision, and difficulty in urination.

Chapter 52: Antiviral Agents and Drugs to Treat AIDS—cont'd

4. See Nursing Implications Summary in text on page 590.

5. Ribavirin is given as an aerosol (it should not be given concurrently with other aerosol drugs). Health care workers should avoid contact with drug if they are wearing contact lenses or may be pregnant.

6. The drug inhibits reverse transcriptase, which is necessary for DNA synthesis. Zidovudine does not cure HIV but delays HIV's effect on the immune system.

7. Opportunistic infections are caused by organisms that would be unlikely to cause infections in persons with normal immune systems; they are common in patients with AIDS.

Chapter 53: Drugs to Treat Protozoal and Helminthic Infections

1. Disease caused by microscopic, single-celled parasitic organism

2. Serious infectious illness transmitted by mosquitos; four species of *Plasmodium: P. falciparum, P. vivax, P. ovale,* and *P. malariae*

3. Small protozoans that live in water and infect the microvilli of the small intestine, causing diarrhea

4. Pinworm infection

5. Opportunistic pathogen, related to fungi; little known of life cycle

6. The life cycle is complex. Sporozites enter the bloodstream and travel to the liver (and may lay dormant for prolonged periods); merozoites (produced in liver) are then released into the blood, where they attack red blood cells, causing them to rupture. This rupture leads to the signs and symptoms of malaria: fever, chills, and sweating.

7. See Pediatric Considerations Box in text on page 597.

8. d

9. a, b

10. d

11. d

12. a

13. a, c

14. b

15. c

16. When ethyl alcohol is ingested, patients experience intense flushing, nausea, headaches, and abdominal cramps. The action of warfarin may be potentiated, resulting in increased bleeding tendencies.

17. See Nursing Implications Summary in text on pages 606-607.

Chapter 54: Introduction to Cancer Chemotherapy

1. First, cancer cells lose the normal property of contact inhibition, which prevents normal cells from dividing when they are crowded together. Cancer cells continue to divide even when the pressure of the surrounding cell mass is considerable. Second, cancer cells are able to spread far from the original site via the blood or lymph. This secondary tumor formation is called metastasis. The single defining property of cancer cells is that they are no longer responsive to appropriate signals controlling cell proliferation.

2. Agents that do not necessarily affect the DNA of a cell but in some other way can influence the fate of a transformed cell, even causing it to become malignant

3. Genes that are activated in human cancers and override normal regulation of gene expression and drive cell proliferation

4. The process by which a normal cell is transformed into a cancerous cell

5. The use of cytotoxic drugs, drugs that are designed to cause cell death, in the treatment of cancers

6. Dose-limiting toxicity is a side effect that limits the dose of a drug that can be given. If the dose of the drug that is needed to kill all the cancer cells is given, then so many normal cells would also be killed that the patient could not survive.

7. Resting phase, G0; RNA synthesis, G1; DNA replication, S; RNA and protein synthesis, G2; mitosis, forming two daughter cells; then back to resting phase, G0, OR immediately reenters G1 and divides again. Refer to Figure 54-1 in text on page 615.

	Normal Cells Attacked	Adverse Response Seen	Interventions
8.	Gastrointestinal tract	Anorexia, nausea, vomiting, and diarrhea	See Nursing Implications Summary in text on page 622.
9.	Bone marrow	Depressed WBC production, causing leukopenia and susceptibility to infections; also, bleeding tendencies	See Patient Problems boxes in text on pages 617 and 618 and Nursing Implications Summary on page 622 regarding anemia.
10.	Hair follicles	Alopecia, or hair loss	See Nursing Implications Summary in text on page 623.
11.	Mouth	Stomatitis	See Patient Problems box in text on page 619.

Chapter 55: Cytotoxic Drugs to Treat Cancer

1. d
2. c
3. b
4. a
5. Severe nausea and vomiting, metallic taste in mouth, renal toxicity, hearing loss and tinnitus, and myelosuppression
6. Bone marrow suppression, gastrointestinal toxicity (nausea and vomiting), alopecia, immunosuppression, suppression of menstrual cycle and sperm formation, hemorrhagic cystitis, cardiotoxicity, pneumonitis, renal toxicity, and uric acid accumulation
7. Severe allergic reactions, impaired renal and hepatic function, hyperglycemia or hypoglycemia, and CNS toxicity (depression, lowered consciousness, coma)
8. Bone marrow depression (anemia, leukopenia, neutropenia, thrombocytopenia), diarrhea, nausea, vomiting, hair loss, peripheral neuropathies (numbness or tingling in limbs), and muscle and joint pain
9. See Nursing Implications Summary in text on page 644. The patient should be warned to avoid the use of alcohol and to avoid foods containing tyramine.
10. Follow recommended guidelines for avoiding contact through inhalation and direct skin contact. Refer to the Nursing Implications Summary section on "Safe Handling of Intravenous Chemotherapeutic Drugs" on pages 623-624.

Chapter 56: Tissue-Specific Anticancer Agents

1. e
2. c
3. b
4. a
5. d
6. b
7. a

Chapter 56: Tissue-Specific Anticancer Agents—cont'd

8. a

9. f

10. Prednisone is lymphocytic; it causes regression of lymphoid tissue and is therefore effective against lymphoid tumors and lymphoblastic leukemias, especially in children, when used in combination with other drugs.

11. Answer should include three of the following: increased blood clotting, water and sodium retention, altered mood, decreased glucose tolerance, elevated calcium levels, nausea and vomiting, breast tenderness, and abdominal cramps.

12. See Nursing Implications Summary in text on page 658.

Chapter 57: Sedative-Hypnotic and Antianxiety Drugs

1. An illness that prevents an individual from coping and that can disrupt daily life; five types are recognized

2. An intense and irrational fear to a specific object, situation, or place

3. Paradoxical, dreaming or rapid-eye-movement sleep

4. Difficulty falling asleep or staying asleep, or waking up early in the morning

5. The nurse should find out what a patient's sleep habits are and how he or she ensures good sleep at home. A thorough sleep history is required including environmental control, physical self-care/relaxation, eating habits, and quiet recreation.

6. In addition to standard aspects of the nursing care plan for antianxiety drugs, the pediatric considerations should include references to the higher susceptibility of children to the CNS depressant effects of benzodiazepines; danger of impaired functions with chronic use of clonazepam; the contraindications in children for buspirone, methyprylon, and—for hyperactive or psychotic children—diazepam; the importance of following manufacturer's dosage instructions; avoiding, when possible, concurrent use of other CNS depressants; and monitoring excessive sedation or lack of coordination; and monitoring for paradoxical reactions with the use of barbiturates.

7. Interventions may include supportive nursing measures such as relaxation therapy techniques, quiet recreation before sleep, a back rub, reduction of environmental stimuli, or a warm drink. Refer to Patient Problems Box in text on page 663.

8. A small dose given to calm an anxious patient is a sedative; a larger dose sufficient to induce sleep is called a hypnotic.

9. Refer to Patient Problems Box in text on page 676.

Chapter 58: Antipsychotic Drugs

1. Causing general quiescence and a state of psychic indifference to the surroundings

2. Emotional disorder in which there is a loss of reality

3. Psychosis caused by damage to brain by disease or injury

4. Psychosis caused from drug or alcohol withdrawal

5. Agents that reduce symptoms of psychosis

6. A potentially fatal syndrome that occurs during neuroleptic therapy

7. See Patient Problems box in text on page 690.

8. Phenothiazines block neurotransmitters dopamine, acetylcholine, and norepinephrine.

9. The terms *acute dystonia, akathisia, pseudoparkinsonism,* and *tardive dyskinesia* are defined in the text in Table 58-3 on page 688.

10. See Nursing Implications Summary in text on page 693.

11. They have a low risk of the disabling extrapyramidal side effects and are effective in treating the negative symptoms of schizophrenia (e.g., as apathy, social withdrawal, blunted affect), which are not relieved by traditional antipsychotics.

Chapter 59: Antidepressant and Antimanic Agents

1. A disorder of mood (affect) that is not a single entity but a syndrome

2. A depression that lasts more than 2 years that is not disabling but keeps the patient from functioning fully

3. Manic-depressive illness that involves cycles of depression and elation or mania

4. Altered mental status with confusion, agitation, disorientation, poor concentration, and restlessness along with muscle spasms, exaggerated reflexes, shivering, and sweating; results from combining MAO inhibitors with any agent that promotes increased serotonin

5. The four categories are selective serotonin reuptake inhibitors (SSRIs), tricyclic antidepressants, heterocyclic (atypical) antidepressants, and monoamine oxidase (MAO) inhibitors. The botanical is St. John's Wort.

6. The SSRIs have greater pharmacologic specificity, fewer side effects, and minimal potential for fatal overdose.

7. Refer to the Dietary Considerations Box in text on page 706.

8. The therapeutic index for lithium is relatively small; testing is done to ensure therapeutic ranges and to avoid toxicity.

9. Several weeks of therapy may be necessary before full effects are noted. The drugs should be continued as ordered, regularly, even if the patient begins to feel better.

10.

Adverse Reaction	Nursing Interactions
a. Sedation	1. Teach about side effect.
	2. Instruct the patient not to operate heavy machinery.
b. Anticholinergic effects	1. Increase fluids and roughage.
	2. Give hard candy and artificial saliva for severe dry mouth.
c. Cardiac effects	1. Assess apical pulse and blood pressure.
	2. Instruct patient to gradually rise to a sitting position.

Chapter 60: Central Nervous System Stimulants

1. Drugs that suppress appetite

2. Drugs that stimulate respiration

3. A disorder with a variety of symptoms that impair one's ability to learn or maintain appropriate social interactions

4. Stimulants of mainly the cerebral cortex

5. Syndrome characterized by excessive drowsiness and uncontrollable sleep attacks during the daytime

6. The patient should be instructed not to self-regulate the dose; habit-forming potential should be stressed. If the effect seems to decrease, the patient should consult the physician. Inform the patient of CNS and cardiovascular side effects; amphetamines may impair functioning in tasks requiring mental alertness and coordination. Instruct the patient to swallow sustained-release tablets without breaking, chewing, or crushing them. Caution the patient to store the drug securely to prevent unintended use by another person.

7. Sympathomimetic drug effects are increased by anorexiants. MAO inhibitors can cause dangerous hypertension. Other drugs that produce CNS stimulation will be potentiated.

8. Nervousness and insomnia are often caused, along with hypertension and tachycardia. Anorexia, nausea, and abdominal pain also may occur. In prepubertal children a temporary slowing of growth may occur.

9. Methylxanthines such as caffeine, aminophylline, and theophylline, and doxapram may be used.

Chapter 61: Anticonvulsants

1. Significant changes in the electric activity of the cerebral cortex
2. Adverse effects include drowsiness, dizziness, ataxia, visual disturbances, and gastrointestinal upset.
3. Valproic acid is a first-line drug for the treatment of many generalized seizures, including simple and complex absence seizures, myoclonic seizures, and tonic-clonic seizures, as well as many partial seizures.
4. a. T
   b. T
   c. F
   d. T
5. In addition to aspects of a general nursing care plan for anticonvulsants, pediatric considerations should include the following: increased susceptibility to gingival hyperplasia, especially with phenytoin or mephenytoin therapy; impaired school performance is reported with high-dose, long-term hydantoin use; when possible, other anticonvulsants should be considered before the hydantoins; risk of serious hepatotoxicity exists with use of valproic acid or multiple anticonvulsant drug use; and coarse facial features and excessive body hair growth are more often reported in young patients.
6. a
7. c
8. d
9. b
10. Gingival hyperplasia, overgrowth of the gums, may occur. The patient needs regular dental checkups and a thorough dental care program that includes flossing, brushing, and rinsing.
11. a. Generalized seizures: Result from the discharge of cells over both sides of the brain
    b. Partial seizures: Begin with specific symptoms that reflect the particular part of the brain in which the seizure originates
    c. Status epilepticus: Seizures that last 30 minutes or longer or that are repeated for 30 minutes or longer and during which consciousness is not regained
    d. Tonic-clonic epilepsy: Formerly called grand mal, involves the contraction of all skeletal muscles and loss of consciousness
    e. Absence epilepsy: Formerly called petit mal, involves loss of consciousness for a few seconds yet the body tone is seldom lost

Chapter 62: Drugs to Treat Parkinson's Disease and Alzheimer's Disease

1. Progressive neurologic disorder of the extrapyramidal system caused by degeneration of dopaminergic neurons
2. Difficulty in initiating any movement
3. Slowness in movement
4. Condition in which muscle tone is greatly increased but reflex activity is not
5. Progressive dementia characterized by the loss of short- and long-term memory
6. Parkinson's disease is a progressively debilitating disorder of the CNS caused by a degeneration of the dopamine-producing neurons of the substantia nigra, which produces a dopamine-acetylcholine imbalance. Symptoms include muscle rigidity and muscle tremor. The muscle rigidity or increased tone appears as "ratchet resistance" or "cogwheel rigidity." The muscle tremors appear to have a "to and fro" movement, and are usually worse at rest and commonly manifested as "pill-rolling" motion of the hands and bobbing of the head.
7. These drugs, which inhibit or block the effects of acetylcholine, are called anticholinergic drugs. They block central cholinergic excitatory pathways, returning the dopamine-acetylcholine balance in the brain (especially, the basal ganglia) to normal.
8. See Nursing Implications Summary in text on page 747.
9. Pharmacologic treatment for Alzheimer's disease is lacking because the cause is unknown. Two acetylcholinesterase

inhibitors (cholinergic drugs) have been specifically approved to improve cognitive functions in the early stages of Alzheimer's disease.

Chapter 63: Centrally Acting Skeletal Muscle Relaxants

1. Result of loss of inhibitory tone in the polysynaptic pathways of the spinal cord so that fine motor control is lost

2. Local muscle contractions initiated by muscle or tendon injury and inflammation

3. Gamma-aminobutyric acid, an inhibitory neurotransmitter

4. Action results from CNS depression in the brain and spinal cord. This CNS depression results in relaxation of striated muscle spasm.

5. Other muscle relaxants work on the CNS; dantrolene works directly on the muscle by interfering with intracellular release of calcium.

6. Mild: Diarrhea, sleepiness, fatigue, muscle weakness

   Severe: Liver damage

7. See Nursing Implications Summary in text on page 74.

8. Do not take with alcohol or other CNS depressants; do not take cyclobenzaprine with MAO inhibitors.

Chapter 64: Introduction to Endocrinology

1. Substance synthesized by a specific cell to act on target tissues elsewhere in the body

2. Organs that produce hormones

3. Body tissues affected by hormones

4. Thyroid-stimulating hormone

5. Antidiuretic hormone

6. Active forms of protein hormones derived from larger protein molecules

7. Located in brain; regulates synthesis and release of hormones

8. As a result of genetic engineering, genes from one species are placed into an unrelated species, thus producing large quantities of human protein

9. First type: Steroid hormones derived from cholesterol; includes hormones of adrenal and sex glands

   Second type: Formed from amino acids; includes all other hormones

10. a. Diagnostic agents: To assess the function of target organs (e.g., ACTH to test adrenal function)

    b. Replacement therapy: To restore normal levels of hormones (e.g., insulin for diabetes)

    c. Pharmacologic agents: Higher dosages of the hormone are given to make use of a function of the compound that is not usually seen at normal physiologic levels (e.g., corticosteroids as antiinflammatory agents for arthritis)

Chapter 65: Drugs Affecting the Pituitary Gland

1. Posterior pituitary

2. Hormone released by the neurohypophysis

3. Antidiuretic hormone

4. Anterior pituitary

5. Regulates length of long bones, which determines adult stature

6. See Figure 65-3 in text on page 766.

7. Growth hormone deficiency in childhood results in adult height that is well below average and is linked to a reduced mass of the left ventricle of the heart.

   Growth hormone excess causes acromegaly and gigantism. Acromegaly results if excessive growth hormone is

Chapter 65: Drugs Affecting the Pituitary Gland—cont'd

secreted after puberty, and results in a thickened fingers, coarse facial features, and a massive lower jaw as well as myocardial hypertrophy. Gigantism results if the excess of growth hormone begins at an early age and can result in growth rates of 3.5 inches a year.

8. Diabetes insipidus results from reduced ADH; urinary concentration is impossible, and large volumes of dilute, sugar-free urine are produced.

9. SIADH is syndrome of inappropriate ADH secretion and results from an excess of ADH. Symptoms of water intoxication, hyponatremia, and low serum osmolality occur.

10. a

11. a

12. a

13. b

14. a

15. b

16. See Nursing Implications Summary in text on page 768.

Chapter 66: Drugs Affecting the Adrenal Gland

1. Hormones produced by the outer layer of the adrenal cortex (zona glomerulosa); cause the kidneys to retain sodium and water and promote potassium loss

2. System involved in regulation of mineralocorticoid synthesis

3. A corticosteroid produced in two inner layers of the adrenal cortex

4. Failure of the adrenal cortex

5. Chronic insufficient amounts of glucocorticoids

6. Released by the adrenocortical zona glomerulosa, slows loss of sodium and water through the kidneys

7. Symptoms include confusion, restlessness, nausea, and vomiting. Circulatory collapse, deep shock, and death may follow rapidly.

8. The outer layer of the adrenal cortex secretes mineralocorticoids; the inner two layers of the adrenal cortex convert cholesterol to corticosteroids, including glucocorticoids and sex steroids. The adrenal medulla is closely associated with the autonomic nervous system at maturity and synthesizes catecholamines such as epinephrine.

9.
Drug	Effect
a. digitalis	Increased digitalis toxicity
b. rifampin and phenytoin	Decreased action of mineralocorticoids

10. Cortisol is the major glucocorticoid produced. Cushing's syndrome is an overproduction of cortisol and may be induced by a variety of factors, including tumors, increased ACTH, and administration of high dosages of glucocorticoid. Symptoms include increased fat stores on the face and shoulders, weak and thin extremities, fragile skin that is easily bruised, bone thinning, and possibly hypertension and diabetes.

11. a

12. b

13. a

14. See Nursing Implications Summary in text on page 777.

Chapter 67: Drugs Affecting the Thyroid Gland

1. T_3 is triiodothyronine, and T_4 is thyroxine. They regulate the primary function of cells by changing the pattern of protein synthesized in organs such as the skeletal muscles, heart, liver, and kidneys. T_3 is considered the most important regulator.

2. TSH (thyroid-stimulating hormone) is released from the anterior pituitary and stimulates the release of the thyroid hormones into the bloodstream.

3. Euthyroid, meaning normal thyroid hormone levels, is the goal of thyroid replacement therapy.

4.

Disease	Excess or Deficiency?	Symptoms
a. Myxedema	A severe form of hypothyroidism	See Table 67-1 in the text on page 782.
a. Graves' disease	A form of hyperthyroidism (also called thyrotoxicosis)	See Table 67-1 in the text on page 782.

5. The thyroid uptake of radioiodine test uses radioactive iodine to distinguish hyperthyroid and hypothyroid conditions from euthyroid states. This test may be affected by dietary intake of iodine or iodine-containing medications or antithyroid agents.

6. See Nursing Implications Summary in text on page 789.

Chapter 68: Drugs Affecting Calcium Metabolism

1. Calcium is needed for proper function of all cells and tissues; the normal range is 4.7 to 5.6 mEq/L.

2. Vitamin D acts like a hormone in the body and works through a variety of methods to increase calcium concentration in the blood. It may be formed from cholesterol in the skin when it is exposed to sunlight or taken in the diet.

3. Deficiency: In children, the condition is rickets; in adults, deficiency can contribute to osteoporosis. In both cases calcium is taken from the bone to supply the necessary element for life-supporting needs.

   Excess: The result is hypercalcemia.

4. Hormone that prevents loss of calcium from bone, lowering serum calcium levels

5. Produced in parathyroid glands; regulates and maintains serum calcium

6. Calcium loss from bones (resulting from insufficient dietary intake) that results in weakened bones

7. Excessive bone resorption that leads to fragile bones

8. a. Excess serum calcium levels; calcium serum level >5.6 mEq/L (see Table 68-1 in text on page 792).

   b. Deficient serum calcium level; calcium serum level <4.7 mEq/L (see Table 68-1 in text on page 792).

9. See Dietary Considerations box in text on page 793. Infants to age 10 years: 400 to 800 mg/day. Adults: 800 to 1200 mg/day and pregnant or lactating women may require more.

10. See Nursing Implications Summary in text on page 798.

Chapter 69: Drugs to Treat Diabetes Mellitus

1. Caused when glucose levels in the blood exceed about 160 mg/dl, which causes glucose to begin appearing in the urine.

2. A serious acute complication of diabetes mellitus, primarily type 1, that is a result of excessive protein and fat metabolism, causing a patient to become ketotic or acidotic

3. The hormone that regulates glucose metabolism and is synthesized in the beta cells of the pancreas

4. Used to stimulate the release of insulin in patients with type 2 diabetes

5. In type 1 diabetes, all insulin production is lost. Type 1 primarily affects the young.
   In type 2 diabetes, insulin production continues but is insufficient to meet the body's demands.

6. See Nursing Implications Summary in text on page 813.

Chapter 69: Drugs to Treat Diabetes Mellitus—cont'd

7. a. HYPO
   b. HYPER, DC
   c. DC
   d. HYPER
   e. HYPO
   f. HYPO
   g. DC
   h. HYPO
   I. HYPER, DC
   j. DC
8. a. 6 to 12 hr
   b. 2 to 4 hr (the only form that can be given intravenously)
   c. 18 to 24 hr
9. See Nursing Implications Summary in text on page 813. Be sure to emphasize to take the ordered doses with the first meal of every day.

Chapter 70: Estrogens, Progestins, and Contraception

1. Occurring in women in their late forties or early fifties, the state in which estrogen levels begin to decrease
2. Compound that stimulates female reproductive tissues
3. Compound that stimulates uterine lining
4. Point in time when menstrual cycles begin
5. Human chorionic gonadotropin
6. d
7. b
8. a
9. c
10. b
11. d
12. a. C
    b. A
    c. A
    d. A
    e. C
    f. A
    g. A
    h. C
13. See Nursing Implications Summary in text on page 830.

Chapter 71: Drugs for Labor and Delivery

1. Derivatives of fatty acids that help in the regulation of myometrial activity
2. Muscle layer in the uterine wall
3. Hormone, produced by the posterior pituitary gland, that induces uterine contractions
4. Produced from a fungus known for vasoconstrictive properties; drugs that have less vasoconstrictive effects and are used to increase the force and frequency of myometrial contractions; used for postpartum

hemorrhage after delivery of the placenta

5. The process of giving birth

6. Adverse reactions include angina, bradycardia, nausea, uterine cramps, myocardial infarction, and severe hypertension.

7. This beta$_2$ agonist causes relaxation of the myometrium and is used to halt premature labor.

8. See Nursing Implications Summary in text on page 838.

9. a. To control premature labor

   b. Intracervical—to induce cervical ripening; intravaginal—for induction of labor or to induce abortion

   c. IV for induction or augmentation of labor, postpartum hemorrhage or abortion, or intranasally to stimulate lactation

   d. To control postpartum bleeding

Chapter 72: Drugs Acting on the Male Reproductive System

1. Testosterone stimulates synthesis and activity of RNA, which results in an increased protein production. Androgens are also potent anabolic agents; they stimulate formation and maintenance of muscular and skeletal protein. They also bring about retention of nitrogen and enhance storage of inorganic phosphorus, sulfate, sodium, and potassium.

2. Testosterone is used in the treatment of androgen deficiency, the treatment of delayed male puberty when not induced by a pathologic condition, the treatment of breast carcinoma, and the treatment of anemia.

3. With oral anticoagulants, anticoagulant effects may be enhanced or increased; with other hepatotoxic medications, the risk of inducing hepatotoxicity is increased.

4. These have androgenic potency: increased libido, priapism, voice changes, acne, personality changes, increased bone growth and closure, and increased muscle growth. In healthy young men, effects are minimal, but they are at risk for severe adverse reactions (altered liver function and decreased spermatogenesis). See Nursing Implications Summary in the text on page 846.

5. Androgens have been used for various conditions in females, such as relief of dysmenorrhea, menopausal symptoms, and postpartum breast engorgement, but other agents are now preferred. Androgens are still indicated for the treatment of certain advanced breast carcinomas. Masculinization, or virilization, may occur, resulting in deeper voice, hoarseness, enlargement of clitoris, decreased breast size, vaginal drying, acne, changes in hair growth patterns, abnormal menstrual periods, or amenorrhea.

Chapter 73: Drugs to Treat Glaucoma

1. Glaucoma is an eye disease caused by increased intraocular pressure that results in damage to the optic nerve and ultimately blindness. Chronic (open-angle) glaucoma is more common, with gradual onset, and is characterized by a slow degeneration of the anterior chamber that impairs the uptake of aqueous humor. Acute (closed-angle) glaucoma is characterized by the iris bulging up to shut off access of the aqueous humor to the anterior chamber.

2. Possible nursing diagnoses are knowledge deficit related to new ophthalmic drug regimen, anxiety related to possible decrease in or loss of vision; alteration in comfort related to ophthalmic disorder, and potential injury related to impaired vision.

3.

Drug	Effect
a. acetazolamide	Decreases the production of aqueous humor
b. glycerin	Immediate but short-term reduction in intraocular pressure by drawing fluid from the eyeball to the hyperosmotic blood
c. mannitol	Same as above
d. urea	Same as above

4. a. Act in the eye to decrease the production of aqueous humor, thus lowering intraocular pressure (e.g., betaxolol, timolol)

Chapter 73: Drugs to Treat Glaucoma—cont'd

b. Stimulates alpha-receptors, resulting in decreased production of aqueous humor and decreased intraocular pressure (e.g., epinephrine)

c. Mimic the action of acetylcholine, causing miosis (constriction of the pupil) and relief of intraocular pressure as a result of the spread of the trabecular spaces of the anterior chamber. (e.g., pilocarpine, carbachol)

5. See Nursing Implications Summary in text on page 855 and refer to Chapter 5.

6. Adverse systemic effects include bradycardia, syncope, low blood pressure, asthmatic attack, congestive heart failure, hallucinations, loss of appetite, headaches, nausea, weakness, and depression.

7. See Nursing Implications Summary in text on page 855, especially the points about preventing overflow of eye medications into the nasal and pharyngeal passages and administering two or more eye medications.

Chapter 74: Other Ophthalmic Drugs

1. Changing the shape of the lens for purposes of focus

2. Opaqueness, or loss of transparency, of the lens with age

3. Inflammation of the eye

4. Constriction of the pupil

5. Dilation of the pupil

6. Paralysis of the ciliary muscle, resulting in loss of near vision

7. Mydriasis and cycloplegia are induced when examination of the eye is necessary, as well as accurate measurement of lens refraction. In addition, these actions may hasten the healing of inflammatory conditions, especially after eye surgery.

8. The adrenergic drug phenylephrine is used as a mydriatic when only the interior structures of the eye are to be examined and cycloplegia is not necessary.

9. Anticholinergic drugs cause mydriasis and cycloplegia.

10. These drugs prevent action of prostaglandin. Prostaglandins cause eye irritation, miosis, and resistance to the action of atropine. These drugs are administered locally before surgery to prevent these actions.

11. See Nursing Implications Summary in text on page 861.